Orthopaedics

Samuel L. Turek, M.D.

Attending Orthopaedic Surgeon
Mount Sinai Medical Center and Miami Heart Institute
Miami Beach, Florida
Formerly, Clinical Assistant Professor
Department of Orthopaedics and Rehabilitation
University of Miami School of Medicine
Miami, Florida
Formerly Chief, Department of Orthopaedic Surgery
St. Francis Hospital
Miami Beach, Florida

Fourth Edition

Orthopaedics

Principles and Their Application

VOLUME 1

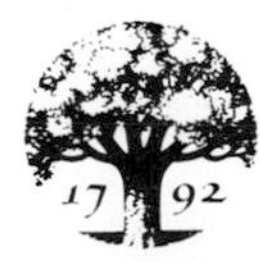

J. B. Lippincott Company
Philadelphia

London, Mexico City, New York,
St. Louis, São Paulo, Sydney

Sponsoring Editor: Darlene D. Pedersen
Manuscript Editor: Delois Patterson
Indexer: Ann Cassar
Art Director: Maria S. Karkucinski
Designer: Patrick Turner
Production Supervisor: N. Carol Kerr
Production Assistant: George V. Gordon
Compositor: Monotype Composition Company, Inc.
Printer/Binder: Halliday Lithograph

The author and publisher have exerted every effort to ensure that drug selection and dosage set forth in this text are in accord with current recommendations and practice at the time of publication. However, in view of ongoing research, changes in government regulations, and the constant flow of information relating to drug therapy and drug reactions, the reader is urged to check the package insert for each drug for any change in indications and dosage and for added warnings and precautions. This is particularly important when the recommended agent is a new or infrequently employed drug.

FOURTH EDITION

6

Library of Congress Cataloging in Publication Data

Turek, Samuel L.
Orthopaedics : principles and their application.

Includes bibliographies and index.
1. Orthopedia. I. Title. [DNLM: 1. Orthopedics.
WE 168 T9340]
RD731.T8 1983 617'.3 82-24961
ISBN 0-397-50604-X

To my dear wife Maxine

Preface

Orthopaedics is a medical and surgical science that continues to encompass an ever-expanding spectrum of subsciences each of which appears to endlessly widen its horizons as new principles evolve and formerly held tenets are modified. Ingenious developments reflect the dynamic state of the art that historically has outmoded the ideas of the past and inevitably will continue to do so in the future. Consequently, controversy is the natural characteristic of probing for irrefutable principles that will guide our approach to orthopaedic problems. This philosophy pervades this book which documents these evolutionary changes. The application of this new information derived from the basic sciences and confirmed by clinical trials is paramount to a thorough grasp of the science of orthopaedics and the development of the sophistication of the orthopaedic surgeon.

The proven format of previous editions that allows easy retrieval of information is followed. The section on the basic sciences has been extensively revised; emphasis has been placed on osteonecrosis, its various forms, physical properties, biologic repair, relevance to bone transplantation, and an emerging concept of osteoarticular allografting. A parallel study of the blood supply of bone has been included, and its relationship to the repair of necrotic bone is described in detail.

A new chapter on "Collagen" has been introduced. A study of this ubiquitous tissue component, including its chemical composition, physical properties, and ultrastructural characteristics, has important relevance to genetic abnormalities, the biophysical properties of bone, cartilage and tendon, and its important relationship to electrical phenomena in bone. A corollary study on the electrical stimulation of osteogenesis has been added.

Previously regarded obscure or recalcitrant conditions are now receiving emphasis because of precise methods of diagnosis and successful treatment. Congenital pseudarthrosis of the tibia now can be managed by preventive and corrective surgery and by electrically induced osteogenesis. Its frequent occurrence and a component part of generalized neurofibromatosis, which has serious implications, is now well documented. The latter condition has been extensively revised to facilitate early diagnosis and appropriate treatment. Congenital dislocation of the hip describes a serious avoidable complication, avascular necrosis of the femoral head.

The section on rheumatoid arthritis has been thoroughly revised to describe modern medical management, early diagnosis, and recognition of potentially serious complications, particularly cervical spine involvement where atlantoaxial dislocation and cord compression may occur. A new section on rheumatoid variants and their orthopaedic implications has been added. Similarly, Paget's disease now deservedly receives intensive study, because it too poses therapeutic problems in various regional locales.

Many topics are discussed in depth in relation to the problems of surgical management about the shoulder, elbow, and hand. For example, the operative treatment of Dupuytren's contracture now embraces the modern method of the "open-palm" technique and the surgical correction of an often associated flexion contracture of the proximal interphalangeal joint.

Acute carpal tunnel compression is now a recognized complication of Colles' fracture that accounts for the untoward residuals of this fracture. Its early recognition and treatment are described.

The complications of total hip replacement and their prevention and management deserve an intensive updating that is paramount to successful management. In addition, procedures that are applicable to high risk situations such as an infected femoral head prosthesis or previously failed total hip replacement are described.

Sports medicine focuses attention on mechanical derangements of the knee. A more detailed description of the anatomy, biomechanics, repair, and reconstruction of the knee ligaments should aid the diagnostic acumen and increase the therapeutic options of the orthopaedic surgeon. Although the precise indications for arthroscopy are not as yet clearly delineated, the use of this instrument is described in situations that are deemed incontrovertibly appropriate.

Within the region of the foot, various topics have been rewritten to reflect modern methods of treatment. The indications and limitations of the many procedures for hallux valgus are defined.

During the past decade, electrical monitoring of spinal cord function has become a reality. It is now possible to detect, by measuring and following changes in the somatosensory potentials (SEPs), early impairment of spinal cord transmission and, conversely, improvement of physiologic function within the spinal cord. This new modality is described, and is especially applicable to the management of spine injuries and during forcible correction of scoliotic curves.

The text on chondrosarcoma has been revised to aid precise identification and classification of the various grades, each of which varies in its outlook. A recently recognized clear-cell variant of chondrosarcoma has been added. Elaborate descriptions of chondromyxoid fibroma and parosteal osteogenic sarcoma, tumors with vastly different prognoses, will aid in precise diagnosis. Modern methods of treatment of Ewing's tumor, adamantinoma, and rhabdomyosarcoma are described.

The compartment syndrome and its potentially serious outcome, often beyond the control of the orthopaedic surgeon, has significant medicolegal implications. The modern methods of early detection, means of reducing the incidence of muscle necrosis and contracture, and treatment are documented. In this manner it can be recorded that generally accepted principles have been followed.

The problems pertaining to the spine and their management are typical of the dynamic changes that continue to evolve. Computed tomography is an important diagnostic tool; chemonucleolysis is undergoing clinical evaluation; identification of various types of spondylolisthesis and their treatment have been clarified; advanced methods of treatment of scoliosis and modifications of the Milwaukee brace; an intensive study of neurofibromatosis and its crippling spinal curves. All these topics are exhaustively reviewed and updated.

The section on amputations emphasizes the need for an objective test that determines the level of amputation, and details the most recent methods. The most advanced methods of forequarter, hindquarter, and Symes' amputations are described and underline their importance in current amputation surgery.

Innumerable additions, deletions, and modifications have been made throughout *Orthopaedics* so that each subject reflects modern views. Again, after surveying voluminous and ever-expanding literature, only clinically proven fundamentals have been stressed. The apparent omission of subjects in which the reader may have an abiding interest is intentional and is the result of my prerogative and judgment that these do not meet the criteria for inclusion.

It is my sincere hope that this lifetime of a continuing effort to crystallize a mountainous and often contradictory accumulation of precepts into logical concepts will help to raise the state of proficiency of both the neophyte and the experienced orthopaedic surgeon. Perhaps this may also engender a need to perpetuate this work so that we may always pride ourselves that orthopaedic surgery represents the model for continuing self-education. This will be sufficient reward for my labors.

SAMUEL L. TUREK, M.D.

Preface to the First Edition

Orthopaedic surgery has progressed from an immature limited specialty to a practice of scientific exactness encompassing a vast field of interrelated medical sciences. This book was born of a desire to compile scientifically accurate information relating to orthopaedic surgery and to formulate a method by which these facts are readily accessible.

Science implies truth. It is not opinion. A man who makes statements based upon opinion and tries to convince others that he is justified because he is entitled to his own opinion lacks the scientific approach. Scientific fact must be based upon documented irrefutable evidence. Only by insisting on truth and accuracy in investigative research can we progress in our diagnostic and surgical techniques.

About 25 years ago, at the outset of my interneship training, the practice of orthopaedic surgery consisted of attempts to treat and rehabilitate patients affected by a variety of ill-understood conditions, including chronic osteomyelitis, poliomyelitic paralysis, "sciatica" and the like. Fractures, hand injuries and peripheral vascular disease came under the care of the general surgeon. The orthopaedic service seemed to be the least attractive to the interne. The literature was replete with opinionated, unsubstantiated reports and treatments which were admittedly empirical.

Nevertheless, a number of dedicated workers, each concentrating upon his own individual interest, labored to bring order out of chaos. In no small measure, tremendous impetus was derived from the efforts of the American Academy of Orthopaedic Surgeons. In certifying graduate students, the American Board of Orthopaedic Surgery recognized the importance of basic science studies. World War II afforded unlimited material for study and improvement of surgical techniques. There remained only the task of collecting and organizing the facts so that the specialty could proceed on a firm footing.

The problem of sifting and correlating the information became apparent to me about 18 years ago. To increase my own efficiency and have ready access to accurate and up-to-date material, I prepared and maintained a classified file of information. First it was necessary to provide a foundation of basic scientific knowledge. Thus was evolved the sections on bone development, histology, physiology and basic pathology. Next there followed the recording of general conditions. Any disease peculiar to a certain location was classified within that particular region. The advantage of this procedure in a differential diagnosis is easily apparent.

Every effort was made to ascertain and record gross and microscopic pathology. The understanding of a disease process is a basic prerequisite to intelligent interpretation of the clinical picture, establishing the prognosis and formulating the treatment. It is a natural steppingstone in the investigation of etiology. The importance of histologic appearance and staining qualities of tissue is reflected in the enormous expenditure of time and effort in reproducing the colored photomicrographs in this book. It has always amazed me that pathologists everywhere confess their lack of knowledge about the musculoskeletal system. Descriptions in textbooks are inadequate. The orthopaedic surgeon was compelled to become a student of orthopaedic pathology and necessarily be self-reliant in making prognoses and surgical decisions. The histologic sections from which the photomicrographs have been prepared were obtained chiefly from the slides used for study by graduate students in the Orthopaedic Laboratory at Northwestern University Medical School.

This work constitutes an effort to record, between two covers, accurate scientific facts necessary to the study and the practice of orthopaedic surgery. The scope of the specialty extends far beyond that of 25 years ago. The study of gross anatomy, histology, pathology and physiology is fundamental to the armamentarium of the orthopaedic surgeon. He must comprehend architectural and engineering principles. He must labor incessantly to improve and perfect surgical techniques. He must be critical and prepared to reject untruths. He is a surgical perfectionist and an authority on the musculoskeletal system. Now he must acquire an understanding of nuclear physics, the newest investigative and therapeutic weapon. Above all, he unselfishly transmits this fund of knowledge and tries to stimulate the enthusiasm necessary to research. If this book creates a degree of interest and curiosity which will encourage investigation, I shall feel doubly rewarded for my efforts.

I wish especially to express my gratitude to Doctors Edward and Clinton Compere who have afforded me the opportunities for completing this work and under whose tutelage a challenging and stimulating world was opened up to me.

The accumulation of this storehouse of knowledge could not have been possible without my studies and associations with Doctors William Cubbins, James J. Callahan, Carlo Scuderi, Kellogg Speed, Vernon Turner, Sam Banks, Robert McElvenney, Newton Mead, Hampar Kelikian, Elven Berkheiser, Harold Sofield, William Schnute and Charles Pease.

I am especially grateful to Dr. Renato Baserga who prepared the sections on Secondary Tumors of Bone, and that on Radioisotopes in Orthopaedic Surgery. Dr. Baserga is a young, talented and dedicated pathologist with a profound interest in nuclear physics. He is representative of our future hopes of clarifying the pathogenesis of disease.

Grateful acknowledgment is extended to Mrs. Evelyn Palmer for skillfully executing the colored photomicrographs in the laboratories of the Mount Sinai Hospital Research Foundation. The superb tissue sections were prepared by Miss Edith Crook, technician in the orthopaedic laboratory of Northwestern University Medical School.

I wish to express my heartfelt thanks to Walter Kahoe and J. Brooks Stewart of the J. B. Lippincott Company, who have encouraged and guided me through troublesome times of authorship.

My dear wife and children deserve more than mere appreciation. They have displayed admirable courage in the face of social restrictions and paternal absenteeism imposed by the demands of writing. My wife, Sally, contributed a laborious effort of preparing the manuscript while at the same time fulfilling maternal duties. With the completion of this project, I expect to be restored to the position of father and husband in good standing.

Samuel L. Turek, M.D.

Acknowledgments

Since the inception of this literary effort, innumerable authorities, many of whom have devoted a lifetime of study to a limited sphere of interest, have participated by contributing their expertise and ensuring that *Orthopaedics: Principles and their Application* represents an accurate portrayal of the fundamentals of orthopaedic surgery. To these people who have unselfishly imparted the benefits of their research and clinical experience, I am deeply indebted.

This fourth edition has continued to reflect the continuing involvement by orthopaedic surgeons of international renown whose chosen fields of endeavor have indelibly inscribed their names in this surgical science.

The new chapter on collagen was possible by the investigative and literary effort of J. M. Davidson, E. D. Harris, Jr., S. M. Krane, M. E. Grant, D. J. Prockop, J. Gross, R. R. Cooper, and others.

Drs. C. A. L. Bassett and C. T. Brighton have given freely of their experience and editorial acumen toward elucidating the electrical properties of bone. The use of this modality has dramatically improved a therapeutic approach for nonunion and congenital pseudarthrosis of the tibia. Its applicability to conditions associated with bone loss continues under investigation.

Dr. Frank Netter and the Ciba Pharmaceutical Company once again have provided superb detailed anatomical illustrations.

A new section on skin grafts was made possible by the contributions of Dr. I. A. McGregor. His innovative development of a full-thickness skin graft of a pedicle with large blood vessels is an important addition to the armamentarium for traumatic and reconstructive procedures. E. M. Burgess has added to his classic work on amputations. His determined and dedicated investigations have produced aids that will more accurately define the proper levels of amputation.

L. L. Wiltse has provided a classification, and diagnostic and therapeutic fundamentals for an exhaustively revised section on spondylolisthesis.

W. P. Blount, already indelibly inscribed in the orthopaedists hall of fame, has once again added to and edited subjects on scoliosis. L. A. Goldstein and R. Winter participated in this effort.

J. F. Holt and H. J. Williams unstintingly assisted in the preparation of the section on neurofibromatasis of the spine.

An extensively revised chapter on the knee was made possible by the efforts of such as D. O'Donoghue, J. Insall, and J. Goodfellow. I have successfully embraced a technique on total condylar replacement arthroplasty devised and continuing under study by Dr. Insall.

I have reviewed at first hand the surgical procedure of H. C. Amstutz on hip resurfacing. I am indebted to him for elaborating current indications and problems that remain to be circumvented.

The biologic processes of bone resorption and repair continue to be elucidated by such as M. R. Urist, R. W. Young, and W. F. Enneking. Their work deserves prominent emphasis throughout the text.

A. Catterall provided superb roentgenograms depicting the prognostically significant features of Legg Perthes' disease. B. Curtis' contributions are appreciated.

An important evolving study of the craniovertebral region and its implications has been thoroughly updated. D. L. McRae's detailed studies have provided important basic concepts, and the prolific writings of J. W. Fielding and R. Shapiro have added prominently to the knowledge of this region.

The Mayo Clinic and D. C. Dahlin made available diagnostic and prognostic significant histopathologic sections on chondrosarcoma and its clear-cell variant. P. H. Roberts and C. G. H. Price made available their roentgenographic studies of chondrosarcoma of the hand. A. G. Huvos contributed detailed histologic sections on reticulum cell sarcoma. S. C. Ahuja clarified the features of juxtacortical (periosteal) osteogenic sarcoma, a unique tumor with a singularly different outlook. H. Mankin gave me the benefit of his experience with allografting for malignant tumors of bone. These are representative of the studies that are being made to improve the interpretation and management of malignant tumors of bone.

The rheumatoid variants have features that resemble rheumatoid arthritis, but have an outlook that require a vastly different therapeutic approach. The work of V. Wright, J. M. H. Moll, A. E. Good, and others have delineated their features.

Hemophilic arthritis is now more amenable to combined orthopaedic and medical treatment. W. D. Arnold and M. W. Hilgartner have contributed the elements of the classic work, the fundamentals of which should be studied.

Miss Allison's drawings as always represent the product of a supremely talented medical illustrator. These works of medical art exemplify anatomical accuracy, clarity, and detail. I am deeply indebted to her for her collaboration.

The production staff at J. B. Lippincott Company, especially Delois Patterson and Darlene Pedersen, provided encouragement and invaluable assistance during this arduous and exhausting literary creation.

Finally, the vicissitudes of this labor and long days of self-discipline have caused my wife Maxine to persevere and coddle this seemingly uncaring family member. I hope that I shall be restored to a loving husband in good standing.

Contents

VOLUME 1

Part One
The Basic Sciences

29 The Foot and the Ankle 1407

30 The Back 1483

Orthopaedics

Part One

The Basic Sciences

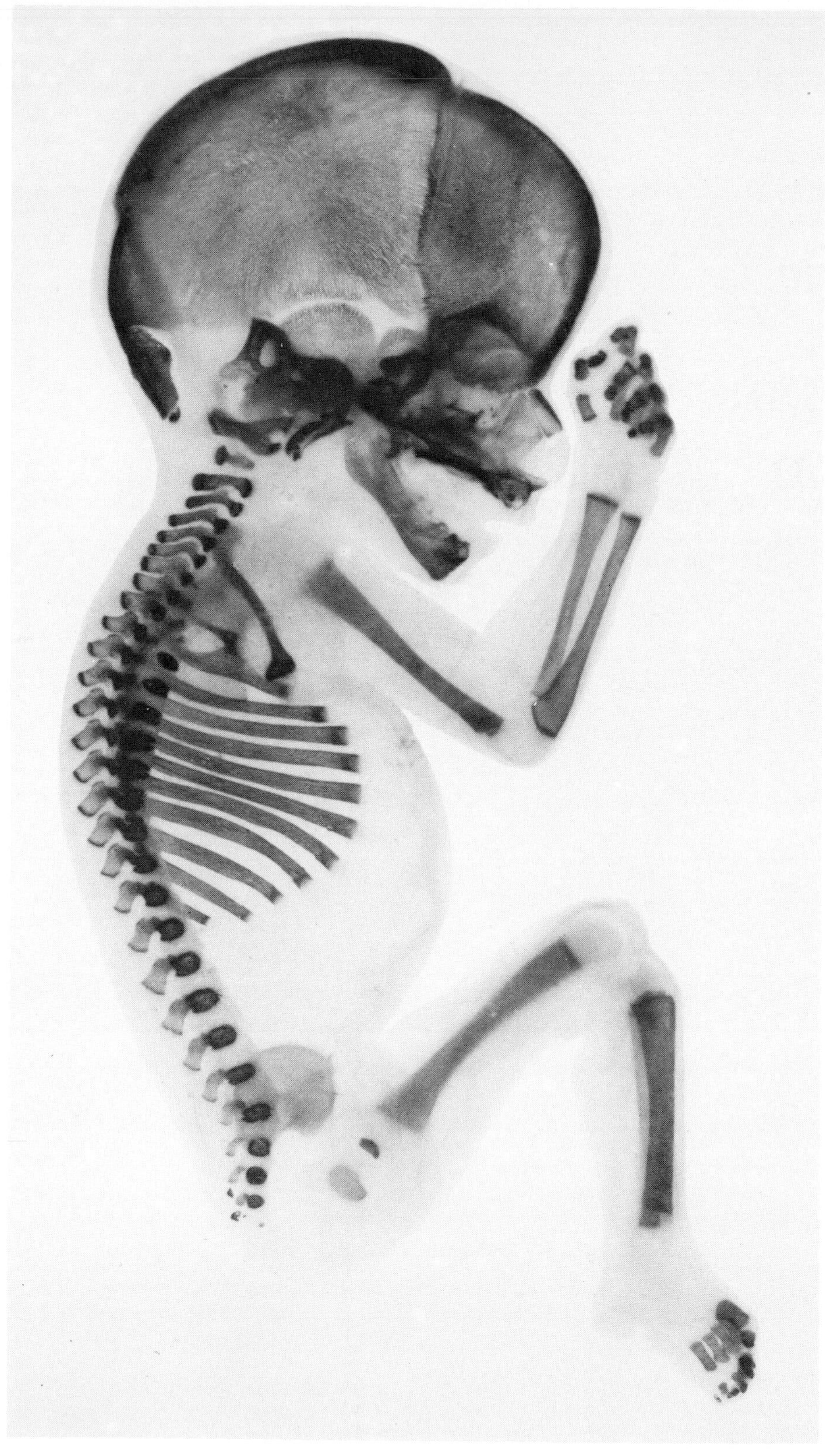

FIG. 1-1. Skeletal development of a 6-month-old fetus.

1

Development of the Skeleton

WITHIN the first few weeks of intrauterine life, the embryo passes through the blastulous and the gastrulous stages and gradually begins to take shape, developing the head, the trunk, and the external protrusions designated as limb buds (Fig. 1-2). Between the ectoderm and the entoderm lies a diffuse, loose, cellular tissue, the mesenchyme, which differentiates into various connective tissue structures including bone, cartilage, fascia, and muscles. The earliest musculoskeletal structures are recognized as dense concentrations of mesenchymal cells that tend to take the shape of the bones of which they are forerunners. Each compact mesenchymal model then is converted into bone, either directly (*e.g.*, cranial and facial bones) or indirectly by first being converted into cartilage that must be replaced by bone (*e.g.*, the long bones).

Each musculoskeletal unit develops most actively during a specific period of early embryonic life. It is at this time that the development is susceptible to external toxic influences. Therefore, a specific congenital anomaly may be related to, for example, an attack of rubella occurring at a time during which that part is being energetically transformed.

CARTILAGE

As early as the 5th embryonic week, mesenchymal cells enlarge, become more compact, and differentiate into a sheet of cells known as *precartilage* (Fig. 1-3). Then matrix is laid down between the cells. The matrix contains fibrils that are peculiar to the type and to the function of the cartilage. In hyaline cartilage the fibrils are not demonstrable by ordinary staining methods, so that the matrix appears clear and homogeneous. In elastic cartilage yellow elastic fibers are seen. In fibrocartilage heavier white fibers are deposited within the matrix. Cartilage increases in thickness by growth, both internally and externally. Internal growth occurs by multiplication of cartilage cells and production of new matrix. Peripheral growth occurs from the investing sheath (the perichondrium), whose inner cells are transformed into cartilage cells.

BONE

Bone first appears after the 7th embryonic week. This bone is of two types: membranous and cartilaginous. Membrane bones are those that form directly in membranous sheets (*e.g.*, facial and cranial bones). Cartilage bones are those in which cartilaginous structures are first formed and then replaced by bone. Although the histogenesis of bone is identical in each instance, in the latter type the cartilage must first be removed before bone can be laid down.

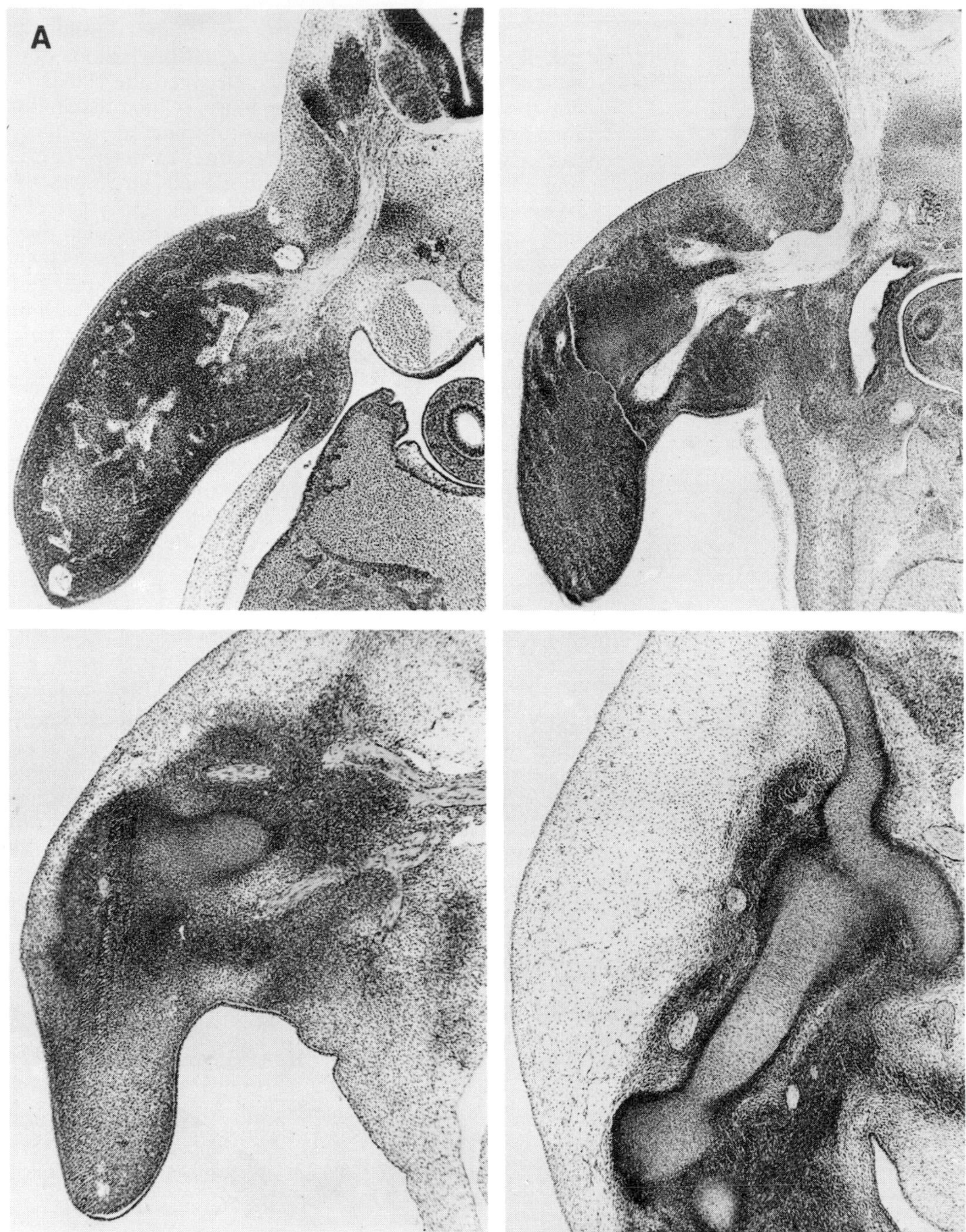

FIG. 1-2. (*A*) Origin of a limb bud. Development of the upper limb bud and histogenesis of the humerus are shown. The limb bud originates as a small elevation of the body wall and at first consists of a condensed mass of proliferating mesoblastic cells. Within a few days, a central condensation of mesoblasts occurs. This is the *skeletomuscle condensation,* so-called because separate muscle and skeleton cannot be identified. At the same time, a broad sheet of branching nerve trunks from the cord and the spinal ganglia stream into the base of the arm bud (*top, left*). A few days later, muscular and skeletal condensations become distinct, and massive nerve trunks enter the center of the muscle condensations (*top, right*). Next section, definite muscle groups can be identified (*bottom, left*) containing conspicuous nerve trunks, and major branches of the brachial plexus are obvious. At the same time, the central part of the skeletal condensation is being

(*Continued on facing page*)

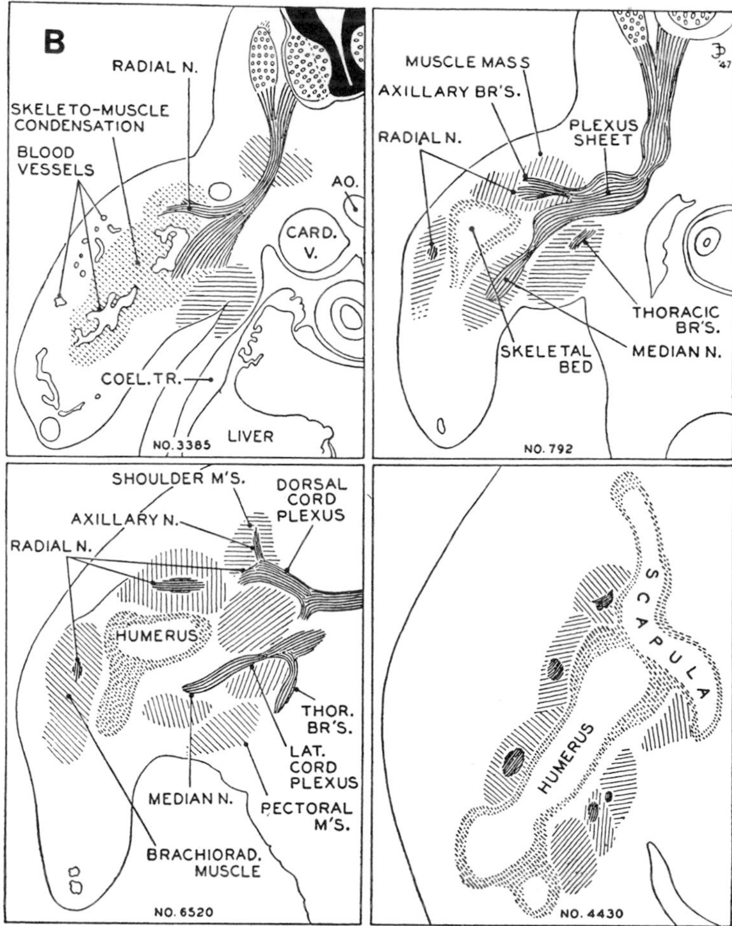

FIG. 1-2. *(Continued from facing page)* transformed into cartilage (this tissue appears lighter in color). The cartilage of different bones is deposited separately in the last section *(bottom, right)* so that these central cartilaginous cores within the skeletal bed acquire the shape of the bones of which they are forerunners. These sections represent developmental periods of about 2 days each. *(B)* These diagram drawings correspond to these sections in *A*. (Streeter GL: Developmental horizons in human embryos. (Pub 583), Contrib Embryol 33:149, 1949. From the Carnegie Institution of Washington)

MEMBRANOUS BONE

The mesenchymal or connective tissue membrane first forms the original model of the facial and the cranial bones. At one or more central points of the membrane, intramembranous ossification begins. These ossification centers are characterized by the appearance of osteoblasts that lay down a meshwork of bony trabeculae spread radially in all directions. The mesenchyme at the periphery differentiates into a fibrous sheath (the periosteum), the undersurface of which differentiates into osteoblasts, which in turn deposit parallel plates of compact bone (the lamellae). This is periosteal ossification, by which the inner and the outer tables of the skull are formed. Trabeculae are arranged mainly along lines of greatest stress.

CARTILAGE BONE

A cartilaginous model of the structure precedes destruction of cartilage and its replacement by bone. Two processes are involved: ossification centrally within the cartilage, or endochondral ossification; and ossification peripherally beneath the perichondrium (or periosteum), or perichondrial or periosteal ossification.

ENDOCHONDRAL OSSIFICATION

In the center of the cartilaginous precursor, the cells enlarge and become arranged radially. Lime salts are deposited in the matrix. This calcified cartilage disintegrates and is destroyed by invading vascular tissue from

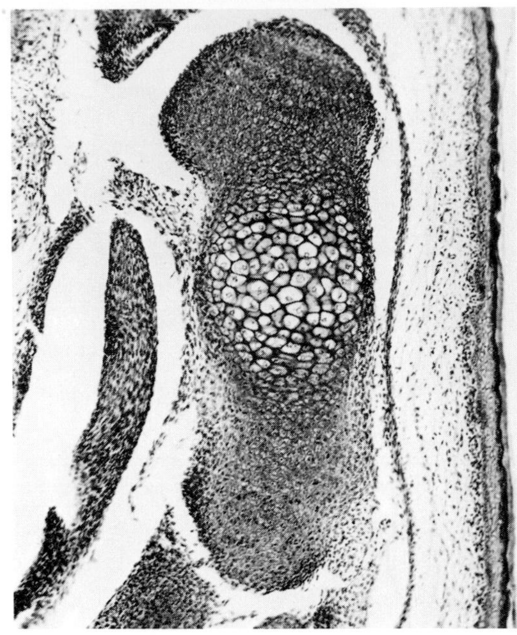

FIG. 1-3. Early fetal anlage of a long bone. It is composed of mesenchyme at the center of which the cells become rounded and assume the appearance of chondrocytes. Later, the peripheral mesenchyme will give rise to vascular tissue that will invade the calcified cartilage and replace the latter with bone.

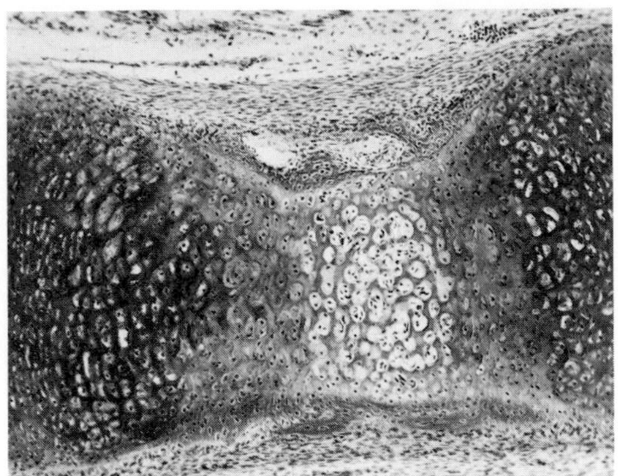

FIG. 1-4. Ossification of a fetal cartilaginous long bone. The cartilage cells at the center of the calcified cartilage have become enlarged, and the matrix is sparse. A bone collar has formed about this level and is gradually replacing the cartilage.

the perichondrium (Fig. 1-4). At the same time the invasive budlike mass gives rise also to osteoblasts that deposit new bone at many points and even on the calcified cartilage. This spongy bone formation continues to replace the cartilage, extending proximally and distally.

PERIOSTEAL OSSIFICATION

At the same time as the process of spongy central bone formation is occurring, the inner layer of perichondrium, (now more appropriately named the periosteum), is laying down parallel layers of compact bone.

The process of endochondral ossification continues throughout the growth period by the persistence of a layer of cartilage near the epiphyses, and it is responsible for growth in length of the structure. Periosteal ossification contributes to growth in thickness of the structure. These processes are described later in this chapter.

JOINTS

Joints occur where bones meet and are of two types: synarthroses, in which little movement is allowed; and diarthroses, in which movement is free.

The *synarthrosis* is formed by the differentiation of mesenchyme into a uniting layer of connective tissue (the suture or syndesmosis), cartilage (the synchondrosis), or bone (the synostosis).

The *diarthrosis* is characterized by a joint cavity that arises from a cleft in the mesenchyme. The capsule forms from the dense external tissue which is continuous with the periosteum. The cells on the inner surface of the capsule flatten into a false epithelium called the *synovial membrane.* Ligaments or tendons which apparently course through the cavity represent secondary invasions covered with synovial membrane reflected on them and, therefore, are really external to the cavity. An articular disk is a fibrocartilaginous plate formed from mesenchyme midway in the cavity.

MORPHOGENESIS OF THE AXIAL SKELETON

The notochord is the primitive axial support. Mesenchymal tissue (designated as sclerotomes) migrate toward the notochord and come to lie in paired segmental masses alongside the notochord. Each sclerotomic mesenchymal mass is separated from similar masses before and behind by the intersegmental arteries. Each sclerotome then differentiates into a caudal compact portion and a cranial less-dense half. The denser caudal half then unites with the looser cranial half of the succeeding sclerotome to form the substance of the vertebra (Fig. 1-5). Both the condensed and the looser portions grow about the notochord to form the body of the vertebra. From the denser (now cranial) half, dorsal extensions pass around the neural tube to form the vertebral arch, and paired ventrolateral outgrowths form the costal processes or forerunners of the ribs. The mesenchymal tissue in the intervertebral fissure gives rise to the intervertebral disk. The nucleus pulposus in the disk constitutes the remnant of the notochord. The two parts

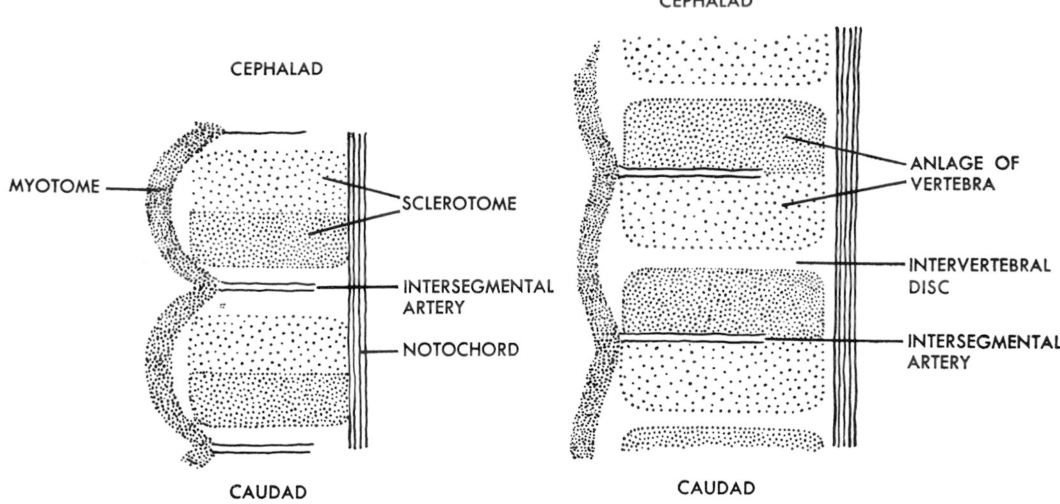

FIG. 1-5. Early stages of differentiation of vertebrae. (Redrawn from Arey LB: Developmental Anatomy. Philadelphia, WB Saunders, 1974)

of sclerotomes, in joining, enclose the intersegmental artery which therefore passes through the center of the vertebral body. In the 7th embryonic week, centers of chondrification appear, two in the vertebral body and one in each half of the vertebral arch. These four centers enlarge and fuse into a complete cartilaginous vertebra. Vertebral ossification starts in the 10th week. A single center in the body and one in each half of the arch appears, but union is not completed until several years after birth (Fig. 1-6).

Continued growth in length of the body occurs by endochondral ossification at the cephalad and the caudad epiphyseal plates. About the rim of the superior and the inferior surfaces, a prominent ring of cartilage exists to which is attached the fibers of the longitudinal ligament of the spine (Fig. 1-7). It does not participate in growth. Gradually, it develops secondary ossification centers that are triangular in cross section but actually skirt the rim of the body. Eventually, this center appears as a line parallel with the upper and the lower surfaces of the body and resembles a plate (Fig. 1-8). The term *plate* is reserved for the growth cartilage that intervenes between the ring and the main body of bone. The secondary centers fuse with the main body by the age of 17. The central artery can be seen up to 6 years of age, after which it is obliterated (Fig. 1-9). It may persist beyond this time in certain conditions (*e.g.*, Scheuermann's disease).

An exception in the development of the vertebra

FIG. 1-6. Development of vertebra. Three primary ossification centers develop *in utero;* three secondary centers appear during the growth period and, with epiphyseal plates, become completely ossified as growth is completed. (After Goss CM: Gray's Anatomy, 28th ed. Philadelphia, Lea & Febiger, 1966)

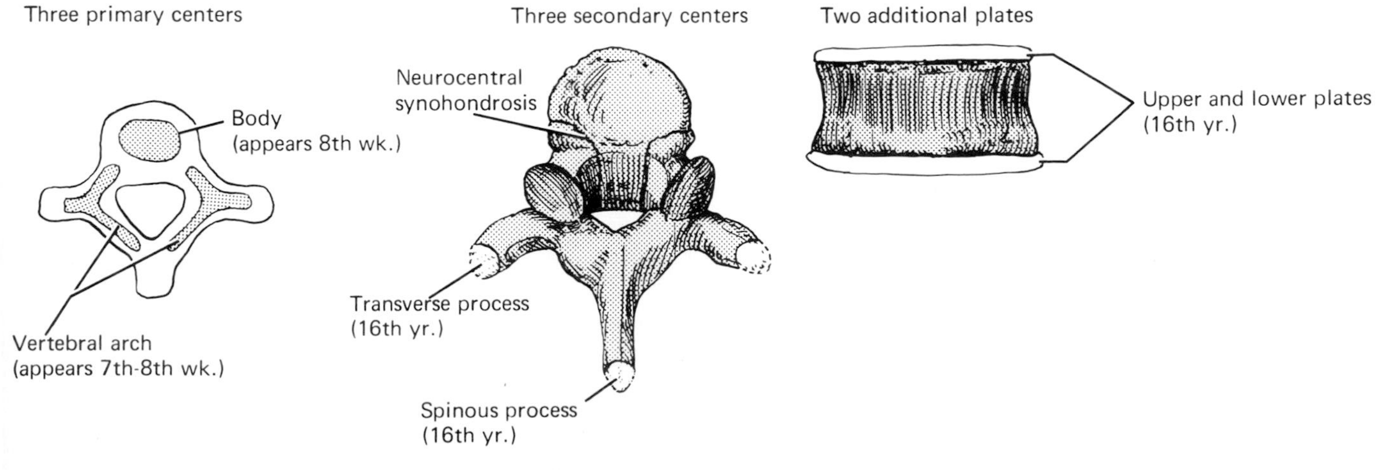

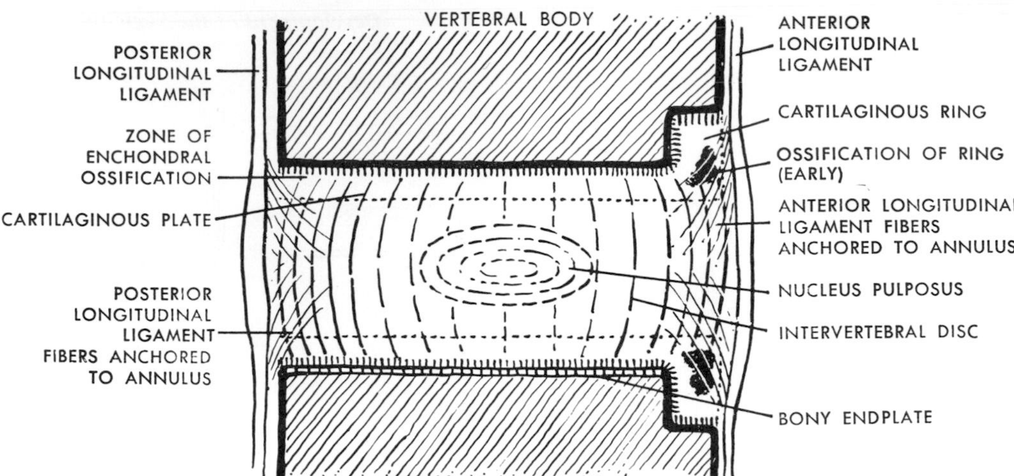

FIG. 1-7. Sagittal section through adjacent vertebral bodies during ossification of the cartilaginous ring. (Redrawn from Schmid P: Zur Entstehung der Adoleszentenkyphose. Dtsch Med Wochenschr 74:798, 1949)

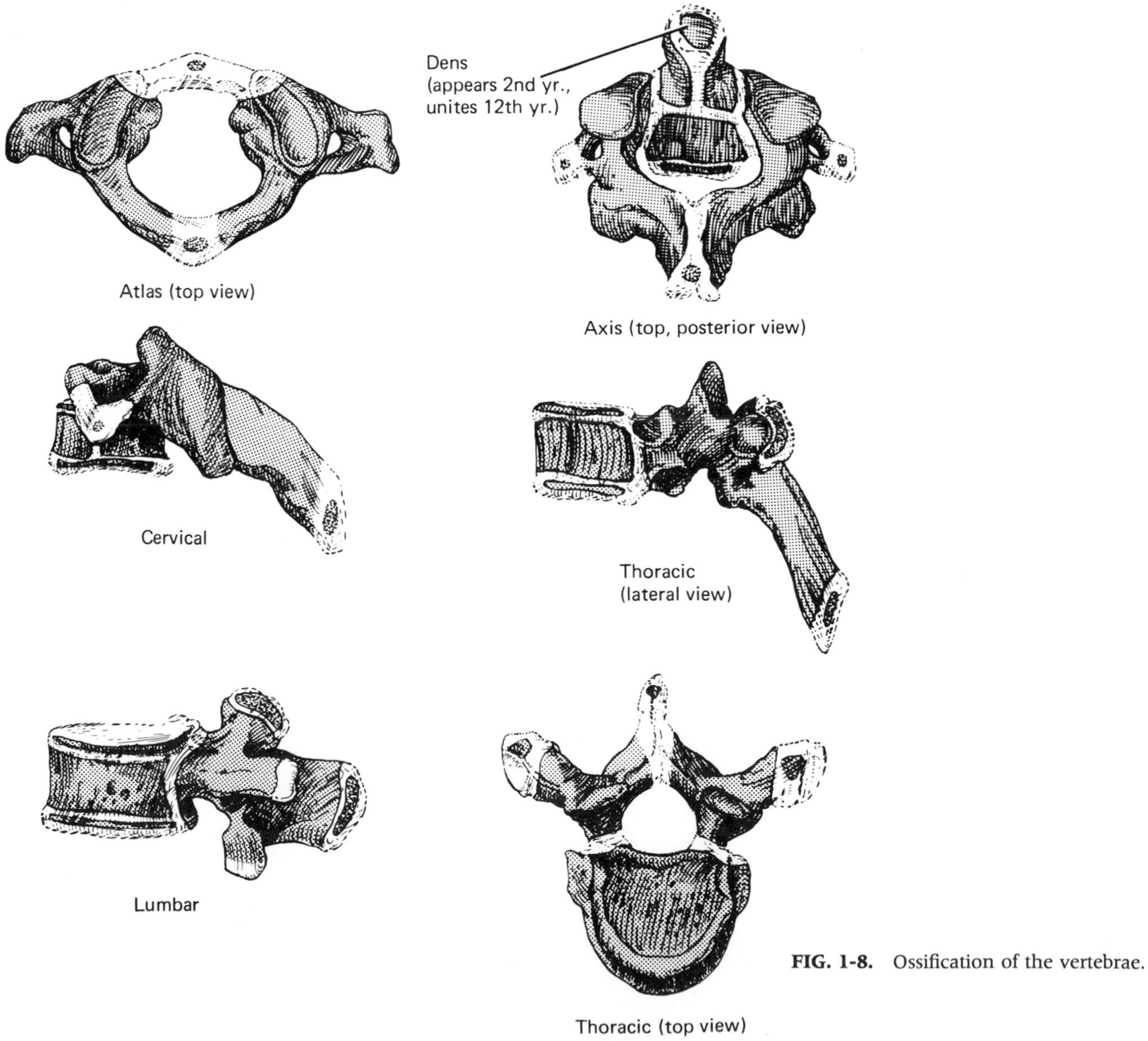

Dens
(appears 2nd yr.,
unites 12th yr.)

Atlas (top view)

Axis (top, posterior view)

Cervical

Thoracic
(lateral view)

Lumbar

Thoracic (top view)

FIG. 1-8. Ossification of the vertebrae.

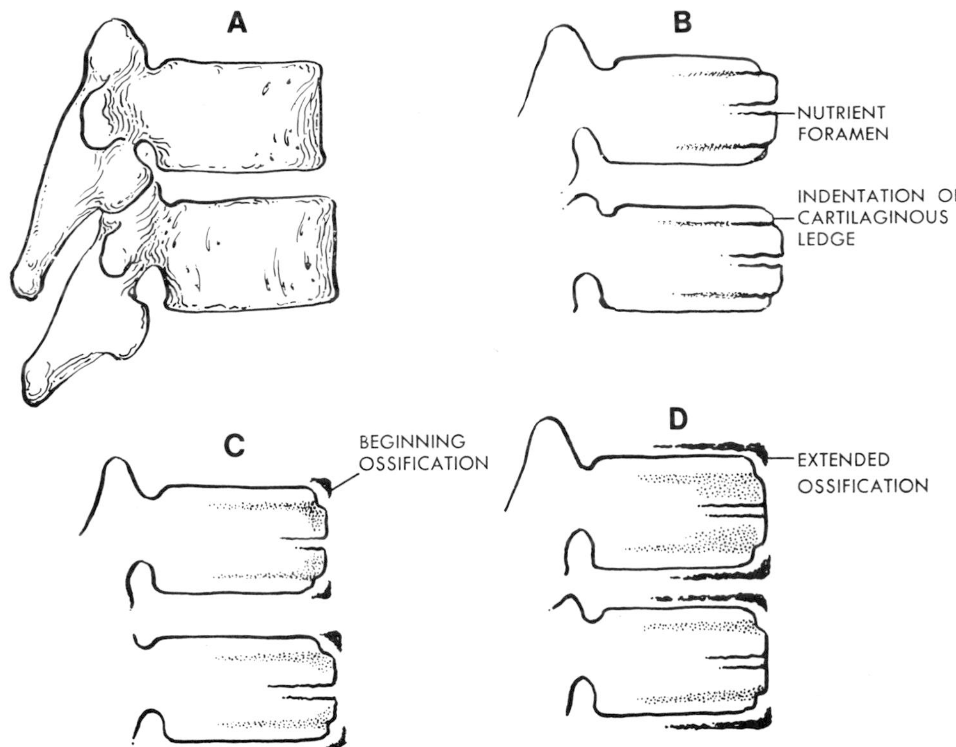

FIG. 1-9. The appearance of normal thoracic vertebrae in children at various ages. (*A*) Normal thoracic vertebrae, fully developed, lateral view. (*B*) Lateral roentgenographic view of vertebral bodies in children under 6 years of age. (*C*) Lateral view in children, 6 to 9 years of age. Ossification starting in the cartilaginous ring is most visible anteriorly. (*D*) At 9 to 15 years of age. Ossification is more extensive in the ring and progresses posteriorly. The nutrient foramen normally is obliterated after 6 years of age.

occurs in the atlas. The body differentiates typically but soon is taken over by the epistropheus (axis) serving as a peglike extension (dens) of the latter, about which the atlas rotates. The atlas is left as a ring. The sacral and the coccygeal vertebrae represent types with reduced vertebral arches. The sacral vertebrae eventually fuse into a single mass. The coccygeal vertebrae exist as rudimentary structures. The entire spine at birth displays one continuous curve convex posteriorly. As the erect posture is assumed after the first year, secondary forward curves develop at the cervical and the lumbar regions. Finally, the lordosis in the cervical and the dorsal regions is balanced by the kyphosis in the thoracic and the sacral regions.

The original union of the costal process with the vertebra is replaced by a joint for the head of the rib. The center of ossification appears at the angle of the rib. However, the distal ends of the long ribs always remain cartilaginous. In the neck the ribs are represented by their tubercles, which are fused with the transverse processes and their heads fused with the bodies; between these processes is an interval, the transverse foramen, through which the vertebral arteries course. When the costal processes are overdeveloped in the cervical region, a supernumerary rib is formed, which may lead to compression of nerve structures.

The sternum originates from the junction of two bars of ventrolaterally placed mesenchyme, which initially have no connection with the ribs or with each other.

At birth, the posterior bony arch is separated from the anterior bony centrum by cartilaginous bridges. The bony arch is completed by the second year. Junction between arch and body occurs between the third and the sixth years.

MORPHOGENESIS OF THE APPENDICULAR SKELETON

Morphogenesis of the appendicular skeleton consists of a cranial and a caudal internal support or girdle and the skeleton of free appendages attached to them. The appendicular skeleton is derived directly from the un-

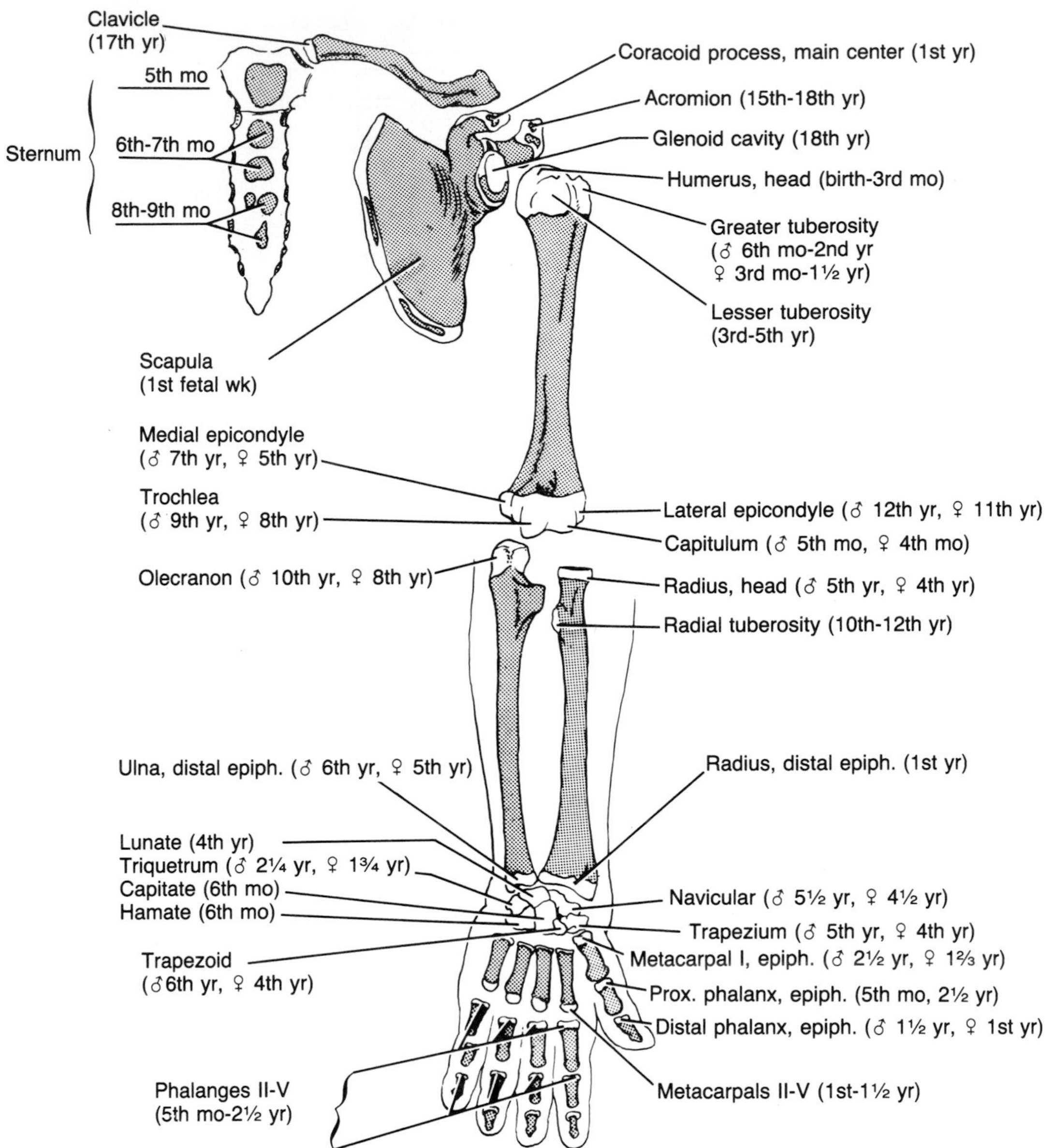

FIG. 1-10. The appearance at birth of the upper extremity. The ages at which the ossification of the epiphyses appear are shown with the differentiation between male and female indicated.

segmented somatic mesenchyme. Definite masses are formed at the sites of the future pectoral and pelvic girdles and limb buds. This is followed by the sequence of bone development through cartilaginous and osseous stages.

The clavicle is the first bone of the skeleton to ossify. Before ossification, a peculiar tissue resembling both membranous and cartilaginous tissue makes it difficult to classify the origin. Two primary centers of ossification appear.

The scapula is a single plate with two chief centers of ossification and several epiphyseal centers that appear later. An early primary center forms the body and the spine. The other, after birth, gives rise to the coracoid process.

The humerus, the radius, and the ulna all ossify from a single primary center in the diaphysis and an epiphyseal center at each end. Additional epiphyseal centers are constant at the lower end of the humerus. Each carpal bone ossifies from a single center. The metacarpals ossify from a single primary center and an epiphyseal center (Figs. 1-10 and 1-11).

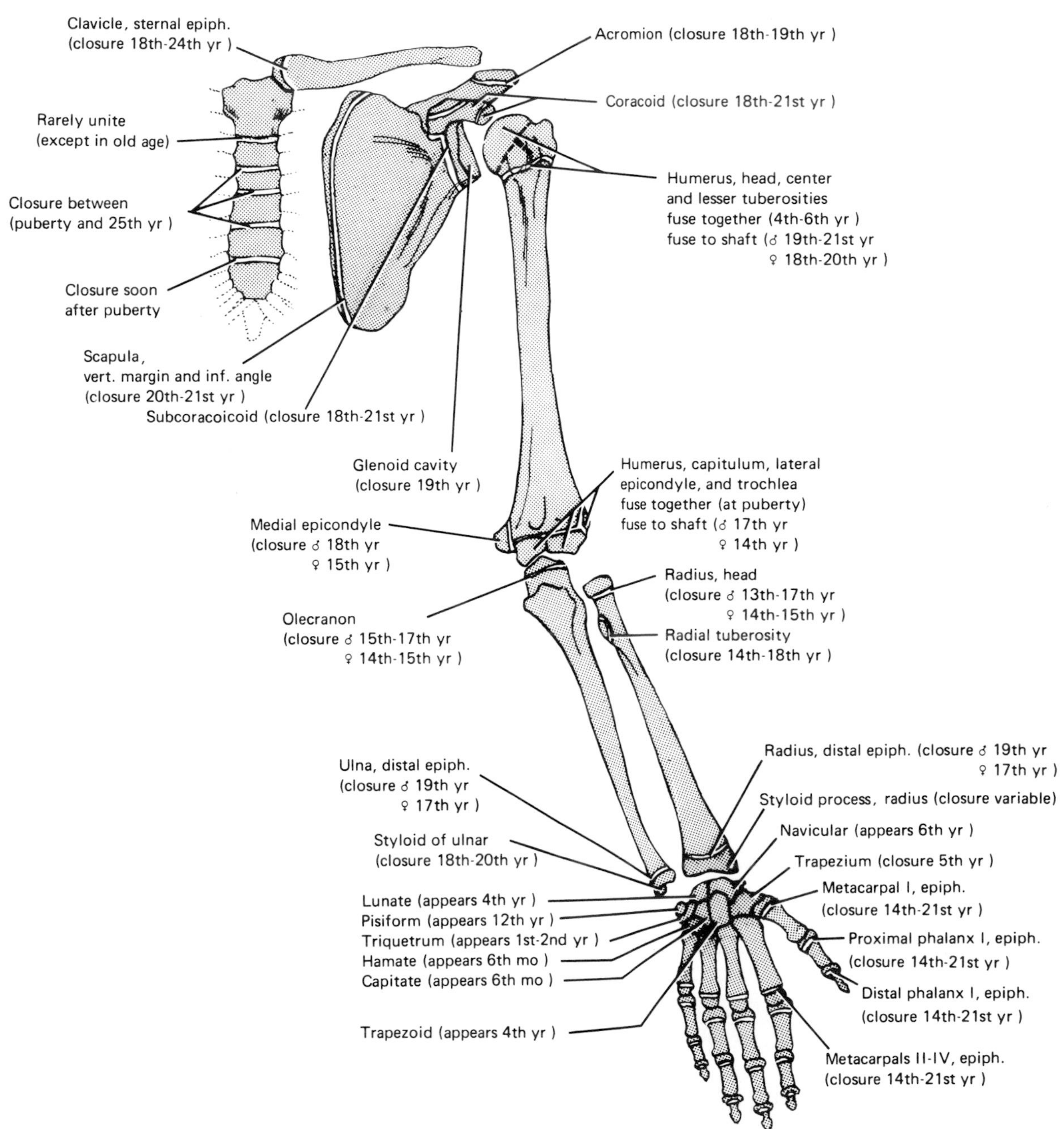

FIG. 1-11. Stages of advancing ossification and epiphyseal closure of the upper extremity.

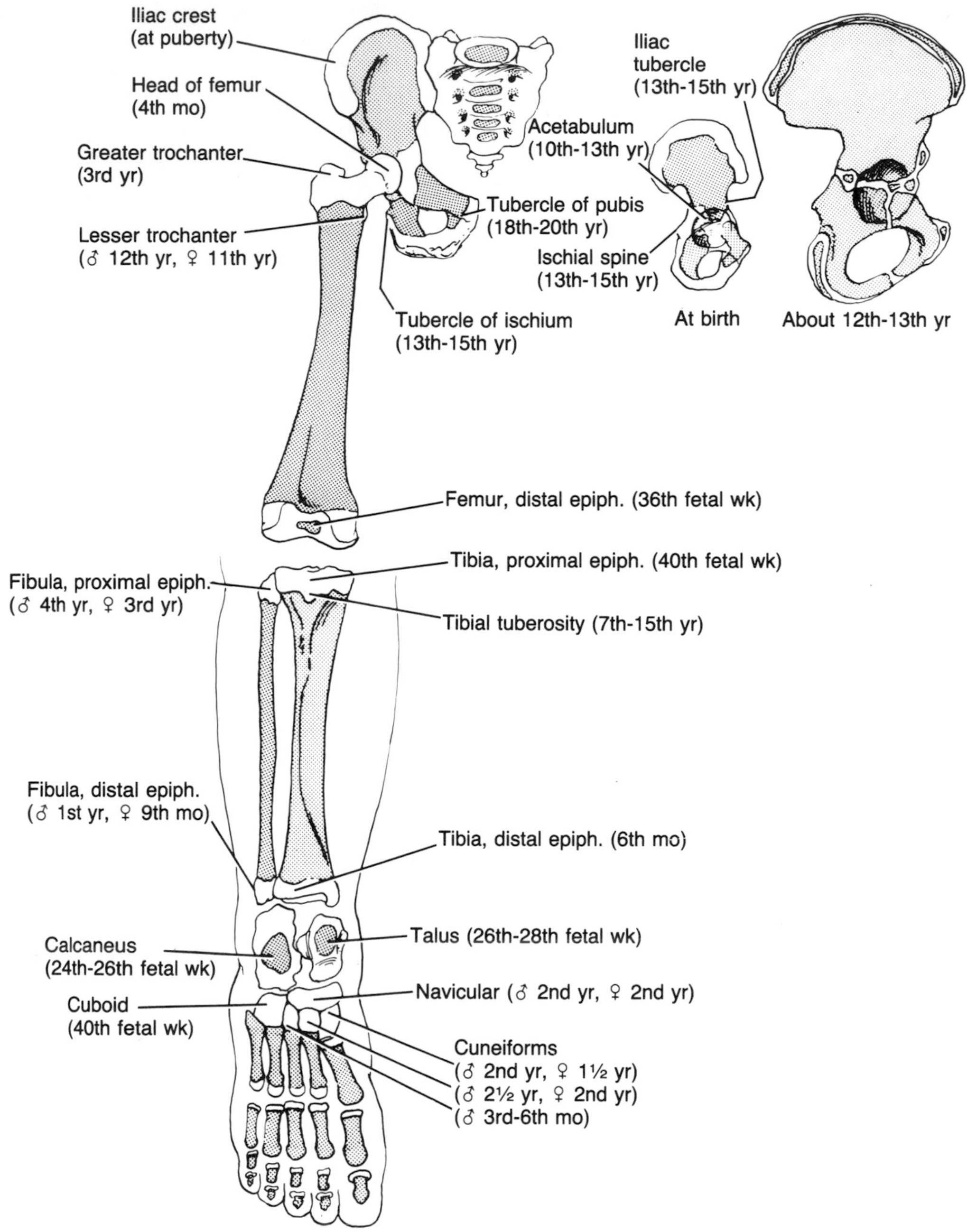

FIG. 1-12. The appearance at birth of the lower extremity. The ages at which ossification of the epiphyses appear are shown with the differentiation between male and female indicated.

At first, the cartilaginous plate of the pelvis lies perpendicular to the vertebral column. Later, it rotates to a position parallel with the vertebral column and in relation to the first three sacral vertebrae. Three main centers of ossification appear for the ilium, the ischium, and the pubis. The three elements join at a cup-shaped depression, the acetabulum, the articulation for the head of the femur.

The development of the femur, the tibia, the fibula, the tarsus, the metatarsals, and the phalanges corresponds to that of the bones of the upper extremity (Figs. 1-12 and 1-13).

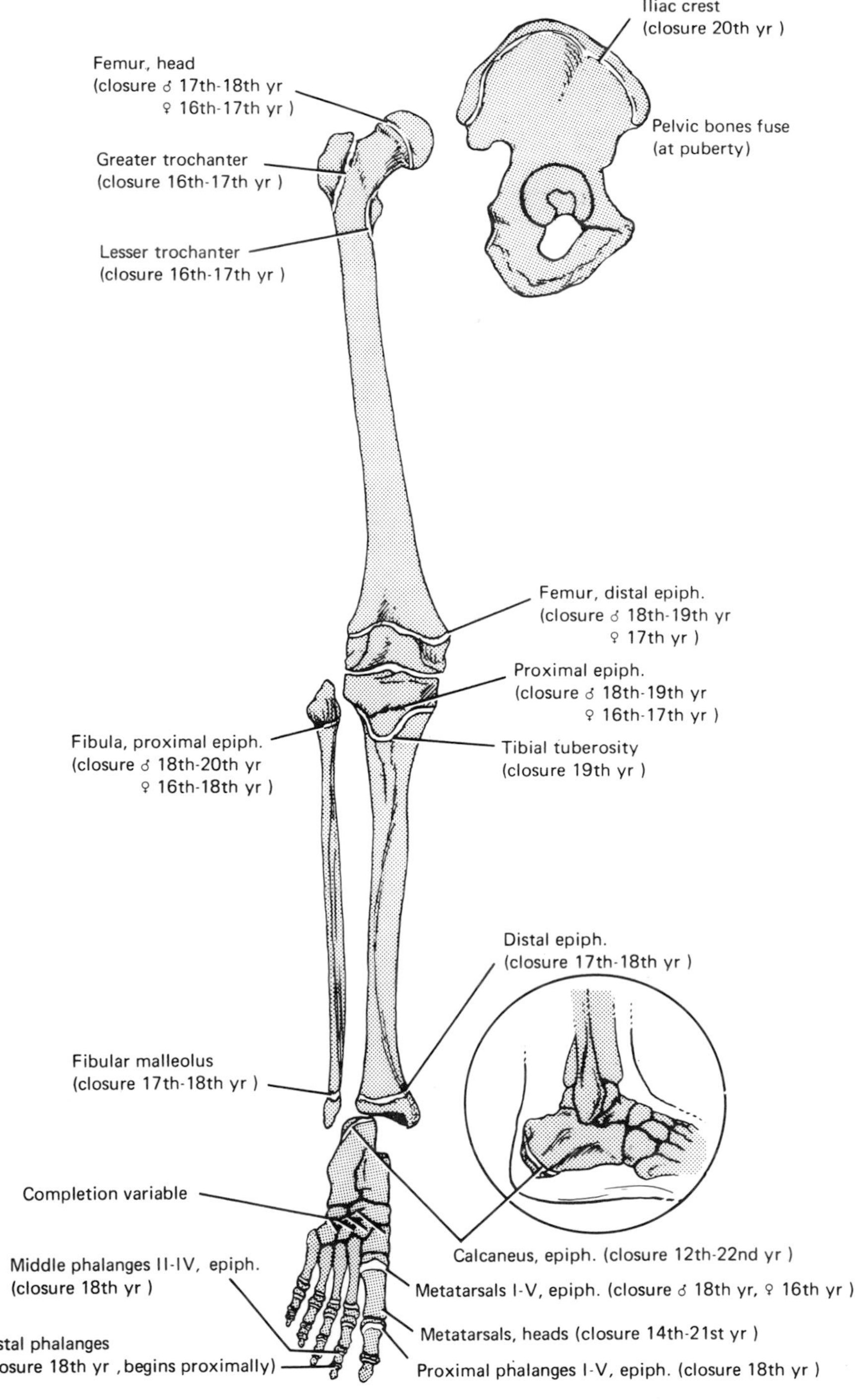

FIG. 1-13. The stage of advancing ossification and epiphyseal closure of the lower extremity.

2

Histology of Cartilage

CARTILAGE is a specialized dense connective tissue that forms the temporary skeleton in the embryo as a model on which bones develop. It persists in the adult animal in joints, respiratory passages, ribs, and ears. The intercellular substance is a hydrophilic gel composed chiefly of chondroitin sulphate within which is embedded a network of collagen fibers. The quantity of intercellular substance is large in contrast with the cavities that contain the cells, the chondrocytes.

HYALINE CARTILAGE

The most widespread type of cartilage is hyaline cartilage which covers the articular surface of bones, forming the anterior portion of the ribs, and providing flexible support for the respiratory passages (*e.g.*, the ringlike structures of the trachea). Hyaline cartilage is flexible, elastic, bluish white, and opalescent. The cells are mainly spherical and occupy the entire lacuna, although in stained sections the cell membrane retracts and the contour appears angular or stellate. Nearer the surface, the cells appear flattened and lie in a plane parallel to the surface (Fig. 2-1). The cytoplasm contains long mitochondria, vacuoles, and, particularly in more mature larger cells, fat droplets, and glycogen. The vacuoles may be large and distend the cell. The nucleus contains one or several nucleoli. Mitotic figures are found only in young, immature animals; in adult cartilage, mitotic figures are rarely found.

Nearer the surface, the cells occur singly or in pairs, often within the same lacuna. Multiple cells are often aggregated into compact groups irregularly placed. A group is formed by rapid multiplication within a cavity. At deeper levels, the cells tend to become oriented into longitudinal columns and are large and rounded. In the immature growing animal, the columns of cells proceed toward advancing bone formation at the epiphyseal plate (see discussion of endochondral ossification, Chapter 3.) In the adult mature animal, the deepest layer consists of partially calcified cartilage resting on the subchondral bone plate.

The interstitial substance appears homogeneous because refractive indexes of both collagen and acid mucopolysaccharide are identical. The acid mucopolysaccharides (glycosaminoglycans, GAG) can be stained by the metachromatic method (*e.g.*, toluidine blue) which colors mucopolysaccharides red, pink, or purple; by alcian blue, a copper phthalocyanin dye which becomes linked to acidic groups of mucopolysaccharides, coloring them blue; and by Hale's colloidal iron method. At a *p*H of 2.5, the acidic groups of mucopolysaccharides bind colloidal iron which can then be stained by a specific method for iron.

In H and E sections, the intercellular substance stains blue because the sulphated mucopolysaccharides combine with hematoxylin.

Collagenous fibers within the interstitial substance are demonstrable by silver impregnation methods or by

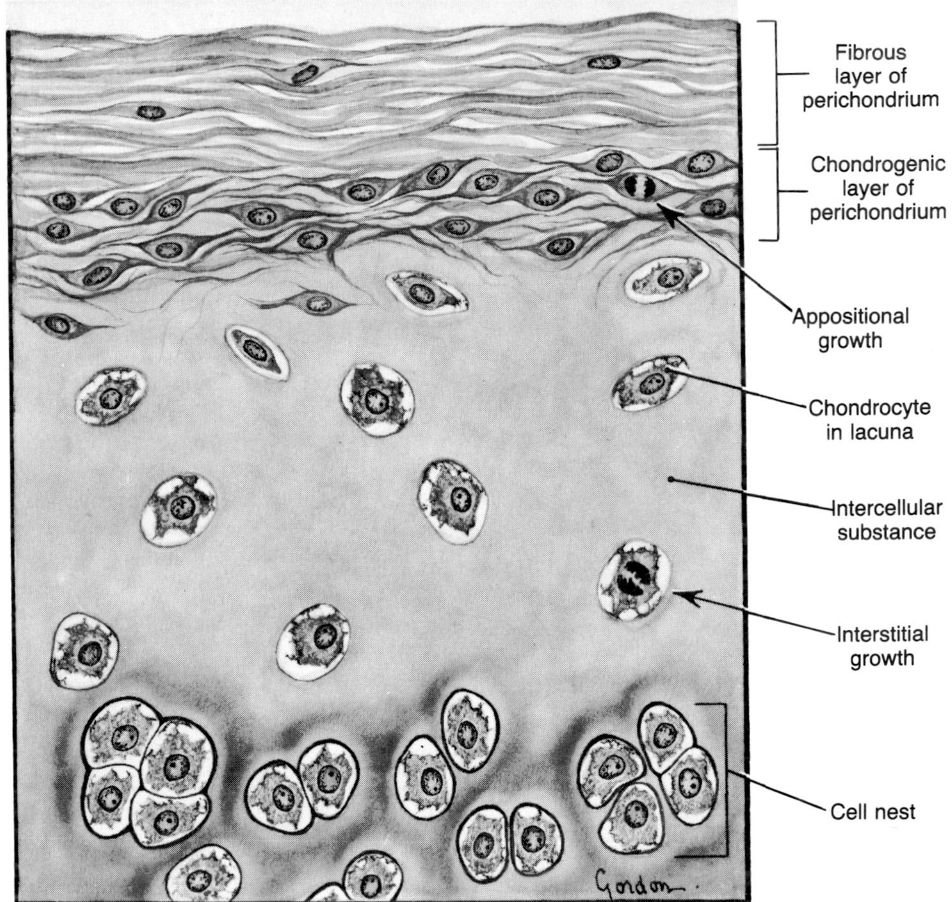

FIG. 2-1. Development of hyaline cartilage from perichondrium. The fibroblastlike cells enlarge into chondroblasts and become encapsulated. They multiply and form groups, then tend toward columnar orientation. The matrix stains more intensely immediately adjacent to the deeper cells reflecting their greater metabolic activity. (Ham AW: Histology, 7th ed. Philadelphia, JB Lippincott, 1974)

digesting the tissue with trypsin, which does not affect the fibers.

Glycosaminoglycans, chiefly chondroitin sulphate, are contained within the interstitial substance and are responsible for the basophilic staining.

Cartilage has no blood vessels except an occasional one passing through to other tissues. Its nourishment is derived from the synovial fluid from which dissolved substances diffuse through the wet intercellular gel to reach the chondrocytes. Where no synovial lined joint exists, diffusion from vascular structures in the perichondrium and the adjacent bone appears to be the source.

ELASTIC CARTILAGE

The difference between hyaline cartilage and elastic cartilage is that the interstitial substance is penetrated in all directions by heavily staining, branching elastic fibers which give the cartilage its yellow color, elasticity, flexibility, and opacity. Elastic cartilage occurs chiefly in the ear (Fig. 2-2).

FIBROCARTILAGE

Fibrocartilage differs from hyaline cartilage by the presence of thick, compact bundles of collagenous fibers within its interstitial substance. These bundles are arranged parallel to each other, separated by clefts in which encapsulated cells are squeezed. Fibrocartilage appears to be a transitional tissue between hyaline cartilage and collagenous tissue and, as such, occurs in special situations (*e.g.*, where the articular cartilage is connected to the dense connective tissue of capsules or ligaments of joints). It also occurs in the intervertebral disks, certain articular cartilages, the symphysis pubis, the ligamentum teres, and in the attachment of certain tendons to bones (Fig. 2-3).

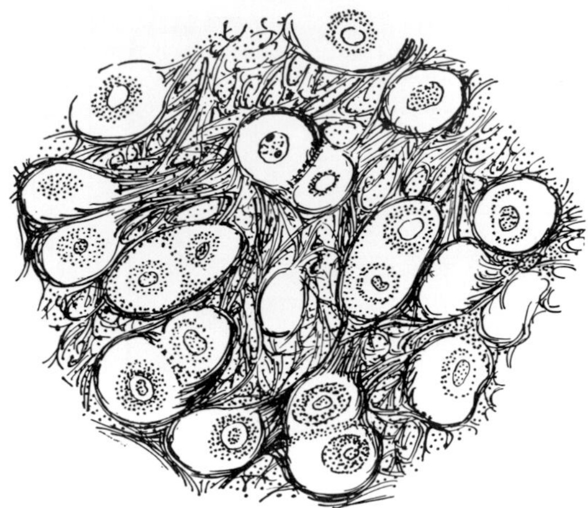

FIG. 2-2. Elastic cartilage of the human ear.

FIG. 2-3. Fibrocartilage is observed at osseotendinous junctions. Note the transformation of rows of tendon cells at the top into cartilage cells surrounded by deeply staining cartilaginous matrix. (Redrawn from Maximow AA, Bloom W: Textbook of Histology. Philadelphia, WB Saunders, 1968)

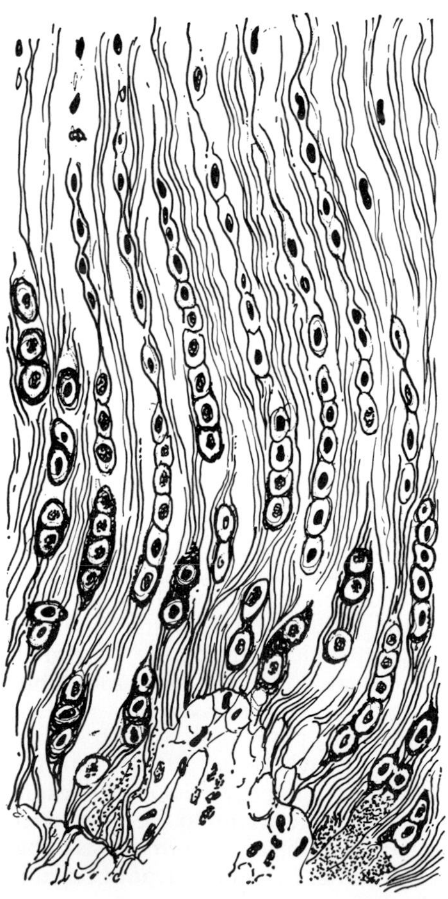

HISTOGENESIS OF CARTILAGE

In the mesenchyme the cells become rounded, and the collagenous fibrils in the intercellular substance become enclosed by a basophilic material (Fig. 2-4). The cells accumulate vacuoles, frequent mitoses occur, and daughter cells in a group are separated only by a thin partition. A thin, shining layer, the capsule, appears about the cell cavity and represents the recently formed intercellular substance. The mesenchyme surrounding the cartilage model of the future bone forms a connective tissue layer covering, the perichondrium. A constant transformation of these layers and their cells into cartilage occurs during embryonic life. In the adult, this connective tissue layer covering becomes the periosteum.

The collagenous fibers are acidophilic flat bundles. They are surrounded by basophilic intercellular substance (acid mucopolysaccharides), while the elongated cells within the perichondrium lose their spindle shape and are transformed to spherical cells (the chondrocytes) surrounded by capsules. This process is termed appositional growth of cartilage as contrasted with interstitial growth wherein the cells within the cartilage multiply within their capsules and add to the surrounding matrix. After embryonic life, appositional growth may continue until the embryonic cartilage model is entirely replaced by bone. Further cartilage growth in the young animal occurs almost exclusively by interstitial growth.

FIG. 2-4. Development of cartilage from mesenchyme. The cells of the mesenchyme (*below*) become rounded, encapsulated, and separated by matrix (*above*).

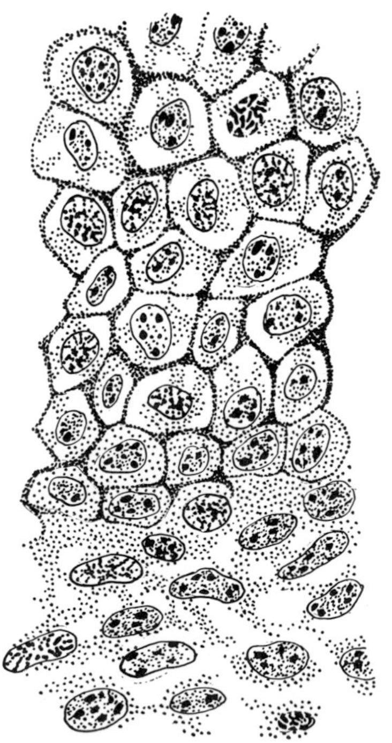

CARTILAGE CHANGES IN GROWTH

Before cartilage can be replaced by bone, the matrix must calcify and resorb, providing the minerals necessary for ossification. At the same time the chondrocytes die. In the chain of events the cartilage cells proliferate, increase in size, and advance toward the zone where ossification will occur. These multiplying cells become arranged in a large group (as in a vertebra or an os calcis) or in columns of cells separated by wide bands of matrix (as in the epiphyseal plate of a long bone). As the cells hypertrophy, they contain an increasing amount of glycogen that will help to make phosphorus available for matrix calcification. In addition, the breakdown of chondrocytes releases large quantities of alkaline phosphatase. Then, under the influence of the enzyme phosphorylase, the glycogen breaks down, forming hexose-phosphoric esters. These organic compounds are hydrolyzed by alkaline phosphatase to liberate inorganic phosphorus. The matrix then becomes calcified, and the chondrocytes lose their glycogen. The cells degenerate as vascular osteogenic granulation tissue penetrates the capsules, and osteoid is laid down about the calcified cartilage and is followed by mineralization of the osteoid.

ADULT ARTICULAR CARTILAGE

In most joints, adult human articular cartilage is of the hyaline type. The thickness of human articular cartilage varies from area to area within a single joint and from joint to joint. In large joints (*e.g.*, the knee) the thickness is 2 mm to 4 mm, and, provided that the surface remains healthy, the thickness remains unchanged during adult life.[10] However, degenerative fibrillation and erosion are extremely common, causing thinning of the cartilage and sometimes exposure of the underlying bone. A study of the normal structural and histochemical characteristics of human adult articular cartilage is basic to interpreting the pathologic changes and alterations of its biochemical and biomechanical properties.

THE MATRIX

Articular cartilage is avascular and lacks nerve structures. The tissue is composed of a relatively small number of cells and abundant extracellular matrix. Chondrocyte activity is necessary for the synthesis of matrix and probably its physiologic degradation and removal.[6] The matrix is responsible for maintaining the homeostasis of the cells' environment[2] and is the main component providing the biomechanical properties of the articular cartilage. The matrix contains a large amount of water, a network of collagen fibers, and a ground substance composed mainly of carbohydrate and noncollagenous protein. A small amount of lipid and inorganic compounds is also present.

Morphology. For descriptive purposes it is convenient to subdivide the tissue into strata or zones aligned parallel to the articular surface (Fig. 2-5).

Zone 1, Superficial or Tangential. At the surface, fibers are oriented tangential to the surface; the cells are ovoid or elongate and are disposed parallel to the surface.

Zone 2, Intermediate or Transitional. Collagen fibers form a coiled interlacing network; cells are more numerous, spheroidal, and dispersed but equally spaced.

Zone 3, Deep or Radial. Fibers are thicker, form a tighter meshwork, and are disposed somewhat radial to articular surface. Spheroidal cells are larger, and are arranged in columnar fashion, often in groups of two to eight cells.

Zone 4, Calcified. Adjacent to the subchondral bone, cells are sparse and smaller, and the matrix is heavily impregnated with calcium salts.

Zones 3 and 4 meet at a basophilic line designated the "tidemark."

Fibrous Components. Collagen accounts for more than one half the dry weight of adult human articular cartilage. Special staining techniques are required to demonstrate the fibrous network in the matrix.[8] Under electron microscopy, most fibers have characteristic electron-dense bands with a periodicity averaging 640 A. The thickness of the fibers increases with the distance from the surface, and in a large joint can range from 300 A to 800 A in diameter.[15] Very slender filaments lacking the typical banded periodicity of collagen are scattered between the large fibers, and are especially prominent adjacent to the chondrocytes. These filaments may represent an early stage of collagen fiber formation.

Ground Substance. Proteinpolysaccharide (PPS) complexes constitute the principal component. Although considered an amorphous material, recent electron micrographic studies have demonstrated a meshwork of fine, branching filaments.[12] However, these may represent artifacts produced by protein precipitation during tissue fixation.[11]

The Pericellular Matrix. The ground substance nearest to the cell stains intensely, the intensity of staining decreasing as the distance from the cell increases. The pericellular matrix contains a delicate meshwork of fine filaments. In mature adult articular cartilage, there is a sharply defined boundary between the pericellular and the intercellular matrix. This zone, corresponding to an abrupt transition between finely and coarsely textured matrix, contains a high concentration of protein and glycoprotein. The collagen fibers at this site are arranged circumferentially to form a strong enclosure about the chondrocyte.[15]

Zonal Characteristics of Collagen Fibers. In Zone 1, collagen fibers are closely packed in bundles with a paucity of intervening ground substance. The fibers are about 300 A in diameter, with typical periodicity, and

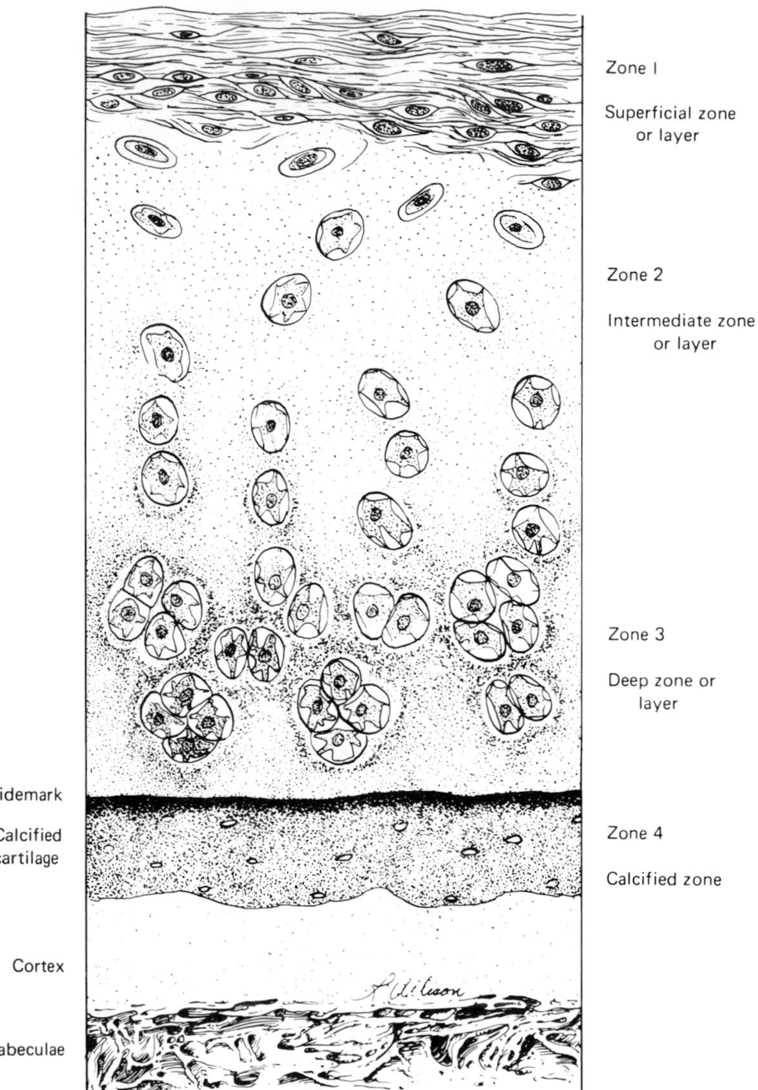

FIG. 2-5. The zones of adult articular cartilage.

lie parallel to the surface. At the periphery, the fibrous components merge with the fibrous periosteum of the adjacent bone.

In Zones 2 and 3, banded fibers are broader (from 300–800 A), are more widely spaced, and intervening ground substance is more abundant. In general, these fibers are randomly oriented and show little tendency to form bundles. They form a strong basketlike enclosure about cells.

In Zone 2, the collagen fibers form a tangled open network. At a deeper level, the fibers are thicker, more tightly packed, and tend toward a vertical arrangement.

When articular cartilage is subjected to a physiologic compressive load for a period of about 12 hours, the open fibrous network in Zone 2 becomes obliterated, the fibers becoming oriented at right angles to the direction of loading. The radial fibers in the deep layer show little change under load.[4,5]

Contour of Articular Surface. The question of whether the articular surface is normally smooth or irregular remains unresolved.

Water Content. The water content of articular cartilage constitutes approximately 75% of the wet weight and does not change with aging. Temporary swelling of the cartilage develops after exercise and is attributed to absorption of water from the joint space. The water content is highest next to the articular surface.[14]

The Ground Substance. Glycosaminoglycans are mainly chondroitin sulfate and keratan sulfate, large molecules with a molecular weight of 50,000 and considerable negative charge. These polyanions are covalently bound to protein forming a PPS complex termed *proteoglycan,* with a molecular weight up to 4×10^6. Proteoglycan molecules aggregate about a specific "link" glycoprotein, forming very large complexes. Closely associated with the PPS complexes are neutral glycoprotein molecules containing a large proportion of protein and only a small carbohydrate moiety; these carry little or no negative charge.

Histochemical Identification of Proteoglycans. Glycosaminoglycans have characteristic ion-binding properties that are used for histochemical identification by using cationic dyes, and often stain metachromatically. Various fixation methods are best avoided because they often cause loss of glycosaminoglycans and thereby adversely affect staining. It is preferable to work with fresh-frozen material stained immediately after sectioning.

Various factors can affect staining qualities. For example, a lesser degree of polymerization of glycosaminoglycan-protein complexes reduces the molecular weight and results in a more orthochromatic reaction.

The immunofluorescent method is useful for determining the degree of polymerization. The more highly polymerized the polysaccharide, the more effective is the exclusion of the antibody protein from the site of the antigen. This causes reduction or loss of immunofluorescence.

The basophilia and metachromasia typical of staining glycosaminoglycans are less intense in the superficial zone than in the intermediate and deep zones. The matrix of the intermediate zone is diffusely stained, but, in the deep zone, intense color is concentrated about the cell groups. Immature cartilage stains evenly throughout the whole thickness of matrix.

Such cationic dyes as alcian blue, azure A, toluidine blue, and safranin act as precipitants of carbohydrate polyanions. Generally, keratan sulfate and chondroitin sulfate are stained together, but it is possible to determine the distribution of the individual components. When sections are previously treated with testicular hyaluronidase to remove the chondroitin sulfate, the residual staining is due to the keratan sulfate and is most intense in the deep zone matrix lying remote from the chondrocytes. Conversely, the chondroitin sulfate stains most intensely in the deeper parts of Zone 3 immediately about the cells.[13]

Histochemical Measurement of Protein Polysaccharides. The concentration of polysaccharides in the ground substance can be quantitatively determined by using safranin O, a cationic dye that binds stoichiometrically to the polyanions (Color Plate 2-1). One dye molecule binds to each negatively charged group of chondroitin sulfate and keratan sulfate (see Chapter 7).

Extracellular Lipid. Lipid constitutes 1% of the wet weight and is mainly pericellular in location. In the superficial zone, it is spread diffusely in the matrix, and under electron microscopy appears as electron-dense granules and membranous bodies.[3] Their function is unknown.

Calcified Zone. The basal zone contains small chondrocytes. The tidemark is the undulating basophilic line which sharply delineates the calcified zone from the deep zone. The calcified zone provides a firm attachment to the subchondral lamellar bone. The calcified cartilage sends extensions into the subjacent bone, while vascular marrow extensions penetrate the basal layer a short distance, but eventually become obliterated with advancing age.

Changes in the Superficial Zone. Since changes in the superficial zone are very important in altering the biomechanical function of articular cartilage, the following facts should be emphasized and correlated with the mechanical properties (see Chapter 7).

Loss of Glycosaminoglycan. Basophilia in this area is normally weaker in adults than in children, reflecting the relatively low glycosaminoglycan in the superficial zone of adult cartilage.[1] Beneath a "histologically intact" surface, a band of pronounced pallor has been described, attributable to further loss of glycosaminoglycan, and may imply the earliest evidence of degenerative change.[9]

Cell Depletion. Changes in nuclear staining and empty lacunae accompany loss of glycosaminoglycan and may imply necrosis of chondrocytes.

Effects of Glycosaminoglycan Loss. The overlying cartilage may be intact but the regressive change may extend deeply, thereby seriously impairing the ability of the articular cartilage to withstand loads. It has also been shown that the regressive change influences the depth to which the zone of low fixed-charge density extends below the articular surface. Therefore, a determination of fixed-charge density reflects the glycosaminoglycan content.[7]

THE CHONDROCYTES

Chondrocytes are involved with the physiologic turnover of extracellular ground substance, which is responsible for the biomechanical and biologic properties of this tissue. The synthesis and degradation of the individual components of the matrix occur not only during the stage of rapid skeletal development but also continue throughout adult life.[17] The metabolic activity occurs within the organelles and cytoplasm, and the morphology of the organelles and other cytoplasmic inclusions reflect the degree of functional activity. Therefore, studies should be carried out chronologically by light microscopy and transmission electron microscopy, supplemented by histochemical techniques and by autoradiography to trace the pathways of the metabolic processes. Moreover, it is essential to define the "norm" before these studies can be interpreted.

Freshly isolated living chondrocytes exhibit ameboid movement, constantly changing their shape by putting out and withdrawing their pseudopodia.[16] Near the articular surface, the cells, in vertical sections, appear elongated, but when a tangential section is viewed en face, they appear discoidal. Superficial cells are less active than those in the deep layers. As its distance from the surface lengthens, the cell becomes increasingly rounded, larger, and metabolically more active,[18] as indicated by prominent, well-defined organelles and by an increased concentration of matrix components in the pericellular area. This is confirmed by autoradiography.

Cells are most numerous near the articular surface, and the number of cells per unit volume diminishes with increasing distance from the surface to a depth of 0.5 mm or more, beyond which the number remains relatively unchanged. There are few cells in the basal calcified zone. In normal human articular cartilage, cell density remains unchanged with advancing age.

Mitotic division can be observed in immature, rapidly growing cartilage, but not in mature adult articular cartilage. However, in adult cartilage, tritiated thymidine (H^3-thymidine) which is incorporated into deoxyribonucleic acid (DNA) just prior to mitotic division, can be demonstrated within the nucleus after its administration. This phenomenon occurs infrequently, explaining why actual mitosis is almost impossible to observe except under certain circumstances. For example, when cartilage is damaged, reactive attempts at repair may be indicated by an increased uptake of H^3-thymidine, signifying increased cell replication.

ULTRASTRUCTURAL CHARACTERISTICS OF CARTILAGE

THE CHONDROCYTE

Basic to a study of the structure and function of the chondrocyte is a review of its component organelles.[20]

Mitochondrion is a threadlike vesicle housing enzymes that catalyze the formation of adenosine triphosphate

FIG. 2-6. A chondrocyte showing nucleus (*N*) with nucleolus (*S*), cytoplasm (*C*), limiting cell membrane (*R*), and cell processes (*P*). Pericellular (*L*) and intercellular (*T*) matrix. Transmission electron micrograph × 10,000. Glutaraldehyde. (Meachim G: The matrix. In Freeman, MA: Adult Articular Cartilage, 2nd ed, p 1. London, Pitman, 1973)

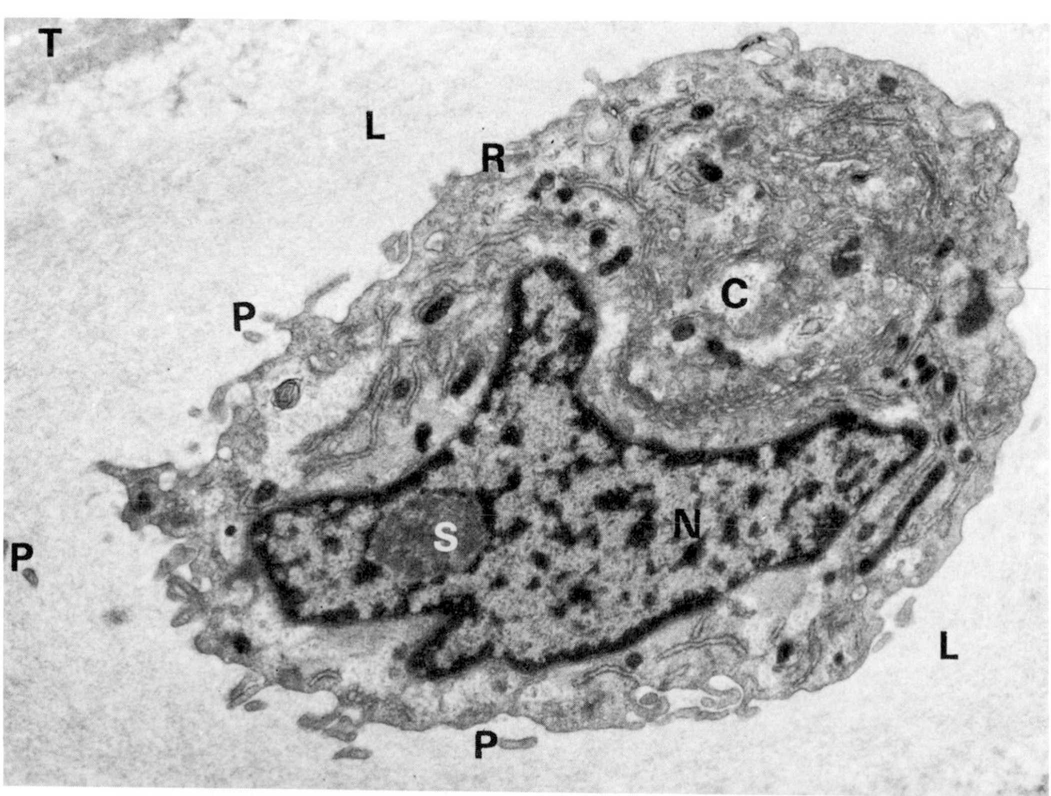

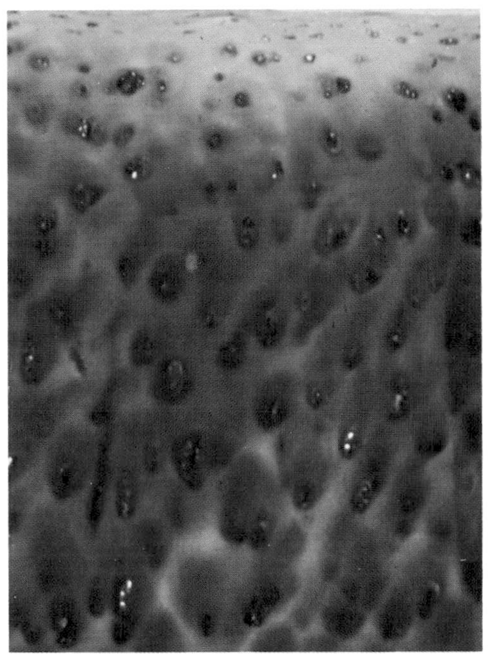

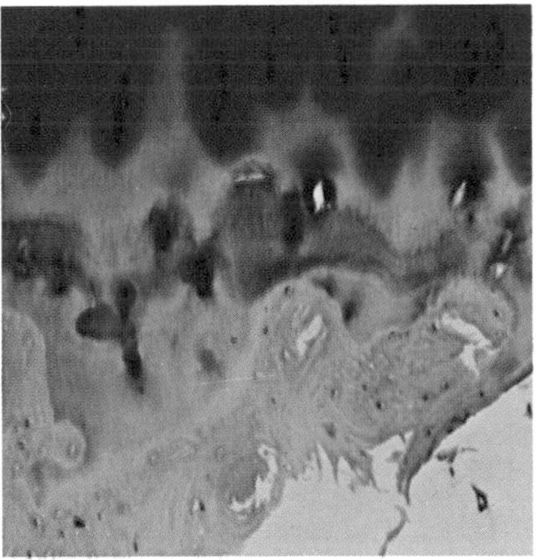

PLATE. 2-1. Normal adult (70-year-old patient) human cartilage stained with safranin-O to specifically demonstrate, by the intensity of the stain, the concentration of glycosaminoglycans; counterstained with hematoxylin. (*Top*) Superficial zone: elongated cells are arranged with the long axis parallel to articular surface. The acellular bright line at the articular surface is the lamina splendens. The matrix does not stain with safranin-O. Transitional zone: rounded cells are in random arrangement; some cells are in pairs. This zone stains with safranin-O. Radial zone: rounded cells are in short columns arranged perpendicular to the articular surface. The zone stains with safranin-O. (*Bottom*) Basilar portion. The cell columns of the radial zone are surrounded by an intensely stained matrix indicating an increased concentration of glycosaminoglycans at this level. The "tidemark" separates the radial from the calcified zone. Calcified zone: rests upon the subchondral bony end plate. (× 100) (Courtesy of Dr. Charles Weiss) (See p. 19.)

(ATP), which provides energy for the synthesis of other compounds by transferring one of its energy-containing terminal phosphate groups to another molecule. The ATP is changed to adenosine diphosphate (ADP), which is subsequently reconverted to ATP within the mitochondrion.

Ribosomes are electron-dense little bodies of nucleoprotein and serve as sites where amino acids are linked together to form protein. Ribosomes are produced in the nucleolus and are composed of ribosomal RNA (rRNA). They are either unattached and strewn throughout the cytoplasm, or are attached to rough-surfaced endoplasmic reticulum, the main site of protein synthesis.

Nucleoli, usually single, have no limiting membrane, and are difficult to see in metabolically inactive cells. They are more prominent, often double, in cells with heightened metabolism. They produce most of rRNA and produce preribosomal particles (ribosomal subunits) which form ribosomes (Fig. 2-6).

Rough-surfaced endoplasmic reticulum are hollow membranous structures, either tubules or bladderlike vesicles. Large flattened vesicles are termed cisternae and are of two types, rough and smooth. The rough type possesses ribosomes responsible for the localized cytoplasmic basophilia. Synthesis of protein occurs at ribosomes sitting on membranous walls of cisternae. The ribosome-studded cisternae are packed closely together and lie parallel to each other. Secretions in the lumens are electron dense (Figs. 2-7 and 2-8).

The *Golgi apparatus* is a membranous structure of flattened saccules resembling stacks of pancakes, three to eight in number. Transfer vesicles budding off from the cisternae of the rough endoplasmic reticulum lose their ribosomes, fuse with the Golgi saccule, and discharge their contents into its lumen. At the same time, vesicles bud off from the mature face of the Golgi stack, becoming secretory granules (Fig. 2-9).

Within the Golgi stack, the PPS molecule, which has

FIG. 2-7. Part of a chondrocyte showing paired membranes of rough endoplasmic reticulum (*R*) with ribosome granules (*arrows*). The rough endoplasmic reticulum contrasts with the smooth membranes of the Golgi apparatus (*G*). Micropinocytotic vesicles (*V*). Limiting cell membrane (*D*). Transmission electron micrograph × 37,500. Glutaraldehyde. (Meachim G: The matrix. In Freeman MA: Adult Articular Cartilage, 2nd ed, p 1. London, Pitman, 1973)

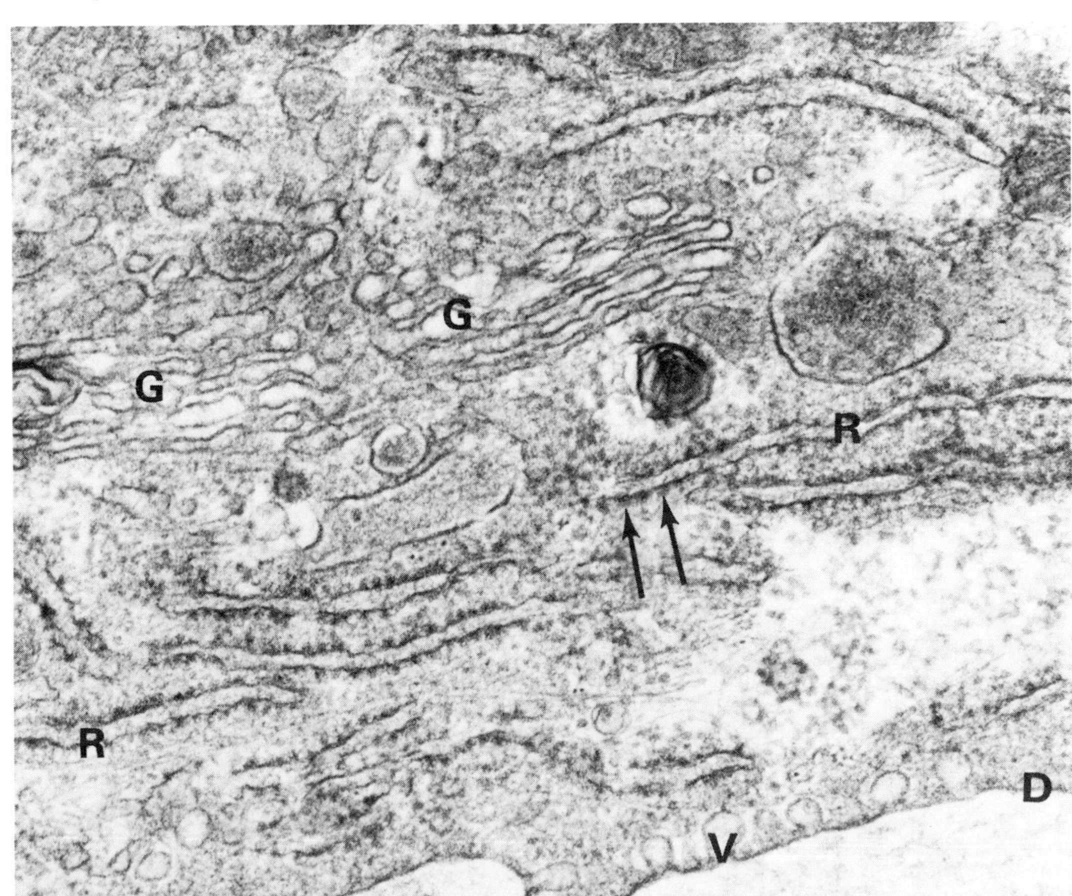

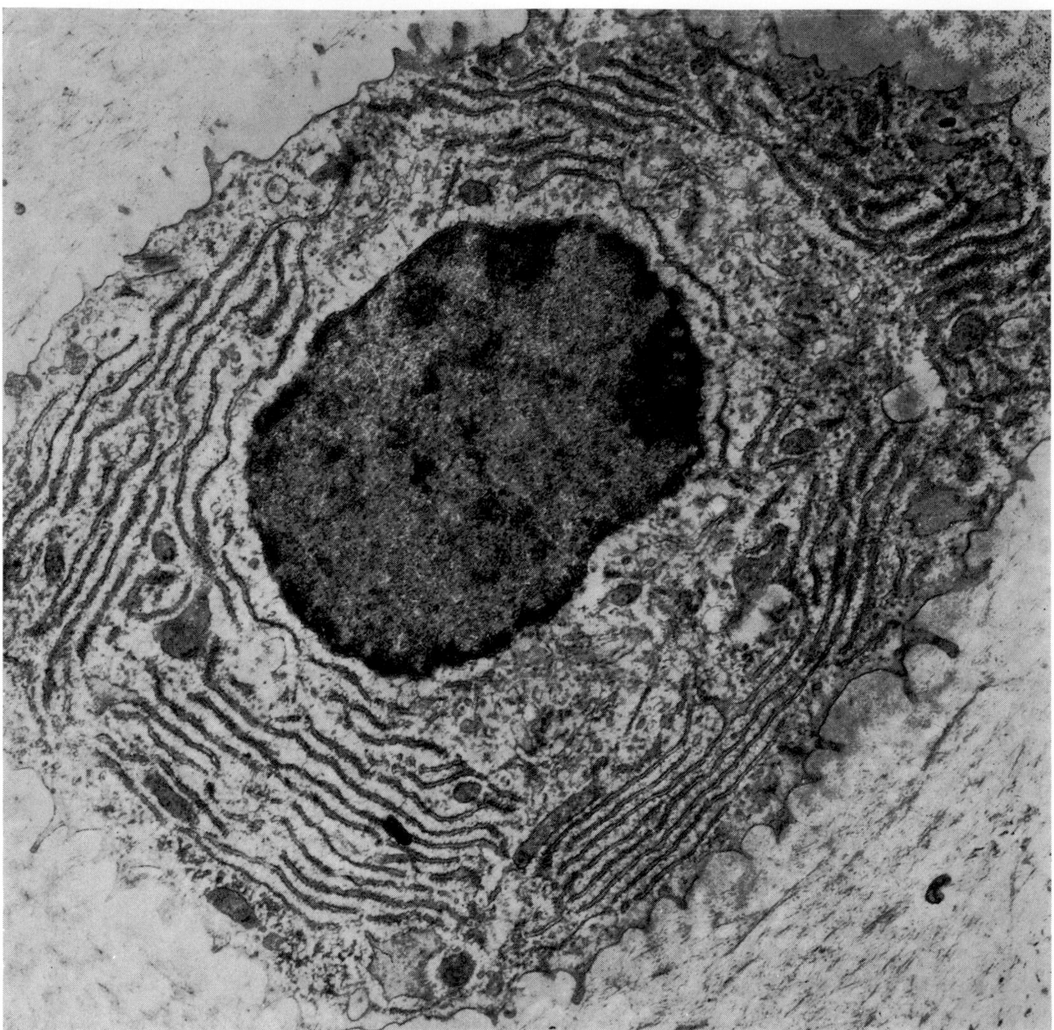

FIG. 2-8. Ultrastructural characteristics of the chondrocyte. The cytoplasm reveals well-developed rough-surfaced vesicles of endoplasmic reticulum and a well-developed Golgi apparatus. The cytoplasmic processes extend off into the intercellular substance (cytoplasmic footlets). As the chondrocyte becomes older and synthesis of protein is less, the rough-surfaced vesicles and Golgi apparatus become less prominent, and glycogen and lipid material accumulate in the cytoplasm. (Ham AW: Histology, 7th ed. Philadelphia, JB Lippincott, 1974)

originated in the organelles prior to entering the Golgi stack, is further modified by the addition of polysaccharide side-chains. The final substance accumulates in the saccules toward the mature face distending them. The secretory vesicles bud off from membranous globules.

Therefore, the function of the Golgi apparatus is to complete the addition of carbohydrate side-chains to glycoproteins arriving from the rough endoplasmic reticulum. This is accomplished by enzymes, the sugar transferases.

The periodic acid-Schiff (PAS) reaction, a stain for polysaccharides, is weakest in the immature saccule. Intense staining occurs within mature saccules, indicating that these contain molecules with the highest number of side-chains.

Lysosomes are vesicles budding off from the Golgi apparatus and contain digestive enzymes, the hydrolases, which break down macromolecules originating either intracellularly or extracellularly. These round or oval bodies of approximately 0.5 μ in diameter are identified by the Gomori technique which causes the precipitation of lead salts. The black electron-dense material results from the presence of phosphatase.

The *nucleus* is either oval or elongated, and its outline is smooth or indented. It contains electron-dense granular nucleoplasm and occasionally a nucleolus can be seen.

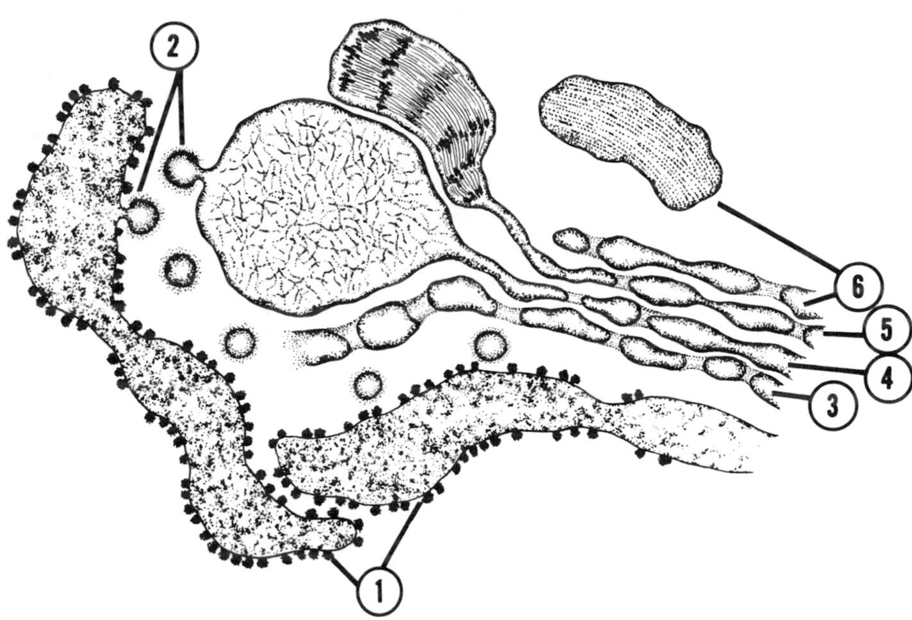

FIG. 2-9. Part of Golgi region of collagen-secreting cell. (*1*) The cisternae of RER with their coating of ribosomes; (*2*) a few intermediate or transfer vesicles, one of which, at left, is being released from a cisterna, while another is connected to the distended portion of a Golgi saccule; (*3*) part of a stack of Golgi saccules at right, the first saccule of which shows the pattern characteristic of fenestrations; (*4*) the second saccule ending in a distended portion filled with entangled threads; (*5*) the third saccule ending in a distended portion filled with parallel threads; (*6*) the fourth saccule showing no connection in the figure, but, above it, a solid structure with discrete striation, which is believed to come from a distended portion which has been separated from it; the parallel threads have aggregated. This is a secretory vesicle (also called secretory granule) that carried its content for release at the cell surface. (Ham A: Histology, 7th ed. Philadelphia, JB Lippincott, 1974. From M Weinstock and C. P. Leblond)

The nucleus is surrounded by two membranes forming the nuclear envelope in which there are small openings termed nucleopores.

The nucleus contains DNA, the genetic material of the cell. The information is stored in this material and is transmitted by messenger chemicals (mRNA) for instructions to the cytoplasm.

CHARACTERISTICS OF CHONDROCYTES IN ARTICULAR CARTILAGE

Zone I, at the surface, shows ellipsoid cells oriented parallel to the articular surface. Mitochondria are few and small. The cytoplasmic volume is small, the rough endoplasmic reticulum is poorly developed, and few ribosomes attest to a low level of protein synthesis.[23] The Golgi apparatus forms numerous flattened saccules devoid of electron-dense material. There is no evidence of synthesis of sulfated polysaccharide. These surface cells resemble relatively inactive fibrocytes.

Zone II cells are rounded and larger than those of Zone I. The cell membrane is scalloped, suggesting that vesicles and vacuoles have merged with the cell membrane to discharge their contents. Micropinocytosis vesicles and acanthosomes are present. An extensive endoplasmic reticulum heavily studded with ribosomes forms concentric lamellae. The Golgi complex is particularly well developed with many vesicles and vacuoles. The vacuoles may contain electron-dense amorphous material. Intracellular fibrils of 40-A diameter lie adjacent to the Golgi complex throughout the cytoplasm and immediately subjacent to the cell membrane. Mitochondria are abundant.

Zone III cells show abundant rough endoplasmic reticulum, ribosomes are plentiful, and there are a large Golgi apparatus and large mitochondria. Glycogen is present. The intracellular cytoplasmic filaments are about 70-A diameter.

In summary, the cells of Zones II and III show abundant cytoplasm, extensively developed endoplasmic reticulum heavily studded with ribosomes, enlarged Golgi complex, and many mitochondria. The degree of protein synthesis closely parallels the development of the granular endoplasmic reticulum and the Golgi complex. The polypeptide protein chain is synthesized by the ribosomes. The carbohydrate side-chains of glycoproteins are built up successively at different sites by transferases, adding sugars one at a time stepwise as the glycoprotein travels through the cisternae of the rough endoplasmic reticulum and from these through the Golgi apparatus, where much of the carbohydrate is added.

The ultrastructural characteristics of the chondrocytes of articular cartilage indicate that the highest degree of metabolic activity occurs in Zones II and III.

FIBROUS ELEMENTS OF ARTICULAR CARTILAGE

The extracellular substance of articular cartilage consists of fibrous elements, only some of which show the characteristic morphology of collagen, embedded in a gel-like matrix.[22,23] The collagen fibers near the articular surface are predominantly parallel to the surface and are densely aggregated. The deeper zones show more random distribution, the density decreasing progressively with the distance from the articular surface (Fig. 2-10).

At the free surface, a thin layer (3 μ thick) is composed of a dense network of randomly oriented fine fibers of 40 A to 120 A in diameter. This layer has no cells.

Zone I consists of large bundles of closely aggregated collagen fibers with the characteristic periodicity of 640 A, each fiber being about 340 A thick, and containing little or no intervening ground substance. The bundles parallel the joint surface and lie at oblique or right angles to each other. This layer has the highest collagen density.

Below Zone I the bundles abruptly disappear and are replaced by widely spaced, randomly oriented, individual collagen fibers, with characteristic periodicity of 640 A, of progressively increasing diameter, from 700 A to 1000 A. Within the broad matrix, between the unit collagen fibers, runs a delicate network of fine fibers lacking characteristic periodicity and 40 A to 100 A in diameter. Large numbers of fibrils, 40 A to 100 A, lie immediately adjacent to each cell.

Within Zone II, the diameter of collagen fibers varies widely, reaching about 600 A. At greater depths, large fibers may reach approximately 1400 A in diameter.

Although the microfibrils are morphologically distinct from mature collagen fibers, being of rough texture and lacking the typical periodicity, they may represent true collagen in a modified physical state.[21]

In the newborn infant, although the articular surface is composed of collagen fibers with characteristic periodicity, which are grouped into bundles, the remainder of the cartilage generally contains smaller fibers that lack periodicity and rarely form bundles.[19]

FIG. 2-10. Electron micrograph of newly polymerized microfibrils of collagen beside a fibroblast, the edge of whose cytoplasm is seen at the top (CYT). Note that the microfibrils closest to the cytoplasm are finer than those that are farther away, showing how microfibrils can increase in diameter after they are first polymerized outside of fibroblasts. (× 76,000) (Fernando NVP, Movat HZ: Fibrillogenesis in regenerating tendon. Lab Invest 12:214, 1963)

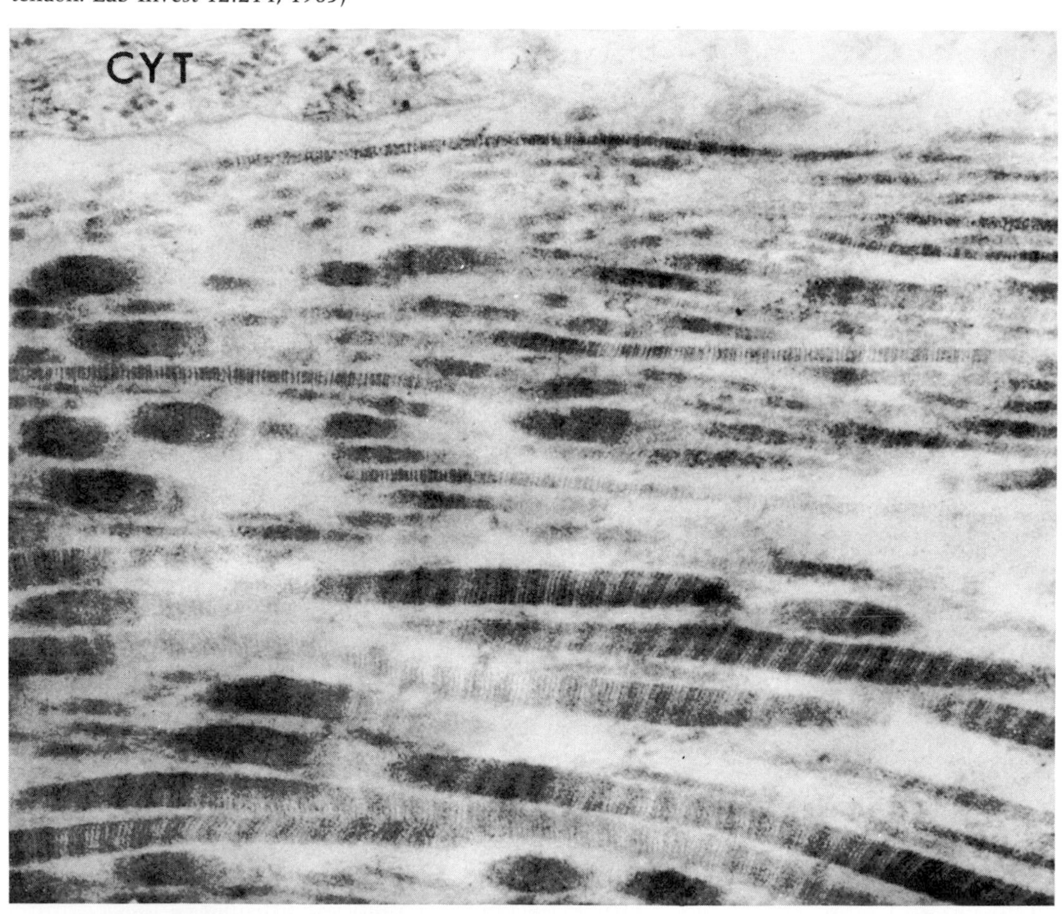

REPAIR OF ARTICULAR CARTILAGE

A traumatic or surgically induced defect in articular cartilage possesses variable potential for repair. The original viewpoint expressed by Hunter,[27] that a defect of articular cartilage is incapable of anatomical restoration, has many supporters. To some extent this is true when the defect is limited to the articular cartilage and does not penetrate the subchondral bone.[25] There is controversy not only concerning whether repair actually occurs, but also, when the defect appears to be filled in and the degree and source of the repair reaction.

Following an injury to articular cartilage, whether or not the defect is repaired, certain changes occur in the adjoining tissue that suggest heightened metabolic activity.

HISTOCHEMICAL CHANGES

The tissue forming the surface of the defect loses its staining qualities (basophilia, metachromasia), and the chondrocytes are absent. Deeply situated chondrons containing many chondrocytes are encircled by intensely stained matrix, suggesting increased production of PPS.

ISOTOPE STUDIES

There is increased uptake of H^3-thymidine (used in formation of DNA prior to mitosis), increased uptake of $^{35}SO_4$ (specific indicator of synthesis of acid polysaccharides), and increased uptake of labeled glycin (used in synthesis of protein for PPS and perhaps for collagen).

ULTRASTRUCTURAL STUDIES

Nucleoli, the site of synthesis of rRNA precursors concerned with protein synthesis, are hypertrophied and often multiple. Fine fibrillary material, the probable precursor of collagen, is produced in large amounts. The Golgi complexes are well developed, suggesting increased polysaccharide synthesis.

At the surface, the superficial thin layer of fine, horizontally disposed, collagenlike fibers appear to proliferate, extending outward to cover the defect, and, from its deep surface, gives rise to cellular tissue extending inward to fill the defect and differentiating into varying amounts of fibrous tissue, fibrocartilage, and hyaline cartilage. When partial thickness defects confined to the articular cartilage are subjected to constant joint motion, the differentiation toward hyaline cartilage is more pronounced.

When a full thickness defect extends into the subchondral bone, granulation tissue rapidly invades from the vascular marrow spaces, and healing is predominantly fibrous or fibrocartilaginous.

The manner of repair of cartilage defects remains controversial, and the following representative concepts have evolved from investigations. (Refer to original articles and study Chapter 7, Physiology of Cartilage.)

No Repair.[26] Defects limited to the articular cartilage adjacent to the synovial attachment, or perichondrium can undergo some degree of healing by proliferation and invasion from the soft tissue. Wounds at a distance from soft tissue do not heal.

Electron Microscopic Studies.[25] At 4 days to 1 month, the tissue bordering the defect loses its staining qualities (necrosis?), and the matrix becomes peppered with cytomembranous remnants and lipidic debris (Fig. 2-11). The surface of the adjacent articular cartilage is covered with debris and encrusted with amorphous electron-dense material. Fine fibrillary material surrounds the chondrocytes adjacent to the defect, and organelles are altered (*e.g.*, Golgi complexes are large or multiple, increased numbers of lysosomes, nucleolar hypertrophy, increased rough endoplasmic reticulum, and unaltered ribosomes; Fig. 2-11).

At 2 to 6 months, the fine filament fibers within the chondrocyte are increased, and the packed fibers within the cytoplasm obscure the organelles. The glycogen content is increased. The fine fibers accumulate on the surface of the defect as a fine feltwork tending toward orientation parallel to the surface. Granular or amorphous electron-dense material covers the surface.

In conclusion, there is no evident repair reaction, but there is evidence of heightened synthesis of matrix components.

Repair of Partial Thickness Defects.[24] Complete repair is attained in approximately 20% of defects induced in experimental immature animals, during a period of extraordinary cellular proliferation and cartilage growth. At first the surface is bridged by the larger of elongated compacted cells in a collagenous stroma. The defect is then filled in rapidly by cellular fibroblastic tissue which changes, as it extends deeply, into chondroid tissues with cells irregularly disposed in a homogeneous matrix. The reparative tissue consistently forms hyaline cartilage which blends with preexisting cartilage (Figs. 2-12 and 2-13).

Repair of Full Thickness Defects.[24,26] Repair of full thickness defects (extending through the subchondral bone) occurs by proliferation of cellular tissue originating from the superficial layer which has bridged the defect at the surface; and from the marrow spaces at the base by rapidly invading osteogenic cells and granulation tissue, resulting in a mixture of bony trabeculae, cartilage, and mostly fibrous tissue (Fig. 2-14). In experimental animals, when the joint is subjected to continuous passive motion for several weeks after creation of the defect, the reparative tissue is composed almost entirely of cartilage.

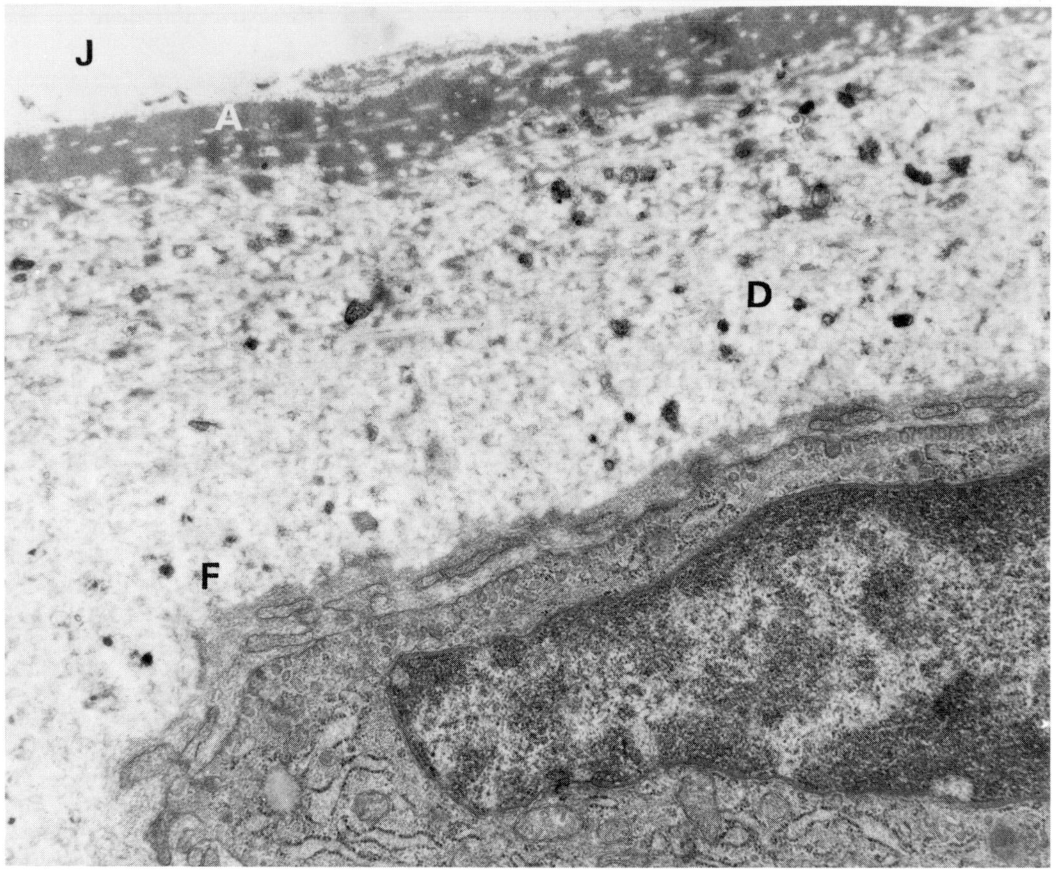

FIG. 2-11. A 4-day specimen showing a Zone 1 chondrocyte lying at the junction between the defect and adjacent cartilage. Note fibrillary collar (*F*) around chondrocyte, lipidic debris (*D*) in matrix, and irregular surface encrusted with amorphous material (*A*). Joint space (*J*). (× 23,000) (Fuller JA, Ghadially FN: Ultrastructural observations on surgically produced partial-thickness defects of articular cartilage. Clin Orthop 86:193, 1972)

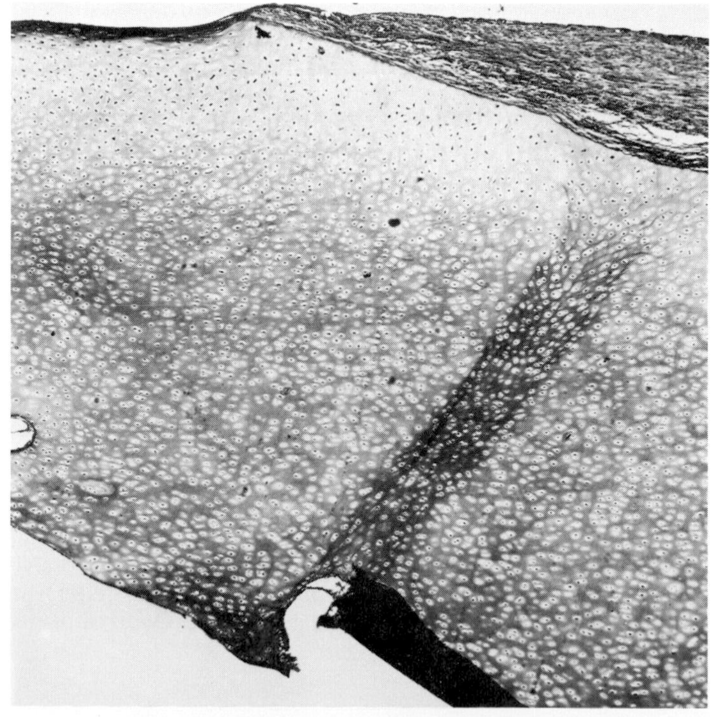

FIG. 2-12. Partial articular cartilage defect at 3 weeks. The surface fibrous layer has extended to fill and obliterate the defect and eventually will assume a "chondroid" appearance. The tissue adjacent to the defect stains poorly and contains necrotic cells and empty lacunae. At a distance from the defect, the tissue is hypercellular, the cells often form groups, and the stain for glycoaminoglycan is most intense in pericelluar areas.

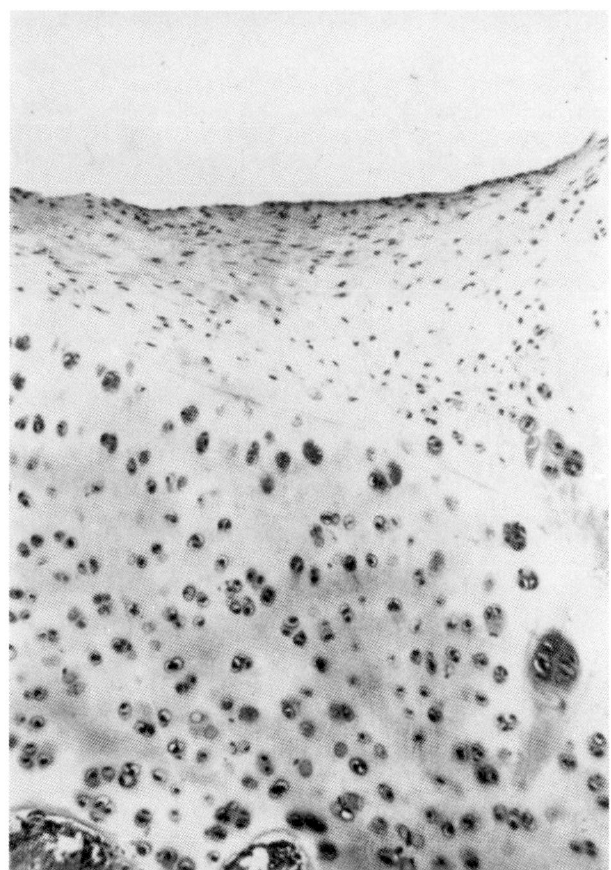

FIG. 2-13. Superficial defect involving about one third the thickness of the articular cartilage after 7 weeks. The defect has been filled by tissue that became progressively more cartilaginous from the surface downward. There is a thin zone of dead cells in the cartilage at the margin of the defect, and just outside the zone numerous new chondrons are present. (× 43) (Calandruccio RA, Gilmer WS, Jr: Proliferation, regeneration, and repair of articular cartilage of immature animals. J Bone Joint Surg, 44A:431, 1962)

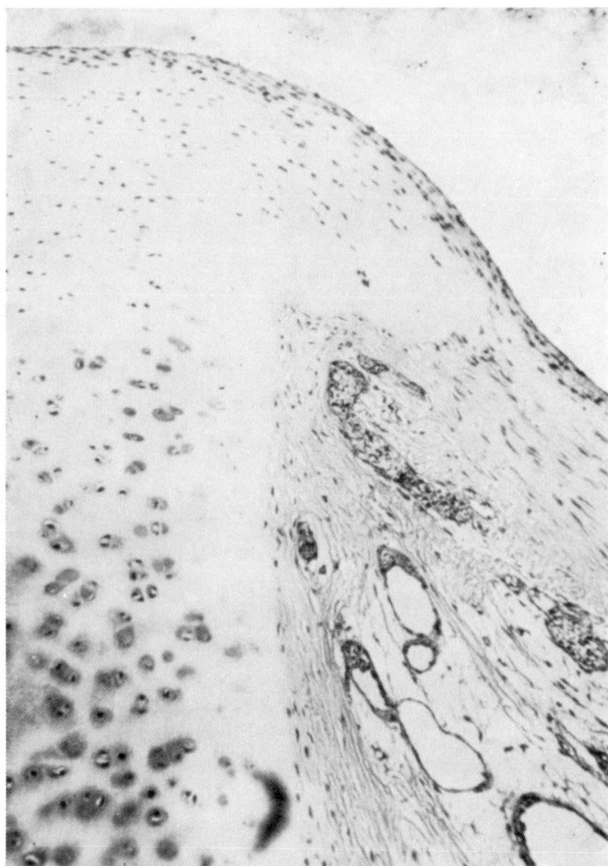

FIG. 2-14. Photomicrograph of the surface (*top, right*) and margin (*top, left*) of a complete defect after 7 weeks. Note the loss of metachromasia and of basophilia and the dead cells in the cartilage at the margin of the defect. Also visible is the marked overhang of cartilage produced by the flow of the matrix and presumably of some of the cells of the upper intermediate layer into the defect. The proliferation and extension of the superficial cell layer (surface layer of compact cells) across the defect are clearly shown as are the reorientation of the chondrocytes toward the defect and the large blood vessels that have entered the defect from the subchondral bone. (× 43) (Calandruccio RA, Gilmer WS, Jr: Proliferation, regeneration, and repair of articular cartilage of immature animals. J Bone Joint Surg, 44A:431, 1962)

The main cartilaginous constituent forms nearer the surface. The tendency to form hyaline cartilage is much greater when the joint is subjected to continuous passive motion than when the joint is immobilized or is actively exercised intermittently (Fig. 2-15).[28]

When the joint is immobilized, the defect fills with primitive connective tissue with little cartilage. Under conditions of continuous motion, the reparative tissue becomes cartilaginous, restores a smooth articular surface, and the intercellular matrix fuses with the original cartilage. The margins of the original cartilage defect remain necrotic over a depth of several cells (empty lacunae, matrix does not stain). At a greater depth, the original cartilage shows evidence of increased cellular multiplication (multicellular chondrons).

REFERENCES

Adult Articular Cartilage

1. Collins DH, McElligott TF: Sulphate ($^{35}SO_4$) uptake by chondrocytes in relation to histological changes in osteoarthritic human articular cartilage. Ann Rheum Dis 19:318, 1960
2. Gersh I, Catchpole MR: The nature of ground substance of connective tissue. Perspect Biol Med 3:282, 1960.
3. Ghadially FN, Meachim G, Collins DH: Extracellular lipid in the matrix of human articular cartilage. Ann Rheum Dis 24:136, 1965

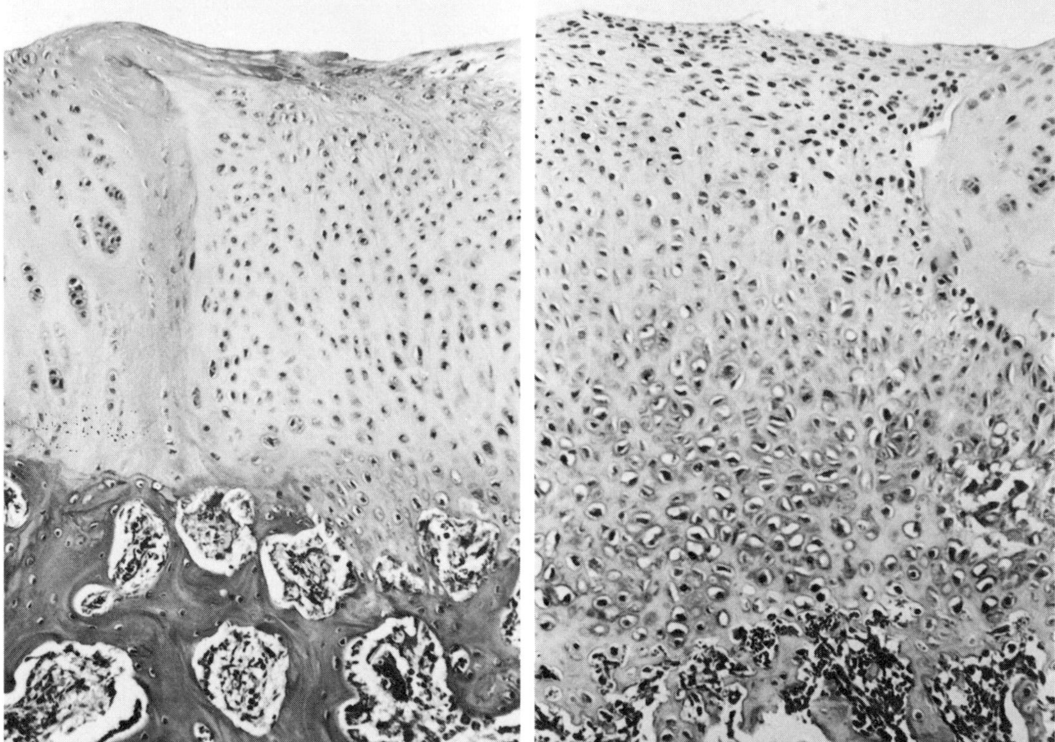

FIG. 2-15. The influence of motion on cartilaginous repair of articular cartilage, full-thickness defect. The knee joint of this animal was subjected to continuous passive motion for 3 weeks after the defect was created. The reparative tissue originating from the bone below is entirely cartilaginous and is fusing with the edges of the original articular cartilage. (Salter RB *et al.* In Ham AW: Histology. Philadelphia, JB Lippincott, 1974)

4. McCall JG: Load deformation response of the microstructure of articular cartilage. *In* Wright V (ed): Lubrication and Wear in Joints, p. 39. London, Sector, 1969
5. McCall JG: Load deformation studies of articular cartilage. J Anat 105:212, 1969
6. Mankin HJ, Lippiello L: The turnover of adult rabbit articular cartilage. J Bone Joint Surg 51A:1591, 1969
7. Maroudas A, Thomas A: A simple physiochemical micromethod for determining fixed anion groups in connective tissue. Biochim Biophys Acta 215:214, 1970
8. Maximow AA, Bloom W: A Textbook of Histology, 5th ed, p 118. Philadelphia, WB Saunders, 1948
9. Meachim G, Ghadially FN, Collins DH: Regressive changes in the superficial layer of human articular cartilage. Ann Rheum Dis 24:23, 1965
10. Meachim G: Effect of age on the thickness of adult cartilage at the shoulder joint. Ann Rheum Dis 30:43, 1971
11. Meachim G: Meshwork patterns in the ground substance of articular cartilage and nucleus pulposus. J Anat 11:219, 1972
12. Rosenberg L, Hellman W, Kleinschmidt AK: Macromolecular models of protein polysaccharides from bovine nasal cartilage. J Biol Chem 245:4123, 1970
13. Scott JE, Stockwell RA: On the use and abuse of the critical electrolyte concentration approach of the localization of tissue polyanions. J Histochem Cytochem 15:111, 1967
14. Stockwell RA: Changes in the acid glycosaminoglycan content of the matrix of aging human articular cartilage. Ann Rheum Dis 29:509, 1970
15. Weiss C, Rosenberg L, Helfet AJ: An ultrastructural study of normal young adult human articular cartilage. J Bone Joint Surg 50A:663, 1968

The Chondrocytes

16. Chesterman RJ, Smith AU: Homotransplantation of articular cartilage and isolated chondrocytes. J Bone Joint Surg 50B:184, 1968
17. Collins DH, Meachim G: Sulphate ($^{35}SO_4$) fixation by human articular cartilage compared in the knee and shoulder joints. Ann Rheum Dis 20:117, 1961
18. Kuhlman E: A microchemical study of the developing epiphyseal plate. J Bone Joint Surg 42A:457, 1960

Ultrastructural Characteristics of Cartilage

19. Cameron DA, Robinson RA: Electron microscopy of epiphyseal and articular cartilage matrix in the femur of the newborn infant. J Bone Joint Surg 40A:163, 1958
20. Ham AW: Histology, 7th ed. Philadelphia, JB Lippincott, 1974
21. Low FN: Microfibrils; Fine filamentous components of the tissue space. Anat Rec 142:131, 1962

22. Muir H, Bullough P, Maroudas A: Distribution of collagen in human articular cartilage with some of its physiological implications. J Bone Joint Surg 52B:554, 1970
23. Weiss C, Rosenberg L, Helfet AJ: Ultrastructural study of human articular cartilage. J Bone Joint Surg 50A:663, 1968

Repair of Articular Cartilage

24. Calandruccio RA, Gilmer WS Jr: Proliferation, regeneration, and repair of articular cartilage of immature animals. J Bone Joint Surg 44A:431, 1962
25. Fuller JA, Ghadially FN: Ultrastructural observations on surgically produced partial-thickness defects of articular cartilage. Clin Orthop 86:193, 1972
26. Ham AW: Histology, 7th ed, p 453. Philadelphia, JB Lippincott, 1974
27. Hunter W: On the structure and diseases of articulating cartilage. Philos Trans B 9:267, 1743
28. Salter RB, Simmonds DF, Malcolm BW et al: The biological effect of continuous passive motion on the healing of full-thickness defects in articular cartilage. J Bone Joint Surg 62A:1232, 1980

3

Histology and Histopathology of Bone

Section I
Histology of Bone

TYPES OF BONE

Bone is a specialized connective tissue with a mineralized collagenous framework for skeletal support of the body. It is either spongy (cancellous) or compact in structure. Spongy bone consists of intercrossing and connecting bone (trabeculae) of varying shapes and thicknesses, between which are spaces filled with bone marrow. Compact bone is a continuous bone mass containing interconnecting vascular channels of microscopic size. Both spongy and compact bone exist in almost every bone.

TYPICAL LONG BONE

The diaphysis (shaft) of a long bone (*e.g.*, the femur) consists of a wall of compact bone enclosing a large cylindrical bone marrow cavity.

The epiphysis (end of the bone) consists of spongy bone with a thin outer wall of compact bone, the articular end of which is covered by articular cartilage. In a growing animal, the epiphyseal cartilage plate, from which longitudinal growth occurs, lies between the epiphysis and the diaphysis.

The metaphysis (spongy bone directly beneath the epiphyseal plate) is composed of the most recently formed bone arising out of the growth process at the plate.

FLAT BONES

Flat bones of the skull are composed of inner and outer compact cortical layers (tables) enclosing spongy bone (diploë).

SMALL BONES

Small bones (*e.g.*, carpals) are of simple construction, an outer wall of compact bone enclosing spongy bone.

STRUCTURE OF BONE

The cortex of bone is composed of compact bone, whereas the medulla contains spongy bone. Spongy bone is made up of a loose network of bone trabeculae that are interconnected but generaly arranged along lines of maximum stress or tension. The trabeculae are made up of a varying number of adjoining bone plates. Osteocytes within the lacunae communicate with each other by canaliculi.

Compact bone consists of lamellae, which are regularly arranged about branching and anastomosing canals through which nutrient vessels pass. These haversian canals communicate with the outer surface of the bone or with the medullary cavity through Volkmann's canals (Fig. 3-1).

The basic structural unit of compact bone is designated the *haversian system,* named for Clopton Havers who originally attempted to define the structure of compact bone in 1691.[2] Since he did not describe the concentric lamellae around vessels, the term *osteon* is regarded by some observers as the appropriate eponym.[1] It consists of lamellae concentrically arranged about the haversian canal (concentric lamellae). Most haversian systems are directed in the long axis of the bone. Therefore, in cross section the canals appear as small rounded openings and the lamellae as circles; in longitudinal section, the canals appear as long slits. Large numbers of canaliculi pass radially from the canal to the lacunae and intercommunicate with each other. Their function is supposedly for diffusion of nutrient fluids toward the osteocytes and waste products toward the nutrient vessels. Compact bone is made up of large numbers of haversian systems between which are interstitial or ground lamellae. The latter constitutes the remains of haversian systems that have only partially resorbed (Figs. 3-2 to 3-4).

On the outer and internal aspects of the compact bone are basic or circumferential lamellae which are arranged circumferentially in relation to the main bone. They are penetrated by Volkmann's canals, through which nu-

Fig. 3-1. A cross section and a longitudinal section of the cortex of a long bone. Note the haversian systems running longitudinally. Volkmann's canals constitute connecting channels between periosteal, haversian, and bone marrow blood vessels. (Redrawn from Ham AW, Cormack DH: Histology, 8th ed. Philadelphia, JB Lippincott, 1979)

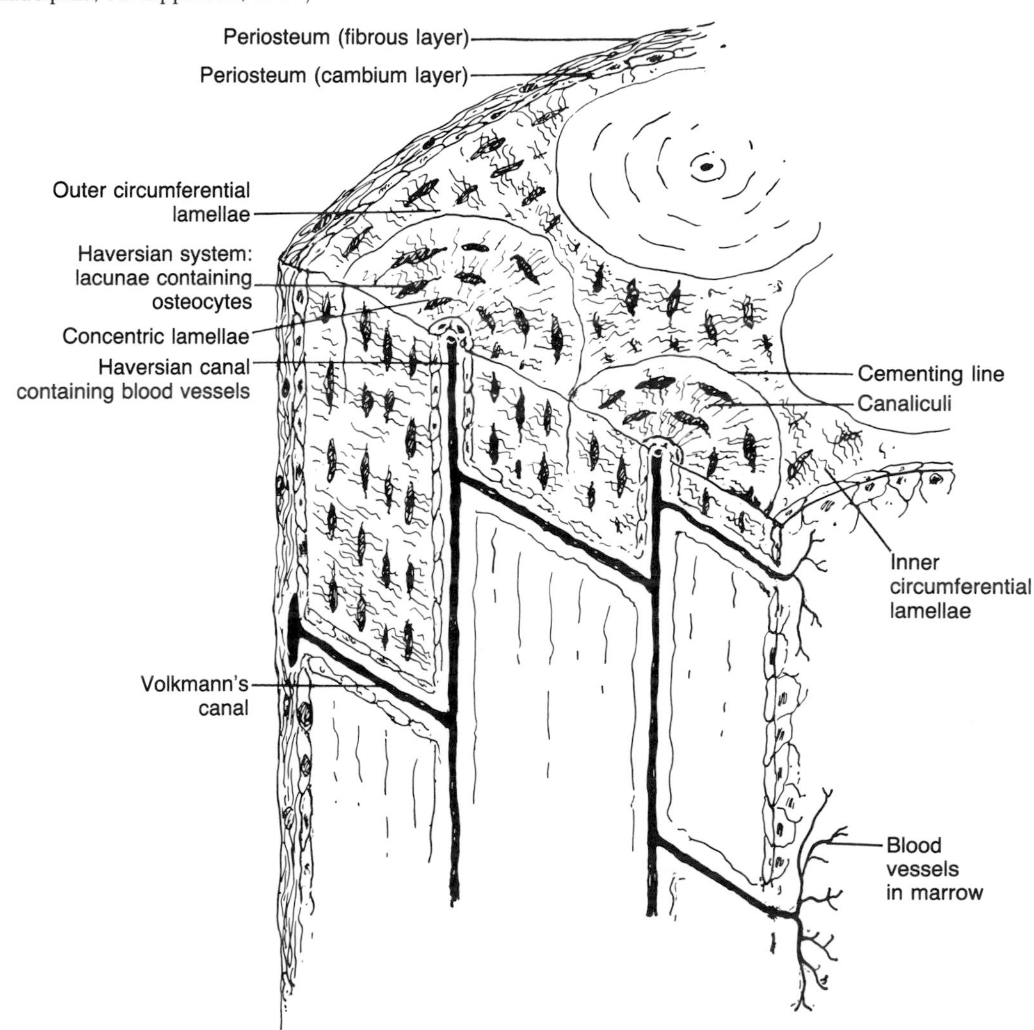

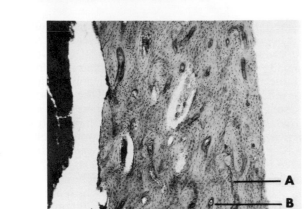

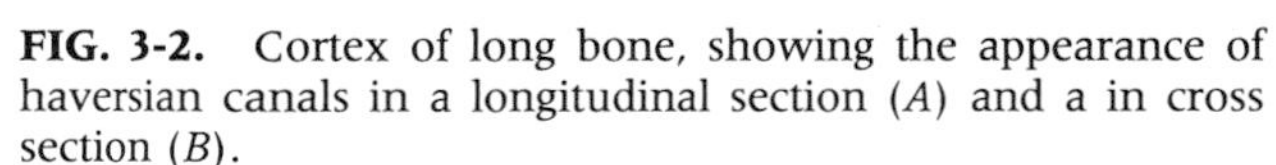

FIG. 3-2. Cortex of long bone, showing the appearance of haversian canals in a longitudinal section (*A*) and a in cross section (*B*).

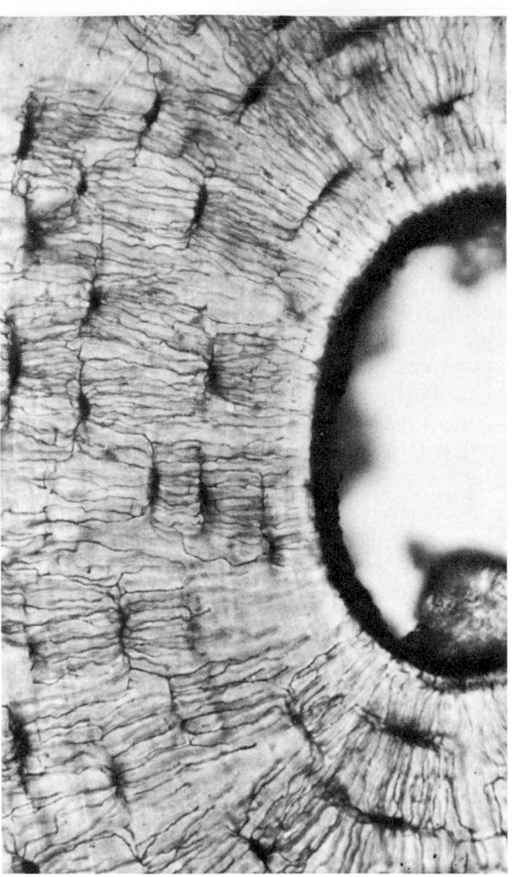

FIG. 3-4. A photomicrograph of a ground bone section. The lacunae in which the osteocytes reside are dark flattened oval structures. The fine lines connecting these are canaliculi. The canaliculi extend to the empty canal on the right. In life this contained blood vessels that supplied tissue fluid to the canaliculi. (Preparation by H. Whittaker. Ham AW, Cormack DH: Histology, 8th ed. Philadelphia, JB Lippincott, 1979)

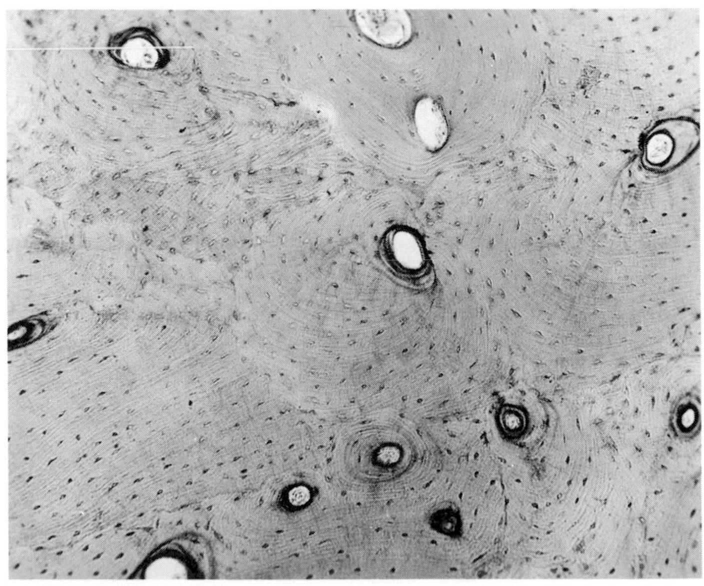

FIG. 3-3. Cross section of the cortex of a long bone. The haversian systems are well displayed.

trient vessels enter the bone to reach the vessels in the haversian canals. They contain large vessels and are not surrounded by concentrically arranged plates.

Sharpey's fibers are thick bundles of collagenous fibers that pass from the periosteum into the basic external circumferential lamellae. They fix the periosteum firmly to the surface of the bone, particularly where tendons and muscles attach, where large blood vessels enter the bone, and at the junction of the epiphysis with the shaft in long bones.

The periosteum consists of dense connective tissue containing blood vessels. Its deepest stratum, the cambium layer, is more loosely arranged and contains spindle-shaped cells (osteogenic cells) and a network of thin elastic fibers.

The endosteum is a thin layer of cellular connective tissue that lines the walls of bone cavities, including the marrow spaces. It is osteogenic and hemopoietic, and perhaps contributes to the formation of osteoclasts.

COMPONENTS OF BONE

PERIOSTEUM

The periosteum, the membrane covering the outer surface of the bone, represents the counterpart of the perichondrium. It is composed of two layers: the fibrous layer, an outer thin layer of dense, irregularly arranged connective tissue containing some fibroblasts; and the osteogenic layer containing osteogenic cells which are flattened, spindle-shaped cells with pluripotential (Fig. 3-5).[3]

OSTEOGENIC CELLS

The osteogenic cells (osteoprogenitor cells) are normally found apposed to the bone surface in the deep layer of resting periosteum, and they also comprise the endosteum where they are likewise apposed to the bone surfaces. During the growth period, the osteogenic cells of the periosteum proliferate and give rise to osteoblasts which add new bone to the surface, accounting for its growth in width. Similarly, the endosteal membrane may give rise to osteoblasts. However, on this surface, frequent bone resorptive cavities containing osteoclasts suggest that these multinucleated cells may arise from fusion of osteogenic cells of the endosteum or from a common stem cell.

The osteogenic cells throughout life retain their potential for differentiating into either chondroblasts or osteoblasts, and perhaps osteoclasts.

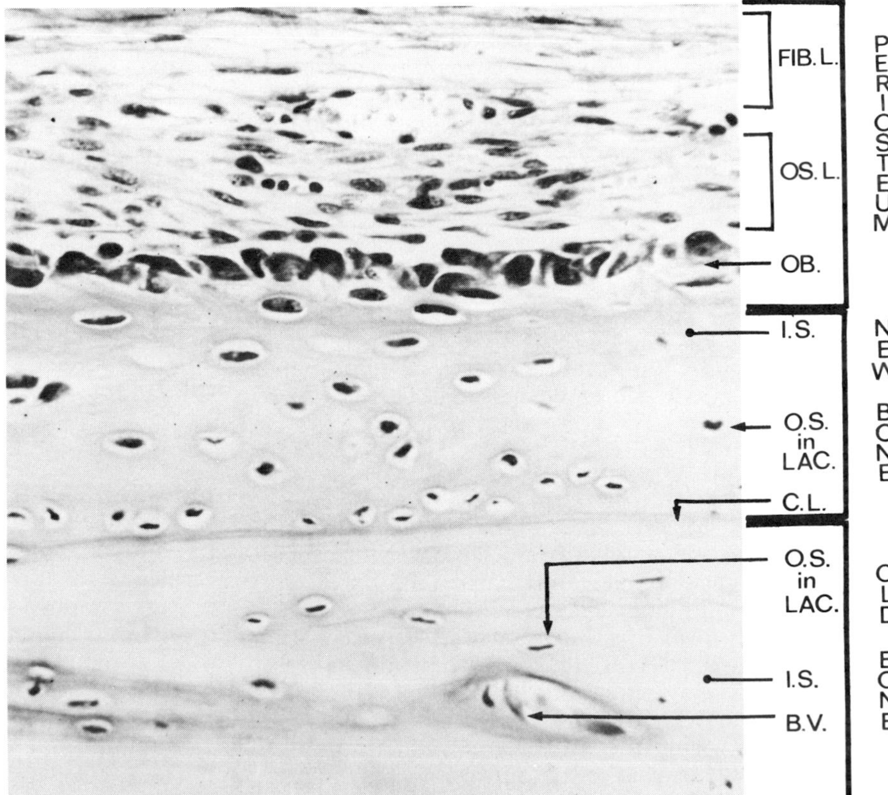

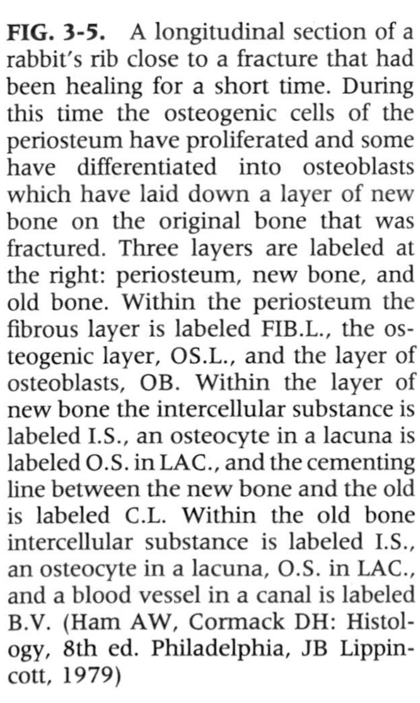
FIG. 3-5. A longitudinal section of a rabbit's rib close to a fracture that had been healing for a short time. During this time the osteogenic cells of the periosteum have proliferated and some have differentiated into osteoblasts which have laid down a layer of new bone on the original bone that was fractured. Three layers are labeled at the right: periosteum, new bone, and old bone. Within the periosteum the fibrous layer is labeled FIB.L., the osteogenic layer, OS.L., and the layer of osteoblasts, OB. Within the layer of new bone the intercellular substance is labeled I.S., an osteocyte in a lacuna is labeled O.S. in LAC., and the cementing line between the new bone and the old is labeled C.L. Within the old bone intercellular substance is labeled I.S., an osteocyte in a lacuna, O.S. in LAC., and a blood vessel in a canal is labeled B.V. (Ham AW, Cormack DH: Histology, 8th ed. Philadelphia, JB Lippincott, 1979)

OSTEOBLASTS

The osteogenic cells of the deep layer of periosteum, and of the endosteum, differentiate into osteoblasts. Beneath the deep layer can be seen relatively large, roughly fusiform cells characterized by abundant cytoplasm staining a deep blue with H and E. The intense staining reaction with basic aniline dyes is due to its high, rough endoplasmic reticulum content, which is responsible for the synthesis of the organic intercellular substance. Osteoblasts line the surface of actively growing bone in large numbers. They measure from 15 μ to 20 μ in diameter, and each contains a large nucleus and one fairly large nucleolus. Under the light microscope, it is difficult to distinguish cytoplasm from nucleus because both stain deeply basophilic. Phosphatase is contained within the organelles. Osteoblasts are often connected with each other by their cytoplasmic processes.

OSTEOCYTES

The osteoblasts synthesize and secrete the organic intercellular substance of bone with which they surround themselves. They come to lie within the lacunae in the intercellular substance and become osteocytes. The osteocyte has a faintly basophilic cytoplasm, a large oval nucleus with large chromatin granules, and one or more nucleoli. The cytoplasm of both osteocytes and osteoblasts contains spherical granules stainable with periodate-leukofuchsin, suggesting a common origin.

Osteoblasts add successive new layers of bone-to-bone surfaces, a process termed *appositional growth,* and the cells become osteocytes as they are enclosed within the new intercellular substance. A watermark or cementing line is observed between each new layer and the layer formed previously.

LACUNAE

These cavities are flat or oval. Cytoplasmic processes from the cell bodies project through fine apertures in the walls of the lacunae and enter the canaliculi.

OSTEOCLAST

The osteoclast consists of a multinucleated giant cell varying in size and number of nuclei. The cytoplasm is pale-staining, acidophilic, and foamy. The nuclei are poor in chromatin, but each has a prominent nucleolus. It is supposedly formed by the fusion of several osteoblasts or from stromal cells of the marrow. It functions to resorb both minerals and intercellular organic substance. The manner in which this is carried out is unknown, but it is noteworthy that osteoclasts are not found in association with osteoid tissue but always with mineralized bone. Several enzymes are contained within the cell, notably β-glucuronidase.

CANALICULI

The canaliculi, tiny canals that permeate the bone, contain the delicate cytoplasmic processes of the osteocytes, together with a certain amount of tissue fluid. They radiate from each lacuna and join with those that radiate from others and the canaliculi from lacunae that are close to the bone surface adjacent to nutrient vessels (*i.e.,* the haversian canal). The canalicular mechanism provides the means by which nutrients from blood vessels can diffuse to osteocytes, and cellular products diffuse in the opposite direction. Canaliculi cannot be seen with the light microscope unless the bone section is undecalcified.

INTERCELLULAR SUBSTANCE

The intercellular substance consists mainly of matrix, inorganic salts, and water.

Matrix[4] is the organic framework consisting chiefly of a unique type of collagen (approximately 90%), differing from other types by its amino acid composition and by its relative insolubility in salt solutions and weak acids; and of a small amount of PPS and some glycoprotein, which diminish as mineralization occurs.

Inorganic salts consist mostly of submicroscopic crystals of hydroxyapatite, the approximate formula of which is $Ca_{10}(PO_4)_6(OH)_2$. The apatite lattice is determined by x-ray spectrograms. Various ions may be situated, presumably on the surfaces, in the crystal lattice and include cations such as magnesium and sodium, and anions such as carbonate, citrate, and fluoride. The bone salt comprises about 75% of the adult dry bone but it is reduced to 30% to 35% in rickets and osteomalacia.

The term ossification refers to the formation of the organic intercellular substance (osteoid tissue) by osteoblasts. Under normal conditions this osteoid tissue is rapidly mineralized.

Water occupies the spaces within the bone, including the nutrient canals of the haversian systems and the ultramicroscopic channels within the molecular aggregates of the collagen fibrils.

HISTOGENESIS OF BONE

In embryonic life most of the skeleton is composed of cartilage, which is absorbed and replaced by bone. This process is termed *endochondral ossification.* It begins prenatally and continues throughout the postnatal period until growth is complete. Basically, the sequence of events is:

1. Mesenchymal cells differentiate into chondrocytes
2. Chondrocytes proliferate and secrete intercellular substance
3. Chondrocytes mature and secrete alkaline phosphatase, and the cartilaginous matrix calcifies

4. Calcified matrix impairs diffusion of nutrients, chondrocytes die, and calcified matrix undergoes disintegration and dissolution
5. Ingrowth of highly vascular and cellular tissue, and osteoblasts surround remnants of calcified cartilage and lay down new bone

In a long bone, this sequence of events forms the diaphyseal ossification center, which extends to replace the entire diaphysis of the model with bone. Next, the epiphyseal ossification center is formed in a similar manner. Finally, between the bony epiphysis and the bony diaphysis, endochondral ossification continues as a persisting layer of cartilage, the growth plate, thereby increasing growth in length of the bone until growth is completed. The cartilage plate itself is then completely replaced by bone.

When bone is formed in the embryo directly from a loose form of connective tissue without intervening stages of cartilage formation, calcification, and resorption, the process is called *intramembranous ossification*. This process occurs in flat bones (*e.g.*, the skull), but the scapula, which is formed in cartilage, is an exception.

ENDOCHONDRAL (INTRACARTILAGINOUS) OSSIFICATION

The process of endochondral ossification is best studied in the limb bud of the developing embryo (Fig. 3-6). The mesenchymal cells proliferate and condense to form the outline of the future bone. These cells soon differentiate into chondroblasts that become chondrocytes as

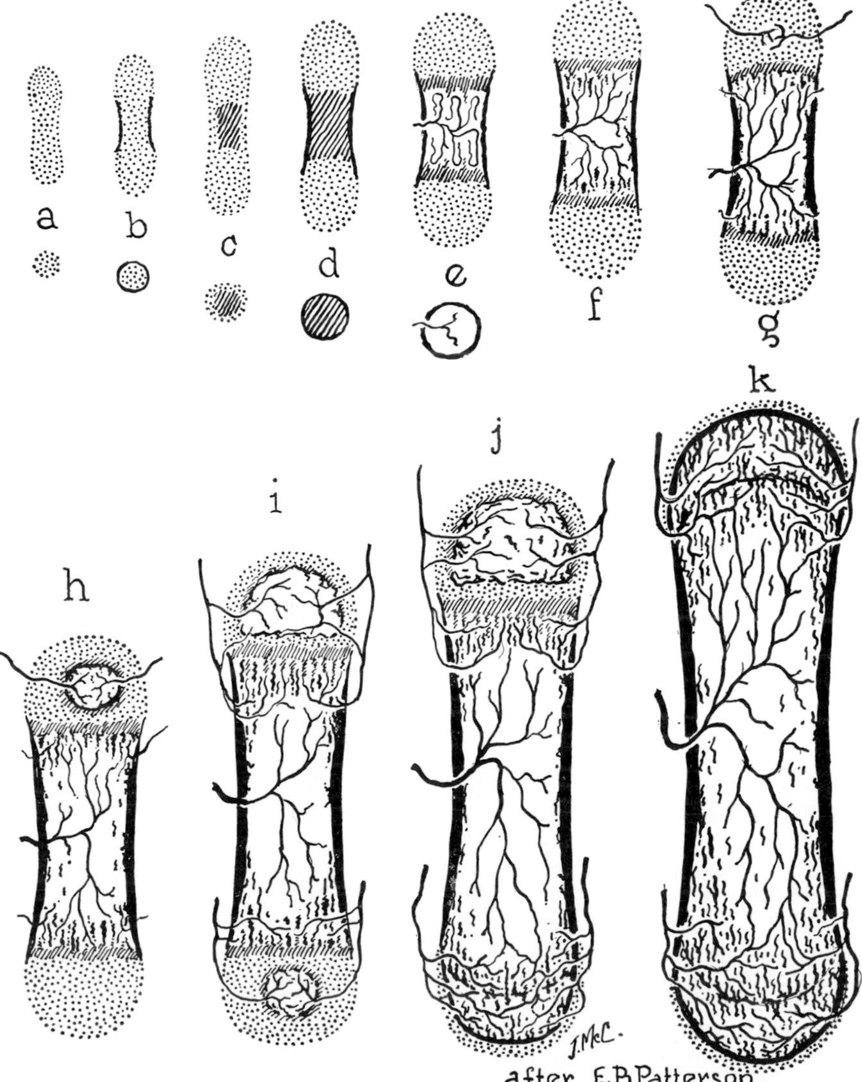

FIG. 3-6. Development of a typical long bone. (*a*) Cartilage model. (*b*) Periosteal bone collar appears. (*c*) Center of calcifying cartilage. (*d*) Further development of calcified cartilage. (*e*) Vascular mesenchyme enters, resorbs calcified cartilage, and new bone is laid down toward either extremity of the model. (*f*) Endochondral ossification is further advanced, bone increased in length. (*g*) Blood vessels and mesenchyme enter upper epiphyseal cartilage. (*h*) Development of epiphyseal ossification center. (*i*) Ossification center develops in lower epiphysis. (*j* and *k*) The lower and then the upper epiphyseal cartilage plates disappear, bone ceases to grow in length, a continuous bone marrow cavity traverses the entire length of the bone, and blood vessels of diaphysis, metaphysis, and epiphysis intercommunicate. (Redrawn from Maximow AA, Bloom W: Textbook of Histology. Philadelphia, WB Saunders, 1968)

they secrete cartilaginous intercellular substance with which they become surrounded. The result is a cartilage model of the bone-to-be. The mesenchyme immediately adjacent to the developing cartilage model becomes arranged into a surrounding membrane, the perichondrium. It is composed of two ill-defined layers: the outer part differentiates into a connective tissue sheath composed of fibroblasts and collagen fibrils; the inner layer (the chondrogenic layer) between the connective tissue sheath and the cartilage model, consists of relatively undifferentiated cells that retain the pluripotential of the mesenchymal cells from which they are derived.

The cartilage model increases in length by interstitial growth. This involves proliferation, maturation, and enlargment of the chondrocytes, which continue to form intercellular substance. The model also grows in width not only by the interstitial growth within the shaft but also by layers of cartilage laid down at the surface by the chondrogenic cells of the perichondrium.

Cell division for interstitial growth actively proceeds from the center of the model toward the ends of the model. Meanwhile, the earliest chondrocytes at the center of the model proceed to mature, enlarge, and secrete alkaline phosphatase into the intercellular substance, which becomes calcified. Because diffusion of nutrient solutes through a calcified matrix is impeded, the hypertrophied chondrocytes die and the calcified matrix in the center of the model disintegrates, forming cavities.

Within the perichondrium, blood vessels invade, and the new vascular environment (raised *p*H?) appears to effect a change in the behavior of the pluripotential cells of the sheath. These cells begin to differentiate into osteoblasts with the result that a thin layer of bone is soon laid down around the cartilage model. The membrane enclosing the model is now called the periosteum.

As the calcified cartilage in the midsection of the model begins to distintegrate, the periosteal bud, vascular hypercellular tissue carrying osteogenic cells and osteoblasts from the periosteum, invades the breaking-down mid section of the cartilage model. Osteoblasts surround and lay down new bone on the surfaces of the remnants of calcified cartilage. A cancellous (lattice) type of bone with interlacing trabeculae is formed. In an H and E section, the new bone stains pink, whereas the cartilage cores stain blue.

While the central process is going on to form a diaphyseal center of ossification in the midshaft, the young cartilage at each end of the model continues to grow and extend by interstitial growth, increasing the length of the model. At some point, however, the rate of ossification equals the rate of production of cartilage, so that the amount of cartilage in the model remains constant. The process of ossification at the center of the shaft extends up and down the model, replacing the cartilage at the ossification front as rapidly as new cartilage is formed at the ends.

As the spread of ossification in the middle of the bone proceeds, a marrow cavity is formed. The model continues to grow in width by osteogenic cells adding further bone to the surface, producing strong, compact walls. The cancellous bone in the central part is mostly resorbed, leaving a cavity (the marrow or medullary cavity) that becomes filled with myeloid tissue. This cavity never extends to the cartilage ends of the model, but instead is separated from each cartilaginous end by a region of longitudinally disposed trabeculae of bone that have cartilage cores.

EPIPHYSEAL CENTERS OF OSSIFICATION

In a long bone, in addition to the formation of a diaphyseal center of ossification, epiphyseal centers of ossification develop in the cartilaginous ends of the bone. The chondrocytes situated near the central part of the cartilaginous epiphysis proliferate and hypertrophy, secrete and become separated by intercellular substance; the matrix calcifies, cavities form as the matrix disintegrates, vascular cellular tissue invades, and bone is laid down about the remnants of calcified cartilage. The process extends peripherally, but ossification stops short of replacing all of the cartilage. A portion remains at the surface for articular cartilage. Between the bony epiphysis and the bony diaphysis, a transverse layer of cartilage remains, the epiphyseal plate or disk, which is concerned with longitudinal growth and which ossifies when growth is complete.

LONGITUDINAL GROWTH

Interstitial growth of chondrocytes within the epiphyseal plate accounts for longitudinal growth of the shaft of a long bone (Fig. 3-7). Continuing proliferation of cells with formation of cartilage matrix constantly tends to thicken the plate, thereby moving the bone of the epiphysis away from the bone of the diaphysis. The thickness of the plate is not increased because a simultaneous process is at work that tends to reduce the thickness of the disk, namely, maturation, calcification of interstitial substance, death of chondrocytes, disintegration and dissolution of calcified cartilage, and replacement by bone on the diaphyseal side of the disk. Appositional bone growth continues to increase the length of the bony shaft (Color Plate 3-1).

MICROSCOPIC STRUCTURE OF GROWTH PLATE

Extending from the epiphyseal to the diaphyseal ends of the growth plate, four zones can be identified. (Fig. 3-8).

The *zone of resting cartilage* is adjacent to the epiphysis. The chondrocytes are of moderate size and are scattered throughout the intercellular substance of the cartilage.

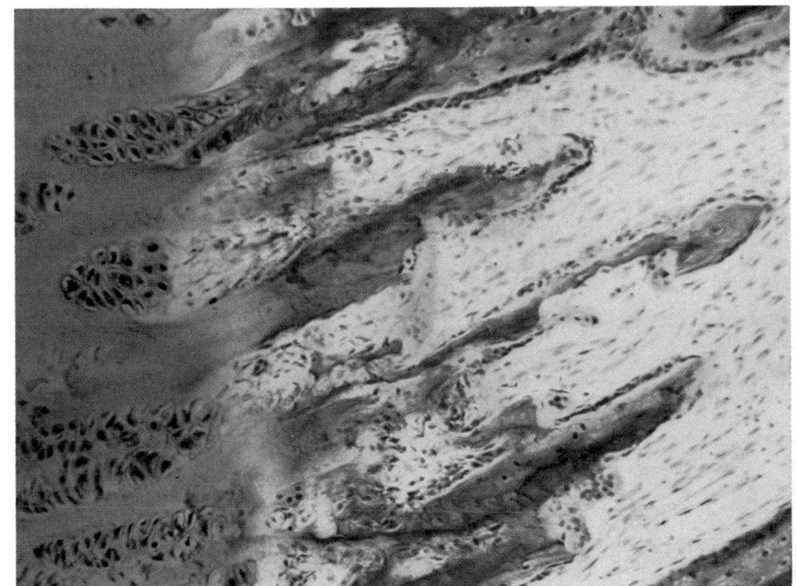

PLATE 3-1. Endochondral ossification. The capillary loops are seen entering and destroying the piled-up cartilage cells. At the left is the layer of proliferating chondrocytes. Proceeding toward the right, one observes calcified cartilage which becomes enveloped with osteoid laid down by a profusion of osteoblasts. The earliest appearance of mature bone is at the extreme right of the section. (See p. 36.)

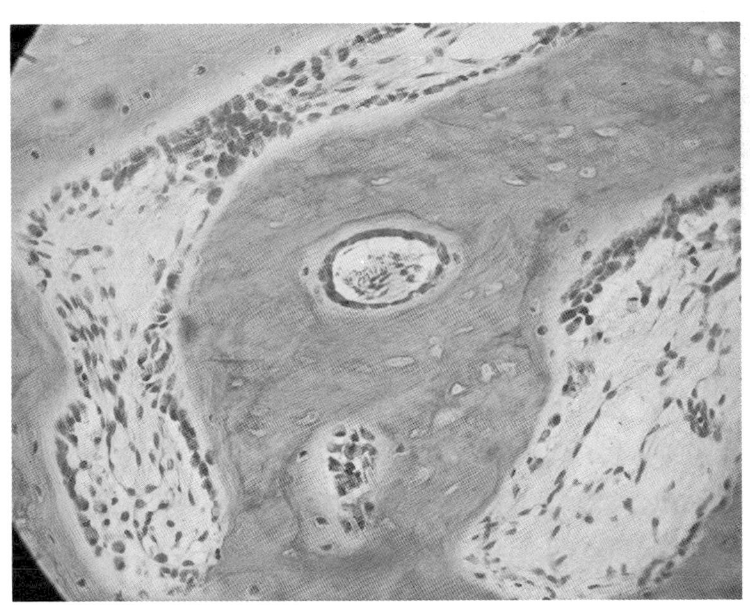

PLATE 3-2. Aseptic necrosis and creeping substitution. Active osteogenesis and osteoclastic resorption are occurring at the same time. Loose vascular osteogenetic granulation tissue occupies the marrow spaces and the enlarged haversian canals. A concentric lamella is being laid down in the haversian canal at the center of the section. (× 160) (See p. 80.)

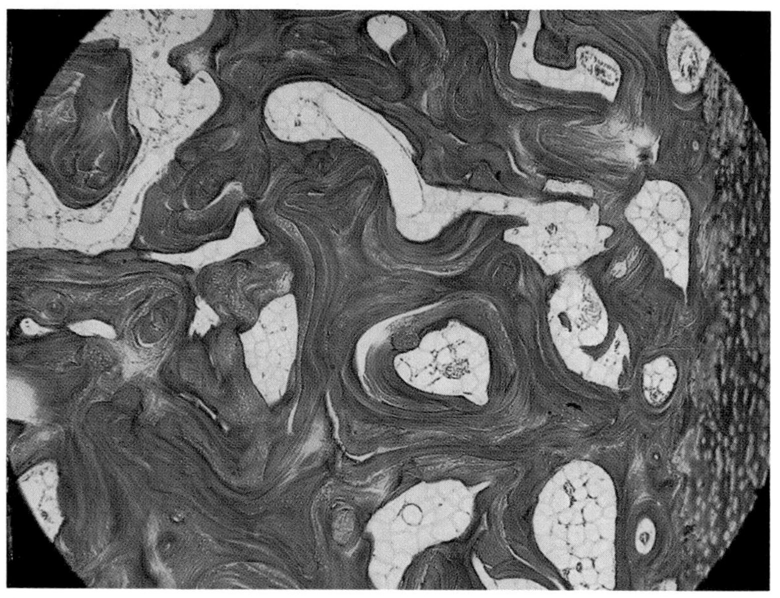

PLATE 3-3. Radiation necrosis of cancellous bone. The characteristic "molasses" appearance is well shown. Marrow spaces are empty or contain fatty tissue. (× 35) (See p. 93.)

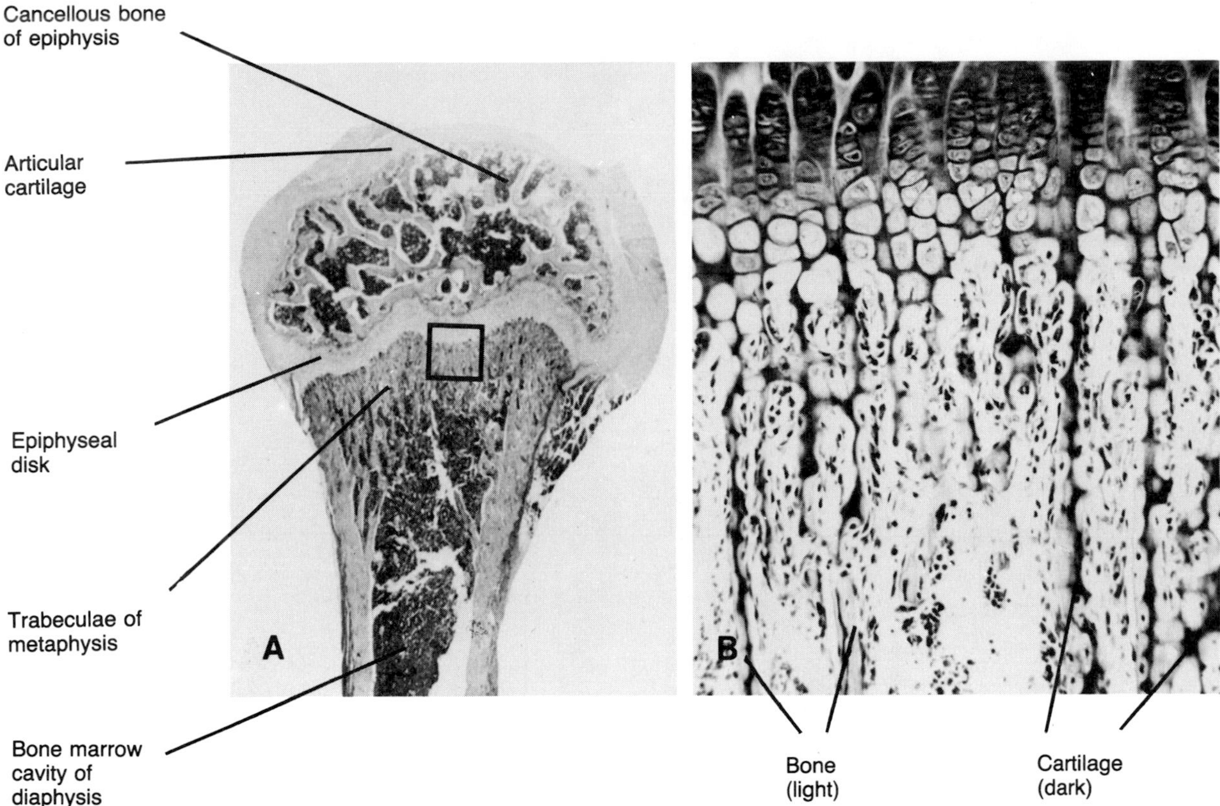

FIG. 3-7. (*A*) A low-power photomicrograph of a longitudinal section cut through the end of a long bone of a growing rat. At this stage of development osteogenesis has spread out from the epiphyseal center of ossification so that only the articular cartilage above and the epiphyseal plate below remain cartilaginous. On the diaphyseal side of the epiphyseal plate are the metaphyseal trabeculae, which (*B*) consist of cartilage cores on which bone has been deposited. (Ham AW, Cormack DH: Histology, 8th ed. Philadelphia, JB Lippincott, 1979)

In some sites the cartilage is separated from the bone of the epiphysis by spaces containing nutrient blood vessels. At this level the epiphyseal plate is firmly anchored to the epiphysis.

The *zone of young proliferating chondrocytes* is made up of thin or wedge-shaped cells stacked in columns whose longitudinal axes parallel that of the main bone.

The *zone of maturing chondrocytes* contains chondrocytes that are still arranged in columns. They gradually mature, grow larger, and accumulate glycogen and alkaline phosphatase. As this zone merges with the next, the intercellular substance becomes increasingly calcified.

The *zone of calcified cartilage* is very thin, at most only one or several cells thick. It abuts directly on the bone of the diaphysis. The cells are necrotic and the calcified substance undergoes cavitation and dissolution. The horizontal partitions between the cells in each column and some of the vertical partitions between adjacent columns melt away. A small portion of the vertical partitions remain and is used as a site of bone deposition. Capillary loops and accompanying osteogenic cells invade the tunnels formed by disintegration of the cell columns, osteoblasts line the remnants of calcified cartilage partitions, and new bone is laid down on them. This results, on the diaphyseal side of the epiphyseal plate (metaphysis) in the formation of longitudinally disposed bone trabeculae with calcified cartilage cores. The cartilage cores are continuous proximally with the partially calcified cartilaginous intercellular matrix of the disk, and in this manner the newly formed bony trabeculae of the metaphysis are firmly united with the cartilaginous plate.

INTRAMEMBRANOUS OSSIFICATION

Intramembranous bone is formed directly from the concentrated mesenchymal model of a flat bone and is best studied in the skull bone of the embryo. Intramembranous ossification is initiated when a cluster of mesenchymal cells accumulate within a rather loose tissue with delicate fibrils between an amorphous fluid substance. The elliptical cells soon differentiate into osteoblasts by enlarging and becoming polyhedral with numerous processes. Bars of dense intercellular substance, the organic

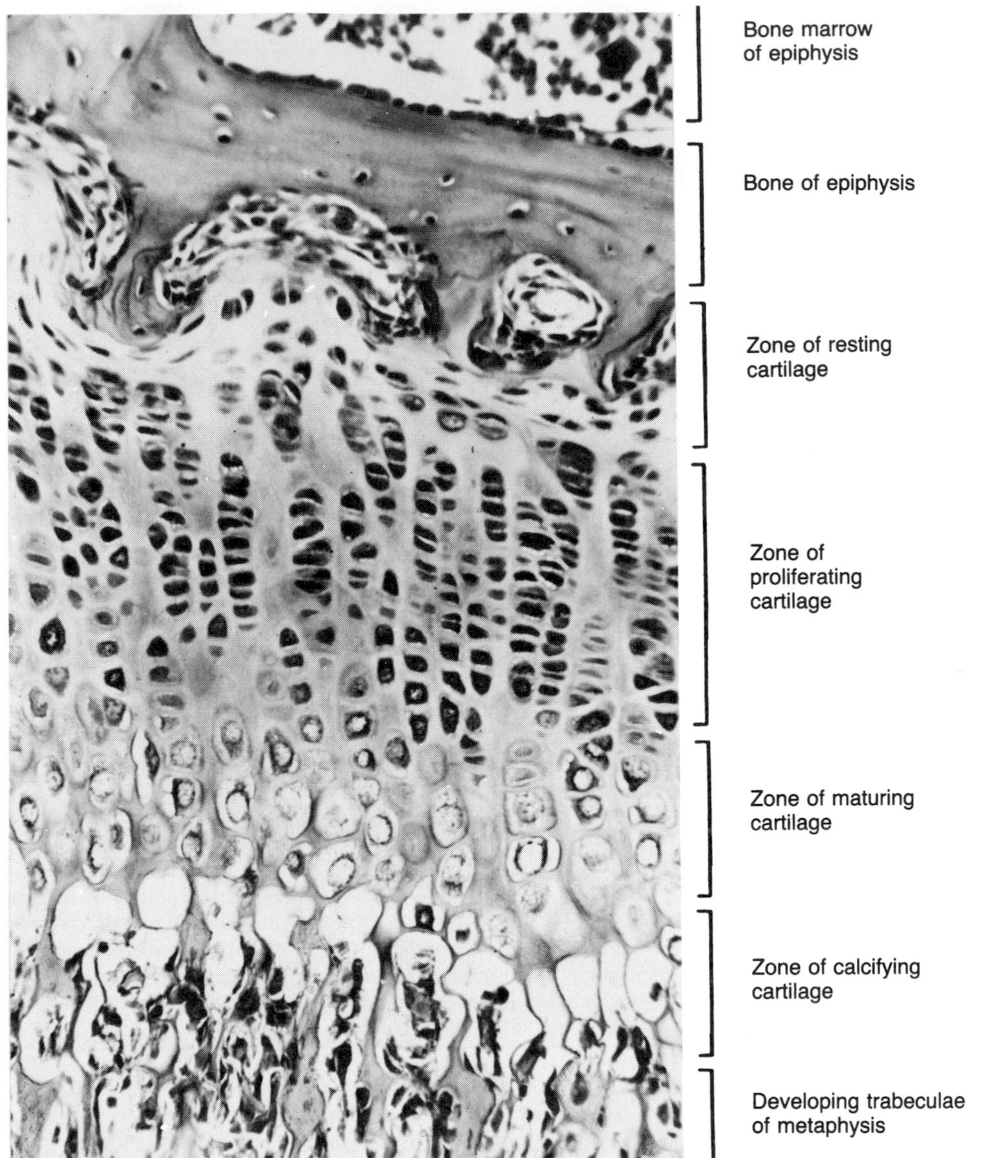

FIG. 3-8. High-power photomicrograph of longitudinal section cut through upper end of tibia of a guinea pig. Note different zones of cells in the epiphyseal plate. (Ham AW, Cormack DH: Histology, 8th ed. Philadelphia, JB Lippincott, 1979)

matrix of bone, appear and become thicker, replacing the amorphous fluid substance and enclose the osteoblasts which are now called osteocytes. Actively secreting osteoblasts profusely line the surfaces of the newly formed matrix spicule, which rapidly mineralizes. The formed spicules of bone continue to grow outward from the center of ossification in a radial manner, producing trabeculae (beams) of bone which branch and join to form a scaffolding. Bone that consists of scaffolding trabeculae enclosing spaces containing vascular myeloid tissue is termed cancellous bone. Each trabecula consists of one to five layers of bone within which are identified intercommunicating canaliculi between osteocytes and lacunae. The surface connective tissue becomes the periosteum whose deep lying cells resemble fibroblasts and potentially are capable of reverting to osteoblasts under certain conditions (Fig. 3-9).

The continued deposition of fresh bone lamellae on trabeculae and appositional bone growth at the surface forms the compact or dense bone of the inner and outer

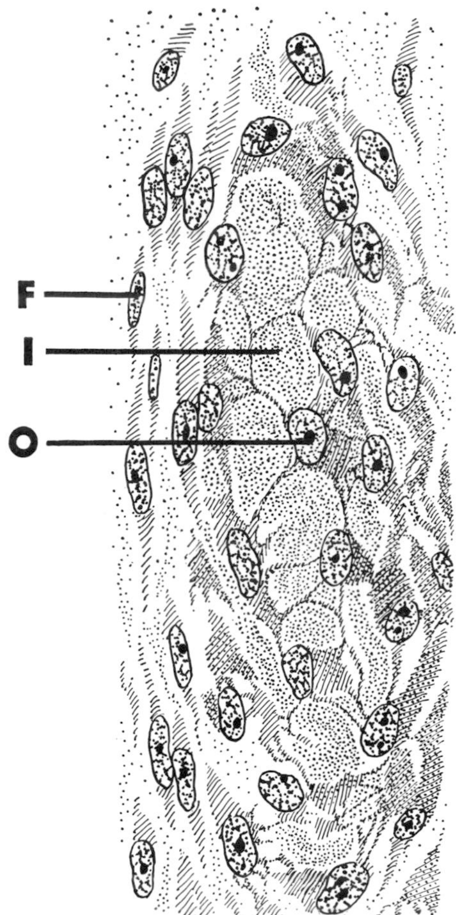

FIG. 3-9. Intramembranous bone formation. Fibroblasts (*F*). Homogeneous interstitial bone substance (*I*), collagenous fibrils no longer visible. Connective tissue cells (*O*) that have developed processes to become osteoblasts and later osteocytes.

cortices. The layer of cancellous bone and marrow between the plates of compact bone is termed the diploë, which contains many large, thin-walled veins (diploic veins).

REMODELING OF BONE

Throughout life bone is constantly being resorbed and reformed, thereby developing and preserving the structure and size of the bone as well as providing a mechanism for maintaining calcium ionic homeostasis in body fluids.[5] Osteoclasts are almost always seen in areas of bone resorption and disappear when bone formation is the primary activity. The osteoclast can be found in a deeply scalloped indentation (Howship's lacuna) of mineralized bone surfaces suggesting erosion, but actual phagocytosis cannot be demonstrated. The rate of bone reconstruction to some degree is related to levels of serum ionized calcium and phosphate, local *p*H (low *p*H favors mineral resorption), parathyroid hormone (PTH) and calcitonin levels, and metabolically active vitamin D. When new osseous matrix is formed, but remains unmineralized, osteoid tissue accumulates, and the wide osteoid seams that stain pink with H and E are characteristic of rickets and osteomalacia.

Some regions of spongy bone are converted into compact bone. Within an area of marrow, osteoblasts lay down a circumferential layer of bone about a blood vessel. Next, another layer (plate) is laid down within the first layer, then successive concentric layers are added, progressively narrowing the central space until a primitive haversian system is formed.

Resorption can occur from within the haversian canal by osteoclasts forming an enlarged, elongated tubular cavity, a resorption cavity within the bone substance (Fig. 3-10).

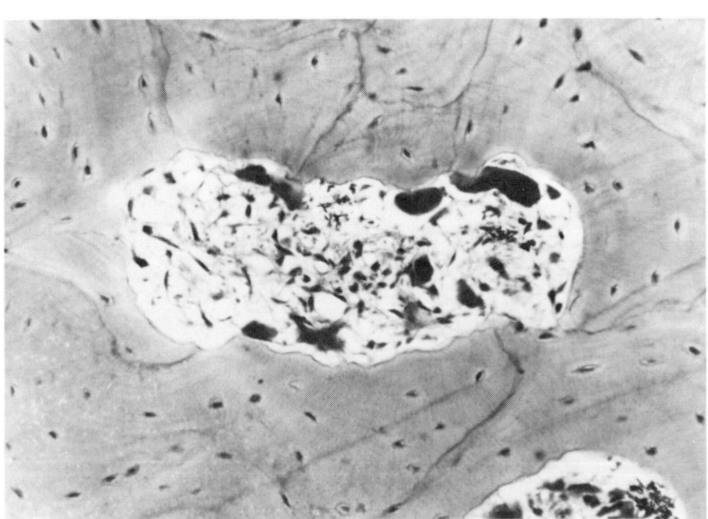

FIG. 3-10. Photomicrograph of a cross section of the shaft of a bone showing a resorption cavity in cross or somewhat oblique section. The large dark cells are osteoclasts; their activity explains the etched-out borders of the cavity. (Ham AW, Cormack DH: Histology, 8th ed. Philadelphia, JB Lippincott, 1979)

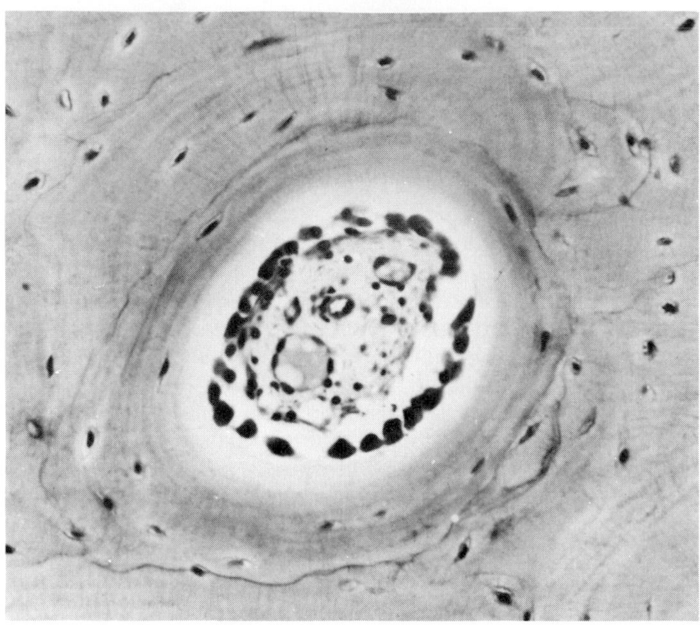

FIG. 3-11. This is the way a former resorption cavity, which is being filled in to make a new haversian system, appears in an H and E cross section of compact bone. The dark cells that ring the cavity are osteoblasts. For details see Figure 3-13. (Ham AW, Cormack DH: Histology, 8th ed. Philadelphia, JB Lippincott, 1979. From C. P. Leblond)

Next, osteoblasts appear, line the inner surface of the cavity, and proceed to produce successive layers of bone. As a new layer of matrix is laid down, it is rapidly mineralized. The border between the edge of a resorption cavity that becomes a new haversian system and the new bone of the system can be identified by a cementing line (Fig. 3-11).

A frontier line is a line seen between what appears to be the most recently formed layer and the layer that had previously been formed. The presence of this bone can

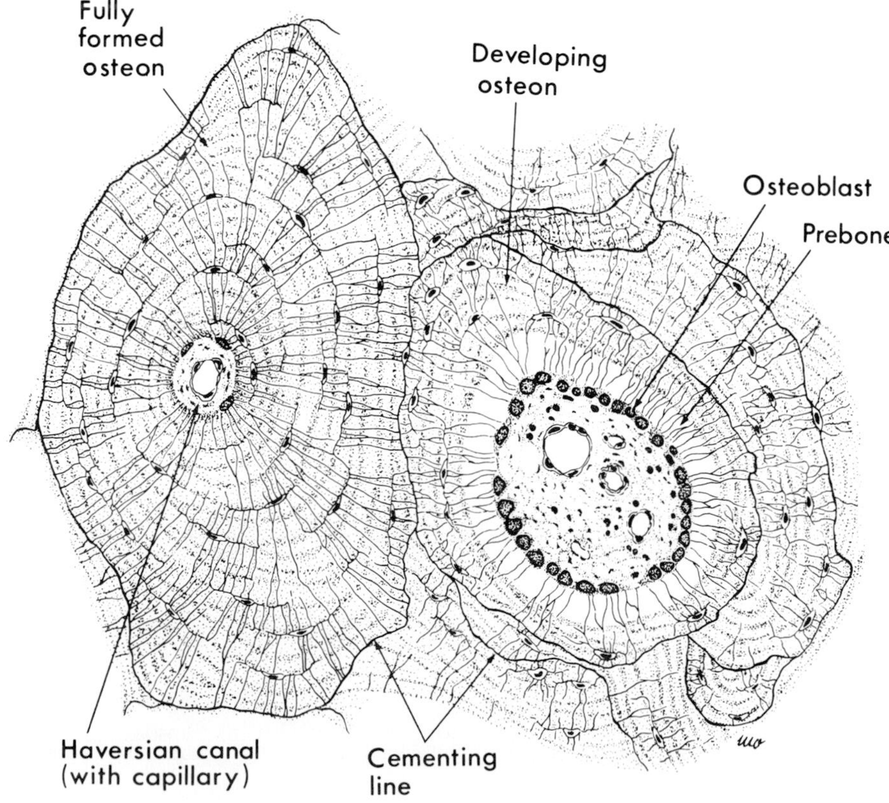

FIG. 3-12. Osteons in the process of formation and the fully formed osteon. The osteoblasts are separated from the mature formed bone by a pale layer of newly formed but as yet unmineralized bone. The material of this layer (*right side of figure*) is called prebone or osteoid tissue. It consists of organic matrix that is not as yet calcified. At its periphery a line called the frontier line (not labeled) marks the site where mineral begins to be deposited. Farther out, cementing lines indicate the borders between new layers of bone that have been formed on older layers. The fully formed osteon (*left*). (Ham AW, Cormack DH: Histology, 8th ed. Philadelphia, JB Lippincott, 1979. From C. P. Leblond)

be explained by the fact that in forming the haversian system a period of time is required for mineralization of each layer. The most recently formed layer (*i.e.*, the layer that abuts on the haversian canal) remains in an uncalcified state as osteoid tissue or prebone for a period of time (Fig. 3-12).

By using various methods of study—vital staining (feeding animals alizarin dyes), autoradiography (labeled calcium or proline), or tetracycline fluorescence—the rate of newly forming matrix can be determined. It appears that cortical bone is replaced at a rate of 5% to 10% a year.

ULTRASTRUCTURAL CHARACTERISTICS OF BONE

OSTEOBLASTS

Because osteoblasts are secretory and elaborate mainly procollagen, PPS, and minerals, their cytoplasm is characterized by extensive development of the rough endoplasmic reticulum (RER) and Golgi stacks. The structure is similar to that of the young fibroblast (Fig. 3-13).

Many osteoblasts are relatively elongated. The nucleus tends to be at one end, the rER at the other end, and

FIG. 3-13. Electron micrograph of an osteoblast from demineralized rat alveolar bone showing the arrangement of the organelles. Numerous collagen fibrils, which these cells secrete, are present in the adjacent prebone and bone (*upper right*). The procollagen, which is the precursor of the collagen fibrils, is carried within secretory granules (*arrowheads*) originating from the Golgi saccules. Procollagen is released into the prebone by fusion of the secretory granule with the apical plasma membrane of the cell. A portion of a cell of the type that gives rise to osteoblasts is seen at lower left. (× 12,000) (Ham AW, Cormack DH: Histology, 8th ed. Philadelphia, JB Lippincott, 1979. From Melvyn Weinstock)

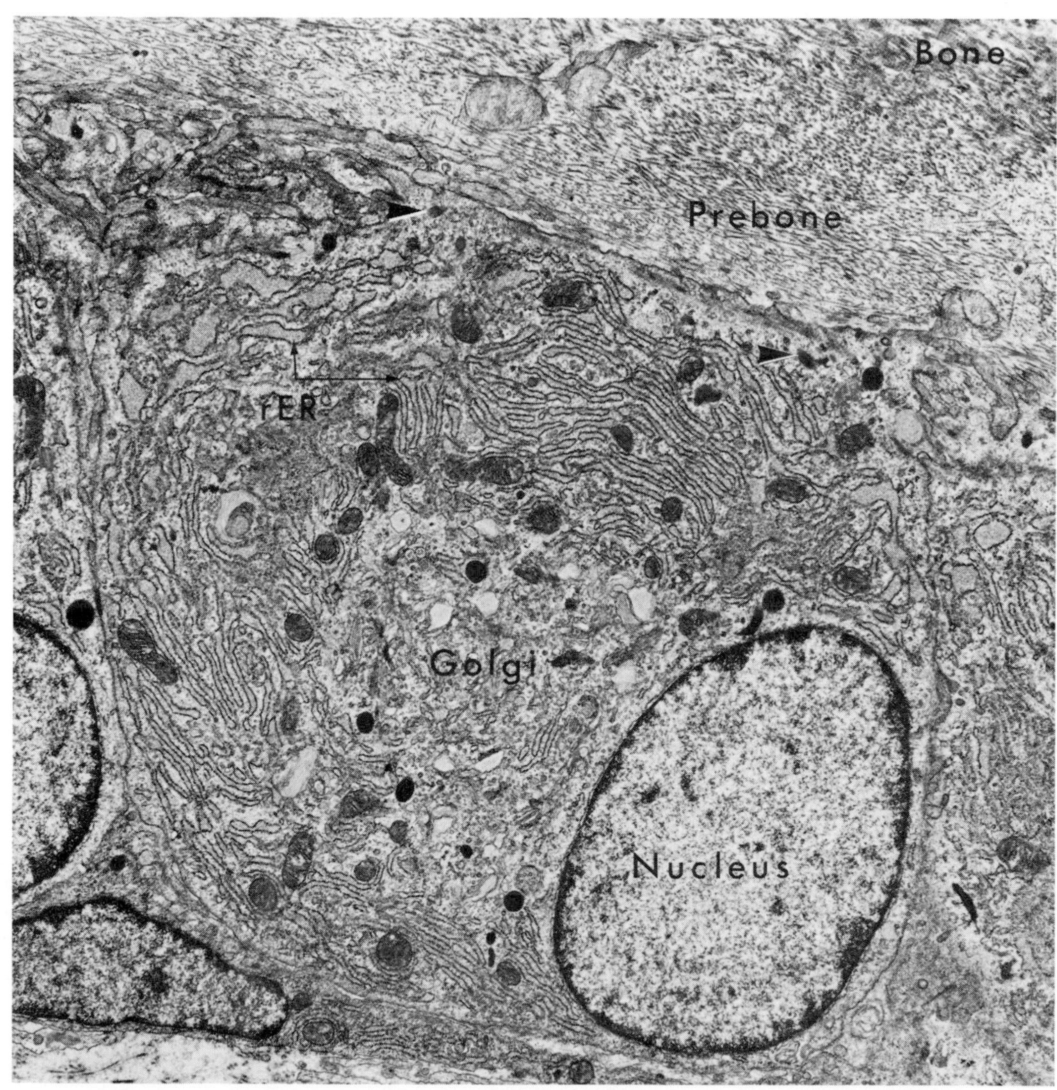

the Golgi in the middle. Procollagen fibrils can be identified in secretory vesicles originating from the Golgi saccules. Collagenic microfibrils lie immediately beyond the cell membrane in the intercellular substance. Under electron microscopy, an undecalcified section shows electron-dense mineral deposits sparsely distributed near the cell, although they accumulate in greater concentration at a distance from the cell.

OSTEOCYTES

Osteocytes may be studied in either decalcified or mineralized bone sections.[6] The cell body and its processes do not fully occupy the lacuna and the canaliculi, thus space is provided for the accommodation of fluid (Fig. 3-14).

Under the electron microscope (EM), the osteocyte in undecalcified bone shows less rER and less cytoplasm, and the cell is surrounded by heavily calcified intercellular substance. The cytoplasmic processes extend from the main cell body into the surrounding canaliculi. The cytoplasm is acidophilic, the staining becoming more pronounced as the cell ages.

OSTEOCLASTS

Under the light microscope, in H and E sections, osteoclasts appear as multinucleated cells containing as many as a dozen nuclei. Mitotic figures are never seen in osteoclasts, and it is believed that, like foreign body giant cells, they develop as a result of fusion of cells. They occupy pits in the bone surface, Howship's lacunae. Typically, the cell surface directly opposite the bone exhibits hairlike processes that appear to extend between the cell and the bone. This is termed the *striated* or *brush border* and may be an appearance created by collagen fibrils of the bone substance freed of mineral in the resorptive process (Fig. 3-15).

Under electron microscopy, the peripheral part of the cytoplasm that abuts on the bone surface consists of innumerable villuslike processes, called the *fluffy* or *ruffled border* (Fig. 3-16).

FIG. 3-14. Low-power electron micrograph of an osteocyte and its processes in a section of decalcified bone. The nucleus (*O*) and an arrow points to a process in a canaliculus. Two processes in canaliculi cut in cross section can be seen, one near the upper right corner and the other toward the lower left corner. (Ham AW, Cormack DH: Histology, 8th ed. Philadelphia, JB Lippincott, 1979. From S. C. Luk and G. T. Simon)

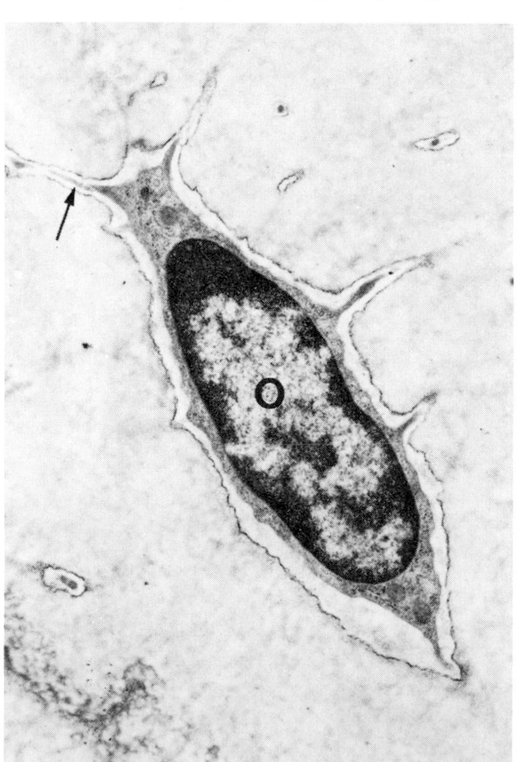

FIG. 3-15. Oil-immersion photomicrograph (taken with the phase microscope) of an osteoclast. This shows that the striations of its striated border continue into the intercellular substance of the bone as collagenic fibers and fibrils. (Ham AW: Some histophysiological problems peculiar to calcified tissues. J Bone Joint Surg 34A:701, 1952)

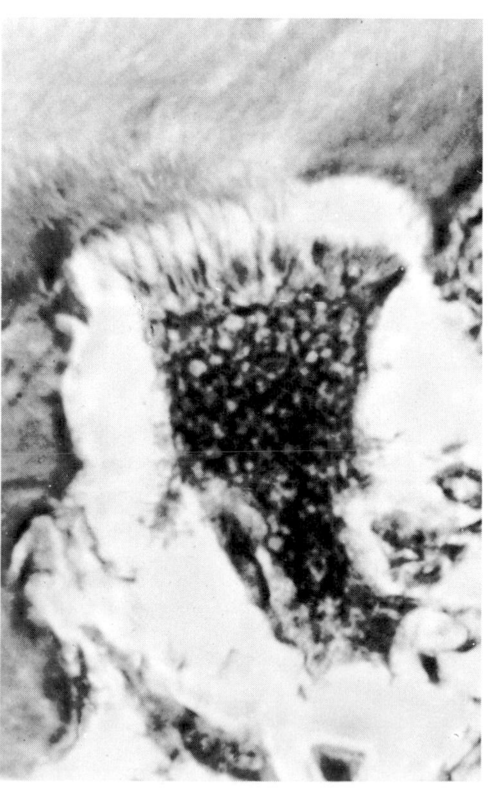

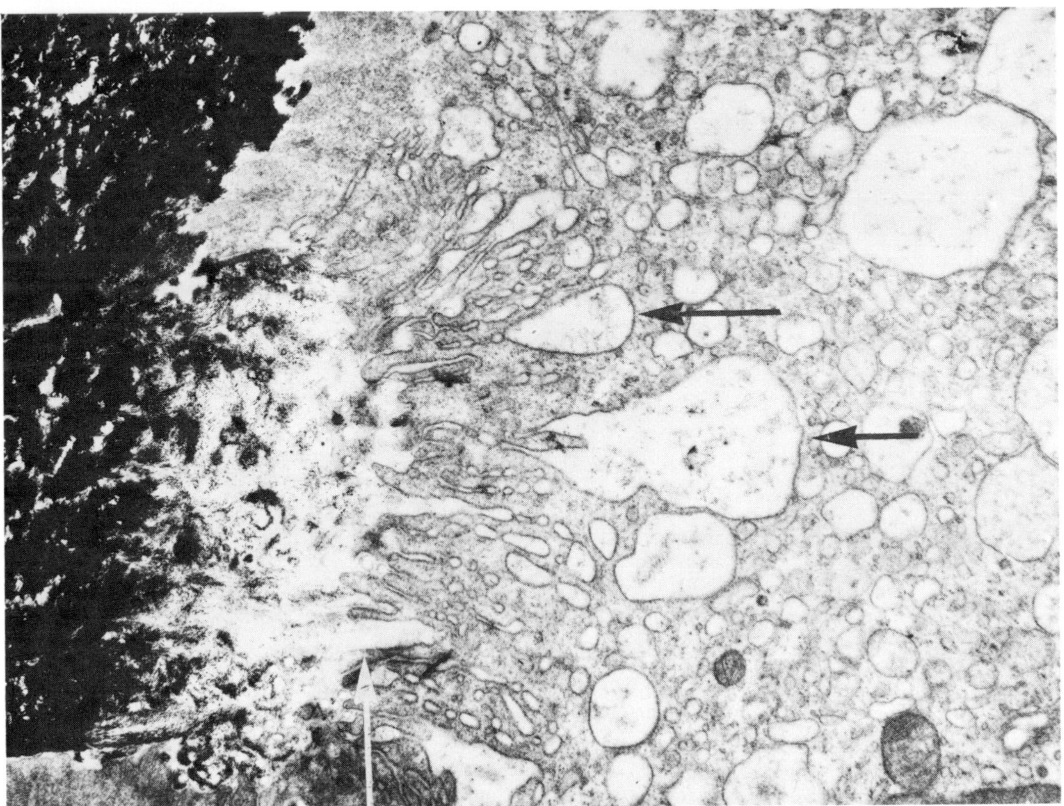

FIG. 3-16. Electron micrograph of a section of a bone surface undergoing resorption. Calcified bone appears black at the left. The main part of the picture is occupied by the cytoplasm of an osteoclast. Extending from the top to the bottom, in the middle of the picture, is the ruffled border of the osteoclast; this consists of complex folds and projections which abut on the bone at the left. Between the ruffled border of the osteoclast and the heavily calcified bone is an area where the calcium content is much less, which suggests that the osteoclast is dissolving or otherwise removing mineral from this area. Black granules of mineral can be seen in some of the large vesicles which are indicated by horizontal arrows, and which probably form because of the bottom of crypts being pinched off. In the original print a collagenic microfibril showing typical periodicity could be seen at this site indicated by the vertical arrow. (× 20,000) (Ham AW, Cormack DH: Histology, 8th ed. Philadelphia, JB Lippincott, 1979. From B. Boothroyd and N. M. Hancox)

Between the bases of the villi, there are tubular-shaped invaginations of the cell membrane that extend into the osteoclast cytoplasm. This portion of the cytoplasm is remarkably free of organelles. However, abundant mitochondria reflect the high degree of resorptive activity. The rER may or may not be well developed. Well-developed Golgi stacks lie close to the nuclei and give rise to various vesicles containing lysosomes and hydrolytic enzymes.

MINERALIZED TISSUE

The relationship of the inorganic minerals to the organic matrix, and the actual location of the solid mineral phase with respect to the structural components of the organic matrix, are important in determining why and how inorganic crystals are deposited in tissues.[9]

Electron microscopic studies demonstrate that inorganic crystals are preferentially oriented with respect to the long axes of the collagen fibrils: the crystallographic *c*-axes of the crystals, corresponding to their long axes, are roughly parallel to the axes of the fibrils (Fig. 3-17).

Electron micrographs of longitudinal sections of undecalcified bone show that the mineral phase is deposited in specific locations corresponding to the axial repeat of the collagen fibril at intervals of 600 A to 700 A, and is disposed along the axial direction of the fibrils. The intervals between adjacent dense mineral-impregnated regions are relatively free of apatite crystals. Electro

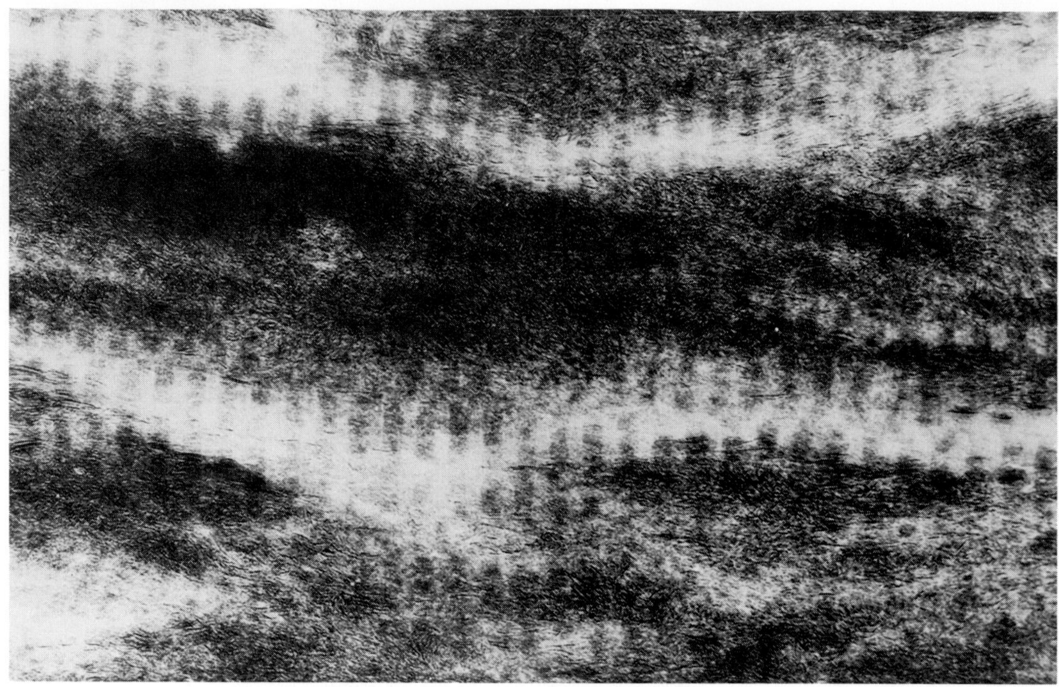

FIG. 3-17. Electron micrograph of an undecalcified unstained section of embryonic chick bone. The ordered disposition of the dense mineral phase along the axial direction of the collagen fibrils is evident. Note also that the mineral phase is in lateral register as well. (× 110,000) (Glimber MJ: A basic architectural principle in the organization of mineralized tissues. Clin Orthop 61:16, 1961)

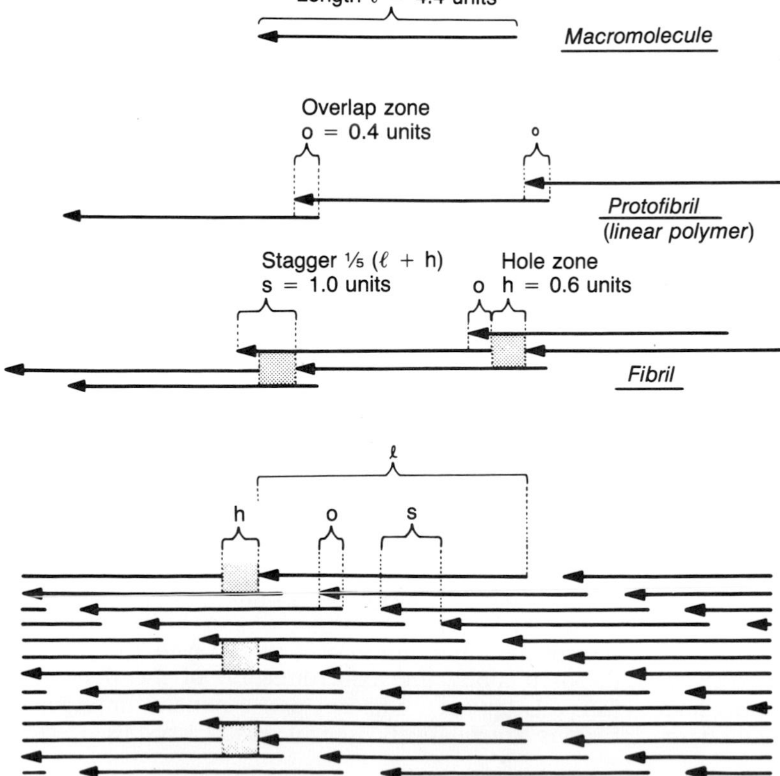

FIG. 3-18. Schematic illustrating how the packing of the collagen macromolecules in the collagen fibril generates a void or hole within the fibril. Note that the overlap (*o*) plus the hole zone (*h*) are equal to the axial repeat of the collagen fibril(s). (Glimcher MJ, Krane SM: The organization and structure of bone, and the mechanism of calcification. In Gould BS, Ramachandran GN (eds): A Treatise on Collagen, Vol II. New York, Academic Press, 1968)

diffraction indicates that the crystals are well oriented with their crystallographic *c*-axes parallel to the fibril axis, whereas their other planes are randomly disposed about the fibrils with which they are associated. The majority of the inorganic crystals are within the collagen fibrils.[8,10] The maximum length of the crystals is 400 A and the average width is 30 A.

The collagen macromolecules within the collagen fibril are closely packed, and yet their volume and organization are undisturbed when the inorganic crystals are added. To accommodate the inorganic crystals, channels or "hole zones" are created by a staggering arrangement of adjacent macromolecules, and it is within these "hole zones" that the inorganic crystals are deposited.[11] The adjacent macromolecules are staggered by approximately one fourth of their length, resulting in the native type of 700-A axial repeat. The "hole zones" are 400 A long and 15 A wide (width of macromolecules) and occur once per axial period (Fig. 3-18). Within the intraperiod fine structure, narrow sub-bands are identified, and the "hole zone" lies between the a_3 and c_1 or c_2 bands, and at least the initial stage of calcification is located here (Fig. 3-19).

Although collagen fibrils lack resistance to compression and are relatively inelastic, and apatite crystals are brittle, their binding together, architecturally and chemically, by both covalent and noncovalent bonds results in a material of superior structural strength. This is a typical two-phase material whose mechanical properties are such that its structural characteristics are greater than the sum of its individual components.

The location of the mineral phase is important for regulating mineral ion constancy in extracellular fluids, facilitating transport, diffusion, and resorption and accretion of mineral ions, mainly calcium and phosphate but also sodium and magnesium.

Under the EM, Bonucci bodies can be identified. Intracellular electron-dense granules, representing calcium complexed to proteins, are contained within vesicles that are extruded from the cell and coalesce to form new mineral.[7] Using autoradiography with ^{47}Ca, the grains localize first in the mitochondria, then the endoplasmic reticulum, shift toward the surface of the cell, and finally arrive within the matrix at calcification sites.[12] The intracellular processes are, therefore, intimately related to the mineralization of bone (see Chapter 6).

BIOLOGIC CONSIDERATIONS

Bone is not a static tissue. The biologic processes, whether biochemical or biophysical, intracellular or extracellular, are poorly understood, and are the subjects of ongoing investigation and controversial interpretation. Nevertheless, many fundamental facts have evolved that should ultimately lead to exact concepts of bone formation and resorption.

The following currently accepted factors should be studied in greater detail.

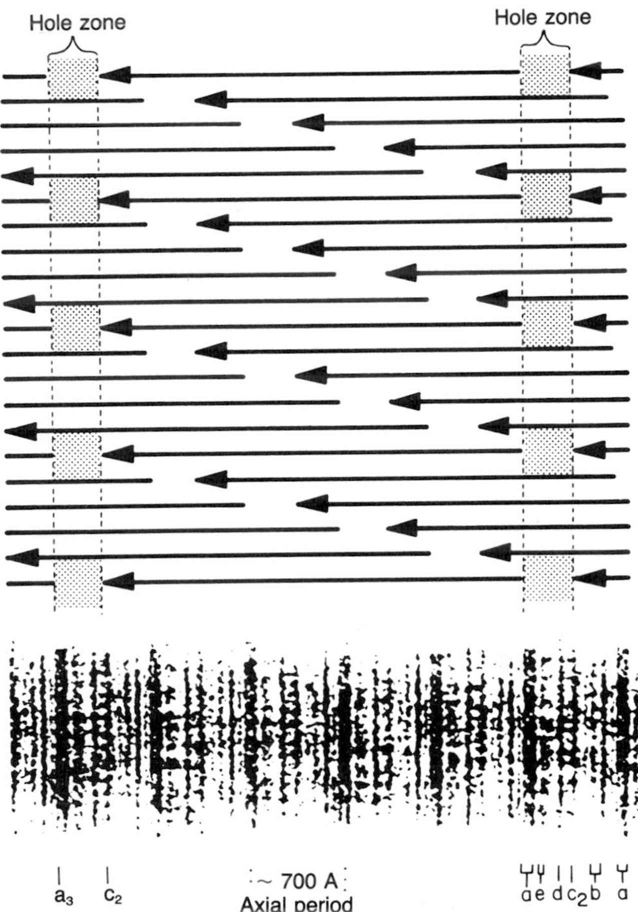

FIG. 3-19. The identification of the location of the mineral phase in bone collagen between a_3 and c_2 bands places the crystals in the hole zone. (Adapted from Hodge AJ, Petruskov JA: Recent studies with the electron-microscope on ordered aggregates of the tropocollagen molecule. In Ramachandran GN (ed): Aspects of Protein Structure. New York, Academic Press, 1968)

Minerals. They are chiefly crystals of hydroxyapatite with the probable formula $Ca_{10}(PO_4)_6(OH)_2$. These crystals are shaped like needles, rods, or plates, and measure approximately 30 A to 50 A in width and up to 600 A long.

Relation of Crystals to Collagen. The relationship is linear along or between fibrils. The probable site is the gap regions between the ends of tropocollagen molecules.

Minerals in the Bloodstream. The minerals calcium, phosphate, and hydroxyl ions diffuse through tissue fluids to be deposited in bone. An increase of $Ca^{2+} \times PO_4^{\equiv}$ product causes precipitation of $Ca_3(PO_4)_2$, especially in an alkaline environment.

Role of Cells. Osteoblasts and osteocytes contain soluble calcium salts within mitochondria and endoplasmic reticulum. Calcium is transported to nucleation sites by vesicles. Cells provide alkaline phosphatase, alkaline phosphorylase, and ATP.

Role of Collagen. It provides nucleation centers at which amorphous calcium phosphate is deposited, then crystals form in relation to the collagen periodicity. Some unknown mechanism produces increased local supersaturation of ions sufficient to cause precipitation.

Role of Sulfated PPS. It acts as an inhibitor of calcification (by binding available Ca^{2+}?). At areas of active mineralization, the concentration of PPS is markedly reduced.

Role of Inorganic Pyrophosphate. It inhibits crystal growth by chemisorbing to apatite.

Lipids. Acidic phospholipids are present in larger than normal amounts where active mineralization is occurring.

Hormonal Influence. PTH and calcitonin are present.

Section II
Histopathology of Bone

OSTEOPROGENITOR CELL PRINCIPLE

During fetal and postfetal life, all connective tissue cells, each of which becomes highly differentiated and destined to perform a specific function, are derived from an undifferentiated, highly prolific cell, the mesenchymal cell. It is now well established that throughout life there is a widespread presence in the circulating blood, hemopoietic tissues, and presumably throughout the vascular channels of all connective tissue systems, of undifferentiated mesenchymal cells that can be induced to form either bone, cartilage, fibrous tissue, or blood.[25] Their ubiquitous distribution implies that they form a pool of true multipotential cells. The bone derived from these undifferentiated cells is temporary, and repeated acts of inductive activity are required for osteogenesis to be maintained; once the inducing agent is removed, the bone disappears.

The morphological appearance of the undifferentiated mesenchymal cell is unknown. It is often referred to as a cell with a pale, vesicular, ovoid, or fusiform nucleus, and inconspicuous cytoplasm, but it may take many forms. Despite its elusive morphology, its indisputable existence is established by consistent radioisotope and histochemical studies and its irrefutable ability, using an appropriate inducing agent in a proper environment, to differentiate into a highly specialized cell with a specific function (*e.g.*, the osteoblast). On morphological grounds alone, it is extremely difficult, if not impossible, to identify the transition of mesenchymal cells into the earliest forms of specialized cells, the precursor cells of bone. These populations of dividing cells are most commonly found near bone surfaces, and since they are the precursors of both osteoblasts and osteoclasts, the two most differentiated cells of bone, they will be termed *osteoprogenitor cells* (Fig. 3-20).[32]

Marrow tissues contain cells capable of bone induction. In this case, the bone formed is more permanent. A self-perpetuating population of bone cells capable of relatively unlimited osteogenesis can be derived from these cells, and the presence of an inducing agent is not necessary. It is suggested, therefore, that these cells are already predetermined along the pathway to osteogenesis (DOPC = determined osteogenic precursor cells).

FIG. 3-20. The osteoprogenitor cells (p) and their derivatives, the osteoblasts (b) and osteoclasts (c). These different cell types represent specialized functional states of the same cell. Note the dark granular (basophilic) cytoplasm and prominent nucleoli, the sites of RNA concentration, both in osteoblasts and osteoclasts. (H and E, × 800) (Young RW: Nucleic acids, protein synthesis and bone. Clin Orthop 26:147, 1963)

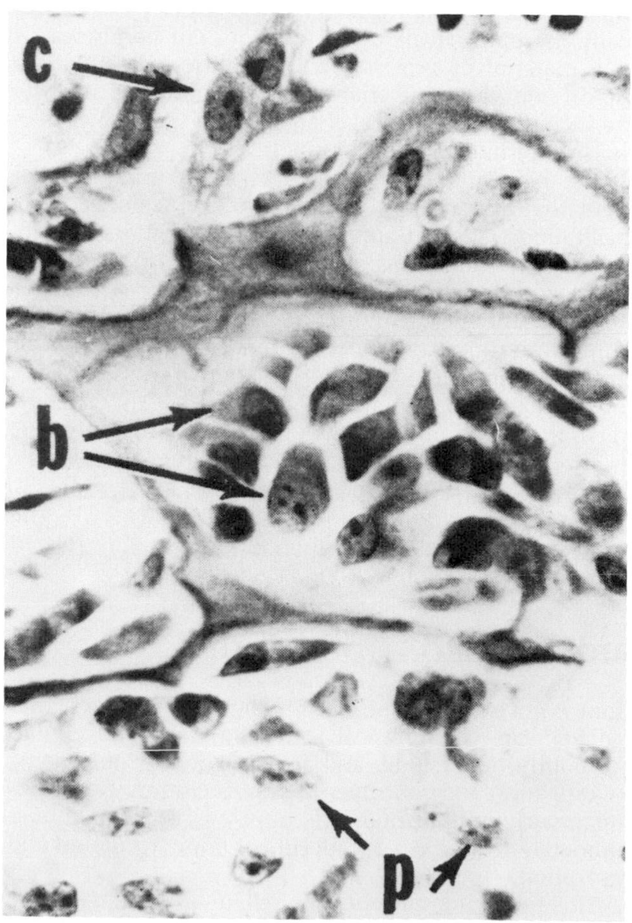

In summary, there appears to be two types of cells capable of induced osteogenesis. These are undifferentiated mesenchymal cells with a widespread distribution, and cells in the marrow tissues that are already predetermined in an osteogenic direction.[20] The superiority of marrow tissues (which contain DOPC) for the purposes of bone grafting is an accepted fact.[16]

The osteoprogenitor cell principle postulates a mesenchymal-like stem cell that is ubiquitous in all connective tissues, and which under various influences can be induced to proliferate rapidly and differentiate into cells with highly specialized function. Once the latter well-differentiated cells have fulfilled their function, apparently within a predetermined period of time, they disappear, whether by autolysis, transformation to another type of differentiated cell, or by reversion to the original mesenchymal state, and, if the osteoblastic process must continue, they are constantly replenished by newly differentiated cells (Fig. 3-21). In the case of bone, this concept is fundamental to the processes of remodeling, fracture repair, and removal and replacement of necrotic bone. Therefore, osseous repair is dependent on the intracellular metabolic activities not only of osteoblasts and osteoclasts but also of their respective precursors.[21] Because well-differentiated cells with specific functions have little or no ability to divide, the processes of bone formation and resorption require constant replenishment of osteoblasts and osteoclasts by primitive connective tissue cells.[13,28,33]

Various studies have demonstrated that already differentiated cells, such as reticulo-endothelial cells lining the sinusoids of bone marrow,[16] endothelial cells,[31] fibroblasts,[23] nucleated erythrocytes,[14] and histiocytes,[29] can undergo further transformation into osteoblasts. Such morphological changes can be demonstrated by electrical stimulation.[26] These observations are compatible with the stem-cell concept, because such cells may represent intermediate steps of differentiation from mesenchymal cells to highly specialized bone cells; or these various daughter cells of the primitive connective tissue cells may be induced to undergo reversion to a mesenchymal state before differentiation to osteoblasts and osteoclasts. Although all such cells may collectively be designated as osteoprogenitor cells, the term within this text will be reserved for the morphologically undifferentiated cells whose metabolic pathways toward bone production or resorption can only be established by radioisotopic and histochemical identification.

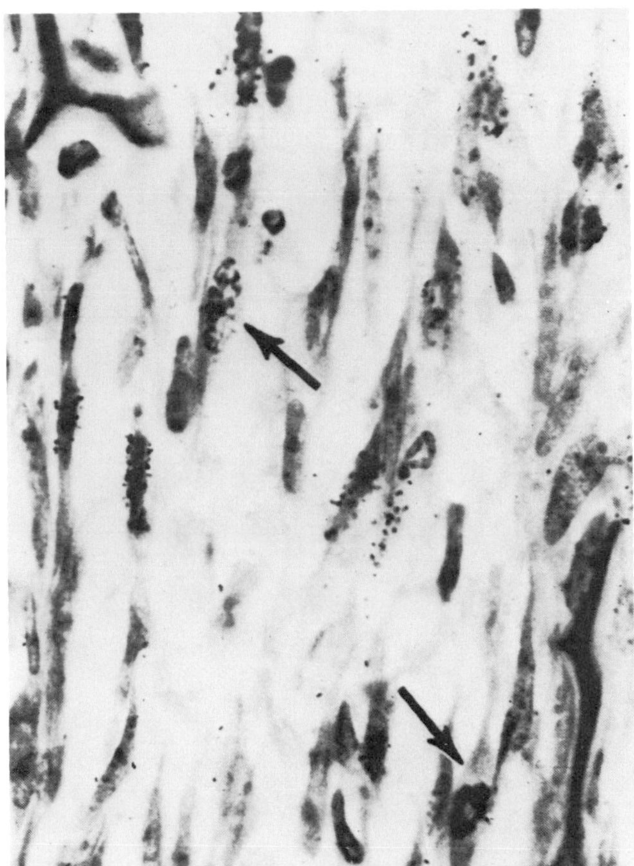

FIG. 3-21. Dedifferentiation of osteoblasts and osteoclasts. Microscopic section of tibial metaphysis of a 6-day-old rat given 4 injections of parathyroid extract, 25 units each, at 3-hour intervals, and sacrificed 24 hours after the first injection. One hour before sacrifice the animal was injected with 1 μC/g thymidine-H^3. Osteoblasts have reverted to the osteoprogenitor state. Many osteoprogenitor cells are engaged in DNA synthesis, prior to mitosis, as indicated by incorporation of thymidine-H^3 (revealed by exposed silver grains overlying nuclei). Note mitotic figures (*arrows*). (Periodic acid-Schiff (PAS) and hematoxylin; autoradiogram × 800) (Young RW: Nucleic acids, protein synthesis and bone. Clin Orthop 26:147, 1963)

DNA AUTORADIOGRAPHIC STUDIES

Thymidine-H^3, the radioactive specific precursor of genetically coded deoxyribonucleic acid (DNA), is rapidly incorporated (within an hour) into the nucleus of cells that are engaged in DNA synthesis immediately prior to mitotic division.[33] Owing to the metabolic stability of DNA, the incorporated radioactivity, detected autoradiographically, is retained within the nuclei as long as these cells survive, except that with each division half of the radioactivity is distributed to each daughter cell. Within the first hour after the tritiated thymidine is injected, neither osteocytes nor osteoblasts incorporate thymidine-H^3, and the excess is rapidly excreted. In bone, the process of DNA synthesis and its sequel mitosis is restricted to cells of relatively undifferentiated morphology (Fig. 3-22). The specialized cells, osteoblasts, osteocytes, and osteoclasts, arise by transformation of osteoprogenitor cells, and are incapable of reproduction. It is only after an extended period of time during which repeated divisions of labeled osteoprogenitor cells have

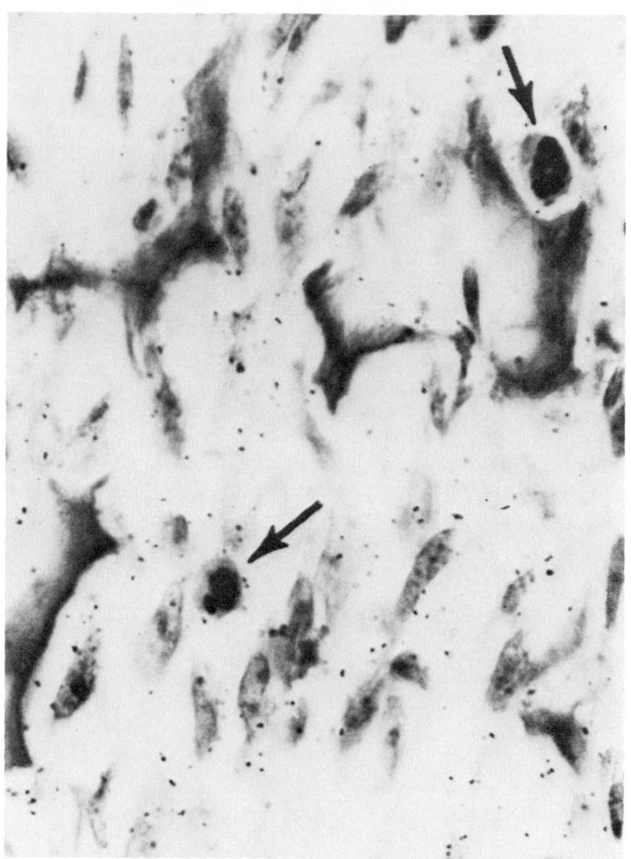

FIG. 3-22. Same conditions as Figure 3-21, except that glycine-H^3 (5 μC/g), rather than thymidine-H^3, was injected 1 hour before sacrifice. The osteoprogenitor cells incorporate very little glycine-H^3 because it does not synthesize collagen. Note mitotic figures (*arrows*). (PAS–hematoxylin; autoradiogram × 800) (Young RW: Nucleic acids, protein synthesis and bone. Clin Orthop 26:147, 1963)

occurred that they give rise to specialized bone cells with their pro rata share of radioactivity. Since these cells do not directly incorporate thymidine-H^3, the only source of such radioactivity is by transformation of the already labeled osteoprogenitor cells.

Osteoblasts and osteoclasts with heavily labeled nuclei do not persist long after their initial appearance. Since death of osteoblasts and osteoclasts is seldom observed, it is logical to assume that they either transform into other specialized cells (osteoblasts to osteoclasts?[30]), or dedifferentiate to rejoin their predecessors, the osteoprogenitor population. The latter probability appears to be confirmed after injections of parathyroid extract (see Fig. 3-21). The osteoblasts disappear, and are replaced by a profusion of osteoclasts and osteoprogenitor cells.

In osteoclasts, after thymidine-H^3 labeling and passing of time, one or more nuclei may be labeled, suggesting their origin from fusion of precursor cells. The studies show that there is continuous incorporation and shedding of nuclei by osteoclasts.[32] Consequently, the average lifetime of the nucleated components is important, and it can be shown that the average lifetime of the nucleus in an osteoclast in the metaphysis in young animals may be as long as 150 hours, while the turnover of osteoclast nuclei in the endosteum and periosteum is slower.[26] This appears to refute the possibility that osteoclasts arise through cell division or through fusion of osteoblasts. The actual lifetime of the osteoclast may be lengthy, perhaps remaining morphologically intact as long as the need for its function exists, and requiring only continual nuclear replenishment during its lifetime.

RNA AUTORADIOGRAPHIC STUDIES

Ribonucleic acid (RNA) can be identified and traced through generations of cells by various techniques. RNA has the characteristic property of absorption of ultraviolet light at 2000 A, the intensely absorbing material first appearing in the nucleolus and then accumulating in the cytoplasm as the osteoblasts develop from osteoprogenitor cells.[22] This can be confirmed by histochemical staining for RNA, and by preventing histochemical identification of RNA by preliminary extraction of RNA by RNase.[18]

Autoradiographic studies are specific means of tracing RNA. Cytidine-H^3 or uridine-H^3 is a specific precursor of RNA. By injecting either of these tritiated substances, measurable amounts of RNA can be traced through stages of osteoprogenitor proliferation and transformation to osteoblasts and osteoclasts, both of which contain significant amounts of RNA (Fig. 3-23). Autoradiographic labeling can be prevented by prior incubation with RNase.

HISTOCHEMICAL STUDIES

Current histochemical investigations of patterns of enzymic activity and cell organelles in different osteogenic cells are as yet not sufficiently revealing in tracing metabolic pathways and tracing cell origin.[17,19,27] However, certain consistent distinctive patterns have emerged:

1. Alkaline phosphatase predominates in cells destined for osteogenesis . . . osteoblasts and preosteoblasts
2. Acid phosphatase and succinic dehydrogenase predominates in cells destined for bone resorption . . . osteoclasts
3. Succinic dehydrogenase is specific for osteoclasts. Since mononuclear cells and binuclear cells are found with strong succinic dehydrogenase activity in bones under hyperparathyroid conditions, this may indicate a preosteoclast origin from osteoprogenitor cells.

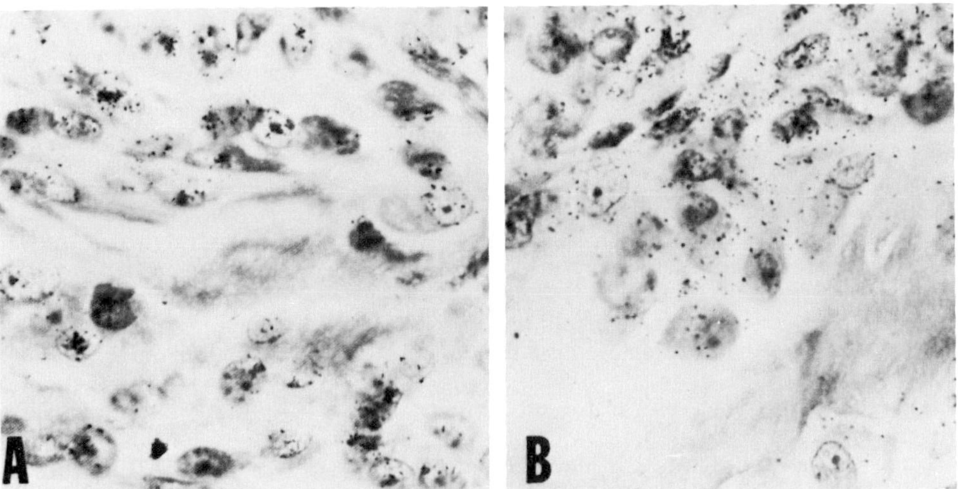

FIG. 3-23. Tibial diaphysis of 6-day-old rat injected with cytidine-H^3 (precursor of RNA), 2 μC/g at different intervals before sacrifice. (*A*) Injected ½ hour before sacrifice. Radioactivity is confined to the nuclei of the osteoblasts. (*B*) Injected 24 hours before sacrifice. The autoradiographic reaction is now concentrated over the cytoplasm. This reaction can be prevented by prior incubation of the sections with RNAase, indicating that the cytidine-H^3 has been incorporated in RNA. (PAS–hematoxylin; autoradiograms × 800) (Young RW: Nucleic acids, protein synthesis and bone. Clin Orthop 26:147, 1963)

THE OSTEOGENIC CELL

BIOLOGIC CHARACTERISTICS

Under conditions of active osteogenesis, which can be induced by a variety of means (*e.g.*, artificially induced electrical potentials), the ultrastructural characteristics of the osteoblast become pronounced and easily visualized by electron microscopy.[40] The morphological changes reflect the enhanced intracellular dynamics during bone formation (see Fig. 3-13).

The *Golgi complex* is a prominent feature of the osteoblast. This organelle is the site of synthesis of glycoprotein[41], sulfated mucopolysaccharides[37], and phospholipids. These substances become encapsulated within membrane-bound vesicles[46] (MBV) which fuse with the cellular membrane, dissolving the latter, and expelling their contents into the extracellular matrix.

Tropocollagen forms within the *rough endoplasmic reticulum* (RER) which becomes swollen and transformed into ribosome-lined cisternae. On encountering the cell membrane, the latter and the cisternal membranes undergo dissolution, and the tropocollagen is expelled into the extracellular matrix.[44]

Usually the *mitochondria* are concerned with electron transport and the formation of high-energy phosphates. Typically these organelles possess a limiting membrane and folded, closely packed intramitochondrial cristae. An additional role is the ability of the mitochondrion to concentrate calcium and phosphate as a tricalcium phosphate.[42] The tricalcium phosphate complex is initially amorphous, and under electron microscopy the mitochondrion becomes distended with an electron-lucid substance, transforming it into a membrane-bound vacuole. Its membrane breaks down in the extracellular matrix. Hydroxyapatite crystals slowly become apparent, either while within the intact vacuole or lying "free" within the extracellular matrix.[43] It has also been suggested that the mitochondria containing tricalcium phosphate form micropackets, and that the tricalcium phosphate is released from the mitochondria by reverse phagocytosis or by diffusion.

LOCAL FACTORS INFLUENCING OSTEOGENESIS

The following are local factors that influence osteogenesis.

Compression Forces.[36] Pressure within the physiologic limits of force exerted by the musculature stimulates or enhances osteogenesis. Excessive pressure causes necrosis with delayed osteogenesis. Absence of compression force fails to stimulate, but does not prevent osteogenesis. Even in the presence of infection, osteogenesis is stimulated by compression. When stresses are applied to a bone, the trabeculae within that bone develop and align themselves to adapt to these lines of stress (Wolff's law). Pressure force exerted perpendicular to the axis of a long bone is more likely to cause resorption of bone. Pressure force acting in the line of the bone axis is more likely to cause osteogenesis.

Circulation. A blood supply within certain limits is necessary for osteogenesis. Hyperemia (congestion, sluggish blood flow) results in reduction of osteogenesis. The bone becomes decalcified and osteoporotic. Theoretically, local decreased *p*H (acidity) effects solution of calcium salts. Deprivation of blood supply results in necrosis of bone. When a section of bone is necrotic, it appears dense in contrast with the surrounding bone which become hyperemic and therefore decalcified.

Disuse or Inactivity. With disuse or inactivity, osteogenesis is reduced, and all bone in the immobilized part become osteoporotic. Sluggish blood flow and lack of muscle forces are the main causative forces.

Inflammation. Injury or infection causes a reactive hyperemia which in turn effects dissolution of calcium salts. Leukocytic proteolytic enzymes cause degradation of matrix and interfere with the formation of osteoid.

Neurotrophic Disturbance (Sudeck's Atrophy; Reflex Sympathetic Dystrophy). Following trauma, reflex vasodilatation may affect the local region of trauma or may extend throughout the extremity. Sluggish blood flow is reflected clinically by cyanosis and coolness of the part, and spotty decalcification of the bone which may be attributed at least in part to local acidosis (increased solubility of bone mineral salts?) and decreased local oxygen tension (decreased bone formation?)

Traction Stress. This force tends to reduce the rate of bone formation. For example, distraction at a fracture site lessens the formation of callus and delays union.

Shearing Stress. Following a fracture, when the opposing ends of the fragments are subjected to shearing stresses, osteogenesis is reduced, and fibrous tissue and cartilage formation is likely.

The Periosteum. The presence of an enveloping periosteum is a major factor, although not absolutely necessary, for osteogenesis. For example, when a rib with its periosteal covering is removed, it does not regenerate. Periosteum, when transplanted, continues to grow bone. Destruction of periosteum (*e.g.*, thermal cauterization) retards osteogenesis. When the periosteum is stripped upward (*e.g.*, by a tumor), a layer of new periosteal bone forms beneath it.

Availability of Local Bone Substance. The presence of bone, whether viable or nonviable, is a major stimulus to osteogenesis. Bone appears to possess a bone morphogenetic principle (BMP) which induces the formation of new bone as old bone is resorbed.[45]

When a fibrous union exists between fragments, a bone transplant laid alongside the pseudarthrosis effects ossification within the fibrous tissue. Therefore, it is unnecessary to remove the fibrous tissue in order to effect a bony union.

Growth Hormone. Growth hormone (somatotropic hormone, STH) causes an increase in bone, mainly endosteal in origin, although periosteal and intracortical bone formation is also increased. The rate of new bone formation and resorption are both rapid, but osteogenesis is more rapid and the net bone mass is increased.[38] Sex hormone does not display the same osteogenic effect.[39]

Bioelectric Phenomena. Hydrated, living bone becomes electrically charged, probably piezoelectrically, when subjected to mechanical stress (*e.g.*, when deformed by compressive loading).[34] Similarly, externally applied weak currents will effect transformation of mesenchymal cells to osteoprogenitor cells, and increased bone formation will occur about the negative electrode.[35]

THE BONE INDUCTION PRINCIPLE

Bone, whether immature[48,50] or mature[47] has the property of inducing osteogenesis. Experimentally, consistently reproducible bone formation has been observed in implants of devitalized bone in various mammalian and laboratory species.[51] The development of bone in nonviable extraskeletal implants conclusively demonstrates the presence of an autoinductive agent in bone matrix. When bone is demineralized in 0.6 N HCl at 6° C within 24 hours, lyophilized and implanted in allogeneic animals, an ingrowth of mesenchymal cells and capillaries, accompanied by wandering histiocytes and macrophages, into old vascular channels occurs. Between the fifth and tenth days, old matrix is resorbed producing enlarged "excavation chambers," and the migratory mesenchymal cells differentiate mainly into osteoblasts which then proceed to lay down new bone on the old matrix (Fig. 3-24).

The organic matrix of bone and dentin, even in the absence of living cells, contains a bone morphogenetic protein (BMP), termed the bone induction principle.[53,54,55] Within the bone, an endogenous neutral proteinase, BMPase, exists which degrades BMP without dissolution of bone collagen. Under conditions of extreme acidity and low temperature of a demineralizing solution, BMPase activity is inhibited, and BMP is protected against degradation.

Undemineralized bone demonstrates poor autoinduction, perhaps because the diffusion of BMP toward the excavation chamber is slowed and the induction principle may be sufficiently degraded before it reaches the site of

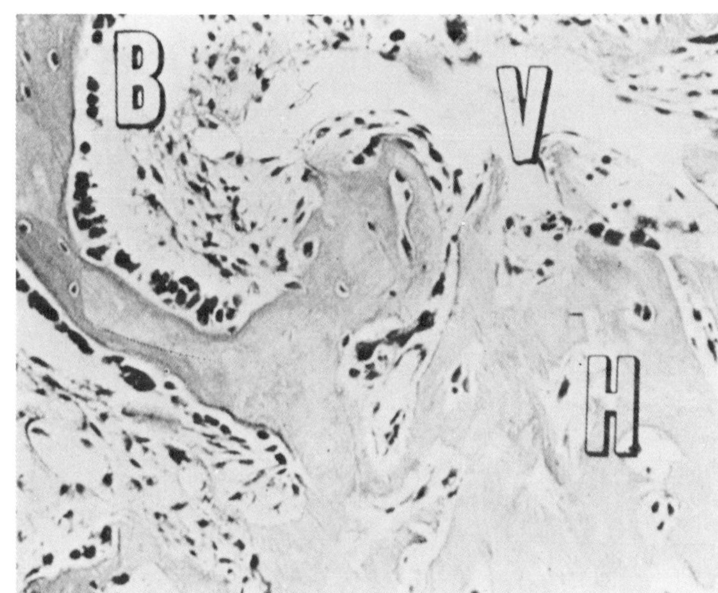

FIG. 3-24. Photomicrograph of an implant 4 weeks after the operation in a rabbit, showing palisades of osteoblasts and the first deposits of new bone (*B*) on the surfaces of old decalcified matrix. The marrow vascular spaces are repopulated with wandering and fixed histiocytes (*H*). Dilated blood vessels (*V*) are surrounded by spindle-shaped mesenchymal cells. (Urist MR, Silverman BF, Büring K et al: The bone induction principle. Clin Orthop 53:243, 1967)

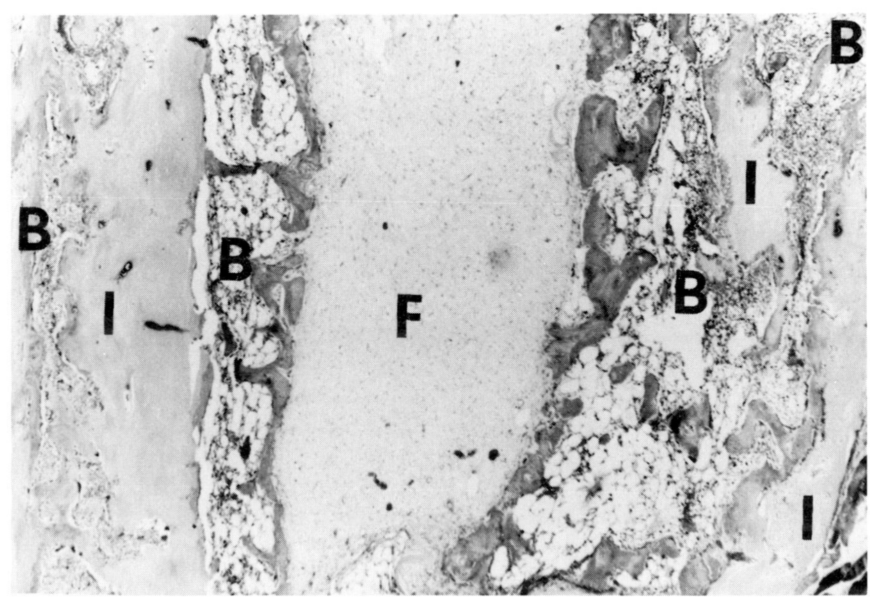

FIG. 3-25. Photomicrograph of an implant of 2°C 0.6 N hydrochloric acid, demineralized bone matrix 28 days after implantation in a muscle pouch. New bone (*B*); implanted matrix (*I*); fibrous connective tissue without any small round cell infiltrate (*F*). (Urist MR, Mikulski A, Stuart DB: A chemosterilized antigen-extracted autodigested alloimplant for bone banks. Arch Surg 110:416, 1975. Copyright, 1975, American Medical Association)

induction. Chemical inhibition of the matrix enzyme (*e.g.*, by iodoacetic acid, IAA) will enhance osteoinduction.[52]

Osteoinduction depends on substrate-cell interaction: histiocytes (macrophages) at first resorb the old dead matrix. Then the primitive connective tissue cells (stem cells) are induced to transform into osteoprogenitor cells and, ultimately, osteoblasts (Fig. 3-25).

The responding cell is a perivascular hypertrophied mesenchymal cell. It differentiates into an osteoblast, a chondroblast, or a hematocytoblast and becomes an induced cell, which later becomes an inducing cell. Induction occurs in two directions: centrifugally, to produce lamellar bone; centripetally, to produce new bone marrow cells (Fig. 3-26).

The bone induction principle works best in demineralized bone. It is preserved by decalcification at low temperatures with 0.6 N HCl or ethylenediaminotetraacetate (EDTA) or 1:1 formic acid and citric acid. Nitric or nitrous acid destroys the bone induction principle. Because lactic acid does not remove all the mineral, bone induction is severely retarded.

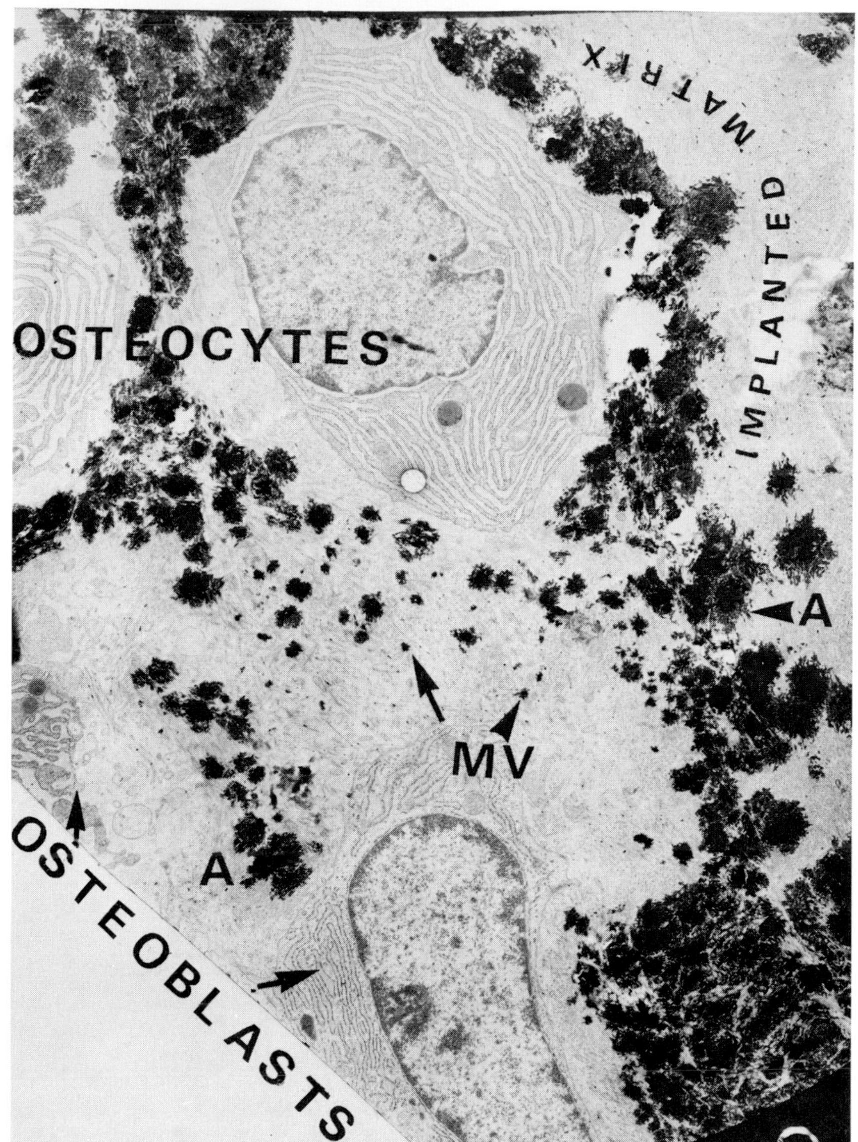

FIG. 3-26. Electron micrograph showing interface between autolysed demineralized acellular implanted matrix and earliest deposits of new bone. Recalcification of the implanted old matrix occurs only at line of contact with newly calcifying deposits of bone. Microvesicles (*MV*); clusters of apatite in areas between young osteocytes and osteoblasts (*A*). (Urist MR, Mikulski A, and Stuart DB: A chemosterilized antigen-extracted autodigested alloimplant for bone banks. Arch Surg 110:416, 1975. Copyright, 1975, American Medical Association)

HISTOLOGIC SEQUENCE OF EVENTS IN EXTRASKELETAL IMPLANT

The histologic sequence of events in extraskeletal implants are as follows (Fig. 3-27):

1. The extraskeletal implant floats in serosanguineous fluid containing leukocytes and wandering histiocytes. After 12 days, the fluid is absorbed.
2. Implant becomes enveloped in inflammatory connective tissue. The cells involved include wandering histiocytes or macrophages, lymphocytes, and fibroblasts.
3. Old matrix swells and becomes amorphous when stained with H and E, and slightly metachromatic with toluidine blue. Collagen fibers are intact.
4. Donor cells undergo autolysis and lacunae become empty or contain remnants of dead cells.
5. Emigrant cells enter the marrow spaces and vascular channels.
6. Proteolytic enzymes, presumably contained in lysosomes from macrophages and multinucleated giant cells of the recipient, resorb the old matrix enlarging the old vascular channels into excavation chambers.[49]
7. By 4 weeks, the proliferating hypertrophied mesenchymal cells differentiate into polygonal cells which become oriented in palisades on the surfaces of the old matrix and lay down new bone on the surface of

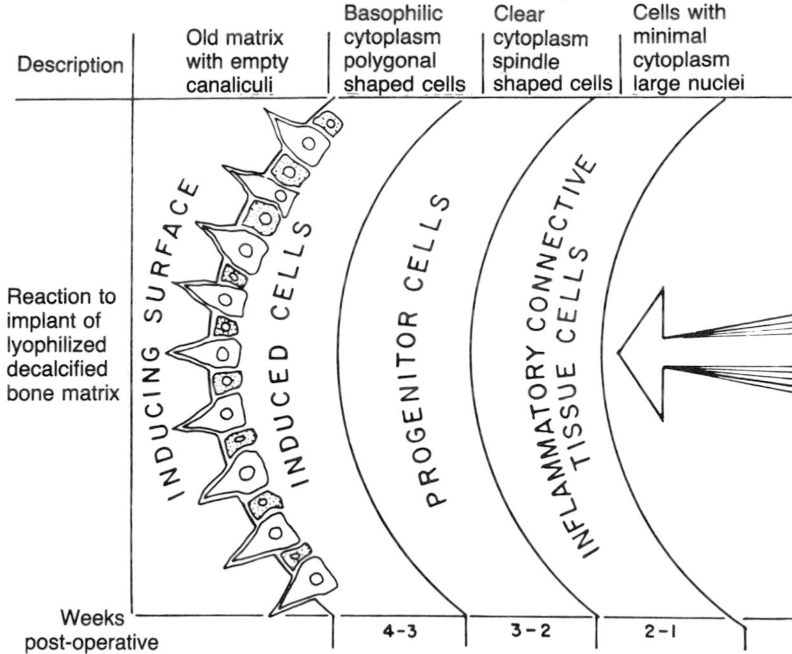

FIG. 3-27. Early stages of bone induction. Cell morphology and time relationships in bone induction by an implant of decalcified lyophilized bone matrix. Urist. MR et al: The bone induction principle. Clin Orthop 53:243, 1967)

the old dead bone matrix, being separated from the latter by a film of cement substance.

8. The new bone is remodeled by osteoclasts and redeposited by new osteoblasts. Eventually a new haversian system is formed with multiple concentric lamellae surrounding the vascular haversian canal. In addition, hematocytoblasts, formed by differentiation from the mesenchymal cells, form marrow centrally.
9. Over a period of 6 months, the induced cells, osteoblasts, osteocytes, and even osteoclasts, become pyknotic. The ossicle formed from allogeneic bone matrix becomes necrotic, and slow absorption and replacement by fibrous tissue is the end result.

FACTORS AFFECTING BONE INDUCTION

THE IMMUNE REACTION Systemic and local manifestations of an immune response to a nonviable foreign tissue inhibit bone induction.
Histocompatibility antigens (H-antigens) incite a prolonged lymphocyte and plasma cell immune reaction in the host bed leading to absorption of the implant. Resorption of an implant of undecalcified bone is slow compared to an implant of decalcified lyophilized bone, probably because in the former, diffusion of H-antigen is impeded by minerals and released in small doses. Decalcifed matrix is resorbed rapidly, since the recipient receives relatively large amounts of H-antigen. The immune response reduces the degree of bone induction. Lyophilizing the implant reduces its antigenicity, lowers the immune response, and bone induction is high.

Xenogeneic bone introduces a large dose of H-antigen, and induction of bone is scanty or absent. This implant is always infiltrated and surrounded by great numbers of lymphocytes and plasma cells and large volumes of serous fluid.

Effect of Cold. The greatest degree of bone induction is obtained by freezing at −70° C in liquid nitrogen. Sterile decalcified nonlyophilized bone matrix stored in sealed containers at room temperatures deteriorates within 3 months. Decalcified (0.6 HCl) and lyophilized bone at −70° C induce bone formation in 96% of implants.

Effect of Heat. Heat denaturation of bone apparently does not impair bone induction until the temperature approaches 100° C. Above 60° C, despite shrinkage of collagen, the bone induction principle is preserved, but bone induction rapidly decreases beyond 80° C, and is nonexistent at 100° C.[53]

Effect of Radiation. Denaturation of lyophilized decalcified bone by gamma rays of radioactive cobalt at levels above 2 million roentgen equivalent physicals (rep) inhibits bone induction. Resorption of the irradiated denatured matrix induces the formation of a mass of fatty fibrous tissue, but never new bone. The exact levels of radiation that reduce antigenicity while enhancing bone induction have not been determined.

Enzymatic Degradation. Only proteolytic enzymes degrade the protein of decalcified bone matrix sufficiently to inhibit bone induction. The hydrolysis of matrix organic phosphates by acid or alkaline phosphatase, and mucopolysaccharides by hyaluronidase does not inhibit bone induction. This indicates that a specific protein macromolecule is responsible for bone induction.

Effect of Minerals. The presence of minerals impedes the process of resorption of matrix, retards the formation of excavation chambers, and delays the onset of bone induction.

REPAIR OF SIMPLE FRACTURE OF A LONG BONE

Interruption in continuity of a long bone, whether traumatic or surgical, is followed by a definite histologic sequence aimed at bridging the defect.[57,58] A basic understanding of this process is necessary for intelligent handling of fractures and osteotomies.

When the bone breaks into two or more fragments, the periosteum is torn, and bleeding occurs forming a clot in and about the fracture site. The blood vessels become sealed off by hemostatic mechanisms, and the circulation stops within these vessels back to the sites where they anastomose with vessels within which blood flow continues. Since haversian blood vessels run predominantly longitudinally in bone, and the vessels in the haversian systems are torn at the fracture site, blood flow stops within them back to sites where they anastomose with functioning blood vessels of other haversian systems. Therefore, blood flow ceases in haversian systems for a variable distance on each side of the fracture line, and the bone immediately adjacent to and extending a variable distance from the fracture line becomes necrotic. Furthermore, the periosteum and marrow bordering on the fracture line also become necrotic. The distance from the fracture line over which avascular necrosis develops varies, depending on the site within the long bone and the particular bone involved.

Blood and plasma infiltrate the surrounding muscles which within a few hours become swollen, edematous and friable.

EARLY STAGES OF REPAIR

A new tissue, callus, develops around and between the fragments, forming a bridge by which the fragments are initially united. The callus that develops around the outer aspects of the opposing ends of the bone fragments is termed external callus, and that which forms between the bone ends is termed internal callus.

Within the first 2 days following the fracture, at a short distance from the fracture site and within the deep layer of the periosteum, the osteogenic cells proliferate and lift the fibrous layer of periosteum farther away from

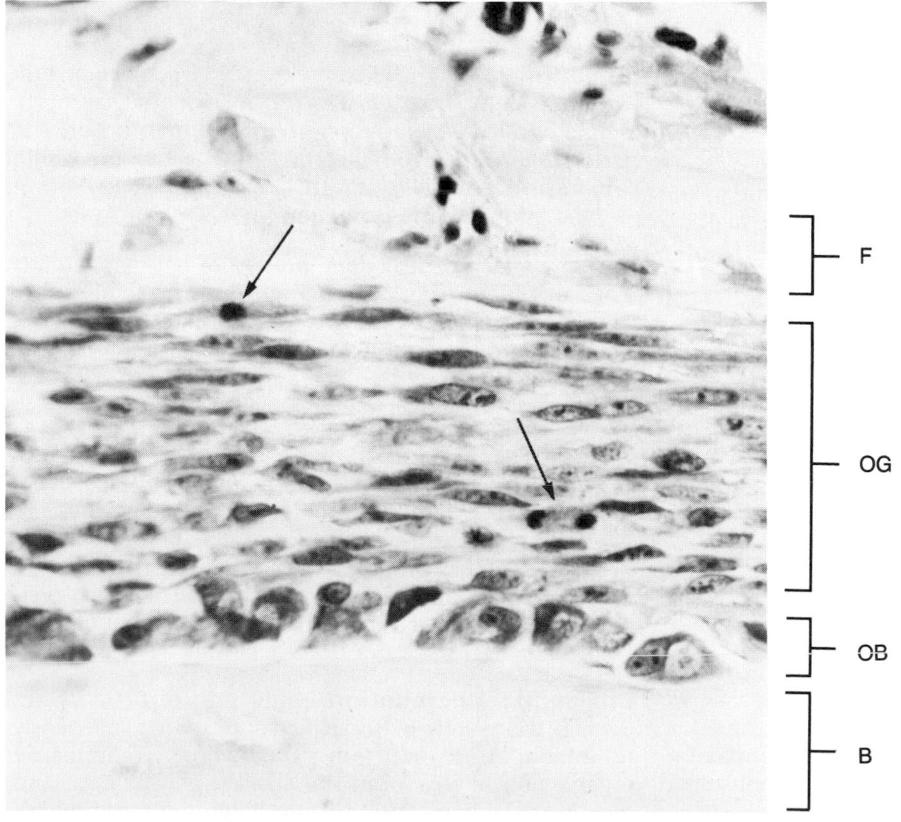

FIG. 3-28. Photomicrograph showing what happens in the periosteum shortly after and close to a fracture. The fibrous layer (F) is lifted away from the bone (B) by the greatly thickened osteogenic layer (OG) in which osteogenic cells are proliferating. Mitotic figures are indicated by arrows. At the bone surface the osteogenic cells have differentiated into osteoblasts which will soon form a new layer of bone on the surface on which they lie. (Ham AW, Harris WR: Repair and transplantation of bone. In Bourne GH (ed): The Biochemistry and Physiology of Bone, Vol 3, 2nd ed. New York, Academic Press, 1971)

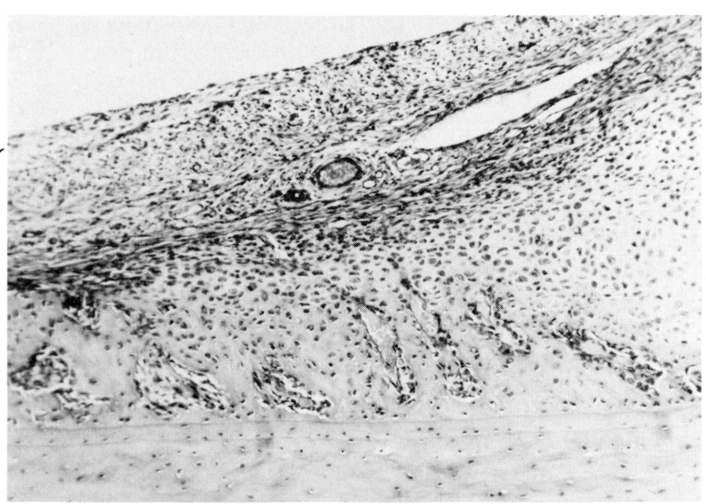

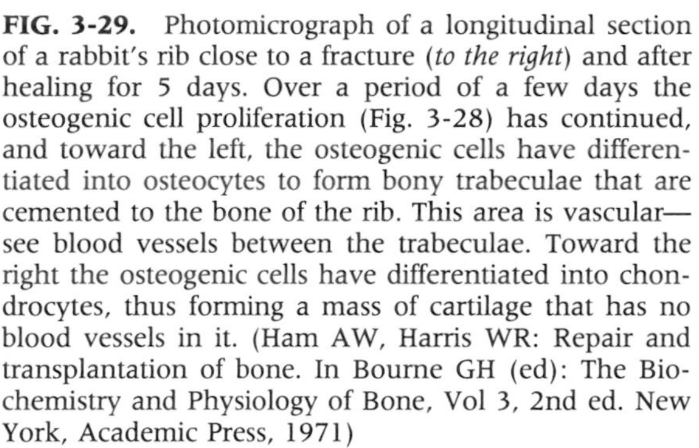

FIG. 3-29. Photomicrograph of a longitudinal section of a rabbit's rib close to a fracture (*to the right*) and after healing for 5 days. Over a period of a few days the osteogenic cell proliferation (Fig. 3-28) has continued, and toward the left, the osteogenic cells have differentiated into osteocytes to form bony trabeculae that are cemented to the bone of the rib. This area is vascular—see blood vessels between the trabeculae. Toward the right the osteogenic cells have differentiated into chondrocytes, thus forming a mass of cartilage that has no blood vessels in it. (Ham AW, Harris WR: Repair and transplantation of bone. In Bourne GH (ed): The Biochemistry and Physiology of Bone, Vol 3, 2nd ed. New York, Academic Press, 1971)

FIG. 3-30. A drawing of a longitudinal H and E section of a rabbit's rib in which a fracture had been healing for 48 hours. The territory encompassed by the drawing was that which could be seen with a very low-power objective, but the detail has been depicted at higher magnification to obviate the necessity of making several drawings at different magnifications. (Ham AW, Harris WR: Repair and transplantation of bone. In Bourne GH (ed): The Biochemistry and Physiology of Bone, Vol 3, 2nd ed, p 338. New York, Academic Press, 1971)

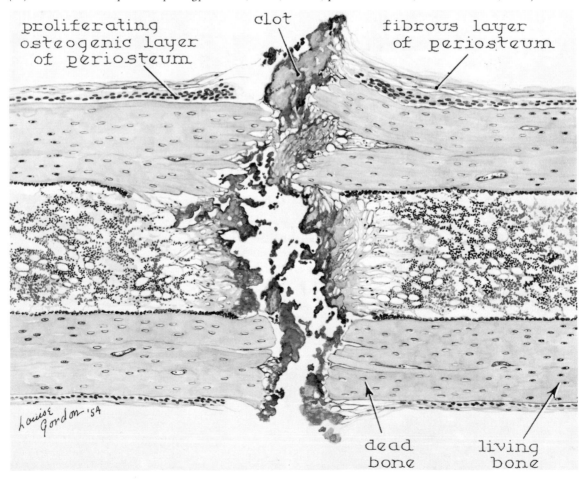

the bone (Fig. 3-28). At the same time, the osteogenic cells lining the marrow cavity also proliferate, but not to the same degree as those of the osteogenic layer of periosteum.

The cells within the deep layer of periosteum proliferate so rapidly that, within a few days, they form a distinct collar around each fragment close to the line of fracture. Simultaneously the capillaries among them also proliferate (Figs. 3-29 and 3-30).

Next, the osteogenic cells differentiate. Those that are situated deeply within the collar adjacent to the bone lie within a highly vascular area. In the presence of an adequate blood supply, they become osteoblasts and form bone trabeculae. These newly formed trabeculae resemble embryonic new bone because they are poorly organized and do not stain as evenly as the more mature bone. They become firmly attached to the matrix of both live and dead cortical bone of the fragment (Fig. 3-31).

The osteogenic cells lying in the areas of the collar remote from the bone have proliferated so rapidly that they are far removed from the slower growing capillaries. Lacking adequate vascularity, they differentiate into chondroblasts and chondrocytes and, consequently, cartilage develops in the outer region of the collars (Figs. 3-32 and 3-33).

The amount of cartilage which forms depends mainly on the rapidity with which the collar forms, since the formation of capillaries lags behind the rate of cell proliferation, and the motion at the fracture site.

The collars when fully developed exhibit three layers. In the deep inner layer, the bone trabeculae are firmly cemented to the bone. The intermediate layer, the car-

FIG. 3-31. A drawing of a longitudinal H and E section of a rabbit's rib in which a fracture had been healing for 1 week. The territory encompassed by the drawing was that which could be seen with a very low-power objective, but the detail has been filled in at higher magnification to obviate the necessity of making several drawings at different magnifications. (Ham AW, Harris WR: Repair and transplantation of bone. In Bourne GH (ed): The Biochemistry and Physiology of Bone, Vol 3, 2nd ed, p. 338. New York, Academic Press, 1971)

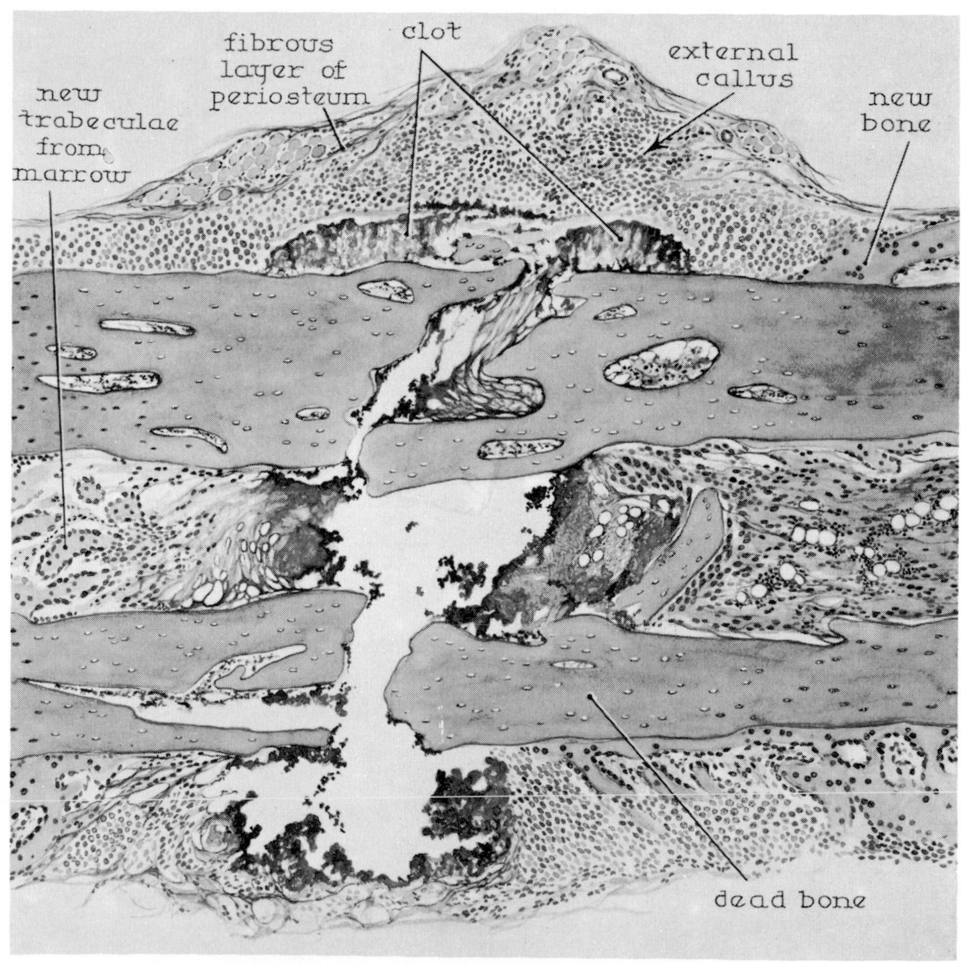

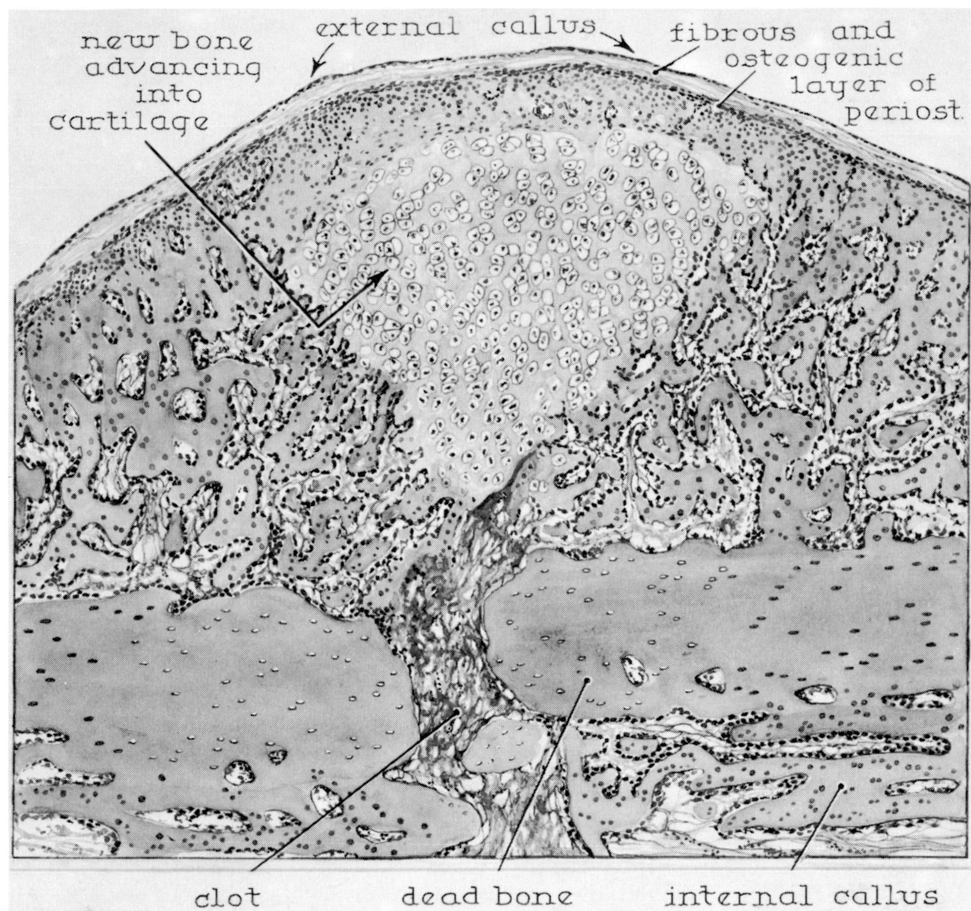

FIG. 3-32. A drawing of part of a longitudinal H and E section of a rabbit's rib in which a fracture had been healing for 2 weeks. (Ham AW, Harris WR: Repair and transplantation of bone. In Bourne GH (ed): The Biochemistry and Physiology of Bone, Vol 3, 2nd ed, p 338. New York, Academic Press, 1971)

tilage, merges imperceptibly with the outer parts of the newly formed bone trabeculae beneath it, and, at its outer aspect, with the proliferating cells of the periosteal deep layer, which constitutes the third and outer layer.

The collars from the two fragments become thicker, advance toward each other, and fuse, with the trabeculae, cartilage, and proliferating cells forming a bridge. Thus, the initial union is achieved.

The cartilage in callus has a temporary existence and is eventully replaced by bone, mainly by the process of endochondral ossification. Those cartilage cells nearest to the newly formed bone mature, the matrix calcifies, the chondrocytes die, and vascular tissue with osteoblasts lay down bone to replace the disintegrating calcified cartilage. The original V-shaped cartilage becomes progressively smaller and eventually is completely replaced by bone. Finally, within the resulting cancellous bone small remnants of calcified cartilage can be seen between the trabeculae.

The internal callus, or medullary callus, is the chief source of union between the fragments. Within the first few days, marked vascular proliferation occurs within the medullary cavity about the fracture site. The marked ingrowth of capillaries and regenerated nutrient vessels is accompanied by infiltration of mesenchymal type of cells that proceed to differentiate into preosteoblasts which in turn are converted to osteoblasts, and new bone trabeculae of an embryonic type are laid down. The process replaces the marrow locally. The vascular cellular tissue then proceeds to invade the interfragmentary interval, laying down immature trabeculae of bone, interspersed with a variable amount of fibrocartilage, and cementing the fragments together. The newly formed internal callus between the fragment ends than undergoes remodeling by which the embryonic bone is replaced by lamellar bone. Finally, vascular sprouts accompanied by osteoclasts invade from the adjacent fragment ends, burrowing enlarging tunnels that extend from one frag-

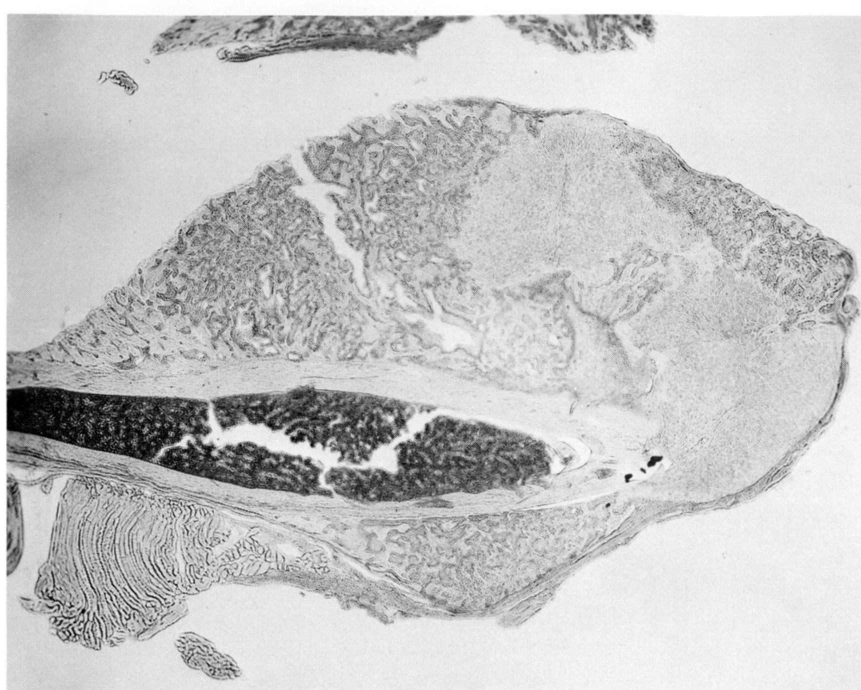

FIG. 3-33. Fracture callus. A cancellous type of bone forms adjacent to the cortex, replaces the cartilage, and extends distally as a bridge to meet the callus formation from the opposite fragment. The other fragment is not seen in this section.

ment to the other. Ultimately, concentric lamellae line these tunnels to form osteons that bridge the fracture site and restore continuity. Once the internal callus has invaded the fracture interval, the osteogenic process within the medulla is resorbed and replaced by hematopoietic marrow or fatty tissue.

REMODELING OF CALLUS

The newly formed trabeculae of bone are firmly cemented to the original bone. Moreover, the fragments are bridged with this cancellous network. Between the trabeculae which are laid down by osteoblasts on dead bone, osteoclasts slowly remove the necrotic bone and create cavities. Osteoblasts then line these deep indentations and lay down viable bone. Thus, almost all the matrix of the dead bone is eventually replaced with new living bone.

The internal callus bridging the fragments has meanwhile developed trabeculae from both the endosteum that lines the marrow cavity and the osteogenic cells of the marrow itself. In addition, a portion of the internal callus originates from osteogenic cells from the external surfaces of the fragments which have grown down into the fracture gap, adding to the cancellous bone joining the bone ends.

With the passing of time, the cancellous bone is remodeled and converted into compact bone.

HEALING BETWEEN CORTICES

When fractures are treated by open operation at which the fragments are joined firmly together by some metallic device until the fracture heals, little or no external callus forms.[58] Repair must, therefore, depend to great extent on the formation of internal callus.

On both sides of the fracture line, back at sites where capillaries and osteogenic cells are viable within the haversian canals, proliferation of vessels and osteogenic cells occurs. The osteogenic cells differentiate into osteoclasts which ream out the walls of the haversian canals, thus enlarging them. Moreover, the osteogenic cells differentiate into osteoblasts which line the walls of the widened canals and lay down, in series, concentric lamellae. This process advances to the fracture line where newly forming osteons extend across the line into the opposite fragment. The process is similar to that which occurs in ordinary remodeling within the shaft of the bone and by which old osteons are replaced by new ones.

Before the new osteons cross the fracture line, the spaces between the fragments must first be joined by bone of an immature type which appears to develop as an internal callus from the endosteum and marrow. This type of union is not strong until remodeling introduces new haversian systems which extend through and replace the immature bone.[56]

DELAYED UNION AND NONUNION

The biologic process of repair of a traumatic or surgically induced interruption in the continuity of a bone may develop slowly or not at all. Delayed union implies that union will ultimately occur but over a longer period than usual, whereas nonunion, by definition, is the complete suspension of the process at some point short of osseous bridging of the defect. Because the bone defect allows unnatural and perpetual mobility, it is termed a *pseudarthrosis*. The fragments are relatively fixed by interfragmentary tissue that permits varying degrees of motion, but at times such unnatural mobility may be slight and defies detection. The question of whether, at any point in time, failure of union represents a delay in the reparative process or is a perpetual nonunion may be difficult to resolve.

CAUSES OF DELAYED UNION OR NONUNION

The principal causes of nonunion or delayed union are as follows.

Extensive Gap. Loss of bone substance at the time of fracture, wide displacement of fragments, and distraction by an improperly applied device may create an interfragment gap that cannot be bridged by osseous tissue.

Loss of Blood Supply. ***Anatomical Susceptibility.*** A prime example is the lower third of the tibia which is devoid of surrounding vascular muscle and is almost wholly dependent on its medullary nutrient vessels. When these vessels are compromised by intramedullary nailing, soft tissue interposition (periosteum), wide displacement of fragments, or ill-advised surgical dissection, delayed union or nonunion is highly probable.

Damage to Surrounding Muscles. When the nutrient arteries of a long bone are disrupted, the surrounding muscles develop compensatory hypervascularity that provides a centripetal blood supply to the bone. If these muscles are damaged by the original trauma or by extensive surgical dissection, revascularization of the bone is poor, and delayed union or nonunion is probable.

Abnormal Biomechanics.[74,75] Shearing, torsional, and bending stresses will counteract the biologic repair process short of osseous bridging. Instead, fibrous or cartilaginous tissue, more suited to movement, occupies the interfragment gap. For example, a vertical fracture of the femoral neck produces shearing stresses and predisposes to nonunion. When the fracture line is horizontal, compressive forces predominate and union is more likely (Fig. 3-34).

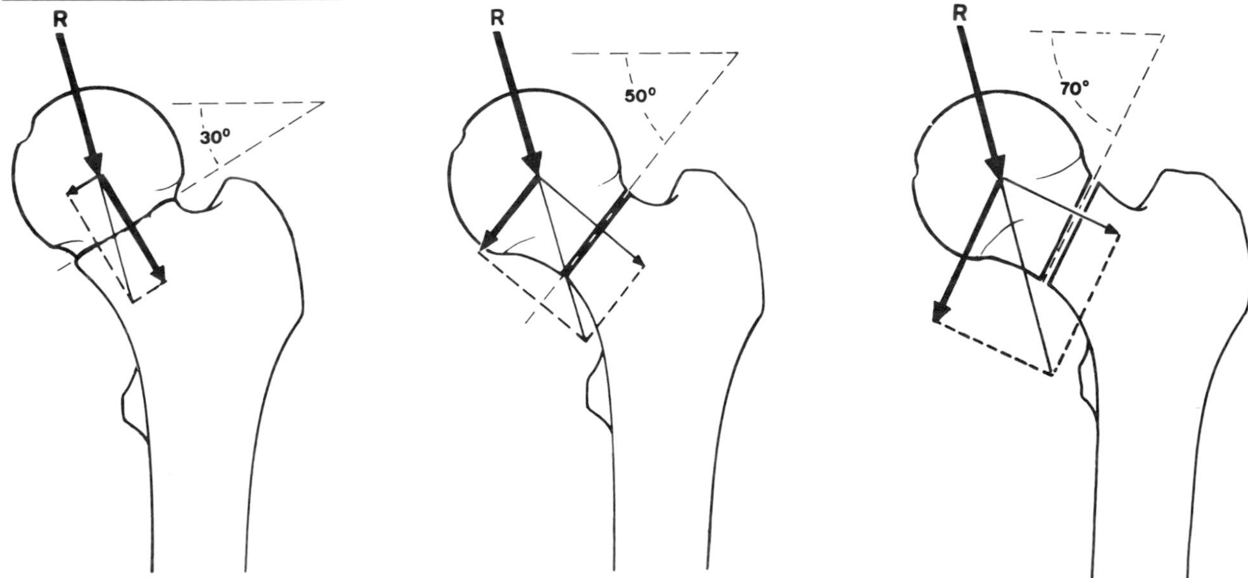

FIG. 3-34. Biomechanics of fractures of the neck of the femur showing stress patterns of different angles of inclination, according to Pauwels. (*Left*) Grade 1 fracture: angle of inclination 30°. Compression component greater than shearing component, is mechanically stable, and conditions are optimal for union. (*Center*) Grade 2 fracture: angle of inclination 50°, compression component less, shearing stress greater, stability reduced, probability of union diminished, yet possible. (*Right*) Grade 3 fracture: angle of inclination 70°. Compression component insignificant, shearing stresses pronounced, stability almost nil, high probability of nonunion. (From Weber BG, Cech O: Pseudarthrosis Bern, Hans Huber, 1976)

Infection. This will often impair the biologic repair process. Compound fractures are predisposed, and a history of an open fracture, despite the absence of overt signs of infection, should arouse suspicion of a smoldering osteomyelitis.

Extensive Comminution. Fragments may be torn from soft tissue attachments and remain necrotic. Wide gaps are created.

Improperly Applied Fixation Devices. Excessive intramedullary reaming will devascularize the diaphyseal cortex (Danckwardt-Lilliestrom). Distraction of fragments may be maintained by a metal plate, external skeletal fixation (*fixateur externe*), or excessive traction.

Individual Bone Susceptibility. Certain bones characteristically form little callus, and union is very slow (*e.g.*, lower third of tibia, neck of femur, carpal scaphoid). On the other hand, other bones possess a strong tendency to unite despite adverse conditions (*e.g.*, the ribs).

Insufficient Immobilization.[71] Absolute and prolonged mechanical rest reduces the need for callus, and even callus-free union (so-called primary union) may occur. This principle forms the basis for early internal fixation, "osteosynthesis" (*e.g.*, by intramedullary nails, compression plates, and so forth) permitting early resumption of function.

Metabolic Disturbance. Physiologic aberrations that adversely affect the availability and use of elements necessary for the formation of bone will impair the osteogenesis of fracture repair (*e.g.*, hyperparathyroidism favors bone resorption and phosphorus excretion, and fracture union is markedly delayed).

PATHOLOGY OF NONUNION

The lower diaphysis of the tibia serves as a prime example of the development of a nonunion. The failure of union represents interruption at some phase of the biologic sequence of fracture repair.[82]

At 6 months the fracture line is firmly enclosed in a spindle-shaped capsule of fibrous connective tissue and periosteum (Fig. 3-35 *Left*). The lateral and posterior aspects (site of soft tissue attachments) of the shaft on the periosteal surface show thin deposits of cancellous new bone beginning 1 cm to 2 cm above and below the fracture site. Similarly, some endosteal new bone is found away from the fracture site. At the fracture line, the bone ends are covered with fibrocartilage and hyaline cartilage. In the center of the fracture gap, an amorphous material and inflammatory connective tissue are found. The amorphous material consists of a mixture of substances—fibrinoid, hyalin, and mucinous fluid—and is surrounded by patches of necrotic fibrous tissue and evidence of chronic inflammatory cells.

Fibrinoid is the principal constituent of the amorphous material. It is acellular, homogeneous or refractile, fibrinlike, eosinophilic, metachromatic (with toluidine blue), pink-staining with the McManus-Hotchkiss procedure, and staining a mixture of orange, brown, yellow, and blue with phosphotungstic acid (which stains collagen), and hematoxylin. Morphologically, fibrinoid appears as a mass of material consisting of collagen and ground substance in all stages of degradation. Experimentally, it can be produced by mechanical trauma with extravasation of plasma into normal connective tissue, and is believed to be the result of precipitation of acid mucopolysaccharides.[81] Subsequently, the fibrinoid undergoes complete disintegration and liquefaction, resulting in the accumulation of a mucinous fluid in the center of the callus. The mucinous fluid of an early pseudarthrosis stains metachromatically with toluidine blue, thus resembling the protein polysaccharide complex found in a bursa. It is postulated that increased friction and motion between the bone ends traumatizes the small vessels increasing capillary permeability and extravasation of fluid into the amorphous material, and the fibrinoid imbibes the water leading to the formation of the pseudarthrosis fluid.

Hyalin is found in patches. It is eosinophilic, homogeneous, and refractile, but does not have the granular or fibrillar appearance of fibrinoid. It does not stain metachromatically with toluidine blue and is negative to the McManus-Hotchkiss procedure. With phosphotungstic acid, it stains multicolored, but lacks blue-staining elements. The quantity of hyalin increases with the age of the callus.

A variable amount of fibrous tissue represents the remains of the original granulation tissue that replaces the fracture hematoma. Fibrous tissue is increased following local sepsis.

At 6 months to 2 years a fibrous capsule envelops the fibrocartilaginous callus (Fig. 3-35 *Center*). Each bone end is freely movable and is capped by fibrocartilage and hyaline cartilage. The gap is occupied by fibrous or fibrocartilaginous tissue with patches of fibrinoid and hyalin surrounding a space with highly mucinous fluid. The fragment ends are densely sclerotic.

At 2 to 5 years the mature pseudarthrosis has eventuated (Fig. 3-35 *Right*). The proximal bone end is expanded and shaped like a metaphysis with a saucerized concave surface. The end of the distal fragment is rounded and often enclosed within the concavity of the proximal fragment. The bone ends are either composed of bare sclerotic bone with a variable amount of covering by fibrocartilage, hyaline cartilage, fibrous tissue, and some amorphous material. The cavity is filled with a highly viscous hydrophilic fluid, and a synovial-like membrane may form. A characteristic feature is the endless laying down of new bone from the rim of the proximal fragment end.

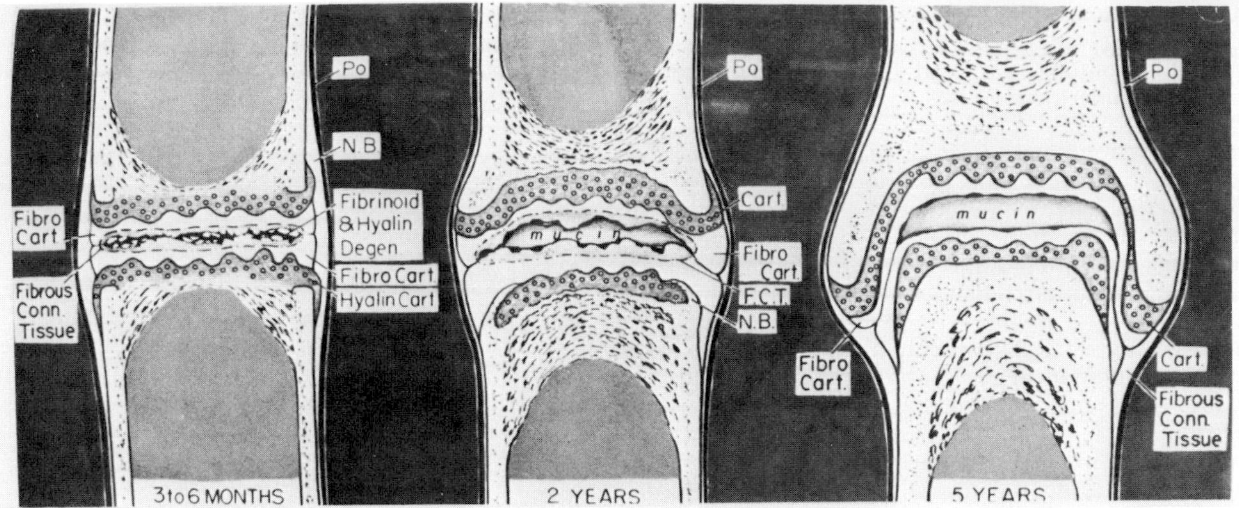

FIG. 3-35. The three stages of formation of pseudarthrosis. (*Left*) An amorphous area of fibrinoid and hyaline degeneration appears in the center of the callus during the first 3 to 6 months of healing. (*Center*) At any time before 2 years of healing have elapsed, a mechanical disturbance of the fracture will result in cleavage of the amorphous area and the formation of extracellular fluid containing mucin. (*Right*) Unrestricted motion at the fracture site, mechanical bruising, and inflammation of tissue is followed by a continual fibrinoid degeneration of callus, overgrowth of bone all around the bone ends, and formation of false joint surfaces. Osteogenesis never actually ceases, it simply fails to bridge the fracture gap. The process of new-bone formation from one fragment seems to make an endless attempt to reach bone produced by the other fragment. (Urist MR, Mazet R, McLean FC: The pathogenesis and treatment of delayed union and non-union. J Bone Joint Surg 36A:931, 1954)

TREATMENT OF DELAYED UNION OR NONUNION

The classical treatment of nonunion consisted formerly of a "bone graft" and prolonged immobilization in a cast without weight bearing. This often required repeated operations and was followed by joint stiffness, muscle atrophy, and scarring. The philosophy was that nonunion represented delayed union that only needed prolonged immobilization (Watson-Jones,[78] Böhler[61]).

The following objectives of modern treatment are restoration of bone continuity and anatomical configuration within a reasonable period of time and restoration of normal muscle and joint function.

It is not necessary to remove the intervening tissue or to resect the bone ends.[64,76] By providing mechanical stability, and providing axial compressive loading rather than disruptive stresses between the fragment ends, primary union (*i.e.*, direct osteonal bridging with little dependence on periosteal or medullary callus) is possible. Various methods to induce osteogenesis, preferably autogenous bone transplants, should be added. Stability between the fragments eliminates the detrimental forces (shear, torque, bending), and permits early exercises that not only preserve joint motion but also induce stress-generated osteogenesis. Necrotic fragments need not be replaced. Necrotic cortical bone will add to strength, will unite to contiguous viable bone, acts as a scaffold about which new bone will be laid down, and will undergo remodeling and substitution by new viable bone. A large defect, especially when it exceeds more than one half the diameter of the bone, usually cannot be spontaneously bridged unless a massive cortical transplant is interposed. During the remodeling period of a large necrotic cortical bone, it is mechanically weakened, and, despite uniting to the adjacent viable cortical fragment, it must be protected by an external support for many months to prevent a fatigue fracture. Untoward stresses during the period of revascularization, resorption, and osteoporosis that precedes ultimate replacement by new bone will fracture the bone and also any fixation device.[79]

Before introducing foreign material and bone transplants, certain basic principles must be observed. Infection must be overcome. Despite the absence of overt signs of infection, it is sound surgical judgement to resect possible osteomyelitic foci. Before deep surgical procedures are attempted, good thick skin covering is mandatory, and transfer of a pedicle flap may be necessary.

Stress-induced electronegative potentials in bone favor osteogenesis. Using this principle, externally applied electrical current may be used in conjunction with surgical methods or as an independent modality to effect union.

PRELIMINARY STUDIES

The objectives are to determine regional pathophysiology: vascularity (medullary, intraosseous, muscle); to determine feasibility of achieving optimum mechanical conditions (coaptation, compression, axial loading, permissible movement of joints); to determine the presence or absence of infection; and to ascertain whether a synovial pseudarthrosis exists.

History. A compound fracture suggests smoldering infection. Iatrogenic factors contributing to delayed or nonunion include inappropriate conservative treatment (*e.g.*, excessive traction, insufficient immobilization), and faulty surgical techniques (*e.g.*, excessive intramedullary reaming, loose internal fixation, distracting bone plate).

Roentgenograms. A markedly displaced fracture may prevent restoration of continuity of medullary nutrient vessels, and implies soft tissue interposition. A wide insurmountable gap may be due to overtraction, a distracting fixation device, or bone loss. Sclerosis of fragment ends may occlude the medullary cavity and impede regeneration of nutrient vessels across the fracture gap. An "elephant foot" configuration of one fragment is the result of high biodynamics and has a good outlook for repair. Atrophic osteoporotic and resorbed bone ends reflect reduced vascularity, poor osteogenic activity, and reduced osteogenic reparative potential. Marked comminution produces open gaps between fragments which are often necrotic and permits excessive motion. A large intermediate fragment is necrotic, will unite to adjacent viable bone, and should be studied by serial roentgenograms to follow the process of remodeling. During the phase of resorption, the bone becomes osteoporotic and is highly susceptible to fatigue fracture and nonunion. Tomograms will define the configuration and disposition of the pseudarthrosis, and may reveal an osteomyelitic focus.

Scintiscan and Scintimetry.[77] Radionuclides measure new bone formation. On the scintiscan, a "hot zone" envelops a biodynamically active pseudarthrosis. If its center shows a "cold" translucent zone, a synovial pseudarthrosis is present. The increased radioactivity about the nonunion site represents hypervascularity and high osteogenic activity, and therefore excellent repair potential. If both fragments are highly reactive and therefore viable, the outlook for achieving union by fragment coaptation, compression, and stabilization is good.

PRINCIPLES OF TREATMENT

Before embarking on a course of treatment, it is imperative to determine whether actual nonunion or a state of delayed union exists. It is possible that the circumstances (axial compressive forces, stability, absence of or improbability of infection, and so forth) favor union, and an additional period of externally applied immobilization is all that is necessary. Watson-Jones has stated that nonunion is rare following a fracture, and continued immobilization will effect a union in nearly all cases. However, an extended period of incapacity may be untenable, and prolonged immobilization often is followed by joint stiffness, muscle atrophy, and lengthy, expensive rehabilitation. Such treatment is warranted only when union can be expected within a reasonable period of time, or when surgical intervention is contraindicated.

Surgical Principles

Correct Biomechanical Factors.[74,75] Eliminate disrupting stresses (torsion, shear, bend). For example, in the neck of the femur, a transposition osteotomy changes shearing to compression forces (Pauwels). Compressive stresses must be physiologic (*i.e.*, cyclic axial loading). Excessive vertical loading is harmful.

Coapt Fragments By A Compressive Device. Compressive devices include the compression plate,[66] intramedullary rod of Kuntscher,[72] external fixation-compression of Charnley (*fixateur externe*),[73] compression lag screw, and tension band wiring (*e.g.*, for the patella and the greater trochanter).

Provide Stability.

Bone Transplants. Bone transplants provide mechanical strength, induce osteogenesis (autogenous cancellous bone preferred), and fill a wide gap. Autogenous cortical bone (*e.g.*, fibula, tibial cortex) provides strength and stability. Transfer a vascular pedicle graft if possible. Autogenous cancellous bone provides maximum osteogenic potential and is readily revascularized and incorporated. For massive replacement, a processed alloimplant is used. It must be protected either by internal fixation or external support for at least 2 years to prevent fatigue fracture and possible nonunion.

Excise Synovial Pseudarthrosis. In other types of pseudarthrosis, resection is not necessary.[76]

Decortication (Shingling) Procedure of Dunn.[65,67,69,70] The objective of decortication is to produce stabilizing periosteal callus. Periosteum is elevated with thin slivers of bone from the superficial layer of cortical bone about the pseudarthrosis. The elevated petals remain attached to the periosteum. Cancellous bone chips may be added (Charnley). The nonunion is stabilized by external skeletal fixation. Intramedullary nailing is contraindicated to avoid compromising the medullary blood supply. As a rule, abundant periosteal callus forms.

Bridge Gaps. The length of bones must be maintained with plates that extend well beyond the osteoporotic portion of the fragments for better fixation. The gap is filled with autogenous cancellous bone and cortical allografts (composite transplants).

External Skeletal Fixation (Fixateur Externe). External skeletal fixation is useful for an extremely unstable nonunion with a wide gap, poor soft tissue covering that requires skin grafting, a nonunion that is adjacent to a joint surface, and for arthrodesis of a large joint. It is especially suitable for *fixation at a distance* when infection of the nonunion is suspected.

Eradicate Infection. Excision of the nonunion site and sequestrectomy may be necessary. Appropriate antibiotics are administered.

Plan Surgical Approaches. Providing an adequate thick skin covering is paramount. The available blood supply must be defined and studiously protected. An intraosseous angiogram may be necessary.

Electrical Treatment

A true nonunion (*i.e.*, a persistent interfragment gap bridged by soft tissue), the predominant elements of which are fibrous tissue and fibrocartilage that permits and is perpetuated by detrimental stresses, can be united in a high percentage of cases (estimated at about 85%), by creating weak electrical currents in the gap. A fibrous union can be converted to fibrocartilage which then undergoes endochondral ossification by inserting cathodal electrodes, each delivering an optimal osteogenic current of 20 μamp within the gap. When fibrocartilage is already present, it only needs to become calcified, and this in turn induces vascular invasion, chondroclastic resorption, and replacement by woven (fibrous) bone. This process can be brought about not only by introducing direct current into the gap but also by noninvasive means (*i.e.*, by producing electromagnetic fields).

Before selecting the appropriate electrical modality, it is essential to define by clinical and laboratory methods, imprecise as they are, whether union is delayed, and, if actual nonunion exists, what is the nature of the bridging tissue. A large gap, one greater than one half the diameter of a long bone, is unlikely to unite by electrical means alone. The pseudarthrosis with sclerotic bone ends with extreme mobility and constantly exposed to shearing, bending, and torsional stresses is generally occupied by fibrous tissue, and may yield to electrical stimulation, but often requires surgical methods.

When scintigrams reveal the "cold" interval of a synovial pseudarthrosis, it will not respond to electrical stimulation. The synovial pseudarthrosis is a grossly mobile lesion and frequently has eburnated rounded bone ends flanking the gap region. Most elements of a true joint are present, including fibrocartilage covering the bone ends, a line of "subchondral bone," viscous fluid similar to that of a joint, and pseudocapsular structures. Surgical excision is required before other modalities, including externally applied currents, can produce a union.

It is important to recognize that nonunion and delayed union are often multifactorial in origin, and these detrimental forces may need to be corrected before using the osteogenetic induction of electrical currents. For example, a wide gap certainly must be bridged by bone transplants while at the same time stabilizing the main fragments by various means. Immobilization by plaster is essential and avoidance of stresses is mandatory during the early phases of electrically induced osteogenesis. Union by electrical means can be lengthy and is not always successful. If rapid and more certain rehabilitation is desired, operative intervention is more applicable.

When union is markedly delayed, the application of electrical current will expedite union and the known consequences of prolonged immobilization in a cast will be avoided. It should be strongly considered in a bone with a known propensity for slow healing.

Before considering electrical stimulation of delayed union or nonunion, the section on electrical properties of bone should be reviewed.

Invasive Method.[68,74] A self-powered, self-contained, and totally implantable electrical stimulator is used (Fig. 3-36).* It consists of three elements: (1) A power unit consisting of 2 zinc/silver oxide cells, series-connected to produce 3 volts which is coupled to the active electrodes by way of a transistorized constant current regulator. The latter produces a constant current output of 20 μamp regardless of bone tissue resistance changes over the range of 0 to 100,000 ohms. The operating life of the unit is 22 to 26 weeks. (2) A single titanium cathode designed to implant it within the nonunion site. (3) A single platinum anode that is placed in the soft tissues adjacent to the generator.

Union is achieved in more than 85% of cases of delayed or nonunion within 12 to 36 weeks, even in the presence of infection.

Procedure: The nonunion site is exposed with a minimum of dissection. The tibia may be approached directly anteriorly. A rectangle of cortical bone measuring approximately 2 cm × 1 cm and centered on the line of nonunion is removed. Sclerotic bone and fibrous tissue are curetted from the medullary cavity to ensure continuity of the cavity across the nonunion site. Proximally through another small incision, the titanium capsule enclosing the stimulator and the anode are placed in an intermuscular plane at least 5 cm from the cathode. The cathode is passed subcutaneously into the nonunion site, formed into a helix, and placed centrally across the defect. The helix must not contact any metallic device that has been placed for fixation. In the case of an intramedullary rod, bone grafts must be interposed between the rod and the cathode. Autogenous cancellous bone grafts are then placed within the rectangular cavity over the helix. Phemister type of bone grafts may be

* Osteostim Division, Telectronics, 8515 East Orchard Road, Englewood, CO. 80111

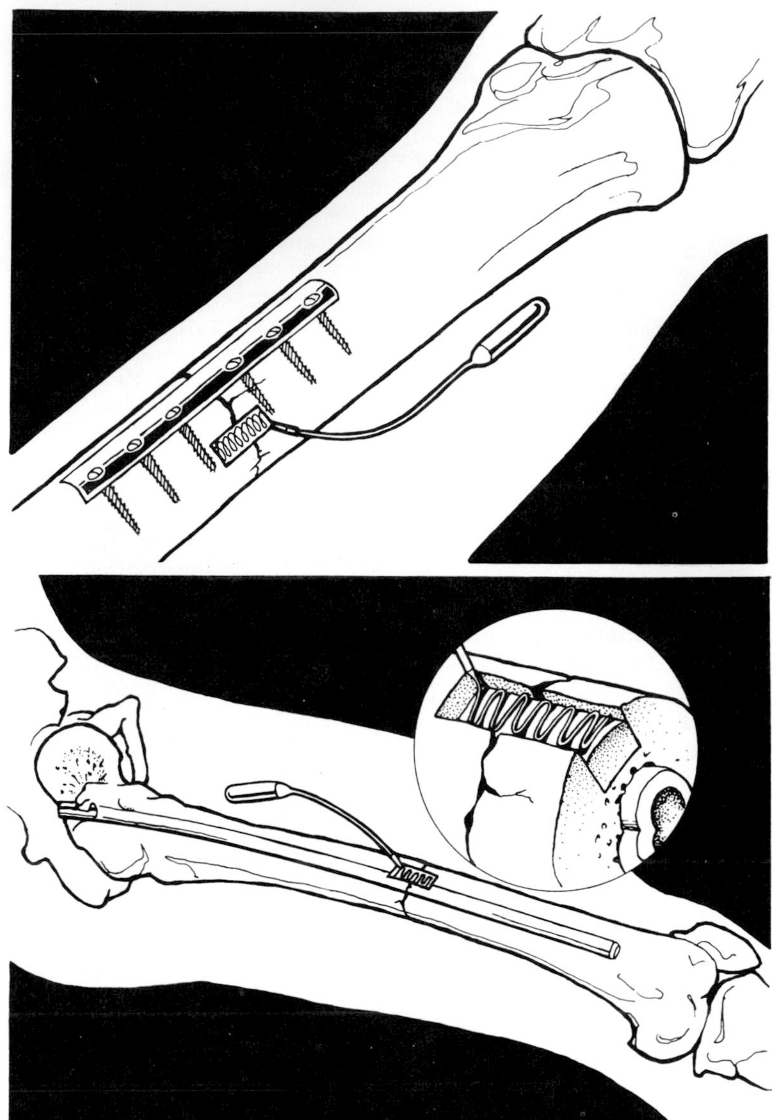

FIG. 3-36. Electrically induced osteogenesis (invasive method). The titanium cathode is formed into a helix and implanted with cancellous bone transplants into a surgically created rectangular defect across the nonunion site. The cathode must not contact the metal of the fixation device. It is connected by a stainless steel lead with the generator, which is enclosed within a hermetically sealed titanium case, embedded in an intermuscular plane at a distance. Instead of a separate anode lead, one end of the generator capsule is composed of platinum and acts as the anode. (*Top*) Plate fixation. (*Bottom*) Intramedullary rod fixation. (Orthofuse™ M, Courtesy of the DePuy Co., Warsaw, Indiana)

inserted about the nonunion site. After wound closure, a plaster cast is applied. After 6 months the generator is removed. It is not necessary to expose the site of nonunion or to remove the cathode helix which is now imbedded within the bone. Titanium is well tolerated.[80]

During the period of electrical stimulation, a telemetry circuit placed over the nonunion site will monitor the delivered current. Electrosurgical equipment should not be used on the patient after implantation because it will damage the electronics. Diathermy must be avoided because it will cause coagulation necrosis about the electrode tips.

Semi-Invasive Method.[62] This method consists of the insertion of cathodes directly into the nonunion site and the continuous application of small amounts of direct current. The success rate is about 85%, and generally early osteogenesis can be detected at 12 weeks (Fig. 3-37). Its advantages are that the pins can be inserted percutaneously on an outpatient basis, the apparatus is portable, and its effectiveness is not compromised by the presence of metallic devices. Its main disadvantages are that iatrogenic infection is possible and the presence of a preexistent infection may be lighted up.

The electrical apparatus consists of a power source of field-effect transistors and resistors in circuit with a 7.5 volt battery delivering a constant current of 20 μamp regardless of changes in resistance using four cathode leads, each delivering 20 μamp.* Each cathode lead contains a clamp-on stainless steel connector on its free

* The Zimmer Co., Warsaw, Indiana.

end into which the Teflon coated stainless steel Kirschner wire is inserted. The anode lead is connected to a disposable, self-adherent, nonmetallic anode. Insulated monitoring leads extend from the power source (Fig. 3-38).[63]

Procedure: The cathodes are inserted percutaneously under local anesthesia under roentgenographic control across a bony cortex at an oblique angle so that the bare tip of each cathode, 1 cm in length, comes to lie directly within the nonunion site. The tips should not touch one another. The extremity is wrapped in cotton-roll bandage. The insulated ends of the cathodes protruding from the skin are bent so that the wires course parallel to the skin, and are then cut off. The cathode connectors are then clamped to the exposed ends of the cathodes. The anode and cathode leads and the power source are encased in further cotton-roll bandage, and a plaster non-weight-bearing cast is applied. The anode lead protrudes from the proximal end of the cast and is snapped to the disposable self-adhering electrode. Monitoring leads also protrude from the cast (Fig. 3-39). The electricity is allowed to flow continuously for 12 weeks. The power source is monitored every 4 weeks. After 12 weeks of direct current application, cast and electrodes are removed, and roentgenograms in various projections are made out of plaster. Usually early evidence of osteogenesis is detected at this time, and immobilization is then continued for an additional 12 weeks, this time in a weight-bearing cast without electricity; complete bone healing ensues.

When all principles are observed, the success rate is high. One cause of failure is the presence of a synovial pseudarthrosis (in 6% of cases). This can usually be detected by ^{99m}Tc scintography. Instead of the usual increased uptake about the nonunion site, the synovial pseudarthrosis is characterized by a cold or nonreactive gap. The synovial pseudarthrosis should be excised prior

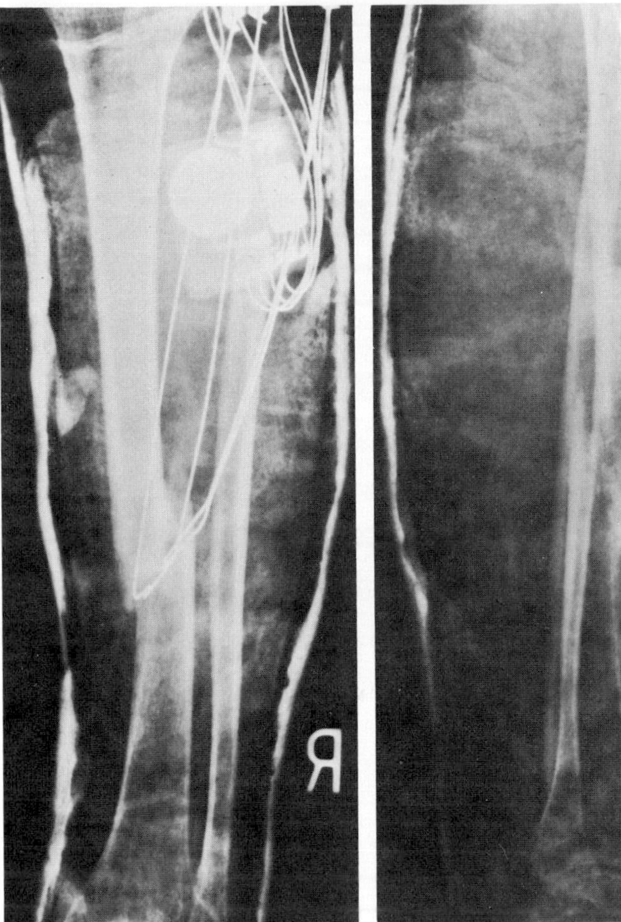

FIG. 3-37. Roentgenograms of electrical stimulation of non-union, (semi-invasive method). The power unit lies outside the leg and beneath the cast. Four electrodes penetrate the cortex on either side of the nonunion enroute to the defect. Solid bony union is achieved within 4 months.

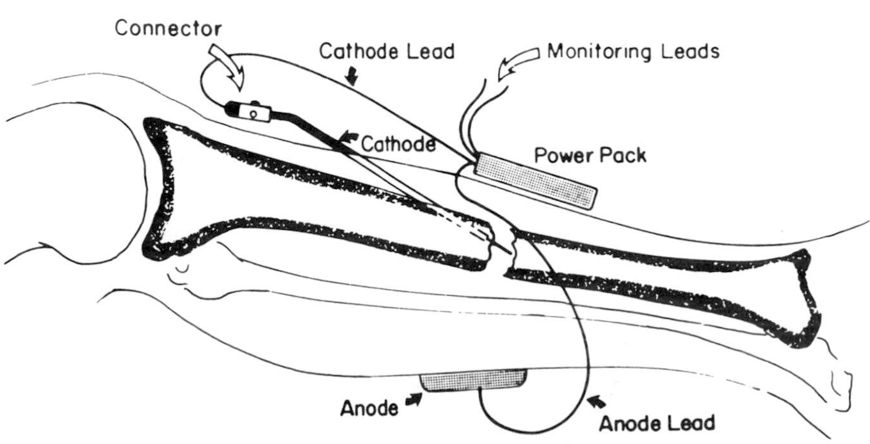

FIG. 3-38. Electrically induced osteogenesis (semi-invasive method). The cathode is covered by Teflon insulation except for 1 cm at its tip. The junction of the bare tip and the Teflon coating is the most active portion of the electrode and should be sited within the pseudarthrosis. The power pack, when tested, should read "80" and four cathodes, each delivering 20 μamp, are inserted. The power pack lies outside and beneath the cast. The anode lead and the two monitoring leads protrude from beneath the proximal end of the cast, and the anode is placed on the skin of the thigh. The cathode must be replaced every few days. (Brighton CT, Friedenberg ZB, Zemsky LM et al: Direct-current stimulation of non-union and congenital pseudarthrosis. J Bone Joint Surg 57A:368, 1975)

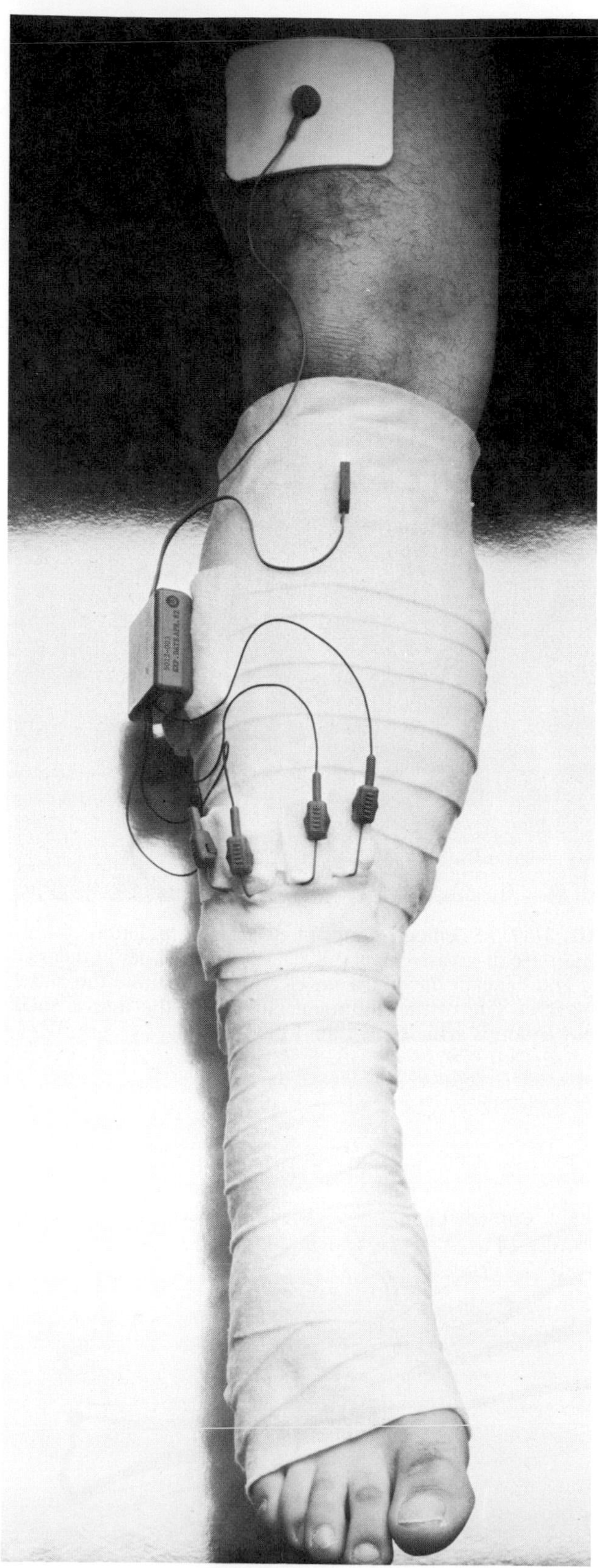

to electrode implantation. Another cause of failure is the lighting up of an unsuspected prior infection.

The main contraindications are a sizable gap, generally one greater than one half the diameter of the bone at the level of the nonunion, and chronic osteomyelitis at the nonunion site. The presence of a metallic device bridging the nonunion site does not compromise the electrical treatment.

Noninvasive Method.[59,60] Weak electrical currents in bone are induced by pulsing electromagnetic fields [PEMFs] (Fig. 3-40). Presumably the fibrocartilage in the gap becomes calcified, and endochondral ossification naturally follows.

The ideal case has neither gross motion nor roentgenographic evidence of a gap in excess of 1 cm. Active drainage or a history of local infection is not considered a contraindication to treatment. The method is not suited for pseudarthroses with a fluid-filled gap, presumed to be present when there is gross instability in all planes and the bone ends are smooth and eburnated.

Procedure: A plaster cast is applied and weight-bearing is forbidden. The pulse-shaping circuits and coils provided by the manufacturer* require an accurate measurement of the intercoil distance. The cast diameter is measured with calipers at the level of the nonunion. This determines the size (diameter) of the coils and the voltage applied to the coils. A cast applied to the leg must be extended to the thigh level with the knee at 40° of flexion. Internal metallic devices are not removed since 316L stainless-steel and cobalt-chromium alloys are not significantly permeable to magnetic flux and are therefore compatible with the electromagnetic field.

The site of nonunion must be accurately identified by placing a block on the cast and directing the roentgenographic beam at the block. If the site is at or proximal to the middle third of the tibia, the block is placed anteriorly. Otherwise the block is placed laterally and is offset anteriorly. The block is then fixed to the cast.

The coils are then fitted to the coil-placement block and adjusted so that each coil of the pair is at 180° to the other, parallel to each other and on opposite sides

* EBI (Electro-Biology, Inc.), 300 Fairfield Rd., Fairfield, New Jersey. Bi-Osteogen System 204

FIG. 3-39. The semi-invasive method of electrical treatment of nonunion showing the clinical appearance of the four cathode electrodes connected to the power pack. From the latter, one lead lying over the infrapatellar area will be attached to the monitoring unit to determine the adequacy of output. The other lead attaches to the anode placed over the lower thigh. This must be changed every few days. A short leg cast encloses the apparatus except for the two proximal leads. When the cathode pins are inserted, the junction of the Teflon insulation and the bared tip of the pin must be sited within the nonunion gap since this is the most active portion of the electrode. (The Zimmer Co., Warsaw, Indiana)

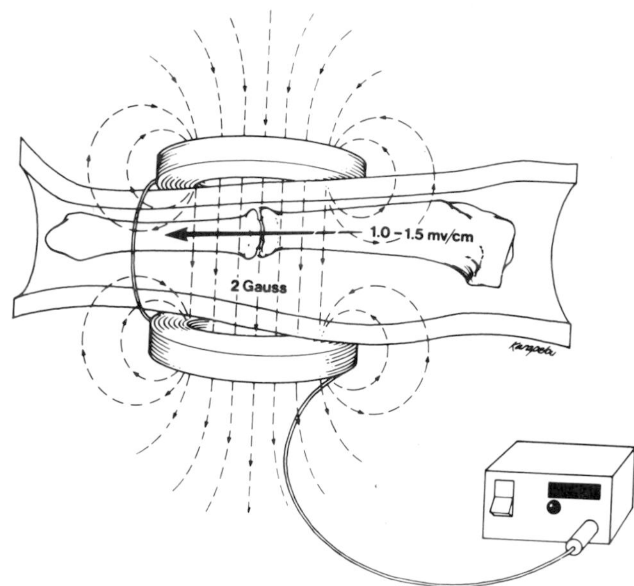

FIG. 3-40. Principles of application in the treatment of nonunion in electromagnetic fields. The pair of coils is mounted anteriorly and posteriorly on the surface of the cast and is plugged into the pulse generator. The generator, which is attached to the 110-volt line, "drives" the coils with 10 to 18 volts, depending in part on the distance between the coils. As current flows in the coils, a pulsing electromagnetic field is established between the pair, penetrating the cast and the soft tissues. The field is weak (average, 2 gauss) and the magnetic flux lines (B field), which are at right angles to the bone in this configuration, induce a voltage drop (E field, at a right cycle to the B field) along the long axis of the tibia of 1 mv/cm to 1.5 mv/cm. (Bassett CAL, Mitchell SN, Gaston SR: Treatment of ununited tibial diaphyseal fractures with pulsing electromagnetic fields. J Bone Joint Surg 63A:511, 1981)

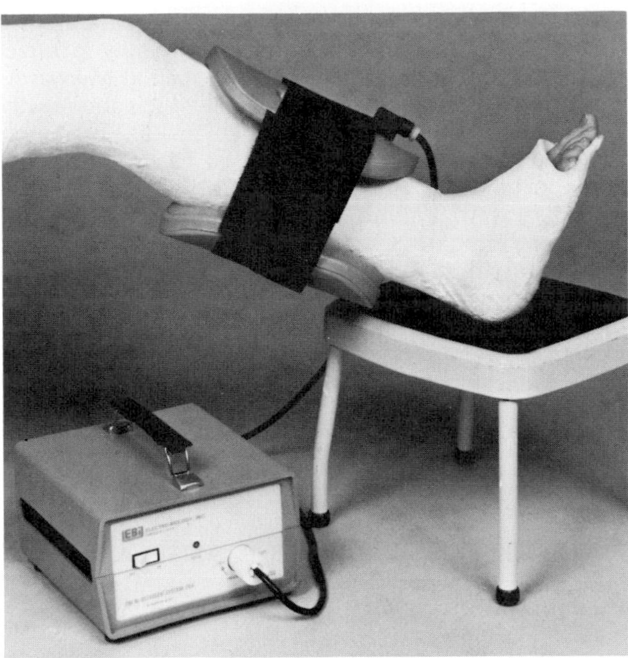

FIG. 3-41. Noninvasive method of inducing osteogenesis. Electromagnetic fields are created about the nonunion site between the pads. For nonunion of the tibia, a thigh-length cast is necessary. Note that the knee is fixed in 30° flexion to eliminate tensile forces. (Electro-Biology, Inc., Fairfield, New Jersey)

of the cast. The final assembly is held with an encircling elasticized Velcro strap (Fig. 3-41).

The pulse-shaping unit is plugged into the standard wall outlet and the coils are attached to the unit. Ten hours of treatment daily are required. The 10 volts of current applied to the coils are nonhazardous even if the coils are inadvertently immersed in water.

Radiographs are made at 4 to 6 week intervals without removing the cast. Tomograms may be necessary. Evidence of healing is not based on external callus which rarely occurs. An increase of radiographic fuzzy density in the gap and patchy loss of density of the sclerotic bone ends may develop within several months. Then the leg is placed in a short cast and axial compression exercises are started. Repeated impactive loads may be measured by bringing the heel down forcibly on a bathroom scale. If the fracture is transverse and hypertrophic, a maximum pressure of 25 to 30 pounds (11–14 kg), 50 times, three times a day is allowed. If no ache develops, the load is doubled for several weeks. Then partial weight-bearing is permitted. For oblique or comminuted fractures, the starting loads are 10 to 15 pounds (5–7 kg).

The appearance of consolidated bone-stress lines that bridge the fracture gap may occur even before partial weight-bearing is instituted. The cast, coils, and crutches are discontinued, and a well-molded fiberglass support is applied, and must be worn until full healing and remodeling are achieved.

BONE TRANSPLANTATION

Removing bone from one site and transplanting it to another is a common surgical procedure. It is employed for the following reasons:[97]

- To fill cavities or defects from cysts, tumors, or other causes (*e.g.*, disease, trauma)
- To bridge joints for arthrodesis
- To bridge major defects and restore continuity of a long bone
- To provide bone block to limit joint motion (arthrorisis)
- To promote union in a pseudarthrosis (nonunion)
- To promote union in delayed union, malunion, fresh fractures, or osteotomies

The use of the term *bone graft* is inaccurate since histologic sections of such bone reveal empty lacunae, indicating necrosis of osteocytes and matrix. Moreover, transplanted bone is invaded by blood vessels and rapidly proliferating multipotential mesenchymal-like cells from surrounding tissues of the host, that enter the marrow and the haversian canals, resorb the old dead matrix from its external surfaces and from within the canals, and replace the dead bone. The transferred bone acts as a scaffold within and about which new bone may form. By its presence it stimulates new bone formation, perhaps by means of a bone induction principle, an as yet undefined protein contained within the implant, inducing the mesenchymal-like cells to differentiate into osteogenic cells. A bone graft placed adjacent to a site of fibrous nonunion encourages ossification within the fibrous tissue bridging the bony defect.

FUNCTIONS OF THE BONE TRANSPLANT

The bone transplant serves the following principal functions:

Immobilization. For immobilization to occur, dense cortical bone is used. Most often it is removed from the subcutaneous aspect of the tibia and is fixed in place by metallic screws. Cortical bone is resorbed and replaced very slowly, and prolonged protection from weight-bearing is necessary.

Osteogenesis. Replacement by new bone is active and rapid when cancellous bone, particularly autologous in origin, is used. Its soft marrow is quickly penetrated by capillaries, and many of the original osteoblasts at the surface of the implant survive and continue to produce new bone. The extensive network of fine trabeculae provides a tremendous surface area about which new bone is laid down while the slender spicules of necrotic bone are rapidly resorbed. The iliac bone is an excellent source of cancellous bone.

Replacement. Extensive loss of the shaft of a long bone may occasionally be suitable for replacement. For large bones, cadaver bone or bone removed from amputated extremities are used. The upper half or two thirds of the fibula, the head of which is covered by articular cartilage, may be used to replace the lower end of the fibula or the distal end of the radius. A vascular pedicle bone graft may be necessary.

TERMINOLOGY

The following designations of the various types of bone transplants are in current use, although the word "graft" as commonly used is not applicable in the strictest sense as a growing tissue.

An *autograft* (autologous graft, autochthonous graft) is transplantation of a tissue or organ from one site to another in the same person.

An *isograft* (isogeneic graft) is a graft exchanged between people with genetically identical characteristics from the same zygote (*e.g.*, identical human twins). Syngeneic describes the relationship between two animals of the same inbred strain. In this situation, the term "isograft" as commonly used is incorrect.

An *allograft* (homograft) is transplantation from one person to another of the same species, but with dissimilar genetic characteristics. When the graft is between members of different highly inbred lines, the allograft is termed "allogeneic."

A *xenograft* (heterograft) is transplantation from one person of one species to a person of another species (*e.g.*, calf bone to human).

Orthotopic is the positioning in an appropriate site (*e.g.*, bone placed in a bed of bone).

Heterotopic is the positioning in an inappropriate site, (*e.g.*, bone placed in a bed of soft tissue such as muscle).

THE IMMUNE RESPONSE

Fate of Foreign Bone Grafts

Fresh autogenous bone is most commonly used. It provides the highest degree of osteogenesis because the surface cells remain viable and participate in the process of replacement. It is nonantigenic, vascularization is quicker, especially in cancellous bone, and bone induction is greater.

In contrast, as a general rule, all homografts are destroyed fairly soon by an allergic reaction invoked against them by the host.[104,115] This type of bone is a weak antigen, and the allergic response to allogeneic transplants can be thoroughly altered by lyophilization or other means so that it is not readily destroyed.[90] Thus, modified bank bone can act as a long-persisting scaffold for invasion from the host of vascular osteogenic tissue which progressively resorbs the old bone and replaces it with new bone. The success of bone grafting leading to osteogenesis, resorption and remodeling, and eventual obliteration and healing of a defect by bone depends mainly on eliminating immunological reactions.[92]

Mechanism of Bone Graft Rejection

Antigens initiating allograft rejection are the protein or glycoprotein structural elements of the cell surface membranes.[126] Cytoplasmic and nuclear components do not evoke the immune reaction. In man, a single major histocompatibility system is governed by the genetic locus, HL-A. A match at HL-A locus (*i.e.*, two people who are matched at this locus) gives a skin graft rejection time of 22 days, as compared with 12 days for nonmatched pairs. Therefore, it must take 22 days in an

HL-A matched pair for the sum of the minor loci to bring about graft rejection.

Various mechanisms are probably involved, including cell-to-cell interaction, cell-mediated immunity, and antibody mediation.

In a cell-mediated response, the lymphocyte is the mediating cell. When a normal lymphocyte contacts the foreign cell surface, it begins a stereotyped series of reactions which result in the destruction of the target cell. The lymphocyte gives off a cytotoxic substance into its immediate environment. These effector molecules kill target cells, immobilize macrophages in the vicinity, and transfer this message to the noncommitted lymphocytes.

The later lymphocytes, termed B-lymphocytes, become differentiated into plasma cells which produce the antibodies specific for the particular antigen. Antibody mediates the cytolytic effects in the presence of complement. Other effects of antibody include chemotaxis, release of anaphylatoxin, which affects capillary permeability, and aggregation of cells. Additional responses include platelet stickiness, sluggish blood flow, leukocyte-platelet thrombi, and vasoconstriction and vasodilatation.

The Immunologically Competent Cells

The immunological defense cells are lymphocytes.[4] They are very small globular-shaped leukocytes with rounded or ovoid nuclei containing condensed chromatin surrounded by a very narrow rim of basophilic cytoplasm. Under phase microscopy, these cells are quite motile, and are drawn out into a racquet shape with a nucleus at one end and a tail of drawn-out cytoplasm. Ultrastructurally, the scarcity of organelles reflects their low metabolic activity (Fig. 3-42).

Lymphocytes can recognize and react to foreign antigens. Under such circumstances, small lymphocytes develop into larger cells that contain large numbers of ribosomes in their cytoplasm. The abundance of RNA in the cytoplasm causes it to stain intensely with pyronin, hence the cell is described as "pyrinophilic." These cells are termed blast cells which actively divide and form larger cells.

Lymphocytes in cell cultures, when exposed to a foreign antigen, are stimulated to enlarge and undergo mitotic division. Within the body, the transformation into blast cells and the proliferation of their progeny occur mainly in lymph nodes and the spleen.

B lymphocytes, probably derived from the bone marrow, are short-lived cells that differentiate into plasma cells. The latter have characteristics of secretory cells (*i.e.*, a great abundance of rough endoplasmic reticulum and a prominent Golgi apparatus) and produce the specific antibody to react with the particular antigen which the B lymphocytes have encountered. The specific immunoglobulin is present on the cell surface in small patches designated as recognition sites or surface receptors.

T lymphocytes, termed memory cells, are long-lived cells derived from the thymus. They serve as killer cells in graft-rejection phenomena. They also give rise to progeny with the appearance of small lymphocytes which are programmed to react to the antigen that caused the mother cell to become a blast cell.

In general, in order for a B lymphocyte to be activated by an antigen to form a blast cell, the antigen must first be picked up by a recognition site (surface receptor) on a T lymphocyte that was programmed to react with it, and subsequently delivered to a properly programmed B lymphocyte. The T lymphocyte, acting as a helper cell, can bring the specific antigen to the specifically programmed B lymphocyte, either directly or indirectly through the surface of reticular cells (Fig. 3-43).

T lymphocytes can recognize, react specifically with, and destroy foreign cells possessing the proper antigen. They act as killer cells by releasing a cytotoxic substance, which in itself is nonspecific, and is termed a cell-mediated reaction. T lymphocytes therefore are the chief cause for the rejection of homologous transplants. The connective tissue bed on which the graft is placed soon becomes infiltrated with graft rejection cells. These are the cytotoxin-elaborating T lymphocytes.

The antibody formed by plasma cells reacts specifically with antigen on body cells, but does damage to body cells only if the antigen-antibody complex on the cells fixes complement. Except for erythrocytes and leukocytes, the antigen on the surfaces of most body cells is not sufficiently close together for complement to be fixed. Therefore, the antibody formed in response to a foreign transplant may not have any deleterious effect on the transplant.

Measures Preventing Homograft Immune Reaction

Measures for preventing homograft immune reaction include:

1. Selection of appropriate donors with mutually common genes and antigens by tissue typing. A practical method is the use of a skin graft; a skin graft that survives about 3 weeks indicates that the donor bone transplant will excite a minimum of immune response.
2. Immunosuppressors. The formation of lymphocytes is inhibited by x-irradiation and drugs. However, these pose the threat of suppressing the host's capability for combating infection.
3. Antilymphocytic serum. Lymphocytes from the recipient are injected into animals, and a serum is prepared and purified so as to contain only antibodies.
4. Modification of antigenicity of homograft. Freeze-drying, lyophilization.
5. Removal of periosteum and marrow.

Immunological Response to Bone

An autologous fresh graft at 3 weeks shows no evidence of an inflammatory reaction, but does show considerable

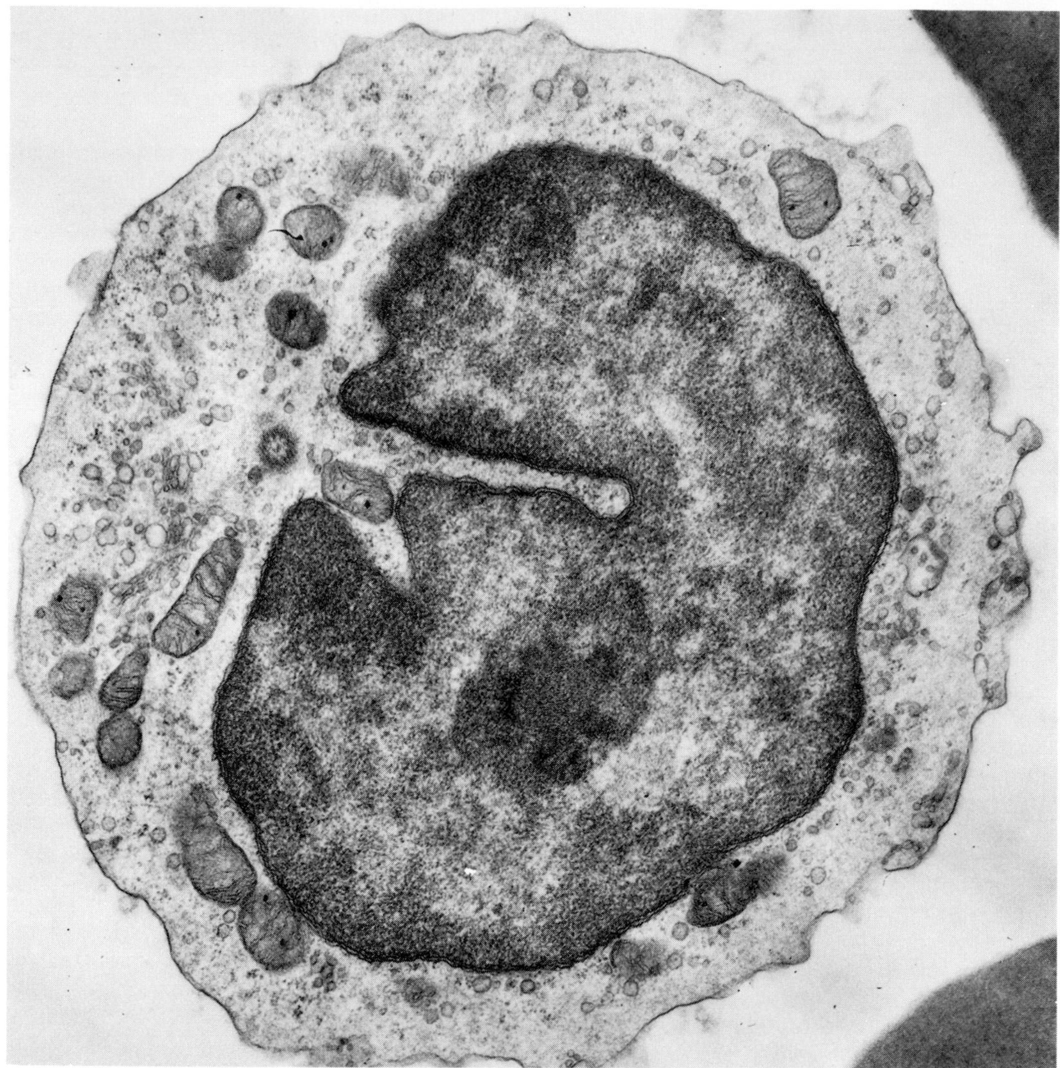

FIG. 3-42. Electron micrograph of section of small lymphocyte from thoracic duct lymph. Note the deep indentation of the nucleus, below which can be seen the nucleolus. Close to the open end of the indentation is a centriole cut in cross section; to its left, components of the Golgi apparatus are visible. About 12 mitochondria can be seen. Note free ribosomes only sparsely distributed in cytoplasm. (approximately × 30,000) (Ham AW: Histology, 7th ed. Philadelphia, JB Lippincott, 1974. Preparation by Dorothea Zucker-Franklin)

periosteal new bone.[89] By contrast, a fresh homologous graft as early as 1 week shows a marked inflammatory response.[104] Surrounding the graft is an exudate consisting of numerous lymphocytes, macrophages, and scattered eosinophils. A minimal amount of periosteal new bone may form, but by 3 weeks, at the peak of the inflammatory reaction, undergoes necrosis and resorption. Host vascular connective tissue surrounds the homograft rather than uniting it with the host cortex. Once the acute inflammation subsides, inflammatory cells in large numbers appear about resorption sites.

When a second homograft is implanted in an animal which has already shown the immune response, the second response is more vigorous, appears earlier, and is prolonged.

When the antigenicity of the homograft has been modified by freezing, a less cellular reaction ensues, it is still quite pronounced and is delayed so that it reaches its maximum intensity at 3 weeks. Although less intense initially, the reaction lasts longer.

The principle that freezing markedly impairs the antigenicity of allogeneic corticocancellous bone,[95,98] has been one of the prime reasons for the clinical use of deep-frozen or freeze-dried bone for allotransplantation.[104,106] However, recent investigations reveal no difference in the degree of induced cellular immunity from

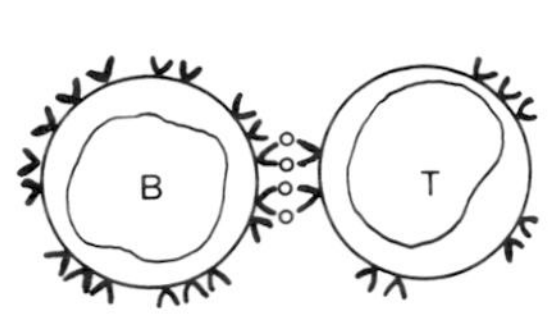

B
T
The antigen may be brought into contact with a B lymphocyte receptor by an encounter between a B and a T lymphocyte; the antigen is attached to the surface of the T lymphocyte through the latter's own specific immunoglobin receptor molecules.
- or -
INDIRECT INTERACTION
The immunoglobin receptor molecule may be set free from the surface of a T lymphocyte after the antigen has become attached to it.
T
B
The free T cell immunoglobin molecule bearing the antigen may then become attached to the surface of a reticular cell. When a B lymphocyte encounters a reticular cell, B lymphocyte receptors can come into contact with the antigen.
Either type of interaction would serve to present the antigen to the B lymphocyte receptors in an optimal configuration, thus increasing the chance of "triggering" the B lymphocyte.

FIG. 3-43. Tentative schemes of B-lymphocyte-T-lymphocyte interaction. (After Mitchison and Feldmann & Nossal. Ham AW: Histology, 7th ed. Philadelphia, JB Lippincott, 1974)

fresh as opposed to frozen bone.[91,113] Therefore, freezing of the graft may not be necessary for protection from immunological rejection. Despite these contrary views that refer to the *degree* (as opposed to the *rate*) of immunogenicity, allotransplantation (*i.e.*, grafting between histoincompatible people or strains) does not necessarily result in graft rejection. Blocking phenomena may prevent rejection and the graft will survive (see Tests of Immunogenicity).

The recipient immune reaction can be reduced by preliminary injection of pooled extracts of donor bone combined with Freund's complete antigen.[103] Low titers of antibody are demonstrable by complement fixation, and such immunization greatly diminishes the cellular reaction. A 3-week specimen from the immunized animal shows cartilaginous and bony union of the homologous graft to the recipient without evidence of a vascular, cellular immune response.

Tests of Immunogenicity

Presently there is no practical and consistently reproducible method for determining the immune response to allogeneic bone and cartilage in human recipients.[93] However, various methods of processing allogeneic (homologous) bone to lessen its immunogenicity may be assessed in laboratory animals by the following representative tests. Because bank bone is allogeneic and most often processed by procedures that encompass deep-freezing or freeze-drying (lyophilization), and frequently include the marrow cells, the major source of transplantation antigens, most investigations on the antigenicity of alloimplants refer to bone processed in this manner, and interpret a locally induced vascular-round cell infiltration as indicative of an immune response. Conversely, the absence of this local vascular-cellular reaction may be interpreted as lack of induced immunity. It must be emphasized, however, that immune phenomena are highly complex and variable, and that the various tests reflect a balanced state between induced immunity and counteracting poorly understood blocking factors. Consequently, no single immunological test can reliably define the immunogenicity of the bone implant or determine its acceptance or rejection.[93,109]

Leukocyte Migration Test.[108,112] This test measures cell-mediated immune reaction. The antigen consists of donor leukocytes obtained from the spleen and placed in culture dishes containing sera of bone graft recipients. Spleen leukocytes share major transplantation antigens with marrow leukocytes, and are used to detect transplantation immunity to bone grafts.[95] The test depends on the natural motility of leukocytes and their ability to migrate out of the open end of a capillary tube in which they have been packed. If the leukocytes have been primed *in vivo* by prior exposure to graft antigen, reexposure to the same antigen will normally result in inhibition of migration and thus a smaller area of accumulation of cells about the open end of the capillary tube. From a comparison of migration areas with and without antigenic stimulation, the migration index is calculated. The migration index therefore varies directly with the amount of inhibition and is a measure of the induced transplantation immunity to the particular transplantation antigen.[101] In other words, the lower the migration index, the greater the immunity to the graft.

Occasionally, if immune blocking factors develop in the recipient sera in which the antigen is suspended, the leukocyte migration will not be inhibited, and instead may be enhanced. The migration index will then be greater than 1. This may be the mechanism that protects the graft from rejection.

Survival Time of Second-Set Allografts. This test assesses the cell-mediated immunity. At various intervals after an allograft, donor skin is placed on the recipient animal. Signs of rejection are sought daily, and the results compared with rejection times in animals that have received allogeneic skin grafts without prior allografts. The second-set skin graft rejection is usually rapid. If the antigenicity of an alloimplant can be reduced by processing in some manner, the rejection time of the second-set skin graft will be prolonged.

Humoral Cytotoxic Antibodies. This test measures the cytotoxicity of recipient lymphocytes to donor cells. The humoral cytotoxic antibodies are detected in the sera of bone allograft recipients by using trypan blue to determine cell viability. Sera are collected from animals at the time of killing and stored at 70° C. Prior to testing, the sera are inactivated at 56° C for 30 minutes. The target cells are lymphocytes isolated from the spleen of the donor, and incubated with antisera, with complement added, and cultured at room temperature. Trypan blue is added to the sediment and the number of dead and live cells are counted. Cytotoxicity is expressed as a percentage of dead cells compared to the total number of lymphocytes.

The principle behind the test is that there wil be lysis of cells when antibody, formed specifically in response to cell surface antigen, is allowed to react with this antigen in the presence of complement. Trypan blue will not stain viable cells, thus determining the degree of cytotoxicity.

A first-set implant of freeze-dried, marrow-containing bone will produce no cytotoxic antibodies. Ten weeks later, the application of a second-set skin graft may be rejected no differently than a first-set skin graft, and little or no cytotoxic antibodies are formed.[98] This implies that freeze-drying reduces the antigenicity of the bone. However, as seen below, the allograft may yet produce a local vascular-cellular response. The contribution, if any, of such cytotoxic antibodies to bone allograft rejection is unknown.[109]

Cellular Changes in Regional Lymph Nodes. The lymph nodes draining the area of the bone alloimplant may exhibit numerous characteristic pyrinophilic lymphoid cells indicative of heightened immunity. Absence of these cells in the regional lymph nodes about implanted freeze-dried alloimplants implies reduced immunogenicity of these grafts.[93]

Histology. Allografts, whether fresh or frozen, produce an inflammatory reaction surrounding the outer cortex starting 1 week after implantation. Vascular hyperplasia is associated with a cellular infiltrate consisting initially of neutrophils, later many lymphocytes and plasma cells, a reaction which peaks in intensity at 3 to 4 weeks, then gradually lessens so that minimal reactive changes are observed at 14 weeks. The cell-mediated reaction interferes with induction of osteogenesis which requires vascular invasion with accompanying mesenchymal cells from the surrounding soft tissues, a necessary prelude to resorption of the necrotic bone and replacement by new bone.

THE VASCULAR RESPONSE

Bone always dies when deprived of its circulation. However, the surface cells associated with bone—in the deep layers of periosteum, in the endosteum, and on the trabecular surfaces—are able to survive for short periods even in the absence of a blood supply.[120] They are apparently preserved by diffusion of nutrient fluids from the recipient. The evidence of such viability includes the ability of the surface cells to proliferate in tissue culture. A common physiologic test: viable cells produce dehydrogenase which effects reduction of methylene blue and the cells fail to stain. If fresh bone is devitalized completely (*e.g.*, by repeated freezing and thawing), the dead cells are intensely stained by the unreduced methylene blue.

The surviving surface bone cells possess the capability of laying down matrix, but the development of haversian systems depends on sufficient vascular ingrowth. Thus, some of the bone cells can survive temporary loss of blood supply and retain their bone-forming capacity, can be preserved by dehydration (*e.g.*, with glycerol) and slow freezing, and subsequently can regain their viability and function and can be grown in tissue culture.

An autogenous bone graft rapidly revascularizes, perhaps by direct anastomosis, from the host bed,[97] and remains permanently so. An allograft initially vascularizes, but after a number of days a host tissue immune reaction sets in and vascularity is lost.[104] Therefore, failure of an allograft to survive is accomplished not only by a cellular response on the part of the host but also by impairment of vascularization.

Thin slices of cancellous bone vascularize within 48 hours after transplantation. If viability of the graft has been previously compromised (*e.g.*, by repeated freezing and thawing), revascularization is delayed or entirely prevented.

CELLULAR BEHAVIOR

Cell reaction is required to unite a bone transplant with the recipient, to increase or decrease the size of the graft, and to precipitate rejection.[85] The surface cells in free, mature, cancellous bone grafts can survive transplantation and participate in osteogenesis, even though the osteocytes within the graft are necrotic. The dead matrix serves a mechanical function, resisting applied forces, and thereby generates electric potentials. The dead matrix is resorbed to a large extent and replaced by newly deposited extracellular matrix, which assumes an orientation corresponding to its mechanical use.

Vessels can invade the osseous graft only when shearing motion between the graft and adjacent surfaces is eliminated. This is accomplished mainly by callus which "glues" the host tissue and graft firmly together. The source of osteogenesis forming this important early callus is perivascular host cells, and, to some degree, an appreciable number of cells on the surface of the transplant. Early callus formation is essential to immobilization of the graft, and this prevents shearing motion thereby permitting penetration of host vessels. The invasion of host capillaries is responsible for an influx of cells which are necessary for matrix resorption and formation.

The pool of mesenchymal-stem cells accompanying

the vascular ingrowth are multipotential and can differentiate into osteoblasts, osteoclasts, chondroblasts, chondroclasts, fibroblasts, and occasionally lipoblasts, depending on nutritional factors and the stimuli of their microenvironment.[84]

Bone formation requires three factors: proper specialized cell, proper nutrition, and proper stimulus.

The proper cell arises from a mesenchymal-stem cell which comes from perivascular cells, reticular cells of bone marrow, cells of trabecular surfaces, and cells of the cambium layer of periosteum. The specialization of cells is influenced by nutritional and electromechanical factors. When cells become compacted and the oxygen supply is adequate, bone formation results. These same stem cells when subjected to low oxygen concentrations (5% or lower), differentiate into cartilage-producing cells. If the outgrowth of vascular cellular tissue is stretched, although oxygen concentration is adequate, fibroblasts develop and highly oriented fibrous tissue resembling that seen in young tendons and fascia is formed. Thus nutritional (O_2) and physical (tension versus compression) factors determine the differentiation of specialized cells. If the concentration of oxygen is significantly elevated in a tissue culture, both osteoclasis and chondroclasis ensue.[123] Perhaps this depends on lysosomal enzymes.[125] Other factors such as PTH, thyrocalcitonin, vitamin A, antibodies, and so forth, introduced into the culture environment affect the differentiation of mesenchymal cells.

There is evidence *in vivo* that chondrocytes can be transformed into osteocytes,[88] and that fibrous tissue can be transformed into bone.[122] The tissues in pseudarthrosis (cartilage and fibrous tissue) can therefore be transformed into bone without the need for surgical excision.[119]

The metabolism of these stem cells determines the type of specialized cell to be formed. Suppression of collagen synthesis and stimulation of the formation of acid mucopolysaccharide is characteristic of chondrogenesis. Conversely, an increase in collagen synthesis and suppression of mucopolysaccharide production by these stem cells result in osteogenesis.

Bone functions as a transducer in converting mechanical energy to electrical. When cultures of fibroblasts are exposed to electrostatic fields, of an intensity well within the physiological range, collagen synthesis is markedly increased.[86] The dedifferentiation of cells, similar to that occurring in fracture healing and collagen synthesis, can be induced by weak electric fields.[87]

Influence of Mechanical Factors

Fibrous tissue develops under the influence of net tensile forces. Cartilage appears in regions of shearing forces. Where continuous increasing tension is applied to a bone graft, osteoclasis occurs, and the middle of the graft is replaced by fibrous tissue. Compression favors specialization into osteoblasts and osteogenesis. Tension favors specialization into osteoclasts and fibroblasts. Stress-generated electrical potentials are thought to control osteogenesis.[135]

When the particle size of autologous bone is reduced below a critical point, a granulomatous foreign body response removes these particles, and therefore does not participate in osteogenesis.

Osteoinduction Role in Bone Graft Incorporation (Urist)

The incorporation of an autologous bone graft occurs in five stages (see Fig. 3-44).

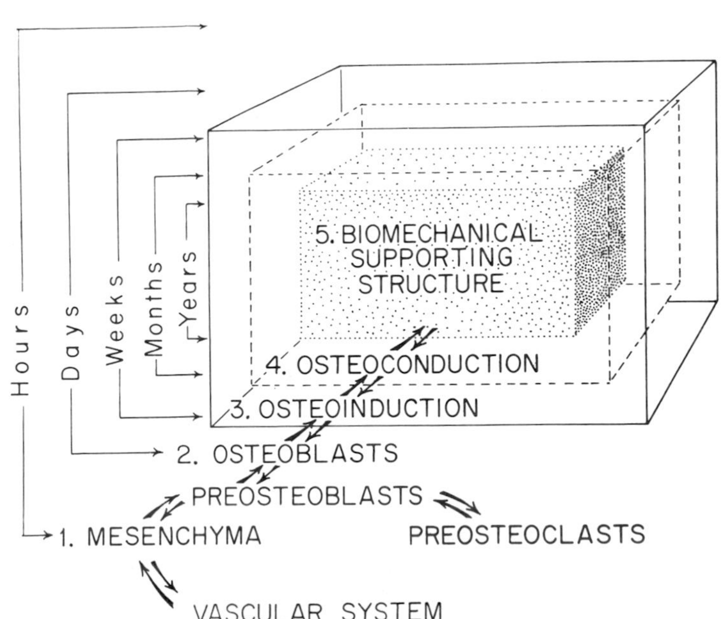

FIG. 3-44. The three-dimensional relationships, time sequences, and equilibria established in the five stages of incorporation of a bone graft. The end point is reached when the inert biomechanical structure of the donor tissue is completely encased in the remodeled lamellar bone deposits of the recipient. (Urist MR: Instructional courses. Am Acad Orthop Surg 1976)

Stage 1. Occurring within minutes to hours after surgical trauma, Stage 1 consists of inflammation, activation of migratory fibroblastlike mesenchymal cells, and proliferation of preosteoblasts and preosteoclasts in the recipient bed. Degradation products of transplanted tissue incite chemotaxis, which evokes directional migration of cells toward all exposed surfaces, outside and within the graft, whether autologous or allogenic, or living or dead.

Stages 2 and 3. Continuous with Stage 1, these stages begin 1 day to a week after inflammation of surgical injury subsides. Stages 2 and 3 are characterized by cell osteoinductive interactions between protein macromolecules of donor bone matrix and cell surface receptor sites on the fibroblastlike mesenchymal cells. In an autograft, osteoinduction is activated immediately by secretions of osteoblasts; in an allogeneic implant, it is initiated by resorption of the organic matrix. The osteoinductive action may be destroyed by improper processing of the implant (*i.e.*, by autoclaving or irradiation), or it may be blocked by a histoincompatibility immune response. When the osteoinductive response is unimpeded, differentiation of cartilage and bone occurs within a few weeks. The inductive response is regulated by a tissue-specific system consisting of a collagen-fiber entrapped bone morphogenetic polypeptide (BMP) and polypeptidase (BMPase).

Stage 4. This stage consists of osteoconduction, occurs over periods of months to years and depends on the growth of new bone by extension from the recipient bed. It is characterized by ingrowth of sprouting capillaries and new bone. It is promoted by contact compression between the donor and host bone structure.

Stage 5. This stage occurs slowly over many years. Both autografts and allografts perform a purely mechanical function, eventually becoming enmeshed in the structure of recipient bone.

BIOPHYSICAL BEHAVIOR

The repair process within and about a bone transplant is temporally a continuing phenomenon by which old necrotic bone is resorbed and new bone is formed and continually remodeled so that the composite of newly formed and old necrotic bone, at any point in time, possesses a certain degree of capability to withstand the various stresses. The mechanical strength of the transplant is related to the amount of resorption as related to bone mass and structural configuration. Although the repairing transplant may be subjected to vertical compressive loading (which encourages osteogenesis and bone hypertrophy), tensile stresses (which may cause bone resorption), bending, shear, and torsion, usually the mechanical strength of such bone is measured by a single type of stress (*e.g.*, torsion). An analysis of forces acting on the recipient site is necessary for predicting the fate of the transplant.

The bone transplant, assuming its antigenic properties are minimal, undergoes resorption over its external and internal surfaces followed by bone accretion. Variable amounts of donor bone are resorbed, and are greater in autogenous cancellous bone than in cortical bone, but less in alloimplants. The process of envelopment and interdigitation of donor necrotic bone with new bone deposited by the recipient is termed *incorporation*, with the end point of incorporation falling short of complete replacement by entirely living bone. Sometimes as much as 90% of the volume of cortical bone transplant may remain unresorbed for many years.[91] When the transplant is subjected to torsional stress, failure is correlated with the degree of porosity of the bone when resorption exceeds accretion.

Necrotic cortical bone retains its breaking strength during the early weeks following transplantation, then gradually loses is resistance to torsional and bending stresses when resorption is at a maximum, then slowly regains its strength as bone mass and structure are restored. These facts are very important where stability must be provided or anatomical parts of long bones replaced by massive segmental or osteoarticular bone transplants.[139]

In the process of incorporation of massive autogenous cortical bone transplants, the major amount of matrix resorption is intra-osteonal, while the interstitial lamellae remain unchanged.[99] In the experimental animal (dog), the transplant loses half of its strength as porosity becomes apparent on the roentgenogram, usually by 6 weeks. Then it regains its normal radiological density and resistance to torsional stress by 1 year. By this time, only 60% of the graft is resorbed and replaced. *In man, a 2 year period is required for completion of internal remodeling of the transplant. Union between the transplant and the recipient bone occurs from 6 to 12 months, and it is only after union takes place that resorption and porosity and susceptibility to stress fracture become apparent. Restoration of mechanical strength requires about 2 years.*[100]

Homogenous cortical bone, when it is not isolated by an immune reaction, undergoes replacement at a slower rate and less completely than autogenous cortical bone.[105,119] Revascularization is slower and is completed after several weeks.[110] Internal resorption and widening of the haversian canals proceed slowly, and by 2 years cortical bone replacement is terminated, although with residual unchanged osteonal and most of the interstitial lamellae. At the periosteal surface, active resorption may continue.

When a homogenous bone transplant is processed to reduce it antigenicity (*e.g.*, by freeze-drying), osteogenesis about and within the transplant is increased in rate and quantity and the transplant readily unites to the recipient bone. Following this, resorption is rapid, the breaking strength is about one half that of normal viable bone,[131] and fatigue fracture may occur.

HISTOLOGIC CHANGES FOLLOWING A SUCCESSFUL BONE TRANSPLANT

When bone is removed from its site of origin, the osteocytes disappear, and empty cell spaces suggest death of the bony matrix. The surface cells (*i.,e.*, those in the cambium layer of periosteum, in the endosteum, and on the trabecular surfaces) survive for short periods provided they are protected from adverse elements (*e.g.*, excessive warmth, sterilizing solutions, drying). When such bone from the same person is immediately transplanted to a bed of adequate nutrition, particularly when the transplant is cancellous, the surface cells' continued survival is ensured by diffusion of nutriments from the host bed. Fine blood vessels rapidly invade the graft carrying perivascular mesenchymal-like cells from the recipient into the graft, and with the surviving viable surface cells of the graft initiate osteogenesis. The old bone is resorbed, and newly formed bone is laid down on the remnants of necrotic bone (creeping substitution). An abundance of medullary elements from the recipient bed enter the implanted bone with the capillaries, and the mesenchymal-stem cells differentiate into osteoblasts. Therefore, transplantation of bone is more effective when placed in a bed of cancellous bone. When the transplanted bone consists chiefly of dense cortex, marrow spaces are lacking, and the haversian canals permit only a limited vascular cellular invasion by which the interiors of the canals are enlarged by resorption and followed by the laying down of new lamellar, concentric layers of bone. This process of osteogenesis and replacement of cortical bone is slower than in cancellous bone grafts. The thick bone is also slowly resorbed and replaced at its periphery. Therefore, dense cortical bone is mainly suitable for mechanical strength. Cancellous bone seems best suited for transplantation when osteogenesis is the major consideration. It is rapidly invaded, and its trabeculae are rapidly resorbed and replaced. Rapid revascularization occurs, and many of the original osteoblasts (surface cells) survive. Cancellous bone containing red marrow is revascularized better than that containing fatty marrow.

When a homologous graft is implanted, its medullary elements quickly disappear, a result of both loss of vascularity and the recipient immune response. The supply of osteoblasts must originate entirely from the invading tissue. Microscopically, this is demonstrated by the fact that, although soft, cancellous, easily penetrated bone is used, new bone formation is more active at the periphery of the implanted bone and rapidly declines in degree toward the center. The degree of protein incompatibility is the main factor delaying or completely preventing osteogenic replacement of homologous bone.

Heterogenous bone, when examined microscopically, is entirely incompatible with human bone. It becomes enveloped with a capsule of connective tissue and is gradually resorbed.

Histologic Sequence of Fresh Autologous Cancellous Transplant

The histologic sequence of fresh autologous cancellous bone is as follows:

Initial inflammatory response occurs about the necrotic transplant.
Macrophages invade narrow spaces and haversian canals and remove necrotic debris.
Capillaries and accompanying mesenchymal cells grow into marrow spaces.
Autolysis of deeply seated osteocytes continues; superficial cells on trabecular surfaces remain viable.
Primitive mesenchymal cells differentiate into osteoblasts, and surface cells participate in osteogenesis.
Osteoblasts line surfaces of dead trabeculae and deposit a seam of osteoid which is annealed to and surrounds a central core of remaining dead trabecular bone.
Entrapped dead cores are eventually resorbed by osteoclasts during remodeling.
Necrotic matrix is eventually replaced by trabeculae of living bone.
Marrow spaces become repopulated by marrow cells.

Histologic Sequence of Fresh Autologous Cortical Bone

The histologic sequence of fresh autologous cortical bone is as follows (Fig. 3-45):

Initial inflammatory response occurs about the necrotic transplant.
Vascular invasion of haversian canals accompanies mesenchymal cells and macrophages.
Proteolytic and osteoclastic resorption of exposed surfaces occurs with enlargement of haversian canals.
Osteoblasts line walls of enlarged excavation chambers (old haversian canals) and deposit concentric lamellae of new bone.
The remaining necrotic bone is sealed off from osteoclasis by the new bone. The necrotic cortical bone thus contains multiple osteons of viable bone.
Osteoclastic resorption and osteoblastic new bone formation continues at a slower rate.

PRACTICAL APPLICATIONS

Bone tissue, whether autogenous or homogenous, with the possible exception of the outermost or surface portion of autogenous cancellous bone, once removed from its site of origin, is necrotic. Therefore, such bone tissue, being incapable of intrinsic growth, cannot be considered as a *graft*. In its true sense, it should be termed an *implant* possessing utilitarian properties of inducing osteogenesis and providing mechanical strength.

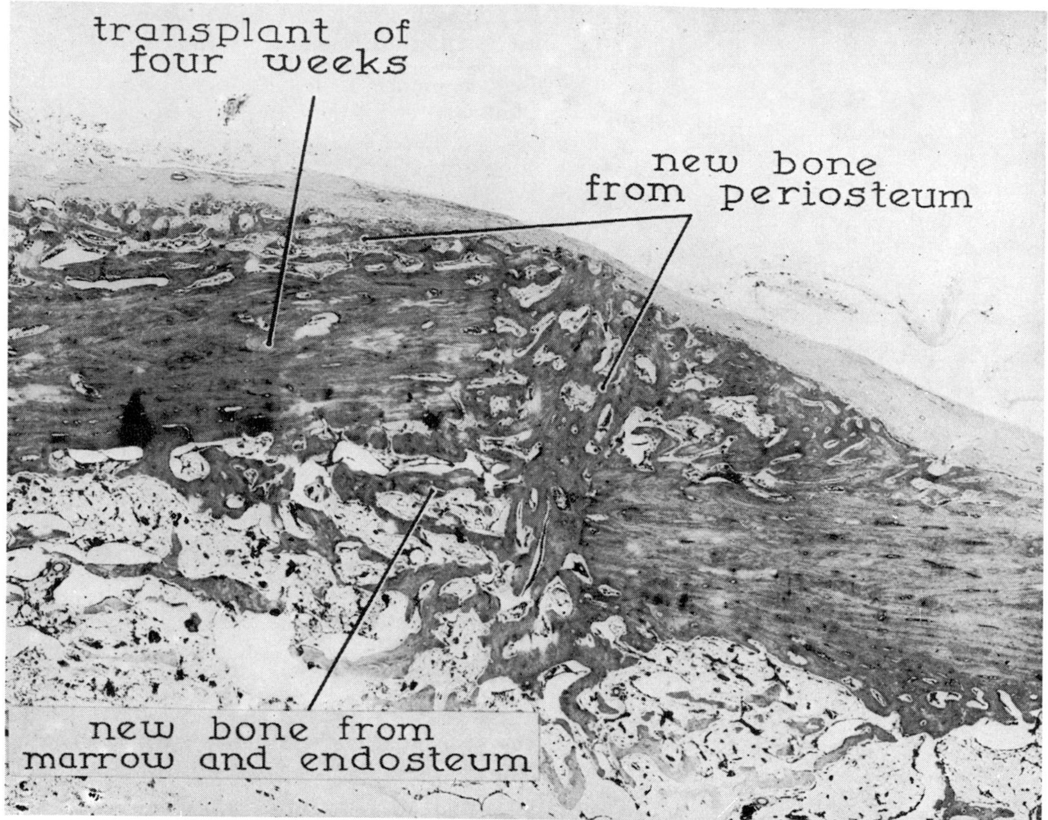

FIG. 3-45. Transplanted bone, 4 weeks old. The transplanted bone is necrotic as shown by empty lacunae. It originally was a solid cortical graft which is now porous by virtue of resorption at its surface and from within the haversian canals which now appear widened. New trabeculae of bone formed from the periosteum and endosteum of the host bone have spread about and become firmly fixed to the necrotic bone. Where new living bone lies in contact with necrotic bone, the latter is being resorbed by the process of creeping substitution. (Ham AW: Histology, 2nd ed. Philadelphia, Lippincott, 1974)

AUTOGENOUS BONE TRANSPLANTS

Fresh autogenous bone is preferred for bone transplants since it is nonantigenic and has superior osteogenic induction properties. Cancellous transplant material is used principally as a filler of small bone defects and to induce osteogenesis about nonunion or delayed union sites. Its main source of supply is from the ilium. Cortical segments of autogenous bone are primarily used as supportive struts, although it too possesses osteogenic inductive capabilities. The proper clinical application of autogenous bone transplants requires an intimate knowledge of the biological processes of transplant repair.

During the first 2 weeks post-transplantation, both cancellous and cortical autogenous transplants display similar histologic features. During the first week, the transplant, or implant, is enveloped by coagulated blood. An initial inflammatory response, consisting of capillary hypervascularity and cellular invasion, at first polymorphonuclear and later mononuclear, surrounds the transplant. By the second week, granulation tissue pervades the transplant bed, the number of inflammatory cells decreases, and osteoclasts appear at the transplant surfaces. At the interior of the transplant, the osteocytes undergo autolysis and disappear leaving vacant lacunae.[99] Some peripheral cells, especially about cancellous bone transplants, may remain viable, perhaps because of diffusion of nutrients from surrounding host vascular tissues.[99] Following the second week, autogenous cancellous bone transplant repair differs from autogenous cortical bone transplant repair.

Autogenous Cancellous Bone Transplant Repair

Autogenous cancellous bone differs from autogenous cortical bone by the rate of revascularization, mechanism of creeping substitution repair, and the completeness of the repair. Within the first 2 days, cancellous bone transplants are entirely covered by blood vessels, and presumably within hours, whether by spontaneous vascular anastomoses or by actual ingrowth of host capillaries into the marrow interstices, revascularization is initiated and completed within 2 weeks. As vascular invasion proceeds, accompanying primitive mesenchymal cells differentiate into osteoprogenitor cells, then these in turn differentiate into osteoblasts that line the surfaces of dead trabeculae and deposit a seam of osteoid which becomes annealed to, and surrounds, a central core of dead bone.[133] Finally, each trabeculum is composed of the original dead trabeculum enclosed by newly deposited viable bone having the appearance of woven bone. The bone mass is increased. Subsequently, the woven bone and the entrapped cores of necrotic bone are gradually resorbed by osteoclasts and the new trabeculum is gradually reformed. The first phase of increased bone mass produces an increased radiodensity within the transplanted area; the second phase of resorption, which goes hand-in-hand with replacement by new lamellar bone restores the original radiodensity.

At the same time, hematopoietic marrow elements are again formed within the intertrabecular spaces. Ultimately, the cancellous transplant is completely replaced by viable, lamellar, trabeculae of bone.

Autogenous Cortical Bone Transplant Repair

The autogenous cortical transplant, in contrast to the cancellous transplant, is revascularized at a slower rate. Blood vessels penetrate the Volkmann's and haversian canals by the sixth day,[119] and complete vascularization occurs by 1 to 2 months. In addition, at the surface of the cortical bone, vascular-cellular tufts, termed "cutter heads," by osteoclastic resorption progressively burrow new tunnels into the bone. Vascularization of the cortical bone transplant requires at least twice the time span than for cancellous bone transplants.

In marked contrast to cancellous bone repair, the process is initiated by osteoclastic resorption rather than by osteoblastic bone deposition. Resorption begins at the outer regions of the transplant. In experimental cortical bone transplants observed in dogs, the rate at which the interior of the haversian canals is widened is significantly increased until the sixth week ("excavation chambers"), a phase correlated with loss of mechanical strength; then the resorptive rate gradually declines to nearly normal levels by the end of 1 year. The active resorptive process is at first preferentially directed toward peripherally located haversian systems (osteons), reaching the interior by the fourth week. The interstitial lamellae remain relatively untouched. When appropriate cavity size is obtained, resorption ceases and osteoblasts appear and rebuild concentric lamellae. The appositional phase occurs initially at 12 weeks after transplantation. The repair is at first greater at transplant-host junctions, and secondarily the repair advances toward the center of the transplant.[128] The ratio of the admixture of necrotic and viable bone in the cortical transplant remains basically unaltered after the process of repair has been completed. In these studies, the proportion of viable new bone to necrotic old bone increases from 2 weeks to 6 months after transplantation, but then the ratio appears to remain unchanged in transplants between 6 months and 2 years. Thus it can be seen that cancellous bone is completely repaired whereas cortical bone is only partially repaired and remains as an admixture of necrotic and viable bone.

Mechanical Strength of Autogenous Bone Transplants

Necrosis *per se* does not alter the mechanical strength of bone. It is the biologic process of repair that modifies the physical properties of the transplant. Because cancellous bone is repaired by a process that adds new bone onto necrotic bone surfaces, such transplants tend to be mechanically strengthened by the addition of new bone.

On the other hand, cortical bone transplants are initially repaired by osteoclastic activity which produces internal porosity, decreased radiodensity, and mechanical weakening. In the experimental cortical bone transplants, within the period from 6 weeks to 6 months post-transplantation, as porosity of the transplant is increased, the bone is approximately 40% to 50% weaker than normal. One to two years after transplantation, the porosity is nearly normal and the mechanical strength and radiodensity are normal. Consequently, segmental cortical bone transplants must be protected during the critical phase when resorption exceeds apposition, and the transplant is susceptible to fatigue fracture and potential nonunion.

Procurement of Autogenous Bone Transplants

Autogenous cancellous bone is best secured from the posterior portion of the iliac bone. Autogenous cortical bone is usually obtained from the subcutaneous aspect of the tibia at the junction of the upper and middle thirds. Ribs provide a source of cortico-cancellous bone of lesser mechanical strength.

Fresh autogenous cancellous bone provides the largest number of surface cells, the viability of which must be protected in order to ensure early incorporation of the transplant into the host bed. The cancellous bone slivers should not exceed 5 mm in thickness to permit rapid and complete revascularization. Exposure of the bone to air for more than 30 minutes results in a significant decrease in the viability of the surface cells.[119] Physiologic saline solution is toxic after long-term immersion. Elevation of ambient temperature above 42° C from exposure to operating room lights kills these cells. Chemical sterilization (*e.g., by mercurials*) is lethal to cells. Antibiotics (*e.g.,* bacitracin and neomycin) destroy cells.

In the interval between procurement and implantation, bone can be wrapped in a blood-soaked sponge; heat must be avoided. For storage at longer intervals up to several days, 10% human serum in 90% balanced saline solution (Hank's, Earle's, or Ringer's Tyrode) at 3° C preserves the surface cells.

Adequate diffusion of nutrients at the recipient site must be facilitated. Interposition of dead space, hematoma, or necrotic tissue between the transplant and its bed must be studiously avoided. A bed of cancellous bone is best. If the thickness of cancellous bone is limited to a maximum of 5 mm, a central core of necrotic bone may be circumvented.[129] The total mass of the transplants must not be so thick and dense as to impede nutrient diffusion from the underlying bone bed.

The bed which actively produces new vessels and bone (*e.g.*, beds which are prepared 2 to 3 weeks prior to transplanting) improves survival of fresh autologous cancellous transplants.[124]

By these precautions, survival of a maximal number of potential osteoblasts is assured.

HOMOGENOUS (ALLOGENEIC) BONE TRANSPLANTS

Fresh allotransplants (homogenous transplants), whether cancellous or cortical, behave initially as fresh autogenous transplants, but ultimately induce an immune response which may reject the bone. Before implantation, allogeneic bone must be processed to reduce its antigenicity, while preserving its osteogenic induction property, and retaining its mechanical strength. By achieving these objectives, an unlimited supply of readily available bone is possible.

Various methods are used to process the bone before storage, and most include freeze-drying (lyophilization) which is generally believed to reduce the bone antigenicity so that the immune response is greatly delayed and reduced, permitting the induced osteogenesis in the recipient to proceed unhindered. Freeze-drying is the process of removing water from a frozen substance under high vacuum. During freeze-drying of tissues, ice crystals are removed as a vapor.[106,111] Freeze-drying is used by the pharmaceutical industry for preservation, storage, and shipping of proteins, enzymes, and vitamins without refrigeration. Such organic materials remain stable for years.[102] Despite freeze-drying, although the immune response is reduced in degree, delayed, and prolonged,[91] it is still immunogeneic since the major transplantation antigens, most of which reside in the marrow, still remain. These need to be removed.[134]

Freeze-drying *per se* is presumed to modify the transplant antigens because the regional lymph nodes do not respond to the implant, antibody formation is not detected, and second-set rejection of skin transplants is not induced. However, histologically, freeze-drying does not completely eliminate the local vascular and round cell infiltration, and varying degrees of rejection intensity may still occur. A disadvantage of lyophilization is the reduction of the mechanical strength of the implant, and fatigue fracture and nonunion are frequent when allogeneic bone is used for massive segmental and osteoarticular implants.* Such grafts must be stabilized both by internal devices and external supports for lengthy periods until union and repair are certain.

Processed and preserved allogeneic bone is not a substitute for autogenous bone except for the following reasons:

To fill large bone defects. These defects are a result of the excision of a locally aggressive bone tumor or traumatic bone loss.

Provide structural stability. Because it is slowly and partially replaced, a transplant of cortical bone maintains length and support while providing a scaffold about which new bone forms.

Induce osteogenesis. This is usually enhanced by combining the alloimplant with autogenous cancellous bone chips (composite transplants).

Crushed freeze-dried cancellous bone chips have been used in arthrodeses and to obliterate small bone defects.[127,138]

PRINCIPLES OF PROCESSING

Unprocessed allogeneic bone contains antigens that may provoke a strong immunological reaction that causes rejection of the transplant. The transplant also contains a substance that induces osteogenesis in the recipient tissues and which is readily destroyed by proteases within hours after death. The bone must be aseptically procured shortly after death and immediately processed, first to remove the antigens, and secondly to nullify the degradative action of the proteolytic enzymes in order to preserve the osteogenic inductive substance. This processed bone is termed an *alloimplant.*

Bone transplantation antigen is a glycopeptide with a molecular weight of about 5000 daltons. It resides within the cell membranes,[114,121] mainly within the marrow, and is responsible for provoking the immune reaction by which the transplant is encircled by vascular-cellular tissue that impedes the ingrowth of the osteogenic vascular-cellular tissue. The antigen can be extracted by an organic solvent (*e.g.*, chloroform-methanol), especially when the bone is demineralized.[109,116,134] As a result, even the minimal immune reaction of freeze-dried bone is absent, and deposits of bone may form within the implant.

Within 48 hours after a fresh alloimplant, the cellular components undergo autolysis and dispersion of nuclear and cytoplasmic proteins. This enzymatic digestive process is duplicated *in vitro.* The bone cells are preserved by freeze-drying, but when observed under electron microscopy they undergo autolysis when the bone is placed in neutral phosphate buffer solution at 37° C, and

* Mankin HJ: Personal communication

the osteocyte lacunae are almost completely emptied before the bone is transplanted. Approximately 90% of the transplantation antigens are removed by repeated washing in buffer.

The second problem, namely, the preservation of the osteogenetic principle, is surmounted by adding enzyme inhibitors, such as sulfhydryl compounds (*e.g.*, iodoacetic acid and sodium azide) to the buffer solution during the autodigestion process.[130,132] Because the protease action is prevented, and the morphogenetic substance is unaffected, new bone forms ten times more frequently and in greater amounts. A more complete efflux of the autolyzed substances occurs when the bone is at least partially demineralized. Thus, by allowing autodigestion to occur in neutral buffer solutions to which sulfhydryl enzyme inhibitors are added, the bone inductive property can be spared from enzymatic destruction.

The osteogenic induction property of bone matrix appears to be due to a trypsin-labile, pepsin-stable, collagenase-stable protein or part of a protein firmly bound to collagen. It is almost as insoluble as the highly cross-linked structure of bone collagen.[136]

The term *AAA bone* is applied to an alloimplant of bone processed by "autodigestion, antigen-extraction, and chemosterilization" to produce allogeneic bone of very low immunogenicity and high osteogenetic properties.[131] The bone is aseptically collected and cut into cylinders 15 cm long or in strips 10 cm × 2 cm in size. Old blood and marrow are washed out by vigorous stirring in cold sterile distilled water. The bone remnants are surface demineralized at 2° C in 0.6N HCl for 24 hours to increase the permeability of the matrix to solutions. Before or after surface demineralization, the bone segments are placed in a 1:1 chloroform-methanol mixture for 4 hours to defat the bone and thereby open up the structure for aqueous solvents. The organic solvent extracts the lipids and cell membrane lipoproteins, including the glycopeptides which constitute the major transplantation antigens. The segments are then transferred to a sterile phosphate buffer solution containing iodoacetic acid and sodium azide (10 mM/L each) for 72 hours at 37° C. Phosphate buffer, *p*H 7.4, activates intra- and extracellular enzymes for autolytic digestion of nearly all intralacunar stainable material.

The segments are then washed in fresh buffer, frozen in liquid nitrogen at −210° C for 15 minutes, and then transferred to a vacuum jar for freeze-drying at −70° C over a period of 24 hours. The segments of AAA bone are stored in sterile double plastic envelopes and outer paraffin or vacuum-sealed, labeled glass containers to prevent rehydration and chemical deterioration.

AVASCULAR NECROSIS OF BONE

Avascular necrosis (aseptic necrosis) of bone is defined as death of bone as a result of deprivation of its blood supply.

CAUSES

Any condition that shuts off the blood supply produces avascular necrosis of bone. Causes include fracture, dislocation (*e.g.*, at the hip joint), extensive stripping of the periosteum from the bone during surgery, dysbaric (caisson) disease, prolonged corticosteroid intake, organ transplantation, bone transplantation, metal corrosion and ionization, and exposure to roentgen rays and radioactive substances. By definition, infection does not cause aseptic necrosis, but, secondarily, accumulation of exudate within unyielding bony walls shuts off the blood supply and thus produces osteonecrosis in osteomyelitis. A prominent cause of iatrogenic osteonecrosis is interruption of the medullary nutrient vessels necessitated by reaming of the medullary cavity prior to insertion of intramedullary rods or prosthetic stems, and introduction of acrylic cement.

SITES OF PREDILECTION

Following are the most common locations of avascular necrosis of bone.

Femoral Head. The blood supply enters by way of the capsular vessels which enter the intracapsular cavity distally and pass proximally beneath a subsynovial reflection toward the head, mainly along the posterior aspect of the neck, meanwhile sending branches which penetrate the neck along their course. A fracture through the femoral neck, especially in its proximal portion, or a severe dislocation which ruptures the capsular and retinacular vessels, is likely to produce avascular necrosis of the femoral head.

Carpal Scaphoid (Navicular). The blood supply that provides the intramedullary nutrient vessels enters the bone mainly at its distal portion. In addition, many vessels penetrate the dorsal aspect of the bone. Therefore, the more proximal a fracture, the more likely the interruption of the blood supply to the proximal fragment. Moreover, surgical exposure along the dorsal aspect will interrupt the penetrating arteries and contribute to an avascular necrosis of the bone.

Astragalus (Talus). The main nutrient vessels enter the bone at the neck and within the tarsal tunnel. Extensive stripping of the bone or a complete dislocation may be followed by avascular necrosis.

Segmental Fractures. A large or a small fragment of the shaft of a long bone may be separated from its blood supply and undergo necrosis.

Other Locations. The capitellum of the humerus, the radial head, and the lateral femoral condyle at the knee are less common anatomical sites predisposed to loss of blood supply.

HISTOLOGIC FINDINGS

The bone architecture and mass are unaltered. The trabeculae, lamellae of osteons, interstitial bone, and circumferential layers of cortical bone retain their original histologic characteristics. However, the lacunae become empty as the osteocytes undergo autolysis, and the marrow contents disintegrate into formless debris. No evidence of vascularity or cellular activity can be found.[151,152]

The adjacent bone, which has retained its blood supply, undergoes reactive hyperemia in preparation for replacement of the dead tissue. Vascular and cellular proliferation is accompanied by osteoclastic resorption and thinning of the osseous elements, and, in addition, reduction in bone mass occurs by other means as yet unknown. Thus the bone structure neighboring on the avascular bone exhibits early characteristic demineralization and trabecular thinning depicted on roentgenograms as osteoporosis. The necrotic bone, lacking in blood supply, cannot undergo such resorption and trabecular thinning during the early stages and therefore retains its mass and architecture until late. By contrast with hyperemic thinned bone, the necrotic bone appears relatively dense, but in reality is unchanged.

REPAIR OF CANCELLOUS BONE

The proliferating capillaries accompanied by a young fibrous cellular stroma then penetrate the marrow spaces of necrotic cancellous bone and phagocytes remove marrow debris. A profusion of osteoblasts encircle the dead trabeculae and lay down immature woven bone that surrounds each necrotic trabeculum. This results in an increase of total bone mass that adds to the roentgenographic density. A minimum of osteoclastic resorption occurs on some bony surfaces at the same time. Later, osteoclastic resorption intensifies, the apposed woven bone and the old trabecular bone are removed and replaced with well-organized lamellar bone, and the trabeculae are reconstituted. The process of apposition of new bone on some surfaces while osteoclastic resorption occurs on other surfaces is termed "creeping substitution" (Color Plate 3-2).

In cancellous bone, early repair is characterized by predominant osteogenesis by which the trabeculae are thickened by a composite of new bone superimposed on old dead bone. Later, remodeling reconstitutes the trabeculae. In cortical bone, osteoclastic resorptive activity is prominent early, the necrotic bone being first removed, and the lamellar bone is laid down later so that the osteons are rebuilt.

REPAIR OF CORTICAL BONE

Excavation of haversian canals of osteons must precede their reconstruction.[157] The initial resorptive process proceeds from without inward during the early weeks.[140,143,152,154,157] Haversian canals are rapidly invaded by proliferating thin-walled vessels enveloped at its front by rapidly dividing mesenchymal-like cells, the osteoprogenitor cells which can differentiate into osteoblasts and osteoclasts.[161] While the vascular cellular tuft advances, osteoclasts line the walls of the haversian canals and active resorption and enlargement occur. The advancing bone-resorptive elements are often termed "cutter heads" which markedly enlarge the canals of old haversian systems. Furthermore, the cutter heads may form new canals as they invade at the periosteal and endosteal surfaces.[140] The initial routes of excavation consistently involve the osteonal systems and do not involve the interstitial lamellae.[145] The excavation cavity ultimately reaches the outermost limits of the osteon before the resorptive process is halted. The effect is to create multiple cavities of rather uniform size throughout the avascular segment, and occasionally adjacent excavated osteons may coalesce to form large dumbbell-shaped cavities. Ultimately, the volume of bone resorbed is so great that extensive porosity becomes visible on roentgenograms.

The vascular cutter heads that invade at the periosteal and endosteal surfaces form channels entering the circumferential lamellae transversely, after which they become oriented longitudinally.[140] In the case of a fracture, the cutter heads excavate channels through the necrotic bone ends and enter the fracture gap.

As the resorptive vascular cellular tufts continue to advance, the earliest points of resorption then undergo reconstruction. A profusion of osteoblasts line the wall of the cavities and proceed to lay down concentric rings of new bone so that the osteon is reconstituted. The bone apposition process must of necessity lag behind the resorptive process. The rate of apposition of new bone appears to increase when stress is transmitted to the revascularized tissue.

Under experimental conditions, after 40 weeks, more than 50 percent of the absolute amount of new bone has been deposited. Repair is never complete, because some of the interstitial lamellae remains as persistently necrotic bone. Some of the enlarged haversian canals may remain so indefinitely.

Necrotic cortical bone retains its intrinsic strength until weakened by the resorptive phase of the reparative process. After 2 weeks, bone strength progressively declines as the reparative process accelerates.[141,145,153] The loss of strength parallels the increasing porosity seen on roentgenograms,[149,159] and after 6 to 12 weeks the decrease in strength continues at an unvarying level (*e.g.*, about 50% of normal), then gradually regains its physical integrity after at least 1 year or more.

Roentgenographic Findings of Osteonecrosis

Necrotic bone, lacking in blood supply, at first retains its original structure and radiographic density. Meanwhile, adjacent viable bone responds by preparing for repair of the necrotic bone, undergoing vascular and cellular proliferation, resulting in local demineralization and osteoclastic resorption of trabeculae of the spongiosa and osteons of the cortical bone. Consequently, the thinning trabeculae and enlarging haversian canals produce diminishing density (osteoporosis) characteristic of the initial phase of the reparative process occurring within the adjacent bone. The contrast between the vascular osteoporotic bone and the unchanged necrotic bone creates an illusion of increased radiographic density of the latter.

Later stages of repair of cancellous bone, best exemplified within the necrotic femoral head, involve continuing accretion of new bone laid down about necrotic trabeculae thereby increasing their size and altering the architecture. Thus a real, rather than an apparent, increase in density develops slowly over a lengthy period of months to several years. This roentgenographic feature of osteonecrosis may not become apparent until the reparative process is well advanced. When the vascular and cellular reparative tissue eventually reaches the cortical bone (*e.g.*, the subchondral bone of an epiphysis), this bone is gradually resorbed and thinned as observed on the roentgenogram. The overlying articular cartilage, deriving its nutrition from the synovial fluid, remains uninvolved until a late date, and the "joint interval" is maintained. Immediately beyond the subchondral necrotic bone, the most recent advancing reparative process forms a point of weakened resistance which yields to axial loading, and subchondral fracture can occur, later followed by collapse. As the reparative tissue ultimately reaches the articular cartilage about the periphery of the necrotic zone, the cartilage is likewise resorbed. In the late stages, the articular cartilage of an epiphysis undergoes osteoarthritic changes, at first revealed roentgenographically by narrowing of the "joint interval," and later readily apparent by the features of degenerative joint disease.

Necrotic cortical bone retains its roentgenographic density and architecture for lengthy periods of time despite early and rapid revascularization of the haversian canals. Although the repair process is initiated within 2 weeks, and strength of the bone undergoing repair is progressively decreased, the osteoporosis related to the continuing osteoclastic resorption and widening of the haversian canals may not be apparent on roentgenograms until the process of repair is far advanced, usually after many months. Noninvasive methods of measurement of bone density may provide the means for early detection. Such bone, despite a roentgenographically normal structure, should be protected against physical stresses.

Histologic Diagnosis of Osteonecrosis

Ischemia of more than 6 to 12 hours duration produces bone death.[147,160] However, osteocytes retain their ability to incorporate radioactive amino acids for 48 hours after the blood supply is lost.[148] In conventionally prepared histologic sections, osteocytes retain their morphological characteristics for 2 to 4 weeks after the onset of ischemia.[142] Consequently, histologic determination of bone death may be delayed, but it is possible to identify osteocyte necrosis at an early stage by using special techniques, particularly by incorporation of labeled amino acids.[144,155] For example, labeled glycine is taken up by osteoblasts and ultimately appear in osteocytes. Histochemical staining for metabolically active intracellular enzymes will identify functioning osteocytes.

When examining a specimen of biopsied bone, the presence of occasional empty lacunae does not necessarily imply that these are the result of avascular necrosis. These may result from improper histologic techniques. Cells that lie farthest from blood vessels may suffer from precarious nutrition, and therefore it is not unusual to observe empty lacunae in interstitial lamellae, the outer concentric lamellae of osteons, and the subchondral cortex. Since the number of empty lacunae increases with advancing age, focal loss of osteocytes is regarded as a physiologic process related to gradually diminishing blood supply.[156] This is true of both cortical and cancellous bone.[146] These foci of osteonecrosis associated with the aging process are greatly increased in the presence of chronic peripheral vascular disease,[158] and, despite extensive involvement of a long bone, there are no clinical or roentgenographic signs.[160] Moreover, such osteonecrotic foci do not impair the strength of the bone.

DYSBARIC OSTEONECROSIS

Bone necrosis is a major hazard in occupations associated with extreme changes in atmospheric pressure conditions (*e.g.*, during tunnel construction, by caisson workers, deep sea divers, and those working under subatmospheric conditions in space exploration). Osteonecrosis is a frequent development of dysbarism, a generalized syndrome known by various names such as caisson disease, decompression sickness, "the bends," and aeroembolism.[169,176] It is generally accepted that the formation of gas bubbles within the tissues and in the bloodstream initiates the chain of reactions that are responsible for decompression sickness and bone necrosis.[173] The symptoms are presumably brought about by liberation of nitrogen within the tissues. Atmospheric nitrogen is absorbed through the lungs and deposited by the blood in various body tissues, particularly those containing fat (bone marrow) and lipid substances (brain, spinal cord). At greater than normal atmospheric pressures, nitrogen absorption is proportionately higher. When environmental pressure is suddenly lowered (*e.g.*, during rapid ascent to higher levels by divers, tunnel workers, and those working in an unpressurized aircraft), nitrogen gas is liberated in a concentration that cannot be readily absorbed by the bloodstream or excreted by the lungs.[167] As a result, gas bubbles accumulate in the tissues, causing local ischemia by extravascular compression, or by accumulation within the bloodstream producing intravascular occlusion.

The precise mechanism of production of bone necrosis is uncertain, but the following factors are relevant:

Rate of decompression. Necrosis of bone is more likely when the decompression rate is rapid.[170] Slow decompression reduces incidence.[165,171] In deep sea divers taking few precautions during decompression, the incidence of osteonecrosis rises to more than 50%.[179]

Magnitude of pressures.[176] Osteonecrosis is unlikely when pressures are below 17 p.s.i.g., or in diving depths of less than 20 meters.[163] Osteonecrosis is more probable during prolonged exposure to more than 30 p.s.i.g. A single short exposure to 55 p.s.i.g. is sufficient to produce bone necrosis.

Duration, number, and frequency of exposure. Frequently repeated exposures or lengthy exposures appear to be cumulative, and the incidence is greater.[176] Likelihood of osteonecrosis increases with the number of decompressions.

Individual susceptibility. An inexplicable susceptibility does exist. Obesity and hyperlipidemia increase the probability of osteonecrosis, perhaps because nitrogen is highly soluble in fat.[166]

Bone necrosis is not correlated with a history of decompression sickness.[175] Many victims of acute decompression sickness do not develop osteonecrosis, and, conversely, bone lesions have been detected in compressed air workers with no history of acute decompression sickness.

Although gas bubbles may act to compress or occlude the small caliber vessels within the unyielding bone, other mechanisms may play a part. Gas-induced denaturation of lipoprotein molecules will free lipids which then coalesce to form lipid emboli.[172] Lipids may also derive from gas disruption of the fatty marrow.

Gas bubbles activate the Hageman factor thus triggering the coagulation mechanism.[164] Disseminated intravascular coagulation associated with a fall in circulating thrombocytes is thought to play an important role in decompression sickness.[180] However, the administration of anticoagulants fails to prevent the development of dysbaric osteonecrosis. The pathogenesis remains obscure.[166]

CLINICAL PICTURE

Symptoms of acute decompression sickness may develop within minutes to hours after decompression.[172] Complaints include severe pain about various joints ("the bends"), vertigo ("the staggers") and diverse neurologic manifestations. These symptoms are usually relieved by prompt treatment. Delayed treatment invites development of tissue necrosis and permanent sequelae, especially paralyses and skeletal lesions. In severe untreated cases, circulatory failure, coma, and death quickly ensue.

Medullary necrotic lesions of bone are asymptomatic, and juxta-articular lesions are seldom painful until deformation of the subchondral cortical bone occurs.

In the shoulder, symptoms may commence suddenly when a subchondral segment collapses, often the result of a trivial type of injury. In some people, subchondral collapse may occur slowly and silently, and symptoms develop insidiously over many months. Movement of the shoulder becomes painful and often radiates toward the deltoid insertion. It is usually intensified by lying on the affected side. As the articular surface becomes slightly deformed, there may be a painful arc within the full range of abduction, usually at about 70° to 90° of abduction. The clinical picture resembles a degenerative lesion of the rotator cuff. After further collapse has occurred, osteoarthritic changes follow, and are associated with persistent pain, stiffness, and progressive restriction of motion.

Juxta-articular lesions of the hip rarely give rise to an acute onset of pain, and may remain asymptomatic for a long period of time. Despite late subchondral collapse, pain usually develops insidiously and may not be noticeable for many months, even years. The initial symptom may be pain over the anterior aspect of the hip joint radiating distally along the anterolateral aspect of the thigh toward the knee. The discomfort at first is thought to be due to a mild episode of the bends, but it is not relieved by recompression. After a variable interval, the pain becomes severe and interferes with sleep. Later, with the advent of osteoarthritic changes of the articular cartilage and deformation, movement at the hip becomes progressively restricted, especially abduction and rotation. A useful range of flexion is retained even after marked deformation of the articular surfaces has developed.

ROENTGENOGRAPHIC FINDINGS

The necrotic lesion is not immediately discernable, and only after revascularization occurs and necrotic trabeculae become thickened by apposition of newly formed viable bone does the true extent of the lesion become apparent, usually about 4 to 5 months after its inception.[162]

Juxta-Articular Lesions. These lesions occur in the head of the humerus or femur, or both, and may be bilateral (Figs. 3-46 and 3-47). They are usually in close proximity to the articular cortex, which may ultimately collapse with distortion or disruption of the unsupported articular cartilage. Small dense areas appear in close relationship to the subchondral cortex. Their margins, unlike those of bone islands, are irregular with thickened trabeculae. These opacities may be shaped like the segment of a sphere. At a late stage, these lesions that involve a portion of the subchondral cortex are prone to collapse or become sequestrated. They may be sharply

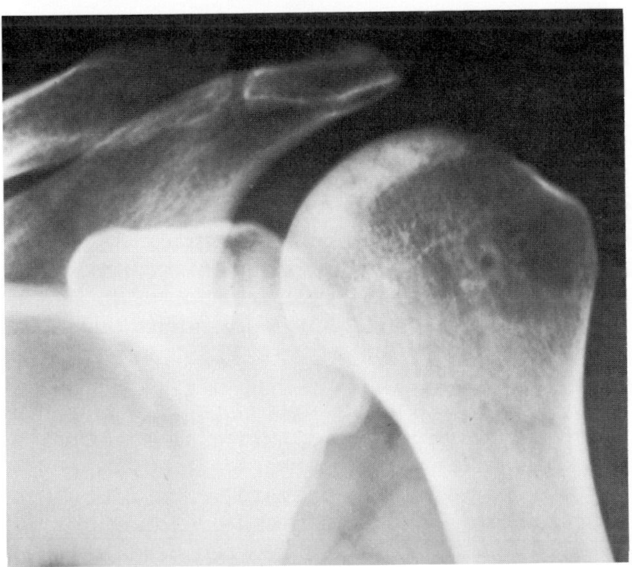

FIG. 3-46. An early roentgenogram of dysbaric osteonecrosis showing the "snow-cap" lesion in the typical location. The "crescent sign" can be seen at the center, immediately adjacent to the articular surface. (Courtesy of Dr. J. R. Nellen)

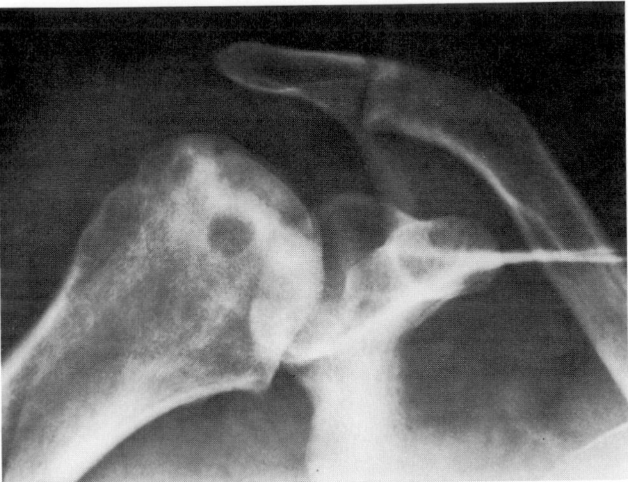

FIG. 3-47. A late roentgenogram of dysbaric osteonecrosis showing the subchondral elliptical segment that has partially collapsed, and is separated by a radiolucent zone ("crescent sign") from surrounding sclerotic bone. The latter is composed of new bone laid down on necrotic trabeculae. (Courtesy of Dr. J. R. Nellen)

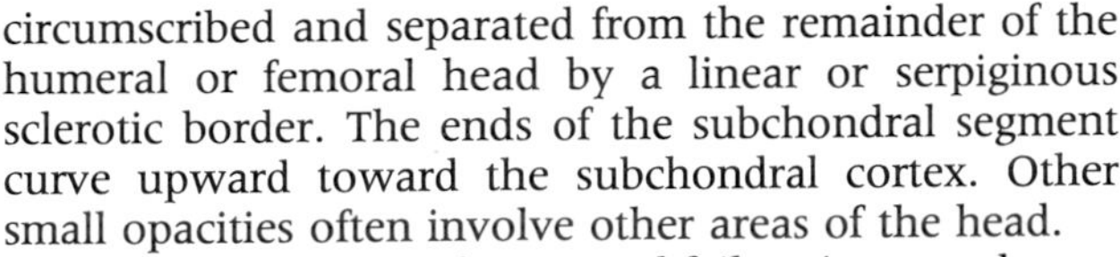

circumscribed and separated from the remainder of the humeral or femoral head by a linear or serpiginous sclerotic border. The ends of the subchondral segment curve upward toward the subchondral cortex. Other small opacities often involve other areas of the head.

The first evidence of structural failure is a translucent subcortical line ("the crescent sign")[178] which probably represents a fracture. Sometimes the middle third of the subchondral cortex collapses. In the humeral head, this generally occurs at a point which lies opposite to the glenoid when the arm is abducted to 90°. In the femoral head, this occurs at the anterior superior load-bearing area. A large intact segment or several smaller segments sink into the subcortical bone. Or these may be extruded into the joint. The remainder of the affected bone shows an irregular increased density.

In the early stages, despite obvious signs of necrosis, the width of the joint interval is maintained, indicating that the articular cartilage is still thick and viable. At a later stage, as osteoarthritic changes in the articular cartilage supervene, the joint interval gradually narrows and marginal osteophytes form.

Combined Head, Neck, and Shaft Medullary Lesions. The initial radiological changes appearing several months after the onset of the necrosis consist of irregular dense areas frequently found within the medulla of the neck and the proximal shaft of the femur and humerus. Less often they are found in the distal shaft of the femur or proximal portion of the tibia (Fig. 3-48). The lesions are multiple, variously sized, and often bilateral. Occasionally, a large region of the bone is involved, but it is more usual to observe small ill-defined lesions that may be difficult to differentiate from bone islands. The latter are composed of uniformly dense compact bone and are ovoid or oblong in shape,[174] whereas the lesions of dysbaric osteonecrosis tend to be irregular in shape with thick enveloping trabeculae.[177]

PATHOLOGY

Medullary Lesions. These lesions vary in size from small foci, a few millimeters in diameter, to extensive lesions occupying the length and breadth of the medulla, sometimes involving the inner cortex.[163] Grossly, the lesions have a pale necrotic center sometimes containing flecks of calcification, and surrounded by a serpiginous border of glistening fibrous tissue. Immediately beyond the fibrous border, the bone is dense and sclerotic. Microscopically, the medullary lesions contain a central mass of architecturally unchanged necrotic trabeculae with empty lacunae, and marrow spaces which are empty or contain cellular debris or fat. The dead central focus is encapsulated by dense collagen beyond which the necrotic trabeculae are broadened by the apposition of newly laid down woven bone or older remodeled lamellar bone.

The appearance suggests that attempts at revascularization and osteoblastic replacement of the necrotic trabeculae have slowed and halted at the point where collagen has been laid down. Within the adjacent region,

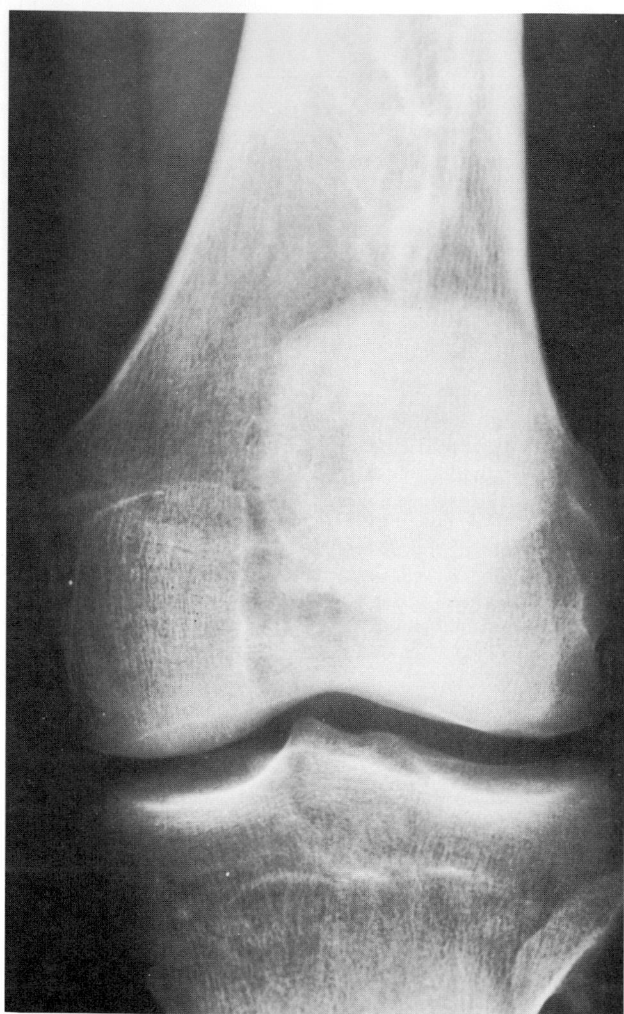

FIG. 3-48. Roentgenogram of dysbaric osteonecrosis showing typical medullary irregular lesion. (Courtesy of Dr. J. R. Nellen)

the trabeculae contain central cores of dead bone on whose surfaces apposition of woven or lamellar bone produces the radiological appearance of blotchy increased density. When thickening of the medullary trabeculae extends to involve the endosteal portion of the cortex, the latter becomes locally thickened.[168] The blood vessels show no evidence of thromboses or recanalization.

Juxta-Articular Lesions Before Collapse. Early, while the joint is yet asymptomatic, the joint contour is normal, and the articular cartilage shows no sign of degenerative change. On cross section, a yellowish opaque necrotic focus is demarcated from surrounding vascularized and living bone by a greyish zone of dense collagen. Beyond the necrotic lesion and adjacent to the encircling wall of collagen, necrotic trabeculae are greatly broadened by the apposition of newly formed woven bone or older lamellar bone, forming a radiologically dense zone that encloses a shallow subchondral saucer-shaped segment of dead bone. The widespread extent of broadened trabeculae composed of both dead and viable bone indicates that originally much of the involved bone had revascularized and undergone creeping substitution, leaving only a shallow necrotic subchondral segment.

Juxta-Articular Lesions with Collapse of Joint Surface. Flattening, fragmentation (fracture), and collapse of the subchondral dead segment occur most often at the superolateral load-bearing region of the femoral head, and in the central dome of the humeral head (*i.e.*, that portion which is apposed to the glenoid when the arm is abducted to 90°). The pattern is identical at both sites. A single compact necrotic subchondral bone mass separates, is depressed, and becomes isolated from the adjacent viable bone by a wall of fibrous tissue. The articular sequestrum is usually covered at first by living articular cartilage which derives its nutrition from the synovial fluid. The fracture between dead and living bone produces an appearance closely resembling that of osteochondritis dissecans. The deep interval between the dead and living bone becomes filled with fibrous tissue, and sometimes fibrocartilage. Later, secondary osteoarthritic changes develop, at first in the cartilage to one side of the articular cartilage overlying the necrotic bone, but eventually spreading to involve all of the articular cartilage. The cartilage initially becomes dull, fissured, soft, and easily depressed. Later, it is eroded exposing the subchondral bone, and marginal osteophytes and subchondral cysts form. The sequestrum may become completely detached and extruded into the joint, or it may be ground away, leaving a cavity lined by fibrocartilage or irregular bone surfaces. Calcification within the dead marrow occurs more readily than it does in avascular necrosis following a subcapital fracture, and this contributes to the increased density observed on roentgenograms. Within the neighboring spongiosa, coarse strands of highly basophilic woven bone continue to be laid down upon necrotic trabeculae, a process that appears to halt short of completion since the necrotic cores or wholly necrotic trabeculae persist indefinitely.[81]

HYPERCORTISONISM OSTEONECROSIS

A state of hypercortisonism, whether endogenous[190] or exogenous[193] may sometimes induce focal necrosis of bone, particularly in the juxta-articular region of the femoral head. Prolonged systemic administration of high doses of corticosteroids may at times produce osteonecrosis of bone adjacent to asymptomatic and radiologically normal joints. The development of bone necrosis may go undetected for months until the typical roentgenographic changes appear and while the articular cartilage is yet unaffected and symptoms are few or nonexistent. It is only after a latent period of several months to a year after the roentgenographic changes first appear, when the subchondral bone and articular cartilage are invaded by the reparative tissue, and early osteoarthritic degeneration develops, that the joint becomes symptomatic. Ultimately, trabecular fracture and collapse of the load-bearing aspect of the articular surface may occur, at times becoming severe and Charcot-like in appearance. Extreme collapse is more likely to occur when the joint is already affected by rheumatoid disease, osteoarthritis, or the ravages of other conditions such as lupus erythematosis, and has been treated repeatedly by intra-articular injections of steroids.[196] Osteonecrosis of juxta-articular bone resulting from the hypercortisonism state which secondarily involves the joint cartilage should be differentiated from steroid-induced arthropathy due to repeated and frequent intra-articular administration of corticosteroids which primarily affect the articular cartilage and secondarily affect the underlying bone (see discussion of intra-articular-steroid-induced arthropathy).

The pathogenesis of bone necrosis induced by hypercortisonism is unknown. The following theories have been propounded:

Fat Emboli Theory. Both experimentally[186] and clinically,[191] fat is known to accumulate in the liver of cortisone-treated people and an increase in serum lipids occurs, giving rise to fat emboli.[192] Such emboli are frequent during high-dose immunosuppressive regimens that include large and fluctuating doses of corticosteroids,[182] and may even be fatal.[185,187] In experimental animals, intravenously administered fat will localize in the subchondral region of the femoral head and in the metaphysis of the femur and tibia adjacent to the knee.[189] During prolonged high-dosage steroid therapy, embolic fat can be demonstrated adjacent to the necrotic bone focus.[183,184,188]

Subchondral Osteoporotic Fracture.[194–197] The protein catabolic effect of corticosteroids is presumed to be responsible for the generalized osteoporosis. This hypothesis supposes that the subchondral osteoporosis, trabecular microfractures and loss of joint pain, lead to bone collapse and aseptic necrosis.

PATHOLOGY

In the early stages of the disease, the articular cartilage is intact but often is dull and yellow over the area of necrotic bone.[183] In later stages, the cartilage is wrinkled, spongy, and soft over the collapsing bone. With complete collapse, the cartilage is lacerated and loosened from the underlying subchondral bone, and sometimes is either fragmented or worn away, and there are secondary degenerative changes. On cut sections, the necrotic portion of the femoral head appears as yellowish white, chalky, and clearly demarcated from normally appearing trabecular bone. Often a fracture separates a flap of necrotic subchondral bone and overlying cartilage. Fibrous tissue is seen at the junction of necrotic and viable bone. Cysts and osteophytes are seen only in advanced cases with collapse and osteoarthritis.

Microscopically, vascular cellular tissue invading at the periphery is seen where osteoblasts are laying down new appositional bone on cores of necrotic trabeculae. Fat stains identify probable fat emboli within the subchondral arterioles in some cases.

CLINICAL PICTURE

Usually the patient is being treated for a disorder (*e.g.*, generalized collagen vascular disease) requiring prolonged systemic administration of corticosteroids in doses far in excess of normal physiologic requirements (*e.g.*, 25 mg–30 mg per day, generally over a period of more than 6 months). The time interval between the initiation of treatment and the onset of symptoms is variable, and averages between 2 and 3 years. The usual complaint is dull aching pain in the medial and anterior aspect of the thigh or knee, sometimes following trauma. Rarely, severe pain in the hip develops suddenly without trauma. The clinical presentation is often modified by the underlying disease (*e.g.*, rheumatoid arthritis involving multiple joints).

LABORATORY FINDINGS

Serum lipids are often increased and liver function studies may be abnormal.

ROENTGENOGRAPHIC FINDINGS

The following sequence of events represents those observed in osteonecrosis associated with systemic hypercortisonism.[194] When there is no arthritic or skeletal involvement as part of the underlying disease, the radiological appearance of the affected joint may continue to be normal for weeks to months after the onset of pain and stiffness. In the subchondral load-bearing portion of the femoral head, the necrotic zone of the head becomes delineated by increasing sclerosis developing within the immediate surrounding bone. This represents appositional new bone which is being laid down on the necrotic trabeculae at the periphery of the necrotic segment. Later, a fine radiolucent line ("crescent sign") develops between the necrotic zone of increasing radiodensity and the surrounding unaffected normal trabeculae. This radiolucent line represents a fracture between the necrotic segment and the normal spongiosa. The earliest evidence of depression of the subchondral segment is flattening of the head outline. Meanwhile, until very late, the articular cartilage remains viable and the radiological joint interval is intact. As articular cartilage undergoes osteoarthritic degeneration and erosion, the joint interval gradually narrows, and fragmentation and progressive destruction of the femoral head occur. The acetabulum is uninvolved until very late when it too develops secondary osteoarthritic changes. The weight-bearing joints are most often involved in this process.

ORGAN TRANSPLANT OSTEONECROSIS

Homotransplantation of an entire organ requires long-term administration of immunosuppressive agents such as azothioprine (Imuran), actinomycin C, and corticosteroids to reduce the possibility of rejection. Renal transplantation is the most commonly performed procedure, and in surviving cases (approximately 12.5% in one series) about one third of these will develop osteonecrosis, most often in the femoral head(s) or about the knee(s), but rarely in other sites.[182,198] The symptoms of osteonecrosis usually develop before roentgenographic evidence is apparent. The affected joint becomes symptomatic from 2 to 10 months postoperatively, and the roentgenographic manifestations develop within the next 2 months. Rarely does osteonecrosis develop more than 2 years after transplantation. Recently, the incidence of homotransplantation osteonecrosis has been markedly lessened by appropriate medical management of the metabolic aberrations and improvement of dialysis technique during the months prior to operation.[199]

ETIOLOGY

The exciting cause of osteonecrosis is unknown. The predisposing factors include the following:

- Renal bone disease leading to secondary hyperparathyroidism, osteomalacia, disuse, and metabolic osteoporosis
- Location—two thirds in proximal femur, often bilateral.[201] Other common locations are the distal femur and proximal humerus. Less common locations are the capitellum, talus, carpal navicular, and phalanges.
- High-dosage corticosteroids—reduction of dosage is associated with reduced incidence of osteonecrosis[198,199]
- Repeated transplantations—increases the incidence

CLINICAL PICTURE

The patient may complain of pain, swelling, limping, or loss of joint motion. Initially, the roentgenograms are negative.

ROENTGENOGRAPHIC FINDINGS

Several months after the onset of symptoms, subchondral changes are seen. Typically, within the femoral head at the lateral, superior, and anterior portion, increasing opacity develops in the subchondral region. On tomography, the sclerosis is revealed within trabeculae encircling the necrotic center. As the subchondral necrotic segment fractures and collapses, it separates from the articular surface creating the pathognomonic radiolucent "crescent sign." This is best seen in the frog lateral view, and is located several millimeters below the joint surface. This represents a fracture that delineates the necrotic bone from the surrounding zone of densely thickened trabeculae. The latter consist of necrotic trabeculae that are enlarged by apposition of newly formed bone. The subchondral collapse is extensive and resembles osteochondritis dissecans. Ultimately, osteoarthritis supervenes.

TREATMENT

Reduction of renal bone disease will greatly lessen the probability of developing osteonecrosis.[210] For at least 1 year preceding transplantation, during the period of hemodialysis, the dialysate should be converted from a solution that withdraws calcium from the patient into one that favors movement of calcium from the bath to the patient. The dialysate levels of ionized calcium should be raised to 6.5 mg/100 cc (3.25 to 3.5 mEq/liter). Patients who are not hyperphosphatemic are given oral calcium supplementation so that the total calcium intake by diet and medication is greater than 1 g per day.

Dihydrotachysterol, 0.125 mg to 0.5 mg per day and multiple vitamins are also given. In addition, oral phosphate binders in the form of aluminum-containing antacids are given regularly to decrease serum phosphate levels and to *lessen the stimulus to the parathyroid glands.* The dialysate bath magnesium is kept constant at 1.5 mEq/liter.

This dialysate protocol has reduced the serum PTH levels from 20 to 30 times greater than normal levels (N = less than 100 μl eq/l) to approximately 2 times normal.

Orthopaedic treatment is directed toward minimizing the stresses on the affected joint and lessening the ultimate deformity while repair continues. Joint replacement arthroplasty is required for the painful deformed hip joint, and arthrodesis or arthroplasty for the knee joint.[201]

CADAVER BONE ALLOGRAFTS—BONE BANKS*

Bone autografts have been used in orthopaedic surgery with great clinical success. However, these grafts are difficult to obtain when large amounts of bone are desired or when a surgeon needs to employ grafts from anatom-

* The section on Cadaver Bone Allografts—Bone Banks was contributed by Theodore I. Malinin, M.D., Professor of Surgery and Pathology, University of Miami School of Medicine, Miami, Fla.

ical sites from which autografts cannot be taken. In addition, excision of bones for autografts is associated with certain morbidity. For these reasons, in a variety of circumstances human cadaver allografts have been used also with considerable success.[203,212] The use of xenografts has been generally unsatisfactory.[214]

The advantages of allografts lie in their availability and the variety of exact anatomical shapes. The biologic nature of these grafts, when properly prepared, allows for their eventual incorporation into the skeletal system and the replacement with host bone. Past experience has shown that the most expeditious way of providing these grafts is through tissue banks.[208] The objective of such banks is to readily provide bone grafts with low antigenicity and maximum osteogenic potential (Fig. 3-49).

TISSUE BANKS

Operation of tissue banks encompasses questions related to the selection of donors, means of procurement of bone, and preservation methodology.

The risk of transmitting disease to the recipient of bone allograft constitutes a potential threat to the patient. However, this can be eliminated entirely by a careful selection of the donor and by adherence to a meticulous technique in the processing and procurement of the bone allograft. The selection of the potential donor is made on the basis of a review of the clinical history. The donor must meet the following criteria:

- No microbial or viral infections
- No malignant disease
- No potentially transmissible diseases of unknown etiology
- No history of administration of long-acting isotopes

The postmortem interval for refrigerated cadavers during which tissues can be excised must not exceed 24 hours.

A complete diagnostic autopsy, bacteriological cultures of blood and tissues, serological test for syphilis, and the determination of an Australian antigen will minimize the risk of a potential transmission of disease.

EXCISION AND PRESERVATION OF CADAVER BONE GRAFTS

The mode of the excision of cadaver grafts depends on whether the grafts are taken and processed aseptically or are sterilized after their removal. In the United States, during the last two decades, the majority of cadaver bone allografts used clinically have been taken under sterile conditions. The bone is obtained under aseptic operating room conditions. The most common sources are the ilium, femur, tibia, humerus, ribs, and vertebrae. Physical injury to the bone should be minimized to prevent denaturation of the protein and to retain its potential osteogenic properties. The saw should be air-cooled or flooded with saline. Cancellous bone is removed with an osteotome. The periosteum is stripped immediately on removal of the bone. The allografts are irrigated copiously with saline and processed immediately thereafter (Fig. 3-49). The sizes and shapes of the grafts vary to suit different types of orthopaedic procedures. Prepared grafts are then placed into sterile heat-proof glass containers and aseptically sealed. All containers are labeled to identify the grafts. Samples from each cadaver bone allograft are taken for bacteriological studies immediately after the excision of the graft and just before it is placed in a storage container.

The bone grafts are frozen rapidly to $-70°$ to $-80°$ C or in the vapor phase of liquid nitrogen (Fig. 3-50). They remain frozen until completion of bacteriological studies. The grafts are then either freeze-dried or released for clinical use in a frozen state. The most extensively used human bone allografts are those preserved by freeze-drying. Freeze-drying offers a double advantage. It is convenient (freeze-dried grafts can be indefinitely stored

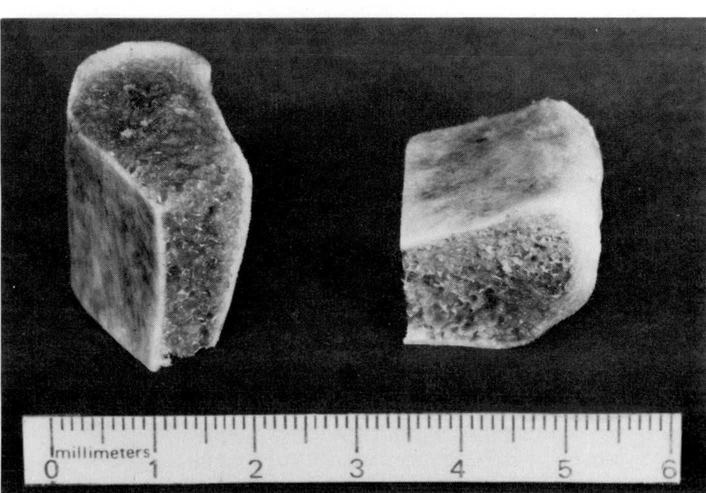

FIG. 3-49. Cleaned and cut cadaver bone grafts.

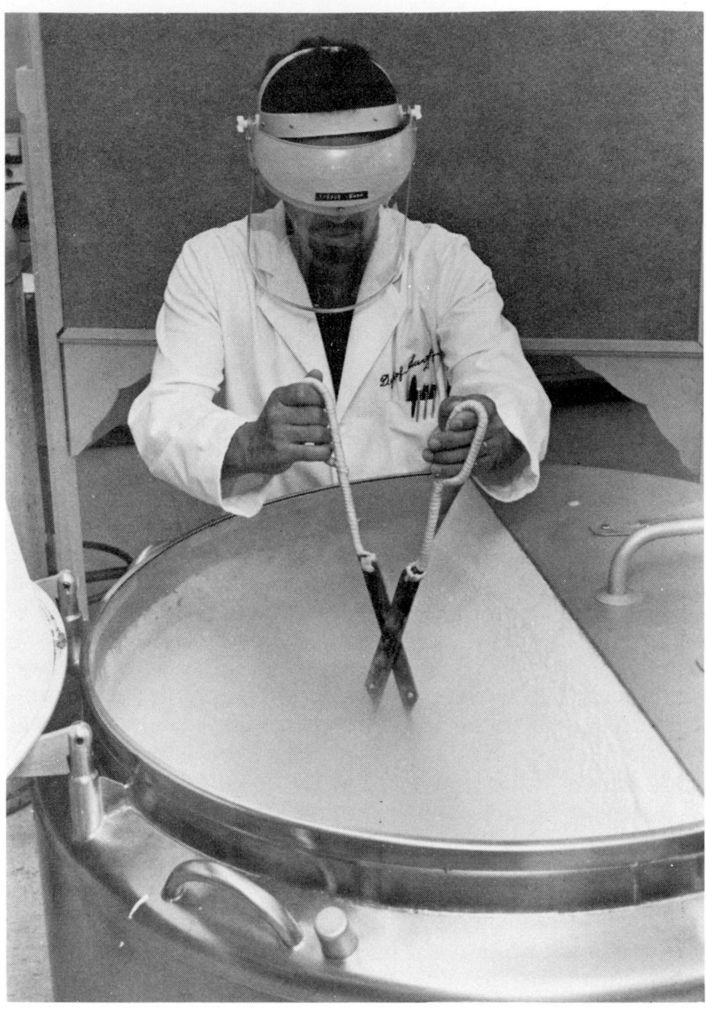

FIG. 3-50. Quick freezing and subsequent storage of cadaver bone grafts in the vapor phase of liquid nitrogen.

at room temperatures), and it apparently reduces bone antigenicity.[202,210]

STERILIZATION OF BONE GRAFTS

When cadaver bone grafts have been obtained under the aseptic conditions described above, it is not necessary to use the various deleterious sterilization precautions which have been employed in the past. These are described below for historical interest.

Boiling is an inefficient method of sterilization. Autoclaving denatures bone protein. Merthiolate-treated bone is washed before use. Under these conditions, no cases of sensitivity to merthiolate have been noted.[211] Urist and co-workers reported that merthiolate at relatively high concentrations had a slight effect on osteogenic inductive capacity of bone matrix at 25° C. However, at 37° C merthiolate caused a decline in the yield of new bone.[215] Benzalkonium chloride was found by the same authors to completely extinguish bone-inductive response. One percent solution of β-propiolactone is much more germidical than difficult-to-use ethylene dioxide. It was found more effective for sterilization of surgical specimens than for cadaver grafts.[205] Antibiotics produce variable microbial inhibition and antibiotic solutions have limited penetration power. Antibiotics inhibit bone osteoinduction.

A dose of a minimum of 2 mrads of ionizing radiation is needed to produce bactericidal effect, but 4 mrads are required to inactivate certain viruses. After such intense irradiation the bone becomes discolored. The solubility of collagen and glycosaminoglycans is proportionally increased with irradiation dose. Ultrastructurally the fibrillar network of bone matrix is destroyed by doses exceeding 2 mrads, as is the bone-inductive capacity of the graft.[204] Ostrowski reported the presence of free radicals of unusual stability in Co^{60} irradiated bone. The long-term effect of such radicals on healthy surrounding tissue is unknown.[210]

ANTIGENICITY, STORAGE, AND FATE OF CADAVER BONE ALLOGRAFTS

The problems associated with antigenicity of bone allografts are not fully understood. Fresh bone allografts are highly antigenic. On transplantation these become surrounded by inflammatory cells, thus diminishing or precluding the incorporation of the graft. The antigenicity of frozen cancellous bone allografts can be demonstrated in animals. Sensitization following transplantation of massive segmental cortical grafts has been noted. Freeze-dried cortical allografts usually do not elicit a demonstrable immune response, indicating a marked reduction of antigenicity. However, the clinical significance of the weak allograft antigenicity has not yet been determined.[207]

Storage of cadaver bone grafts can be accomplished by maintaining these in conventional mechanical freezers (−15° to −30° C), in mechanical deep freezers (−65° to −90° C), in dry ice (−76° C), or in refrigerators with cryogenic gases (−150° C or below). Since ice crystals grow rapidly at −15° to −30° C and mechanically destroy the tissues, storage of bone grafts in home type freezers is least desirable. The growth of ice crystals is slower at temperatures near −70° C. Bone grafts can be maintained at these temperatures for about 1 year. Long-term storage requires liquid nitrogen.

To be freeze-dried, the tissue is first frozen, usually to about −70° C, and then sublimated in vacuum (Fig. 3-51). Drying occurs because of the temperature differential between the specimen and the condensor. Bone grafts are freeze-dried until residual moisture is reduced to 5% or below. Freeze-dried grafts can be stored in vacuum at room temperature (Fig. 3-52). Freeze-dried bone must be reconstituted before use. This is accomplished by injecting saline into the container with the graft. The time required for reconstitution is about 2 hours for cancellous bone and up to 24 hours for cortical bone.

The radiological fate of freeze-dried cortical allografts is divided into three phases. During the first 3-to-6 weeks the graft appears dense and does not change morphologically. The second phase is that of peripheral graft resorption and replacement with host bone. The third phase, which lasts for several years, is continuation of bone resorption and replacement.[207] Cancellous bone allografts are subject to the same fate, save for the fact that the process moves ahead much more rapidly, with bone allograft being incorporated in about 1 year (Fig. 3-53). Histological changes consist of peripheral revas-

FIG. 3-51. Sterile cadaver bone grafts in the process of being freeze-dried. Before placing sterile frozen containers with bone into freeze-dryer, the freeze-drying chamber had been sterilized with ethylene oxide.

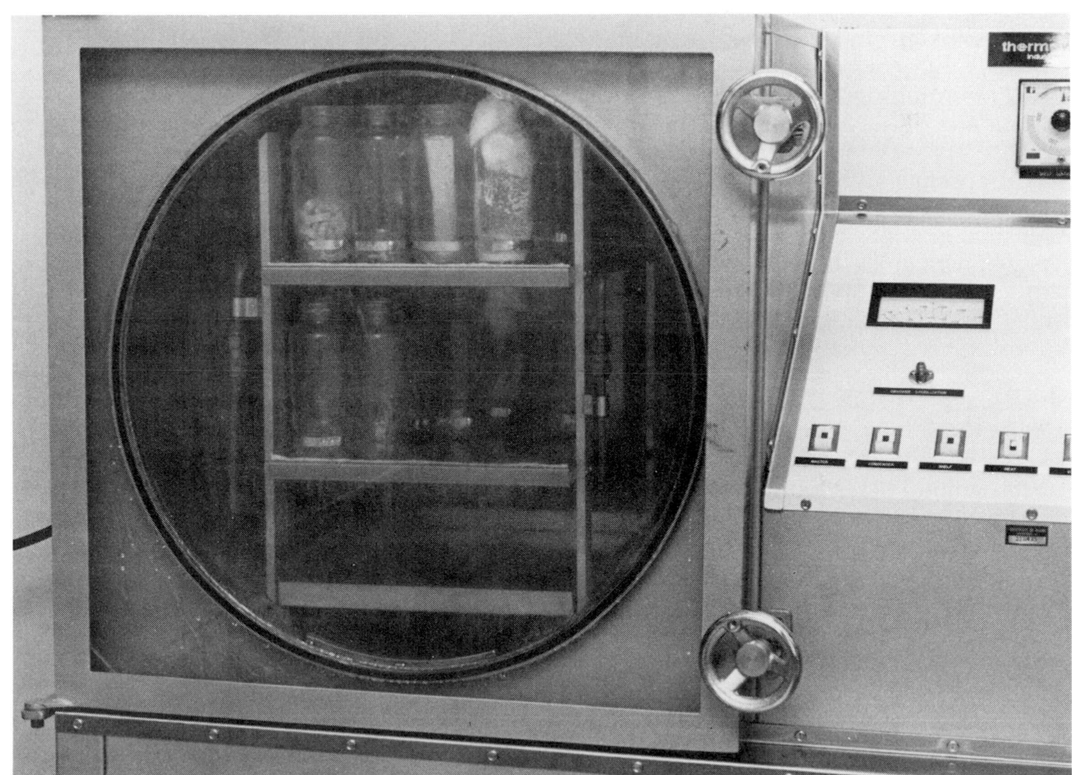

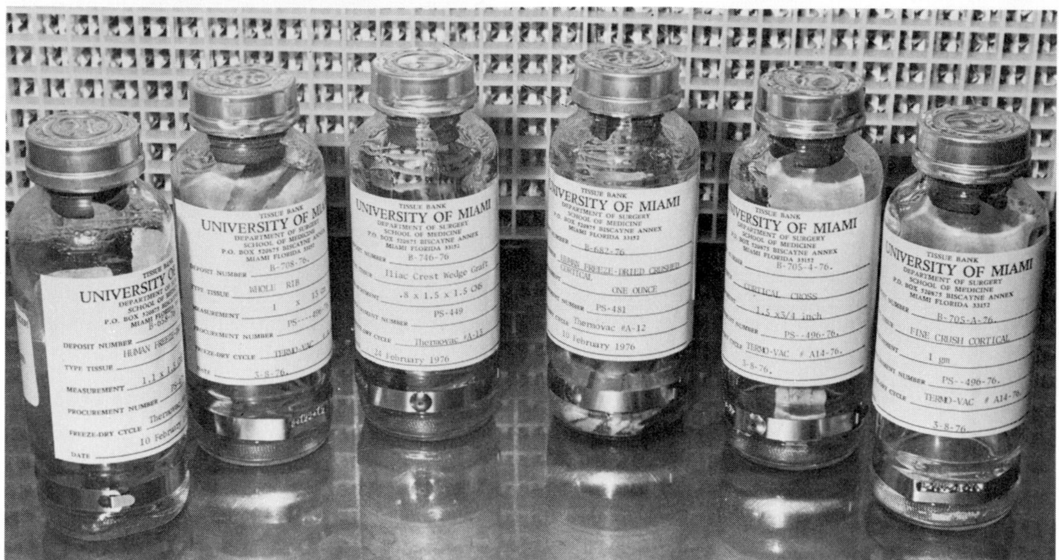

FIG. 3-52. Packaged freeze-dried cadaver bone grafts. Before packaging, the tissues are subjected to final bacteriologic study. Freeze-dried bone can be stored at room temperature for an indefinite time period. Before use, these grafts must be reconstituted by immersion in saline.

cularization, and resorption and replacement of graft by immature ossified bone. This process of gradual allograft bone replacement has been referred to as "creeping substitution."

In summary, tissue bank technology has progressed to the point at which cadaver bone allografts can be obtained routinely and transplanted into patients without risk of transmitting disease. Although several methods of bone processing and preservation have been used in the past, the best clinical results seem to be obtained with aseptically excised freeze-dried bone, which, by circumstance, would appear to be the least antigenic. With smaller grafts, equivalently good results have been obtained with quick-frozen bone. The current experience with freeze-dried and frozen bone does not preclude further efforts in the study of graft preparation.

EFFECTS OF IONIZING RADIATION ON BONE*

The recognition of the hazards of exposure to radioactive substances, and their late effect on bone and other tissues, has led to preventive measures which make the injury one rarely seen in clinical practice. Lesions, when encountered, are usually due to external radiation received by the patient in the course of treatment for malignant disease. However, the changes observed are similar, whether the source of radiation is a bone-seeking radioactive substance or external radiation, and depend on the age of the patient at the time of exposure, the part of the skeleton irradiated, and the dose given. The physiopathology and clinical sequelae differ depending on whether growing or adult bone is irradiated.

* The section on "Effects of Ionizing Radiation on Bone" is contributed by Ivor Fix, M.D., F.A.C.R., Chairman, Dept. of Radiotherapy, Mount Sinai Medical Center; Associate Professor, University of Miami School of Medicine, Miami Beach, Fla.

EFFECTS OF IONIZING RADIATION ON GROWING BONE

PHYSIOPATHOLOGY

Growing bone and cartilage are relatively radiosensitive. Irradiation of growing bone and cartilage may cause retardation and cessation of growth.[228–230,237,240] The degree of stunting depends on the extent of damage to the proliferating cartilage cells in the zones of endochondral ossification and on the fine vasculature of the marrow. The recovery of the latter is essential for regeneration and resumption of growth after injury. It has been well documented in animal studies that the greater the radiosensitivity of the cells and growth potential of the cartilage, the greater is the degree of skeletal retardation. Treatment given to an infant has a more profound effect than that given to an older child. In adolescense the cartilage becomes more radioresistant and higher doses of radiation are required to bring about growth retardation.

Clinically noted alteration in bone growth has been reported at doses as low as 500 rads—a dosage level previously used in treating benign lesions such as hemangiomata. Generally, however, doses below 1200 rads rarely give rise to clinical problems of growth retardation.[240] As the dose is increased above this level—the usual dose given to the blastemic tumor, for instance, is between 3000 and 4000 rads—there is an increasing incidence of severe change, depending on the age of the patient, to complete cessation of growth (Fig. 3-54).[240,244]

Irradiation of an epiphysis causes arrest of chondrogenesis and more shortening than does exposure of the metaphysis or diaphysis. Metaphyseal irradiation leads to failure of the absorptive process, resulting in widening of the shaft. Diaphyseal irradiation produces alteration in periosteal activity, resulting in modeling errors. As the dose is increased there is an increased incidence of sclerosis and fracture. These changes are, in the main, applicable to tubular bone but similar changes occur in vertebrae where the maximum change due to irradiation is on the epiphyseal plate. The mechanism of the late changes resulting in cartilaginous exostosis and malignant tumors in the irradiated field is unknown.

CLINICAL PICTURE

Second only to accidents, malignant tumors have become a significant cause of death in childhood. The widespread use of radiation in the treatment of these malignancies, with the gradual but significant improvement in survival, makes recognition of the effects of radiation on growing bone increasingly important. The acute and subacute phases of the radiation injury do not give rise to clinical, biochemical, or radiological changes. The clinical and radiological features seen are those of the chronic or late effects following radiation therapy. Approximately 1 year after exposure early abnormalities may be noted, followed by slowly progressive changes depending on the site treated.

It is the vertebral column that is most often subtended by the treatment beam in the therapy of Wilms' tumors, neuroblastoma, and medulloblastoma; the ilium is less often treated. The skull is irradiated in the treatment of intracranial lesions and the leukemias, and more rarely the tubular bones are treated in such lesions as Ewing's sarcoma, reticulum cell sarcoma, metastatic disease, and osteosarcoma.

Vertebral Column.[215,232,235,241,246,248] Irradiation of the vertebral column, when it leads to arrest of growth, causes curvature of the spine. Two types of deformity are seen, a lateral flexion curve and a rotary scoliosis. The curvatures are essentially minor and are not progressive as in idiopathic scoliosis.[241] The scoliosis becomes evident approximately 1 year after therapy. Pronounced limp is rare since pelvic tilt compensates for the curvature. Gross cosmetic defects (*e.g.*, gibbus) are rarely seen.

Roentgenographic Findings.[232,240,244] These depend on site treated, dose delivered, age of the child at the time of treatment, and time after irradiation. The initial change is that of subcortical lucent zones. These progress to growth-arrest lines parallel to the epiphysis of the vertebral body, eventually giving rise to the "os-in-os" appearance. These growth-arrest lines are similar to those

FIG. 3-53. Roentgenogram of a 57-year-old man with cervical spondylosis taken 4 months after insertion of a freeze-dried cylindrical cadaver femoral head allograft.

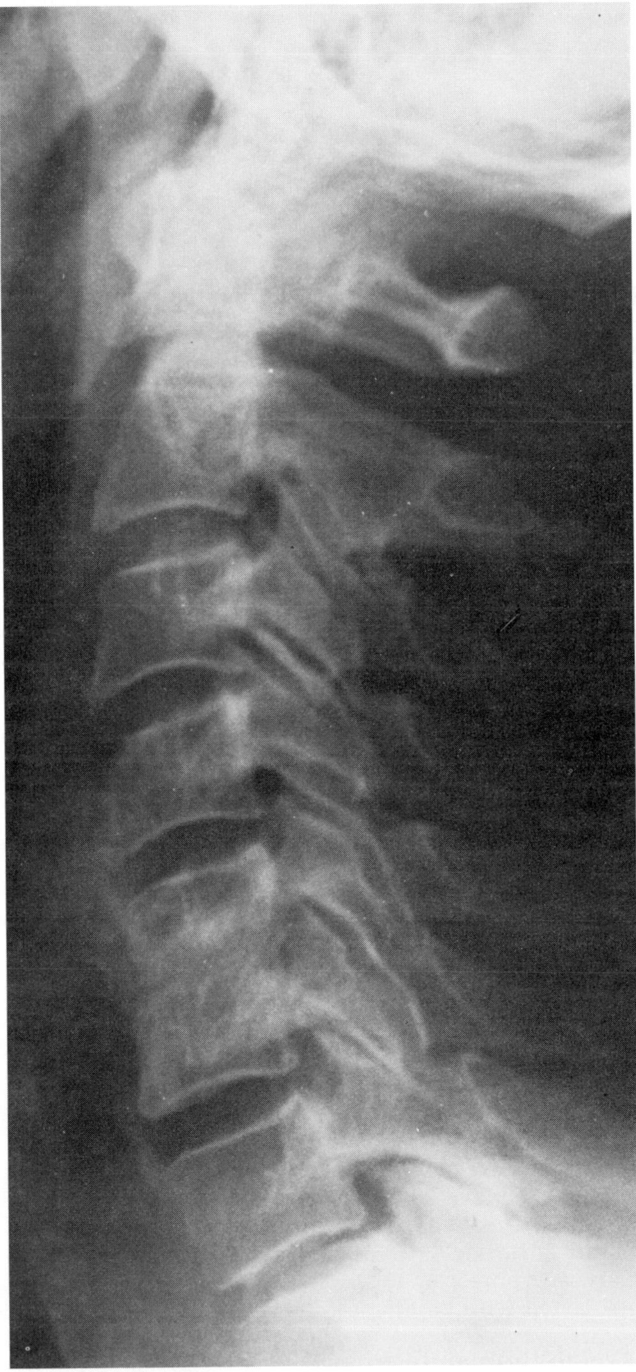

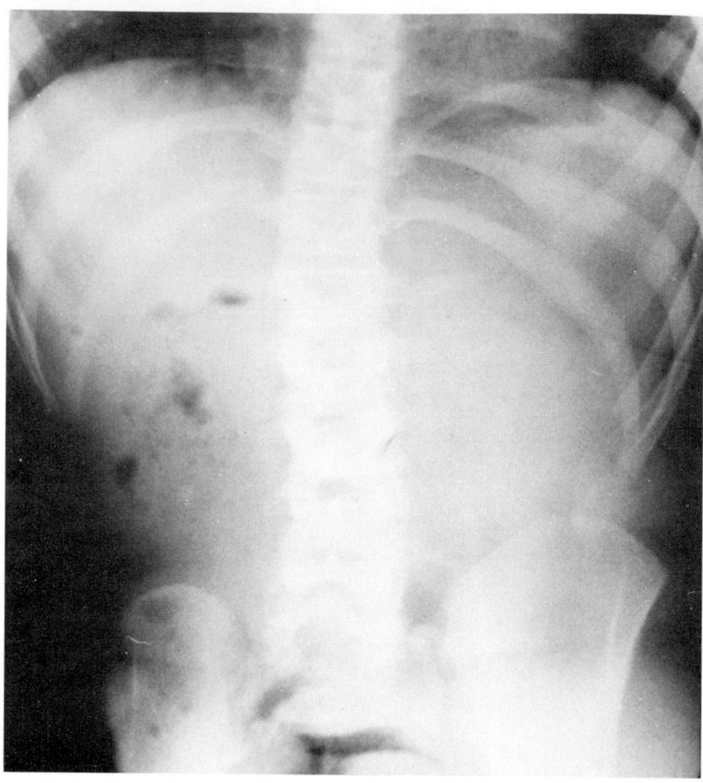

FIG. 3-54. Roentgenogram of an 8-year-old patient who received postoperative radiotherapy for Wilms' tumor at age 4 months. Note the hypoplasia of the right ilium and sacrum. There is also unilateral wedging of lumbar vertebrae and compensatory scoliosis, despite the inclusion of full width of the spinal column in treatment fields.

arising elsewhere in the skeleton from other causes and may occur at a dose between 1000 and 2000 rads. Higher doses—between 2000 and 3000 rads—may produce gross irregularity and scalloping of the epiphyseal plates. Gross contour changes resembling osteochondrodystrophy may be seen.

Treatment. Because the chronic bony changes when manifest are irreversible, treatment is directed either toward the prevention of the radiation-induced scoliosis or corrective measures. Prophylactic measures entail subtending the entire width of the vertebra in the treatment field to avoid a unilateral wedge effect.[235] However, unilateral changes in the pedicle do not necessarily give rise to a severe curvature, nor does treatment of the entire vertebra exclude unilateral changes.[240,241] Corrective measures are rarely required. If, however, the scoliosis is severe and progressive it should be treated as if it were an idiopathic scoliosis.

Ilium and Ribs.[232,240,241,243,244] The ilium and lower thorax are not infrequently included in the radiation field in the treatment of Wilms' tumor and neuroblastoma. Whenever possible they should be excluded; however, this is not always feasible in treating a larger tumor adequately. Treatment of the crest of the ilium causes hypoplasia and adds to the pelvic tilt when associated with a radiation-induced scoliosis.

Acetabulum and Femur.[232,240,241,244] Irradiation of the acetabulum and femur may lead to moderate to severe deformities. Acetabular dysplasia, coxa valga, and coxa vara, with dislocation of the hip and leg shortening have been reported. These usually can be avoided because inclusion of this area in a treatment field for Wilms' tumor or neuroblastoma is usually unnecessary.

Skull and Orbit.[240,244] Irradiation of this area in the therapy of lesions of the orbit or brain leads to arrest of growth of the bones in the treatment field. In the case of the treatment of orbital tumors, it may lead to marked facial asymmetry.

Tubular Bones.[239,240,244] When irradiated, the extremity may be shortened or bowed. The degree of deformity again depends on the amount of radiation and the portion of the bone irradiated. Inclusion of the epiphysis in the irradiated field gives rise to metaphyseal flaring similar to the hypoplastic form of achondroplasia and results in dwarfing. Metaphyseal irradiation causes shortening and bowing. In diaphyseal irradiation the length of the bone is minimally affected, but there is narrowing because of the interference with periosteal new bone formation.

POSTRADIATION SARCOMA OF BONE

Malignant tumors can develop in a bone exposed to ionizing radiation, and constitute approximately 1.5% of primary malignant tumors of bone. Following radiotherapy, it is only after a prolonged latent period, averaging about 15 years, that a recognizable sarcoma develops.[216,247] These tumors form following radiotherapy for a wide variety of neoplastic and non-neoplastic conditions, and they may arise both in preexisting osseous lesions and in bones that were normal but lay in the path of external irradiation administered for a nonosseous condition.[227]

The criteria for the diagnosis of postradiation sarcoma of bone are:[216,221]

1. There must be microscopic or roentgenographic evidence of the benign nature of the initial lesion, or malignant tumors devoid of osteoblastic activity (*e.g.*, Ewing's tumor, malignant lymphoma)
2. Irradiation must have been given and the sarcoma that subsequently developed must have arisen in the area included within the radiotherapeutic beam
3. A relatively long latent period must have elapsed before the clinical appearance of the bone sarcoma. A period of at least 5 years has been suggested.
4. All sarcomas must be proved histologically.

The history will often reveal that excessive radiation therapy was given as evidenced by, for example, actinic proctitis, severe actinodermatitis, and radiation osteonecrosis. The recent change from orthovoltage to megavoltage therapy has not as yet reduced the incidence of radiation-induced sarcoma. No case has been reported following linear accelerator radiation therapy.

PATHOLOGY

Postradiation sarcoma can occur in any bone. The preexisting lesions are highly variable. Approximately 90% of postradiation sarcomas are osteosarcomas and fibrosarcomas. Osteosarcoma predominates in tumors arising in normal bone; fibrosarcomas account for the majority of tumors arising in preexisting osseous lesions, many of which having documented radiotherapy for giant cell tumors and fibrous dysplasia. Since such tumors have a well-known propensity for malignant change on exposure to ionizing radiation, radiotherapy is best avoided.

CLINICAL PICTURE

The onset of symptoms is rather abrupt and progression is rapid. Pain and swelling are the most common symptoms. A mass may be palpable when the tumor extends beyond the confines of the bone.

TREATMENT

Postradiation sarcomas are relatively radioresistant tumors and prompt radical surgery is the preferred treatment. Ablative surgery can effect a 5 year survival in approximately 30% of cases. The outlook for tumors affecting the craniofacial bones, and those of the shoulder girdle, spine, and pelvis is poor. Local irradiation can effect temporary symptomatic relief.

EFFECTS OF IONIZING RADIATION ON ADULT BONE

PHYSIOPATHOLOGY

The acute effects of ionizing radiation on growing bone and adult bone differ.[219,222,226,240] In the former, there is damage to both the proliferating cells and vasculature; in the latter, damage is primarily to the fine vasculature with resultant degeneration of cells secondary to the interference with the blood supply. The sequence of events following the initial vascular damage depends on the degree of damage and on whether there is secondary infection and trauma. If the vascular damage is slight there will be recovery; if not, necrosis will ensue. This osteoradionecrosis is simple or "aseptic" in the absence of infection; however, if the heavily irradiated area is infected, "complicated osteoradionecrosis" results (Color Plate 3-3).

In simple osteoradionecrosis the findings are no different from aseptic necrosis from any other cause. The progressive occlusion of the damaged blood vessel leads to loss of parenchymal cells, disorganization of the matrix, porosis, fibrosis, and eventually necrosis. Large resorption cavities fill with gelatinous material, and the "molasses" appearance results.

Osteoradionecrosis complicated by infection leads to destructive septic lesions—radiation osteomyelitis. The damage to the vasculature results in slow formation of a sequestrum and delayed healing when the sequestrum is removed.

The dose required to bring about aseptic necrosis and fracture is 6000 rads or above, as opposed to the lesser dosage which brings about abnormalities in growing bone.[219,240] Whereas of minor importance in the treatment of growing bone, the quality of radiation is of major importance when mature bone is irradiated. The dose in rads to a mature bone exceeds by a factor of 3 the dose in roentgens at 250 kv. At supervoltage energies, however, the rad and roentgen are essentially interchangeable and the differential absorption is not a significant factor. The general use of high-energy radiation has markedly reduced the incidence of aseptic necrosis.

CLINICAL PICTURE

The clinical presentation may be acute, subacute, or chronic, depending on the area irradiated and the presence or absence of infection and trauma. The bones most often involved are the mandible, pelvis, femur, and ribs. With the exception of the mandible and occasionally the ribs, the clinical presentation is usually chronic and is due to an aseptic necrosis.

Mandible. In irradiating cancers of the mouth[225,236] and oropharynx, dental caries and osteonecrosis may result. The process is more often acute when a persistent tumor is present and occurs more frequently when the tumor is contiguous or involves the bone. The clinical presentation is usually that of progressive pain with or without persistent tumor and dental caries. Roentgenograms will show an ill-defined lytic lesion, but sequestrum formation is rare.

If a tumor is present the treatment is surgical. In the absence of a tumor, conservative measures may be successful.[233] Early excision at the onset of necrosis has, however, been proposed.

In the chronic presentation—in those patients in whom the cancer has been controlled and some time has elapsed since the completion of radiation therapy—dental caries not infrequently precede the development of osteoradionecrosis. To prevent this complication, prophylactic measures prior to radiation therapy are recommended. These range from total dental extraction[223] to preservation of healthy teeth with fluoride gel applications. Chronic necrosis usually heals with the conservative measures, surgery only occasionally being necessary.

Femur and Pelvis. Radiation-induced changes in the femur and pelvis are the result of chronic changes occurring 5 months to 5 years after radiation. Trauma, due to the stress of weight bearing on the irradiated bones, rather than infection is the precipitating factor. The secondary changes due to vascular impairment lead to sclerosis and occasionally spontaneous fracture.

Femur.[217,234,240,245] Pain in the groin or knee, occasionally incapacitating, may indicate incipient necrosis prior to roentgenographic changes. Once fracture has occurred, the clinical findings are similar to those which follow fracture due to trauma with pain, limitation of movement, and leg shortening. Aseptic necrosis of the femoral head is rare and, fracture is usually through the femoral neck. Roentgenograms show gradually progressive sclerotic changes.[219,222]

It is important to differentiate between radionecrosis and metastatic disease. In the former, osteolysis is rare. Metastatic disease to the femur from carcinoma of the cervix is rare and in a patient previously treated with radiation for this disease, spontaneous fracture through the neck of the femur is regarded as a postradiation fracture until proven otherwise.

If there is no major displacement or if found in patients with impending fracture, these lesions will heal by rest and restriction of weight bearing.[217] With displacement, the usual orthopaedic procedures are undertaken, and the results of the treatment are similar to those obtained in post-traumatic fractures without radiation.

Pelvis. Irradiation may lead to sclerosis and fracture of the ilium and pubic bones. Roentgenograms show typical sclerosis with fracture. In patients previously treated for carcinoma of the cervix, the lesion must be differentiated from progressive pelvic disease.[240,241,242,243]

Ribs and Clavicle. Osteoradionecrosis of these bones may follow irradiation of the chest wall following surgery for carcinoma of the breast. Pain and point tenderness in a rib or the clavicle in a previous field of radiation should arouse suspicion as to the diagnosis. There are usually accompanying skin changes, and the effects of radiation can be seen on the underlying lung. There may be difficulty in differentiating the sclerotic roentgenographic changes caused by blastic metastases from those due to the previously treated breast carcinoma; however, if the lesions are confined exclusively to the treatment area, they are more likely to be due to radiation. Since the general use of supervoltage, this problem is seldom encountered.

THERAPEUTIC USE OF IONIZING RADIATION IN BONE TUMORS

The use of radiation therapy, either alone or in conjunction with surgery and chemotherapy, is well accepted in the treatment of metastatic carcinoma, myeloma, malignant lymphoma involving bone and in Ewing's sarcoma. The role of radiation therapy in the treatment of osteogenic sarcoma of tubular bones is less clear.

The most common malignant lesion involving bone is metastatic carcinoma. Radiation therapy is valuable in alleviating pain and promoting bone healing. When metastatic disease causes pathologic fracture of a long bone and radiation therapy is given, callous formation at the fracture site rarely occurs and remodeling of the bone is delayed or absent.[218] In the management of incipient or known pathologic fractures, therefore, internal fixation is required. Radiation therapy may be given either pre- or postoperatively. Since callous formation cannot be expected, the patient should be mobilized within approximately 2 weeks of the pinning, because further immobilization is unlikely to result in increased stability of the bone.

Preoperative radiation therapy, either as primary radiation with selective delayed amputation or followed immediately by surgery, has been proposed in the treatment of osteogenic sarcoma. This has been advocated, since the disease is usually rapidly lethal because of early pulmonary metastases. A series of reported patients is generally small in number. It is difficult to arrive at a valid conclusion. Some series show that preoperative radiation therapy give better results than surgery alone,[238] others show little or no difference in the survival rate.[220,224,231]

REFERENCES

Structure of Bone

1. Cooper RR, Milgram JW, Robinson RA: Morphology of the osteon: An electron microscopic study. J Bone Joint Surg 48A:1239, 1966
2. Havers C: Osteologia Nova (treatise). London, Smith, 1961

Components of Bone

3. Ham AW, Cormack DH: Histology, 8th ed. Philadelphia, JB Lippincott, 1979
4. Herring GM: Chemistry of the bone matrix. Clin Orthop 36:169, 1964

Remodeling of Bone

5. Lacroix P: The internal remodelling of bones. In Bourne G: The Biochemistry and Physiology of Bone, Vol 3, 2nd ed, p 119. New York. Academic Press, 1972

Ultrastructural Characteristics of Bone

6. Baud CA: Submicroscopic structure and functional aspect of the osteocyte. Clin Orthop 56:277, 1968
7. Bonucci E: Fine structure and histochemistry of calcifying globules in epiphyseal cartilage. Z Zellfrch 103:192, 1970
8. Glimcher MJ: The molecular biology of mineralized tissues with particular reference to bone. Res Mod Physics 31:359, 1959
9. Glimcher MJ: A basic architectural principle in the organization of mineralized tissues. Clin Orthop 61:16, 1961
10. Glimcher MJ, Daniel EJ, Travis DF et al: Electron optical and x-ray diffraction studies of the organization of the inorganic crystals in embryonic bovine enamel. J Ultrastruct Res (Suppl) 7:1, 1965
11. Hodge AJ, Petruska JA: Recent studies with the electron-microscope on ordered aggregates of the tropocollagen molecule. In Ramachandran GN (ed): Aspects of Protein Structure, p 289. New York, Academic Press, 1963
12. Martin JH, Matthews JL: Mitochondrial granules in chondrocytes. Calcif Tissue Res 3:184, 1969

Osteoprogenitor Cell Principle

13. Bassett CAL: Current concepts of bone formation. J Bone Joint Surg 44A:1217, 1962
14. Becker RO, Murray DG: The electrical control system regulating fracture healing in amphibians. Clin Orthop 7:169, 1970
15. Burwell RG: Studies in the transplantation of bone. VII. The fresh composite homograft-autograft of cancellous bone: An analysis of factors leading to osteogenesis in marrow transplants and in marrow-containing bone grafts. J Bone Joint Surg 45B:402, 1963
16. Burwell RG: Studies on the transplantation of bone. VII. The fresh composite homograft-autograft of cancellous bone. J Bone Joint Surg 46B:110, 1968
17. Cabrini R: Histochemistry of ossification. Int Rev Cytol 11:283, 1961
18. Cappellin M: Contributo all'indagine eitochimica degli acidi nucleini negli osteoblasti. Chir Organi Mov 33:410, 1949
19. de Voogd van der Straaten WA: Proceedings of the Third European Symposium on Calc. Tissues, Davos, Switzerland, 1966, p 10. New York, Springer–Verlag,
20. Friedenstein AJ: Induction of bone tissue by transitional epithelium. Clin Orthop 59:21, 1968
21. Frost H: Bone biodynamics. Henry Ford Hospital International Symposium. Boston, Little, Brown, 1964
22. Hambergere CA, Hyden H: Cytochemical studies on experimental bone fistulae. Acta Otolaryngol 35:479, 1947
23. McLean FC, Bloom W: Mode of action of parathyroid action on bone. Science 85:24, 1937
24. Owen M: In Budy AM (ed): Biology of Hard Tissue. Proc. Second Conf. p 147. Washington, DC, National Aeronautics and Space Administration, 1968
25. Owen M:The origin of bone cells. Int Rev Cytol 28:213, 1970
26. Pilla AA: Electrochemical information transfer at living cell membranes. Ann NY Acad Sci 238:149, 1974
27. Pritchard JJ: In Bourne GA (ed): The Biochemistry and Physiology of Bone, p 179. Academic Press, New York, 1956
28. Scott BL: ^{3}H-thymidine electron microscopic radioautography of osteogenic cells in the fetal rats. J Cell Biol 35:115, 1967
29. Seeman H: Über die entstehungsbedingungen metaplastischer Knochenbildungen. Deutsche Zeitschrift für Chirurgie 217:60, 1929
30. Tonna EA, Cronkite EP: Use of tritiated thymidine for the study of the origin of the osteoclast. Nature 190:459, 1961
31. Trueta J: The role of vessels in osteogenesis. J Bone Joint Surg 45B:402, 1963
32. Young RW: Cell proliferation and specilization during endochondral osteogenesis in young rats. J Cell Biol 14:357, 1962
33. Young RW: Nucleic acids, protein synthesis and bone. Clin Orthop 26:147, 1963

The Osteogenic Cell

34. Bassett CAL, Becker RO: Generation of electric potentials in bone in response to mechanical stress. Science 137:1063, 1962
35. Bassett CAL, Pawlek RJ, Becker RO: Effects of electrical currents in bone *in vivo*. Nature 204:652, 1964
36. Eggers GWN, Shindler TO, Pomerat CM: Osteogenesis: Influence of the contact-compression factor on osteogenesis in surgical fractures. J Bone Joint Surg 31:693, 1949
37. Fewer DJ, Threadgold J, Sheldon H: Studies on cartilage. V. Electron microscopic observations on the autoradiographic-localization of S35 in cells and matrix. J Ultrastruct Res 11:166, 1964
38. Harris WH, Heaney RP: Effect of growth hormone on skeletal mass in adult dogs. Nature 223:403, 1969
39. Koskinen EVS: The influence of hormone treatment and orchiectomy, oophorectomy and thyroidectomy on experimental fractures. Acta Orthop Scand Suppl 80, 1965
40. Lavine L, Lurstin I, Rinaldi R et al: Clinical and ultrastructural investigations of electrical enhancement of bone healing. Ann NY Acad Sci 238:552, 1974
41. Leblond C, Weinstock A: Radioautographic studies of bone formation. In Bourne GH (ed): Biochemistry and Physiology of Bone, Vol 3, p 181. New York, Academic Press, 1971
42. Lehninger AL: Mitochondria and calcium ion transport. Biochem J 119:129, 1970
43. Posner AS: Crystal chemistry of bone mineral. Physiol Rev 49:760, 1969
44. Rohr H: Die Kollagensynthese in ihrer Beziehung zur submikroskopischen Struktur des Osteoblasten (electronen mikroskopisch-autoradiographische Untersuchung mit Tritium markieter Proline). Virchows Arch Pathol Anat Physiol 338:342, 1965
45. Urist MR, Strates BS: Bone morphogenetic protein. J Dent Res (Supple 60) 50:1392, 1971
46. Weinstock A: Elaboration of enamel and dentin matrix glycoproteins. In Bourne GH (ed): Biochemistry and Physiology of Bone, Vol 2, p 121. New York, Academic Press, 1972

The Bone Induction Principle

47. Büring K, Urist MR: Transfilter bone nduction. Clin Orthop 54:235, 1967
48. Hellstadius A: Studies on osteogenesis around autoplastic bone transplants in bony defects. Acta Orthop Scand 24:278, 1955
49. Lapiere CM, Gross J: Animal collagenase and collagen metabolism. In Sognnaes RF (ed): Hard Tissue Destruction, pp 663–694. Washington, DC, Am J Adv Sci Publ No. 75, 1963
50. Post RH, Heiple KG, Chase SW et al: Bone grafts in diffusion chambers. Clin Orthop, p 44:265, 1966
51. Urist MR: Bone: Formation by autoinduction. Science 150:893, 1965
52. Urist MR: Osteoinduction in underminearlized bone implants modified by chemical inhibition of matrix enzymes. Clin Orthop 87:132, 1972
53. Urist MR, Silverman BF, Büring K et al: The bone induction principle. Clin Orthop 53:243, 1967
54. Urist MR, Iwata H: Preservation and biodegradation of the morphogenetic property of bone matrix. J Theor Biol 38:155, 1973
55. Urist MR, Strates BS: Bone morphogenetic protein. J Dent Res (Suppl 6) 50:1392, 1971

Repair of Simple Fracture of a Long Bone

56. Grant CG: An Investigation of the Mechanical Aspects of Long-term Fracture Healing Following Rigid Fixation, Ph.D. thesis, Institute of Medical Science, University of Toronto, 1973
57. Ham AW, Harris WR: Repair and transplantation of bone. In Bourne GH (ed): The Biochemistry and Physiology of Bone, Vol 3, 2nd ed, pp 377–399. New York, Academic Press, 1971
58. Schenk R, Willenegger H: Morphological findings in primary fracture healing. Symp Biol Hung 7:75, 1967

Delayed Union and Nonunion

59. Bassett CAL: The electrical management of ununited fractures. In Gossling HR, Pillsbury SL (eds): Complications in Fracture Management. Philadelphia, JB Lippincott, 1982
60. Bassett CAL, Mitchell SN, Gaston SR: Treatment of ununited tibial diaphyseal fractures with pulsing electromagnetic fields. J Bone Joint Surg 63A:511, 1981
61. Böhler L: Technik der Knochenbruchbehandlung, p 12. Aufl Maudrich, Wien, 1957
62. Brighton CT, Friedenberg ZB, Black J: Evaluation of the use of constant direct current in the treatment of nonunion. In Brighton CT, Black J, Pollack SR (eds): Electrical Properties of Bone and Cartilage, p 519. New York, Grune & Stratton, 1979
63. Brighton CT, Friedenberg ZB, Mitchell EI et al: Treatment of nonunion with constant direct current. Clin Orthop 124:106, 1977
64. Burrows HJ: Treatment of ununited fractures by bone grafting without resection of the bone ends. Proc R Soc Med (Section on Orthopaedics) 33:157, 1940
65. Charnley J: Editorial: Surgical treatment of ununited fractures. J Bone Joint Surg 42B:3, 1960
66. Danis R: Theorie et pratique de l-ostéosynthèse. Paris, Desoer, Liège, Masson, 1949
67. Dunn R: Treatment of ununited fractures. Br Med J 2:221, 1939
68. Dwyer AF, Wickham GG: Direct current stimulation in spinal fusion. Med J Aust 1:73, 1974
69. Jarry L, Uhthoff HK: Activation of osteogenesis by the "petal" technique. J Bone Joint Surg 42B:126, 1960
70. Judet R: La décortication. In Actualités de Chirurgie Orthopédique. IV. Paris, Masson, 1965
71. Krompecher S: Die Knochenbildung. Jena, Fischer, 1937
72. Küntscher G: Die Schenkelhalsbruch. Ein mechanisches Problem. Beilh Z für Orthop Chir Stuttgart, Ferdinand, Enke, 1935
73. Müller ME, Allgower M: Zur Behandlung der Pseudarthrose. Helv Chir Acta 25:253, 1958
74. Pauwels F: Der Schenkelhalsbruch. Ein Mechanisches Problem. Stuttgart, Ferdinand Enke, 1935
75. Pauwels F: Grundriss einer Biomechanik der Frakturheilung. Verh Dtsch Orthop Ges 34:62 1940
76. Phemister DB: Treatment of ununited fractures by onlay bone-grafts without screw or tie fixation and without breaking down the fibrous union. J Bone Joint Surg 29:946, 1947
77. Segmüller G, Čech O, Bekier A: Die osteogene Aktivität im bereich der Pseudarthrose langer Röhrenknochen. Z Orthop 106:599, 1969
78. Watson–Jones R: Fractures and Joint Injuries. Edinburgh, Livingstone, 1955
79. Weber BG, Čech O: Pseudarthrosis. Bern, Hans Huber, 1976
80. Williams DF: Titanium as a metal for implantation. Part 2: Biological properties and clinical applications. J Med Eng Technol 1 (5):266, 1977
81. Wu TT: Über Fibrinoidbildung der Haut nach unspezifischer Gewebsschädigung bei der Ratte. Virchows Arch Pathol Anat 300:373, 1937
82. Urist MR, Mazet R, McLean FC: The pathogenesis and treatment of delayed union and non-union. J Bone Joint Surg 36A:931, 1954

Bone Transplantation

83. Anderson K, LeCocq JF, Akeson WH et al: End points results of processed heterogenous, autogenous, and homogenous bone transplants in the human. Clin Orthop 33:220, 1964
84. Bassett CAL: Environmental and cellular factors regulating osteogenesis. In Frost H (ed): Bone Biodynamics, pp 233–244. Boston, Little, Brown, 1964
85. Bassett CAL: Clinical implications of cell function in bone grafting. Clin Orthop 87:49, 1972
86. Bassett CAL, Herrmann I: The effect of electrostatic fields on macromolecular synthesis by fibroblasts *in vitro.* J Cell Biol 39:96, 1968
87. Bassett CAL, Murray DL: A method for producing cellular differentiation by means of very small electrical currents. Trans NY Acad Sci 29:606, 1967
88. Bohatirchuk FP: Metaplasia of cartilage into bone. A study by stain historadiography. AM J Anat 126:243, 1979
89. Bonfiglio M, Jetter WS: Immunological response to bone, Clin Orthop 87:19, 1972
90. Brooks DB, Heiple KG, Herndon CH et al: Immunologic factors in homogenous bone transplantation. IV. The effect of various methods of preparation and irradiation on antigenicity. J Bone Joint Surg 45A:1617, 1963
91. Burchardt H, Jones H, Glowczewski F et al: Freeze-dried allogeneic segmental cortical-bone grafts in dogs. J Bone Joint Surg 60A:1082, 1978
92. Burwell RG: Biological mechanisms in foreign bone trans-

plantation. In Clark JMP (ed): Modern Trends in Orthopaedics, p 138. London, Butterworth, 1964
93. Burwell RG: The fate of bone grafts. In Apley AG (ed): Recent Advances in Orthopaedics, p 115. London, Churchill, 1969
94. Burwell RG: The fate of freeze-dried bone allografts. Transplant Proc (Suppl 1) 8:95, 1976
95. Burwell RG, Gowland G, Dexter F: Studies in the transplantation of bone. VI. Further observations concerning the antigenicity of homologous cortical and cancellous bone. J Bone Joint Surg 45B:597, 1963
96. Crenshaw AH (ed): Campbell's Operative Orthopaedics, 5th ed. St Louis, CV Mosby, 1971
97. Deleu J, Trueta J: Vascularization of bone grafts in the anterior chamber of the eye. J Bone Joint Surg 47B:319, 1965
98. Elves MW: Humoral immune response to allografts of bone. Int Arch Allergy Appl Immunol 47:708, 1974
99. Enneking WF, Burchardt H, Puhl JJ et al: Physical and biological aspects of repair in dog cortical-bone transplants. J Bone Joint Surg 57A:237, 1975
100. Enneking WF, Eady JL, Burchardt H: Autogenous cortical bone grafts in the reconstruction of segmental skeletal defects. J Bone Joint Surg 62A:1039, 1980
101. Falk RE, Thorsby E, Moller E et al: *In vitro* assay cell-mediated immunity: The inhibition of migration of sensitized human lymphocytes by HL-A antigens. Clin Exp Immunol 6:445, 1970
102. Flosdorf EW: Changes in products during desiccation from the frozen state and storage. In Freeze-Drying (Drying by Sublimation). New York, Reinhold, 1949
103. Freund JT, McDermott K: Sensitization to horse serum by means of adjuvants. Proc Soc Exp Biol Med 49:548, 1942
104. Hammack BL, Enneking WF: Comparative vascularization of autogenous and homogenous bone transplants. J Bone Joint Surg 42A:811, 1960
105. Herndon CH, Chase SW: The fate of massive autogenous and homogenous bone grafts including articular surfaces. Surg Gynecol Obstet 98:273, 1954
106. Hyatt GW, Butler MC: Bone grafting: The preservation, storage, and clinical use of bone homografts. In Instructional Course Lectures, Vol 14, p 343. Ann Arbor, JW Edwards, 1957
107. Immaliev AS: The preparation, preservation and transplantation of articular bone ends. In Apley AG: Advances in Orthopaedics, pp 209–269. London, Churchill, 1969
108. Kaliss N: Immunological enhancement of tumor homografts in mice: A review. Cancer Res 18:992, 1958
109. Kandutsch A, Stinfling J: Partial purification of tissue isoantigens from mouse sarcoma. Transplantation 1:201, 1963
110. Kingma MS, Hampe JF: The behaviour of blood vessels after experimental transplantation of bone. J Bone Joint Surg 46B:141, 1964
111. Kreuz FP, Hyatt GW, Turner TC et al: The preservation and clinical use of freeze-dried bone. J Bone Joint Surg 33A:297, 1974
112. Langer F, Gross AE: Immunogenicity of allograft articular cartilage. J Bone Joint Surg 56A:297, 1974
113. Langer F et al: The immunogenicity of fresh and frozen allogeneic bone. J Bone Joint Surg 57A:216, 1975
114. Manson LA: Membrane associated histocompatibility antigens. In Nowotny A (ed): Cellular Antigens, pp 235–247. New York, Springer–Verlag, 1972
115. Medawar PB: The immunology of transplantation. Hervey Lect 52: New York, Academic Press, 1958
116. Mikulski A, Urist MR: Control of bone morphogenesis by a matrix glycopeptide and protease (abstr). J Dent Res (Suppl) 1:138, 1974
117. Nilsonne U: Homologous joint transplantation in man. Acta Orthop Scand 40:429, 1969
118. Phemister DB: Biologic principles in the healing of fractures and their bearing on treatment. Ann Surg 133:433, 1951
119. Puranen J: Reorganization of fresh and preserved bone transplants. An experimental study in rabbits using tetracycline labelling. Acta Orthop Scand (Suppl) 92:1, 1966
120. Ray RD: Vascularization of bone grafts and implants. Clin Orthop 87:43, 1972
121. Reisfeld RA, Kahan BD: Transplantation antigens. Adv Immunol 12:117, 1970
122. Rued TP, Bassett CAL: Repair and remodeling in millipore-isolated defects in cortical bone. Acta Anat 68:509, 1967
123. Shaw JL, Bassett CAL: An improved method for studying osteogenesis in vitro. J Bone Joint Surg 49A:73, 1967
124. Siffert RS, Barash ES: Delayed bone transplantation: An experimental study of early host-transplant relationships. J Bone Joint Surg 43A:407, 1961
125. Sledge CB, Dingle JT: Activation of lysosomes by oxygen. Oxygen induced resorption of cartilage in organ culture. Nature (Lond) 205:140, 1965
126. Smith RT: The mechanism of graft rejection. Clin Orthop 87:15, 1972
127. Spence EF, Sell KW, Brown RH: Solitary bone cyst: Treatment with freeze-dried cancellous bone allografts. A study of one hundred seventy seven cases. J Bone Joint Surg 51A:87, 1969
128. Stevenson JS, Bright RW, Dunson GL et al: Technetium 99m phosphate for bone imaging. Radiology 110:391, 1973
129. Stringa G: Studies on the vascularization of bone grafts. J Bone Joint Surg 39B:395, 1957
130. Urist MR: Enzymes in bone morphogenesis: Endogenous enzymic degradation of the morphogenetic property in bone in solutions buffered by ethylenediaminetetraacetic acid (EDTA). In Hard Tissue Growth, Repair and Remineralization. Ciba Symposium 11, p 143. Amsterdam, Associated Scientific Publications, 1983
131. Urist MR: Practical applications of bone research on bone graft physiology. Instructional Course Lectures, American Academy of Orthopaedic Surgeons 25:1, 1976
132. Urist MR, Iwata H: Preservation and biodegradation of the bone morphogenetic property of bone matrix. J Theor Biol 38:155, 1973
133. Urist MR, McLean FC: Osteogenic potency and new bone formation by induction in transplants to the anterior chamber of the eye. J Bone Joint Surg 34A:443, 1952
134. Urist MR, Mikulski A, Boyd SD: A chemosterilized antigen-extracted auto-digested alloimplant for bone banks. Adv Immunol 12:117, 1970
135. Urist MR, Dowell TA, Hay PH et al: Induction substrates for bone induction. Clin Orthop 59:59, 1968
136. Urist MR et al: Bone morphogenesis in implants of insoluble bone gelatin. Proc Natl Acad Sci USA 70:3511, 1973
137. Volkov M: Allotransplantation of joints. J Bone Joint Surg 52B:526, 1970
138. Wilber MC, Hyatt CW: Bone and cysts—Results of surgical treatment in two hundred cases. J Bone Joint Surg 42A:879, 1960
139. Wilson PD Jr: A clinical study of the biomechanical behavior of massive bone transplants used to reconstruct large bone defects. Clin Orthop 87:81, 1972

Avascular Necrosis of Bone

140. Albrektsson B: Repair of diaphyseal defects: Experimental studies on the role of bone grafts in reconstruction of circumferential defects in long bones. Göteborg, Sweden, University of Göteborg, 1971
141. Bechtol CO: Bone as a structure. In Bechtol CO, Ferguson AB Jr, Laing PG (eds): Metals and Engineering in Bone and Joint Surgery, p 127. Baltimore, Williams & Wilkins, 1959
142. Bonfiglio M: Aseptic necrosis of the femoral head: Intact blood supply is of prognostic significance. In Proceedings of the Conference on Aseptic Necrosis of the Femoral Head, p 155. St. Louis, Nat. Inst. Health, 1964
143. Brooks M, et al: A new concept of capillary circulation in bone cortex: Some clinical applications. Lancet 1:1078, 1961
144. Enneking WF: In discussion of paper by Johnson LC, p 78. In Proceedings of the Conference on Aseptic Necrosis of the Femoral Head. St Louis, Nat. Inst. of Health, 1964
145. Enneking WF, Burchardt H, Puhl JJ et al: Physical and biological aspects of repair in dog cortical-bone transplants. J Bone Joint Surg 57A:237, 1975
146. Frost HM: In vivo osteocyte death. J Bone Joint Surg 42A:138, 1960
147. Henard DC, Calandruccio RA: Experimental production of roentgenographic and histological changes in the capital femoral epiphysis following abduction, extension and internal rotation of the hip. Proc Orthop Res Soc, J Bone Joint Surg 52A:601, 1970
148. Kenzora JE, et al: Tissue biology following experimental infarction of femoral heads, Part I. Bone studies. Proc Am Acad Orthop Surg, J Bone Joint Surg, 51A:1021, 1969
149. Petrokov V et al: Bridging over of large diaphyseal defects. Symp Biol Hung 7:87, 1967
150. Phemister DB: The fate of transplanted bone and regenerative power of its various constituents. Surg Gynecol Obstet 19:303, 1914
151. Phemister DB: Repair of bone in the presence of aseptic necrosis resulting from fractures, transplantations, vascular obstruction. J Bone Joint Surg 12:769, 1930
152. Phemister DB: Lesions of bones and joints arising from interruption of the circulation. J Mount Sinai Hospital 15:55, 1948
153. Puhl JJ, Piotrowski G, Enneking WF: Biomechanical properties of paired canine fibulas. J Biomech 5:391, 1972
154. Rhinelander FW: The normal microcirculation and its response to fracture. J Bone Joint Surg 50A:784, 1968
155. Rösingh GE, James J: Early phases of avascular necrosis of the femoral heads in rabbits. J Bone Joint Surg 51B:165, 1969
156. Rutishauser E, Majno G: Physiopathology of bone tissue. Bull Hosp Joint Dis 12:468, 1951
157. Schenk R, Willenegger H: Morphological findings in primary fracture healing: Callus formation. Symposium on Biology of Fracture Healing. Symp Biol Hung 7:75, 1967
158. Sherman MS, Selakovich WG: Bone changes in chronic circulatory insufficiency. J Bone Joint Surg 39A:892, 1957
159. Wilson PD, Lance EM: Surgical reconstruction of the skeleton following segmental resection in bone tumors. J Bone Joint Surg 47A:1629, 1965
160. Woodhouse CF: Anoxia of the femoral head. Surgery 52:55, 1962
161. Young RW: Nucleic acids, protein synthesis and bone. Clin Orthop 26:147, 1963

Dysbaric Osteonecrosis

162. Bell ALL, Edson GN, Hornick N: Characteristic bone and joint changes of compressed-air workers: A survey of symptomless cases. Radiology 38:698, 1942
163. Catto M: Pathology of aseptic necrosis. In Davidson JE (ed): Aseptic Necrosis of Bone, pp 3–100. Amsterdam, Excerpta Medica, 1976
164. Chryssanthou CP, Waskman M, Kousoyiannis M: Generation of SMAF activity in blood by gas bubbles. Undersea Biomed Res 1:A9, 1974
165. Chryssanthou CP: Dysbaric osteonecrosis in mice. Undersea Biomed Res 3:67, 1976
166. Chryssanthou CP: Dysbaric osteonecrosis. Clin Orthop 130:74, 1978
167. Coburn KR: Preliminary investigation of bone changes associated with decompression sickness. Aviat Med 27:163, 1956
168. Davidson JK, Griffiths PD: Caisson disease of bone. X-Ray Focus 10:2, 1970
169. Decompression Sickness Panel, Medical Research Council: Decompression sickness and aseptic necrosis of bone. Br J Ind Med 28:1, 1971
170. Editorial: Bone necrosis in divers. Lancet 2:263, 1974
171. Elliot DH, Harrison JAB: Bone necrosis—An occupational hazard of diving. JR Nav Med Serv 56:140, 1970
172. Elliot DH, Hallenbeck JM, Bove AA: Acute decompression sickness. Lancet 2:1193, 1974
173. Harvey CA: Decompression tables in relation to dysbaric osteonecrosis: Dysbarism related osteonecrosis (symposium proceedings), p 47. Washington, DC, U.S. Department of Health, Education and Welfare, 1974
174. Kim SK, Barry WF: Bone island. Am J Roentgenol 92:1301, 1964
175. Kindwall ED: Aseptic necrosis due to occupational exposure to compressed air: Experience with 62 cases. Fifth International Hyperbaric Congress Proceedings, p 863. Burnaby, Canada, Simon Fraser University, 1974
176. McCallum RI, Walder DN, Barnes R et al: Bone lesions in compressed-air workers. J Bone Joint Surg 48B:207, 1966
177. Mosinger M, Jullien G: L'expertise des ostéoarthroses consécutives aux accidents de décompression. Annales de Médicine Légale, Criminologie, Police Scientifique et Toxicologie 41:597, 1961
178. Norman A, Bullough P: The radiolucent crescent line—An early diagnostic sign of avascular necrosis of the femoral head. Bull Hosp Joint Dis 24:99, 1963
179. Ohta V, Matsunaga H: Bone lesions in divers. J Bone Joint Surg 56B:3, 1974
180. Philp RB, Schacham P, Gowdy CW: Involvement of platelets and microthrombi in experimental decompression sickness: Similarities with disseminated intravascular coagulation. Aerospace Med 42:494, 1971
181. Welfling J: Hip lesions in decompression disease. In Zinn WM (ed): Idiopathic Ischemic Necrosis of Femoral Head in Adults, p 103. Stuttgart, Georg Thieme, 1971

Hypercortisonism Osteonecrosis

182. Bravo JF, Herman JH, Smyth CJ: Musculoskeletal disorders after renal homotransplantation. Ann Intern Med 66:87, 1967
183. Fisher DE, Bickel WH: Cortisone-induced avascular necrosis:

A clinical study of seventy-seven patients. J Bone Joint Surg 53A:859, 1971
184. Fisher DE, Bickel WH, Holley KE et al: Cortisone-induced aseptic necrosis. II. Experimental study. Clin Orthop 84:200, 1972
185. Hill RB: Fatal fat embolism from steroid-induced fatty liver. N Engl J Med 265:318, 1961
186. Hill RB, Droke WA: Production of fatty liver in the rat by cortisone. Proc Soc Exp Biol Med 114:766, 1963
187. Jones JP Jr, Engleman EP, Narajian JS: Systemic fat embolism after renal homotransplantation and treatment with corticosteroids. N Engl J Med 273:1453, 1965
188. Jones JP Jr, Engleman EP, Steinbach HL et al: Fat embolism as a possible mechanism producing avascular necrosis. Arthritis Rheum 8:449, 1965
189. Jones JP Jr, Sakovich L: Fat embolism of bone: A roentgenographic and histological investigation, with use of intraarterial Lipiodol, in rabbits. J Bone Joint Surg 48A:149, 1966
190. Modell SH, Freeman LM: Avascular necrosis of bone in Cushing's syndrome. Radiology 83:1068, 1964
191. Moran TJ: Cortisone-induced alterations in lipid metabolism. Arch Pathol 73:300, 1962
192. Owens G, Sokal JE: Liver lipid as a source of embolic fat. J Appl Physiol 16:1100, 1961
193. Pietrogrande V, Mastromarino R: Osteopatia du prolongata trattamento cortisonico. Ortop e Traumatol dell' Apparato Motore 25:791, 1957
194. Solomon L: Drug-induced arthropathy and necrosis of the femoral head. J Bone Joint Surg 55B:246, 1973
195. Storey GO: Bone necrosis in joint disease. Proc Soc Med 61:961, 1968
196. Sweetnam DR, Mason RM, Murray RO: Steroid arthropathy of the hip. Br Med J 1:1392, 1960
197. Zinn WM: Idiopathic ischaemic necrosis of femoral head in adults. In Hill AGS (ed): Modern Trends in Rheumatology, Vol 2, p 348. London, Butterworth, 1971

Organ Transplant Osteonecrosis

198. Cruess RL, Blennerhassett J, MacDonald FR et al: Aseptic necrosis following renal transplantation. J Bone Joint Surg 50A:1577, 1968
199. Harrington KD, Murray WR, Kountz SL et al: Avascular necrosis of bone after renal tranaplantation. J Bone Joint Surg 53A:203, 1971
200. Kenzora JE, Glimcher MJ: The role of renal bone disease in the production of transplant osteonecrosis. Orthopedics 4:305, 1981
201. Kenzora JE, Sledge CB: Hip arthroplasty and the renal transplant patient. In The Hip (Proceedings Third Meeting Hip Society), p 35. St Louis, CV Mosby, 1975

Cadaver Bone Allografts—Bone Banks

202. Boyne PJ: Review of the literature on cryopreservation of bone. Cryobiology 4:341, 1968
203. Brown MD, Malinin TI, David PB: A roentgenographic evaluation of frozen allografts versus autografts in anterior cervical spine fusions. Clin Orthop 119:231, 1976, 1977
204. Büring K: In Sterilization and Preservation of Biological Tissue by Ionizing Radiation. Vienna, International Atomic Energy Agency, 1970
205. Burwell GR: The fate of freeze-dried bone allografts. Transplant Proc (Suppl 1) 8:195, 1976
206. Friedlander G: Antigenicity of freeze-dried allografts. Transplant Proc (Suppl 1) 8:195, 1976
207. Gresham RB: The freeze-dried cortical bone homograft: A roentgenographic and histologic evaluation. Clin Orthop 37:194, 1964
208. Malinin TI: University of Miami tissue bank. Transplant Proc (Suppl) 8:53, 1976
209. Ostrowski K: Current problems of tissue banking. Transplant Proc 1:126, 1969
210. Pappas AM: Current methods of freezing and freeze-drying. Cryobiology 4:358, 1968
211. Reynolds CF, Oliver DR, Ramsey R: Clinical evaluation of the merthiolate bone bank and homogenous bone grafts. J Bone Joint Surg 33A:873, 1951
212. Rish BL, McFadden JT, Penix JO: Anterior cervical fusion using homologous bone grafts: A comparative study. Surg Neurol 5:119, 1976
213. Sell KW, Billingham R, Russell P et al: (eds): Principles of Transplantation. Chicago, AMA, 1977
214 Urist MR, Mikulski A, Boyd SD: A chemosterilized antigen-extracted autodigested Allo-implant for bone banks. Arch Surg 110:416, 1975

Effects of Ionizing Radiation on Bone

215. Arkin AM, Simon N: Radiation scoliosis: Experimental study. J Bone Joint Surg 32A:396, 1950
216. Arlen M, Higinbotham NL, Huvos AG et al: Radiation-induced sarcoma of bone. Cancer 28:1087, 1971
217. Bickel WH, Childs DS, Poretta CM: Post-irradiation fractures of the femoral neck: Emphasis on the results of treatment. JAMA 175:204, 1961
218. Bonarigo BC, Rubin P: The non union of pathological fractures after radiation therapy. Radiology 88:889, 1967
219. Bragg DG, Schidnia H, Chu FCH et al: The clinical and radiographic aspects of radiation osteitis. Radiology 97:103, 1970
220. Caceres E, Zaharia M: Massive preoperative radiation therapy in the treatment of osteogenic sarcoma. Cancer 30:634, 1972
221. Cahan WG, Woodard HQ, Higinbotham NL et al: Sarcoma arising in irradiated bone: Report of eleven cases. Cancer 1:3, 1948
222. Dalinka MK, Edeiken J, Finkelstein JB: Complications of radiation therapy: Adult bone. Semin Roentgenol 9:29, 1974
223. Del Regato JA: Dental lesions observed after roentgen therapy in cancer of buccal cavity, pharynx and larynx. Am J Roentgenol 42:404, 1939
224. Friedman MA, Carter SK: The therapy of osteogenic sarcoma: Current status and thoughts for the future. J Surg Oncol 4:482, 1972
225. Grant BP, Fletcher GH: Analysis of complications following megavoltage therapy for squamous cell carcinomas of the tonsillar area. Am J Roentgenol 96:28, 1966
226. Gratzek FR, Holstrom FG Rigler LG: Post-irradiation bone changes. Am J Roentgenol 96:26, 1966
227. Hatcher CH: The development of sarcoma in bone subjected to roentgen or radium irradiation. J Bone Joint Surg 27:179, 1945
228. Hinkel CL: Effect of roentgen rays upon growing long bones

of albino rats: Quantitative studies of growth limitation following irradiation. Am J Roentgenol 47:439, 1942
229. Hinkel CL: The effect of irradiation upon composition and vascularity of growing rat bones. Am J Roentgenol, 50:516, 1943
230. Hinkel CL: The effect of roentgen rays upon growing long bones in albino rats; histopathological changes involving endochondral growth centers. Am J Roentgenol 49:321, 1943
231. Jenkin RDT, Allt WEC, Fitzpatrick PJ: Osteosarcoma: An assessment of management with particular reference to primary irradiation and selective delayed amputation. Cancer 30:393, 1972
232. Katzman H, Waugh T, Berdon W: Skeletal changes following irradiation of childhood tumors. J Bone Joint Surg 51A:825, 1969
233. MacComb WS: Necrosis in treatment of intraoral cancer by radiation therapy. Am J Roentgenol 87:431, 1962
234. McCrorie WDC: Fractures of the femoral neck following pelvic irradiation. Br J Radiol 23:587, 1950
235. Neuhauser RB, Wittenborg MH, Berman CZ et al: Irradiation effects of roentgen therapy on the growing spine. Radiology 59:637, 1952
236. Ng E, Chambers FW Jr, Ogden HS et al: Osteomyelitis of the mandible following irradiation: An experimental study. Radiology 72:68, 1959
237. Phillips RD, Kimeldorf DJ: Acute and long-term effects of x-irradiation on skeletal growth in the rat. Am J Physiol 207:1447, 1964
238. Royster RL, King ER, Ebersole J et al: High dose preoperative supervoltage irradiation for osteogenic sarcoma. Am J Roentgenol 114:536, 1972
239. Rubin P, Andrews JR, Swarm R et al: Radiation induced dysplasias of bone. Am J Roentgenol 82:206, 1959
240. Rubin P, Casarett GW: Clinical Radiation Pathology, Vol II. Philadelphia, WB Saunders, 1968
241. Rubin P, Duthie RB, Young LW: The significance of scoliosis in post-irradiated Wilms' tumor and neuroblastoma. Radiology 79:539, 1962
242. Rubin P, Prabhasawat D: Characteristic bone lesions in post-irradiated carcinoma of the cervix. Radiology 76:703, 1961
243. Rubin P, Squire L: Clinical concepts in bone modeling. Am J Roentgenol 82:217, 1959
244. Rutherford H, Dodd GD: Complications of radiation therapy: Growing bone. Semin Roentgenol 9:15, 1974
245. Stephenson WH, Cohen B: Post-irradiation fractures of the neck of the femur. J Bone Joint Surg 38B:830, 1956
246. Vaeth JM, Levitt SH, Jones MD, et al: Effects of radiation therapy in survivors of Wilms' tumor. Radiology 79:560, 1962
247. Weatherby RP, Dahlin DC, Ivins JC: Postradiation sarcoma of bone: Review of 78 Mayo Clinic cases. Mayo Clin Proc 56:294, 1981
248. Whitehouse WM, Lampe I: Osseous damage in irradiation of renal tumors in infancy and childhood. Am J Roentgenol 70:721, 1953

4

Histology of Skeletal Muscle

MUSCLES are built up of fibers about 1 mm in diameter. The contractile material within the fibers consists of myofibrils which are long thin structures, usually about a micrometer or so in diameter, many thousands of which act in parallel. The myofibrils have a very characteristic pattern of bands along their length, repeating at intervals of about 2.5 μm (Fig. 4-1*A*). The details of the structures that give rise to the bands can only be resolved by electron microscopy (EM) and x-ray diffraction data.

In the resting state the muscle is soft and extensible. When stimulated electrically by means of its motor nerve, the contractile process is brought about by a series of events the nature of which is the subject of ongoing research. The current concept suggests that calcium ions are rapidly liberated throughout the muscle fibers and activate an enzyme, an ATPase, located in the structural protein complex of muscle, actomyosin. The contractile material then undergoes a very rapid change in its properties. It becomes much more rigid, develops a large tension—several kilograms per square meter—and shortens rapidly, often at a rate equivalent to many times its own length per second.

MICROANATOMY

Surrounding the muscle, there is a connective tissue sheath, the epimysium, from the deep surface of which septa pass into the muscle at irregular intervals.[1] These septa, the perimysium, invest bundles, the fasciculi, of muscle fibers, the bundles being of somewhat angular outline in section and of varying sizes. Subdivision of the larger bundles into two or three smaller bundles may be observed. From the perimysium, very delicate extensions of fine connective tissue, the endomysium, extend inward to surround each muscle fiber (Fig. 4-1*B*).

The size of the fasciculi composing a muscle determines its texture. In muscles designed for fine movements (*e.g.*, ocular muscles) fasciculi are small and texture is fine, whereas in muscles which require less precision but greater power (*e.g.*, gluteal muscles) fasciculi are larger and texture is coarse.

Where the deep fascia is well developed (*e.g.*, fascia lata), it is separated from the underlying muscle by areolar tissue. Where muscles take origin from the deep fascia, the epimysium is a direct extension of the deep fascia.

The connective tissue elements of muscle include collagen fibers, elastic fibers, and several varieties of cells such as fibroblasts, histiocytes, and fat cells. The amount of elastic tissue is greatest in those muscles attached to soft parts (*e.g.*, tongue muscles). Between individual muscle fibers, the connective tissue is scanty, consists of reticular fibers and fine collagen fibers, and contains capillaries and fine nerves. The larger blood vessels and nerves lie within the perimysium between adjacent fasciculi, the site where muscle spindles are found. When

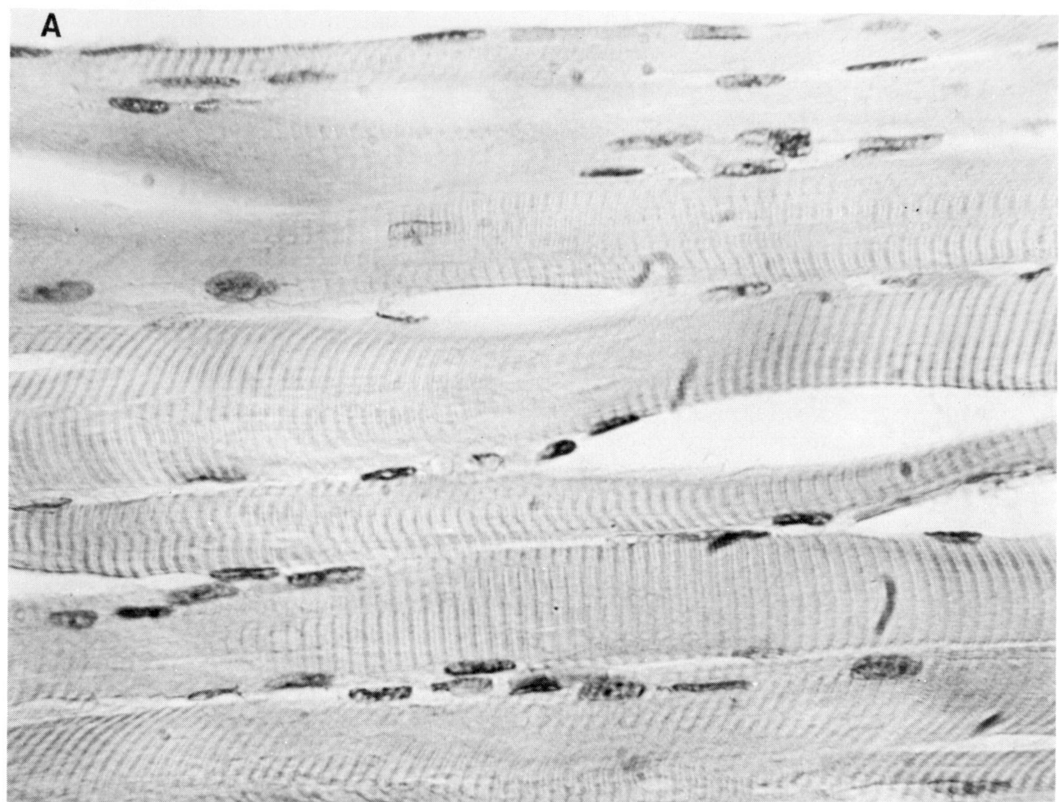

FIG. 4-1. (*A*) Striated muscle, longitudinal section. Note that the fibers do not branch or anastomose. Invisible sarcolemma envelops muscle substance. Each fiber has many flattened, slender sarcolemmal nuclei lying peripherally beneath the membrane and oriented parallel with the long axis of the fiber. In muscle disease these nuclei come to occupy a central position. Large numbers of axially disposed myofibrils are contained within the fiber. (× 670), (*B*) Striated muscle, cross section. An enlargement of a muscle fiber is depicted. The myofibrils are separated by sarcoplasm.

a muscle is extended beyond its relaxed, resting length, the tension develops solely within its connective tissue. During muscle regeneration, the endomysial sheaths of individual muscle fibers (*i.e.*, their investing connective tissue tubes) act as cylindrical guides that direct the formation of new fibers as they sprout from the old.

STRUCTURE OF MUSCLE FIBERS

The basic contractile unit of muscle is the fiber (Fig. 4-2).[5] Each fiber is an assembly of contractile material enclosed within an electrically polarized membrane. Muscle fibers vary in diameter from 10 μ to 100 μ. Their lengths vary depending on the type and construction of the entire muscle.

Each fiber is a multinucleate cell formed during embryonic development by the coalescence of a large number of mononucleated myoblasts. In addition to the contractile material, muscle fibers contain the normal constituents of other cell types—mitochondria, ribosomes, storage granules, and glycogen particles. They contain an elaborate system, the sarcoplasmic reticulum, which is concerned with turning on and off the contractile mechanism, probably by controlling the level of calcium ions in the muscle.

THE MYOFIBRILS

The myofibrils are 1 μ to 2 μ in diameter and extend the entire length of the fiber. They have a banded appearance and are arranged in register within the fiber, giving rise to the characteristic cross-striated appearance of the muscle fiber (Fig. 4-3). These fibrils of muscle show a periodic system of transverse bands which results from a variation of density along their lengths. The individual repeat pattern is called the *sarcomere.* In vertebrate muscles at resting length, the sarcomere measures 2.3 μ to 2.8 μ.

The ends of the sarcomere are bounded by narrow dense lines or disks termed Z lines. Within each sarco-

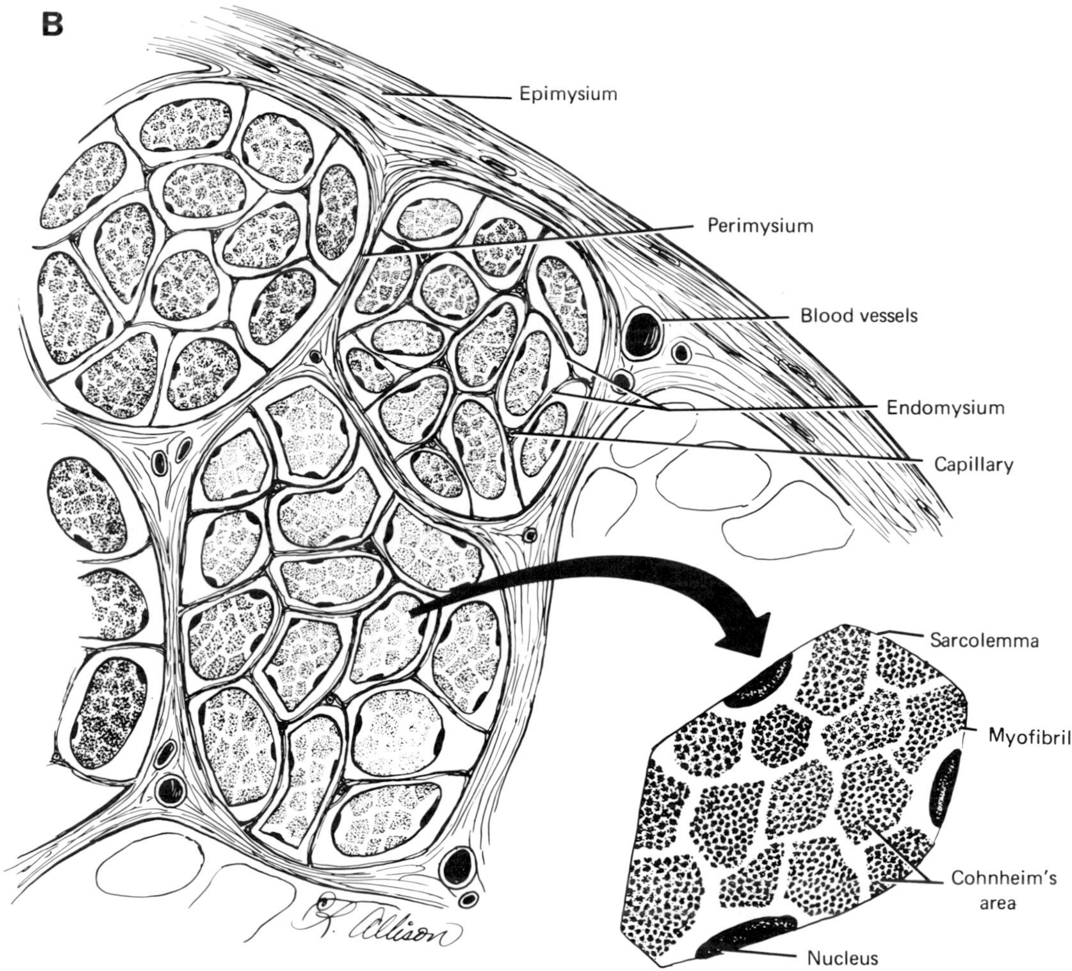

mere, under polarized light, a central birefringent zone is known as the A (anisotropic) band. To either side of the A band and separating it from the Z bands are zones of lower density which are weakly birefringent and are known as the I (isotropic) bands. The central region of the A band in a relaxed muscle is somewhat less dense than the lateral regions of the band. This central lighter area is known as the H zone. A narrow dense line, the M line, about 400 A to 800 A in width, extends across the center of the H band, flanked on either side by narrow zones of lighter density than the rest of the H zone; the width of the whole central H zone is about 1500 A (Figs. 4-4 and 4-5).

THE FILAMENTS

The band pattern arises because the myofibrils are composed of a long series of partially overlapping arrays of longitudinal protein filaments. Under the EM, one can observe only thin filaments, about 50 A to 70 A in diameter, corresponding to the I bands; both thin and thick filaments are situated in the outer portions of the A bands.[4]

The thick filaments are continuous from one end of the A band to the other; the thin filaments, on the other hand, extend into but not as far as the center of the A band, terminating at a point corresponding to the boundary of the H zone. In any single animal species, all the thick filaments have the same characteristic length and are arranged in register; all the thin filaments also have the same lengths and are arranged in register. Consequently, the overlapping perfectly arrayed filaments give rise to sharply defined variations in density along the length of the fibrils, resulting in the characteristic banded appearance.

When cross sections of striated muscle are visualized under the EM, the appearance depends on the portion of the sarcomere through which the section has passed and the relative content of thick and thin filaments.

In the I band region, only thin diameter (50–70 A) filaments are seen. Near the central region of the A band,

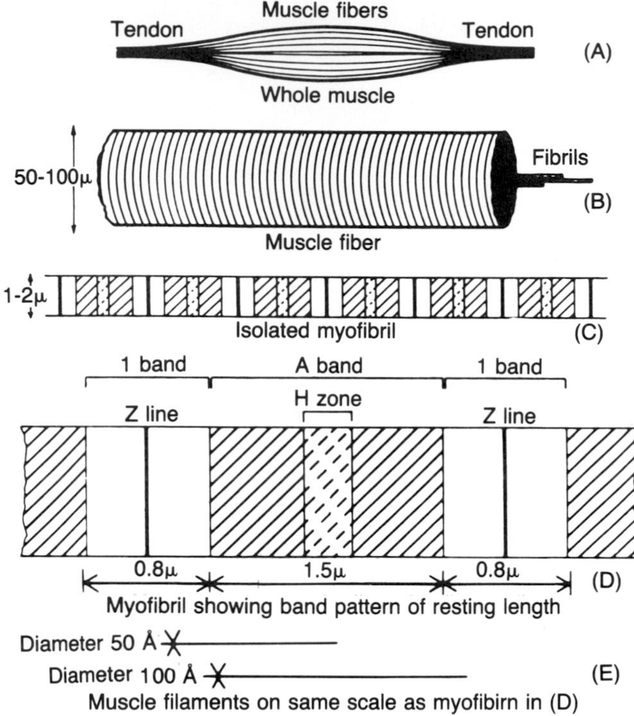

FIG.4-2. The dimensions and arrangement of the contractile components in a muscle. The whole muscle (*A*) is made up of fibers (*B*) which contain cross-striated myofibrils (*C, D*). These are constructed of two kinds of protein filaments (*E*) that overlap and interdigitate in a stereospecific manner. (Huxley HE: The molecular basis of contraction. In Bourne GH (ed): The Structure and Function of Muscle. New York, Academic Press, 1972)

within the H zone, only thicker filaments are seen, arranged a few hundred Angström units apart in a very regular hexagonal lattice. If the section is passed through the denser lateral parts of the A band, a double array of filaments is seen, with the thicker filaments at the points of the hexagonal lattice and the thinner filaments lying between them. The latter lie at the trigonal points of the hexagonal lattice (*i.e.*, symmetrically between three thick filaments).

The thick filaments taper at either end, over the last 1500 A or so of their length. At the very center of the A band, they are especially thickened, and cross-bridges between the thick filaments can be observed at this point.

In very thin sections, cross-bridges extend from the thick filaments to the thin filaments alongside them. These occur at intervals of about 400 A between a given thick and thin filament. Since there are six thin filaments around each thick one, there must be six cross-bridges leaving each thick filament for every 400 A of its length. The cross-bridges extending outward from the thick filaments are especially visible in the H zone where there are no thin filaments. On the other hand, no such projections are seen on the thin filaments in the I bands. The cross-bridges projecting from the thick filaments are about 50 A wide and 100 A long (Fig. 4-6).

PROTEIN COMPONENTS OF FILAMENTS

The two principal proteins in skeletal muscle are myosin and actin. Myosin can be extracted from muscles by strong salt solutions (*e.g.*, 0.47 M, 0.16 M phosphate

FIG. 4-3. A single muscle fiber from human muscle, fixed, sained, embedded in plastic, sectioned longitudinally, and viewed at relatively low magnification in the EM. The striations of the muscle fiber can be seen to arise from the characteristic band pattern of the myofibrils, visible here, with diameters of about 1 μ. The diameter of this fiber is about 55 μ. At the edge of the fiber, several nuclei can be seen just below the surface membrane (sarcolemma). (× 1600) (Huxley HE: The molecular basis of contraction. In Bourne GH (ed): The Structure and Function of Muscle. New York, Academic Press, 1972)

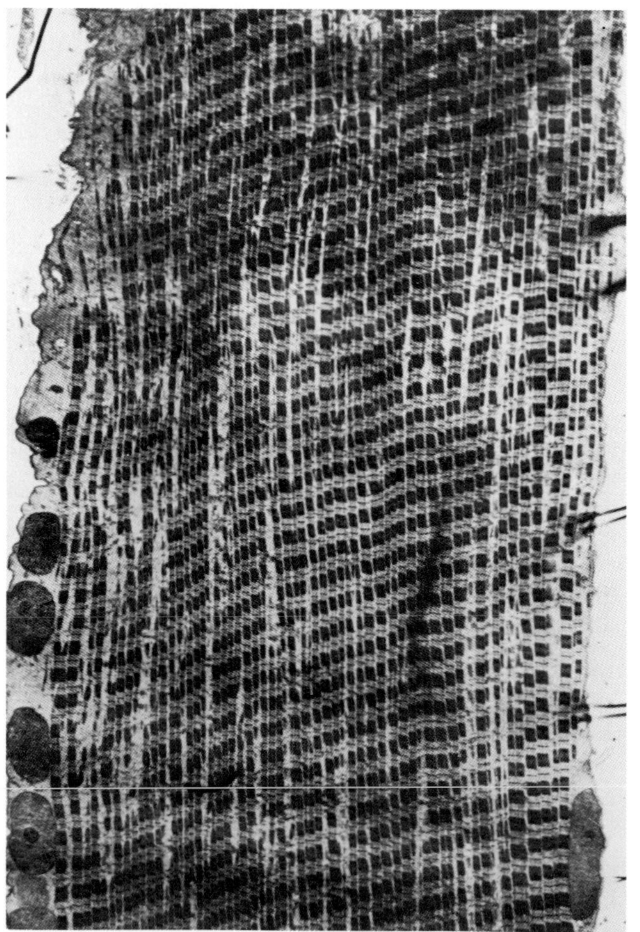

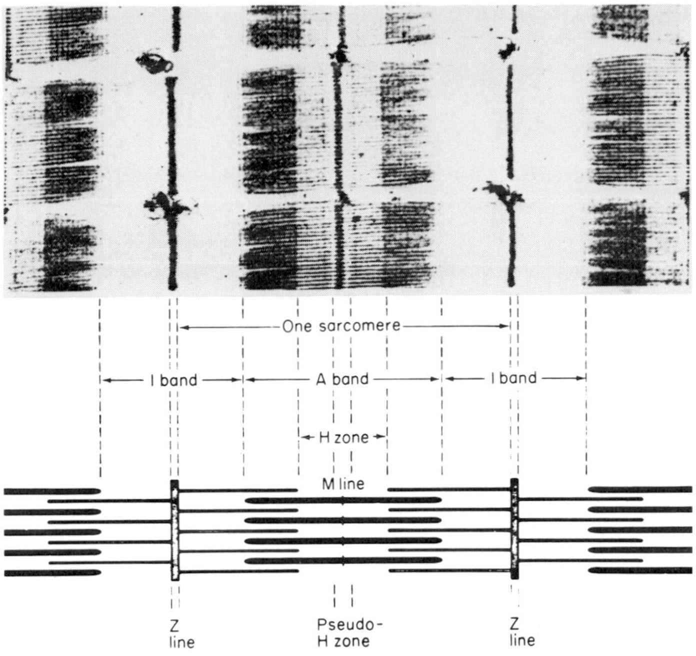

One sarcomere
I band
A band
I band
H zone
M line
Z line
Pseudo-H zone
Z line

FIG. 4-4. Longitudinal section of frog sartorius muscle (*top*) together with a diagram showing the overlap of filaments that gives rise to the band pattern. The A band is most dense in its lateral zones where the thick and thin filaments overlap. The central zone of the A band (the H zone) is less dense, since it contains thick filaments only. The I bands are less dense still because they contain only thin filaments. The sarcomere length here is about 2.5 μ. (Huxley HE: The molecular basis of contraction. In Bourne GH (ed): The Structure and Function of Muscle. New York, Academic Press, 1972)

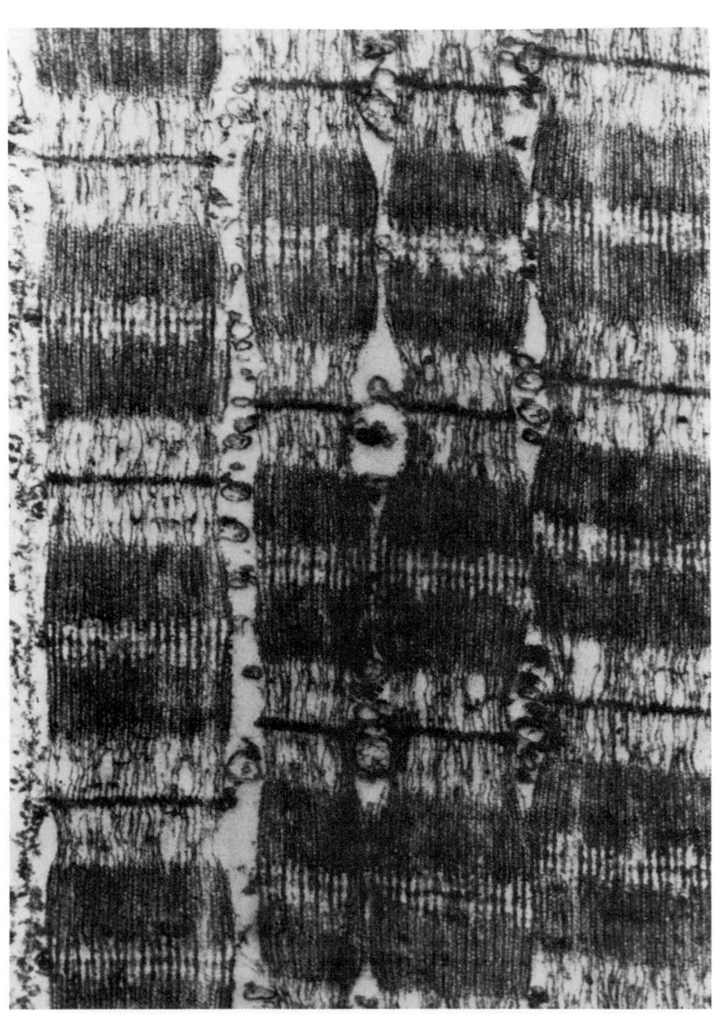

FIG. 4-5. Longitudinal section of muscle cut sufficiently thin so that only single layers of filaments lie within the plane of the section. The thick and thin filaments can be clearly seen, thick filaments in the A bands, and thin filaments in the I bands and extending into the A bands. (× 53,000) (Huxley HE: The molecular basis of contraction. In Bourne GH (ed): The Structure and Function of Muscle. New York, Academic Press, 1972)

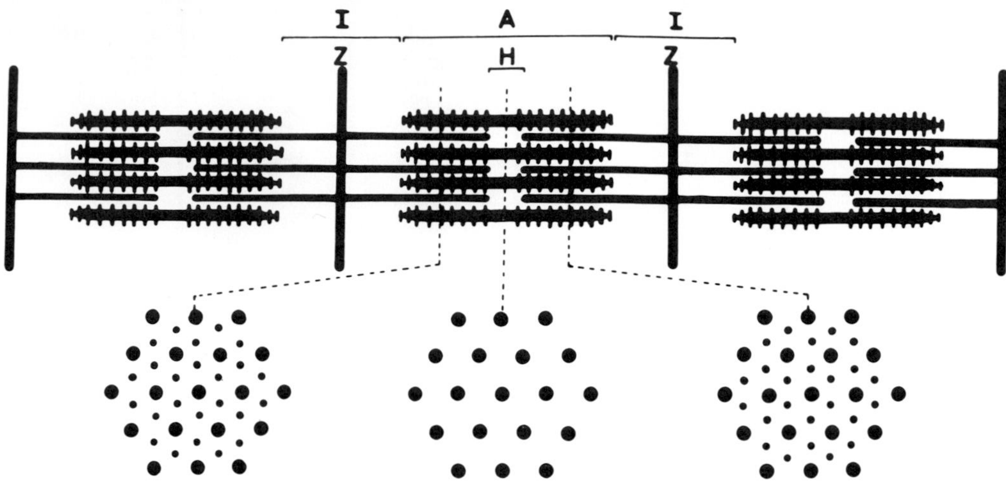

FIG.4-6. Structure of striated muscle, showing overlapping arrays of actin- and myosin-containing filaments, the latter with projecting cross-bridges on them. To facilitate showing the relationships, the diagram is drawn with considerable longitudinal foreshortening, with filament diameters and side-spacings as shown. The filament lengths should be about five times the lengths shown. (Huxley HE: The molecular basis of contraction. In Bourne GH (ed): The Structure and Function of Muscle. New York, Academic Press, 1972)

buffer) in the presence of agents that keep myosin and actin dissociated from each other, either the indigenous ATP present in recently dissected muscles or added pyrophosphate (10 mM) plus magnesium. With a short extraction time, not much actin is removed. Once extracted, the myosin can be precipitated at low ionic strength and estimated.[8] Under the phase-contrast microscope, it can be seen that the dense A bands of the fibrils dissolve and leave a ghost fibril, consisting of Z lines and segments to either side of each Z line with the density of I bands. These I segments extend from the Z lines to the position of the edges of the original H zone. The thick filaments have been dissolved and only the thin filaments containing actin remain.

These biochemical estimations and interference microscope measurements indicate that all the myosin is located in the thick filaments.

After myosin has been extracted, actin can be extracted by 0.6 M potassium iodide. Following this, examination of the myosin-free fibrils under the phase-contrast LM will show that a large portion of the residual I segments will have been extracted.

Actin and myosin *in vitro* form a complex actomyosin, which contracts when treated with ATP. Neither protein by itself is contractile.[3]

The structural protein myosin is also an enzyme, an ATPase necessary to an energy-yielding reaction, the splitting off of the terminal phosphate of ATP.

CHANGES IN THE BAND PATTERN DURING CONTRACTION AND STRETCH

Over a wide range of muscle lengths, whether fibers are subjected to passive stretch or contraction (isometric, isotonic), the length of the A band does not change perceptibly. Changes in the length of the sarcomere occur within the I band alone.

When the muscle has contracted down to about 60% of its resting length, the I bands disappear and the A bands come into contact with the adjacent Z lines. If contraction proceeds beyond this point (which under physiological conditions it does not), contraction bands form around the Z lines. The thick filaments making up the A band remain at constant length during both stretch and contraction, as indicated by the unchanging A band.

In stretched myofibrils, the H zones become wider, and during shortening the H zones become narrower and disappear at about 85% of rest length, being replaced on further shortening by a dense line. In myosin-extracted fibrils, these different lengths of the H zone are duplicated by the lengths of the gap between the ends of the thin filaments. In extreme contraction, where the H zone is replaced by a dark line, this line remains after extraction of myosin. The conclusion is that the two sets of filaments do not change their lengths perceptibly over a considerable range of muscle lengths and must slide past each other. In extreme contraction, a double overlap of the thin actin-containing filaments occurs at the center of the A band, thus accounting for a central zone which is denser than the rest of the A band.

THE HUXLEY HYPOTHESIS OF MUSCLE CONTRACTION

Since the principal muscle proteins, myosin and actin, are involved in contraction and are organized into separate filaments that slide past each other during contraction, a relative sliding force must be developed between the filaments. The chemical reaction involves splitting off the terminal phosphate of ATP, a basic energy-yielding reaction. The splitting of ATP by the enzymelike myosin is strongly activated by actin.

When a muscle is activated, an interaction occurs between myosin molecules in the thick filaments and actin molecules in the thin filaments. This enables myosin to split ATP at a rapid rate, thereby providing the energy for the force which causes the filaments to slide past each other.

Cross-bridges on thick filaments are visible under the EM and their presence is confirmed by low-angle x-ray diffraction studies. These projections represent the parts of the myosin molecules that interact with actin.[4] These structures allow direct physical contact between myosin and actin, activating ATPase, and developing the relative sliding movement between filaments of the order of several thousand Angströms during shortening. The reasonable assumption is that cross-bridges function repetitively during contraction, each one going through many cycles of enzymatic and structural change as the muscle shortens. In such a model, the cross-bridge attaches to a monomer in the actin filament in one configuration; the structural change draws the actin filament a certain distance. The cross-bridge then releases and returns to its starting position (Fig. 4-7).

Meanwhile, other bridges become attached and a steady force develops. Each time a cross-bridge goes through a cycle, one (or two) molecules of ATP ar split. When activation is ended, interaction between cross-bridges and actin filaments ceases, ATP splitting falls to a low level, no sliding force develops, and the muscle once again is extended to its resting length.

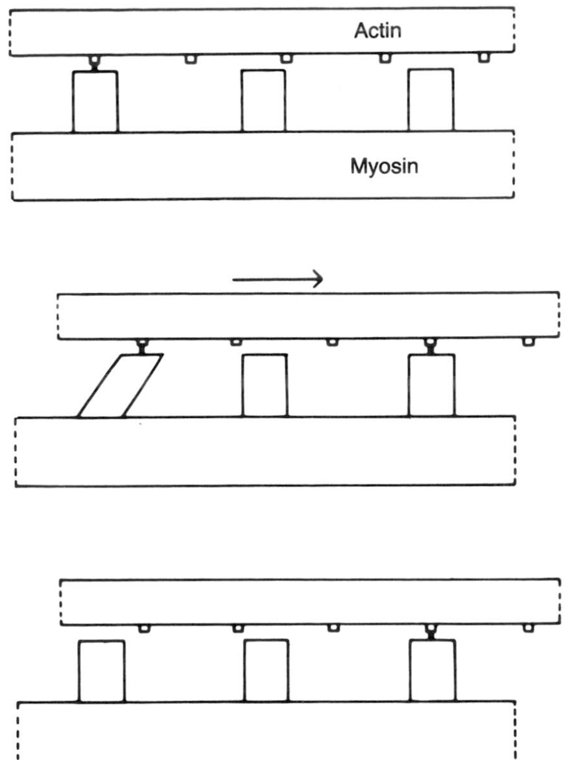

FIG. 4-7. Possible mode of action of cross-bridges. A cross-bridge attaches to a specific site on the actin filament, then undergoes some configurational change that causes the point of attachment to move closer to the center of the A band, pulling the actin filament along in the required manner. At the end of its working stroke, the bridge detaches and returns to its starting configuration in preparation for another cycle. During each cycle, probably one molecule of ATP is dephosphorylated. Asynchronous attachment of other bridges maintains steady force. (Huxley HE: The molecular basis of contraction. In Bourne GH (ed): The Structure and Function of Muscle. New York, Academic Press, 1972)

MOLECULAR STRUCTURE OF FILAMENTS

THE MYOSIN FILAMENT

The molecular weight of myosin is approximately 475,000 and the number of myosin molecules in each thick filament is about 384. Under EM, the number of cross-bridges is approximately 216 (about 18 sets of six bridges in each half of an A band). This is confirmed by x-ray diffraction which indicates that there are six cross-bridges in each interval of 429 A along the thick filaments. The number of cross-bridges may represent the active part of either one or two myosin molecules.

Under the EM, individual myosin molecules are seen as long rod-shaped structures with a globular region at one end.[6] The rods are about 20 A in diameter and 1500 A in length, and the globular region appears to be about 50 A in diameter and 100 A to 200 A in length. The globular region consists of two separate subunits (Fig. 4-8).

Proteolytic digestion cleaves the myosin into two well-defined subfragments. Tryptic digestion breaks myosin into two large pieces, called heavy meromyosin (HMM) and light meromyosin (LMM).[7] HMM carries the biologic activity of myosin, (*i.e.*, its ATPase activity and actin-binding activity) and is soluble at all ionic strengths. LMM carries the self-assembly properties (*i.e.*, the ability to aggregate into filaments at physiologic ionic strengths).

Under the EM, LMM is seen to be a simple rod-shaped structure, having the same diameter as the rod part of intact myosin, and about 960 A in length. HMM appear as a double-headed tadpole-shaped structure (*i.e.*, two globules sharing a short tail) about 400 A to 500 A in length. A satisfactory model for myosin, therefore, places these two subfragments end to end, with a short-trypsin-sensitive junction between them.

Using papain as a cleaving agent, the globular portion can be separated from the rod portion, and is found to consist of identical subunits, the S1 subfragments. Each of the S1 subfragments has a molecular weight of about 117,000 and has actin-activated ATPase activity and actin-binding ability like the parent myosin. The rod part of HMM (S2) is soluble at all ionic strengths.

The myosin molecule is built out of two probably identical polypeptide chains wound around each other to form a two-chain α-helix in the long rod part of the molecule, and then continuing on and folding up separately in the two S1 head units.

X-ray diffraction observations suggest that the LMM parts of the myosin molecules are arranged with their long axes parallel to the long axis of the muscle. This implies that the backbone of the filaments is made up of LMM, with the HMM projecting out sideways at regular intervals to interact with the actin filaments alongside.

In summary, the myosin molecules are placed in pairs, one on either side of a thick filament, and successive pairs are situated at 143-A intervals and rotated relative to each other so as to place the projecting cross-bridges on a 429-A helix. If the entire rod part of myosin is about 1500 A in length, a cross section of a filament will include about 20 molecules. The terminal ends of the filaments are tapered. The cross-bridges extend outward to a radius of about 130 A from the center of the thick filaments, and extend about 70 A from the surface of the thick filaments. Therefore, in resting muscle, the linear portion of HMM (*i.e.*, the S2 rod) is likely to be closely applied to the backbone.

In a thick filament, the central portion is bare of projections. All the myosin molecules in one half of the filament are oriented in one direction, and all those in the other half of the filament are oriented in the other direction. The length of the bridge-free central region is determined by the packing arrangements in which antiparallel molecules overlap. In other words, the polarity

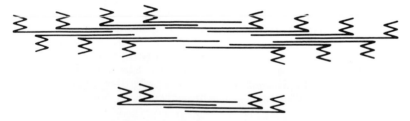

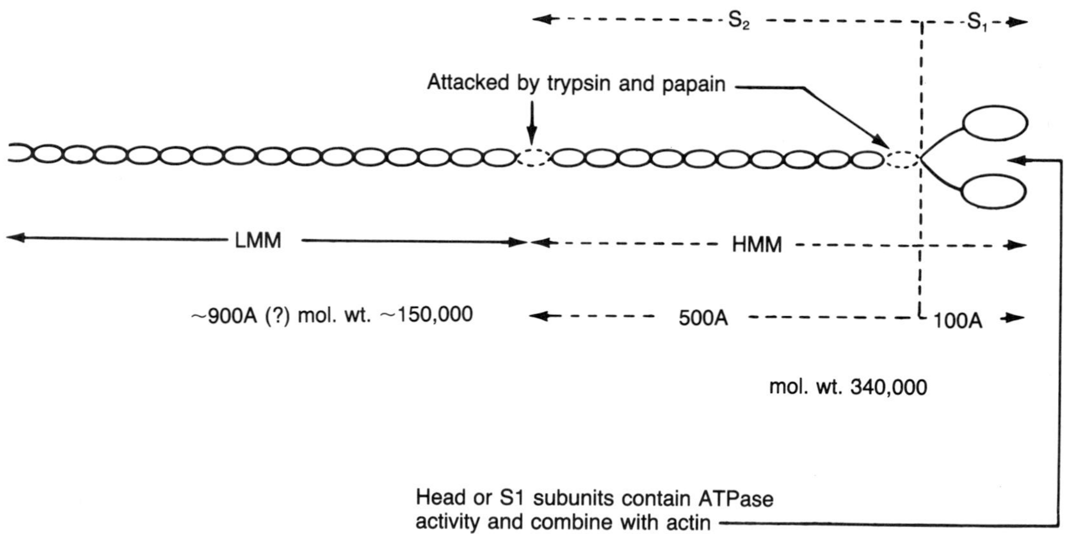

FIG. 4-8. A myosin molecule. (After Lowey S et al: Substructure of the myosin molecule. J Mol Biol 42:1, 1969)

FIG. 4-9. (*Top*) Possible arrangement of myosin molecules, with globular region at one end only, to produce short filaments of type observed, with globular region at either end and straight shaft in center. The polarity of the myosin molecules is simply reversed on either side of the center. (*Bottom*) Possible arrangement of same myosin molecules to produce longer filaments in which the straight shaft in the center is still present, but in which a longer region on either side now has globular projections on it. The polarity of the myosin molecules is reversed on either side of the center, but all the molecules on the same side have the same polarity. (Huxley HE: The molecular basis of contraction. In Bourne GH (ed): The Structure and Function of Muscle. New York, Academic Press, 1972)

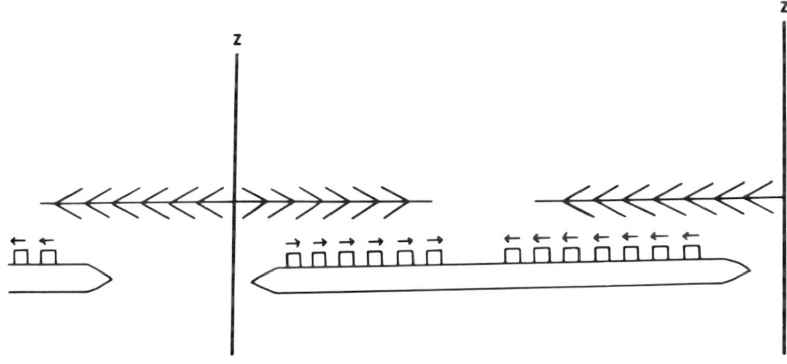

FIG. 4-10. Structural polarity of cross-bridges on myosin filaments and of molecules of actin in the thin filaments, showing how their interaction could produce sliding forces that would move the actin filaments toward each other in the center of the sarcomere. (Huxley HE: The molecular basis of contraction. In Bourne GH (ed): The Structure and Function of Muscle. New York, Academic Press, 1972)

of the myosin molecules is reversed on either side of the center, but all molecules on the same side have the same polarity (Fig. 4-9).

The significance of this arrangement is to generate forces by cross-bridges that draw the actin filaments toward the center of the A band. Thus two actin filaments are drawn toward each other and provide the shortening mechanism (Fig. 4-10).

THE ACTIN FILAMENTS

The actin filaments form a two-chain helical structure with a subunit repeat of 54.6 A along either chain and a helical repeat of 360 A to 370 A. These I filaments extend from the Z line, to which they are attached, to the H zone, and are about 1 μ in length. Each I filament contains about 360 to 370 actin monomers. The molecular weight is 47,600. Actin forms a tight complex with the regulatory protein system, tropomyosin and troponin.

The tropomyosin forms a continuous structure along the thin filaments, is a fibrous molecule of molecular weight about 70,000, a length of about 450 A, and follows a helical path in the actin filament, perhaps in the two grooves between the subunits.[2] It consists of two identical polypeptide chains. Approximately one tropomyosin period (385 A) corresponds to the spacing occupied by seven actin monomers (Fig. 4-11).

Troponin binds to I filaments by an approximate 400-A periodicity, corresponding to a specific binding site for troponin on the tropomyosin molecules.

Actin monomers are globular units of protein molecules with very specific myosin-binding and ATPase-activating sites on their surfaces, and embracing regulatory proteins. Actin enters into a very stereospecific combination with the S1 subunits of myosin. The polarity of the actin filaments is reversed on either side of the Z lines, corresponding with the reversed orientation of the cross-bridges. All the monomers in both chains of an actin filament are oriented in the same direction, and this polarity reverses at the Z lines.

The actin filaments are not continuous through the Z line, but are joined there to some other structure providing mechanical stability to hold them in register and ensuring reversal of polarity.

MOLECULAR CHANGES DURING CONTRACTION

ACTIVATION OF MYOSIN ATPase BY ACTIN

ATPase of purified myosin at neutral *p*H and in the presence of magnesium acts on its own but at a relatively low rate. However, in the presence of actin, under conditions of ionic strength that favor the association of

FIG. 4-11. A model for the fine structure of the thin filament. In this model it is assumed that two molecules of tropomyosin and troponin exist in each period (cf. Ebashi, *et al.*, 1968). The pitch of the double helix in the thin filament formed by the actin molecules is considered to be 360 A to 370 A, which is slightly shorter than the period due to troponin. (After Ebashi: Quart Rev Biophysics 2:351, 1969)

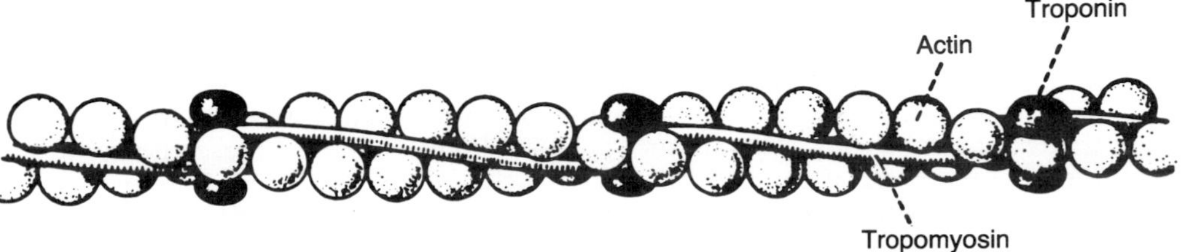

myosin and actin (*i.e.*, the physiological range), the ATPase activity is greatly increased.

When the myosin cross-bridge is not attached to the actin filaments, the enzyme site of the myosin splits ATP very slowly, but when attachment occurs the splitting is greatly accelerated. Only those cross-bridges attached to thin filaments are able to complete the cycle of splitting of ATP, and this provides the mechanism by which the use of energy by the muscle can be regulated.

ALTERATION OF CONTRACTION BY CALCIUM IONS

A regulatory protein complex in actin filaments consists of tropomyosin and troponin. In the absence of calcium, this regulatory complex prevents actin from activating the myosin ATPase. This inhibition is removed when calcium is supplied by release from the reticulum.

Under *in vitro* conditions, in the absence of the tropomyosin-troponin complex, actin activates myosin ATPase whether calcium is present or not. The manner by which this inhibitory mechanism is exercised has not yet been clearly established.

SUMMARY OF MECHANISM OF MUSCULAR CONTRACTION

The contraction of striated skeletal muscle is brought about by some mechanism that generates a relative sliding force between partly overlapping arrays of actin and myosin filaments. Strong evidence indicates that cross-bridges projecting from the myosin filaments, and carrying ATPase and actin-binding sites, are involved in the generation of this force in some cyclical process. The actual force-generating structure, the two subunits of myosin, is attached to the backbone of the myosin filaments by a linkage, 400 A long, which has flexible couplings at either end; the force-generating structure can therefore attach itself to the actin filament, in a constant configuration, and undergo the same structural changes, and produce the same longtitudinal force over a wide range of interfilament separations. The muscle structure is arranged so that the linkage is under tension, not compression, when a contractile force is being generated. A feature of the contraction mechanism is the rigid attachment of the globular head of the myosin molecule to the actin filament, perhaps an active change in the angle of attachment, and splitting of ATP.

In the relaxed fiber, thin filaments are composed of two helicoidal rows of G-actin molecules, with two strands of tropomyosin between the rows and, at 400 A intervals, the troponin complex. The troponin complex combines with tropomyosin which in turn combines with the G-actin molecules. At a distance of 135 A from the thin filaments are the thick filaments which are composed entirely of myosin molecules. The space is bridged, but only partly, by the protruding globular heads of myosin molecules which approach, but do not make contact with, the G-actin molecules.

Calcium ions are absent. Troponin combining with tropomyosin appears to prevent G-actin from interacting with the myosin heads. When the fibril contracts, calcium ions appear within the myofibril and interact with troponin, freeing the latter from tropomyosin. The inhibitory influence on the G-actin is thereby removed, and the latter then combines with the myosin heads.

The extent of sliding of actin filaments along myosin filaments is greater than the distance between any two successive myosin heads on the thick filaments. This suggests that the myosin heads alternately disconnect and reconnect to new sites along the actin filaments.

The source of energy for muscle contraction may be summarized as follows: As calcium ions release the inhibitory effect of troponin through tropomyosin, actin and myosin combine to trigger the contraction. The energy required for the reactions is provided by splitting of ATP to ADP and free phosphate ions, a reaction that releases large amounts of energy. However, there is no great amount of ATP in muscle. Therefore, the ATP broken down during contraction must be rapidly restored. This is provided by splitting phosphocreatine, a process which occurs at the same time. The amount of phosphocreatine is limited and must also be replenished. Consequently, other sources of energy are required for the resynthesis of phosphocreatine and ATP. This is provided by the combustion of glycogen and other metabolites in the presence of oxygen, but only after the contraction has been completed. The store of glycogen is large, and its oxidation yields sufficient energy for as much as 10,000 contractions. When the supply of oxygen is insufficient, as may occur during exercise, energy may still be obtained from glycogen anaerobically. In this case glycogen is not oxidized but instead is transformed into lactic acid, but the energy thus produced is sufficient only for a very limited number of contractions.

COMPONENTS OF SARCOPLASM

The muscle fiber is the unit cell of striated muscle and therefore contains the basic intracytoplasmic components. Within the sarcoplasm (cytoplasm) adjacent to each one of the nuclei scattered along the periphery of the fiber, a few ribosomes and a small Golgi apparatus are observed. The most prominent organelles are mitochondria, transverse tubules that extend into the fiber from the sarcolemma, and the smooth-surface endoplasmic reticulum which, in striated muscle fiber, is termed the *sarcoplasmic reticulum*.

Mitochondria are numerous, particularly in red fibers, are disposed in rows between myofibrils and are involved in the ATPase energy-producing reaction.

Glycogen in numerous particles is seen between myofibrils, generally within the sarcoplasm surrounding the tubules.

Transverse tubules (T-tubules) begin as funnel-like invaginations of the sarcolemma; or the tubules originate from vesicles at the surface. The vesicles, known as caveolae, are numerous below the plasma membrane. The tubules enter the substance of the fiber more or less at a right angle to the surface. They then branch so as to surround every myofibril, while remaining in the same plane as the Z lines (in frog muscle).

In mammals, the tubules surround the sarcomeres at the sites of the junctions between A and I bands. The opening of the transverse tubules at the surface of the fiber or in caveolae can be demonstrated under the EM by injection of ferritin, an electron-dense material. After injecting the material outside the fiber, it is seen to pass into the lumina of transverse tubules. The system of transverse tubules therefore represents complex extensions and invaginations of the sarcolemma.

The electrical charge on the outer surface of the sarcolemma is approximately the same as that on the outer surface of a nerve fiber. When a nerve impulse arrives at a motor nerve ending in a fiber, the sarcolemma at this site becomes depolarized, and as a result a wave of depolarization progresses rapidly along the sarcolemma and the fiber contracts. The system of transverse

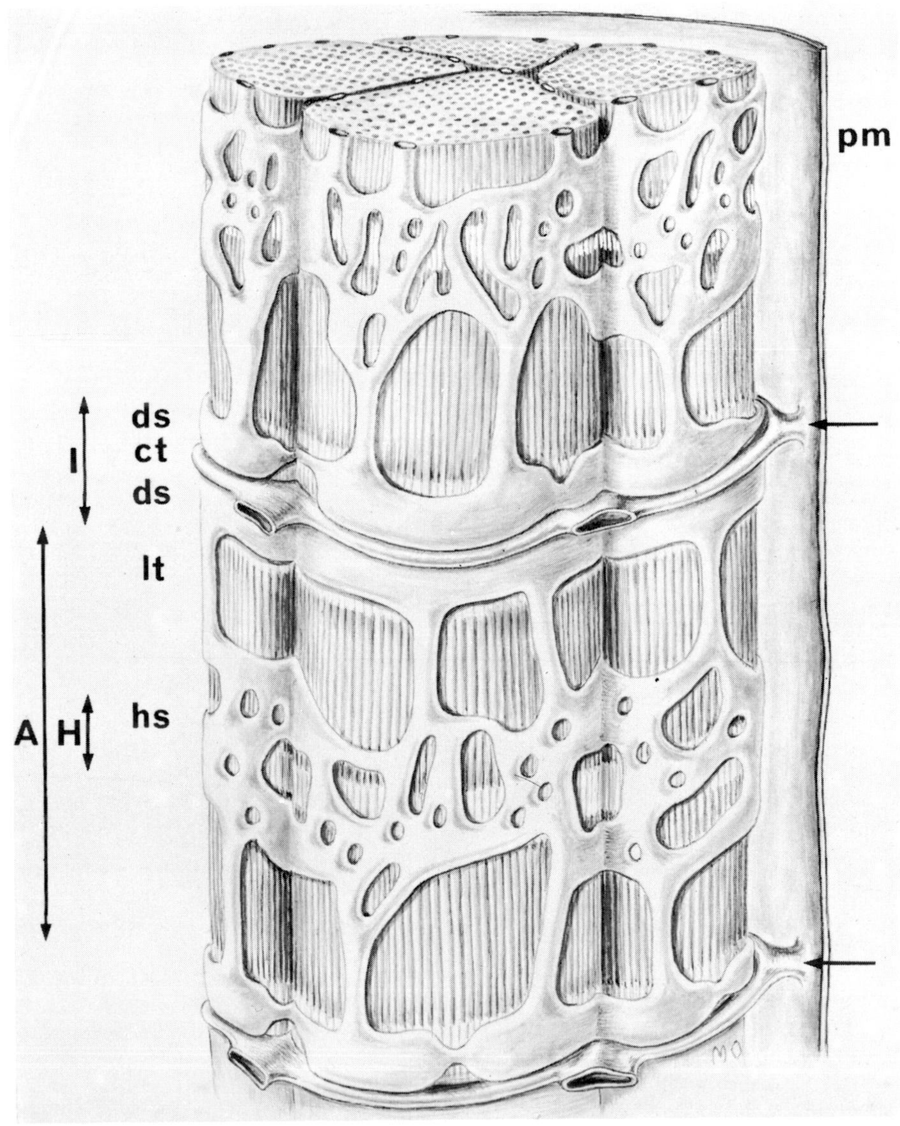

FIG. 4-12. Three-dimensional drawing of parts of four myofibrils to illustrate (1) the sarcolemma (labeled *pm* on the right), (2) the transverse tubules that etend into the substance of the fiber from the sarcolemma (from points indicated by arrows on the right) and (3) the sarcoplasmic reticulum which is interposed, and so lies between myofibrils, over their I, A, and H portions (labels for the latter on left). The transverse tubules are delicate tubules which are invaginations of the sarcolemma; hence their walls are composed of cell membrane, and their lumens open onto the outer surface of the sarcolemma. Transverse tubules (in the frog) enter the fiber at the level of Z line (indicated by arrows on right side), and each one branches as it extends across the fiber so as to surround myofibrils whose Z lines are in register with the site where it entered, as is shown by following the two tubules in this illustration, from right to left. The sarcoplasmic reticulum consists of cisternae and channels of smooth-surfaced endoplasmic reticulum that lie between and so surround myofibrils. In the region of the I band, the extent of which is indicated at the left of the illustration, the cisternae, known as terminal cisternae, are large and flattened, but they may be more or less distended (*ds*); they lie to either side of the transverse tubule (*ct*). The cisternae, by means of channels which run longitudinally (*lt*) over the A band to the region of the H-zone, connect with a network of more or less flattened sacs called the H sacs (*hs*). The site of the H-zone in the A band is indicated at the left of the illustration. (Ham AW: Histology, 7th ed. Philadelphia JB Lippincott, 1974. From C. P. Leblond)

tubules thus provides the means for rapid transmission of the impulse into the fiber quickly enough for all of its parts to contract simultaneously.

THE SARCOPLASMIC RETICULUM

The smooth endoplasmic reticulum consists of an array of connected membranous vesicles and channels that lie in the sarcoplasm around the myofibrils (Fig. 4-12). These membranous structures are of various shapes and sizes. Flattened cisternae at each end of the sarcomere are in contact with the transverse tubules. They connect with tubular channels running longitudinally toward the middle of the sarcomere where they connect with an irregular branching system of channels surrounding the myofibrils at the level of the H zone, where they are termed H sacs.

Theoretically, the wave of depolarization conducted by a transverse tubule causes the sacs of sarcoplasmic reticulum to release calcium that diffuses among the filaments and initiates contraction when the calcium ions combine with troponin. This process releases the blocking by tropomyosin on active sites of G-actin.

REFERENCES

Microanatomy

1. Gould RF: The microanatomy of muscle. In Bourne GH (ed): The Structure and Function of Muscle Vol II, p 186. New York, Academic Press, 1973

Structure of Muscle Fibers

2. Hanson J, Lowy J: The structure of F-actin and of actin filaments isolated from muscle. J Mol Bio 6:46, 1963
3. Hayashi T, Rosenbluth B, Satir P et al: Actin participation in actomyosin contraction. Biochem Biophys Acta 28:1, 1958
4. Huxley HE: The double array of filaments in cross-striated muscle. J Biophys Biochem Cytol 3:631, 1957
5. Huxley HE: Molecular basis of contraction. In Bourne GH (ed): The Structure and Function of Muscle Vol I, p 302. New York, Academic Press, 1972
6. Lowey S, Slate HS, Weeds AG, Baker H: Substructure of the myosin molecule. J Mol Biol 42:1, 1969
7. Szent–Györgyi AG: Meromyosins, the subunits of myosin. Arch Biochem Biophys 42:305, 1953
8. Szent–Györgyi AG, Mazia D, Györgyi A: On the nature of the cross-striation of body muscle. Biochem Biophys Acta 16:339, 1955

5

Collagen

FUNCTION OF COLLAGEN

Collagen is probably the most abundant protein in the human body, and it is the major constituent of most connective tissues.[1] The other major components are elastin, a related fibrous protein, and the class of sugar polymers known as *mucopolysaccharides* or *proteoglycans.* Tissues such as skin and tendon are composed of 70% of collagen by dry weight. Collagen represents about 23% of the total dry weight of whole bone, but it comprises almost 90% of the organic matrix. Since collagen constitutes the major component of most connective tissues, it makes a major contribution to their properties. However, the different properties of such tissues are in large part accounted for by the varying amounts of elastin and mucopolysaccharides associated with collagen (*e.g.*, cartilage has a 50% collagen content, but is more resilient to pressure than other tissues, probably because of a high content of mucopolysaccharides).

The function of collagen is to provide strength and structural integrity of various tissues and organs. It has appreciable tensile strength. Rupture of a collagen fiber 1 mm in diameter requires a load of 10 kg to 40 kg.[2] Such physiologic stability is in contrast to disruption of collagen fibers by nonphysiologic conditions. For example, when collagen fibers are heated in water at *p*H 7, they undergo an abrupt decrease in length at a characteristic temperature (the shrinkage temperature or T_s). When the fiber is heated to its T_s at an acid or alkaline *p*H, it not only shrinks but also goes into solution as gelatin. Commercial gelatins are generally prepared from connective tissues, such as bone, by boiling in water under either acidic or alkaline conditions. The resulting protein represents collagen that has been both denatured and partially degraded by hydrolysis of some of its cross-links and peptide bonds.

STRUCTURE OF COLLAGEN MOLECULE

The collagen molecule consists of three polypeptide chains, each of molecular weight of about 95,000 daltons and containing slightly more than 1000 amino acids.[13] In some collagens, the individual (α) chains may be linked intramolecularly by covalent cross-links producing dimers (β components). The major determinants of the triple helical structure of the collagen molecule are the occurrence of glycine (Gly) in every third position of the amino acid sequence and the high content of the amino acids proline (Pro) and hydroxyproline [Hypro] (Fig. 5-1).[27] The component polypeptide chains are characteristic for their tissue source. Skin and bone collagen consist of two α1 (I) chains and one α2 chain. Collagen from cartilage is composed of three identical chains called α1 (II) that are similar in molecular weight to α1 (I) chains but have a different primary structure as well as increased hydroxylation of lysine (Lys) residues and

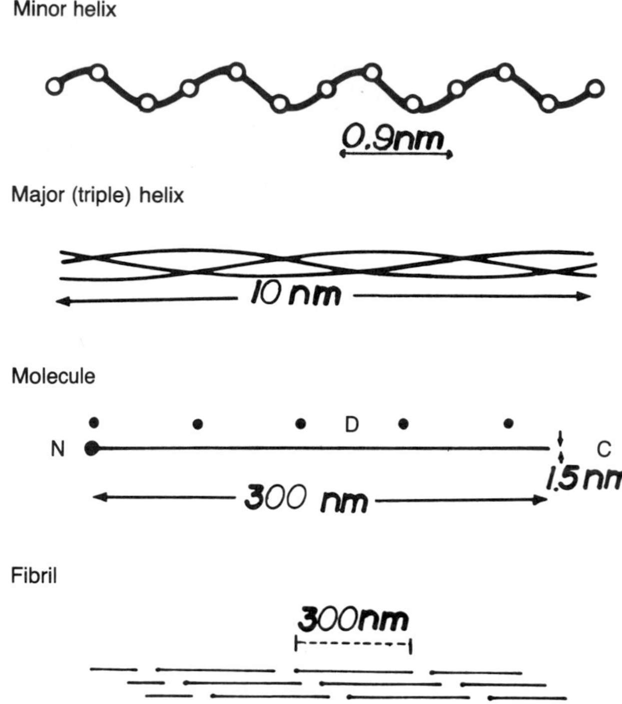

FIG. 5-1. Structure of collagen showing steps of development from the polypeptide chain to the fibril (modified from Piez). In the typical polypeptide sequence, Gly occurs in every third position throughout most of the chain. There are large amounts of Pro and Hypro. *X* and *Y* represent any amino acid. In the completely native collagen molecule, each α chian has a polyproline II-type helical conformation. This is the minor helix. In the diagram, only the alpha-carbon atoms (*O*) of the amino acids are indicated. The three α chains in each molecule are then wound about each other to form a coiled-coil structure, the major (triple) helix. One turn of the major helix is shown. The completed molecule, after the additional peptide from procollagen has been cleaved away, has short nonhelical regions at the amino-(*N*) terminus and (probably) at the carboxy-(*C*) terminus. The additional piece or registration peptide of the procollagen molecule is not shown in these diagrams. The distribution of amino acids along the molecule is unique throughout its length but, because of the manner in which molecules are stacked into the fibril, there is a pseudorepeat (*D*) seen on electron microscopy of native fibrils at 64 nm to 70 nm (640–700 A). (Harris ED Jr, Krane SM: Collagenases. N Eng J Med 291: 557, 1974)

greater glycosylation of hydroxylysines (Hylys).[24] Collagen molecules with the chain composition $[\alpha 1(III)]_3$ have been found in blood vessels and dermis, and, unlike α1 (I), α2, or α1 (II) chains, α1 (III) collagen contains cysteine that results in cross-linking within molecules through disulfide bonds.[20] Collagen from other sources (*e.g.*, basement membranes) has even different amino acid sequences.

The molecules of collagen are synthesized within fibroblasts, osteoblasts, and chondroblasts, and have additional nonhelical segments at one or both ends that may facilitate registration of the polypeptide α chains to form triple helical molecules. Once secreted into the extracellular space, the excess nonhelical terminal segments of these procollagen molecules are cleaved off, leaving characteristic triple-helical molecules that aggregate with one another to form fibrils (Fig. 5-2). After the fibrils are formed, cross-links develop within single molecules and among adjacent molecules.[8]

PHYSICAL CHARACTERISTICS

The native molecules have dimensions of 1.5 nm × 300 nm (15 × 3000 A). As long rigid rods in solution, the collagen molecules have a high viscosity and a strong negative optical rotation. If a solution of collagen is heated, a sharp transition occurs within a narrow temperature range, with lessening of viscosity and loss of negative optical rotation (Fig. 5-3). This melting temperature (T_m) is the midpoint of the denaturation curve as the helical structure melts to random coil configuration of gelatin. For fully hydroxylated native collagen near neutral *p*H, the T_m is 37° C. It appears that the chief function of Hypro in collagen is to stabilize the triple helix.[20] Since denatured collagen or gelatin is readily degraded by most tissue proteases, it follows that the presence of Hypro in collagen determines the resistance of collagen to general proteases. Moreover, when collagen molecules are aggregated into fibril form, they are not denatured until temperatures of 55° C to 60° C are reached. Thus, even during febrile illness, denaturation of collagen *in vivo* is unlikely.

ULTRASTRUCTURAL CHARACTERISTICS

The electron micrographic appearance of collagen fibrils, when negatively stained with phosphotungstic acid (PTA), a method that causes the stain to penetrate gaps or "holes" within the structure, shows them to consist of smaller identical and parallel microfibrils having a characteristic pattern of cross-striations or bands. The most prominent cross-striations are about 680 A apart and are accounted for by a specific alignment of the basic molecular units of collagen (Fig. 5-4). These units, known as *tropocollagen,* have the dimensions of a rod 15 A in diameter and 3000 A in length. The periodicity of the cross-striations in the microfibril is explained by the fact that each tropocollagen molecule has five charged regions 680 A apart that under appropriate conditions appear as stained bands. These bands are placed in register by the tropocollagen molecules aligning themselves in an exact arrangement in which neighboring tropocollagen molecules are displaced longitudinally with respect to one another. A gap or "hole" of about 410 A occurs between the end of one tropocollagen molecule and the beginning

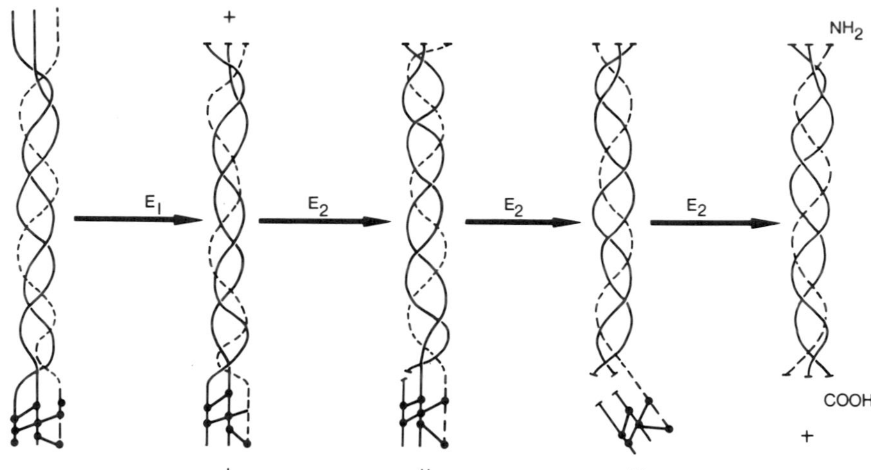

FIG. 5-2. Procollagen. Steps of enzymatic cleavage of NH- and COOH- nonhelical extensions, and conversion to protcollagen. (Courtesy of Jeffrey M. Davidson, Ph.D)

of the next on the same line.[17] This hole has been shown to be the site of initial formation of the inorganic solid phase of mineralization of bone.

The molecules in a microfibril are arranged in a parallel but staggered fashion, with each molecule overlapping the one beside it by one fourth of its length. Molecules in the same line are separated from one another by an interval of 410 A. The gap separates each molecule from the one ahead of it and also from the one behind it. The side-by-side staggered array of molecules causes the fibril to have less dense and more dense cross-bands that alternate along the length of the microfibril. One dark plus one light band forms one period. The gaps between tropocollagen molecules fall within the dark bands. The light bands represent multilayered molecules without gaps. The longitudinal striations seen in negatively stained microfibrils probably represent small bundles of staggered tropocollagen molecules.

CHEMICAL COMPOSITION

Throughout most of each polypeptide chain, every third amino acid is Gly, and collagen can be considered a polymer of tripeptide units with the formula: Gly-X-Y. The X and Y represent other amino acids in the two positions between each pair of Gly residues. Since Gly is the smallest possible amino acid, it can pack tightly into the center of the triple-stranded tropocollagen molecule and provide HN-groups for hydrogen bonding to O=C groups in the peptide bonds of the other chains. The amino acid in the "X" position immediately after Gly in the repeating tripeptide structure is frequently Pro. The third amino acid in the repeating tripeptide structure is frequently Hypro. There is only one hydrogen bond per triplet, and this bond is always formed between HN-groups of Gly in one chain and an O=C group of Pro or some other amino acid in the "X" position of the second chain.[28]

The high percentage of Gly in collagen (33% of all amino acid residues) distinguishes it from all other known proteins with the exception of the closely related fibrous protein elastin. Other unique features of amino acid composition are the high content of the amino acids Pro and Hypro (approximately 22%), the presence of Hylys,

FIG. 5-3. Mechanisms of action of collagenase. The melting point (T_m) of collagen in solution is the midpoint of the transition from native collagen to its denatured form, gelatin. The decrease in viscosity (ηsp) is shown to parallel the decrease in negative optical rotation (α). If the collagen molecule is cleaved at a temperature well below T_m, ηsp decreases but α remains constant, indicating that although the fragments are shorter, they still are in a triple helical conformation. In its native triple-helical state collagen is resistant to general tissue proteases; as gelatin, it is very susceptible to breakdown by these same enzymes. *In vivo* any gelatin formed (as when skin is burned) is immediately degraded enzymatically. (Harris ED Jr, Krane SM: Collagenases. N Eng J Med 291:557, 1974)

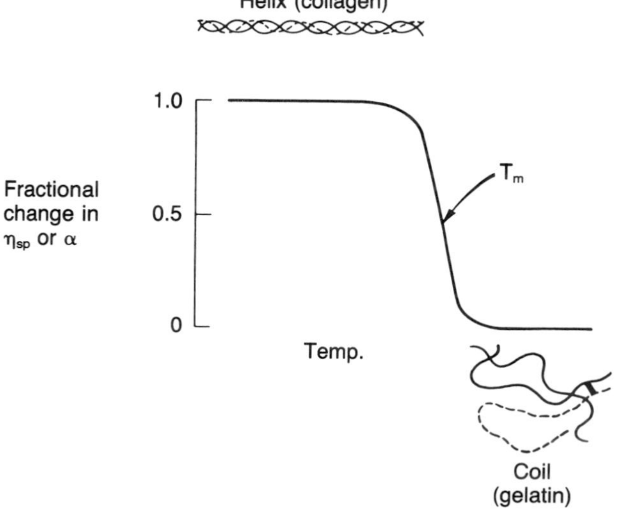

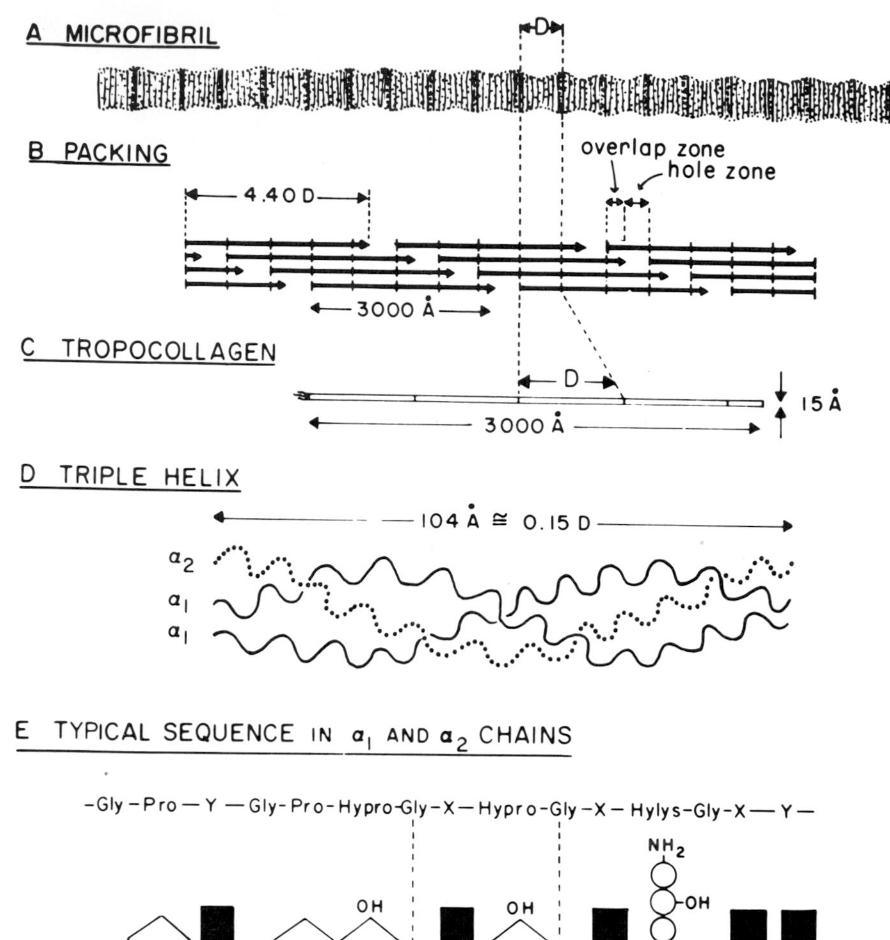

FIG. 5-4. Collagen structure (abbreviations as given in the text). (*A*) A stained microfibril of collagen exhibiting characteristic cross-striations with a regular repeat period (*D*) of approximately 680 A. (*B*) A two-dimensional representation of the packing arrangement of tropocollagen macromolecules in the microfibril. The drawing indicates the lateral displacement of tropocollagen molecules, but not the three-dimensional geometry of the microfibril. Veis and Bhatnagar discuss the limits imposed on the size of the microfibril by the three-dimension geometry. (*C*) Each tropocollagen molecule has large numbers of darkly staining bands, and five of these, which are separated by a regular distance of 680 A, account for the repeat period (*D*) in the microfibril. The H_2N-terminal and probably the HOOC-terminal ends of the molecule are atypical and nonhelical in structure and are called "telopeptides." (*D*) Each tropocollagen molecule consists of three polypeptides, two with identical amino acid sequences (α_1 chains) and one with a slightly different amino acid sequence (α_2 chain). Each α chain is coiled in a tight left-handed helix with a pitch of 9.5 A, and the three chains are coiled around each other in a right-handed "super-helix" with a pitch of about 104 A. (*E*) Gly occurs in every third position throughout most of the polypeptide chains, and there are large amounts of Pro and Hypro in the other two positions. *X* and *Y* represent any amino acid other than Gly, Pro, Hypro, Lys, or Hys. (Grant ME, Prockop DJ: The biosynthesis of collagen. N Eng J Med 286:194, 242, 291, 1972)

the relatively low content of tyrosine, and the absence of tryptophan. Moreover, in most collagen, cysteine is absent, eliminating the possibility of disulfide cross-links in the molecule. The exceptions are the α1(III) molecules that have been found in blood vessels and dermis, contining cysteine and disulfide bonds. The collagens isolated from basement membranes also contain cysteine.

A small amount of carbohydrate is found in collagen. This is accounted for by galactose and glucosylgalactose in O-glycosidic linkage to the hydroxyl group of Hylys.

INTRACELLULAR BIOSYNTHESIS OF COLLAGEN

The biosynthesis of collagen occurs in a definite sequence of events: assembly on ribosomal complexes of a polypeptide precursor of collagen termed "protocollagen"; hydroxylation of appropriate Pro and lysine (Lys) residues in protocollagen to Hypro and Hylys; and substitution of some of the Hylys residues with galactose or glucosylgalactose in an O-glycoside linkage before the molecule is extruded through the cell membrane into the matrix.[11]

Protocollagen is an intermediate in collagen synthesis prior to hydroxylation by hydroxylases and before glycosylation. The pure enzyme Pro hydroxylase has been isolated in pure form from chick embryo.[3] The affinity of the enzyme increases as the polymer length of the polypeptide increases to over one tenth of the length of an alpha chain.

Cofactors considered essential for enzymatic hydroxylation include atmospheric oxygen,[14] ferrous iron,[18] ascorbic acid or other reducing compound,[14] and α-ketoglutarate.[14]

A second enzyme, Lys hydroxylase, is responsible for the hydroxylation of Lys, and requires similar cofactors.

Some of the Hylys in collagen are substituted with

galactose or glucosylgalactose.[19] A uridine diphosphate (UDP) galactose transferase and a UDP-glucose transferase appear to be specific for Hylys.[22,23] Both enzymes require Mn^{2+} and they act in sequence so that galactose is added to the Hylys and then the glucosylgalactose is added by glycosidic bonds. Not all Lysyl residues are hydroxylated; depending on the type of collagen, from 2 to 20 Lysyl residues of the polypeptide chain are hydroxylated. Moreover, some hydroxylated Lys residues are not linked to any hexose, others are linked to galactose, and still others are linked to the disaccharide glucosylgalactose.[4]

The entire α_1 and α_2 chains are assembled simultaneously on unusually large complexes of messenger ribosomes (m-RNA).[9]

The triple helix may possibly form while the chains are being synthesized on ribosomes or at some later stage. The first polypeptide chains of collagen synthesized by cells are larger than α chains.[7] Electron microscopy (EM) of segment-long-spacing aggregates of the first collagen extruded by cells has shown that the molecule has an extension of about 130 A at the NH-terminal end of the tropocollagen molecule. Each of the three polypeptide chains has an extension.[15] These extensions might facilitate the formation of the triple helix.

After the collagen polypeptides are released from ribosomal complexes, they probably pass into the cisternae of the rough endoplasmic reticulum.

Hydroxylation is not necessary for extrusion through the cell membrane. Inhibition of hydroxylation does not cause accumulation of protocollagen within the cell.

The cells extrude partially hydroxylated and glycosylated protocollagen probably by reverse pinocytosis. It appears that since no intracellular protein contains an appreciable amount of hexose, and whereas most extracellular proteins contain one or more residues of hexose per molecule, glycosylation appears to be necessary for extrusion.[8] Prior hydroxylation is necessary for the molecule to acquire carbohydrate in the form of Galactosyl-hydroxylysine or Glucosyl-galactosyl-hydroxylysine. When an analogue of Pro is incorporated into collagen, the collagen is not extruded from the cell.[21] The cell membrane must possess some sensing mechanism that determines that it extrudes only the appropriate molecules: trans-Hypro of 90 to 102 residues per 1000. This may have therapeutic implications. In diseases associated with excessive collagen formation, the administration of an analogue of Pro will result in intracellular accumulation of a product that cannot be extruded. A viral hepatitis may be prevented from progressing to the cirrhotic state by administering an analogue to specifically prevent deposition of new collagen.

One may speculate that in diabetes, derangement of glucose metabolism might produce overglycosylation of specific collagens. Such collagens may be resistant to degradation and consequently accumulate in tissues such as blood vessels, thus explaining the thickening of basement membranes seen in diabetes.[3,16]

INTRACELLULAR REGULATION ELEMENTS

The factors governing intracellular synthesis of collagen are as follows:

Atmospheric Oxygen. This is necessary for hydroxylation. However, anoxia for a few hours does not appear to prevent formation of the polypeptide. It has been demonstrated that under anaerobic conditions, connective tissue cells can produce sufficient amounts of adenosine triphosphate (ATP) to support energy-requiring synthetic reactions. The source of ATP must be anaerobic glycolysis by which glucose is converted to lactate. Lactate increases the activity of protocollagen Pro hydroxylase, which subsequently, as oxygen becomes available, increases the rate of hydroxylation.[6,10]

Ascorbic Acid. The source of the reducing agent in hydroxylation of protocollagen. In scurvy, a small but appreciable amount of underhydroxylated collagen is found in connective tissues.

α-ketoglutarate. This salt probably, but not conclusively, regulates hydroxylase activity.

Ferrous Iron. Chelation of iron by α,α'-dipyridyl specifically inhibits hydroxylation of protocollagen. However, iron deficiencies have not been shown to delay wound healing or collagen synthesis.

Enzymes. The cellular levels of the hydroxylating and glycosylating enzymes can affect the rate of collagen synthesis. For example, in experimentally produced hepatic fibrosis by carbon tetrachloride or a choline-deficient diet, there is a fourfold increase in protocollagen Pro hydroxylase in the liver.[25] Similar increases have been noted in other conditions, such as in the synovial tissues of rheumatoid arthritis.[29]

FORMATION OF COLLAGEN FIBRILS

Collagen is an insoluble crystalloid under physiologic conditions. From 1% to 10% of the collagen in a tissue (*e.g.*, skin or tendon) is present as "tropocollagen" and can be solubilized by extraction of the tissue with sodium chloride solutions or dilute acid at 4° C.

"Soluble collagen" is that type of collagen that exists as un-cross-linked tropocollagen, a solid under physiologic conditions, but which can be solubilized with cold sodium chloride solutions or cold dilute acid.

If the solution of tropocollagen is restored to the physiologic conditions of *p*H 7 and warmed to 37° C, it forms an opalescent gel that consists of microfibrils (Fig. 5-5). Once the tropocollagen molecule is synthesized and extruded from the cell, aggregation of such molecules into fibrils does not occur until several processes take place. The initially synthesized soluble transport form of the molecule referred to as "procollagen"[30] does not

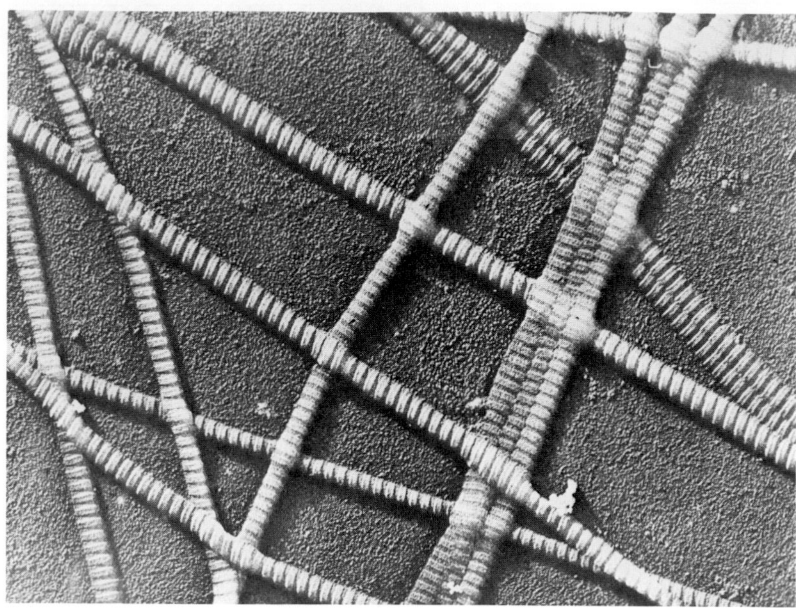

FIG. 5-5. Collagen fibrils deposited from a suspension and shadowed with chromium. This is the electron microscopic appearance of reconstituted collagen fibrils that form spontaneously when an acid solution of native collagen is neutralized. The bands are spaced about 700 A apart, and the length of the molecule is four times greater. (× 70,000) (Courtesy of Dr. Jerome Gross)

aggregate into fibers. It is a larger molecule than tropocollagen, possessing nonhelical extensions, a NH-terminal extension at one end, and a COOH-terminal extension at the other. These extensions are cleaved off enzymatically after the molecule leaves the cell.[33] Therefore, the location of the enzyme determines where the fiber forms. The formation of fibers is prevented until the short nonhelical extensions are cleaved off.

The spontaneous aggregation of tropocollagen into fibrils is produced by the interaction of charged side groups of adjacent molecules. Fibril formation is influenced by salt concentration and *p*H. The interactions between charged side groups of tropocollagen are specific since they produce the precisely overlapped array seen on EM. After the terminal nonhelical extensions are cleaved from the transport form of molecule, the terminal regions (telopeptides) of the helical tropocollagen molecule appear to direct the aggregation of the molecules into fibrils.

The small amount of Galactosyl-hydroxylysine and Glucosyl-galactosyl-hydroxylysine in collagen may also be important in directing fibril formation.[31] The greater the number of glycosylated Hylys residues, the less the tendency for fibril formation and formation of periodic striations. This suggests that carbohydrate content controls the type of fibrils formed.

The amount of glycosaminoglycans (*e.g.*, chondroitin sulfate and keratan sulfate) and proteoglycans may have effects on the rate of fibril formation *in vivo.*[32]

CROSS-LINKING IN COLLAGEN

Tropocollagen molecules spontaneously aggregate to form microfibrils which have little tensile strength until covalent bonds or "cross-links" form between adjacent tropocollagen molecules and between adjacent microfibrils.

The first step in the cross-linking of collagen is the enzymatic synthesis of aldehydes by removal of the terminal amino groups of several of the Lysyl or Hydroxylysyl residues in the tropocollagen:[34]

$$R—CH_2—NH_3 \rightarrow R—CHO + NH_4^+$$

An amine oxidase enzyme catalyzes the reaction. This enzyme is specifically inhibited by nitriles that produce lathyrism, a condition characterized by deformities of the spine, demineralization of bone, dislocation of joints, and aortic aneurysm.[42] The aldehydes obtained from Lys and Hylys form cross-links by two types of reactions: (1) Schiff base formation by condensation of the aldehyde with an amino group of Lys or Hylys in another α chain, and (2) Aldol condensation between aldehydes on adjacent alpha chains.[40]

The Schiff base is not an entirely stable bond, and the same agents that solubilize collagen probably reverse this reaction. An aldol condensation is a stable bond. Most of the cross-links involve an amino group or aldehyde from the telopeptide end of the tropocollagen.

Nitriles inhibit the first reaction required for the cross-linking of collagen. When young animals under experimental conditions are fed diets of sweet peas (*Lathyrus odoratus*) or by administering nitriles (R≡N) such as beta-amino-propionitrile, the active component of sweet peas, lathyrism develops. Significantly, the aorta normally contains large amounts of elastin whose cross-links are formed from aldehydes derived from Lys.

CLINICAL IMPLICATIONS

The clinical implications of cross-linking in collagen are as follows:

Aging.[43] Cross-linking continues indefinitely and may account for the characteristic stiffness that develops in skin, blood vessels, and other connective tissues with age. However, inhibiting cross-linking in collagen does not appear to affect the aging process.

Marfan's Syndrome. This condition is the result of a defect in cross-linking of collagen that is secondary to a genetic defect such as a deficiency of the amine oxidase required to form aldehydes. The clinical picture includes skeletal deformities and aortic aneurysms similar to those seen in lathyritic animals. Since un-cross-linked collagen is easily degraded by collagenases, an increased urinary excretion of Hypro-containing peptides is found in many patients.[38]

Homocystinuria. The chemical structure of homocysteine is similar to the structure of penicillamine. The latter drug prevents cross-linking by reacting with aldehydes so that they are unavailable for cross-linking.[36] The manifestations of homocystinuria are similar to Marfan's syndrome because the high levels of homocysteine present in connective tissues may react with the aldehydes. In the one study reported, the skin of two of four patients with homocystinuria were found to contain an increased amount of tropocollagen extractable with cold dilute acetic acid.[37]

Scleroderma.[41] This condition is characterized by deposition of increased amounts of collagen in subcutaneous tissues, in the submucosal layer of the esophagus, in cardiac and striated muscle, and perhaps in basement membranes. This may be due to increased collagen synthesis, or decreased degradation perhaps by decreased activity of collagenases. A certain type of collagen or increased cross-linking may make the collagen more resistant to collagenases.

Therapeutic approaches using penicillamine, 1 g to 3 g per day, is based on various rationales: (1) inhibiting cross-linking causes more pliability of collagen; (2) un-cross-linked collagen is degraded at a relatively rapid rate; (3) causes an increase in un-cross-linked tropocollagen, reflecting failure of cross-linking.[44] However, there is no evidence that penicillamine halts progression of the disease.

Tendon Healing.[35,39] Tendon repair is effected by ingrowth of vascular fibrogenic tissue from peritendinous tissues. The peritendinous collagen restricts tendon gliding. The physical properties of this scar tissue may be modified experimentally by the induction of lathyrism. By administering β-amino-propionitrile, intramolecular and intermolecular cross-linking is prevented by inhibiting lysyl oxidase activity during the stage of active collagen synthesis.

Pro analogues (*e.g.*, cis-Hypro) reduce the amount of collagen deposited around tendons. The Pro analogues are incorporated into newly synthesized collagen where they act as "collagen breakers." Collagen in which imino acids are replaced by Pro analogues are incapable of forming a triple helix, and nonhelical collagen lacks the tensile strength of newly synthesized collagen. Nonhelical collagen is probably removed by collagenolytic enzymes before being incorporated. The use of Pro analogues in experimental animals appears to be hampered by toxic side-effects.

BONE COLLAGEN

Collagen is the major organic constituent (94% of the organic fraction) of bone, comprising about 19% of the weight of whole compact bone.[50,60,67] By determining the amount of Hypro in bone samples, the total amount of bone collagen can be calculated in bone samples by the known proportions of Hypro in collagen. This imino acid is found in large quantities in collagen and is almost exclusively confined to that protein in mammalian tissues.[47] Most of the minor organic fraction is composed of protein polysaccharides (chondroitin sulfate and keratan sulfate). The amount of the latter is calculated by the known proportions of uronic acid in chondroitin sulfate and the glucosamine in keratan sulfate.

Collagen of bone differs from that of cartilage in its amino acid composition. It contains two highly anionic amino acids, serine and glycine, and much of the serine is present as serine phosphate, pointing out the importance of phosphate bound to bone collagen in the mechanism of calcification. Furthermore, bone collagen also contains the monosaccharide galactose to which calcium ions are bound and prevented from participating in the formation of hydroxyapatite crystals. It has been postulated that this constitutes a balanced regulatory system: the available serine-bound phosphate against the calcium held bound to the galactose.

Bone collagen also differs from soft tissue collagen because it is difficult to solubilize in cold salt solutions and weak acids. This property may be due to the fact that bone collagen is covalently cross-linked more rapidly and to a greater degree than the collagen of most soft tissues. The rapid introduction of cross-links appears to play a role in stabilizing the tissue prior to mineralization.

PREPARATION OF BONE TISSUE FOR COLLAGEN STUDIES

EM will elucidate the fine structure of bone collagen as well as the size, shape, and position of the apatite crystals within the largely collagenous matrix. To prepare bone suitable for ultramicroscopic study, it is necessary to prepare ultrathin sections of developing primary spongiosa of young animals or the cranial bone of fetal animals so that the embedding media can thoroughly permeate the mineralized tissue of compact bone. Mineralized bone is stained with lead acetate or uranyl acetate. For demineralized bone, thin sections are floated on phosphotungstic acid which not only demineralizes the tissue but also stains the collagenous component of the matrix.[49,62]

VARIATIONS OF BONE COLLAGEN SIZE AND ARRANGEMENT

The collagen fibers in bone vary in arrangement and size depending on the age and the particular bone from which samples are taken. Fibers in infant cortex are arranged less compactly than the cortex of a mature adult rib, and have a width ranging from 150 A to 620 A. In the cortex of rib bone and the diaphyseal regions of long bones of aged people, fibers with diameters up to 1500 A are routinely observed.[63] The collagen fibers in various bones of the human embryo seem to be generally smaller (150–500 A) and more widely and randomly distributed than those observed in infant rib cortex. The fibers tend to be of wider diameter when they are closely packed and occupy a larger proportion of the total area. Newly formed collagen (*i.e.,* those nearer the osteoblast) have the smallest diameter, suggesting gradual enlargement by steady accretion of additional molecules as the fibers move away from the cell.

COLLAGEN IN WOVEN (NONLAMELLAR) BONE

Woven bone, the earliest developing bone of the fetus, and the initial bone tissue to form during the repair of bone, has loose, sparse, and randomly arranged collagen fibrils.

COLLAGEN IN LAMELLAR BONE

In lamellar bone there is a well organized, closely aggregated arrangement of collagen fibrils whose axes are parallel in each layer. The direction of the fibrils in each layer differs from its neighboring layer, and is either longitudinal, oblique, or transverse, so that each lamella forms a discrete and easily identified structure (Fig. 5-6).

COLLAGEN OF EPIPHYSEAL GROWTH CARTILAGE

Within the epiphyseal unossified cartilage of the newborn, a loose, widely separated network of thin fibrils courses through an amorphous electron-lucent ground substance.[64–66,68] Numerous fine fibrils measuring 100 A to 200 A in width are observed, and some exhibit a periodicity of about 200 A. Later, as the cartilage matrix approaches the developing cartilaginous septa of the physis, the fine fibrils tend to assume a longitudinal orientation. The process of calcification of the cartilaginous septa begins distally where the concentration of polysaccharides are reduced while the collagen fibrils enlarge. An inverse relationship seems to exist between the width of the collagen fibrils and the concentration of polysaccharides. In contrast to the thin fibrils within proximal regions of high chondroitin content, the distal regions of beginning calcification of cartilage contain a small amount of chondroitin sulfate and rather large fibrils.

The process of calcification at the physis begins at the periphery of the longitudinally disposed cartilaginous

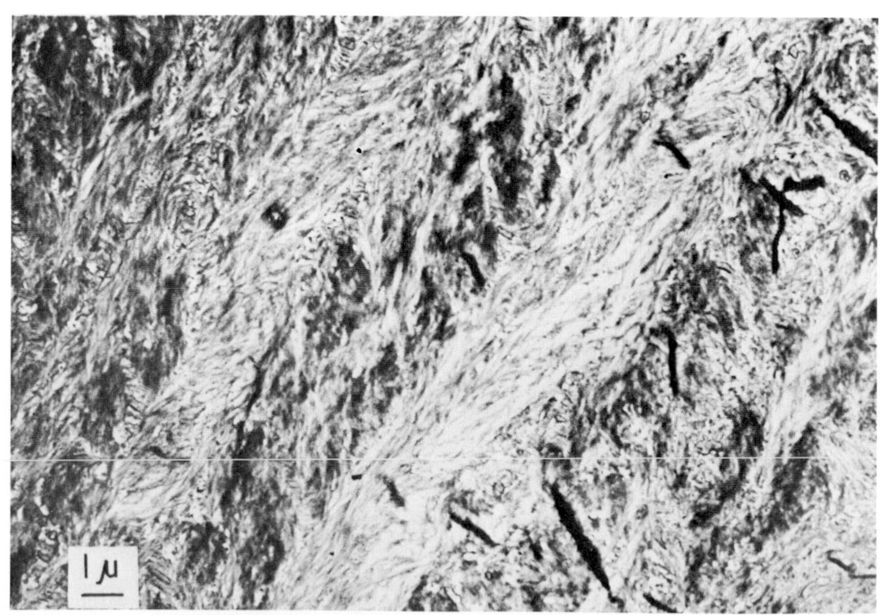

FIG. 5-6. A demineralized section of bone collagen showing the arrangement of the collagen fibrils in the alternating lamellae, electron microscopic appearance, stained with phosphotungstic acid. (Cooper RR, Milgram JW, Robinson RA: Morphology of the osteon. J Bone Joint Surg 48A:1239, 1966)

septa at the level of the third chondrocyte from the metaphysis. The crystals accumulate in irregular aggregates without any consistent relationship to the fibrils. Distally, in areas of advanced calcification, crystals are deposited throughout the septa giving rise to spicules of calcified cartilage, although the central zone of each septum is less densely calcified than its periphery. Mineral is deposited in areas previously occupied by amorphous ground substance between the fibrils.

COLLAGEN AND OSTEOGENESIS AT PHYSIS

The bone matrix forms around the calcified cartilage septa. Osteoblasts surround the septa and elaborate collagen fibrils of greater width (500–700 A) with a typical periodicity of 680 A. There is a lag period, represented by a narrow zone of osteoid, between the laying down of collagen fibrils and eventual calcification.

Extracellular osteoid matrix is at first composed of a loose network of randomly arranged fibrils set in a ground substance, forming a fine uncalcified layer measuring 500 A to 2 μ in width, too narrow to be visualized by ordinary light microscopy. The second zone beyond the osteoblasts forms a clear-cut layer of earliest mineralization. The crystals are deposited with their long (*c*) axes parallel with the long axes of the fibrils, and are not concentrated at 680 A intervals along the fibrils, which at this stage still tend to form a loose, randomly distributed network of fibrils. In the third zone beyond the osteoblasts, the fibrils become better organized and grouped in an orderly parallel fashion close together. The crystals again lie with their long axes parallel with the long axes of the fibrils and are now concentrated in rows at 680 A intervals along the fibrils. The rows of crystals are in register with the periodic bands of the fibrils. Although crystals appear to localize at discrete areas at regular intervals within or on the fibrils as nucleation centers, extremely rapid crystal growth ensues to lengths of 400 A to 500 A, almost two thirds of the distance of the major collagen periods.

COLLAGEN IN THE OSTEON

The fine collagen fibrils of compact lamellar bone surrounding the haversian canal measure 700 A to 800 A in average width, have typical periodicity, and are oriented preferentially in the direction of the osteon axis.[45,49] The lamellar pattern is due to the differing orientation of fibrils in adjoining lamellae (Fig. 5-6). Toward the haversian canal, the lamellar collagen fibrils average about 600 A in width and are generally arranged with their long axes parallel to the long axis of the canal. Immediately encircling the canal as many as three layers of unmineralized collagen fibrils are observed in which the collagen fibers are arranged alternately in a circumferential, longitudinal, or oblique manner with respect to the long axis of the canal.

Within the haversian canal, two vessels resembling capillaries are seen, one usually being thicker than the other. The larger vessel is usually surrounded by collagen fibrils simulating an adventitia. In the human adult, unmyelinated nerve fibers are contained within the canal, and are composed of neurofilaments surrounded by endoneurial collagen fibrils.[49] Osteoblasts line the periphery of a developing osteon. These cells are surrounded by well-developed prominent fibrils that form the major component of a narrow layer of osteoid that forms between the osteoblast and the mineralized matrix. The fibrils within the newly formed osteoid layer are loosely and randomly arranged, but toward the mineralizing front the fibrils become aggregated into well-organized bundles of fibers with a typical periodicity.

Small fibrils of collagen are often seen throughout the space of the haversian canal strewn about undifferentiated mesenchymal cells.

ROLE OF BONE COLLAGEN IN MINERALIZATION

Collagen synthesis and mineralization in bone are closely coordinated. The crystal hydroxyapatite is initially deposited within the "holes" that correspond to the electron-dense bands of the aggregated molecules that make up the microfibrils, but the manner in which this is carried out has not yet been established. On EM, the mineral appears to be deposited within or on recently formed collagen fibrils.

Different rates of synthesis of collagen are noted in different bones and in different areas of the same bone.[51] Bone collagen differs from other collagens in that it is rapidly and more extensively cross-linked immediately after synthesis, resists solubilization, and its resulting stability is therefore uniquely suitable for mineralization. Such cross-linking may be blocked by oxidative deamination of the lysyl residues by lathyrogens such as β-aminopropionitrile, thereby increasing the solubility of bone collagen and preventing its mineralization.[57]

The following are the theories of the mode of mineralization:

Nucleation Hypothesis. The manner of stacking of collagen molecules creates spaces or "holes" within which crystal formation develops from stable or metastable extracellular fluids.

Stereochemical Hypothesis. A stereochemical configuration results from interaction between collagen and protein-polysaccharide complexes.[71] The nucleation site appears to be anionic and the sulfate groups of chondroitin sulfate may provide the nucleating site.

Phosphorylation Hypothesis. The collagen is enzymatically phosphorylated prior to mineralization creating specific regions in the molecules which are suited for initial crystal formation by epitaxy (see Mineralization of Bone).[55]

FACTORS AFFECTING SYNTHESIS AND DEGRADATION

Bone collagen is formed and removed in a nonuniform and complex fashion, and the rate of collagen synthesis undergoes diurnal variation.[69] These may be influenced by diurnal fluctuation of activity of the parathyroid and adrenal glands. Moreover, collagen synthesis decreases in bone with advancing age.[52,58,59,61]

Parathyroid hormone (PTH) administered to experimental animals increases the rate of resorption and also inhibits the rate of synthesis of bone collagen.[48,53,73] However, in hyperparathyroidism in humans the rate of collagen synthesis is increased.[54]

Corticosteroids decrease the rate of collagen synthesis,[72] and hypercortisonism is reflected in decreased levels of hydroxyproline in bone.[46] In hypercortisonism, the rate of collagen degradation is unaffected.

When collagen is resorbed, whether bone mineral or matrix is removed first is unknown. A specific collagenase has not yet been isolated from bone. Acid cathepsin proteases, which are active at about *p*H 3.0, are said to cause degradation of collagen,[70,74] but in bone it appears more likely that they effect tissue resorption after the collagen has been degraded by collagenase into smaller fragments. The actual mechanism by which collagen is degraded is unknown.

COLLAGEN OF ARTICULAR CARTILAGE

The biophysical properties of articular cartilage that allow joints to serve as bearings in locomotion are at least partly related to the unique composition of the extracellular matrix. Collagen constitutes approximately 10% of the wet weight and 50% of the dry weight of cartilage.[82] Noncollagenous material constitutes approximately the other 50% of the dry mass of articular cartilage matrix, of which the bulk is composed of heterogeneous proteoglycan complexes.[85]

Articular cartilage biophysical properties are a consequence of the interaction of the collagen and proteoglycans. The chain extensions of the proteoglycans and the electrostatic charges provide the molecular basis for the mechanical matrix stiffness.[87] The interaction of the proteoglycan with collagen causes the matrix to behave like a gel. The collagen acts as a discontinuous membrane to resist the flow of proteoglycans while preserving its colloidal properties.[76] The collagen is relatively inextensible, existing as a taut structure because of the swollen ground substance, functioning as an immediate elastic element in sustaining compressive loads. The collagen fibrils extend directly through the calcified cartilage matrix, and by their fixation to the subchondral bone serve as anchors of the ground substance.

Articular cartilage collagen is associated with proteoglycans in such a manner that, unlike tendon, skin, or bone, it is almost impossible to demonstrate distinct morphological characteristics of microfibrils (*i.e.*, banding and periodicity, either at the light microscopic or ultrastructural levels). The diameter of the microfibrillar unit in articular cartilage varies with the species, age, and depth from the surface. In general, their diameters vary from 10 nm to over 100 nm.

Otherwise, the typical basic-banded pattern, the dimensions and structure of the single "tropocollagen" molecular unit, the numerical amino acid composition, the molecular weight, the repeating triplets of Gly-X-Y where X is frequently Pro and Y is Hypro, the presence of Hylys, an amino acid unique to collagen, and Lys, and the intramolecular and intermolecular cross-linkages, are essentially similar to other types of collagen.

Articular cartilage contains a distinct type of collagen.[81] Unlike interstitial collagen, cartilage collagen has three identical $\alpha 1$ chains (Fig. 5-7). These $\alpha 1$ chains of cartilage collagen are designated as $\alpha 1$ (Type II) because their amino acid composition and therefore their chromatographic properties are similar to the $\alpha 1$ (Type I) chains from interstitial collagen.[79,80] In addition to the higher Hylys content and glycosylation of the Hylys, there are sufficient differences to allow a separation of cartilage $\alpha 1$ (II) chains from interstitial $\alpha 1$ (I) chains by chromatographic techniques. The cyanogen bromide peptides derived from bone and cartilage collagen differ only by the substitution of a threonine and aspartic acid for the serine and leucine in the bone peptide. Cartilage collagen $[\alpha 1(II)]_3$ is quite difficult to solubilize, and is the main, unique collagen of normal articular cartilage.

In embryonic chick articular cartilage, two types of collagen are synthesized.[86] The amount of interstitial $[\alpha 1\ (I)]_2\alpha 2$ collagen synthesis decreases from 60% in the 8-day embryo to nearly 10% in the newly hatched chick. This suggests the coexistence of both collagen types in the same tissue, and a developmental transformation

FIG. 5-7. Genetic types of collagen found normally in connective tissue. Bone, skin, and tendon contain $[\alpha 1\ (I)]_2\alpha 2$ collagen, and articular cartilage and epiphyseal plate contain $[\alpha 1\ (II)]_3$ collagen. (Lane J, Weiss C: Review of articular cartilage research. Arthritis Rheum 18:553, 1975)

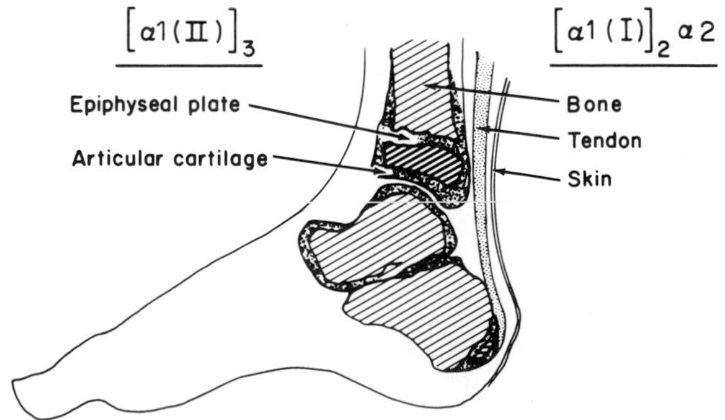

from predominantly interstitial $[\alpha 1\ (I)]_2\alpha 2$ synthesis to cartialge $[\alpha 1\ (II)]_3$ as the articular cartilage matures. The $[\alpha 1\ (II)]_3$ molecules are cross-linked at the amino- and carboxy-terminal ends and the predominant form of cross-linking involves the Schiff base condensation of a Hylys and an oxidatively deaminated Hylys.[81] The unique morphological pattern of cartilage collagen is therefore related to differences in the primary structure, glycosylation and cross-linkage of $[\alpha 1\ (II)]_3$ collagen rather than its relationship to the associated proteoglycans.

ULTRASTRUCTURAL CHARACTERISTICS OF CARTILAGE COLLAGEN

Prior to EM investigations, x-ray diffraction studies have demonstrated that the collagen fibrils are arranged tangential to the articular surface in the superficial or tangential zone; those of the deeper zones are arranged in random fashion, and in the calcified zone of older articular cartilage they are arranged perpendicular to the articular surface (Figs. 5-8 to 5-10).[78]

Transmission and scanning EM studies have confirmed this pattern.[83,90] In the immediate vicinity of cells, collagen fibrils sweep in capsular fashion about the lacunae. In general, the diameter of the collagen fibril ranges from 10 nm to over 100 nm. Under the scanning EM, the fibrils appear to be about three or four times thicker because of the adhering proteoglycans. This same coating is probably responsible for partially obscuring the periodicity and banding of mature collagen fibrils. In the various species studied, the collagen fiber diameter increases with age[89] as well as with depth of the cartilage (Fig. 5-11).[77,83]

COLLAGEN IN OSTEOARTHRITIS

Until recently, the collagen content in osteoarthritis has been regarded as virtually unchanged, particularly since Hypro synthesis and content remains unchanged.[75] However, it has been conclusively demonstrated that osteoarthritic cartilage synthesizes, in addition to the normal $[\alpha 1\ (II)]_3$ cartilage collagen, a collagen with the characteristics of $[\alpha 1\ (I)]_2\alpha 2$.[84] This not only represents an alteration in collagen synthesis but a reversion to the immature type.

The collagen fibrils in advanced osteoarthritis are oriented parallel to the surface of clefts that extend into the middle and deep zones. In the middle zone, the fibrils retain their usual random arrangement until the advanced stages of osteoarthritis, at which time they are arranged perpendicular to the joint surface.[88]

In moderately advanced osteoarthritis, the collagen fibrils are of smaller diameter. Their periodicity and subbanding appear more distinct, perhaps reflecting the diminution of proteoglycan or perhaps the synthesis of the more immature $[\alpha 1\ (I)_2\alpha 2$-type] collagen. In areas of degenerating cells or microscars, collagen fibrils of exceptionally large diameter (up to 450 nm) with altered periodicity may be found. Such fibrils may also be seen in aging cartilage in the vicinity of degenerating chondrocytes or cell remnants.

COLLAGENASE

Collagenases are enzymes capable of degrading native helical collagen in fibril form under physiologic conditions.[113] The need for specific collagenases is dictated by

(Text continues on p. 126.)

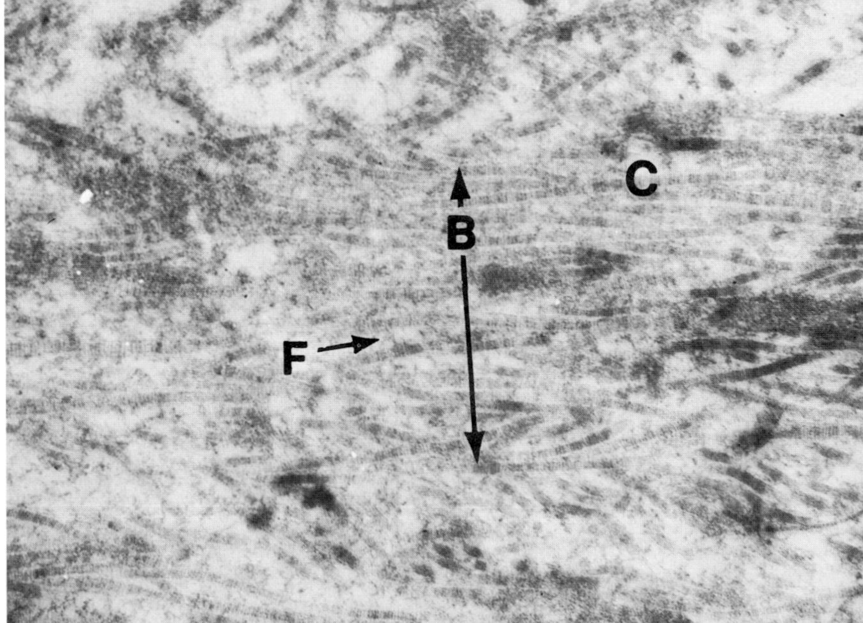

FIG. 5-8. Ultrastructural characteristics (electron micrograph) of the tangential zone adjacent to the surface of normal human articular cartilage. Collagen fibrils (*C*) of approximately 32 nm diameter are arranged in large bundles (*B*) which run parallel to the articular surface. Periodicity of 640 A and sub-banding are present but obscured by overlying fine fibers (*F*), 4 nm to 10 nm located over and between individual collagen fibrils. (× 60,000) (Lane J, Weiss C: Review of articular cartilage research. Arthritis Rheum 18:553, 1975)

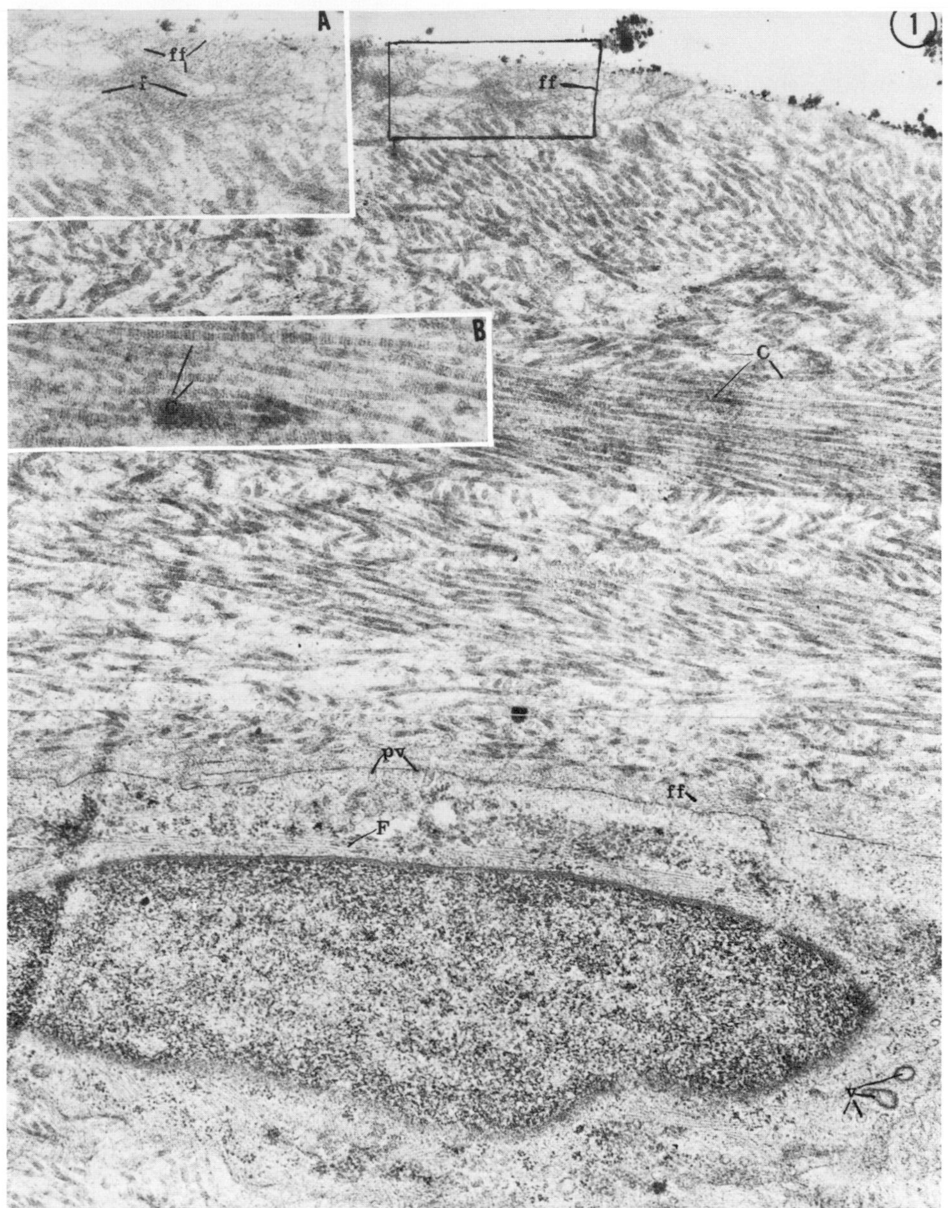

FIG. 5-9. Zone IS, the superficial tangential layer under electron microscopy (× 31,200). The articular surface is covered at the top by a layer probably corresponding to the lamina splendens, consisting of a dense network of filamentous fibrils (*ff*) and fine fibers (*f*) (× 62,400 in inset A). Closely packed unit collagen fibers (320 A ±50 A diameter) are arranged in bundles (*C*) which run parallel to the surface. The fibers have a distinct 640 A periodicity (*arrows*) and subbanding (inset B: × 60,000). Filamentous fibrils (*ff*) surround the surface cell. Pinocytosis vesicles (*pv*) are present. The cell membrane is partially obscured by filamentous fibrils. Intracellular filaments (*F*) of 70 A diameter are abundant. At the summit of the medial femoral condyle, this layer extends to a depth of 200 μ. The superficial tangential layer increases in thickness toward the peripheral nonweight-bearing area to approximately 600 μ. The collagen bundles run parallel to the surface at an oblique or right angle to one another, and are closely packed with little intervening matrix as compared to the deeper zones. Little or no anionic polysaccharide can be detected. The ellipsoid cell has the following characteristics: the cell membrane has few cytoplasmic processes and numerous micropinocytosis vesicles and acanthosomes on its surface. Its secretory vacuoles often contain material similar to the filamentous fibrils of the extracellular matrix. The intracellular filaments (70 A in diameter) are common in the perinuclear area. The rough endoplasmic reticulum is less well developed than in Zone II, mitochondria are small, and the Golgi apparatus forms numerous flattened saccules. (Weiss C, Rosenberg L, Helfet AJ: An ultrastructural studyof normal young adult human articular cartilage. J Bone Joint Surg 50A:663, 1968)

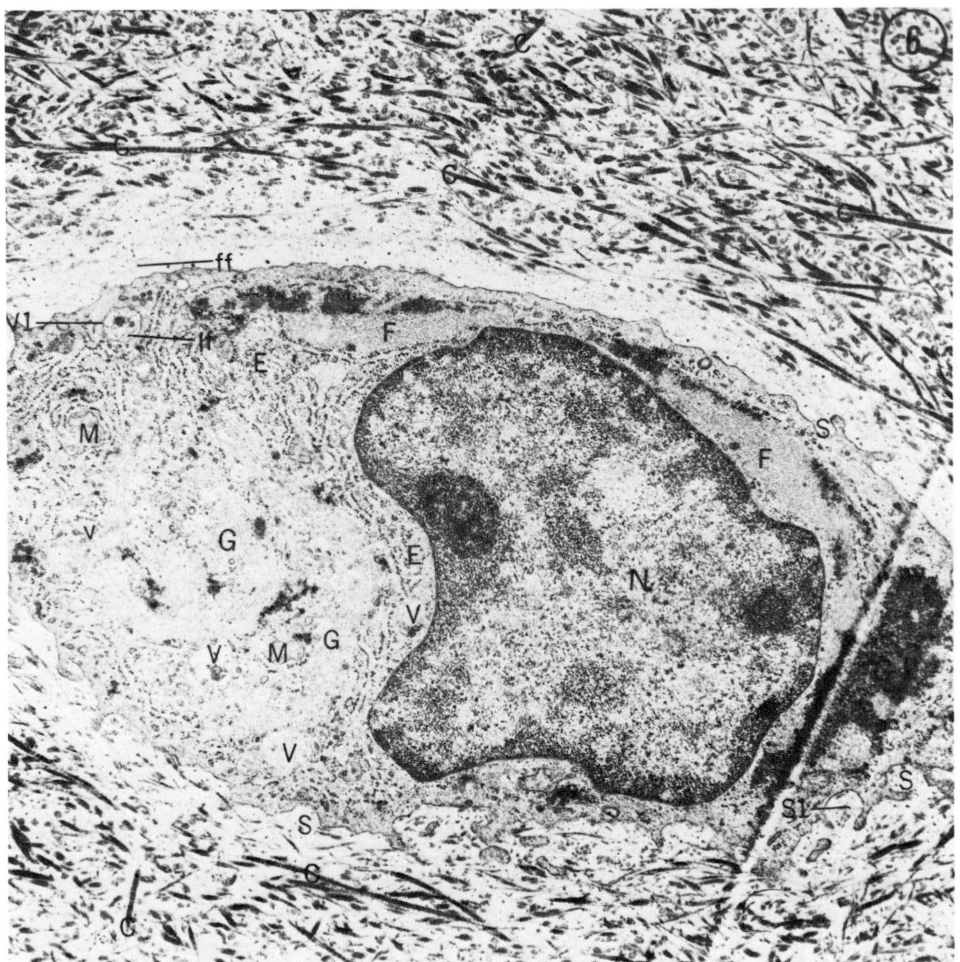

FIG. 5-10. Electron microscopic appearance of Zone II. The chondrocytes of this zone are large and have a scalloped appearance. The endoplasmic reticulum (*E*) is extensively developed, heavily studded with ribosomes, and forms rows of concentric lamellae. The Golgi apparatus (*G*) is highly developed and occupies a large portion of the abundant cytoplasm. Glycogen (*GL*), intracellular filaments (*F*), and many mitochondria (*M*) are present. Intracellular fibrils (*If*) within Golgi vesicles and vacuoles resemble the filamentous fibrils (*ff*) in scalloped areas (*Sl*). Filamentous fibrils (*ff*) immediately surround the cell. At greater distances, unit collagen fibers, more widely separated by increased amounts of amorphous ground substance, appear to run parallel to the surface. The collagen fibers are randomly oriented, show the typical 640 A periodicity, have a diameter ranging from 300 A to 600 A, and show little tendency to form bundles. The fine fibers and filamentous fibrils not only surround the cell but occupy the matrix between the larger collagen fibers. Abundant amorphous ground substance of low to moderate electron density occupies the spaces between the fibers. Cells are usually in pairs or groups. The appearance of the chondrocyte suggests that it is actively engaged in the synthesis of collagen molecules which then are extruded from the cell and undergo the processes by which they aggregate and are progressively transformed into structures of larger dimensions as they move farther away from their point of origin. (× 13,500) (Weiss C, Rosenberg L, Helfet AJ: An ultrastructural study of normal young human articular cartilage. J Bone Joint Surg 50A:663, 1968)

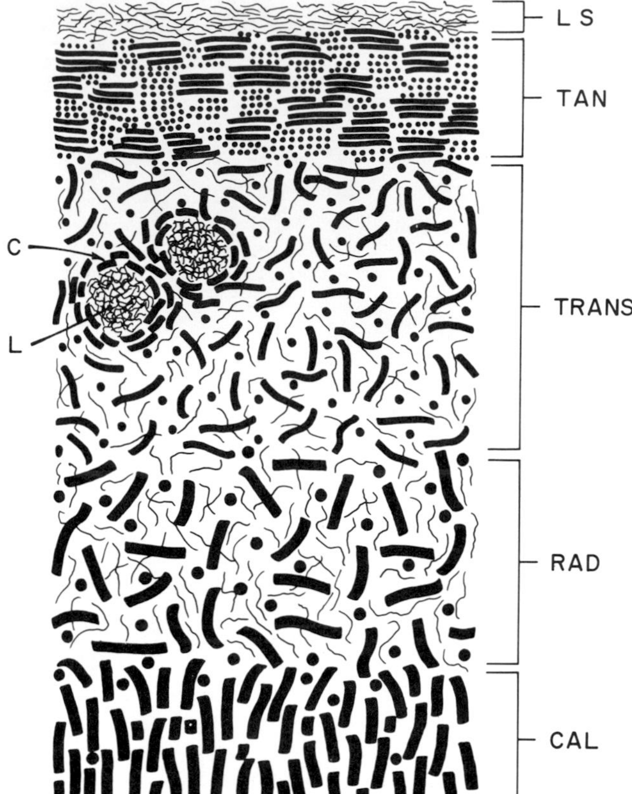

FIG. 5-11. The fibrous architecture of human articular cartilage. The lamina splendens (*LS*) is a layer several micra deep composed of fine fibers (4–10 nm in diameter) that cover the articular surface. Beneath this layer lies the tangential zone (*TAN*), which consists of tightly packed bundles of individual collagen fibrils arranged parallel to the articular surface and often at right angles to each other. This essentially fibrous zone is thickest at the periphery of the joint and thinnest at the center of the joint. The transitional zone (*TRANS*) contains significant amounts of proteoglycans as well as collagen. The collagen fibrils are approximately 60 nm in diameter and are randomly arranged. Fine fibers fill the interfibrillar space and often appear attached to the collagen fibers. The area between the cell membrane and the lacunar rim (the pericellular halo) contains a dense network of fine fibers. (*L*). Mature collagen fibers comprise a capsule about the lacunae (*C*). The collagen fibrils of the radial zone (*RAD*) are also randomly arranged and of large diameter. The calcified zone (*CAL*) constitutes the basal layer of articular cartilage and contains mature collagen fibers that are arranged perpendicular to the articular surface. (Lane JM, Weiss C: Review of articular cartilage collagen research. Arthritis Rheum 18:553, 1975)

the inherent resistance of native collagen to degradation by general tissue proteases. This resistance of collagen fibers to enzymatic degradation by existing tissue proteases is attributed to several factors:

Intramolecular Covalent Cross-Links. These cross-links exist between individual α chains which produce dimers (β components), and between molecules making up the fiber (intermolecular cross-links).

Triple Helical Structure of Collagen Molecule. Following extrusion from the cell, the molecules of newly synthesized collagen contain additional nonhelical extensions at one or both ends that facilitate registration of the polypeptide α chains to form the triple helical molecules. Once secreted into the extracellular space, the excess nonhelical portions of these procollagen molecules are cleaved off, leaving characteristic triple-helical molecules that aggregate with one another to form fibrils. After fibrils are formed, cross-links develop within single molecules and among adjacent molecules.

Physical Characteristics. Collagen in solution is related to the mechanics of action of collagenase. The native molecules have dimensions of 1.5 nm × 300 nm (15 A × 3000 A), are long rigid rods in solution, have a high viscosity, and a strong negative optical rotation. Heating a solution of collagen results in a sharp loss of the viscosity and negative optical rotation that occurs over a narrow temperature range. This melting temperature (T_m) is the midpoint of the denaturation curve as the helical structure melts to a random coil conformation of gelatin. After the collagen is denatured and becomes gelatin, it is readily degraded by most tissue proteases. For fully hydroxylated native collagen near the neutral *p*H, the T_m is very close to 37° C (see Fig. 5-3). The chief function of Hypro in collagen is stabilization of the triple helix.[119,121] Since denatured collagen or gelatin is readily degraded by most tissue proteases, it follows that the presence of Hypro is an important determinant of the resistance of collagen to tissue proteases.

Native collagen molecules are aggregated into fibril form, and are not denatured until temperatures of 55° to 60° are reached. Consequently, collagen is not denatured *in vivo*. In summary, the resistance of native collagen to proteolytic attack is determined first by the primary structure that directs the formation of the triple helix.

Factors that decrease the stability of the helix renders the molecule more susceptible to proteolytic attack. Certain regions of the molecule are more susceptible than others to proteolytic cleavage. For example, trypsin in high concentration slowly attacks collagen from the carboxy-terminus resulting in a fragment approximately 75% of the original length of the molecule.[116] Proteases such as chymotrypsin and pepsin cleave the short nonhelical region of the amino terminus in such a way as to render the molecules soluble in aqueous extracts and yet leave them in native helical form.[96,99]

Prior to 1962, the only known enzymes that could attack the helical backbone of the collagen molecule in solution of fibril form were the collagenases extracted from *Clostridium histolyticum*. In contrast to mammalian collagenases, these clostridial endopeptidases cleave collagen at multiple sites, producing many small peptides.

By lowering the temperature of the reaction, bacterial collagenases clip off short segment-long-spacing (SLS) segments sequentially from each end of the molecule.[125]

FIRST MAMMALIAN COLLAGENASE

When tadpole-tail sections are cultured *in vitro* on collagen gels reconstituted from solution at neutral *p*H by warming to 37° C, collagen adjacent to the explants are lysed.[115] Viable cells produce collagenase, an enzyme which is most active at neutral *p*H or slightly alkaline *p*H.

Most of the collagenase exists in an inactive or latent form, and the question of whether its activation is brought about by certain activators (enzymes) or by removal of inhibitors has not been resolved. For example, the latent collagenase (proenzyme) may be activated by limited proteolysis of its molecule by another protease (*e.g.*, trypsin or chymotrypsin). On the other hand, collagenase activity requires the presence of calcium, and is inhibited by EDTA, cysteine, or serum. It is activated by purified lysosomes between *p*H 5.5 and *p*H 7.4. Collagenase attacks native collagen at about neutral *p*H when it is in solution, in reconstituted fibrils or as insoluble fibers, producing two fragments representing 75% and 25% of the molecule. Both fragments retain the triple-stranded helical conformation of collagen as evidenced by the maintenance of the optical rotation during a fall in viscosity when collagen is incubated with the enzyme, and the ability to reconstitute the individual fragments into segment-long-spacing (SLS) aggregates.[123]

Helical collagen molecules or portions of molecules precipitate from a cold dilute acid solution in the presence of adenosine triphosphate (ATP) in such a manner that the molecular segments are aggregated and aligned in perfect register. These limited length aggregates as viewed under EM correspond in length to that of the tropocollagen (TC) molecule, and are termed *segment-long-spacing aggregates*. When stained with uranyl acetate or phosphotungstic acid, the packing arrangement in lateral register of charged groups on the side chains of the molecules interacting with the stains results in a characteristic banding pattern. By means of this technique, it was demonstrated that the mechanism of action of tadpole enzyme on the native tropocollagen in solution was unique: the molecule underwent scission (cleaved) into two pieces, an amino-terminal 75% fragment ($TC^{A}75$) and a carboxy-terminal 25% fragment ($TC^{B}25$). The collagenase cleaves the molecule between interbands 39 and 41. Although the viscosity falls, the high negative optical rotation does not change. Thus the fragments retained their triple-helical conformation and were resistant to further degradation.[104] However, although remaining in helical conformation after cleavage, the reaction products have a lower T_m and are more susceptible to degradation by trypsin than is intact tropocollagen. Although never proven, further degradation into smaller peptides and free amino acids by collagenase under physiologic conditions of temperature and *p*H has been postulated.[124]

It has therefore been suggested that "the collagenolytic enzyme produced and secreted by the cell attacks collagen molecules within the fibril in the extracellular space. The fibril frays and the reaction products, because of their higher solubility, disperse in the surrounding tissue fluid. In a dispersed state, the denaturation temperatures are considerably lower than when aggregated as fibrils. The fragments lose their helical structure spontaneously at body temperature and become susceptible to degradation either by collagenase, which can degrade gelatin extensively, or by other cellular proteases."[120] It is important to emphasize that other mammalian collagenases discovered will attack the collagen molecule in the same manner as tadpole collagenase.

BIOLOGY OF MAMMALIAN COLLAGENASE

Synthesis of collagenase has been identified in various cells which are not highly differentiated as well as in highly differentiated cells.[102] In normal human skin, most collagenase is produced by cells in the upper papillary dermis. The rheumatoid nodule,[94] a granuloma of fibroblasts and collagen surrounded by foci of chronic inflammatory cells, produces significant amounts of collagenase. It is probable that mesenchymal cells synthesize this enzyme.[108] The method of harvesting collagenase in a culture medium of viable cells is best exemplified by a culture of rheumatoid synovium.

If primary explants of synovial tissue are placed in a sterile culture medium, changed daily, and incubated at 37° C in 95% oxygen and 5% CO_2, collagenolytic activity is absent in the medium during the first few days, appears in appreciable quantity on the third day, and persists for 7 to 10 days. Freezing or thawing the tissue inhibits enzyme production, as does the addition of actinomycin D or iodoacetate in concentrations sufficient to inhibit respectively new messenger RNA-directed protein synthesis and carbohydrate metabolism.[111]

It is now known that a wide variety of tissues contain collagenase, because collagenolytic activity can be demonstrated in homogenates or extracts of these tissues by methods that free the enzyme from both substrate and inhibitory proteins. A procollagenase may need to be activated before collagenolytic activity can be demonstrated (*e.g.*, an inactive proenzyme of leukocytes can be activated by a substance contained within rheumatoid synovial fluid).[114] Rheumatoid synovial fluid is known to possess marked collagenolytic activity.[107]

Various protein inhibitors of collagenase are present in extracellular fluids, and may be the reason why enzymatic activity is not readily detectable in tissue homogenates or extracts. Alpha$_2$-macroglobulin (α_2M) is an example of such an inhibitor,[100] and may form an α_2M-collagenase complex that is dissociable.[91] Thus serum containing these inhibitors will inhibit the production of active collagenase. When trypsin is added to a serum-collagenase mixture, the activity of collagenase is restored. Whether trypsin destroys α_2M, or α_2M binds preferentially to trypsin freeing the collagenase has not been resolved.[92] α_2-macroglobulin will bind and inhibit various proteases including serine proteases, thiol proteases (*e.g.*, cathepsin B1), carboxyl proteases (*e.g.*, cathepsin D), and metalloenzymes like collagenase.[92]

Non-cross-linked or poorly cross-linked fibrils are highly susceptible to degradation by collagenase. This explains why recently synthesized collagen is readily and rapidly degraded. The substrate *in vivo* for collagenase is the collagen fibril and fiber, not single molecules in solution, and collagen in fibril form with its intermolecular cross-linking is resistant to degradation. In the process of aging, the greater introduction of stable intermolecular cross-links results in accumulation in tissues of collagens which are more resistant to breakdown and remodeling by enzymes.

Certain compounds appear to increase the rate of collagenase synthesis or release from cells: Colchicine stimulates synthesis of collagenase in rheumatoid synovium,[111] rheumatoid nodule,[110] and carrageenin granuloma.[118] Dibutyryl adenosine cyclic 3′5′-monophosphate increases collagenase production by explants of tadpole tissue.[116] Heparin added to bone fragments in culture increases collagenase production.[122]

MECHANISM OF COLLAGENOLYSIS

The initial enzymatic step in the breakdown of collagen fibrils occurs within a *p*H range of 7 to 8.6, with an optimum of about 8.0[124] Collagenase cleaves through the collagen helical molecule at one locus only: at the 39 to 40 interband (Fig. 5-12).[97] The products of primary collagenolysis are TC^A and TC^B pieces, which can be thermally denatured at temperatures above 32° C to random coil gelatin polypeptides (Fig. 5-13). In this state of thermally denatured fragments, these can then be cleaved by potent proteases, the enzymes which are released into the extracellular space and which act under physiologic conditions of *p*H and temperature (Fig. 5-14).[117]

An alternative method for the degradation of collagen fibrils is as follows: Purified cathepsin B1 is capable of degrading collagen fibrils, but only at an acid *p*H.[98] This enzyme has a *p*H optimum for degradation of fibrils of less than 4, a state which is said to exist within lysosomes. Macrophages are observed to contain vacuoles (phagolysosomes) within which are seen collagen fibrils in various stages of disintegration.[117] The first cleavage of collagen by cathepsin B1 is at the nonhelical region containing the intramolecular cross-link, and is followed by multiple cleavages of the helical region. This enzyme could conceivably be responsible for lysosomal breakdown of collagen at an acid *p*H.

Cathepsin D, an acid hydrolase believed responsible for proteoglycan degradation in cartilage, is incapable of degrading collagen even at acid *p*H, and has no effect on gelatin.

In summary, collagenases or procollagenases are released into the extracellular space. The active enzymes cleave at a specific locus through all three chains in each

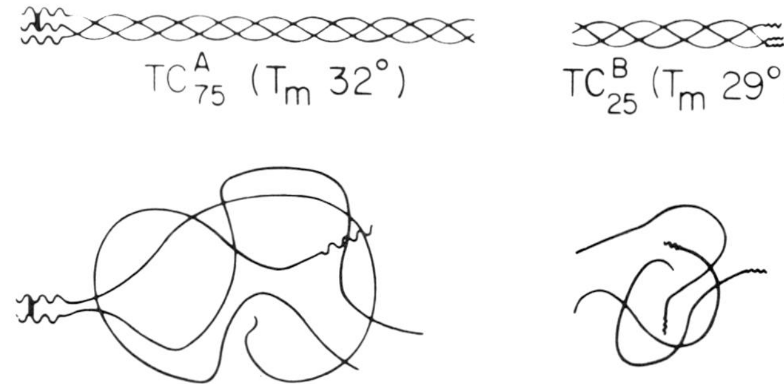

FIG. 5-13. Collagenolysis—step II. If the cleaved molecule is not bound by intermolecular cross-links to other molecules in the fibril, it is immediately solubilized and thermally denatured to random coil gelatin polypeptides. This process happens *in vivo* because the melting temperature (T_m) is lower for framgents of collagen than for the intact molecule and less than usual physiologic temperatures. (Harris ED Jr, Krane SM: Collagenases. N Eng J Med 291:605, 1974)

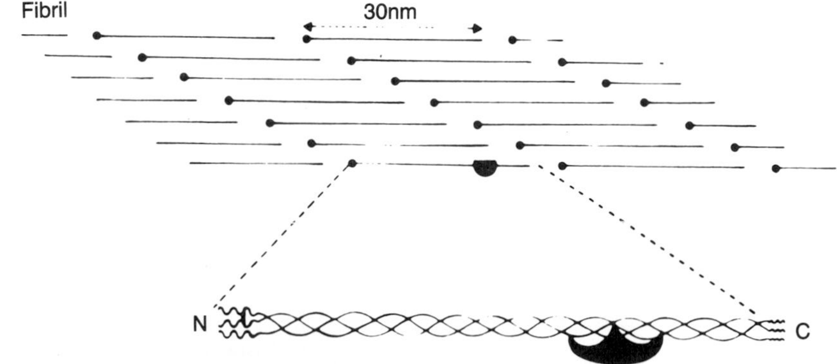

FIG. 5-12. Collagenolysis—step I. The collagenase cleaves through all three α chains at a specific locus in the helical portion of the molecule in fibril form. The triple-helix facilitates recognition or cleavage (or both) by the enzyme. In some species (*e.g.*, rat), the same enzyme apparently has the capacity to make two additional clips producing a 67% and a 62% fragment from the original 75% fragment. In this diagram the nonhelical portions of the collagen molecule at the amino-terminus (*N*) and carboxy-terminus (*C*) are indicated by ≋. (Harris ED Jr, Krane SM: Collagenases. N Eng J Med 291:605, 1974)

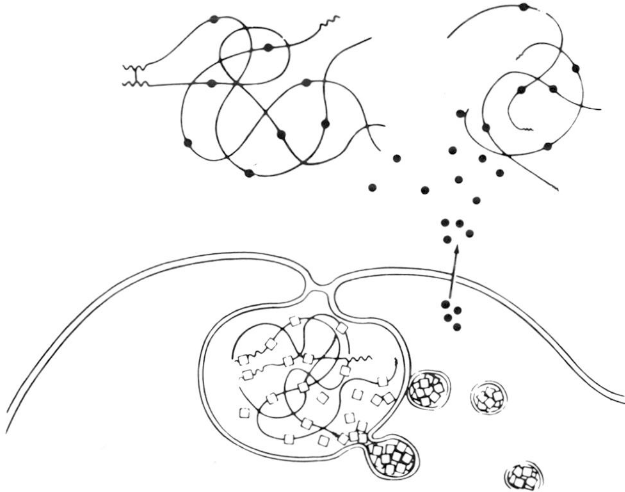

FIG. 5-14. Collagenolysis—step III. Once cleaved, solubilized, and denatured, the collagen 75% and 25% fragments (now gelatin) can be degraded by enzymes released into the extracellular space (*e.g.*, the rheumatoid synovial endopeptidase), or else they can be phagocytosed and degraded within phagolysosomes at acid *p*H (*e.g.*, cathepsin B1). ● = extracellular, neutral protease; □ = lysosomal protease (Harris ED Jr, Krane SM: Collagenases. N Eng J Med 291:605, 1974)

molecule, and at temperatures above 32° C both reaction products are thermally denatured. As gelatin polypeptides, they are cleaved in a second step by neutral proteases in the extracellular space or possibly by intracellular degradation by lysosomal enzymes after phagocytosis.

In situations where collagen absorption is rapid (*e.g.*, within the uterus after parturition), an additional intracellular degradation process occurs; intralysosomal hydrolysis of large segments of insoluble collagen presumably occurs by cathepsin B1.

The substrate *in vivo* for collagenase is the collagen fibril and fiber, not single molecules in solution. Collagen in fibril form is more stable than molecules in solution, as demonstrated by increased resistance to thermal denaturation. Increased intermolecular cross-linking is associated with even further increased stability. Recently reconstituted fibrils (without intermolecular cross-links) are easily solubilized in aqueous solutions and are readily cleaved by collagenases. If, on the other hand, intermolecular cross-links are introduced among the molecules in fibril form, the collagen becomes both insoluble and resistant to degradative effects of enzymes. This change has been demonstrated by the use of methylene cross-links formed by incubating fibrils in dilute solutions of formaldehyde.[109]

Normal fibrils and those artificially cross-linked with formaldehyde are degraded by synovial collagenase at a greater rate only when the temperature of the reaction is raised from 37° C to 38.5° C or 40° C. Since inflammation in rheumatoid joints is associated with an increased temperature within the joint space, this may account for the increased rate of degradation.[103]

In bone, the presence of hydroxyapatite minerals confers a resistance of bone collagen to thermal denaturation.[95] Moreover, mineral protects bone collagen from lytic enzymes.[126] Therefore, mineral must first be removed before collagenase can degrade the matrix.

PATHOLOGIC EFFECTS OF COLLAGENASE

RHEUMATOID ARTHRITIS

One postulated mechanism of breakdown of articular cartilage is enzymatic. At the synovium-articular cartilage junction a zone of amorphous material, degraded collagen fibers, and macrophages containing numerous mitochondria and granules may be seen. The degradation of insoluble collagen fibrils may be the effect of collagenase produced by rheumatoid synovium, whose peak of activity is between *p*H 7 and *p*H 8, and is inhibited by serum, EDTA, and cysteine. Rheumatoid collagenase can be shown to degrade normal human articular cartilage at 37° C with release of Hypro-containing peptides.[131]

Purified preparations of rheumatoid synovial tissue and joint fluid collagenases are capable of degrading the $(\alpha_1\ [II])_3$ cartilage collagen molecules.[112]

RHEUMATOID NODULE

The rheumatoid nodule consists of proliferation of fibroblasts which assume a radial polarization, and a central focus of necrosis containing disintegrating cells, fragments of collagen, and fibrin.[93] The lesion expands centrifugally with enlargement of the necrotic center and fibroblastic proliferation and deposition of new collagen about the periphery. The lesion is often surrounded by lymphocytes suggesting an immune mechanism.

A neutral protease and a collagenase similar to rheumatoid synovial enzymes can be isolated from cultures of these nodules.[108] This suggests that the central focus of necrosis may be the result of collagenolytic destruction.

RHEUMATOID SYNOVIAL FLUID COLLAGENASE

In spite of the greater content of α_2M in both serum and synovial fluid in rheumatoid patients than in normal people, active free enzyme is contained in rheumatoid synovial fluid. The source of this collagenase is not clear, although evidence indicates that it originates from granules of polymorphonuclear leukocytes (PMN). The PMNs of rheumatoid synovial fluid seem different from the buffy-coat PMNs taken from peripheral blood; the former degrade collagen gels *in vitro*, whereas the latter do not.[130] Rheumatoid synovial fluid contains a component that is capable of neutralizing protein inhibitors of collagenase, and the procollagenase synthesized by the PMN becomes an active free enzyme.

SEPTIC ARTHRITIS

In septic arthritis, the synovial fluid contains free, active collagenase during the early days, and this decreases in activity as the patient improves and the PMN count decreases below 50,000/mm^3.[109] It is poorly inhibited by serum. The collagenase is capable of degrading human articular cartilage $(\alpha_1 [II])_3$ in soluble and native form, although at a rate less than that of soft tissue collagens. This suggests that the active, free collagenase originates from PMNs, and is capable of degrading collagen in the presence of serum and synovial tissue fluids, and supports the rationale for frequent arthrocentesis.[109]

COLLAGENASE AND BONE

In both normal bone resorption (*e.g.*, remodeling) and pathologic resorption (*e.g.*, hyperparathyroidism), a carefully regulated collagenolytic system is operative. Lysosomal enzymes are particularly involved in regulating bone resorption, perhaps by acting as inhibitors,[129] or as activators of latent collagenase (procollagenase).[129]

Inactive precursors of collagenase are found in bone.[129] These are apparently bound by an inhibitor[122,123] from which it can be separated by fractional precipitation by ammonium sulfate.[124] Heparin and dextran sulfate, which possesses a charge distribution similar to heparin, enhances the specific activity of the enzyme when collagen in solution is used as a substrate. The effect of heparin in producing osteoporosis must be considered in light of the fact that substances apparently released by mast cells enhance the collagenolytic activity of many tissue collagenases.[127] Lysozyme, in high concentration, appears capable of inhibiting bone collagenase from degrading collagen fibrils,[123] and thus may act to regulate bone resorptive activity.

HYDROXYPROLINE EXCRETION: AN INDICATOR OF COLLAGEN METABOLISM

Protocollagen is the term applied to the polypeptide chains that are synthesized intracellularly in ribosomes. After the protocollagen is released from the ribosomes, hydroxylation of Pro and Lys residues occurs as one of the terminal reactions before the molecule is extruded through the cell membrane into the matrix where it is termed *procollagen.*[139]

SOLUBLE AND INSOLUBLE COLLAGEN

The most recently extruded single polypeptide chains combine to form three-stranded helical molecules, which aggregate and develop intramolecular and intermolecular cross-links to form more stable and less soluble *tropocollagen.* Although newly synthesized tropocollagen molecules aggregate in precise register to form fibrils, which appear insoluble under physiologic conditions, they are readily extracted with cold electrolyte solutions and are therefore regarded as "soluble collagen." Later, the newly synthesized tropocollagen molecules become cross-linked both within the three-stranded complex and between adjacent molecules forming "insoluble collagen."

The result of molecular aggregation in precise register is a three-dimensional crystalloid accounting for most of the fibrils in the body, and which is insoluble unless the collagen is denatured to gelatin (*e.g.*, by heat). Progressively, later stages in the formation of collagen fibers are characterized by an increasing degree of cross-linking, less solubility, and a requirement for stronger electrolyte solutions for extraction.[141]

Collagen normally is subject to a slow but continuous process of degradation of procollagen, tropocollagen, and mature collagen. As a result of the presence of Hypro and Hylys in the tissues, plasma and urine reflect the products of this degradation. The process can be studied by assays of Hypro.

HYPRO EXCRETION AND TURNOVER OF COLLAGEN

Under normal conditions, urinary Hypro is derived from the degradation of collagen in different tissues. Most of the Hypro originates from a single tissue such as bone.[132,136] Essentially all of the Hypro is in a peptide-bound form, and more originates from the degradation of more mature insoluble collagen and less from newly synthesized soluble forms of collagen. Approximately 5% to 10% of Hypro released by degradation of insoluble collagen is excreted, and the rest may be metabolized to other amino acids and ultimately to carbon dioxide and urea.[138]

An increase in the amount of Hypro in urine does not necessarily indicate an increase in the *rate* of collagen degradation. Factors affecting Hypro excretion include:

- Collagen pool is increased, while rate of degradation is normal
- Increased rate of collagen synthesis results in increased excretion
- Conversion of soluble to insoluble fibers is impaired
- Increased rate of degradation from insoluble to soluble forms
- Increased rate of degradation of all forms, soluble and insoluble
- Decreased rate of degradation to carbon dioxide and urea

Hypro Excretion Under Normal Conditions. A specific assay demonstrates the amount of Hypro in urine.[134]

Normal Values: Over 95% of Hypro is in a peptide-bound form, and assays estimate the increase in free Hypro after hydrolysis samples are taken on Hypro-free diets (Table 5-1).

Children excrete more Hypro than adults. The ratio of soluble collagen to insoluble collagen increases, and the rates of collagen synthesis and degradation are accentuated during periods of rapid growth. In older animals, the rate of synthesis is slow and degradation decreases so markedly that the excretion of Hypro may be one tenth of that seen in young animals.

TABLE 5-1 Urinary Excretion of Hydroxyproline in Normal Children and Adults

Age	mg/24 hr	Age	mg/24 hr
0–12 mo	19–56	11–14 yr	63–180
1–5 yr	20–65	18–21 yr	20–55
6–10 yr	35–99	over 21 yr	9–43

Kivirikko KI, Laitinen O, Prockop DJ: Modification of a specific assay for hydroxyproline in urine. Anal Biochem 19:249, 1967

Effect of Disease on Hypro Excretion. Because many factors influence rates of protein synthesis and degradation, changes in Hypro excretion are not specific for any single disease, but nevertheless reflect changes in collagen metabolism.

Growth Hormone. This increases the rate of collagen synthesis, increasing the *amounts* of collagen, both soluble and insoluble, subject to degradation (rate normal).

Hypopituitarism. Hypro excretion is diminished. A favorable response to growth hormone therapy may be measured by an increased excretion of Hypro.

Acromegaly. Hypro excretion is increased. A favorable response to x-irradiation therapy is indicated by decreased Hypro excretion.

Hyperparathyroidism.[137] This causes marked degradation of bone collagen; Hypro excretion is significantly increased. Following parathyroidectomy, the rate of Hypro excretion is diminished.

Paget's Disease. In extensive active involvement, the rate of new bone (and therefore collagen) synthesis and degradation is increased, resulting in extremely high levels of Hypro excretion.

Hypothyroidism. The rate of synthesis and degradation is decreased, resulting in reduced Hypro excretion.

Hyperthyroidism. The rate of synthesis is decreased, but degradation is significantly increased, resulting in increased Hypro excretion.

Hypercortisonism. Hypro excretion levels are normal. When large doses of cortisone are administered for prolonged periods of time, the collagen content of tissues is decreased,[140] and likewise the incorporation of amino acids into newly synthesizing collagen is impaired.[135] Consequently, the synthesis of collagen is decreased. The decrease of Hypro excretion in young animals may be explained by a reduction in the size of the soluble collagen pool. Older animals have small amounts of soluble collagen, which normally arise from the slowly synthesized new collagen or from degradation of insoluble collagen. Therefore, Hypro excretion remains unchanged and the depletion of collagen in long-term steroid therapy is the result of an imbalance between slow degradation and slower synthesis.

Marfan's Syndrome and Lathyrism. Some cases of Marfan's syndrome or arachnodactyly excrete increased amounts of Hypro. This is comparable to lathyrism. After administering a lathyrogenic agent, cross-linking is reduced, and the content of soluble collagen increases.[133] The principal defect is the failure of conversion of newly synthesized but as yet un-cross-linked, soluble collagen to more stable, cross-linked, insoluble forms of collagen. Degradation and excretion of excess collagen occurs.

Collagen Diseases. Reports of excretion levels are conflicting. High levels of Hypro excretion are exceptional.

Malabsorption Syndrome. Normally, following the ingestion of gelatin, it hydrolyzes to dialyzable peptides for absorption, and increased amounts of Hypro are excreted in the urine. In pancreatic insufficiency and in adult celiac disease, failure of conversion of gelatin to absorbable forms occurs, and the urinary Hypro excretion fails to rise.

In malabsorptive states and tropical sprue, failure of absorption of vitamin D, calcium, and phosphorus through the gut wall results in a compensatory hyperparathyroidism to maintain serum calcium levels. Increased resorption of bone results in an increase of urinary Hypro excretion.

REFERENCES

Function of Collagen

1. Grant ME, Prockop DJ: The biosynthesis of collagen. N Eng J Med 286:194, 242, 291, 1972
2. Harkness RD: Biological functions of collagen. Biol Rev 36:399, 1961

Structure of Collagen Molecule

3. Beisswenger PJ, Spiro RG: Human glomerular basement membrane: Chemical alteration in diabetes mellitus. Science 168:596, 1970
4. Butler WT: Structural studies in collagen. In Balarzs EA (ed): Chemistry and Molecular Biology of the Intercellular Matrix, Vol I, p 149. London, Academic Press, 1970
5. Chung E, Miller EJ: Collagen polymorphism: Characterization of molecules with the chain composition $\alpha 1(III)_3$ in human tissues. Science 183:1200, 1974
6. Comstock JP, Udenfriend S: Effect of lactate on collagen proline hydroxylase activity in cultured L-929 fibroblasts. Proc Nat Acad Sci USA 66:552, 1970
7. Dehm P, Prockop DJ: Synthesis and extrusion of collagen by freshly isolated cells from chick embryo tendon. Biochem Biophys Acta 240:358, 1971
8. Eylar EH: On the biological role of glycoproteins. J Theor Biol 10, 89, 1966
9. Fernandez-Madrid F: Collagen Biosynthesis: A review. Clin Orthop 68:181, 1970
10. Green H, Goldberg B: Collagen and cell protein synthesis by an established mammalian fibroblast line. Science (Lond) 204:147, 1964
11. Grant ME, Prockrop DJ: The biosynthesis of collagen (second of three parts). N Engl J Med 286 (5):242, 1972
12. Halme J, Kivirikko KI, Simons K: Isolation and partial characterization of highly purified protocollagen proline hydroxylases. Biochem Biophys Acta 198:460, 1970
13. Harris Ed Jr, Krane SM: Collagenases. N Eng J Med 291:557, 1974
14. Hutton JJ Jr, Tappel AL, Udenfriend S: Cofactor and substrate requirements of collagen protease hydroxylase. Arch Biochem Biophys 118:231, 1967
15. Jiminez SA, Dehm P, Prockop DJ: Further evidence for a transport form of collagen: Its extrusion and extracellular conversion to alpha chains in embryonic tendon. FEBS Lett 17:245, 1971
16. Kefalides NA: Chemical properties of basement membranes. Int Rev Exp Pathol 10:1, 1971
17. Petruska JA, Hodge AJ: a subunit model for the tropocollagen macromolecule. Proc Nat Acad Sci USA 51:871, 1964
18. Rhoads RE, Udenfriend S: Purification and properties of collagen proline hydroxylase from newborn rat skin. Arch Biochem Biophys 139:329, 1970
19. Robert AM, Robert B, Roper L: Chemical and physical properties of structural glycoproteins. In Balarsz EA (ed): Chemisry and Molecular Biology of the Intercellular Matrix, Vol I, p 237. London, Academic Press, 1970
20. Rosenbloom H, Harsch M, Jimenez S: Hydroxyproline content determines the denaturation temperature of chick tendon collagen. Arch Biochem Biophys 158:478, 1973
21. Rosenbloom J, Prockop DJ: Incorporation of cis-hydroxyproline into protocollagen in place of proline and trans-hydroxyproline is not extruded at a normal rate. J Biol Chem 246:1549, 1971
22. Spiro MJ, Spiro RG: Studies on the biosynthesis of hydroxylysine-linked disaccharide unit of basement membranes and collagens. II. Kidney galactosyletransferase. J Biol Chem 246:2910, 1971
23. Spiro RG, Spiro MJ: Studies on the biosynthesis of hydroxylysine-linked disaccharides unit of basement membranes and collagens. I. Kidney glucosyltransferase. J Biol Chem 246:4899, 1971
24. Strawich E, Nimni ME: Properties of collagen molecule containing three identical components extracted from bovine articular cartilage. Biochemistry 10:3905, 1971
25. Takeuchi T, Prockop DJ: Protocollagen proline hydroxylase in normal liver and hepatic fibrosis. Gastroenterology 56:744, 1969
26. Tanzer ML: Cross-linking of collagen: Endogenous aldehydes in collagen react in several ways to form a variety of unique covalent cross-links. Science 180:561, 1973
27. Traub W, Piez KA: The chemistry and structure of collagen. Adv Protein Chem 25:243, 1971
28. Traub W, Yonath A, Segal DM: On the molecular structure of collagen. Nature (Lond) 221:914, 1969
29. Uitto J, Lindy S, Rockkannen P et al: Increased protocollagen proline hydroxylase activity in synovial tissue in rheumatoid arthritis. Clinica Chemica Acta 30:741, 1970

Formation of Collagen Fibrils

30. Bellamy G, Bornstein P: Evidence for procollagen, a biosynthesis precursor of collagen. Proc Nat Acad Sci USA 68:1138, 1971
31. Grant HE, Freeman IL, Schofield JD et al: Variations on the carbohydrate content of human and bovine polymeric collagens from various tissues. Biochim Biophys Acta 177:682, 1969
32. Jackson DS, Bentley JP: Collagen-gylcosaminoglycan interactions. In Gould BS (ed): Treatise on Collagen, Vol 2A, Biology of Collagen, p 189. New York, Academic Press, 1968
33. Jiminez SA, Dehm P, Prockop DJ: Further evidence for a transport form of collagen: Its extrusion and extracellular conversion to alpha-chains in embryonic tendon. FEBS Lett 17:245, 1971

Cross-Linking in Collagen

34. Bailey AJ, Peach CM, Fowler LJ: Chemistry of the collagen cross-links, isolation and characterization of two intermediate intermolecular cross-links in collagen. Biochem J 117:819, 1970
35. Craver JM, Madden JW, Peacock EE Jr: Biologic control of physical properties of tendon adhesions: Effect of beta-aminopropionitrile in chickens. Ann Surg 167:697, 1968
36. Deshmukh K, Nimni ME: A defect in the intramolecular and intermolecular cross-linking of collagen caused by penicillamine. J Biol Chem 244:1787, 1969
37. Harris ED Jr, Sjoerdsma A: Collagen profile in various clinical conditions. Lancet 2:707, 1966
38. Kivirikko KI: Urinary excretion of hydroxyproline in health and disease. Int Rev Connect Tissue Res 5:93, 1970
39. Lane JM, Bora FW Jr, Black J et al: Cis-hydroxyproline limits work necessary to flex a digit after tendon injury. Clin Orthop 109:193, 1975
40. Partridge SM, Elden DF, Thomas J et al: Incorporation of labelled lysine into the desmosine cross-bridges in elastin. Nature (Lond) 209:399, 1966
41. Rodman GP: Progressive systemic sclerosis (diffuse sclerodermal immunological diseases). In Samter M (ed): Immunological Diseases, p 769. Boston, Little, Brown, 1965
42. Siegal RC, Martin GR: Collagen cross-linking: Enzymatic synthesis of lysine-derived aldehydes and the production of cross-linked components. J Biol Chem 245:1653, 1970
43. Sinex FM: The role of collagen in aging. In Gould BS (ed): Collagen, Vol 2B, p 409. New York, Academic Press, 1968
44. Uitto J: Collagen biosynthesis in human skin: A review with emphasis on scleroderma. Ann Clin Res 3:250, 1971

Bone Collagen

45. Ascenzi A, Bonucci E, Bocciareli DS: An electron microscopic study of osteon calcification. J Ultrastruct Res 12:287, 1965
46. Birkenhager JC, van der Sluys Veer J, Vander Heul RO et al: Studies of iliac crest bone from controls and patients with bone disease by means of chemical analysis, tetracycline labeling and histology. In Fleisch H, Blackwood HJ, Owen M (eds): Calcified Tissues, p 73. New York, Springer-Verlag, 1966
47. Campo RD, Tourtellotte CD: The comparison of bovine cartilage and bone. Biochim Biophys Acta 141:614, 1967
48. Cooper CW, Talmage RV: A comparison of exogenous and endogenous parathyroid hormone effects on bone collagen synthesis. Gen Comp Endocrinol 5:534, 1965
49. Cooper RR, Milgram JJ, Robinson RA: Morphology of the osteon. J Bone Joint Surg 48A:1239, 1966
50. Eastor JE: The amino acid composition of mammalian collagen and gelatin. Biochem J 61:589, 1955
51. Firschein HE: Collagen turnover in calcified tissues. Arch Biochem Biophys 119:119, 1967
52. Flanagan B, Nichols G Jr: Metabolic studies of human bone in vitro. I. Normal bone. J Clin Invest 44:1788, 1965
53. Flanagan B, Nichols G Jr: Parathyroid inhibition of bone collagen synthesis. Endocrinology 74:180, 1964
54. Flanagan B, Nichols G Jr: Metabolic studies of human bone in vitro. II. Changes in hyperparathyroidism. J Clin Invest 44:1795, 1965
55. Glimcher MJ, Krane SM: Studies on the interactions of collagen and phosphate. In Lacroix P, Budy AM (eds): Radioisotopes and Bone, p 393. Oxford, Blackwell, 1962
56. Glimcher MJ, Andrikedes A, Kossiwa D: The alteration of amino acid side chain groups of collagen and its effect on in vitro calcification. In Jackson SF, Harkness RD, Partridge SM et al (eds): Structure and Function of Connective and Skeletal Tissues, p 342. London, Butterworth, 1965
57. Glimcher MJ, Friberg UA, Orloff S: The role of inorganic crystals in the solubility characteristics of collagen in lathyritic bone. J Ultrastruct Res 15:74, 1966
58. Kao K–Y T, Hilker DM, McGarack TH: Connective tissue. V. Comparison of synthesis and turnover of collagen and elastin in tissues of the rat at several ages. Proc Soc Exp Biol Med 106:335, 1961
59. Kao K–Y T, Hitt WE, Dawson RL et al: Connective Tissue. VII. Changes in protein and hexosamine content of bone and cartilage of rats at different ages. Proc Soc Exp Biol Med 110:538, 1962
60. Miller EJ, Martin GR: The collagen of bone. Clin Orthop 59:195, 1968
61. Neuberger A, Slack HGB: The metabolism of collagen from liver, bone, skin and tendon in the normal rat. Biochem J 53:47, 1953
62. Robinson RA, Watson ML: Collagen-crystal relationship in bone as seen in the electron microscope. Anat Rec 114:383, 1952
63. Robinson RA, Watson ML: Crystal-collagen relationships in bone as observed in the electron microscope. III. Crystal and collagen morphology as a function of age. Ann NY Acad Sci 60:596, 1955
64. Robinson RA, Cameron DA: Electron microscopy of cartilage and bone matrix at the distal epiphyseal line of the femur in the newborn infant. J Biophys Biochem Cytol (Suppl) 2:253, 1956
65. Robinson RA, Cameron DA: The organic matrix of bone and epiphyseal cartilage. Clin Orthop 9:16, 1957
66. Robinson RA, Cameron DA: Electron microscopy of the primary spongiosa of the metaphysis of the distal end of the femur in the newborn infant. J Bone Joint Surg 40A:687, 1958
67. Rogers HJ, Weidmann SM, Parkinson A: Studies on the skeletal tissues. 2. The collagen content of bones from rabbits, oxen and humans. Biochem J 50:537, 1952
68. Scott BL, Pease DC: Electron microscopy of the epiphyseal apparatus. Anat Rec 126:465, 1956
69. Simmons DJ, Nichols G Jr: Diurnal periodicity in the metabolic activity of bone tissue. Am J Physiol 210:411, 1966
70. Sherry S, Troll W, Rosenblum ED: "Collagenase" activity of cathepsins. Proc Soc Exp Biol Med 87:125, 1954
71. Sobel AE, Penni AL, Burger M: Nuclei formation and crystal growth in mineralizing tissues. Trans NY Acad Sci 22:233, 1960
72. Vaes GM, Nichols G Jr: Metabolism of glycine-1-C^{14} by bone *in vitro:* Effects of hormones and other factors. Endocrinology 70:390, 1962
73. Vaes GM, Nichols G Jr: Effects of massive dose of parathyroid extract on bone metabolic pathways. Endocrinology 70:546, 1962
74. Woessner JF Jr, Brewer TH: Formation and breakdown of collagen and elastin in the human uterus during pregnancy and post-partum involution. Biochem J 89:75, 1963

Collagen of Articular Cartilage

75. Collins DH McElligott TF: Sulphate ($^{35}SO_4$) uptake by chondrocytes in relation to histological changes in osteoarthritic human articular cartilage. Ann Rheum Dis 19:318, 1960
76. Fry A, Robertson W: Interlocked stresses in cartilage. Nature 215:53, 1967
77. Lane J, Weiss C: Review of articular cartilage research. Arthritis Rheum 18:553, 1975
78. Little K, Pimm LH, Trueta J: Osteoarthritis of the hip. J Bone Joint Surg 40B:123, 1958
79. Miller EJ: Identification of 3 genetically distinct collagens by cyanogen bromide cleavage of insoluble human skin and cartilage collagen. Biochem Biophys Res Commun 42:1024, 1971
80. Miller EJ: Isolation and characterization of a collagen from chick cartilage containing 3 identical alpha chains. Biochemistry 10:1652, 1971
81. Miller EJ: A review of biochemical studies on genetically distinct collagen of the skeletal system. Clin Orthop 92:260, 1973
82. Matthews BF: Composition of articular cartilage in osteoarthritis: Changes in collagen/chondroitin sulfate ratio. Med J 2:660, 1953
83. McCall JG: Ultrastructure of human articular cartilage. J Anat 104:586, 1969
84. Nimni M, Deshmukh K: Differences in collagen metabolism between normal and osteoarthritic human articular cartilage. Science 181:751, 1973
85. Rosenberg L, Johnson B, Schubert M: Protein polysaccharides from human articular and costal cartilage. J Clin Invest 44:1647, 1965
86. Seyer JM, Vinson WC: Synthesis of type I and type II collagen by embryonic chick cartilage. Biochem Biophys Res Commun 58:272, 1974
87. Sokoloff L: The Biology of Degenerative Joint Disease. Chicago, University of Chicago Press, 1960
88. Weiss C: Ultrastructural characteristics of osteoarthritis. Fed Proc 32:1459, 1973

89. Weiss C: An ultrastructural study of aging human articular cartilage. J Bone Joint Surg 53A:803, 1971
90. Weiss C, Rosenberg L, Helfet AJ: An ultrastructural study of normal young adult human articular cartilage. J Bone Joint Surg 50A:663, 1968

Collagenase

91. Abe S, Nagai Y: Evidence for the presence of a complex of collagenase with α_2-macroglobulin in human rheumatoid synovial fluid; a possible regulatory mechanism of collagenase activity *in vivo*. J Biochem (Tokyo) 73:897, 1973
92. Barrett AJ, Starkey PM: The interaction of α_2-macroglobulin with proteinases: Characteristics and specificity of the reaction, and a hypothesis concerning its molecular mechanism. Biochem J 133:709, 1973
93. Bauer EA, Eisen AZ, Jeffrey JJ: Regulation of vertebrate collagenase activity *in vivo* and *in vitro*. J Invest Dermatol 59:50, 1972
94. Bennett GA, Zeller JW, Bauer W: Subcutaneous nodules of rheumatoid arthritis and rheumatic fever: A pathologic study. Arch Pathol 30:70, 1940
95. Bonar LC, Glimcher MJ: Thermal denaturation of mineralized and demineralized bone collagens. J Ultrastruct Res 32:545, 1970
96. Bornstein P, King AH, Piez KA: The limited cleavage of native collagen with chymotrypsin, trypsin, and cyanogen bromide. Biochemistry 5:3803, 1966
97. Bruns RR, Gross J: Band pattern of the segment-long-spacing form of collagen: Its use in the analysis of primary structure. Biochemistry 12:808, 1973
98. Burleigh MC, Barrett AJ, Lazarus GS: Cathepsin B_1; a lysosomal enzyme that degrades native collagen. Biochem J 137:287, 1974
99. Drake MP, Davison PF, Bump S et al: Action of proteolytic enzymes on tropocollagen and insoluble collagen. Biochemistry 5:301, 1966
100. Eisen AZ, Bauer EA, Jeffrey JJ: Human skin collagenase: The role of serum alpha globulins in the control of the activity *in vivo* and *in vitro*. Proc Natl Acad Sci USA 68:248, 1971
101. Eisen AZ, Bloch KJ, Sakai T: Inhibition of human skin collagenase by human serum. J Lab Clin Med 75:258, 1970
102. Evanson JM, Jeffrey JJ, Krane SM: Human collagenase: Identification and characterization of an enzyme from rheumatoid synovium in culture. Science 158:499, 1967
103. Gross J, Bruschi A: The pattern of collagen degradation in cultured tadpole tissues. Dev Biol 26:36, 1971
104. Gross J, Nagai Y: Specific degradation of the collagen molecule by tadpole collagenolytic enzyme. Proc Natl Acad Sci USA 54:497, 1965
105. Harper E, Gross J: Collagenase, procollagenase and activation relationships in tadpole tissue cultures. Biochem Biophys Res Commun 48:1147, 1972
106. Harper E, Toole BP: Collagenase and hyaluronidase stimulation by dibutyryl adenosine 3′,5′-monophosphate. J Biol Chem 248:2625, 1973
107. Harris ED Jr, DiBona DR, Krane SM: Collagenases in human synovial fluid. J Clin Invest 48:2104, 1969
108. Harris ED Jr: A collagenolytic system produced by primary cultures of rheumatoid nodule tissue. J Clin Invest 51:2973, 1972
109. Harris ED Jr, Dimmig TA: Collagenolytic enzyme in septic arthritis: Potential significance for joint destruction. Arthritis Rheum 17:498, 1974
110. Harris ED Jr, Farrell ME: Resistance to collagenase: A characteristic of collagen fibrils cross-linked by formaldehyde. Biochim Biophys Acta 278:133, 1972
111. Harris ED Jr, Krane SM: Effects of colchicine on collagenase in cultures of rheumatoid synovium. Arthritis Rheum 14:669, 1971
112. Harris ED Jr, Krane SM: Cartilage collagen: substrate in soluble and fibrillar form for rheumatoid collagenase. Trans. Assoc. Am. Physicians 86:82, 1973
113. Harris ED Jr, Krane SM: Collagenases. N Engl J Med 291:557, 605, 652, 1974
114. Kruze D, Wojtecka E: Activation of leukocyte collagenase proenzyme by rheumatoid synovial fluid. Biochim Biophys Acta 285:436, 1972
115. Lapiere CM, Gross J: Animal collagenase and collagen metabolism. In Sognnaes RF (ed): Mechanism of Hard Tissue Destruction, p 663. Washington, DC, Am. Assn. Adv. Sci., 1963
116. Olsen BR: Electron microscopic studies of collagen. III. Tryptic digestion of tropocollagen macromolecules. Z Zelforsch 61:913, 1964
117. Parakkal PF: Macrophages: The time course sequence of their distribution in the postpartum uterus. J Ultrastruct Res 40:284, 1972
118. Perez–Tomayo R: Collagen resorption in carrageenin granulomas. I. Collagenolytic activity in *in vitro* explants. Lab Invest 22:137, 1970
119. Rosenbloom J, Harsch M, Jiminez S: Hydroxyproline content determines the denaturation temperature of chick tendon collagen. Arch Biochem Biophys 158:478, 1973
120. Sakai T, Gross J: Some properties of the products of reaction of tadpole collagenase with collagen. Biochemistry 6:518, 1967
121. Sakakihara S, Inouye K, Sudo K et al: Synthesis of (Pro-Hyp-Gly) of defined molecular weights: Evidence for the stabilization of collagen triple helix by hydroxyproline. Biochim Biophys Acta 303:198, 1973
122. Sakamoto S, Goldhaber P, Glimcher MJ: Mouse bone collagenase: The effect of heparin on the amount of enzyme released in tissue culture and on the activity of the enzyme. Calcif Tissue Res 12:247, 1973
123. Sakamoto S, Sakamoto M, Goldhaber P et al: The inhibition of mouse bone collagenase by lysosome. Calcif Tissue Res 14:291, 1974
124. Shimizu M, Glimcher MJ, Travis D et al: Mouse bone collagenase: Isolation, partial purification, and mechanism of action. Proc Soc Exp Biol Med 130:1175, 1969
125. Stark M, Kuhn K: Molecular fragments of rat skin collagen obtained on collagenase digestion. Eur J Biochem 6:542, 1968
126. Stern B, Golub L, Goldhaber D: Effects of demineralization and parathyroid hormone on the availability of bone collagen to degradation by collagenase. J Periodonl Res 5:116, 1970
127. Taylor AC: Collagenolysis in cultured tissue. II. Role of mast cells. J Dent Res 50:1301, 1971
128. Vaes G: Lysosomes and the cellular physiology of bone resorption. In Dingle JT, Fell HB (eds): Lysosomes in Biology and Pathology, Vol 1, p. 217. New York, American Elsevier, 1969
129. Vaes G: The release of collagenase as an inactive proenzyme by bone explants in culture. Biochem J 126:289, 1972
130. Wegelius O, Klockars M, Vaino K: Collagenolytic activity in synovial fluid cells in rheumatoid arthritis. Ann Clin Res 2:171, 1970

131. Woolley DE, Glanville RW, Crossley MJ, et al: Purification and some properties of rheumatoid synovial collagenase. Scand J Clin Lab Invest (Suppl 123) 29:37, 1972

Hydroxyproline Excretion: An Indicator of Collagen Metabolism

132. Dull TA, Henneman PH: Urinary hydroxyproline as an index of collagen turnover in bone. N Engl J Med 268:132, 1963
133. Jasin HE, Ziff M: Relationship between soluble collagen and urinary hydroxyproline in the lathyritic rat. Proc Soc Exp Biol Med 110:837, 1962
134. Kivirikko KI, Laitinen O, Prockop DJ: Modification of a specific assay for hydroxyproline in urine. Anal Biochem 19:249, 1967
135. Kivirikko KI, Laitinen O, Aer J et al: Studies with ^{14}C-proline on the action of cortisone on the metabolism of collagen in the rat. Biochem Pharmacol 14:1445, 1965
136. Klein L, Lafferty FW, Pearson OH et al: Correlation of urinary hydroxyproline, serum alkaline phosphatase and skeletal calcium turnover. Metabolism 13:272, 1964
137. Ney RL, Gill JR, Keiser HR et al: Regulation of hydroxyproline excretion in hyperparathyroidism. J Clin Endocrinol 26:815, 1966
138. Prockop DJ: Isotopic studies on collagen degradation and the urine excretion of hydroxyproline. J. Clin Invest 43:453, 1964
139. Prockop DJ, Kivirikko KI: Relationship of hydroxyproline excretion in urine to collagen metabolism. Ann Intern Med 66:1243, 1967
140. Siuko H, Savela J, Kulonen E: Effect of hydrocortisone on the formation of collagen in guinea pig skin. Acta Endocr (Kbh) 31:113, 1959
141. Veis A, Anesy J: Modes of intermolecular cross-linking in mature insoluble collagen. J Biol Chem 240:3899, 1965

6

Physiology and Mineralization of Bone

Section I
Physiology of Bone

BIOCHEMISTRY

The inorganic constituents of bone by dry weight comprise 65% to 70%, and the organic constituents comprise 30% to 35%, of which 90% to 95% is the extracellular matrix consisting of the fibrous protein collagen.[1] Other organic constituents include small amounts of proteinpolysaccharides (PPS) and lipids, particularly phospholipids.

COLLAGEN

Collagen forms a highly ordered system of collagen fibers with the typical axial periodicity of 640 A to 700 A and a unique protein composition of about one third glycine residues, one fifth amino acid residues, a large number of alanine residues, and very few aromatic amino acids; cysteine is completely lacking.

A single collagen fibril is a three-stranded coil composed of three adjacent left-handed helices (designated collagen polymers $\alpha 1$, $\alpha 1$, $\alpha 2$) bound together by intermolecular and intramolecular cross linkages and twisted about a common axis.

When newly synthesized (young) collagen is denatured, it separates into two $\alpha 1$ chains and one $\alpha 2$ chain, each with a molecular weight of about 100,000. Older collagen gives rise to two double and one triple chain ($\beta 11$, $\beta 12$, and $\gamma 112$) whose molecular weights are 200,000 and 300,000, respectively.

Although the composition is similar to other types of collagen, bone collagen differs from most of the soft tissue collagens in certain respects. Bone collagen is insoluble in solvents used to extract collagens from other tissues (neutral salt solutions and weak organic acids). This characteristic is thought to be due to the presence of strong intermolecular bonds between and along the length of adjacent macromolecules.[2]

The theoretical sequence of events in the synthesis of collagen from the intracellular formation of polypeptide chains to the extracellular development of the mature collagen fibril is represented in Figure 6-1.

PROTEINPOLYSACCHARIDES

Proteinpolysaccharides (PPS) comprise 4% to 5% of the organic constituents of bone. They are compounds consisting of a polypeptide chain to which side-chains of highly sulfated polysaccharides are covalently bound. The principal polysaccharide of bone is chondroitin-4-sulfate (chondroitin sulfate A). Its role is not clear, but it appears to inhibit mineralization of bone by strongly complexing with Ca^{2+} ions.

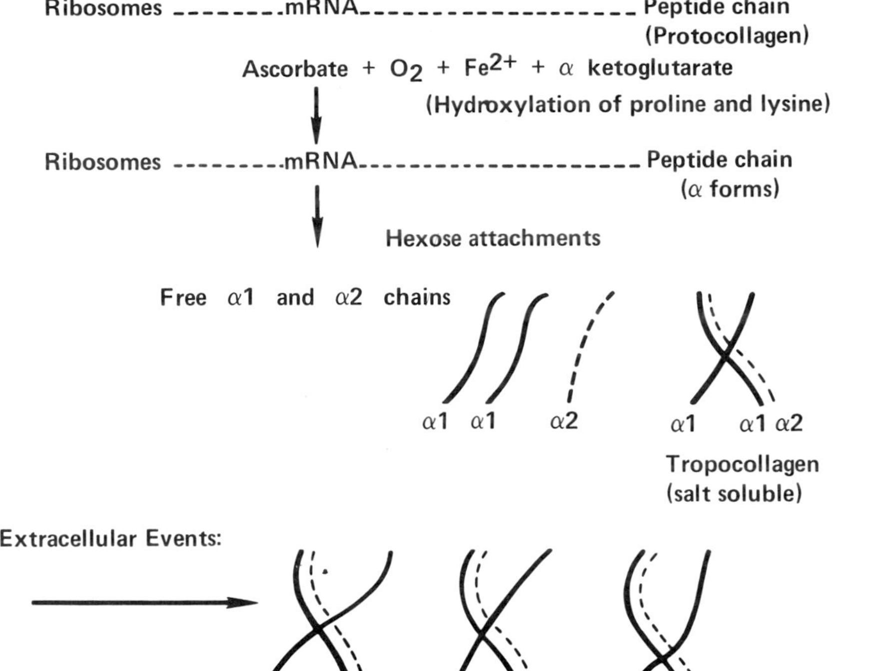

FIG. 6-1. Biosynthesis of collagen fibrils. (Clark I: Biochemistry of bone. In Wilson FC (ed): The Musculoskeletal System. Philadelphia, JB Lippincott, 1975)

In certain diseases (*e.g.*, the mucopolysaccharidoses), increased urinary excretion of polysaccharides takes place. The loss of polysaccharides from bone and cartilage results in specific skeletal deformities.

Noncollagenous protein amounts to about 0.5% of the organic constituents, but most of this fraction represents the protein core of PPS.

LIPIDS

Less than 0.1% of the organic constituents of bone is composed of lipids, consisting of triglycerides, free fatty acids, phospholipids, and cholesterol. Under electron microscopy, it can be observed that phospholipids disappear just before mineralization takes place. Moreover, lipids are absent in the epiphyseal growth plate of rachitic animals and reappear after the administration of vitamin D. This suggests that lipids participate in some unknown manner in the process of mineralization.

INORGANIC CONSTITUENTS

The dry weight of bone is composed of 65% to 70% inorganic mineral, 95% of which is a calcium and phosphate solid. An "amorphous" Ca-P solid is present in greater amounts in young, newly formed tissue (40%

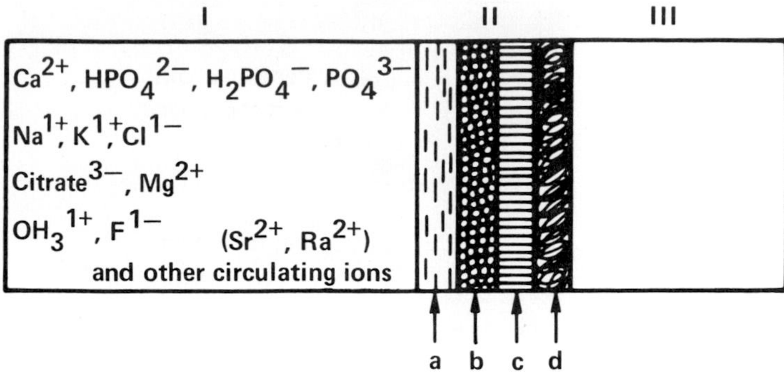

I. Bulk solution
II. Hydration shell
   a) Loosely bound water
   b) Tightly bound water
   c) Hydrated ion layer
   d) Crystal surface
III. Crystal interior

FIG. 6-2. Schematic representation of a hydroxyapatite crystal in contact with an aqueous solution containing various ions. (Neumann WF, Neuman MW: The Chemical Dynamics of the Bone Mineral. Chicago, University of Chicago Press, 1958)

to 50%) than in older, more mature bone (25% to 30%). The chemical composition and structure of this physically amorphous phase has not been elucidated, but studies suggest that the amorphous substance is either $CaHPO_4 \cdot 2H_2O$, or $Ca_3(PO_4)_2 \cdot 3H_2O$.

The main Ca-P solid is a poorly crystalline hydroxyapatite having the unit cell formula $Ca_{10}(PO_4)_6(OH)_2$. According to some investigators, it may be octacalcium phosphate with the formula $Ca_8H_2(PO_4)_6 \cdot 5H_2O$. The theoretical molar ratio of Ca:P is 1.67, but it rarely equals this value in bone.

Roentgen diffraction patterns of synthetic hydroxyapatite and bone crystals are similar. The size of the hydroxyapatite and bone crystals are similar. The size of the hydroxyapatite crystals varies, the approximate dimensions being 25 to 50 A × 400 A × 200 to 350 A. The direction of the long axis (C-axis) of the crystal is parallel to that of the collagen fiber.

Only about 0.65% of human bone calcium is part of a readily exchangeable pool. The sites where rapid exchange takes place can be identified by radionuclides and appear to be the lining of the haversian canals and resorption cavities. Sites of bone deposition do not appear to participate in these exchange reactions.

All crystals in a liquid are surrounded by a layer of water, a hydration shell. Figure 6-2 is a representation of the exchange mechanism.

Theoretically, ions can easily pass to and from an aqueous phase and exchange rapidly. At the surface of the crystal, ions are held by electrostatic charges. Only those ions with chemical properties similar to those elements composing the crystal can actually enter and become part of the crystal. Thus, strontium and lead can replace and substitute for calcium positions of the apatite; fluoride or chloride can replace the hydroxyl ion. These substitutions occur at a slow rate as compared with the rapid rate of exchange at the water layer. Other ions, such as potassium or magnesium, are believed to be adsorbed on the crystal surface.

The gradient between the mineral content in bone and the extracellular fluid (ECF) can reasonably be explained by the hypothesis of Neuman.[3]

The minor mineral constituents of bone are magnesium, sodium, potassium, and a number of trace elements, including zinc, manganese, fluoride and molybdenum. The trace elements are considered to be adsorbed on the bone surface and probably play no role in bone metabolism.

BASIC PHYSIOLOGIC PROCESSES

Calcium salts are relatively insoluble, especially as phosphates and carbonates. The secondary form of calcium phosphate, $CaHPO_4$, has a solubility of greater than 10^{-3} M, and the ions of this form circulate in the ECF at approximately half this concentration. When tertiary calcium phosphate, such as bone apatite crystals, is added to a solution of Ca^{2+} and HPO_4-ions, the ions will be attracted to the bone crystals.[5]

Calcium is complexed by many organic compounds, particularly proteins. This characteristic is essential to strengthening and regulating the permeability of the cell membrane. For the normal functioning of cells, intracellular Ca^{2+} ion concentration must be maintained in the range of 10^{-7} M. A normal *p*H must be maintained, and concentrations of Ca^{2+} and HPO_4-ions must not exceed the range of 10^{-3} M to avoid calcium phosphate precipitation within the cell.

Intracellular homeostasis of calcium shown in Figure

6-3 demonstrates the major difference between the ionic calcium concentration of ECF as compared with intracellular fluids. It also illustrates the relative impermeability of cell membranes to this divalent ion. Nevertheless, calcium continuously enters the cell where mechanisms, probably mitochondria, exist for the precise control of internal ionic calcium concentrations. Some type of biological mechanism, termed the *calcium pump*, must be located in cell membranes functioning to transfer calcium against a chemical gradient to the outside of the cell.

The calcium ion, when absorbed by the intestinal mucosa, or during renal tubular resorption after glomerular filtration, must be transported through the cell itself and pumped out of the cell with sufficient rapidity to avoid disturbing the cellular processes. Theoretically, rapid entry through a more permeable membrane, mitochondrial control, and rapid extrusion by "pumping" permit transcellular transport without raising the intracellular concentration of this ion above permissible limits.

Calcium concentration in plasma is approximately 10 mg/dl. The diffusible ionized portion that is not complexed with nondiffusible plasma proteins is slightly greater than 50% of the total, or 5 to 6 mg/dl, or approximately 1.5×10^{-3} M. This keeps the concentration of ionic calcium below the solubility product of the calcium phosphate salt.

The constancy of extracellular ion concentrations is maintained by an equilibrium between these ions and those complexed to cell membranes. The net movement of ions extruded through cell membranes toward the ECF and of those moving in the reverse direction produces, when this equilibrium is altered, hypercalcemia or hypocalcemia characteristic of the causative pathologic state.

Calcium levels in the blood are influenced by factors other than those that disturb equilibrium exchange processes. The ions are absorbed from the upper small intestine, are continuously resorbed by the renal tubules after glomerular filtration, and incessantly move in and out of bone fluid compartments. All plasma calcium exchanges with bone fluid calcium every 20 minutes (Fig. 6-4).

The dominant role in the maintenance of calcium homeostasis is played by the constant resorption and deposition of bone minerals throughout life. To a lesser degree, other internal factors such as hormonal (parathyroid hormone [PTH], calcitonin), renal (tubular resorption), and vitamin D metabolites exert roles that help to maintain constant plasma calcium concentration. Since bone is the major source of calcium, a cellular interface at the surface of bone appears to be the logical means through which an equilibrial control between the ECF and the solid is accomplished. It has been demonstrated that the fluid bathing the extracellular components of bone (*i.e.*, matrix and apatite crystals) has a different ionic composition than ECF and plasma. The

FIG. 6-3. Intracellular calcium homeostasis. (Talmage RV: Physiological processes in bone. In Wilson FC (ed): The Musculoskeletal System. Philadelphia, JB Lippincott, 1975)

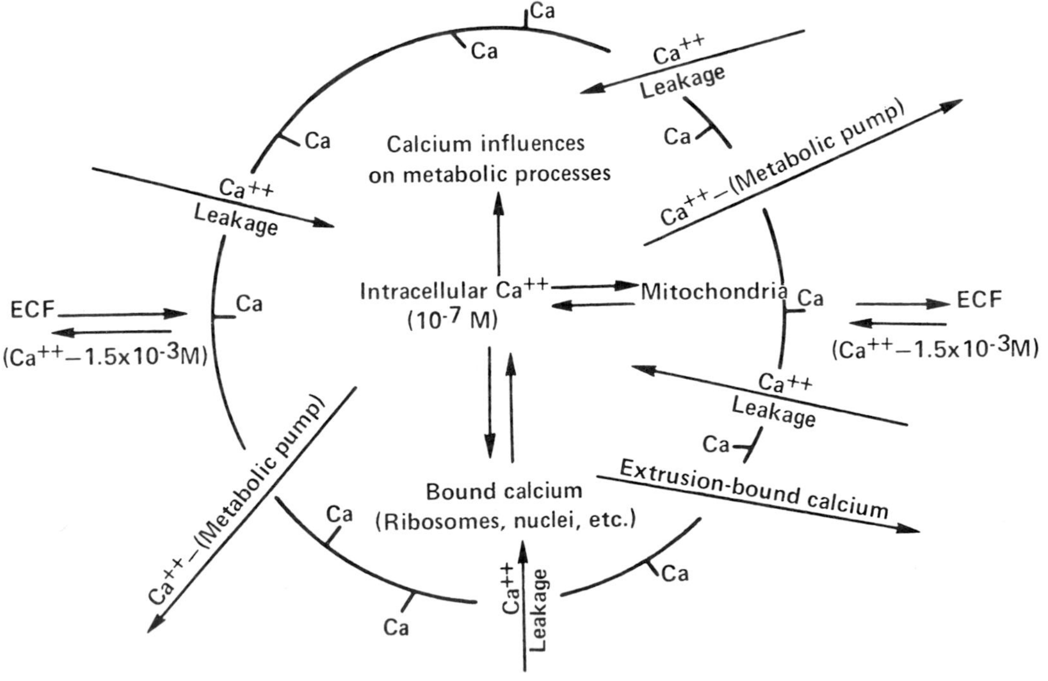

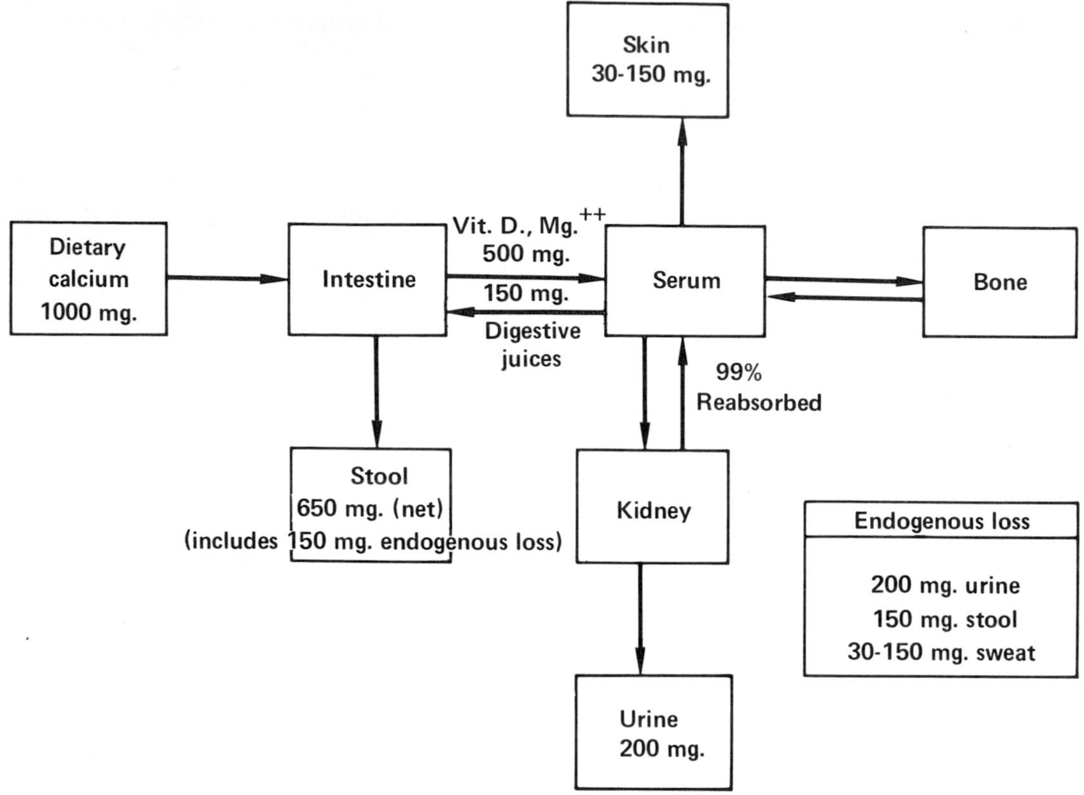

FIG. 6-4. Calcium transfer in the body (24-hour period). (Talmage RV: Physiological processes in bone. In Wilson FC (ed): The Musculoskeletal System. Philadelphia, JB Lippincott, 1975)

primary differences include a very high potassium ion content (20 times that of ECF) and a low calcium content (one third that of ECF). This suggests that bone fluid compartments are maintained distinct and apart from ECF.[4]

The surfaces of active bone tissue are covered by a layer of cells that forms a dynamic interface between the fluid in contact with the intercellular components of bone and the ECF. In the young animal, almost 100% of all bone surfaces are covered. In the old, about 40% of the bone surfaces are uncovered, areas presumably not involved in depleting the calcium content of ECF.

The manner in which the cellular interface functions to maintain the calcium ion differential between the two fluid compartments (bone fluid and ECF) is shown in Figure 6-5. The surface cells are considered to act as "calcium pumps," returning the ions to the ECF as fast as they filter between the cells into the bone fluid compartment.

Calcium ions in bone, intestine, and kidney are transported through the cell toward the ECF. The source of ions in the gut is the dietary intake; ions transported through the renal tubule are derived from the glomerular filtrate; those transported by lining cells of the bone surface are derived mainly from the calcium entering the bone fluid through the intercellular channels.

Intestinal absorption depends on dietary sources plus factors that influence this absorption (*e.g.*, vitamin D metabolites), bile salts to emulsify the fats (to facilitate fat-soluble vitamin D absorption), PTH, and calcitonin. Renal tubular absorption can never exceed 100% of the calcium from glomerular filtration. Bone fluid, when necessary, can call on resorption of bone if the source from ECF is limited. The bone fluid, being in physicochemical equilibrium with bone crystals and other precipitated forms of calcium phosphate, has a limited supply of calcium, which can readily be drawn on and transported to the ECF to maintain the required levels.

In the absence of adequate oral intake, the renal tubular absorption approaches 100%, whereas the bone surface returns more than 100%.

FACTORS AFFECTING THE FATE OF BONE MINERALS

Because bone is constantly being formed and destroyed, its maintenance depends on an adequate supply of its components, both organic and inorganic, and the ability to use them. The main minerals are calcium and phosphorus, in the form of phosphate, and are ingredients of the diet and are excreted mainly in the feces and urine.

The ultimate fate of these minerals is affected by many factors; the principal ones are listed below but are more fully discussed later in this chapter.

The form in which they exist in food. Human milk contains the more soluble and easily absorbed form of calcium lactose. Calcium in green vegetables exists as insoluble oxalates and therefore is not a suitable source.

Food substances affecting solubility and absorption. Excessive intake of phosphates in relation to calcium or, conversely, excessive intake of calcium in relation to phosphates, encourages precipitation of and excretion of insoluble phosphates. Excessive ingestion of fatty acids causes formation of insoluble calcium soaps. Excessive carbonates will precipitate insoluble calcium carbonate. The calcium and the phosphorus thus precipitated become unavailable for absorption.

Condition of the digestive tract. Gastric acidity is necessary for solubility of calcium and phosphorus. Pancreatic enzymes digest fats completely so that fatty acids are not available for formation of insoluble calcium soaps. Bile salts are essential for emulsification of fats and their absorption; absorption of fat-soluble vitamin D requires normal fat absorption. Short-circuiting operations (*e.g.*, gastric resection followed by a gastrojejunostomy) causes rapid propulsion of intestinal contents and diminished absorption in the upper regions of the small intestine. Any disease process of the small intestine interferes with the absorption of minerals.

Vitamin D. Vitamin D is necessary mainly for the absorption of calcium and phosphorus in the upper portion of the small intestine. The metabolites of vitamin D are the most active substances that are essential to formation and mineralization of bone.

Parathyroid hormone. The hormone of the parathyroid glands controls the serum level of calcium by effecting resorption of bone, increasing absorption by the gut, and increasing tubular resorption. It lowers the serum phosphate level by promoting its urinary excretion and diminishing its tubular resorption.

Calcitonin is the serum calcium–lowering hormone that acts by inhibiting resorption of bone.

Condition of the kidneys. Phosphorus and, to a lesser extent, calcium are filtered through the glomeruli

FIG. 6-5. A lining cell on the surface of bone. This figure demonstrates a possible mechanism for the entrance of calcium into bone and a system for its transport back into the extracellular fluid. (From Talmage RV: Physiological processes in bone. In Wilson FC (ed): The Musculoskeletal System. Philadelphia, JB Lippincott, 1975)

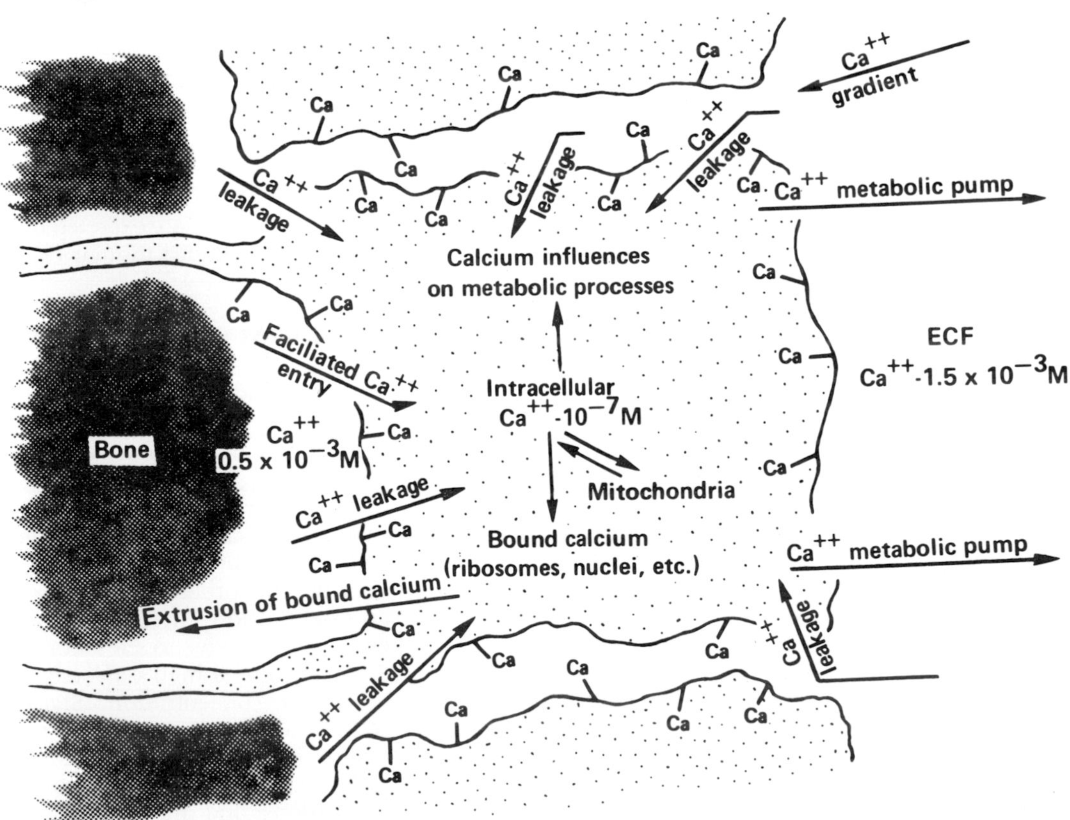

and resorbed by the tubules. Disease at either of these renal levels accordingly interferes with serum levels of these elements, which must rise or fall correspondingly.

Protein metabolism. Destruction of protein throughout the body (catabolism) implies that the protein matrix of bone is likewise involved. As a consequence the mineral content of bone is lessened. An adult, after the age of bone growth is completed, will be in normal calcium and phosphorus balance (*i.e.*, he will excrete the same amount of minerals that he ingests). A growing person, on the other hand, will be in positive balance. The intake will be greater than the excretion. When the person is in negative balance, with the output exceeding the intake, a diseased state is said to exist.

PHOSPHORUS

Phosphorus exists as a completely ionized inorganic phosphate in the bloodstream. Eighty percent of the mineral in the body resides in the skeleton, where it is combined with calcium as a complete hydroxyapatite, the formula for which is approximately $Ca_{10}(PO_4)_6(OH)_2$. Phosphate in bone consists of a labile fraction, which is in equilibrium with the phosphate ions in the blood stream, and a stable fraction, which is fixed in the skeleton.

The minimum daily requirement in the normal adult is 0.88 g and is slightly more for growing children and pregnant women. The main food source of phosphorus is milk, with smaller amounts obtained from meat, cheese, eggs, nuts, and whole cereal. White flour and rice have a small content. Phosphorus exists in food in both organic and inorganic forms.

Absorption takes place from the small intestine in the form of soluble inorganic phosphate. The complex organic phosphorus-containing nucleoproteins must first be broken down by enzymes of the pancreas and succus entericus. The resultant phosphoric acid is hydrolyzed by phosphatase, which occurs in abundance in the intestinal wall. The phosphate ions are then transported across the cell membrane in combination with calcium. Absorption depends on vitamin D.

An excess of ingested calcium encourages the precipitation of insoluble phosphates within the intestinal lumen, thereby lessening the absorption of phosphate. As a result the serum phosphate level is lowered, leading to hypophosphatemic rickets or osteomalacia.

When ingested calcium is inadequate, a relative excess of serum phosphates exists. Serum calcium levels must be restored chiefly by compensatory hyperparathyroidism, which causes bone resorption, increases phosphate urinary excretion and decreases its tubular resorption, and increases calcium tubular resorption. A proper balance of these ions in the ECF must be maintained to ensure solubility and to provide proper levels of Ca^{2+} for normal physiological function.

The normal level of serum phosphates as ionized inorganic phosphate is 3 mg to 4 mg/dl in the adult and 5 mg to 6 mg/dl in the infant.

Excretion takes place principally in the urine as monosodium (acid) or disodium (alkaline) phosphates and in lesser amounts as a salt of potassium, ammonium, calcium, and magnesium. Ninety percent of excreted phosphate is in the inorganic form.

There is normally a wide variation in the daily urinary excretion of phosphate. Excretion may be increased by dietary intake such as a high protein diet, by protein catabolism from energetic exercise, by gout, and by hyperparathyroidism.

Low urinary excretion occurs in low-phosphorus rickets and osteomalacia, renal glomerular disease (associated with hyperphosphatemia), pregnancy, and hypoparathyroidism.

The urinary excretion of phosphate mainly depends on dietary intake, which must be carefully controlled for several days before determinations can be made of intake, output, serum levels, and renal tubular resorption rates. The normal range of urinary excretion for adults is 340 mg to 840 mg/day, whereas that for children is 530 mg to 840 mg/day. Values above or below these levels are considered abnormal.

All inorganic phosphate filtered through the glomerulus is in the ionized state, and over 90% of the phosphate is resorbed in the proximal tubule. The rate of resorption is influenced by PTH, vitamin D, and calcitonin.[6] Resorption is diminished by PTH, 11-oxysteroids, estrogens, deficiency or massive excess of vitamin D, a rise of plasma bicarbonate, acidosis, and various medications.

PTH effects diuresis of phosphate by decreasing its resorption. This results in a diminished serum phosphate level.

Calcitonin inhibits bone resorption, thereby lowering the serum phosphate level, which in turn reduces the amount of phosphate excreted by the kidneys. Calcitonin also directly inhibits tubular resorption of calcium.

CALCIUM

Calcium is indispensable to life. The total calcium content in the body is about 1 kg. Only about 1 g is found in plasma and ECF, whereas most of the remainder is in the skeleton as phosphates, carbonates, and hydroxides.

The cation Ca^{2+} is the physiologically active portion that is necessary for blood coagulation, for neuromuscular excitability, in muscular contraction, as a constituent of mucoproteins and mucopolysaccharides, and as an essential ion for many enzymes. Neural function is especially sensitive to Ca^{2+} concentration. Excitability is diminished by a high Ca^{2+} concentration and increased by a low concentration. Signs of an elevated Ca^{2+} concentration include muscular flaccidity and weakness, dulling of consciousness, and stupor. Increased excitability caused by a low Ca^{2+} concentration causes tetany, convulsions, and muscle cramps.

The normal daily requirement for a normal adult of 70 kg is 0.65 g; 1.0 g is required for growing children and pregnant women. Larger amounts are necessary especially during the last trimester of pregnancy and during lactation. Only milk and milk products provide satisfactory dietary sources of calcium. Certain green vegetables, such as spinach, although high in calcium content, are not suitable sources, because their oxalic acid content forms insoluble compounds with calcium.

Most people on a balanced diet ingest between 0.6 g and 1.0 g/day. About 200 mg to 250 mg are absorbed in the average adult, who ingests 1 g/day, and the remainder is lost in the feces.

Absorption takes place from the upper small intestine. The absorption of calcium from the intestine depends on vitamin D, PTH, and calcitonin. Other factors may modify absorption. An acid *p*H will favor absorption by increasing the solubility of calcium salts; conversely, an alkaline *p*H (*e.g.*, during high intake of alkalies) diminishes absorption. Calcium may be complexed, chelated, or precipitated by a variety of substances in the diet, rendering it unavailable for absorption. These include phytate, oxalate, citrate, and excessive amounts of phosphate.[7] Bile salts increase absorption by emulsifying ingested fat, thus decreasing the loss of fat-soluble vitamin D and diminishing the formation of insoluble calcium–fatty acid soaps, which render the calcium nonabsorbable. Rapid motility or bypass operations, which in effect shorten the rate of passage through the bowel, diminish absorption. Various diseases of the bowel, such as sprue, tuberculosis, and ileitis, interfere with the absorptive process.

The normal level of serum calcium in adults is maintained at 8.8 mg to 10.8 mg/dl (4.4 to 5.4 mEq/kl), with somewhat higher values in children. It occurs in a nondiffusible form, which is mainly bound to proteins, and a diffusible form, most of which is ionized.[8]

The amount of available physiologically active ionic calcium is necessarily related to the degree of calcium-protein binding, which in turn is related to the total serum protein level. Since the present methods of measuring ionized calcium are not reliable for routine use, determining the total protein, particularly albumin, will provide an indirect estimate of Ca^{2+}. About 40% of serum calcium is bound to protein (4/5 albumin, 1/5 globulin), 47% is ionized, and 13% is complexed to PO_4, HCO_3, and citrates.

Excretion of calcium occurs mainly through the kidneys. A small portion is excreted by the colon. Renal excretion of calcium varies considerably with the diet, the person, and other factors. The usual level of renal excretion is 400 mg/day in adults, and generally 4 mg to 6 mg/kg body weight in children.[8] Values above or below these ranges are abnormal, provided that dietary intake of calcium is carefully controlled for several days beforehand.

Both ionized and nonionized calcium filters through the glomerulus and is then resorbed in both the proximal and distal tubules. The resorptive rate for calcium depends on vitamin D and PTH. Normally, over 95% of filtered calcium is resorbed. PTH and certain diuretics increase the resorptive rate.[9]

FATE OF PHOSPHORUS AND CALCIUM

The internal metabolism and homeostasis of calcium and phosphate are controlled by PTH, calcitonin, and vitamin D, all of which act to maintain concentrations of physiologically active ionized calcium and phosphate at levels consistent with normal muscle and nerve function and that do not exceed the solubility product of $CaHPO_4$.[6,10]

PTH effects diuresis of phosphate by decreasing its resorption and mobilizes calcium and phosphate from the bone. This hormone also aids intestinal absorption of calcium, plays a role in the exchange of mineral between bone crystal and ECF, and promotes tubular resorption of calcium.

Calcitonin is a hypocalcemic principle that counteracts the effect of PTH by inhibiting resorption of bone as well as renal tubular resorption of calcium.

The rate of production of PTH and calcitonin depends on the response to the level of ionized calcium in the serum. Hypocalcemia results in elaboration of PTH, which in turn increases the serum calcium level by mobilizing bone calcium, thus increasing intestinal absorption of calcium and tubular resorption. The hormone also acts to diminish serum phosphate levels by decreasing tubular resorption.

Hypercalcemia induces elaboration of calcitonin, which lowers serum calcium levels by diminishing bone resorption and perhaps by decreasing intestinal absorption.

Normally, calcium and phosphorus ions in serum exist in a ratio of 2.5:1. The minerals are continually being excreted and replaced from the bony reservoir and foodstuffs. Calcium phosphate in bone undergoes dissociation under the influence of PTH. The ions are in constant equilibrium with solid calcium phosphate and therefore subject to the law of dissociation. Therefore, an increase of phosphate ions results in a fall of calcium ions and consequent deposition of calcium phospate in the bone. Conversely, a fall of phosphate ions produces a rise of calcium ions by withdrawal from the bone, and the excess of calcium is excreted in the urine. This latter chain of events occurs when increased PTH levels cause increased urinary excretion of phosphorus. An increase of both calcium and phosphate, particularly in the presence of vitamin D, causes deposition of calcium phosphate in cartilage or bone matrix.

Calcium and phosphorus after filtration through the renal glomeruli are resorbed by the tubules. Excessive PTH inhibits tubular resorption of phosphorus (TRP). Similarly, in nephrosis, tubular damage permits abundant excretion of these minerals as well as serum proteins.

Calcium varies directly with the serum protein level and inversely with the phosphorus level. It is excreted in the urine, with only a small amount of absorbed calcium being excreted in the feces. The major portion of calcium in the feces represents unabsorbed calcium. In hyperparathyroidism, the high urinary excretion of calcium often produces renal stones. In hyperthyroidism, there is an increased excretion of both calcium and phosphorus, but the blood levels of these elements remain normal. Ionized calcium may actually be increased in the face of a normal serum calcium level, because the serum protein level may be decreased.

Hypercalcemia results from hyperparathyroidism, invasion of bone by neoplasm (lung, breast, kidney, thyroid), production of parathyroidlike hormone by isolated neoplasms (ovary, kidney, lung), sarcoidosis, multiple myeloma, hyperproteinemia from any cause, vitamin D intoxication, and bleeding.

Hypocalcemia results from hypoparathyroidism, chronic renal insufficiency, rickets and osteomalacia, malabsorption syndrome, nephrosis, celiac disease and sprue (faulty fat digestion), and allergy. Active rickets may show a normal serum calcium level with a low phosphorus level; other cases will show a low calcium level with a normal or high phosphorus level.

The Sulkowitch test for calcium in the urine is used in following urinary calcium excretion qualitatively. It may be used in conjunction with quantitative measurements.

Method: Mix equal parts (about 5 ml each) of urine and reagent and observe for turbidity.

Reagent: This contains oxalate radicals buffered at such *p*H that calcium will almost immediately come down as a fine white precipitate.

Oxalic acid	2.5 g
Ammonium oxalate	2.5 g
Glacial acetic acid	5.0 ml
Distilled water q.s.	150.0 ml

Significance: The serum calcium level of a normal person is from 9.5 mg to 11.5 mg/dl, which is above the kidney threshold of 7.5 mg to 9.0 mg/dl; of a completely parathyroidectomized person, from 5.0 to 7.0 mg/dl. If there is no precipitate, the serum calcium level is below 7.5 mg/dl. With the normal range of serum calcium, the test shows a moderate amount of turbidity. When the serum level is about 11.5 mg/dl or above, the turbidity is greater; and when the reaction looks like milk, there is danger of hypercalcemia. If tetany is due to hypoparathyroidism, the test is negative, since the urine contains no calcium; if tetany is due to alkalosis (hyperventilation, excessive alkali intake), the test is positive.

The test is also used in controlling the treatment of hypoparathyroidism with dihydrotachysterol. The drug is given in amounts sufficient to keep calcium excretion within the normal range. Occasionally, a normal person may show no calcium in a single (random) specimen when on a low-calcium diet or an increased amount of calcium just after drinking a large amount of milk. Additional specimens should be examined.

MAGNESIUM

The divalent cation magnesium belongs to the same family of elements as calcium. However, its salts are more soluble, it does not complex to the same degree with organic molecules, but it nevertheless is fractionally bound to plasma proteins.

Magnesium is not readily absorbed through the intestinal mucosa. In the body, about two thirds is situated in bone and half of the remainder is in muscle. In bone it is found only on the surface of crystals, where it is in equilibrium with magnesium ions in the ECF. Its concentration in body fluids is relatively low (0.75×10^{-4} M).

Dietary deficiencies of magnesium are considered rare. Clinical conditions resulting from magnesium deficiencies are related to muscle hyperactivity such as tetany.

Magnesium is a cofactor for numerous intracellular enzymatic reactions, particularly in various steps of the glycolytic cycle. In many processes it acts as an antagonist to the action of calcium. In other reactions, the two ions can be exchanged or can act synergistically.

PTH affects plasma magnesium concentrations, but the effect is considered incidental to the control of calcium. Its involvement in intracellular metabolic processes, ion transport, and ECF ionic control is unknown.

VITAMINS

VITAMIN A

Vitamin A is found in greatest abundance in animal and fish liver, egg yolk, butter, and cream. Yellow or green vegetables contain provitamin A, which is converted to vitamin A in the animal. Absorption of vitamin A from the gastrointestinal tract depends on and parallels fat absorption. Therefore, conditions that will impair fat absorption will decrease vitamin A absorption and include idiopathic steatorrhea, pancreatic cyst, obstruction of the biliary passages, and hepatic disease. These diseases display decreased plasma vitamin A values below the normal 33.2μg/dl. When vitamin A is dissolved in an aqueous medium (water–propylene glycol mixture), it is absorbed readily, regardless of the degree of fat absorption.

Vitamin A deficiency is characterized by retardation of skeletal growth and maturation, epithelial hyperkeratosis, and impaired ability to see in the dark (nyctalopia).

The normal daily requirement of vitamin A for infants and young children is from 1500 IU to 2500 IU. When over a period of months, large amounts are ingested (*e.g.*, 100,000 IU to 500,000 IU daily), certain clinical phenomena appear. This condition is known as *hypervitaminosis A.* Tender, painful swellings develop over the course of long bones, commonly the ulna, the tibia, and the metatarsals. These swellings are firmly fixed to the bone. The overlying skin is freely movable, and inflammatory signs are conspicuously absent. Limitation of movement probably is a result of protective muscle spasm. The patient invariably is an infant over 12 months of age or a young child.

Roentgenographic investigation reveals that the swellings correspond to areas of periosteal ossification. Usually several bones are involved (most frequently the ulna and the metatarsals). After vitamin A is discontinued, the hyperostosis shrinks over a period of several months and the bone resumes its normal appearance.

The plasma vitamin A level exceeds the normal upper limit of 33.2μg (150 IU).

The condition must be differentiated from infantile cortical hyperostoses because both conditions are featured by similar tender swellings of ossification. Infantile cortical hyperostosis develops before the 4th month of infancy, whereas hypervitaminosis A occurs after the 12th month. The former always affects the face and jaws; the latter does not. Fever is an invariable accompaniment of infantile cortical hyperostosis, whereas the infant with hypervitaminosis A is afebrile. The plasma vitamin A level in infantile cortical hyperostosis is normal; in vitamin A excess it is high.

Treatment requires discontinuing the vitamin. The symptoms and the findings subside within a week.

VITAMIN B

Certain clinical states produced by vitamin B deficiency are of interest to the orthopaedic surgeon. The vitamin is necessary to the integrity of the central and the peripheral nervous systems. Vitamin B_1 (thiamine) and B_{12} deficiencies are common causes of peripheral neuritis.

Vitamin B deficiency, particularly of riboflavin, during pregnancy may produce congenital deformities. Experimentally, the defects can be produced almost invariably in animals by withholding riboflavin. The anomaly most likely to obtain occurs in the limb bud that is in the most active state of development at the time.

VITAMIN C

Vitamin C is found in citrus fruits, tomatoes, and certain vegetables, (*e.g.*, potatoes). Heat, sunlight, and oxidation processes easily destroy it. A synthetic form of ascorbic acid can be administered to ensure adequate intake.

When vitamin C intake is restricted, the plasma level may be maintained while the tissues are being depleted. Therefore, single plasma vitamin C level determinations are of no value. Multiple determinations are necessary. When vitamin C is being excreted in detectable amounts, the tissues are regarded as satisfied, and the excreted ascorbic acid represents the excess. The daily recommended intake varies from 30 mg/day for infants to 100 mg/day for adults. Under periods of stress and fever, daily requirements are greater.

Vitamin C is necessary for the production of intercellular cement substances. Therefore, a deficiency results in a reduced capacity of fibroblasts, osteoblasts, and odontoblasts to form collagen, osteoid, and dentin. Matrix formation is poor. Insufficient collagen formation is reflected in slow organization of hematomas and delayed wound healing. Failure to produce osteoid interferes with endochondral ossification. At the epiphyseal plate, calcified cartilage piles up but is not replaced by osteoid and bone. The bone that does form is slender and fragile. Blood vessels, particularly capillaries, are fragile and easily ruptured, since multiple capillary hemorrhages are a feature of vitamin C deficiency.

Formation, growth, and calcification of cartilage do not depend on ascorbic acid.

VITAMIN D

The two principal vitamin Ds are calciferol (D_2) and cholecalciferol (D_3). Both D_2 and D_3 are fat-soluble sterols similar in structure to cholesterol, and both have high antirachitogenic potency.

Ergosterol, derived from exogenous sources, and 7-dehydrocholesterol, synthesized endogenously from cholesterol, are stored in the skin. By the action of ultraviolet light on the skin, ergosterol is converted to D_2 and 7-dehydrocholesterol is converted to D_3. Then D_2 and D_3 undergo metabolic conversion in the liver to 25-hydroxy vitamin D, a more active form. The latter substance is next converted to two other forms in the kidney. The 25-hydroxy vitamin D, under the influence of PTH (elaborated in response to hypocalcemia), is converted to 1,25-dihydroxy vitamin D (calcitriol), which is highly active in increasing absorption of calcium across the intestinal wall, mobilizing calcium from bone, and resorbing calcium by the renal tubule. Under the influence of calcitonin (which is elaborated in response to hypercalcemia), 24,25-dihydroxy vitamin D, a far less active metabolite, is produced, with the formation of the more active form being suppressed (Fig. 6-6).

Ingested vitamin D is absorbed in the upper intestine, a process materially aided by bile salts. Therefore, absorption of the sterol is diminished in patients with biliary and pancreatic disease.

The three endogenous hormones, 1,25-dihydroxy vitamin D, PTH, and calcitonin, act together to maintain levels of calcium and phosphate within the narrow range required for normal neuromuscular function and at concentrations below the critical solubility product of $CaHPO_4$.

Vitamin D aids absorption of calcium from the intestine and is necessary for deposition of the mineral in bone. Its lack results in failure of the process of calcification of cartilage and mineralization of osteoid tissue necessary to bone growth and produces rickets and osteomalacia. On the other hand, an excess of vitamin D, perhaps by stimulating the parathyroids, results in resorption of

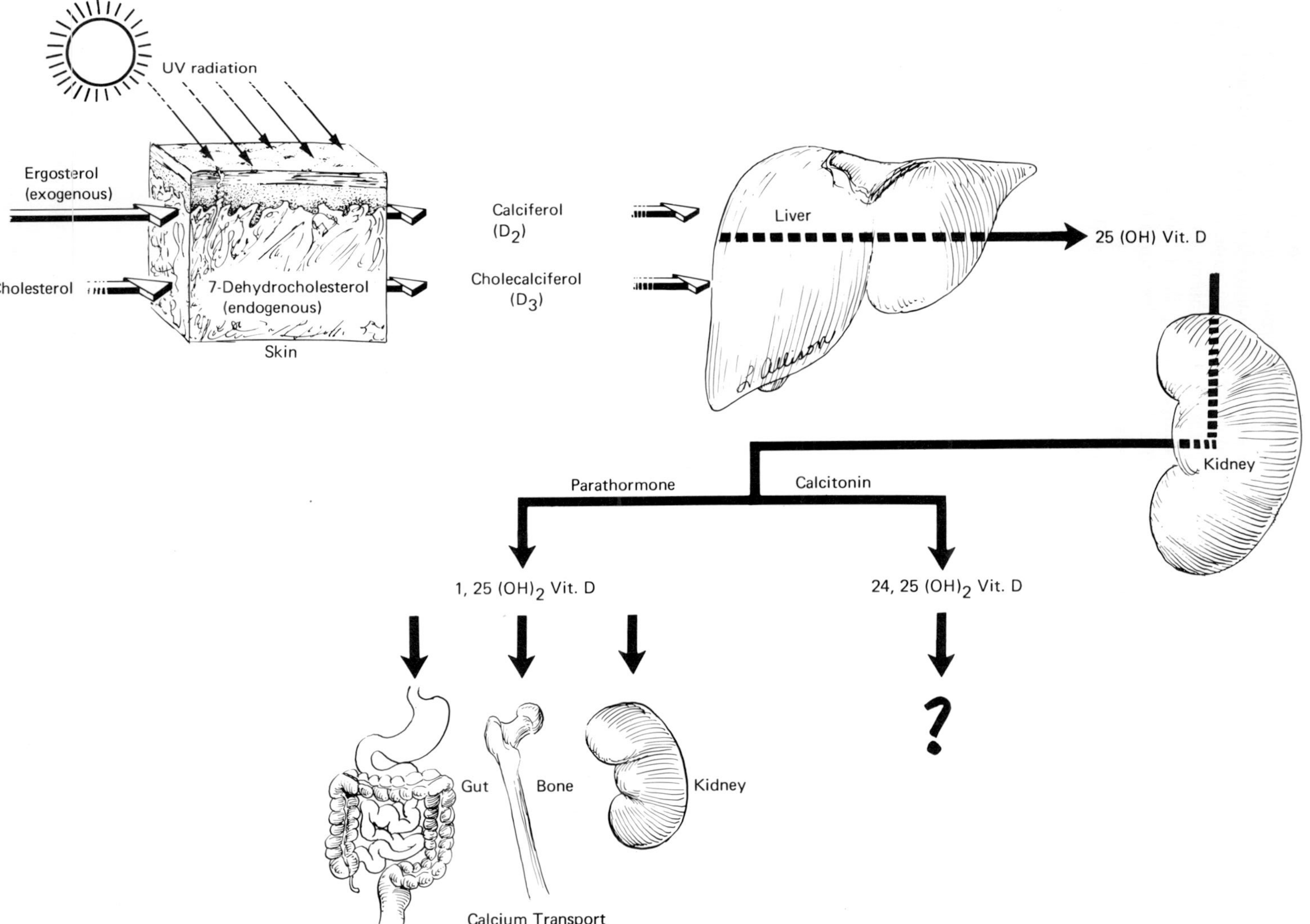

FIG. 6-6. A diagram of the metabolism and action of vitamin D. Ergosterol, from exogenous sources, and 7-dehydrocholesterol, synthesized endogenously from cholesterol, are stored in the skin. These sterols are inactive, but under the influence of ultraviolet light they are converted to calciferol and cholecalciferol and then undergo metabolic conversion in the liver to 25-hydroxy vitamin D, a more active form. The latter is again converted in the kidney to two other forms. In the presence of parathormone (PTH), which is elaborated in response to hypocalcemia, the 25-hydroxy vitamin D is converted to 1,25-dihydroxy vitamin D, which is highly active, increasing the absorption of calcium across the gut wall, mobilizing calcium from bone, and reabsorbing calcium by the renal tubule. Under the influence of calcitonin (CT), which is elaborated in response to hypercalcemia, 24,25-dihydroxy vitamin D, a far less active metabolite, is produced and suppresses the formation of the more active form.

bone, elevation of serum calcium levels, metastatic calcium deposits, and increased urinary excretion with formation of calcium phosphate casts and stones. Albright believes that this sequence of events is secondary to increased phosphorus excretion with reduced tubular resorption caused directly by vitamin D. Ingestion of excessive amounts of vitamin D, for example, in treating vitamin D–resistant rickets, must be carefully monitored by laboratory tests. A positive Sulkowitch reaction and the finding of calcium phosphate urinary casts indicate hypercalcemia. A serum calcium value of 13 mg/dl or above indicates that the dose of the vitamin should be reduced.

VITAMIN E

Vitamin E (the tocopherols), because of its effect on sexual development, naturally influences the production of sex hormones. Consequently, deficiency of this vitamin may be related to growth disturbances. The vitamin also inhibits the formation of collagenous connective tissue. However, its efficacy in the treatment of diseases associated with hyperplasia of collagenous tissue is questionable.

GLANDS OF INTERNAL SECRETION

PARATHYROID GLANDS

The parathyroid glands are small, brownish red bodies measuring about 5 mm × 3 mm × 1 mm. They resemble flattened oval disks. They are located in the posterior capsule of the thyroid gland and usually consist of two superior and two inferior glands, although their number often varies and may be as high as ten. Aberrant parathyroid tissue may be found in the neck and in the upper mediastinum. The hormone, PTH, has the following functions.

- Maintains blood calcium levels by resorption of bone, promoting tubular resorption of calcium and acting with vitamin D to promote intestinal absorption of calcium
- Lowers serum phosphorus levels by inhibiting tubular resorption of phosphate from the glomerular filtrate
- Encourages glomerular filtration of calcium and phosphate ions
- Stimulates osteoclasis
- Directly effects dissolution of bone
- Increases solubility of calcium and phosphate
- Inhibits the mineralizing effect of vitamin D

Symptoms of hypoparathyroidism most often follow accidental removal of the glands during a thyroidectomy. Hyperparathyroid symptoms are caused by adenoma, hyperplasia, or neoplasm.

MECHANISM OF CALCIUM HOMEOSTASIS BY PTH

The ionized calcium level in extracellular fluids is the main factor regulating parathyroid function (*i.e.*, hormone synthesis and release are inversely related to the level of serum calcium).[50] In normal subjects, a rise in serum calcium level above 10.5 mg/dl completely turns off parathyroid secretion. When the serum calcium level reaches or exceeds this point, and the hypercalcemia is caused by a condition other than hyperparathyroidism, the PTH level is zero.[60]

The hormone maintains calcium homeostasis as follows:

- Promotes transfer of mineral from the bone to the ECF through its action on the lining cells (inactive osteoblasts)
- Promotes resorption of calcium in the kidneys by the tubules from the glomerular filtrate, thus elevating the serum calcium level
- Inhibits tubular resorption of phosphate, thus lowering the serum phosphate level, which in turn encourages elevation of serum calcium
- Acts with vitamin D to promote intestinal absorption of calcium
- Interferes with excretion of the hydrogen ion and resorption of amino acids (resulting in hypochloremic acidosis)

Calcium homeostasis requires both PTH and calcitonin, each acting in opposite ways on bone resorption. In addition, the buffering action of bone itself and the serum proteins play minor roles in determining the levels of ionized calcium.

The precise maintenance of serum calcium is largely the result of the reciprocal relation of PTH secretion to the serum calcium level. Elevation of the serum ionized calcium level turns off the parathyroid, reduces the rate of bone resorption, and thereby restores the serum ionized calcium level to normal. Conversely, lowering of serum calcium by only 0.3 mg/dl stimulates parathyroid secretion, increases resorption, and restores the blood calcium level to normal.

Normally, PTH stimulates the lining osteoblasts to release calcium from bone. With an excess of PTH, one observes increases in the osteoclasts as well, but presently it remains unresolved as to whether osteoclasts remove calcium from bone or whether they represent a disposal mechanism.

PTH is not alone in maintaining calcium homeostasis. Even in the absence of PTH, calcium homeostasis is not entirely abolished. This homeostatic mechanism may be attributed to other factors, including the buffering capacity of the bone itself, blood proteins, and calcitonin.

Serum calcium consists of two major fractions, one bound to protein and the other free. Normally, under physiological conditions, these fractions approximately equal each other.

Hypoproteinemia causes a reduction in total serum calcium because of reduced binding protein. The ionized calcium concentration is normal so that patients lack the symptoms of hypocalcemia.

Calcitonin inhibits bone resorption but has short-lived action.

CYCLIC 3′5′-ADENOSINE MONOPHOSPHATE (AMP)

Many peptide hormones act by stimulating hormone-specific, membrane-bound enzymes, the adenyl cyclases, which catalyze the conversion of adenosine triphosphate to cyclic AMP. The cyclic AMP formed is the "second messenger," which induces the cellular responses attributed to the hormone. The rise in serum calcium produced by PTH can also be produced in parathyroidectomized animals by cyclic AMP. PTH-induced inhibition of renal tubular resorption of phosphate (TRP) likewise depends on cyclic AMP.[19]

In pseudohypoparathyroidism, PTH secretion is elevated as a compensatory effort by the parathyroids. However, the renal tubules congenitally lack cyclic AMP and therefore fail to respond to the inhibitory effect of the hormone on phosphate resorption. This can readily be demonstrated by the failure to induce a phosphate diuresis when parathyroid extract is administered intravenously or intramuscularly (Ellsworth-Howard test).

PTH–VITAMIN D INTERRELATIONS

Both PTH and vitamin D are required for calcium homeostasis. When either is lacking, hypocalcemia ensues. In vitamin D–deficient animals, bone is refractory to the action of PTH, but the refractoriness can be overcome by large doses of hormone.

The metabolic effects of vitamin D depend on PTH. In the absence of PTH, the action of vitamin D on intestinal calcium absorption and on bone resorption is diminished.[24]

The conversion of vitamin D to the more metabolically active forms at the liver and at the kidney is stimulated by PTH. Therefore, the metabolic activity of PTH may be mediated in large measure by the ultimate production of the active vitamin D metabolite.

The conversion of 25-OHD_3 to 1,25$(OH)_2D_3$ is specifically stimulated by PTH.[51] Thus is explained the resistance of bone to the action of PTH in vitamin D deficiency.

PTH-MAGNESIUM INTERRELATIONS

When PTH secretion is studied in parathyroid tissue cultures, a reduction in the concentration of magnesium in the culture medium stimulates PTH secretion, an effect identical to that of reducing the calcium concentration. In this system, within certain limits, the sum of the magnesium and calcium concentrations appears to determine the PTH secretory rate. Below a certain critical concentration of magnesium, PTH secretion ceases.[61] Therefore, magnesium deficiency makes hypocalcemia resistant to treatment with calcium. On the other hand, the administration of magnesium restores normal calcium levels.

When an intestinal defect impairs magnesium and calcium absorption, the hypocalcemia can only be restored to normal by treatment with magnesium.

PTH-LIKE SUBSTANCES

Some malignant tumors, notably bronchogenic carcinoma and carcinoma of the kidney, elaborate a PTH-like peptide that gives rise to hypercalcemia and a clinical syndrome indistinguishable from hyperparathyroidism.[58] When the original tumor is not apparent, immunoassay can differentiate the true from these so-called ectopic parathormones.

ACTIONS OF PTH ON BONE

PTH mobilizes calcium from bone and causes a phosphate diuresis, with both actions ultimately depleting the mineral reservoirs of bone. Resorption of bone is best observed in subperiosteal areas and typically is pronounced over the radial aspect of the phalangeal cortices. Resorption of bone takes place mainly through the lining osteoblasts, although microscopically osteoclasts appear to lie within what appears as scalloped eroded areas (Howship's lacunae). PTH also directly dissolves the bone. At the same time, compensatory increases of bone formation by active osteoblasts take place. When the balance is disturbed in favor of resorption in hyperparathyroid states, increased urinary hydroxyproline (Hypro) excretion and increased serum alkaline phosphatase levels are evident.[29]

Although 90% of hyperparathyroid patients fail to exhibit roentgenographic evidence of bone resorption, special techniques will show increased bone resorption rates.[57] Resorption that is extensive and prolonged enough to produce cystic bone disease is rare.

MEASUREMENT OF PARATHYROID ACTIVITY

Serum PTH levels reflecting the degree of activity of the parathyroid glands are variable and will depend on the pathologic state that either stimulates or suppresses intraglandular synthesis of the long-chain polypeptide hormone or cleavage of the latter into smaller peptides that circulate in the bloodstream.[35] PTH assay is primarily concerned not only with defining parathyroid gland activity but also with differentiating disorders of calcium metabolism that produce abnormal serum calcium levels.

It is most often used to identify primary hyperparathyroidism. The assay must be correlated with serum phosphate and creatinine levels. Occasionally, the prednisone-suppression test may be necessary.

PTH Species

PTH is synthesized within the chief cells of the parathyroid glands as a molecule consisting of a single polypeptide chain of 115 amino acid residues termed *Pre-Pro-PTH.* Then by enzymatic cleavage, 25 amino acid residues are removed from the N-terminal end, leaving *Pro-PTH,* which is then converted to *matured PTH* by removal of an additional 6 amino acid residues. The remaining 84 amino acid residues constituting the matured or functional PTH are stored in the Golgi complex before being secreted into the circulation. The biologic activity of matured PTH lies in the region that contains the first 34 amino acids. After this molecule is secreted into the bloodstream, PTH is cleaved at the amino acid 34 region into two major fragments. The N-terminal biologically active fragment containing amino acid residues 1 to 34 has a very short half-life, and the C-terminal fragment containing amino acid residues 35 to 84 has a longer half-life. The latter fragment has no biologic activity.[31]

Radioimmunoassay

Antibodies are prepared against either bovine or porcine PTH because purified human PTH is not available as an antigen.[34,55] Usually serum containing antibodies to beef PTH is developed either in guinea pigs or in chickens. Highly purified beef PTH (B-PTH) labeled with iodine^{125} is added with antiserum to B-PTH and is incubated at 4°C for 4 days, increasing the binding of antiserum to antibody. By adding unlabeled human PTH (H-PTH) to the system, the amount of PTH-^{125}I that is bound to antibody is reduced, and this is read as an increase in the free PTH (Fig. 6-7).[13]

A modification using GP-235 (obtained from guinea pigs injected with porcine PTH) reduces the incubation time to 2 days and accurately identifies primary hyperparathyroidism.[35] The average normals are 39μEq/ml. The upper limit of normal is 70μEq/ml.

Clinical Applications

Patients with hyperparathyroidism tend to have low serum phosphate concentrations (less than 3.0 mg/dl). The phosphate concentrations are normal in neoplastic disease and drug-induced (*e.g.*, thiazides) hypercalcemia. Phosphate levels should be interpreted with caution because chronic intake of alumina gels will inhibit absorption of phosphate and result in hypophosphatemia. Moreover, children have higher phosphate levels than adults.

Patients with chronic renal failure with low serum calcium levels will have high concentrations of PTH, phosphate, and creatinine. The hyperparathyroid state is a compensatory phenomenon that attempts to restore serum calcium levels and induces phosphate excretion.

Hypercalcemia associated with malignancy is generally associated with suppressed or undetectable PTH. However, some cases may demonstrate a marginally high PTH, and it may be necessary to perform special tests, such as the prednisone-suppression test. A decrease in the serum calcium value to the normal range after daily oral administration of prednisone indicates that the cause of the hypercalcemia is unlikely to be primary hyperparathyroidism.[38]

Elevated PTH levels may also be caused by parathyroid carcinoma or, ectopically, by hypernephroma and pulmonary malignancy.

The highest values of PTH are found in the serums of uremic patients with renal osteodystrophy. Descending values of PTH are found in uremic patients without osteodystrophy, in those with primary hyperparathyroidism, and then in those with euparathyroidism. The

FIG. 6-7. Immunoassay. Antisera to partially purified beef parathyroid hormone (*B PTH*) can be developed either in guinea pigs (*GP*) or in chickens (*CH*). Highly purified B PTH is labeled with iodine 125 and added together with antiserum to B PTH in a test tube for incubation at 4°C for 4 days, increasing the binding of the antigen to antibody. Addition of unlabeled B PTH of human PTH (*H PTH*) to system reduces the amount of PTH-^{125}I that is bound to antibody (*Ab*), and this is read as increase in the free PTH. The decrease in initial B/F can be equated to that produced by known amounts of beef or human PTH. Usually a standard curve is obtained by adding a range of increasing amounts of B PTH to the system and plotting the B/F. (Goldman L, Gordan GS, Roof BS: The parathyroids: Progress, problems, and practice. In Current Problems in Surgery. Chicago, Year Book Medical Publishers, 1971)

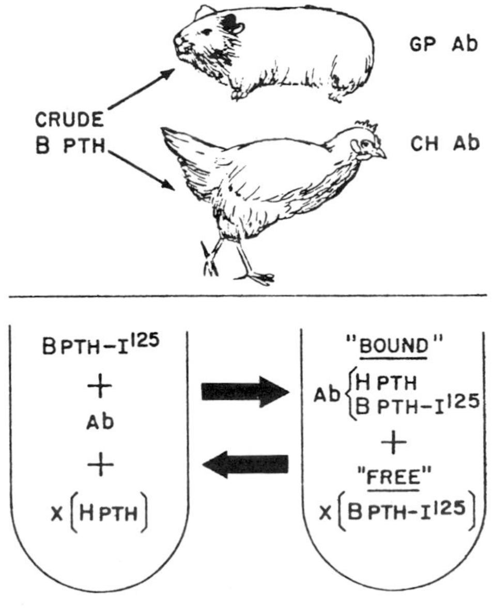

TABLE 6-1 The Components of Total Plasma Calcium

Component	%
Protein-bound (nondialyzable)	45
Dialyzable (ultrafilterable)	55
Ionic	45–50
Complexed (phosphate, citrate, carbonate, sulfate)	5–10

lowest values of PTH occur in hypoparathyroidism or in the hypercalcemia of nonparathyroid causes.

Serum Calcium

There are three major components of the total plasma calcium.

Ionic calcium is the only fraction that is biologically active and represents about 45% of the total. This can be accurately measured by a calcium-sensitive electrode.[44] Approximately 45% of the total serum calcium concentration is bound to protein, primarily albumin, when the plasma protein concentration is normal. Ordinarily it is unnecessary to measure the ultrafilterable fraction, unless assessment of renal handling of calcium is necessary. The calcium filtered by the renal glomerulus comprises only the ultrafilterable portion of plasma calcium.

Pathology

Hypercalcemia.

Significance of Hypercalcemia. The main causes of hypercalcemia are hyperparathyroidism and cancer, representing resorption of calcium from the skeleton. In hyperparathyroidism, hypercalcemia may be masked or abolished, most often by a high dietary phosphate intake.[25] A single normal serum calcium level on an uncontrolled diet, therefore, is not sufficient to exclude hyperparathyroidism. The hypercalcemia is generally mild. The diet should be low in phosphate over 3 days (300 mg daily plus aluminum hydroxide (Amphogel) three times daily).

Differential Diagnosis. Hypercalcemia results from osteolytic metastases (*e.g.*, carcinoma of the breast) or pseudohyperparathyroidism with ectopic hyperparathyroidlike hormone. Skeletal survey or bone scan may reveal osteolytic metastases.

The hypercalcemia of sarcoidosis presumably results from increased absorption of calcium from the gastrointestinal tract secondary to increased sensitivity to vitamin D. Hypercalcemia of sarcoidosis is a manifestation of severe involvement and disseminated disease. Therefore, the chest film may reveal a diffuse fibronodular infiltrate and/or prominent hilar adenopathy. The blood γ-globulin level may be elevated. The noncaseating granulomas are demonstrated by liver biopsy or lymph node biopsy. Contrary to the hypercalcemia of hyperparathyroidism, serum calcium levels are lowered by administration of glucocorticoids.

The hypercalcemia seen in approximately 40% of patients with multiple myeloma presumably is caused by erosion of bone by the neoplastic cells. Typical punched-out bone lesions are detected roentgenographically. Glucocorticoids lower the blood calcium level within several days and act by direct tumor suppression.

Vitamin D intoxication is caused by chronic ingestion of vitamin D in excess for many months. Excessive quantities are stored in the body and are released slowly, so that the hypercalcemia may persist for weeks or months after vitamin D ingestion is stopped. Cortisone inhibits the formation of the active forms of vitamin D and should be used not only for the suppression test but also for treatment to prevent irreversible renal damage due to the persistent hypercalcemia.

Milk-alkali syndrome (Burnett's syndrome) of hypercalcemia and renal failure is rare and is due to long-term ingestion of large amounts of milk or calcium and absorbable antacids. Alkalosis encourages deposition of calcium phosphate in abnormal locations. The syndrome is much less prevalent, since the nonabsorbable antacids are used in ulcer therapy.

Some miscellaneous causes of hypercalcemia include the following:

- Thyrotoxicosis, which is rare and related to bone resorption
- Adrenal insufficiency. Hypercalcemia can occur as a transient phenomenon in acute adrenal failure. Lowering of serum calcium levels by glucocorticoids may act by preventing formation of active forms of vitamin D. However, the cause of hypercalcemia remains undetermined.
- Idiopathic hypercalcemia of infancy which is associated with multiple congenital, cardiovascular lesions
- Prolonged immobilization

Hypocalcemia.

Significance of Hypocalcemia. The main cause of hypocalcemia is uremia associated with chronic renal failure with osteodystrophy. The osteodystrophy is represented by osteomalacia, a consequence of failure of the kidney to convert vitamin D to the metabolically active form, 1,25-dihydrocholecalciferol, thereby impairing intestinal absorption of calcium. Increased TRP leads to an elevated serum phosphorus level, which in itself depresses the serum calcium level.

Hypocalcemia of any cause tends to increase the secretion of PTH, a compensatory mechanism to restore serum calcium levels and excrete phosphate. This secondary hyperparathyroidism leads to osteitis fibrosa. Therefore, bone specimens exhibit evidence of both osteitis fibrosa and osteomalacia.

Differential Diagnosis. The combination of hypocalcemia and hyperphosphatemia, when renal function is normal, must be differentiated from the following disorders:

True hypoparathyroidism. By radioimmunoassay, the serum PTH is low or zero. Deficiency of PTH is said to cause increased density of the skeleton.

Pseudohypoparathyroidism. Serum PTH level is high, but the congenital absence of renal adenyl cyclase permits excessive TRP, resulting in hyperphosphatemia, which in turn lowers the serum calcium level. The mechanism is termed *target organ resistance* to action of the hormone. Clinically, the condition is characterized by round face, stocky body build, and brachydactyly due to foreshortened metacarpals. Failure of the end organ to respond to PTH is determined by the classic Ellsworth-Howard test.

Vitamin D deficiency. Inadequate intake, intestinal malabsorption, and hepatic inability to hydroxylate vitamin D_3 to 25-hydroxycholecalciferol results in rickets and osteomalacia.

Serum Phosphorus. The serum phosphorus level displays a circadian variation and is influenced by dietary carbohydrate and phosphorus intake. Therefore, it is best determined on fasting blood.

Hyperphosphatemia. Hyperphosphatemia occurs in renal insufficiency, hypoparathyroidism, and pseudohypoparathyroidism. In these cases, it is associated with hypocalcemia. The serum phosphorous level tends to rise during immobilization. A high rate of TRP plus a high dietary intake of phosphorus causes elevation of serum phosphate levels. High serum phosphate levels may greatly increase the Ca × P product despite a hypocalcemia, leading to precipitation and ectopic calcification, most commonly seen in the basal ganglia of the brain and the media of large arteries (Mönckeberg's sclerosis).

Hypophosphatemia. In association with hypercalcemia, hypophosphatemia indicates primary hyperparathyroidism. However, this combination may occur as a result of a PTH-like peptide secreted by some malignant tumors and also in sarcoid and myeloma.

It may also be a consequence of malabsorption, vitamin D deficiency, and the Fanconi syndrome (multiple tubular defects, including excess phosphorus loss). Rickets or osteomalacia is the rule.

At least one half of the patients with hyperparathyroidism have normal serum phosphate levels. This is often due to high phosphate dietary intake.

Serum Alkaline Phosphatase. An elevated serum alkaline phosphatase level is a cardinal feature of primary hyperparathyroidism, representing increased osteoblastic activity that compensates for increased bone resorption. The alkaline phosphatase levels correlate well with urinary hydroxyproline excretion, a reflection of bone resorption.[64]

Urinary Calcium. Hypercalcemia increases the glomerular filtration of calcium, and if renal tubular handling of calcium remains unchanged, urinary calcium excretion increases out of proportion to the increase in the serum calcium level. PTH increases tubular resorption of calcium, so that primary hyperparathyroidism is characterized by less of an increase in urinary calcium excretion than would be expected from the degree of hypercalcemia.

In contrast, in sarcoid, a greater increase of urinary calcium excretion occurs for the same degree of hypercalcemia. Urinary calcium rarely exceeds 400 mg/day in primary hyperparathyroidism; hypercalciuria is well above this level in sarcoid, vitamin D intoxication, and cancer.

Renal insufficiency reduces the glomerular filtration rate and therefore results in a significant decrease in urinary calcium excretion. This is the case in the milk-alkali syndrome, which is characterized by renal insufficiency.

The urinary calcium level should be measured only after several days on a low calcium diet. Urinary calcium excretion is influenced by phosphorus intake (inverse relationship). The ingestion of phosphorus-binding substances, such as aluminum hydroxide antacids, should be strictly avoided during the collection of urine.

Urinary Phosphorus. The urinary excretion of phosphorus is a consistent proportion (65% to 70%) of the dietary intake, regardless of the disease state. Therefore, the urinary phosphorus level indirectly assesses dietary intake.

Tubular resorption of phosphorus is decreased by PTH, and measurement of the TRP is an indirect indication of hormone levels in the bloodstream and the renal handling of phosphate. Hyperphosphaturia reflects a subnormal TRP.

Various methods are used to make these determinations, which are affected by many factors. Phosphate intake must be controlled. The normals for each procedure must be determined before the results can be interpreted. The following procedure is typical:

Urine is collected from 8 PM to 8 AM and fasting blood is drawn at the end of the 12-hour collection.[28] Creatinine and phosphorus concentrations are measured in the serum and urine.

$$TRP = 1 - \left[\frac{UP \times SCr}{UCr \times SP}\right]$$

TRP = tubular resorption of phosphate
UP = urine phosphate, mg/dl
UCr = urine creatinine, mg/dl
SCr = serum creatinine, mg/dl
SP = serum phosphate, mg/dl

The TRP is useless in mild renal insufficiency, since phosphate clearance is well preserved with moderately reduced creatinine clearance levels. It is essential to have normal reference standards for TRP under the dietary conditions employed. Thus the TRP may be rendered apparently normal in hyperparathyroid patients whose diets are restricted in phosphate or who are taking aluminum-containing antacids.

Urinary Cyclic AMP. During the activation of renal tubular adenyl cyclase by PTH, cyclic AMP is released into the tubular lumen and is excreted in the urine. This measures the renal responsiveness to PTH. It differentiates hypoparathyroidism from pseudohypoparathyroidism, since the latter disease is characterized by a congenital deficiency of adenyl cyclase, thus explaining the renal unresponsiveness to PTH.

When PTH is administered, one of its first effects in both bone and kidney is to cause an increase of cyclic AMP concentration, which leads to an increase in the urinary excretion of this nucleotide.

Phosphorus Deprivation Tests. Phosphorus intake may mask the chemical manifestations of primary hyperparathyroidism. Phosphorus deprivation may be used as a provocative test to unmask borderline cases and reveal hypercalcemia, hypophosphatemia, and hypercalciuria. Phosphorus deprivation is accomplished by combining a low phosphate intake (avoidance of all dairy products) with ingestion of aluminum hydroxide (phosphorus-binding antacid) prior to each meal. It is necessary to continue this regimen for several weeks in order to produce the desired effects. Calcium levels are monitored to prevent sudden life-threatening hypercalcemia.

Urinary Hydroxyproline Excretion. Excretion of hydroxyproline is increased in hyperparathyroidism, reflecting increased bone resorption.

CALCITONIN

The hormone calcitonin is a hypocalcemic principle elaborated by so-called C cells, which are situated in the thyroid in the perifollicular areas but are known to exist elsewhere, such as in the parathyroids and thymus, although they are difficult to demonstrate.[22] In lower animal forms the C cells apparently have their counterpart in the ultimobranchial body.[47]

The principal functions of calcitonin are to inhibit resorption of bone[42] and to reduce tubular resorption of calcium.[21]

The stimulus to production and release of hormone from the C cells is hypercalcemia. Its hypocalcemic effect counteracts the hypercalcemic effect of PTH. When calcitonin activity is high, hypocalcemia may ensue and may induce a compensatory hyperparathyroid response. When parathyroid activity is high (*e.g.*, in primary hyperparathyroidism), hypercalcemia will induce high plasma levels of calcitonin.

The outstanding condition in which hypercalcitonism is found is medullary carcinoma of the thyroid. In spite of high plasma calcitonin levels, normal serum calcium levels are maintained, presumably by the PTH-calcitonin balance.

The hormone's property of inhibiting bone resorption appears to have therapeutic value in conditions characterized by an excessive rate of bone resorption (*e.g.*, senile osteoporosis,[17] Paget's disease, and renal osteodystrophy).

GONADS

Estrogens and androgens are present in both the male and female. In the adult female, androgen values are almost as abundant as in the male. Although the main functions of these hormones are related to the development of the genitalia and secondary sex characteristics, they also have certain important influences on the skeletal system.

ESTROGEN

Estrogen is produced by the ovarian follicle. Secretion of estrogen is controlled by pituitary secretion of gonadotropin. Estrogen stimulates the formation of bone by its protein anabolic effect. The hormone accelerates longitudinal growth but also speeds up skeletal maturation so that epiphysiodiaphyseal fusion occurs prematurely. Therefore, administration of the hormone will cause an initial spurt in growth, but such growth is halted early and the overall stature will be less than normal.

In primary hypogonadism, a deficiency of estrogenic hormone permits the epiphyseal plates to remain open for years beyond the usual time of closure, with active longitudinal growth continuing. The characteristic clinical picture of a long, slender, poorly muscled, hypogonadal person is produced. The eunuch is the rarely seen extreme form of this condition.

In contrast, an excess of pituitary growth hormone causes a rapid growth rate without influencing maturation and epiphyseal closure.

Therefore, the skeletal effects of gonadal insufficiency include excessive long bone growth, delayed epiphyseal plate closure, thinned trabeculations, and thinned cortices.

ANDROGEN

In embryologic development the testes and the adrenal cortices arise from adjacent structures, thus explaining the production of similarly acting hormones from these two sites. Androgens are responsible for the development of masculinizing characteristics (*e.g.*, hirsutism, well-developed muscles, deep voice). The testis is under the control of gonadal-stimulating hormones from the anterior pituitary. Pituitary adrenocorticotropic hormone controls the adrenal cortex. Adrenal and testicular androgens are metabolized and excreted in the urine as 17-ketosteroids.

Human androgen has a protein anabolic effect that is exerted on muscles, skeleton, sex organs, and other structures. When androgen is administered, it causes the retention of nitrogen, sodium, potassium, and chlorides. The protein anabolic effect is reflected in an increased size of muscles, stimulation of growth, and premature epiphyseal closure. When testosterone is administered to a child, an early spurt of growth occurs, but skeletal maturation is accelerated so that epiphyseal fusion is premature, resulting in shortened stature.

USES OF SEX HORMONES

The main uses of androgen and estrogen are in situations requiring the protein anabolic effect for osteoblastic activity. The treatment is effective in generalized osteoporosis, particularly of the menopausal type. Slipped upper femoral epiphysis often occurs in the hypogonadal type of person. The epiphyseal separation takes place through an area in the epiphyseal plate weakened by excessive proliferation of chondrocytes. Sex hormones can be used to accelerate epiphyseal fusion.

Administration of sex hormones should not be indiscriminate. Estrogen can stimulate the formation of breast tumors and often causes uncontrollable menorrhagia. Testosterone can inhibit pituitary secretion and thereby suppress adrenal cortical function. This explains the reduction of urinary 17-ketosteroids occurring during androgen therapy.

PITUITARY GLANDS

The glandular cells of the pars anterior of the pituitary are composed of equal numbers of chromaphobes and chromaphils. The chromaphobes are smaller and take the stain poorly. The chromaphils, by their staining reactions to hematoxylin and eosin, are composed mainly of centrally located eosinophils (pink-staining) and a lesser amount of peripherally situated basophils (blue-staining). It is generally agreed that cells can transform from chromaphobes to chromaphils and vice versa. The clinical picture produced by an increase of either acidophils or basophils indicates that these cells are the source of the hormones. Three hormones are produced: growth hormone (GH), lactogenic hormone, and tropic hormones. The tropic hormones are of several types, corresponding to their effects on other glands: thyrotropin, adrenocorticotropin, gonadotropin, and lesser understood hormones affecting in some way the parathyroids and the pancreas.

GROWTH HORMONE

In the epiphyseal growth plate, proliferation and hypertrophy of chondrocytes are controlled by GH, which is secreted by the acidophilic cells of the pituitary gland. Complete deprivation of GH (*e.g.*, after the removal of the pituitary gland) causes the epiphyseal plate to become very thin, and growth stops. With the administering of extracts of the anterior lobe, longitudinal growth is restored, provided that the epiphyseal plate has not closed.

An abnormally increased amount of GH is produced by an increased number of acidophils, and longitudinal growth becomes rapid. Proliferation of cartilage cells in the epiphyseal plate continues even beyond the usual time of skeletal maturation and epiphyseal closure. An eosinophilic adenoma occurring before the growth period has been completed means that longitudinal growth can continue until 20 years of age. All skeletal parts become enlarged, resulting in the picture of gigantism.

When excessive eosinophilism occurs after growth has ceased, the epiphyseal plates have closed, endochrondral ossification no longer takes place, and acceleration of bone growth is confined to sites of membranous ossification, particularly the mandible and the vault of the skull (Fig. 6-8). Subperiosteal ossification is increased, with the result that the long bones become thick. This is the clinical picture of acromegaly.

FIG. 6-8. Acromegaly. Massive type of bone enlargement, enlarged sella turcica, prominent lower jaw, and large paranasal sinuses, especially the frontal sinuses.

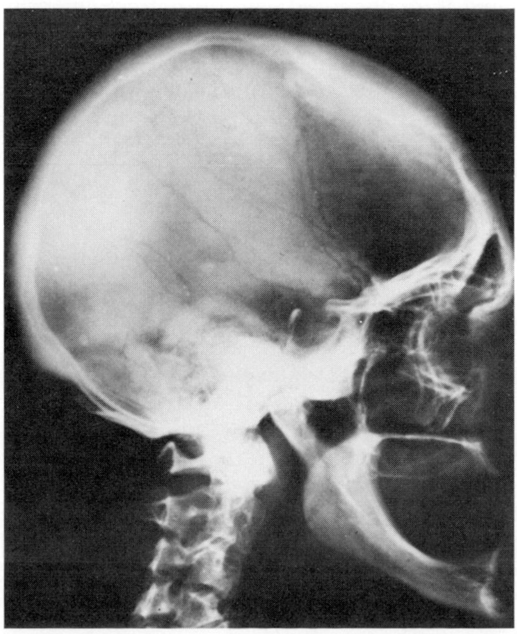

TROPIC HORMONES

The tropic hormones control the secretory activity of other glands of internal secretion. When the latter glands produce an excessive amount of their respective hormone, it will suppress the secretion of the corresponding tropic hormone. A high level of sex hormone will suppress not only gonadotropic hormone but also growth hormone and lactogenic hormone.

The basophils are responsible for producing adrenocorticotropic hormone. When hyperplasia of basophils or a basophilic adenoma occurs, the signs of adrenal cortical hyperactivity ensue. This is Cushing's disease, which is characterized by hypertension, glycosuria, adiposity, sodium retention, and protein breakdown. Protein catabolism is reflected in generalized osteoporosis and pathologic fractures. Treatment is by x-irradiation.

CHORIONIC GONADOTROPIN

Chorionic gonadotropin is found in large amounts in the urine of pregnant women. It is a potent stimulator of the interstitial cells of the testicle, increasing the formation of male sex hormone and encouraging descent of the testicle. It also causes a spurt in growth. Pituitary dwarfs are deficient in GH and usually are deficient in gonadotropic hormone. Consequently, they are underdeveloped sexually. Slipped epiphysis, which frequently occurs in the Fröhlich syndrome, is benefited by gonadotropic hormone.

PITUITARY DISTURBANCES

The pathogenesis is concerned with the chromophil cells of the anterior lobe. The basophils control the adrenals and possibly the sex glands. The acidophils control skeletal growth. Excessive secretion causes gigantism and acromegaly. Diminished secretion produces dwarfism.

Pituitary dwarfism is caused by a tumor or a suprasellar cyst that compresses the gland. Although the epiphyseal line is thin, the plate often remains separated and the metaphysis ends in a line of dense bone. Two types of pituitary dwarfism have been identified: Fröhlich's adiposogenital type, which is characterized by obesity, genital hypoplasia, and mental retardation; and Lorain type, in which the only feature is skeletal retardation.

Gigantism is produced when excessive GH is present before the epiphyses are fused. The typical features of gigantism include thickening of the skull and of the jaw, subnormal mentality, and poor muscle power. All bones are increased in thickness and length. Excessive growth occurs both at the epiphyseal plate and in the subperiosteal area.

Acromegaly develops under the influence of excessive GH after longitudinal growth has ceased. It is caused by an eosinophilic adenoma or hyperplasia and is characterized by exaggeration of ossification unevenly distributed throughout the body.

The osteoblasts are stimulated to overfunction beneath the periosteum but particularly at points of stress and pull (muscle and ligament attachments) and points of compression (ends of the long bones). The growth of bone is greatly exaggerated characteristically in the mandible, the malar bone, and the skull (especially at the frontal area) and at the extremities of the long bones. Bony prominences may protrude inward from the inner table of the skull. The thorax is massive. The vertebral bodies are enlarged, particularly anteriorly. The pituitary fossa may be enlarged because of the expanding pressure of the pituitary tumor. Acromegalic arthritis resembles osteoarthritis in that the subchondral bone is thickened and the articular cartilage is worn away at points of greatest compression. Histologically, the greatest activity of osteoblasts is seen at the points of attachment of ligament or muscle where it seems that bone production is stimulated by the intermittent pull of these structures. In contrast, gigantism has the element of excessive longitudinal growth and a more diffuse increase in size of all the bones.

ADRENAL GLANDS

The adrenals play a prominent role in new bone formation, endochondral ossification, and skeletal maturation.[66] Although the severe type of adrenal hyperfunction is rare, the mild type with few symptoms is quite common and can be identified by appropriate laboratory procedures. An investigation into the cause of osteoporosis, frequent fractures, and delayed union of a fracture should include evaluation of blood and urinary 17-ketosteroids and 17-hydroxycorticoids. The following sections deal only with those adrenal conditions affecting the musculoskeletal system.

ADRENAL HORMONES

According to present concepts, the normal human adrenal cortex secretes three types of hormones.

1. *Glucocorticoids.* These hormones inhibit protein anabolism (or encourage catabolism), increase gluconeogenesis (by breakdown of protein), decrease pituitary secretion of adrenocorticotropic hormone (ACTH), and increase in large amounts the urinary excretion of potassium and tubular resorption of sodium. These hormones are the probable precursors of 17-hydroxycorticoids found in the blood and urine. Hydrocortisone is the most important glucocorticoid in humans.
2. *Androgens.* The androgens stimulate protein anabolism, accelerate endochondral ossification and skeletal maturation (early closure of epiphyseal growth plates), and, in excessive amounts, cause virilization. Andro-

gens are the probable precursors of 17-ketosteroids in the urine.

3. *Mineralocorticoids.* An electrolyte-regulating hormone, aldosterone, increases tubular resorption of sodium, increases excretion of potassium, and influences the distribution of potassium and sodium throughout the body.

DETERMINATION OF CORTICAL FUNCTION

Glucocorticoids and androgens are secreted in appreciable quantity only in response to elaboration of ACTH by the pituitary. The determination of 17-ketosteroids and 17-hydroxycorticoids in the blood and urine is used to assess adrenal cortical function. A quantitative estimation of adrenal cortical reserve and responsiveness can be measured by administering ACTH and noting changes in the blood and urine steroids. When hyperactivity of the adrenal cortex primarily is due to pathology within the adrenal itself, removal of pituitary stimulation will have no great effect on the secretion of 17-ketosteroids and 17-hydroxycorticoids. These substances will remain at high levels in spite of suppression of endogenous ACTH activity by administering fluorohydrocortisone. On the other hand, if adrenal hyperactivity is due to pituitary stimulation, suppression of ACTH activity results in a marked drop of steroid levels.

CLINICAL SYNDROME OF ADRENAL HYPERFUNCTION

Hypersecretion of adrenal steroids is due to pituitary or adrenal hyperplasia or to tumors, either benign or malignant. The syndrome produced depends on the relative amounts of these hormones and may even reflect an excess of a single hormone. Thus, excessive glucocorticoid secretion produces loss of tissue protein, manifested as muscle atrophy, osteoporosis, and striae. On the other hand, excessive androgen secretion, while causing hirsutism, tends to counteract protein catabolism so that the muscles remain well developed, bone structure is adequate, and striae are absent.

The following syndromes are of orthopaedic importance.

Cushing's Disease. A basophilic adenoma or hyperplasia of the basophilic components of the anterior lobe of the pituitary gland produces the classic picture of hypertension, diabetes, osteoporosis, abdominal striae, moon facies, buffalo hump, truncal obesity, and hirsutism. Treatment consists of high-voltage irradiation of the gland, hypophysectomy, or a combination of these procedures.

Cushing's Syndrome. In the vast majority of instances, excessive glucocorticoid production is a result of pathology in the adrenal cortex, either hyperplasia, adrenal carcinoma, or a benign adenoma. Preoperative diagnosis to determine the type of lesion is extremely difficult. Steroid determinations are helpful. Benign hyperplasia or adenoma usually displays a high basal level of 17-hydroxycorticoids and normal or slightly increased 17-ketosteroids. Carcinoma is characterized by markedly increased levels of both hormones. Finally, one can demonstrate that the hyperfunction is independent of the pituitary; suppression of endogenous ACTH by administration of cortisone or fluorohydrocortisone fails to reduce the blood and urine steroid levels materially. Occasionally, roentgenographic examination by intravenous pyelograms and presacral air insufflation may reveal the location of the tumor.

Treatment depends on the intensity of the symptoms. For mild Cushing's syndrome, pituitary irradiation is indicated. Response to x-irradiation is slow but results in a temporary or permanent remission. Surgical treatment is recommended for patients suspected of having an adrenal tumor as well as for those with severe symptoms and for those who fail to respond to irradiation. In the absence of an adrenal tumor, total bilateral adrenalectomy followed by hormonal replacement therapy appears to be the treatment of choice. Postoperatively, a daily high level of cortisone is maintained and then gradually is reduced to less than 75 mg, when a sodium-retaining hormone is added. Testosterone must be given to counteract osteoporosis and muscle atrophy. Cortisone therapy is continued indefinitely after bilateral extirpation.

A unilateral adenoma is associated with atrophy of the contralateral gland. Following removal of the adenoma, cortisone and ACTH are administered until the suppressed gland is restored.

Patients with Cushing's syndrome are susceptible to compression fractures, because of protein loss and osteoporosis. Testosterone must be given to encourage protein anabolism. Potassium replacement is mandatory and reduces sodium retention. Steroid diabetes is resistant to insulin but fortunately does not cause acidosis.

Congenital Adrenal Hyperplasia. The defect in the adrenals of patients with congenital adrenal hyperplasia is the inability to produce normal amounts of hydrocortisone. Consequently, the pituitary secretes excessive amounts of ACTH. Increased amounts of androgenic steroids are produced, resulting in virilization and excessive urinary excretion of 17-ketosteroids. This adrenogenital syndrome causes precocious puberty in the male and pseudohermaphroditism in the female. Growth is rapid, but premature epiphyseal plate closure results in short stature.

Treatment requires correcting hormonal deficiency. Cortisone or hydrocortisone will suppress ACTH production and lessen stimulation of the adrenal cortex to produce androgenic substances. Adequacy of dosage is determined by the reduction of urinary 17-ketosteroids to the normal level and resumption of the normal growth curve.

RELATIONSHIP OF THE ADRENALS TO STRESS

Stress, such as that produced by trauma or infection, is counteracted by hyperfunction of the adrenal cortex. Selye has observed that hypertrophy of the adrenal cortex is invariably associated with the "alarm reaction." Adequate response of the adrenal gland to injury is reflected in a drop in the level of eosinophils in the circulating blood. During eosinopenia, the patient is ill and, as improvement sets in, the eosinophil count rises. Eosinopenia persisting beyond the usual stress period (*e.g.*, for many days after a compound fracture or surgery) suggests a complication, such as an infection. If, after operation or a severe injury, eosinophilia persists and the course is unsatisfactory, adrenal insufficiency is highly probable and demands urgent measures. Cortisone must be administered in large doses. As the patient's condition improves, ACTH is given to stimulate adrenal function.[46]

PHYSIOLOGICAL EFFECTS OF CORTISONE AND HYDROCORTISONE

A summary of the physiological actions of compounds E and F is described in Chapter 13.

THYROID GLAND AND ITS HORMONES

Thyroid hormones have a direct or indirect effect on longitudinal bone growth and maturation. When hormone levels are excessive, the rates of both bone deposition and resorption are increased, but the degree of bone loss always exceeds bone formation, resulting in an osteopenic state.

Deficient levels of thyroid hormone during the growth period are reflected in the skeleton by reduced proliferation and maturation of chondrocytes and slowed endochondral ossification. When the hypothyroid state exists in the newborn, the condition is termed cretinism (Fig. 6-9). Initially, the infant may appear normal, but within the ensuing weeks or months the characteristics of cretinism become manifest and include anorexia, obstinate constipation, protuberant abdomen, umbilical hernia, failure to gain weight, sluggishness, and a hoarse cry. The face appears simian, dull, and pale. The lips are thick and the tongue protrudes. The bridge of the nose is flattened, and dentition is delayed. Longitudinal growth is slowed, resulting in dwarfism. Fontanelle and suture closure of the skull are delayed. Mental development is retarded. The orthopaedic surgeon may be the first to discover early signs of improper skeletal development and should alert the pediatrician to the urgent need for hormone replacement to prevent mental retardation and to encourage longitudinal growth.

Myxedema is the term applied to the state of hypothyroidism developing after birth. During childhood and adolescence, symptoms and findings may be so mild (*e.g.*, retarded longitudinal growth) as to escape notice.

PHYSIOLOGY

Thyroid gland activity is under the control of thyroid-stimulating hormone (TSH), which is produced by the anterior pituitary under the control of the hypothalamus.[52] The basic raw material of thyroid hormone is inorganic iodide. Thyroid hormone synthesis begins when inorganic iodide is extracted from the blood by the thyroid. Within the thyroid, inorganic iodide is converted to organic iodide as one iodine atom is incorporated into a tyrosine molecule to form monoiodotyrosine (MIT). MIT then incorporates a second iodine atom to form diiodotyrosine (DIT). DIT then condenses with itself to form thyroxine (T_4) or with MIT to form triiodothyronine (T_3). T_4 is stored in the thyroid acini as thyroglobulin, to be reconstituted and released when needed. In the bloodstream, T_4 is the main component of thyroid hor-

FIG. 6-9. A cretin infant.

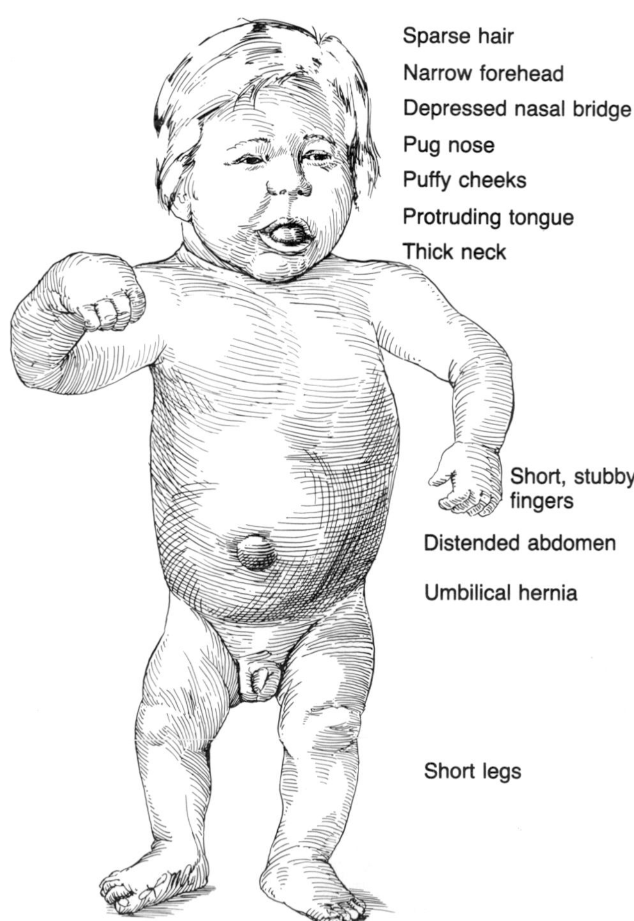

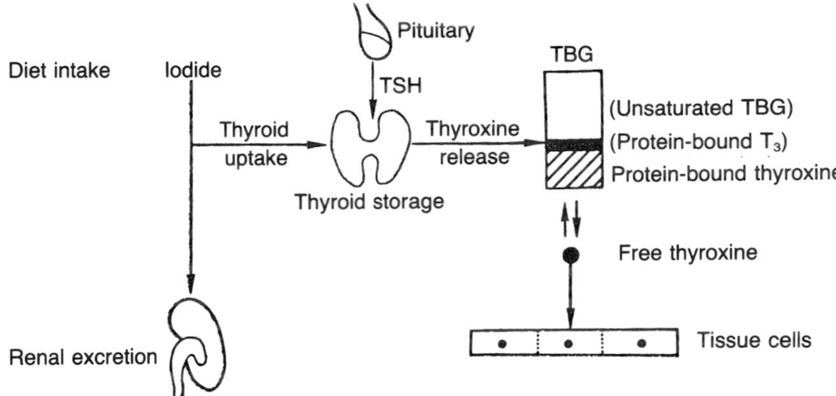

FIG. 6-10. Iodine and thyroxine metabolism. (Ravel R: Clinical Laboratory Medicine. Chicago, Year Book Medical Publishers, 1973)

mone. The iodine of T_4 accounts for about 95% of total serum iodine. T_4 is mostly bound to serum proteins. Inter-α-globulin (thyroid-binding globulin, TBG) carries the majority; a lesser amount is bound to prealbumin and albumin molecules. A very small amount of T_4 is present in the unbound or free form (free thyroxine, T_F); this amounts to less than 1%. The quantity of T_F depends to some extent on the degree of saturation of TBG. TBG saturation depends on the quantity of T_4 available plus the total quantity of TBG available to bind T_4. Normally, TBG is 15% to 30% saturated. Besides T_4, T_3 is present in small quantities. T_3 is much more active, weight for weight, than T_4; it is not yet established whether T_3 is the metabolically active form of T_4 or merely accompanies it from the thyroid storage depot. If T_3 is not the active substance, T_F probably is, because it correlates better with thyroid hormone activity (Fig. 6-10).

EFFECTS OF THYROID HORMONE ON BONE AND MINERAL METABOLISM

Thyroid hormone promotes the release of calcium from bone.[12] Hyperthyroidism causes excessive bone resorption,[12] and, as a consequence, hypercalcemia and hyperphosphaturia can develop.[11] The effect of thyroid hormone is independent of the presence of PTH, but increase in serum calcium level, by negative feedback, depresses PTH secretion.[15] Urinary calcium excretion is increased.

Patients with hyperthyroidism have increased fecal and urinary excretion of calcium and phosphorus. Although daily calcium urinary excretion may exceed 1,000 mg, the formation of renal stones is uncommon. A negative calcium balance is further aggravated by increased calcium loss in the sweat.

By radioisotope studies, it has been shown that the decline of blood levels is not related to increased excretion of the isotope (^{45}Ca) in the urine and feces. Instead the rates of flow into the various calcium compartments were increased. The rates of calcium deposition and resorption in bone increased severalfold, and returned to normal with treatment of the hyperthyroidism. However, resorption always exceeded formation. In the hyperthyroid state, calcium excretion can be decreased by administration of testosterone.[36]

In hypothyroidism, the serum calcium and inorganic phosphate ion concentrations are normal but decrease significantly on low calcium intake. In hypothyroidism, a state of secondary hyperparathyroidism develops and renal tubular resorption of phosphate is decreased. Although there is a lessened release of calcium from the bone in hypothyroidism, the serum calcium ion concentration is maintained at normal levels, probably because of increased intestinal absorption.

Increased urinary excretion of hydroxyproline supports the concept that bone destruction is increased in hyperthyroidism. This reflects, to some extent, the degree of collagen breakdown.[37] Treatment of hyperthyroidism results in a marked decrease in hydroxyproline excretion. Similarly, the treatment of cretins or hypothyroid adults produces a striking increase in hydroxyproline excretion.

An increase of the serum alkaline phosphatase level, which is frequently found in hyperthyroid patients, supports the premise that osteoblastic activity is increased in this disease and may represent a compensatory attempt to deposit new bone.[16]

SKELETAL EFFECTS OF THYROID HORMONES

Principles

During the prenatal and postnatal growth periods, decreased thyroid function retards growth and delays maturation of the skeleton. Growth retardation may, however, be due to secondary deficiency of GH.[20] In the hypophysectomized animal, very little growth can be induced by T_4 alone. In contrast, growth can be stimulated in the thyroidectomized animal by GH alone.

In thyroidectomized animals, with secondary deficiency of GH, the GH levels can be restored to normal by small doses of levothyroxine, which restores vigorous endochondral ossification.

Maturation of the skeleton depends largely on thyroid hormone. In experimental animals that have been thyroidectomized and hypophysectomized, T_4 alone will reactivate chondrogenesis to a moderate degree, followed by endochondral ossification. Striking acceleration of the process occurs when GH and thyroid hormone are administered together.[71] The growth action of GH is potentiated by T_4.

Histologic studies of the effects of T_4 deficiency and excess indicate that T_4, by acting in synergism with GH, encourages the process of endochondral ossification but seems to have the opposite effect on periosteal appositional bone growth.[62] It stimulates the proliferation of chondrocytes and appears to be necessary to the orderly steps of matrix formation and calcification, cartilage degeneration and invasion by vascular osteogenic tissue, and ultimate ossification.

It should be emphasized that thyroid hormone and pituitary GH act together to influence skeletal growth and maturation. Dwarfism may result from hypofunction of either gland. The two glands are interdependent: removal of the pituitary results in atrophy of the thyroid; removal of the thyroid is followed by hypoplasia of the acidophilic cells of the pituitary.

The main effect of T_4 (maturation) and that of GH (linear longitudinal growth) are interrelated and can best be studied in immature animals that have been hypophysectomized and thyroidectomized.[53] The advance of skeletal age in such animals is delayed and unaffected by injections of GH. When injected with T_4, skeletal age advances at a rate approaching control animals.

The maturation effect is best observed in the epiphysis, where the developing ossification center at a certain chronological age comes to occupy most of the epiphysis, and cartilage is found only at the articular surface and at the growth plate. Without T_4, the ossification center is small, spotty, and poorly developed, containing very little bone amid imperfectly formed chondrocytes and matrix, and the marrow is primarily adipose. At the growth cartilage, the chondrocytes are small, sparse, and, on approaching the metaphysis, are less hypertrophied and vacuolated than normal. Vascularity is minimal, and trabeculae are sparse and truncated at the ossifiying zone.

In the animal deprived of thyroid and pituitary hormones, when GH is injected, the epiphyseal ossification center increases in size but never attains the degree of maturity and size in T_4-treated animals.

To summarize, GH produces increase in longitudinal skeletal growth but has little effect on maturation. Both thyroid and pituitary hormones are necessary to coordinate skeletal growth and maturation.

Skeletal Effects in Individual Clinical States

The Cretin. The term *cretin* is applied to the newborn who is congenitally deficient of thyroid hormone. The characteristic skeletal effects are delayed longitudinal growth, which may not be apparent for many weeks or months postnatally, and delayed bone maturation, which can be detected on roentgenograms in one half of the congenital cretins by evaluating bone age, even in the newborn. The proximal tibial and distal femoral epiphyseal ossification centers are present in nearly all full-term newborns weighing in excess of 2500 g. Their absence should arouse a suspicion of intrauterine thyroid hormone deficiency. The appearance of epiphyseal ossification centers is delayed. Endochondral bone formation is defective, resulting in dwarfism.

The fault lies in conversion of cartilage to bone. Intramembranous bone formation is delayed but proceeds. Therefore, the frontal suture is wide and the anterior fontanelle is exceptionally prominent. The sutures at the base of the skull remain unossified for long periods, and the base of the skull is short.

Subperiosteal bone formation (*i.e.*, appositional bone growth) continues at a normal rate, so that the long bones become disproportionately wide relative to their subnormal length.

Juvenile Hypothyroidism (Juvenile Myxedema). The hypothyroid dwarf develops infantile skeletal proportions.[69,70] Growth is stunted. Appearance of epiphyseal ossification centers is delayed, and as each develops it appears as multiple scattered foci that finally coalesce to form a stippled, fragmented configuration. The abnormality is termed *epiphyseal dysgenesis.* When adequate thyroid hormone is administered, the ossification center rapidly regains its normal size and appearance. All cartilaginous centers are involved, but changes are most pronounced in the femoral heads and tarsal naviculars.

Juvenile hypothyroidism is acquired thyroid deficiency developing during childhood or adolescence. The finding of dysgenesis in a given epiphysis indicates the time of onset of the condition. For example, if stippled epiphyses are found in the femoral heads of a 6-year-old child, the thyroid deficiency had its origin before 9 to 12 months of age, the period when these ossification centers usually develop. Moreover, absence of ossification or dysgenesis in centers that normally ossify before birth indicates that the hypothyroidism developed prenatally. Normal infants born of hypothyroid mothers do not show retardation of skeletal maturation.

Epiphyseal dysgenesis may resemble osteochondritis deformans juvenilis (Legg-Perthes disease) but these patients do not develop the typical deformities of the latter condition.

Delayed dentition is characteristic. The size of the crowns is little affected, but eruption is delayed. Shedding of deciduous teeth is delayed, and growth of roots is slowed.

A decreased serum alkaline phosphatase level reflects a slower rate of bone formation. With treatment, the level of alkaline phosphatase rises to normal.

Adult Myxedema. Myxedema is a hypothyroid condition characterized by a unique increase in the water-binding capacity of collagen. There is a colloidal bond between the collagen protein and the water, which causes swelling of all collagenous structures.

In adult myxedema, bone resorption is decreased out of proportion to bone formation. The bones appear denser and have thick cortices.

Hyperthyroidism. In normal bone, remodeling is a continuous process in which bone deposition and resorption are about balanced. In hyperthyroidism, the rates of both deposition and resorption are increased, with bone resorption exceeding bone formation.[11,27]

Microscopically, the trabeculae are thinner and fewer in number. Multiple small eroded areas along only one surface of any single trabecula produce a "sawtooth" appearance. Occasional larger defects are occupied by osteoclasts, and some surfaces are sparsely covered by osteoblasts. Osteoid borders are rare.

The involvement, similar to osteoporosis, chiefly affects the spine and pelvis and, less commonly, the skull, long bones, and hands. Compression fractures of vertebral bodies and hip fractures are occasional complications.

Thyroid Acropathy. Thyroid acropathy is a rare syndrome characterized by clubbing of fingers and toes, subcutaneous swelling of the extremities, and periosteal bone abnormalities.[41] It occurs in less than 1% of hyperthyroid patients, is usually associated with exophthalmos and pretibial myxedema, and makes its initial appearance many weeks to several years following treatment of the primary disease.

It begins as a diffuse swelling of the fingers and dorsum of the hands. Bone abnormalities, most marked in the metacarpals and proximal phalanges, consist of subperiosteal bubbles with marked new bone formation. Inflammatory signs and symptoms are absent, thus differentiating it from hypertrophic pulmonary osteoarthropathy. Treatment is unknown.

CONGENITAL HYPOTHYROIDISM

Congenital hypothyroidism (cretinism, thyroid dysfunction of the newborn) is due to thyroid agenesis or dysgenesis in nongoitrous, nonendemic regions of the world. These hypothyroid infants and children have residual thyroid tissue in the usual position or in ectopic areas, which is detectable by careful neck counting or scanning after radioiodine administration. Ectopic tissue is almost always situated in the midline, and about one half is at the base of the tongue. Such tissue is not usually palpable. The vestigial tissue may be adequate for some degree of hormone production, and maternal thyroid hormone may yet be circulating through the blood of the newborn, so that the signs and symptoms of thyroid deficiency may be milder and more delayed in appearance.

Detection of the hypothyroid state in the immediate postnatal period is extremely important, since early treatment will prevent irremediable mental deficiency. Moreover, adequate thyroid function is essential to normal rates of bone formation, resorption, maturation, and longitudinal growth. The orthopaedic surgeon can help to prevent cretin dwarfism by early recognition of the skeletal manifestations, and by knowledge of multiple etiologic factors, clinical course, and differentiation from other causes of retarded longitudinal growth (*e.g.*, achondroplasia) and by treatment. Collaboration with the clinician and endocrinologist is essential.

The etiology of dysgenetic cretinism in the nongoitrous regions is unknown. It may involve arrest of development of the thyroidal primordium as it descends from the foramen cecum at the base of the tongue. The disorder is sporadic in the vast majority of cases.

Other Causes of Congenital Goiter

There are a number of other causes of congenital goiter.

Inborn Defects of Hormone Synthesis or Metabolism. The synthesis and secretion of thyroid hormones depend on several enzymatic conversions from tyrosine to T_4. Deficiency of one or more of these enzymes and the resulting block of hormone synthesis or release result in hypothyroidism; compensatory TSH hypersecretion produces thyroid hyperplasia. The degree of hypothyroidism, termed *goitrous hypothyroidism* or *familial goiter* determines the effect on the central nervous system and skeletal growth and development.[65,73]

Various defects of steps in the synthetic pathway have been described, such as decreased coupling of iodotyrosines, presence of abnormal circulating iodoproteins in patients with inability to synthesize thyroglobulin, and inability of the thyroid to organify iodide with deafness (Pendred's disease).

In most instances of inborn defects of thyroid hormone synthesis, the patients are described as cretins, and mental and growth retardation suggest that hypothyroidism was present from birth.

Inborn Abnormalities of Thyroid Hormone Transport. Infants with heritable absence of, deficiency of, or excess of TBG do not manifest thyroid dysfunction. These abnormalities are detectable only by studies of hormonal iodine concentration and measurement of maximal binding capacity of TBG.

These defects appear to be transmitted as autosomal dominant or sex-linked dominant traits, and a history of abnormal protein-bound iodine (PBI) levels in other immediate family members is suggestive.

Maternal Drug Ingestion. A large number of drugs and chemicals are goitrogenic in humans.[30] Mainly the thionamides, especially thiouracil, propylthiouracil (PTU), methylthiouracil (MTU), carbimazole, and iodides, have been implicated. The thionamides are the most potent goitrogenic agents used, and fetal goiter occurs as a complication of their use in the therapy of maternal thyrotoxicosis. Prolonged administration of large doses of thionamide drugs to pregnant women increases the risk of, but does not necessarily induce, the development of fetal goiter. Fetal hypothyroidism may also develop without goiter as a result of the use of thionamide drugs.

Iodide is not a potent goitrogen and rarely produces goiter, even after prolonged administration of large doses. Maternal doses associated with congenital goiter have generally exceeded 300 mg daily. Such doses are generally employed in the treatment of chronic respiratory disease.

The administration of therapeutic doses of radioiodine to pregnant women with hyperthyroidism or thyroid cancer can cause fetal thyroid ablation. The fetal thyroid is most susceptible to radioactivity between 3 and 5 months' gestation, a time when the fetal thyroid is known to be able to concentrate iodide.[48]

Congenital Endemic Goiter. Endemic goiter occurs in most major land areas of the world. Iodine deficiency, dietary goitrogens (*e.g.*, soybean milk or flour), and endemic heritable defects in thyroid hormone synthesis have been implicated. Endemic areas of dietary iodine deficiency are statistically lacking in goiter of the newborn. Instead the maximum incidence is observed at about 12 years of age. The majority of endemic goiter patients are euthyroid.

Clinical Picture

The degree of influence on the central nervous system and skeletal structures is related to the time of onset, severity, and duration of hormone deficiency.[63] The presence of thyroid hormone deficiency is judged by the delay of bone maturation at birth, early onset of signs and symptoms of infantile hypothyroidism, and delay of treatment. Early diagnosis and treatment are essential.

Symptoms in an athyroid cretin usually appear by 6 weeks of age. In perhaps one half of such infants, intrauterine T_4 deficiency occurs, and clinical manifestations are present at birth or appear during the first 3 weeks of life. Nonspecific symptoms include lethargy, feeding difficulty, constipation, and persistent neonatal jaundice. Respiratory distress symptoms include noisy respiration, persistent nasal stuffiness, hoarse cry, and intermittent cyanosis. Respiratory symptoms result from myxedema of the tongue, epiglottis, posterior pharynx, and larynx.

Cretins classically present with a large protruding tongue, abdominal distention, umbilical hernia, puffy facies, dry hair and skin, and hypotonia.

Growth alteration and delayed mental development in cretinism are not early prominent findings. Weeks or months elapse before delay in linear growth, bone maturation, and development becomes significant.

Roentgenographic Findings in Infantile Hypothyroidism

Endochondral bone formation is delayed. Epiphyseal growth plates may remain open for many years. Ossific nuclei in the epiphyses are multiple and appear fragmented among persistent cartilaginous islands. The characteristic multiple foci of epiphyseal ossification is designated as cretinoid epiphyseal dysgenesis.[54,71,72]

The ossification centers appear late and, when they do, appear fragmented, mottled, and smaller than usual. These characteristic changes are frequently found at the hip joint and often simulate Legg-Perthes disease or multiple epiphyseal dysplasia. Carpals and tarsals do not exhibit ossific foci until quite late.

The epiphyseal growth plates are widened and irregular, suggesting rickets. They may remain open for many years.

Ossification is delayed in the spine. Characteristically, the anterior surfaces of the vertebral bodies remain persistently notched until adulthood. Typically, the second lumbar vertebra is wedge shaped. The bony endplates of the vertebral bodies are convex. In the newborn, ossification of the membranous bones of the skull is delayed and fontanelle closure is late. Pneumatization of sinuses is delayed and incomplete.

The outlook for normal skeletal development and maturation and normal mental development is good when thyroid hormone therapy is initiated early. If the disorder is not treated, mental retardation worsens and dwarfism and skeletal deformities are inevitable.

Diagnosis

Confirmation of the diagnosis can be made by PBI or serum T_4 measurement. Thyroidal radioiodine uptake using the new isotopes of iodine, ^{123}I or ^{125}I, can be used in infants, since their radioactivity is infinitesimal, as compared with ^{131}I. This will confirm the presence or absence of the thyroid or of dysgenetic thyroid tissue. An uptake of less than 10% of the administered dose after 24 hours indicates thyroid agenesis or dysgenesis.

Scanning often reveals ectopic dysgenetic tissue. When doubt exists because of borderline PBI or serum T_4 concentration and a questionable radioactive iodine uptake, the TSH test is done; that is, 0.25 units/kg or a minimum of 2 units of TSH is administered intramuscularly after a PBI and radioiodine uptake test is done, and the measurements are repeated 24 hours after administration of TSH. An increase of PBI of 2.0 μg/dl or more and an increase of radioactive iodine uptake of 20% to 50% indicates functioning thyroid tissue. A butanol-extractable iodine method (BEI) before and after TSH administration will aid in detection of a small functioning residue of dysgenetic tissue.

Treatment

Delaying treatment in the hypothyroid infant will increase the risk of irreversible central nervous system damage. Sodium L-thyroxine or a preparation combining T_4 and T_3 (liothyronine) in a ratio of 4:1 is the medication of choice; T_3 is two to four times as potent as T_4. Correcting for gastrointestinal losses during oral treatment (60% to 70% absorption), the estimated daily oral T_4 requirement is 9μg to 14μ/kg daily. The serum thyroxine-iodine concentration is kept in the range of 7μ/dl to 10μ/dl. This results in normal growth and development.

HYPOTHYROIDISM IN CHILDHOOD AND ADOLESCENCE

Hypothyroidism developing after 6 years of age (juvenile hypothyroidism) frequently is the result of chronic lymphocytic (Hashimoto's) thyroiditis.[40] In most cases the original thyroiditis has been asymptomatic and remained unrecognized, and the diagnosis has been made in retrospect on the basis of significant titers of antithyroid antibodies. The disease predominates in females and is thought to be autoimmune.[74]

Clinical Picture

Of orthopaedic importance is that such children manifest delayed skeletal growth and maturation and delayed dental development. When of long duration, hypothyroidism can eventuate in severe growth retardation. When the onset of the hypothyroid state can be accurately defined, bone maturation can be shown to slow markedly at the same time. Changes in the appearance of the ossification centers (*e.g.*, stippling), termed *epiphyseal dysgenesis*, are diagnostic of the hypothyroid state in children.

Mental deficiency does not appear to develop when the onset of hypothyroidism occus beyond 2 to 3 years of age. Other manifestations, related to pituitary dysfunction, are variable and include delayed menarche and sexual infantilism, probably a result of insufficient gonadotropin.

Diagnosis

Low PBI values, low radioiodine uptake, and response to administration of thyroid hormone are diagnostic. Primary and secondary (hypopituitary TSH) hypothyroidism can be differentiated by the TSH response test.

Other Causes of Juvenile Hypothyroidism

Less common causes include delayed development due to thyroid dysgenesis, defect in thyroid hormone synthesis, the post-thyroidectomy state, thyroiditis, goitrogens, or hypopituitarism.

DIAGNOSTIC PROCEDURES

Establishing thyroid dysfunction is generally the responsibility of the clinician. As an active participant in recognizing the early signs that may prevent an important cause of mental deficiency and stunted growth and in differentiating a prominent cause of osteopenia and susceptibility to fractures, the orthopaedic surgeon must become knowledgeable regarding basic laboratory procedures.

An extraordinary number of tests have been devised, each of which poses difficulties in performance and interpretation. A few of the more commonly performed procedures that continue to be supplanted by others aimed at reducing diagnostic inaccuracies include the following:

Radioactive Iodine Uptake (RAI)

A small tracer dose of ^{131}I is administered intravenously, and the amount extracted by the thyroid gland from the bloodstream indicates the degree of thyroid hormone production. Thyroid uptake is measured 24 hours after the isotope has been given. However, an occasional patient with thyrotoxicosis has an unusually fast iodine turnover, so that maximal gland iodine concentration is reached before 12 hours, and then falls to within the normal range before 24 hours. Therefore, a 2-hour, 4-hour, or 6-hour determination is preferred.

The RAI is affected by any substance or condition altering thyroid demand for iodine. For example, previously administered organic iodine preparations used in radiographic studies will saturate the thyroid and produce low RAI values.

Normal range:
24-hours = 15% to 49% uptake
2-hours = 1.5% to 15% uptake

Direct Serum Thyroxine (T_4) Measurements

These procedures attempt to directly measure serum T_4 and therefore directly measure hormonal activity of the thyroid. Actually, however, many of these tests measure iodine, not T_4; but since over 95% of serum iodine forms a part of T_4, iodine measurement approximates T_4 measurement unless some contaminant markedly increases the free serum iodine.

The principal substances that falsely influence T_4 levels are listed below:

Long-term steroids; depress T_4 levels
Estrogenic hormones and antiovulatory drugs: increase T_4 levels
Sulfonamides; act like thioureas (*e.g.*, thiouracil) on the thyroid and decrease T_4 levels
Salicylates: in high dosage, decreases T_4 levels
Dilantin: decreases T_4 levels

Protein-Bound Iodine (PBI)

The PBI method precipitates serum proteins and measures the iodine present, providing an indirect estimation of T_4. The test supposedly has a clinical accuracy of 90% to 95%.[18,39] Spuriously high or low levels (*e.g.*, organic iodides in x-ray contrast media will falsely increase PBI values) obtained by this method have caused it to be discarded in favor of procedures with a greater degree of specificity.

Normal range: 4μg to 8μg/dl

Butanol-Extractable Iodine (BEI)

At an acid *p*H, T_4 is insoluble in water, is less ionized, and can be extracted from acidified serum with butanol. The butanol undergoes an alkaline wash to remove inorganic iodide, MIT, and DIT. It is then evaporated to dryness, and the residue ashed and analyzed for iodide.

In the BEI method, T_4 is recovered quantitatively, iodinated proteins are insoluble in butanol and therefore are not extracted, and iodide, MIT, and DIT are eliminated by the alkaline washes. Thus the contaminants that artificially raise the PBI are eliminated. Unfortunately, most of the exogenous forms of organic iodine encountered in clinical situations are soluble in butanol, are not removed by alkaline washes, and continue to be a major problem.

Normal range: 3 mg to 6 mg/dl

Thyroxine by Competitive Binding (CPB-T_4 Method)

This T_4 measurement depends on T_4-binding by serum protein and not on iodine, so that exogenous iodinated materials do not interfere.[45] It is the simplest method for measuring thyroid hormones in the blood, and no interfering substances have been encountered. Because it involves the counting of radioactivity, any radioactivity remaining from a recent radioisotope study negates the value of this test.

Normal range: 4.6μg to 11.2μg/dl

Thyroid Scan

The thyroid uptake of radioactive isotopes is counted by a special device that produces a visual image whose varying areas of density correspond to sites of increased or decreased radioactivity. Generally ^{131}I is used, but in infants and children ^{123}I and ^{125}I produce an innocuous amount of radioactivity. The procedure demonstrates whether increased radioactivity reflects a diffusely hyperfunctioning gland or whether the increased thyroid function is confined to an isolated nodule; that there is a hypofunctioning gland if there is diffusely diminished or entirely absent uptake; an isolated area of absent uptake corresponding to a nonfunctioning localized zone, the "cold nodule" (a single cold nodule has a 10% to 20% incidence of malignancy); and the localization of ectopic thyroid tissue.

Thyroid-Stimulating Hormone Radioimmunoassay (TSH-RIA)

The thyroid participates with the anterior pituitary in feedback control. The hypothalamus secretes thyrotropin-releasing hormone (TRH), which acts on the pituitary to synthesize and release TSH, which, in turn, stimulates the thyroid gland to synthesize and release T_3 and T_4. The latter suppress the release of TSH by a negative feedback mechanism. Therefore, decrease of serum T_3 and T_4 causes increased secretion of TSH; increase of T_3 and T_4 causes decrease of TSH. Radioimmunoassay for TSH can help to assess thyroid function. A TSH assay in conjunction with TRH stimulation gives information not only as to thyroid function but also whether a case of thyroid deficiency is due to a defect of the thyroid, pituitary, or hypothalamus.

The TSH determination differentiates between primary (thyroid) and secondary (pituitary) hypothyroidism.[32]

In primary hypothyroidism, because of decreased thyroid hormone feedback, TSH secretion is increased and the serum TSH levels are higher. The TSH serum levels are normal or undetectable in secondary hypothyroidism due to hypothalamic or pituitary disorders.

Testing TSH response to exogenous synthetic TRH will differentiate pituitary and hypothalamic varieties of secondary hypothyroidism. Injected intravenously, TRH normally produces a prompt rise in serum TSH that peaks between 20 and 40 minutes. When a previously undetectable or normal level of serum TSH in a hypothyroid patient responds to TRH stimulation, the defect is at the hypothalamic level; if it does not respond, the defect is at the pituitary level.

The TRH stimulation test may also be used to measure pituitary TSH reserve.[23,26] If serum T_3 levels are followed after TRH stimulation, thyroid reserve is assessed.[59]

In hyperthyroidism, except in TSH-secreting tumors, serum TSH levels are undetectable or in the normal range. The response of serum TSH to TRH is inhibited by thyroid hormone, and thus the lack of response of serum TSH to TRH stimulation is an excellent confirmatory test of thyrotoxicosis.

The quantitation of serum TSH is valuable for avoiding undertreatment of primary hypothyroidism and overtreatment of hyperthyroidism.

Normal range: up to 10μU/ml.

Modified TSH Test

To differentiate primary from secondary thyroid hypofunction, an RAI is performed, both before and after administration of TSH. In pituitary insufficiency, the thyroid will respond to TSH; if hypofunction is primary, a result of disease of the thyroid, the administration of TSH will not significantly increase the RAI uptake.

T_3 by Radioimmunoassay (T_3-RIA)

In spite of extremely small quantities present in the serum, the activity of T_3 is many times that of T_4 and plays a major role in pathologic states. In the peripheral tissues, T_4 is converted to $T_{\_}$ by removal of an iodide atom, suggesting that T_4 may represent a "prohormone."

The measure of T_3 is important for detecting a variant of hyperthyroidism in which T_3 levels are elevated, although T_4 levels are normal. It is therefore mandatory that serum T_3 levels be done in all cases suspected of having thyrotoxicosis.

In hypothyroidism, T_3 values are low to normal. The technique used is that in which radioactive T_3 is bound to antibody.[20,43]

Normal range: 110 ng to 230 ng/dl

T_3 Suppression Test

Administration of thyroid hormone in adequate doses suppresses radioiodine uptake of the *normal* thyroid, but it has no influence on the uptake of the thyroid gland in thyrotoxicosis.[68] The test is used to differentiate thyrotoxicosis from other diseases and features that suggest thyrotoxicosis. T_3 is usually administered in preference to T_4, because its action is more rapid and its iodine content less.

Free Thyroxine (T_F)

Over 99% of circulating T_4 is protein bound. A very small quantity of T_4 is free (unbound), T_F. The amount of T_F depends mainly on the ratio of protein bound T_4 to the total amount of serum protein-binding capacity available (*i.e.*, degree of saturation of TBG). Free thyroxine more accurately reflects the true thyrometabolic status. It is not affected by TBG abnormalities, since TBG acts as a storage depot.

Direct measurement of T_F is available in only a few reference laboratories.

ENZYMES

Normally, alkaline phosphatase occurs in greatest concentration at the intestinal mucosa, in bone, and in the kidney.[75] In other words, it functions principally at sites of absorption, deposition, and excretion of calcium and phosphorus. In bone, it is concentrated at the main points of ossification (*i.e.*, the epiphyseal line and the subperiosteal area). During active bone destruction, a compensatory stimulation of osteoblasts to replace bone is reflected in an increased intracellular content of alkaline phosphatase and increased levels in the bloodstream. Because it is present in large concentration at points of active bone formation, the Gomori phosphatase stain may be used to identify areas of energetic new bone formation.

The normal range of blood alkaline phosphatase relates to the method used for assaying the enzyme. The following are the normal ranges for the most commonly used procedures:[52]

1–4 units/dl (Bodansky)
4–13 units/dl (King-Armstrong)
0.8–2.5 units/dl (Bessey-Lowry)
30–115 U/liter (SMAC)

In children, the normal ranges are higher (*e.g.*, 5.0 to 14.0 Bodansky units/dl). A marked increase as high as 135 Bodansky units is found in patients with Paget's disease. Hyperparathyroidism is associated with a moderate rise, as is active rickets. A slight to moderate rise in osteoblastic osteogenic sarcoma is proportionate to the amount of new bone formation. Diseases of the liver typically show an elevated level of serum alkaline phosphatase, most of which is heat stabile, and can be differentiated from heat-labile alkaline phosphatase that originates in bone.

The counterpart of alkaline phosphatase is acid phosphatase, an enzyme found in various tissues but principally in the adult human prostate. The normal serum level of acid phosphatase is 0.0 to 1.0 Bodansky unit/dl. An increase occurs in carcinoma of the prostate with metastases.

ALKALINE PHOSPHATASE

DIFFERENTIATION OF ISOENZYMES

Serum alkaline phosphatase is composed of a group of isoenzymes that primarily originate from liver and bone and, to a minor extent, from the intestine and the placenta. The following methods help to define the main source of the increased serum levels.

Fractionation Test by Heating

Heating will destroy the heat-labile portion, which is of osseous origin.

The level of alkaline phosphatase is determined on the unheated serum specimen and then on a serum specimen that has been heated to 56°C for 10 minutes.

If the level of the heat-stabile alkaline phosphatase remaining after heating is greater than 30% of the total (or unheated level), the indication is that the increase is the result of liver disease. If the level of heat-stabile alkaline phosphatase remaining after heating is less than 17% of the total (or unheated level), the indication is that the serum level increase is due to skeletal disease.

Serum γ-Glutamyl Transpeptidase Activity (Serum GGT)

GGT activity is above normal in all forms of liver disease and normal in cases of bone disease.[76] Measurement of

GGT activity offers a means for determining whether bone or liver is the source of increased alkaline phosphatase.

Gel Electrophoresis

Rarely is it necessary to analyze and identify each isoenzyme, and this can be accurately ascertained by gel electrophoresis.

PATHOLOGIC PHYSIOLOGY

Experimental work has demonstrated that the formation of alkaline phosphatase is closely related to young fibroblasts involved in the deposition of the fibrocollagenous framework or matrix of bone rather than to impregnation of this framework with mineral salts. By stains that are specific for this enzyme, the position and concentration of alkaline phosphatase can be detected in the tissues. Thus, fibroblasts in the outer layers of periosteum are lacking in this enzyme, whereas those in the cambium layer, where they are being differentiated into osteoblasts, contain large amounts of this enzyme. Stains identify the sites where the enzyme is located as being intranuclear, intracellular, or extracellular. The fibrils that are formed within the cell and extruded to become the precursors of the collagenous matrix (osteoid) are intensely stained.

Staining of the enzyme is useful for studying osteoblastic activity. For example, osteoblasts and their precursors, both containing alkaline phosphatase, can be followed about a bone transplant in which creeping substitution is taking place. When new fibrocollagenous matrix is formed, osteoblasts can be traced to their ultimate destiny. They become surrounded by matrix that becomes mineralized, the cells persisting as osteocytes. Others become cells within the matrix where they are not demonstrable by ordinary hematoxylin and eosin stain, because the nucleus loses its basophilic staining but retains its affinity for the alkaline phosphatase stain. As the osteoid forms, this cell disappears, and alkaline phosphatase is no longer demonstrable. It appears that the next stage, namely mineralization, does not depend on alkaline phosphatase.[77]

Alkaline phosphatase is closely linked with the formation of a fiberlike material, whether or not these fibers become part of bone. It is related to young fibroblasts and the building material between the cells, both normal and pathologic. The enzyme is present in large quantities in fibrosarcoma, in polyostotic fibrous dysplasia, and in the fibrous matrix of the bone in Paget's disease.

ACID PHOSPHATASE

Acid phosphatase is capable of hydrolyzing hexose diphosphate at a *p*H of 5. It is found in large concentration in the prostate and in lesser amounts in the seminal vesicles, the testes, the epididymis, and the spermatic duct. It appears in large amounts in the bloodstream in metastatic carcinoma of the prostate, even before bone involvement is apparent on roentgenographic examination. The level of alkaline phosphate may also rise in this condition.

Sometimes the osteoblastic phase of Paget's disease or the osteoblastic type of osteogenic sarcoma may be confused roentgenologically with metastatic prostatic carcinoma. In Paget's disease, only the level of alkaline phosphatase shows a marked increase. In osteogenic sarcoma the alkaline phosphatase level may rise slightly or moderately. In metastatic prostatic carcinoma, both alkaline and acid phosphatase values are increased, especially the latter.

Section II
Mineralization of Bone

THEORIES OF MINERALIZATION

Mineralization of bone involves biochemical and biophysical processes that are extracellular and intracellular.

Chemical processes produce nucleation, the incorporation of calcium and phosphate into clusters of hydroxyapatite, the formula of which is $Ca_{10}(PO_4)_6(OH)_2$. At first this is composed of amorphous (noncrystalline) calcium phosphate, from which evolves the crystalline form. Amorphous and crystalline calcium phosphate are embedded in the interstitial matrix together with collagen, a minimal amount of elastin, proteinpolysaccharides (PPS), and traces of lipids. A layer of water, the hydration shell, is believed to be bound to the surface of the crystals, and through it ions are transferred to and from the crystal surfaces.[92,98,102]

Hydroxyapatite crystals are in the shape of needles and plates, 27 A to 75 A thick, 40 A to 75 A wide, and 50 A to 400 A long. Each crystal consists of a lattice composed of thousands of polyhedral units, with some of the positions on the lattice available for substitution by molecules containing sodium, potassium, magnesium, carbonate, citrate, fluoride, and other trace materials. The individual apatite crystals are extremely small. The bone salts comprise 60% of the solid mature cortical bone. An increase in the size and number of particles of amorphous or crystalline mineral at the expense of ions in the fluid environment is termed *mineral growth.* Calcium and phosphate ions are considered to be in equilibrium with amorphous and crystalline calcium phosphate. The equilibrium is affected by many factors, both local (*e.g.*, *p*H) and systemic (*e.g.*, PTH, calcitonin). The transition of mineral ions to nuclei of hydroxyapatite deposited about collagen fibrils is under the regulatory control of osteoblasts.

The key event in mineralization is nucleation of

hydroxyapatite, presumably by two pathways, supersaturation and activation by fibrillar proteins.

In *supersaturation,* amorphous calcium phosphate is precipitated from supersaturated solutions of ions and transformed at neutral *p*H to the complex salt hydroxyapatite. In *activation by fibrillar proteins,* cell-synthesized macromolecules contain bound calcium or phosphate and provide energy to organize relevant ions from a nonsaturated solution into the crystalline phase.

THEORY OF COLLAGEN NUCLEATION

A specialized fibrous matrix, consisting chiefly of collagen, is synthesized, Nucleational sites on the collagen are exposed to tissue fluid, when shielding compounds such as PPS are removed from the fibrous matrix. Phosphate and calcium become bound to the nucleational sites, and from these initial clusters of ions, growth of the mineral phase ensues in a precise manner, determined by the nature of the limiting surface of the collagen fibrils.

Certain evidence for this theory shows that in a solution with adequate concentrations of calcium and phosphate ions, reconstituted collagen is shown by electron microscopy to acquire mineral clusters in regular spaced sites on collagen fibrils.[90] Clustering of mineral develops in relation to specific periodic areas in the collagen fibrils. Collagen can bind covalently to a small amount of phosphate, preferentially by serine or by carbohydrate.

Calcium is believed to be bound to PPS,[93] perhaps by phospholipids or sialoproteins. Theoretically, the ions are stored in intracellular-synthesized carrier molecules, which release them as mineral particles are formed.

The Urist theory postulates that calcium first binds to anionic groups in degraded protein. Calcium phosphate is subsequently released from a calcium phosphate, protein complex.[110]

Under the electron microscope, intracellular electron-dense granules are seen. These may represent calcium complexed to proteins and are contained within vesicles that are extruded from the cell and coalesce to form new mineral.[82] With the use of ^{47}Ca for autoradiographic studies, the grains are observed to localize first in the mitochondria, then in the endoplasmic reticulum, shifting toward the surface of the cell, and finally within the matrix at calcification sites.[100] The intracellular processes are therefore closely correlated to mineralization of bone.

Hydroxyapatite crystals will continue to grow relentlessly in the presence of calcium and phosphate solutions. Certain factors that inhibit this process are described in the following discussion on individual components.

COLLAGEN

Collagen of bone differs from that of cartilage in its amino acid composition. It contains two highly anionic amino acids, serine and glycine, and characteristically much of the serine is present as serine phosphate, thus pointing out the importance of phosphate bound to bone collagen in the role of mineralization.[106,108] Bone collagen also contains the monosaccharide galactose to which calcium ions bind.

GLYCOSAMINOGLYCANS

These large molecules of PPS have high viscosity and form the basis for ground substance. Besides a minute amount of chondroitin sulfate, several PPS complexes have been described in bone.[91] These mucosubstances compose 9.5% of bone organic matrix. These complexes retard mineral growth and at sites of mineralization appear to decrease in amount as they undergo enzymatic degradation.[96]

The free anionic groups of acid PPS may well inhibit calcification by selectively binding calcium ions and making them unavailable for crystallization.[88] PPS extracted from cartilage will inhibit precipitation of calcium phosphate from solution.[83] When the PPS are enzyme digested, their inhibitory action is lost.

INORGANIC PYROPHOSPHATE

Inorganic pyrophosphate will inhibit apatite crystal growth *in vitro,*[85] and a polymer, Graham's salt, will inhibit ectopic calcification.[97] This substance normally exists in ECF and is found in the urine of normal people. It chemisorbs to apatite.[107]

Pyrophosphate increases the minimum product ($Ca \times P$) required to induce precipitation of calcium phosphate from solution. Now diphosphonates, which are stable when administered orally, can be used to prevent calcification *in vivo.*

The most likely mechanism of action of the diphosphonates both *in vivo* and *in vitro* is strong chemisorption on hydroxyapatite. Since diphosphonates resist chemical and enzymatic hydrolysis, and are of low toxicity, they can be used against diseases in which calcium salts deposit in soft tissues.

LIPIDS

Although the lipid content of bone is very low (6 mg to 13 mg/100 g dry wt), acidic phospholipids are increased at the mineralization front. These are present in a larger amount and in a different form where calcification is being initiated.[94]

CELLULAR ACTIVITY

Mitochondria will accumulate calcium *in vitro*[84] and might produce local increased levels of mineral ions and a matrix capable of being calcified.[105] The element has been found in osteoblasts, osteocytes, and chondrocytes. The level of calcium in the cell is closely correlated with the degree of mineralization in the adjacent matrix.[104] There remains unanswered the question as to whether the calcium phosphate in these cells may represent the result of bone resorption.

In growth cartilage, an increasing gradient of inorganic granules within the mitochondria of chondrocytes occurs up to the zone of provisional calcification, where the granules disappear, presumably used up in the process of calcification. In rickets, the granules are scarce but reappear with the administration of vitamin D.

As the zone of provisional calcification is approached, the mitochondrial enzyme content increases, including alkaline phosphatase, alkaline pyrophosphatase, lysozymes, and lactic dehydrogenase.[79]

VESICLES

At areas of active mineralization, very minute membrane-bound bodies are observed, appearing to bud off osteoblasts and containing the earliest formations of crystals and enzymes such as alkaline phosphatase, alkaline pyrophosphatase, and adenosine triphosphate (ATP).[78,82] As the crystals extend beyond their boundaries, they coalesce and become intimately associated with collagen fibrils. These vesicles are chiefly lipid in nature. Lipids can bind calcium, at first, and then phosphate; phosphate binding depends on prior binding of calcium.[80] Vesicles are important for raising the local content of orthophosphate, leading to the formation of hydroxyapatite, and for providing the mechanism for ATP-dependent transport of calcium and phosphate.

SPECIFIC THEORIES OF MINERALIZATION

The intermediate mechanisms between calcium, phosphate, and hydroxyl ions in the bloodstream and the eventual formation and organization of hydroxyapatite are subjects of ongoing investigations that have never been resolved.[99] The following theories represent attempts to interpret the results and are intended to provide a basis from which further inquiry will be pursued.

URIST HYPOTHESIS

The Urist hypothesis involves a triphasic local mechanism.[109]

Phase 1

Protein and calcium form a soluble calcifying substrate complex within the ground substance gel. Calcium disrupts hydrogen cross linkages in fibrous protein and PPS; it forms calcium complexes with anionic groups.

Phase 2

Formation of soluble protein-calcium-phosphate complex takes place. The concentration of phosphate ions must not exceed physiological levels; otherwise, calcium phosphate precipitates out of solution and calcification of tissue is prevented. The initial binding of large concentrations of calcium to serum protein is followed automatically by binding of inorganic phosphate into a nonultrafilterable complex.

Phase 3

In the solid phase, nucleation and crystal growth occur. A reaction occurs between protein-calcium-phosphate complex in the tissues and active Ca^{2+} and HPO_4^{2-}. The reaction takes place only with chemically active calcium and phosphate ions, $A_{Ca^{2+}}$ and $A_{HPO_4^{2-}}$. This may be represented by the following formula:

$$\underset{\text{(solid)}}{CaHPO_4} \rightleftharpoons \underset{\text{(undissociated in solution)}}{CaHPO_4} \rightleftharpoons \underset{\text{(dissociated in solution)}}{Ca^{2+} \times HPO_4}$$

or

$$\frac{[Ca]^{2+}\,[HPO_4]^{2-}}{[CaHPO_4]} = K$$

The product of the ionic concentrations of calcium and phosphate, divided by the concentration of the undissociated salt, is a constant. Since the concentration of the undissociated salt in solution at any one time is transitional, it may be disregarded, and the following formula may be substituted:

$$[Ca^{2+}] \times [HPO_4^{2-}] = K$$

or the solubility product constant. Because the chemically active phosphate is approximately half that of the diffusible phosphate in adult serum, the formula may be restated:

$$A_{Ca^{2+}} \times A_{HPO_4^{2-}} = K$$

Therefore, blood plasma is undersaturated with respect to $CaHPO_4$, on the borderline of solubility of the earliest deposits of bone mineral, but slightly metastable or supersaturated with respect to mature deposits. It would appear that the ECF and blood plasma must be undersaturated with respect to the initial deposit. The theory currently may be summarized as follows:

The first ion to be bound is calcium, which is the activating principle for the following:

- Formation of calcifiable matrix
- Uptake of phosphate by ion association
- Overcoming energy barrier to nucleation
- Formation of ultramicroscopic spaces in tissues by efflux of protein

Formation of tripartite calcium phosphate complex for nucleation
Formation of nucleation centers of apatite mineral by compartmentalized precipitation
Crystal formation

GLIMCHER HYPOTHESIS

This theory postulates the presence of nucleation centers that are related to the physical organization and stereochemistry of collagen components of bone matrix.[89,90]

Structure of Inorganic Phase of Calcium and Phosphate

The first solid deposited in bone is physically amorphous and "noncrystalline," as shown by x-ray diffraction and spectroscopic analyses; it is present in greater amounts in young, newly formed tissue (40% to 50%) than in older, more mature bone (25% to 30%). Its actual chemical composition and structure have not been elucidated. Amorphous Ca-P solid converts slowly to poorly crystalline hydroxyapatite, having the unit cell formula, $Ca_{10}(PO_4)_6(OH)_2$.

Organic Matrix

At least 90% to 95% of extracellular matrix consists of the fibrous protein collagen. This collagen appears similar to soft tissue collagen by wide- and low-angle x-ray diffraction, amino acid analysis, and electron microscopy. However, unlike most soft tissue collagens, bone collagen is insoluble in solvents used to extract collagens from other tissues (*e.g.*, neutral salt solutions and weak organic acids). This is thought to be caused by strong intermolecular bonds between and along the length of adjacent macromolecules.

In addition to collagen, a small amount of mucoprotein, sialoprotein, and lipid, including phospholipid, are present.

Organization of Collagen and the Ca-P Solids (Amorphous and Crystalline) in Bone

Electron microscopy shows inorganic Ca-P deposited in an orderly fashion along the axial dimension of the fibrils, and located primarily within the fibrils.

Crystal deposition within the fibrils takes place without changing the volume or disrupting the closely packed macromolecules in the fibrils. This is attributed to the presence of "holes" or channels in the fibrils owing to a 9% to 10% linear overlap of the individual monomers (Figs. 6-11 through 6-14).

Electron diffraction shows that the long axes of the inorganic crystallites (c-axes) are essentially parallel with the long axes of the fibrils within which they are located.

The inorganic crystals are small, lathelike platelets, 10 A to 30 A thick, 400 A long, and about 100 A wide; they are larger with increasing age. Because of their

FIG. 6-11. An electron micrograph of an undecalcified, unstained, longitudinal section of young, embryonic chick bone. The dense mineral phase appears to "stain" the collagen fibril at regular intervals along its axial length. In some areas, the inorganic crystals can be seen on edges as dark lines (*1*). Most of the mineral phase is not resolvable into individual crystals and has the appearance one might expect from an "amorphous" phase (*2*). (× 320,000) (Glimcher M, Hodge AJ: A basic architectural principle in the organization of mineralized tissue. Clin Orthop 61:16, 1968)

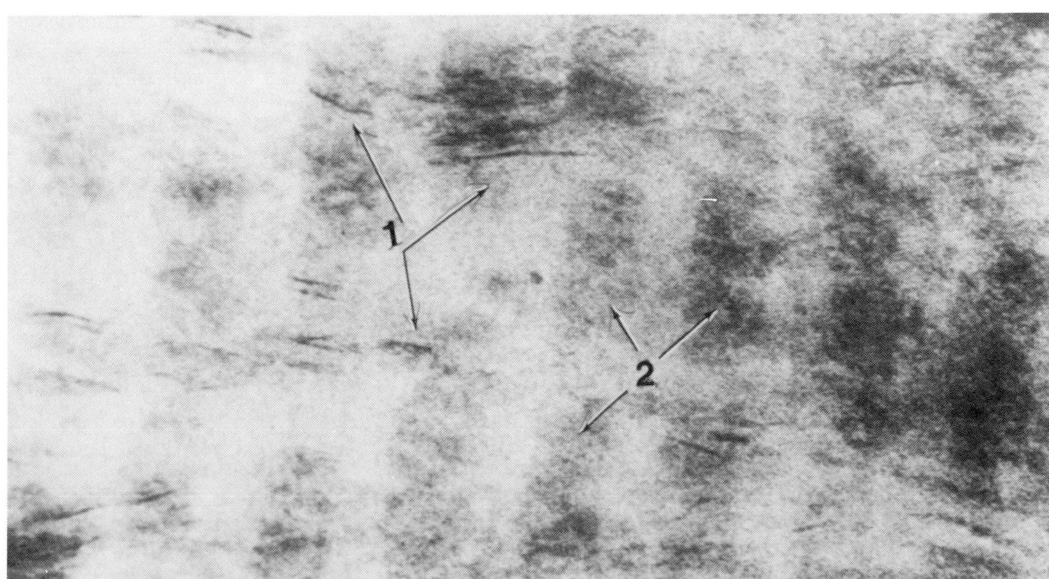

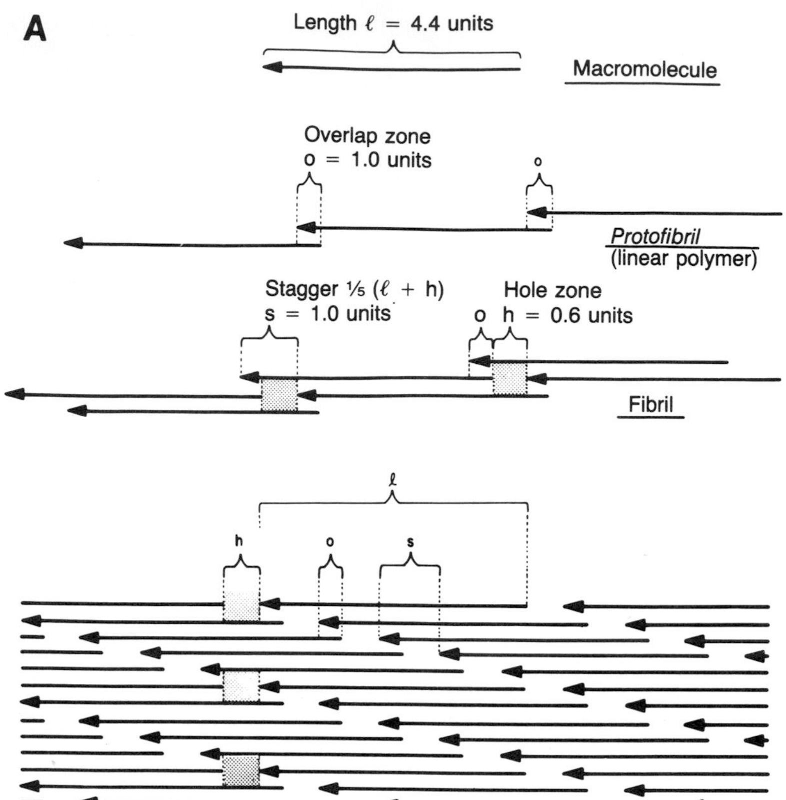

FIG. 6-12. (*A*) This schematic illustration shows how the packing of the collagen macromolecules in the collagen fibril generates a void or hole within the fibril. Note that the overlap (*o*) plus the hole zone (*h*) are equal to the axial repeat of the collagen fibril(s). (Glimcher MJ, Krane SM: In Ramachadran GN (ed): Aspects of Protein Structure, New York, Academic Press, 1963)

(*Continued on facing page*)

extremely small size, their surface area is extremely large. Since the thickness of the crystals represents only two or three unit cells, it is clear that an enormous number of calcium and phosphate ions are available for exchange with the ions of the ECF. This potential surface for exchange helps to maintain ionic homeostasis of the ECF, especially since 30% to 40% of the total body sodium and 60% of total body magnesium is associated with the bone mineral.

Bone represents a two-phase material, the structural and mechanical properties of which are greater than the total of such properties of its individual two major components (Ca-P and collagen).

Current Theories of Mechanism of Calcification

Physical Chemical Concepts. In a metastable equilibrium, solutions in such an equilibrium can remain stable indefinitely, but are capable of forming new phases under special conditions without completely changing the properties of the system.

Mechanisms in Phase Transformation. A change in state from the metastable solution results in the formation of the initial fragments of a new more stable phase called *nucleation,* which is followed by growth of the initial fragments. This phenomenon of recrystallization, the growth of larger crystals at the expense of smaller ones, occurs after the solid state has been achieved.

Homogeneous nucleation is the formation of a new phase in the bulk of the metastable (unstable) phase in the absence of foreign inclusions. It is considered to arise by the formation of clusters of molecules of ions of the original phase as a result of local transient fluctuations in certain properties of the system such as its concentration.

The initiation or induction of a new phase on or by the introduction of a foreign inclusion is referred to as *heterogeneous nucleation.*

An example of both homogeneous and heterogeneous nucleation is provided by the change in state characterized by the crystallization of ice from water. Water may be undercooled to about −39°C to −41°C, if all dust and foreign particles are excluded, and then spontaneous formation of ice crystals is noted. Now if silver iodide crystals are added to the system before undercooling has begun, the water need only be supercooled to about −4°C to −6°C before crystallization of ice begins. In this case, the crystallization of ice starts on the surface of the silver iodide crystals.

Thus a crystallographic theory of heterogeneous nucleation can be proposed based on a similarity between the atomic arrangement and lattice spacings of the nucleation catalyst and the crystals being nucleated. It

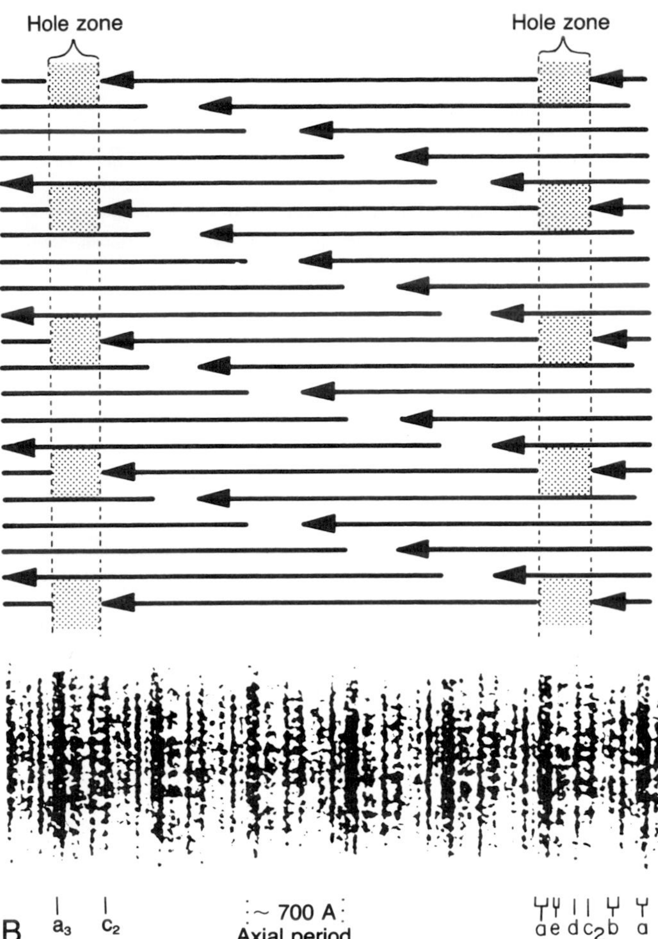

FIG. 6-12 (*Continued*). (*B*) The relationship between the position of the hole zone, the axial period of the collagen fibril, and the "head" (A end) and "tail" (B end) of the collagen macromolecule. The hole zone falls between the a_3 and c_2 bands (Adapted from Hodge AJ, Petruska JA: In Ramachandran GN (ed): Aspects of Protein Structure. New York, Academic Press, 1963)

predicts that the order of catalytic potency should be proportional to the reciprocal of the disregistry between a catalyst and the forming crystals on certain low-index planes of similar atomic arrangement. Thus silver iodide, whose lattice structure closely resembles that of ice, is the most potent catalyst known for the nucleation of ice crystals. This is the basis for cloud seeding experiments.

The similarity of atomic structure and lattice spacings is emphasized in this theory. However, other factors must undoubtedly enter into a quantitative formation, such as the presence of surface defects and specific interactions that depend on the nature and type of chemical bond between nucleation catalyst and nucleation crystal.

Mechanism of Crystal Induction in Biologic Tissues. Since the source of mineral ions for crystals derives from body fluids, and since spontaneous precipitation normally does not take place, some mechanism must exist in mineralizing tissues to initiate the formation of crystals and control further growth and orientation.

Nucleation hypothesis: The physicochemical mechanism initiating mineralization is based on the stereochemistry of the major organic component. The hypothesis proposes that the precise juxtaposition of certain reactive groups in the organix matrix creates highly specific regions both chemically and spatially that act as sites for the heterogeneous nucleation of the appropriate crystals from metastable (or unstable) solutions of body fluids.

Such a mechanism permits localization of crystals to specific regions in the organic matrix at a molecular level and is consistent with the structural order found in mineralized tissues and with the intimate relationships between the organic and inorganic components of these tissues.

Regulation of Calcification *in Vivo*.
Changes in Metastability of the ECF or in Formation of Ca-P Clusters. *Cellular Control of Calcium.* Electron-dense granules appear in the mitochondria of cells of skeletal and dental tissues and in tissues undergoing pathologic calcification. Because mitochondria are capable of concentrating Ca and P, it is postulated that the electron-dense particles represent a solid phase of Ca-P.

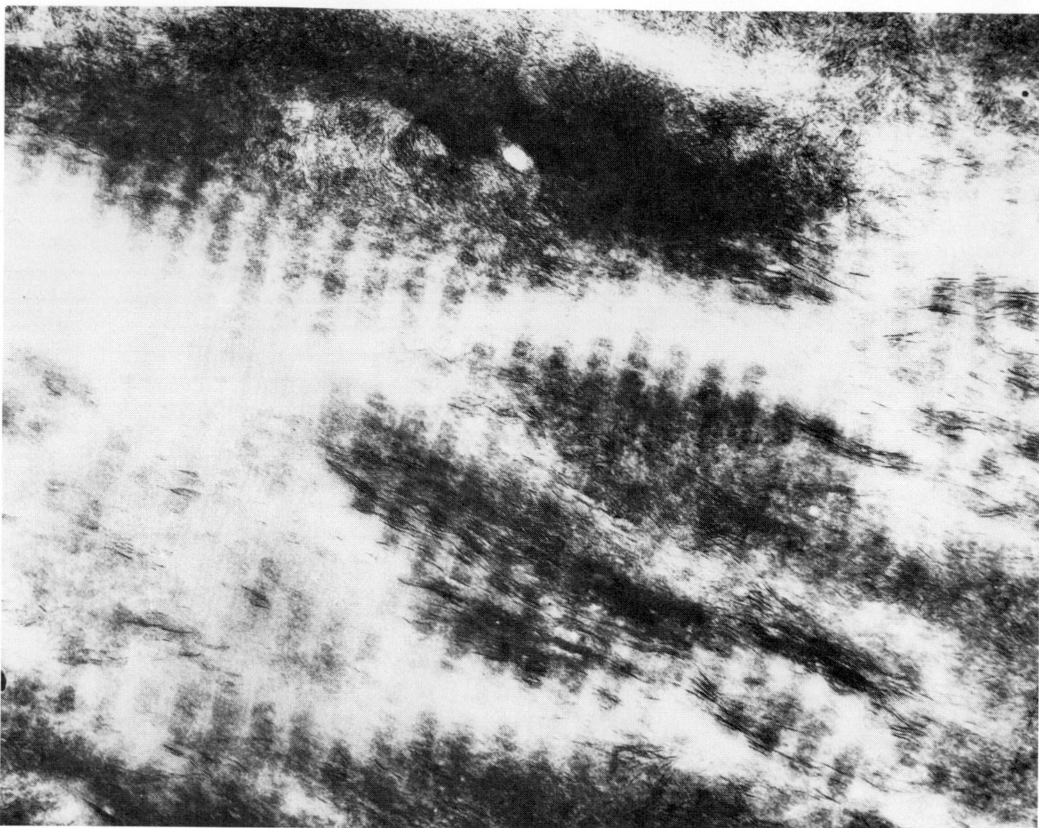

FIG. 6-13. Electron micrograph of undecalcified, embryonic chick bone stained with osmium only. Note the accentuation of the axial period of collagen by the amorphous-appearing density of the mineral phase, the bands and interbands of the collagen fibrils devoid of crystals, and the regions in the collagen fibrils where mineral is just beginning to form. From the position of the mineral phase in relation to the collagen bands, the mineral can be located between the a_3 and c_2, corresponding to the hole zone. (×82,000) (Glimcher MJ, Hodge AJ: A basic architectural principle in the organization of mineralized tissue. Clin Orthop 61:16, 1968)

In addition to intracellular deposits of mineral, extracellular electron-dense material corresponding to the mineral phase is seen in close association with irregularly shaped membrane-bound vesicles in the organic matrix of cartilage and bone. These vesicles are distinct from lysosomes and contain enzymes capable of increasing the local concentration of orthophosphate. They may also provide a mechanism for the ATP-dependent transport of calcium or phosphate into the lumen of the vesicles, facilitating the nucleation of the mineral within the vesicles.

It is therefore postulated that the initiation of mineralization is at least partially controlled by the concentration and subsequent deposition of Ca^{2+} and P^{2-} ions as small granules or clusters within the mitochondria of osteoblasts (Fig. 6-15). The particles or clusters may then be either excreted as such or in packages (vesicles) and act either by dissolving and increasing the local concentration of Ca^{2+} and P^{2-} ions in the ECF surrounding the collage fibrils (or enamel tubules) or by being deposited within specific sites in the organic matrix as niduses of the initial solid phase.

Pyrophosphate and Polyphosphates. Pyrophosphate and polyphosphates have been demonstrated in serum and have been shown to inhibit mineralization by decreasing the metastability of Ca-P solutions. The concentrations of such substances in the ECF surrounding the organic matrix elements may be controlled by the enzyme alkaline phosphatase, which hydrolyzes both pyrophosphate and polyphosphates.

Regulation of Mineralization by Specific Changes in Collagen, or Synthesis and Incorporation of Specific Peptides or Other Organic Compounds. *Possible Role of Protein or Peptide-Bound Organic Phosphate.* Organic phosphate is present in bone and dentin collagen. Serine phosphate and peptide-bound sugar phosphates, as well as non–covalently bound phosphorylated peptides, have been identified. It seems possible that enzymatic phos-

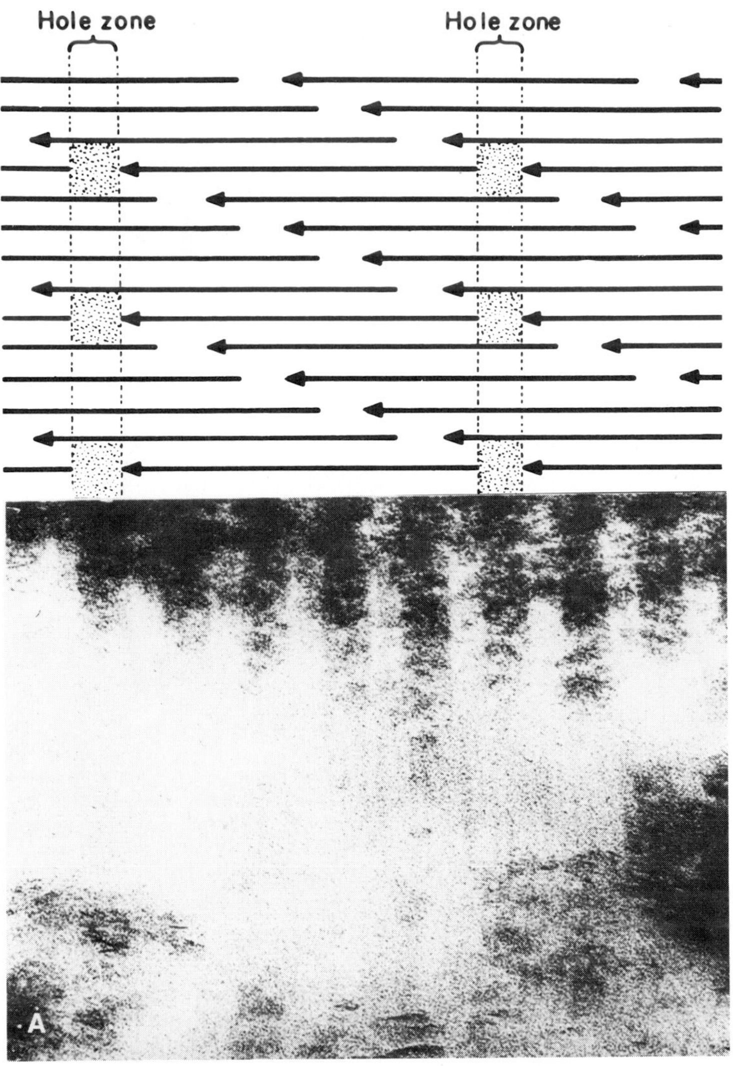

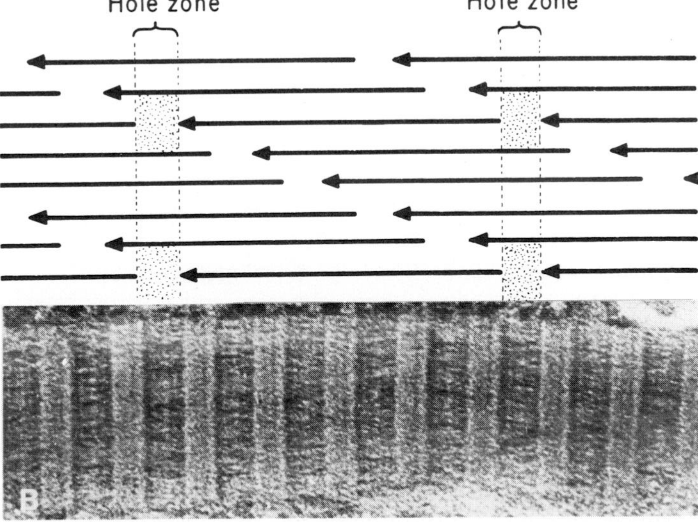

FIG. 6-14. (*A*) The identification of the location of the mineral phase in bone collagen between the a_3 and c_2 bands places the crystals in the hole zone. (*B*) Correlation of the packing of the collagen macromolecules in the fibril, the generation of the hole zone, and the appearance of reconstituted bone collagen negatively stained with PTA to show the hole zone. Note the similarity between the fibrils negatively stained with PTA and bone collagen "negatively stained" with the mineral phase. (Glimcher MJ, Hodge AJ: A basic architectural principle in the organization of mineralized tissue. Clin Orthop 61:16, 1968)

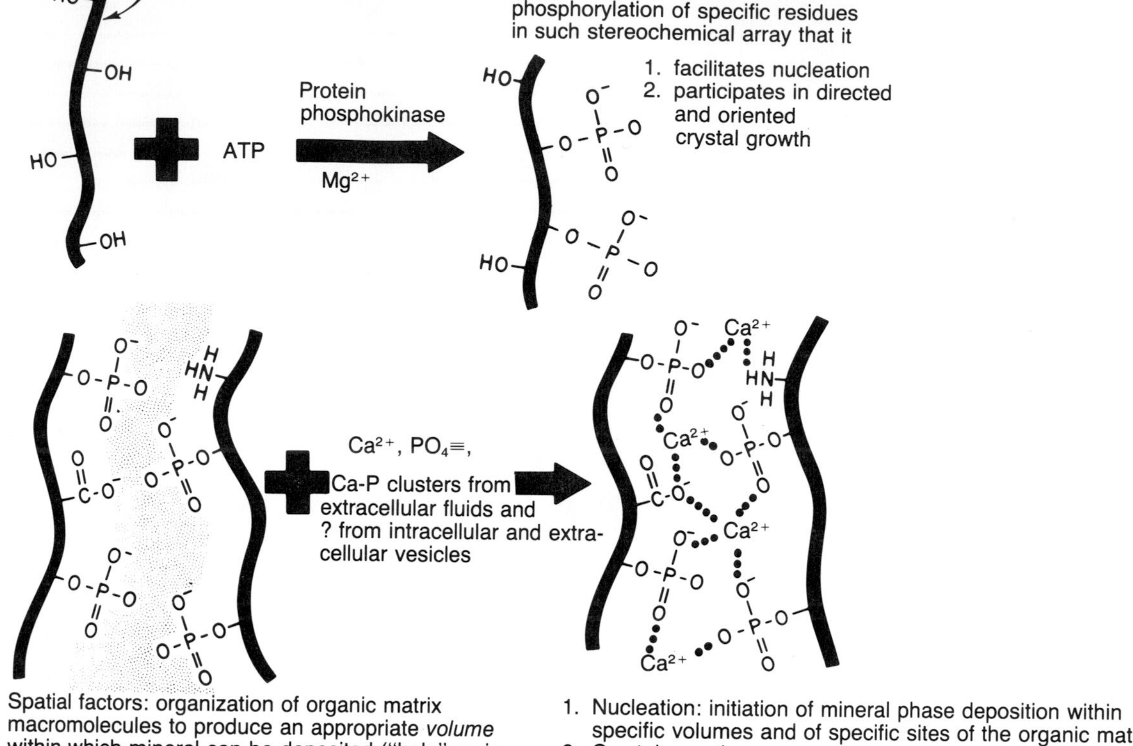
Organic matrix protein
Protein phosphokinase
ATP
Mg^{2+}
Chemical modification of matrix: phosphorylation of specific residues in such stereochemical array that it
1. facilitates nucleation
2. participates in directed and oriented crystal growth
Ca^{2+}, $PO_4^{\equiv}$,
Ca-P clusters from extracellular fluids and ? from intracellular and extracellular vesicles
Spatial factors: organization of organic matrix macromolecules to produce an appropriate *volume* within which mineral can be deposited ("hole" regions of collagen, enamel "tubercles")
1. Nucleation: initiation of mineral phase deposition within specific volumes and of specific sites of the organic matrix
2. Crystal growth

FIG. 6-15. Diagram of the Glimcher hypothesis of mineralization of bone.

phorylation of serine and residues of various structural components from ATP and other high energy phosphate compounds may provide a common biochemical pathway for mineralization.

Covalently bound phosphate possesses the requirements for a mineral ion to participate in the nucleation process: a covalently bound phosphate has fixed direction, energy, and distance and is sterically organized by the structure of collagen. Moreover, covalently bound phosphate would still be reactive and could form bonds with Ca^{2+}, a step necessary for the initial phase. On the other hand, covalently bound or chelated calcium ions would be unavailable for further reaction with phosphate ions.

Phosphoprotein kinases have been isolated from connective tissues, including bone, cartilage, and enamel. These are capable of transferring the terminal phosphoryl group from ATP to both collagen and enamel proteins.

The Proteinpolysaccharides. In their native state of aggregation, the proteoglycans act as inhibitors of calcification by virtue of their ability to bind calcium, exclude phosphate ions, and decrease the diffusion of ions into the interstices of the tissue. Depolymerization of the proteoglycans by enzymes synthesized by the appropriate cells and the eventual removal of the degradation products would not only remove these barriers and release Ca^{2+} and P^{2-} ions previously bound to the proteoglycans (booster portion of theory), all of which would then permit and facilitate nucleation of Ca-P by other structural components in the tissue spaces such as the collagen fibrils but would also provide the extrafibrillar extracellular space needed for additional mineral deposition.

Electron Microscopic Studies

The Glimcher hypotheses should be correlated with a review of electron microscopic studies of mineralized bone (see below).

BONE FORMATION, RESORPTION, AND MINERALIZATION

The determination of bone turnover (formation, resorption) and mineralization is essential for evaluating the metabolic state of the skeleton and differentiating various pathologic states, such as osteoporosis, osteomalacia, and parathyroid abnormalities.[119,121] Such studies may also be used to monitor the effect of treatment.

The procedures used for assessing metabolic bone

disease in conjunction with other requirements for evaluation of these diseases include a careful history and physical examination, roentgenographic studies, and serum calcium, phosphate, and alkaline phosphatase evaluation.

Bone formation and resorption can be accurately measured by microradiography. The following facts are fundamental to interpretation. Bone formation is a two-stage process: first, collagen is laid down, and then it is mineralized. The presence of unmineralized collagen (osteoid) does not mean that bone formation is taking place. In osteomalacia or rickets, little or no bone formation occurs. The little bone that does form is poorly mineralized, resulting in wide osteoid seams.

Only the bone surfaces are in the process of bone formation or resorption, which is recognized by characteristic contours and mineral distribution over these surfaces. The lengths of these active surfaces can be accurately measured, thus determining the degree of bone formation and resorption. The bone biopsy is taken from the anterior iliac crest where a high turnover rate reflects the general metabolic state. A more convenient site is a rib from which a 1-cm biopsy specimen can be taken.

Before the findings can be properly interpreted, the normal values of bone formation and resorption at various ages must be known. In the very young, bone turnover, both formation and resorption, is very active. Between 20 and 40 years of age, the levels of formation and resorption are low but constant. In older subjects, resorption increases whereas formation remains at a level comparable to that in young adults. This eventuates in depletion of bone mass (osteoporosis). Excessive resorption ceases and appears to balance formation in those over 80 years of age.

MICRORADIOGRAPHIC MEASUREMENTS

Fundamentally, the formation and resorption of bone tissue take place only on the surface of bone tissue. The microradiograph is produced by passing soft x-rays through a 100μ section of undecalcified bone held against a glass slide coated with a high-resolution emulsion. The x-rays are differentially absorbed by the mineralized tissue. Darkening of the microradiograph is inversely proportional to the mineral content of the bone tissue. When the microradiograph is viewed through the light microscope, surfaces actively forming or resorbing bone are recognized by characteristic morphological features (Fig. 6-16).

A haversian system or osteon appears distinct from interstitial bone and neighboring osteons by differences in mineral density, as well as by the concentric arrangement of osteocytes in their lacunae. Osteons of low density are those in which new bone tissue is being laid down, with the lamellae of low density (appear dark gray) running parallel to a smooth surface. If such a section were stained, this area surface would be lined

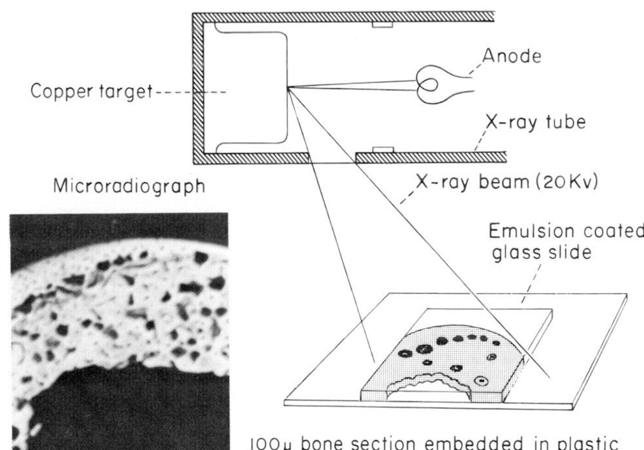

FIG. 6-16. Technique of producing microradiograph. (Jowsey J: In Zipkin I (ed): Biological Mineralization. New York, John Wiley & Sons, 1970)

with osteoblasts and osteoid tissue[116] and would concentrate isotopes of radiocalcium and radiostrontium after an *in vivo* injection, because such radioisotopes are retained during mineralization of newly formed matrix. Other osteons appear less dark because they contain more mineral; when fully mineralized, they appear almost white. Characteristically, mineralization of the osteon begins about the central canal and proceeds toward the cement line of the osteon. The first indication that bone formation has ceased and increasing mineralization is proceeding is a line of increased density (white) immediately adjacent to the vascular space. This line widens and eventually reaches the cement line as increased mineral density develops throughout the osteon.

When resorption of bone tissue is occurring, both in cortical and trabecular bone, the surfaces are rough and uneven, and the bone tissue has a high density (appears white) (Fig. 6-17). On a stained section, the surface would be lined with osteoclasts, and on autoradiographs from animals given an *in vivo* injection of yttrium 91, the isotope is concentrated on this surface, because ^{91}Y is taken up in areas of resorption. When the resorbing surfaces become inactive, a line of increased density appears on the edge of the vascular space and becomes smooth.

Measurements of the balance between formation and resorption give an indication of bone turnover that may define the disease process. The lengths of the bone surfaces undergoing formation or resorption are measured and expressed as a percentage of the total surface in the same area.

OSTEOID TISSUE

An osteoid seam is unmineralized collagen tissue of bone.[115,116] Healthy skeletons at all ages contain osteoid

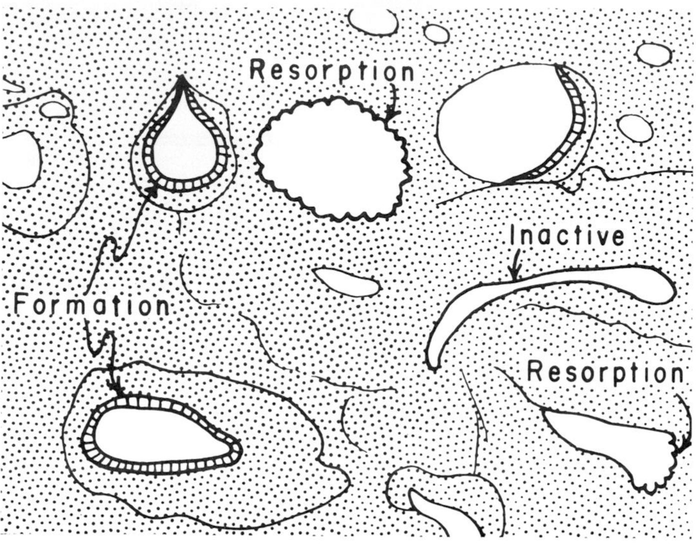

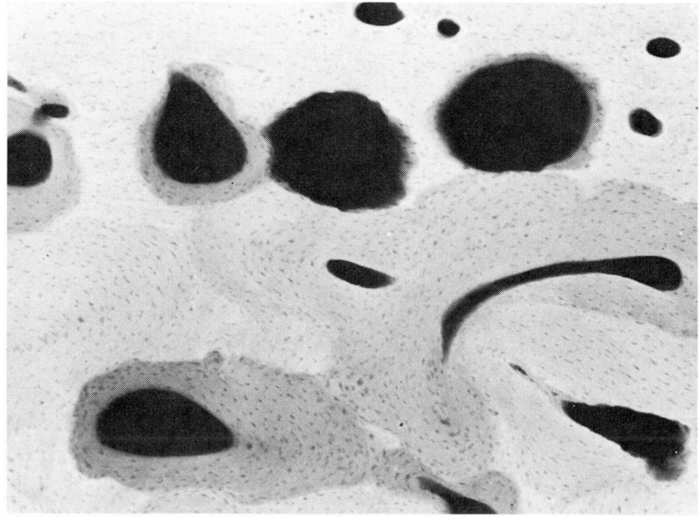

FIG. 6-17. Typical microradiograph of bone. The bone-forming areas are of low mineral density and appear dark on the microradiograph. Their smooth surfaces are not bounded by sclerotic line. Bone-resorbing surfaces are irregularly crenated. (Jowsey J: Quantitative microradiography: A new approach in the evaluation of metabolic bone disease. Am J Med 40:485, 1966)

seams reflecting newly formed matrix but are difficult to visualize in routinely stained sections. Normally, these osteoid seams are 5μ to 30μ thick and are usually applied on preexisting bone surfaces.

The initial phase of bone formation involves the laying down of osteoid tissue on bone surfaces. After a latent period of about 2 weeks, mineralization begins on the interior surface, and during this process, any given bone-forming surface is bounded by a border of osteoid. When an undecalcified, unstained, or Paragon-stained bone section is viewed microscopically, osteoid tissue is easily recognized. The width is measured with the calibrated eyepiece, and values exceeding 20μ, particularly in older subjects, are considered abnormal.

Measurements of osteoid thickness can be made from a specimen taken under local anesthesia from the outer cortex of a rib. In certain diseases (*e.g.*, those associated with vitamin D deficiency or a lowered C × P product), malabsorption, or renal osteodystrophy, mineralization of osteoid is impaired, and thick osteoid seams characteristic of osteomalacia extend over many bone surfaces (Fig. 6-18).

RADIOISOTOPE STUDIES

Bone Resorption

Radioactive yttrium is deposited in high concentration in bone tissue undergoing resorption.[120] It is also taken up throughout the remainder of the mineralized tissue but in a lower concentration, thus being easily distinguishable from the high concentrations at the resorbing surfaces. ^{91}Y is therefore used to demonstrate resorption of bone.

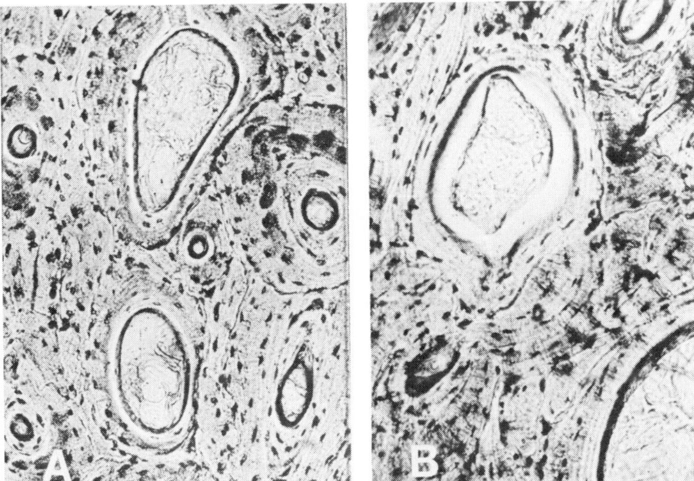

FIG. 6-18. Osteoid borders at the calcification front: (*A*) In health, narrow osteoid borders; (*B*) in osteomalacia, wide osteoid borders. Appearance of undecalcified sections. (Riggs BL et al: Special procedures for assessing metabolic bone disease. Med Clin North Am 54:1061, 1970)

Bone Formation

Accretion of radiocalcium has been equated with bone formation. However, some portion of the retained radioisotope is concerned not with bone formation but with long-term ion exchange.

In osteoporosis, the question of decreased bone formation has not been resolved, with the results of investigation varying from normal accretion to reduced accretion.[113,118] Complicating interpretation, a reduced accretion rate may be related to an already reduced bone tissue mass in this condition.

URINARY HYDROXYPROLINE

Hydroxyproline (Hypro) is a constituent almost exclusively of collagen and is synthesized by hydroxylation of large polypeptides intracellularly as a terminal step in the formation of collagen before the collagen is extruded from the cell. Considerable amounts of Hypro, mostly in a peptide-bound form, are excreted in the urine in normal human subjects throughout life and reflect degradation of collagen of all tissues, including bone collagen.[124] Such degradation of collagen involves both newly synthesized collagen and mature collagen.

During the active growth period, urinary Hypro excretion is high, reflecting increase in the rates of synthesis and of degradation of all forms of collagen. In older human subjecs, both of these rates are considerably slower, even though the total amount of body collagen is much greater, so that excretion of Hypro peptides is one third to one tenth the values seen in children (Table 6-2).

Measurement of urinary Hypro is done while gelatin-containing foods are excluded from the diet. Although changes in Hypro excretion are not specific for any given

TABLE 6-2 Urinary Excretion of Hypro in Normal Children and Adult Subjects

	Jasin and Associates			**Kivirikko and Laitinen Laitinen and Associates**		
		HYPRO EXCRETION			HYPRO EXCRETION	
Age	NO. SUBJECTS	mg/24 hr*	mg/24 Hr/M²†	NO. SUBJECTS	mg/24 hr*	mg/24 hr/M²†
0–12 months	9	21–52	53–141	24	19–56	40–191
1–5 years	} 23	24–102	43–85	22	20–65	} 37–95
6–10 years				21	35–99	
11–14 years	12	68–169	55–112	25	63–180	40–113
18–21 years	} 12	15–55	9–31	22	20–55	13–28
>21 years				48	15–43	9–24

* Range.
† Limits for mean ± 2 sd.
(Data from Jasin HE, et al: J Clin Invest 41:1928, 1965; Kivirikko KI, Laitinen O: Ann Paediat Fenn 11:148, 1965; and Laitinen O, et al: Acta Med Scand 179:275, 1966)

disease, such assays are useful for determining the effects of any condition on collagen metabolism. It may provide, in certain conditions, an index of disease activity and response to treatment. Hypro excretion is increased in any disorder involving extensive lysis of bone, such as:

Hyperparathyroidism. PTH causes increased degradation of collagen and markedly increases Hypro excretion.

Paget's disease. During the phase of very active bone turnover, extremely high levels of urinary Hypro excretion result.

Malabsorption syndrome. In normal subjects, after its ingestion, gelatin undergoes hydrolysis to dialyzable peptides, and increased amounts of Hypro appear in the urine. Impaired hydrolysis of gelatin occurs in pancreatic insufficiency and adult celiac disease, and the urinary Hypro fails to rise after intake of gelatin.

In a calcium–phosphate–vitamin D metabolic defect, a compensatory hyperparathyroidism develops to restore the serum ion levels. PTH causes increased degradation of collagen, and increased levels of urinary Hypro ensue.

HISTOCHEMICAL STUDIES

To study the distribution and density of minerals in bone, fresh, undecalcified, thin bone sections must first be prepared. Special staining techniques then form a pattern of stain that reveals the features of mineralization. Theoretically, the ionized sites of undecalcified bone unite with ions of the dye or other staining agent to form a visible precipitate. For instance, basic fuchsin 1% in 30% alcohol stains the bone at 48 hours at 22°C.[115] Sections should be approximately 75μ thick. At the end of the staining period, the specimen is washed in tap water or

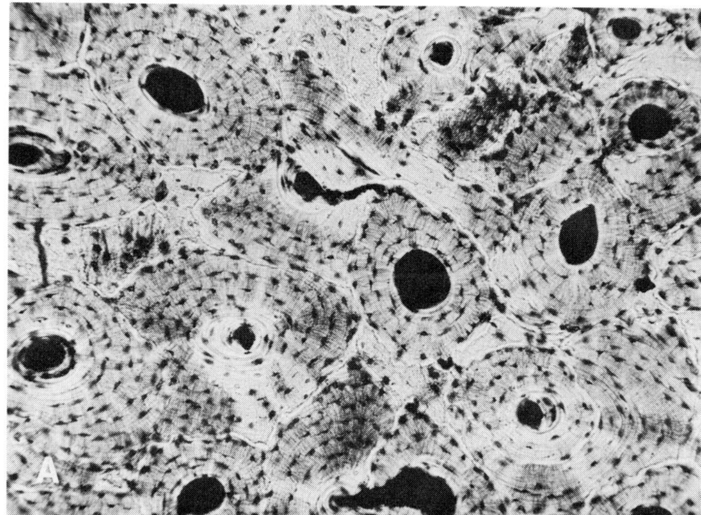

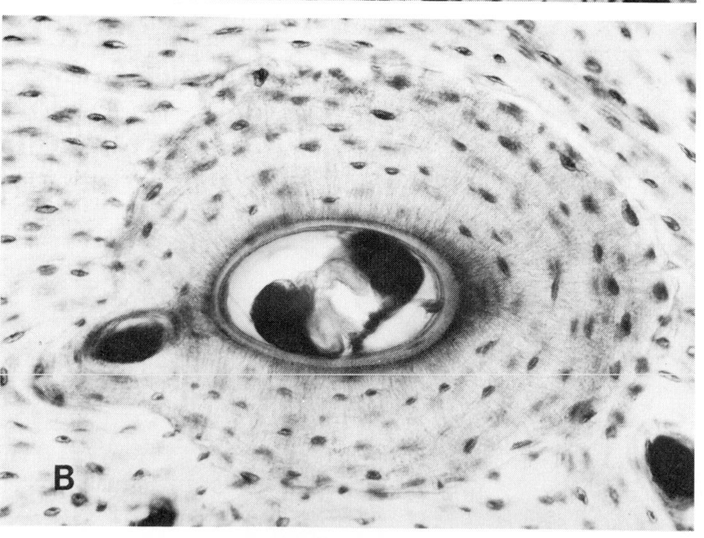

FIG. 6-19. Undecalcified sections of bone stained with basic fuchsin (normal adult appearance). The circumferential lamellae of the haversian system and the interstitial lamellae fail to stain, indicating that this is a completely mineralized mature matrix. The dye occupies the haversian canals, the canaliculi, and the lacunae. (*A*) Low-power section; (*B*) high-power section. (Courtesy of H.M. Frost)

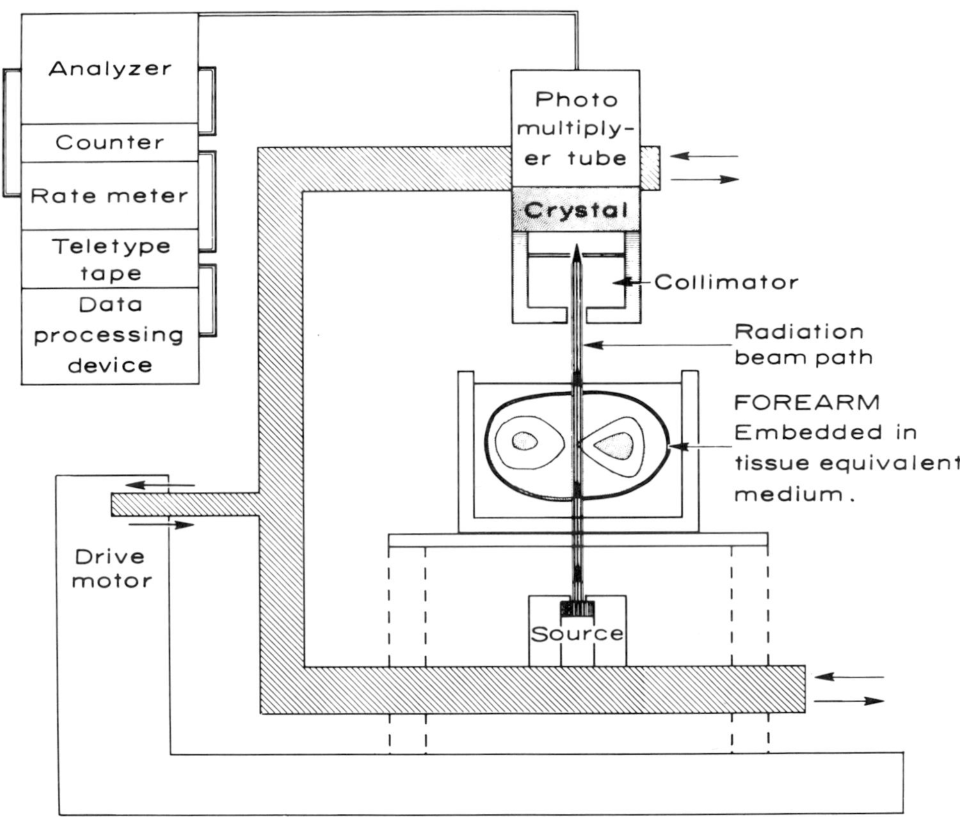

FIG. 6-20. Apparatus for bone-density determination. Photon beam is moved across forearm at 4.5 cm/min, printing a count every 1.5 seconds. Data can be processed by planimetry or computer. Amount of bone material in path of beam is related to transmission count rates according to equation:

$$m_B = \rho_B \ln(\overset{*}{I_o}/I) \Big/ (\mu_B \rho_B - \mu_S \rho_S)$$

where ρ_B and ρ_S are the density of compact bone and soft tissue respectively. $\overset{*}{I_o}$ is the transmission counts through constant thickness of soft tissue, and I, through soft tissue and bone; μ_B and μ_S are the mass attenuation coefficients of compact bone and soft tissue. Beam is scanned across bone, and m_B can be integrated to give mass of bone mineral per unit length of bone in units of g/cm. (Sinaki M, Opitz JL, Wahner HW: Bone mineral content: Relationship to muscle strength in normal subjects. Arch Phys Med Rehab 55:508, 1974)

distilled water that has been made alkaline by the addition of a small quantity of ammonia. While still immersed in this liquid, the top and bottom surface of the section should be removed by grinding.[114] The section is then washed in 0.2% detergent solution, dried in air, and mounted in an ordinary synthetic resin mountant.

In normal, fully mineralized bone, the dye cannot diffuse through the matrix and the fuchsin will be found in a thin layer on the walls of spaces (haversian canals, lacunae, canaliculae) in the bone. There is no permeation of the fuchsin into the mineralized substance of normal bone (Fig. 6-19).

In various stages of deficient mineralization, or during the early phases of mineralization of new bone, there is diffuse permeability of the affected bone. The intensity and extent of staining is directly proportional to the lack of mineral deposition. Therefore, fuchsin is an excellent indicator of the degree of mineralization of bone.

NONINVASIVE IN VIVO MEASUREMENT OF BONE DENSITY

The count derived from passing a monochromatic photon beam from a ^{125}I-isotope source through a specific area of bone is measured directly with a collimated scintillation counter and reflects the amount of bone mineral in the path of the beam (Figs. 6-20 and 6-21)[127]. The extremity

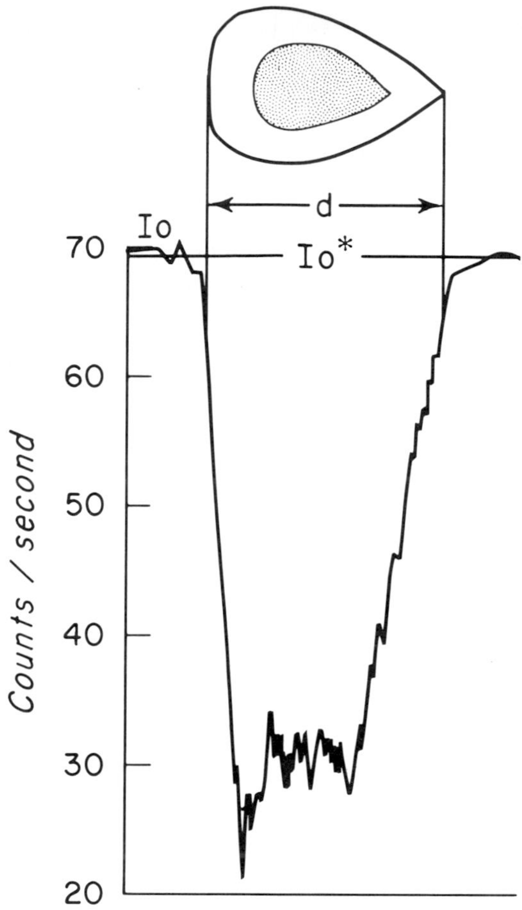

FIG. 6-21. Derivation of bone density from scan. Logarithm of counts/1.5 sec. is plotted on graph paper by recorder, and area of logarithmic plot is proportional to bone mineral content in scanning path. This can be expressed in computer units or converted to bone mineral (g/cm) by an experimentally obtained factor. Calculation of bone mineral content and bone diameter can be performed graphically with a planimeter or by a programmed small desk computer. An automatic readout device relieves the investigator of doing any calculation. (Sinaki M, Opitz JL, Wahner HW: Bone mineral content: Relationship to muscle strength in normal subjects. Arch Phys Med Rehab 55:508, 1974)

is wrapped in a tissue-equivalent material of constant thickness and is scanned by driving the rigidly linked isotope source and detector across it at right angles to its axis. The amount of bone mineral in the path of the photon beam is related to the integrated transmission count rates for this scanning path. Bone mineral per unit length of bone (g/cm) is obtained by calibration procedures and calculations.

The method may be helpful in monitoring decrease or increase of bone mass in disease or in determining response to treatment. The distal radius is generally used for measurement.

TETRACYCLINE DEPOSITION

Tetracycline administered *in vivo* becomes fixed in new-forming mineralizing bone and exhibits a characteristic fluorescence when viewed by ultraviolet light.[117,122] The tetracycline-labeled bone fluoresces a strong yellow to orange color on a faint magenta background, and mature bone fluoresces a faint blue. After intake of tetracycline, serum levels remain sufficiently elevated for adequate uptake by new-forming bone. Under fluorescent microscopy, narrow bands of fluorescence are observed where bone was actively being formed while exposed to the recently administered tetracycline. When two doses of tetracycline are given a number of days apart, two bands of fluorescence will be separated by an interval of unlabeled new bone that has formed during the period between doses. In this manner new bone formation can be accurately measured and normally takes place at a rate of 1μ/day (Fig. 6-22).

By using two types of tetracyclines (*e.g.*, giving oxytetracycline initially and, several days later, dimethyl-chlortetracycline), each type produces its distinctive fluorescent colors, which are easily identified, thus simplifying measurement of new-formed bone. The yellowish green fluorescence of oxytetracycline and the bright yellow fluorescence of dimethyl-chlortetracycline form distinctive layers separated by unlabeled new bone.[113]

Within 30 minutes after intraperitoneal injection in the experimental animal, a diffuse yellow fluorescence develops throughout the undecalcified bone. After 24 hours, the diffuse fluorescence disappears but remains permanently localized as bright yellow bands at sites of very active new bone formation. In the diaphysis, bands 5μ to 10μ in thickness form at the subperiosteal and endosteal surfaces and in cross section appear as concentric rings.

At the metaphysis in the immature rapidly growing animal, a wide band 30μ to 80μ thick develops immediately adjacent to the growth plate and within days moves away from the growth plate as additional new bone forms. The fluorescent band becomes less distinct and finally disappears as this bone is resorbed during the remodeling process. During the time interval between the administration of the antibiotic and the examination of the bone section, the distance the fluorescent band lies beyond the growth plate represents the growth rate of that epiphyseal plate.

Tetracycline labeling is a method of determining the effect of various factors on bone growth and accurately measuring it. For example, when tetracycline labeling is applied to bone transplants within a few days after fresh autogenous cancellous bone has been transplanted (before ingrowth of vascularity is possible), intense uptake of tetracycline is demonstrable, suggesting continuing viability of bone-producing cells. When the autogenous cancellous bone is exposed to air or immersed in normal saline solution, even for short periods of time before transplantation, uptake is markedly reduced. Moreover, homogenous bone grafts show no tetracycline fluores-

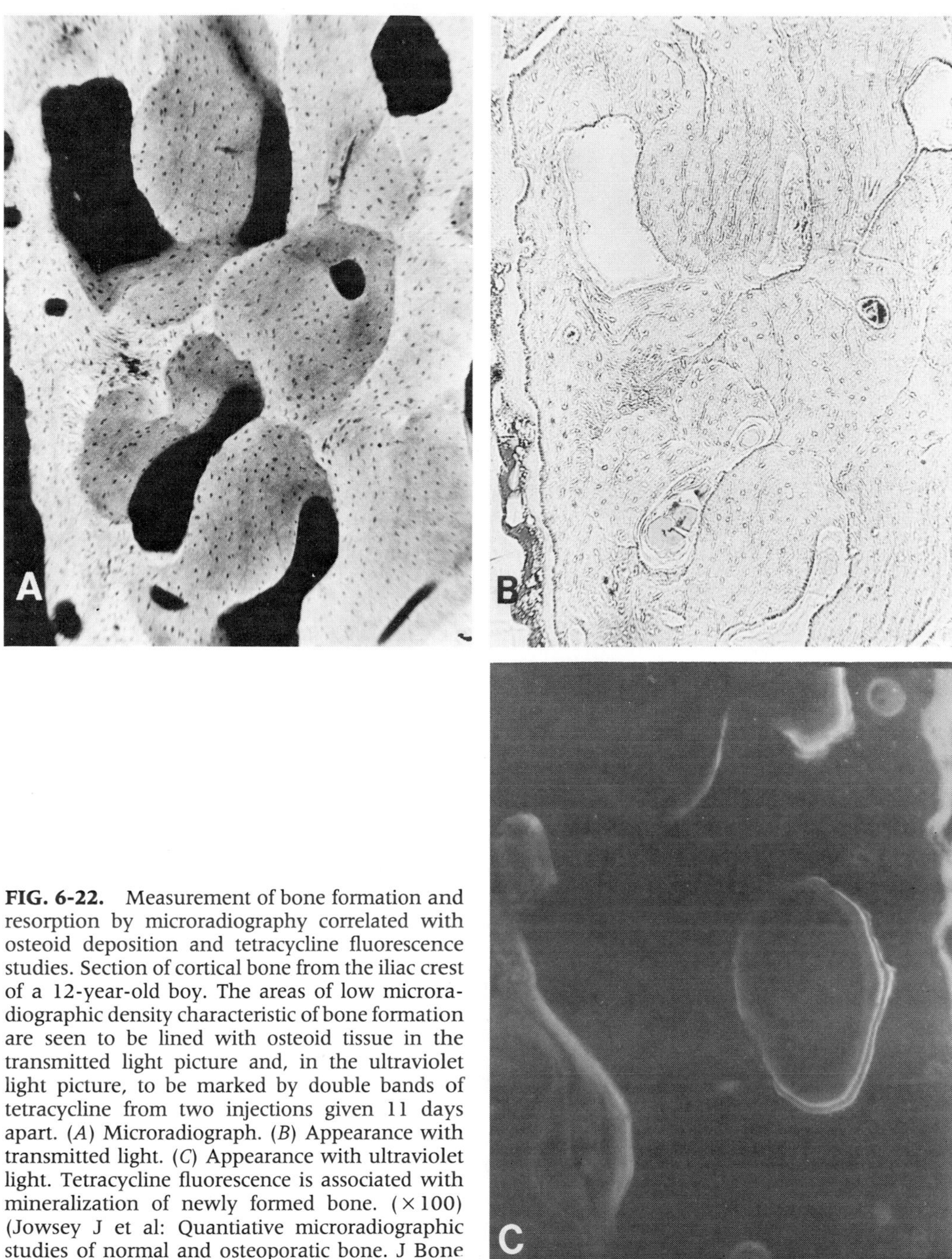

FIG. 6-22. Measurement of bone formation and resorption by microradiography correlated with osteoid deposition and tetracycline fluorescence studies. Section of cortical bone from the iliac crest of a 12-year-old boy. The areas of low microradiographic density characteristic of bone formation are seen to be lined with osteoid tissue in the transmitted light picture and, in the ultraviolet light picture, to be marked by double bands of tetracycline from two injections given 11 days apart. (*A*) Microradiograph. (*B*) Appearance with transmitted light. (*C*) Appearance with ultraviolet light. Tetracycline fluorescence is associated with mineralization of newly formed bone. (×100) (Jowsey J et al: Quantiative microradiographic studies of normal and osteoporatic bone. J Bone Joint Surg 47A:785, 1965)

cence, indicating that autogenous bone is superior for transplantation, especially when done immediately.[125]

TRIPLE FLUOROCHROME LABELING[123]

Bone remodeling can be studied by using various fluorochromes, which produce easily identified different colors. Tetracycline produces a yellow color; hematoporphyrin, a bright red color; and a purified form of calcein, identified as 2,4-*bis* [N, N'-di-(carbomethyl) aminomethyl] fluorescein (DCAF), a green color. Alizarin has been used but is not recommended because it is very toxic to bone formation. It can be used in experimental animals but only as a last label before the animal is sacrificed.

Section III

Blood Supply of Long Bones

THE MATURE LONG BONE

Long bones have three sources of blood supply: (1) vessels at the ends of the bone, the epiphyseal and metaphyseal; (2) usually one or two main arteries, the proper nutrient arteries, entering the diaphysis; and (3) the periosteal vessels (Fig. 6-23).

After entering the diaphysis, the nutrient artery divides into a major ascending and a descending branch; each branch sends lateral (radial) oriented arteriolar branches, most of which lead directly to the cortex while others go to sinusoids within the marrow (Fig. 6-24). The terminal vessels of the main ascending and descending branches contribute to the blood supply at the ends of the long bone, where they anastomose with the epiphyseal and metaphyseal vessels.

The cortical arterioles originating from the main medullary nutrient artery are directed radially and enter the cortex singly or in bundles of two to six arterioles. Within the cortex they give rise to branches, some extending longitudinally along the axis of the bone, while others proceed radially; these branches ultimately form capillaries within the haversian systems (Fig. 6-25). Some arterioles traverse the entire cortex to reach and anastomose with the periosteal arteriolar network (Fig. 6-26). Within the marrow, some arterioles are short and profusely branched to supply the capillaries for the marrow.[143]

The haversian canals usually contain two thin-walled vessels, one smaller than the other, suggesting that one carries arterial blood while the other is a vein and that blood flows in both directions. The walls of these small vessels are composed of a single layer of endothelial cells, but rarely one vessel appears to display the histologic characteristics of an arteriole.[151]

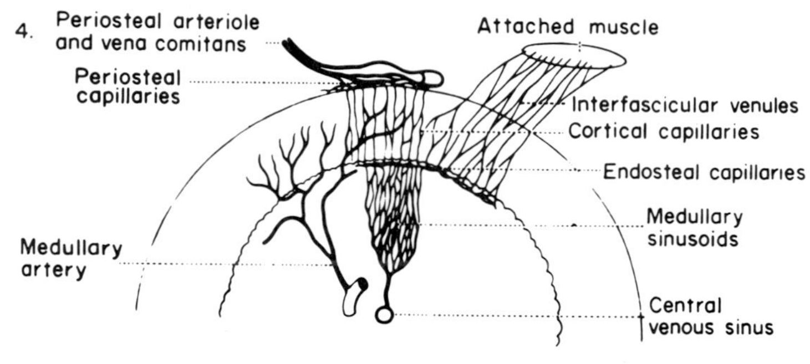

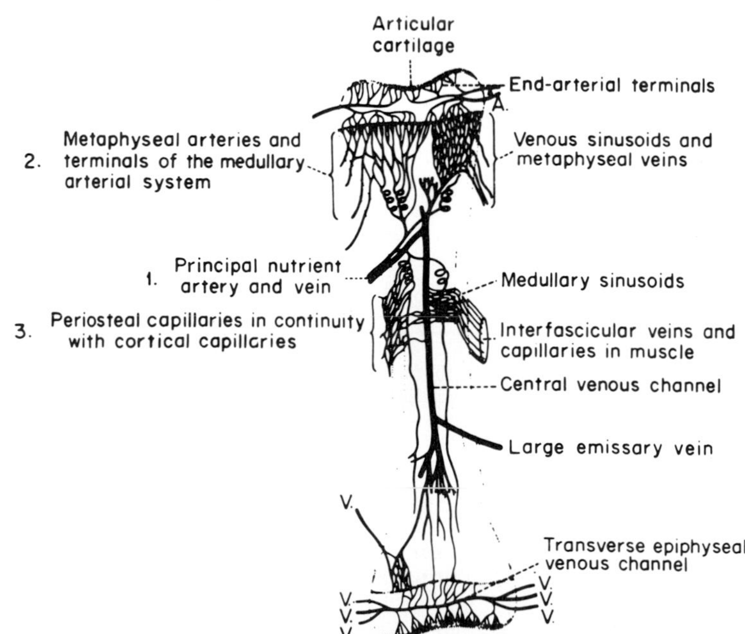

FIG. 6-23. Blood supply of a long bone. Three basic blood supplies are shown: (*1*) nutrient; (*2*) metaphyseal, which anastomoses with epiphyseal after epiphyseal closure; and (*3*) periosteal. The numerous metaphyseal arteries arise from periarticular networks and anastomose with terminal branches of ascending and descending medullary arteries. Periosteal capillaries emerge from the cortex (efferent blood flow). (*4*) A periosteal arteriole feeds capillaries that provide afferent blood flow to a limited outer layer of cortex. (Rhinelander FW: Circulation of bone. In Bourne GH (ed): Biochemistry and Physiology of Bone, 2nd ed, p 2. New York, Academic Press, 1972)

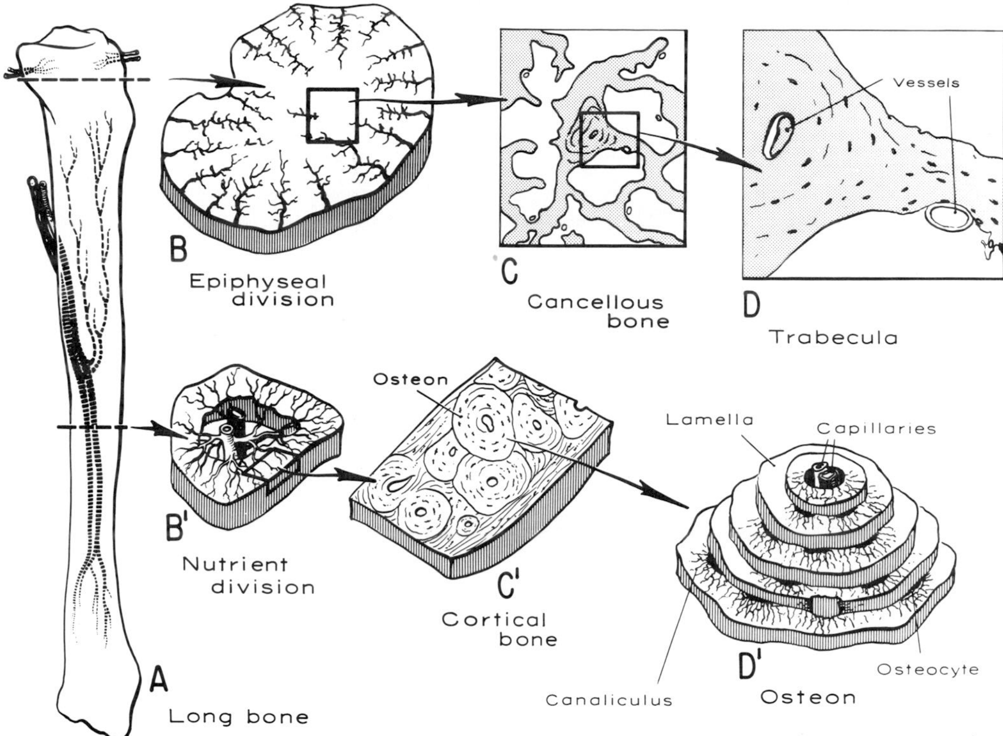

FIG. 6-24. Distribution of nutrient blood supply to the diaphyseal and epiphyseal regions of a long bone. (*A*) Basic pattern of nutrient circulation to a long bone (human tibia). (*B*) Pattern of circulation in epiphyseal-metaphyseal region. Arteries perforate thin cortical shell to enter cancellous bone. (*C*) Structure of cancellous bone. (*D*) A trabecula of bone. Capillaries abut against thin trabecula. In thicker trabecula, an osteon can be seen. (*B'*) Cross section of mid diaphysis. Here there is a single nutrient artery and vein. Lateral branches arise from the artery to supply the cortical bone. (*C'*) Cortical bone. Osteons and interstitial bone between osteons. (*D'*) Diagrammatic concept of a single osteon. Canaliculi of the osteocytes are canals in which the processes of the osteocytes are located. It is by way of these canaliculi that nutrition if derived from the vessels in the haversian canal. (Kelly PJ, Peterson LFA: The blood supply of bone. Heart Bull 12:96, 1963)

THE NUTRIENT MEDULLARY SYSTEM

All long bones have one or more nutrient arteries that enter through a nutrient foramen without branching within the foramen and that are accompanied by several thin-walled veins and a myelinated nerve. In the humerus, a single artery, rarely a double one, enters the humerus anteromedially; usually this occurs at the junction of the middle and lower thirds, but the point of entry is variable.[131,141] The femoral shaft usually has two nutrient arteries arising from perforating branches of the profunda femoris. The area of entry is the linea aspera.[140] In the radius and ulna, the nutrient foramen is located proximally and directed toward the elbow.[149] In the tibia, the nutrient artery arises from the posterior tibial artery and penetrates the posterolateral cortex at a point just below the oblique line of the tibia, the site of origin of the soleus.[145]

The nutrient artery and its ascending and descending medullary branches form the important sources of blood supply to at least the inner two thirds or more of the cortex. Their radially oriented branches supply capillaries to the marrow and provide capillaries within the cortical bone. Approximately 30% of their blood flow goes to the marrow capillary beds and about 70% supplies the cortical capillary beds.[143] The marrow and cortical capillary beds are independent of one another, and the effluent blood flow of each drains separately. The arterioles that enter the marrow sinusoids originate from lateral branches of the nutrient artery, while other arterioles penetrate the endosteal surface of the cortex.

The diaphyseal cortical bone is said by some observers be totally supplied by the transversely directed vessels of the medullary nutrient artery;[144] others describe a divided supply, with the nutrient artery branches supplying the inner one half to two thirds of the cor tex and the remainder being supplied by the periosteal vessels.[139]

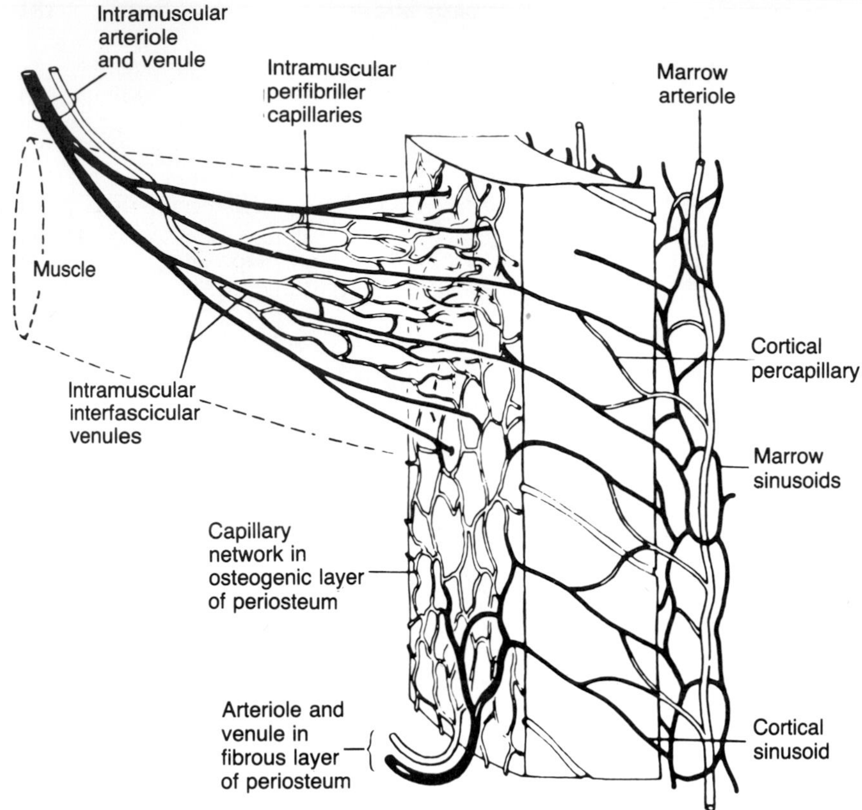

FIG. 6-25. Cross section of a longitudinal section of the cortex of a long bone. The haversian systems (osteons) run longitudinally. Interstitial lamellae fill the intervals between the haversian systems, and at the periphery of the long bone they form the circumferential lamellae. Volkmann's canals are connecting channels that provide conduits for vessels and unmyelinated nerve fibers between periosteum, haversian systems, and marrow. (Redrawn from Ham AW: Histology. Philadelphia, JB Lippincott, 1974)

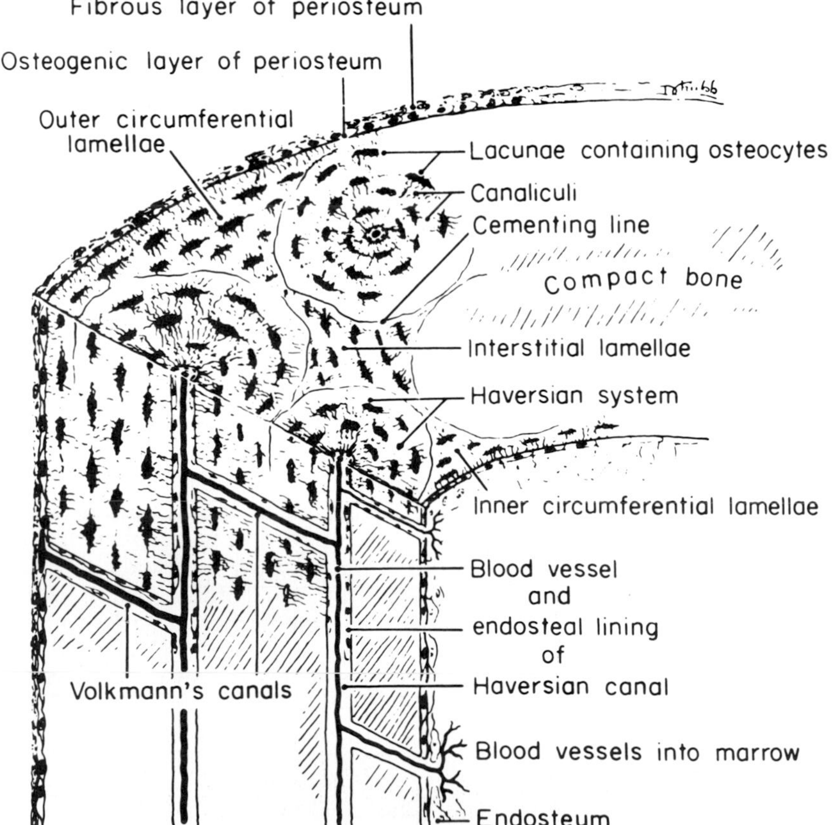

Fig. 6-26. Brookes concept of microcirculation in cortical bone. The direction of flow through normal cortex is centrifugal, with perfusion of intravital dyes passing slowly from medulla to periosteum. Periosteal arteries play only a minor part in the nutrition of mature cortex. The capillary network along the external surface of the cortex is continuous with the intracortical capillaries and, externally, with the general periosteal circulation. A limited number of large caliber arteries of the periosteum, known as the accessory nutrient arterioles, enter the cortex only where surrounding muscles gain strong tendinous attachments to the bone (*e.g.*, linea aspera) and supply only the extreme outer portion of the cortex. (Brookes M: The blood supply of bone. In Clark JMP (ed): Modern Trends in Orthopaedics, Vol 4, Science of Fractures, p 91. Washington, DC, Butterworth, 1964)

VENOUS DRAINAGE

Long bones possess a large central venous sinus.[134,135] It receives transverse venous channels that transport effluent blood from marrow capillary beds (sinusoids); each channel accompanies a transversely directed nutrient arteriole that enters the endosteal aspect of the cortex. These transverse venous channels may either drain directly into the central venous sinus or drain into a larger venous tributary and then into the central venous sinus.[130] The central venous sinus then emerges from the diaphysis through the nutrient canal as the nutrient vein (Fig. 6-27).

The major venous drainage from a long bone is into the periosteal venous complex, with only 5% to 10% of the effluent blood leaving by way of the nutrient vein.[132] Much of the venous drainage leaves the bone at the bone ends, especially through the metaphyseal vessels, which can be considered as part of the periosteal venous system. Emerging from the diaphyseal cortex at the periosteal surface is a profusion of endothelial tubes that have been interpreted as venules.[145] Despite the current belief that little of cortical blood flow drains back into the endosteal veins, an *in vivo* study indicates that the capillaries, after leaving the haversian canals, may swing back into the marrow and enter the marrow sinusoids.[128]

BLOOD FLOW

The direction and extent of blood flow within the diaphyseal cortex remains controversial. One theory favors centrifugal flow, with the blood entering the endosteal aspect from the medullary nutrient system and flowing out through the periosteal surface.[129,130,146] In the event that the medullary nutrient system is interrupted, the periosteal system provides a reserve supply and blood flow becomes centripetal.[145] This concept appears to be substantiated by microangiographic studies.[143]

The role of periosteal vessels has not been clearly defined. The periosteal system originates mainly from the surrounding muscles, and it appears to provide a blood supply to the outer one third to one half of the cortex.[139,152] However, despite anastomotic connections between periosteal vessels and cortical vessels originating from medullary vessels, many investigators deny that the periosteal system provides more than a minimal blood supply to the cortex[129,130] At the outer aspect of the cortex, many thin-walled vessels within the haversian canals are observed to be in continuity with arterioles within the periosteum. This forms the basis for an assumption that this forms an important auxiliary source of blood flow to the entire cortex when the intramedullary nutrient blood supply is interrupted (*e.g.*, by severely displaced fractures).[142]

The ends of long bones are supplied by vessels that enter the epiphysis and metaphysis through small foramina at the periphery. After entering the bone, these arterioles branch into arterial arcades, forming a dense interlocking network, the vessels becoming progressively smaller in caliber as they approach the subchondral zone, where they terminate as small capillary loops.[138] The epiphyseal-metaphyseal arterioles anastomose with terminal twigs of the medullary nutrient arteries and contribute 20% to 40% of the total blood supply of the entire bone.[151]

VARIATIONS IN CORTICAL BLOOD FLOW

There are great variations in blood flow through normal cortical channels mediated through unknown control mechanisms. In a normal extremity, not all blood vessels are functioning at the same time. Blood transport occurs through a limited number of vessels, the others being considered "in a resting state." Under certain conditions (*e.g.*, fracture of the opposite extremity), a greater number of blood vessels become actively functional and demonstrable by microangiographic methods.[146]

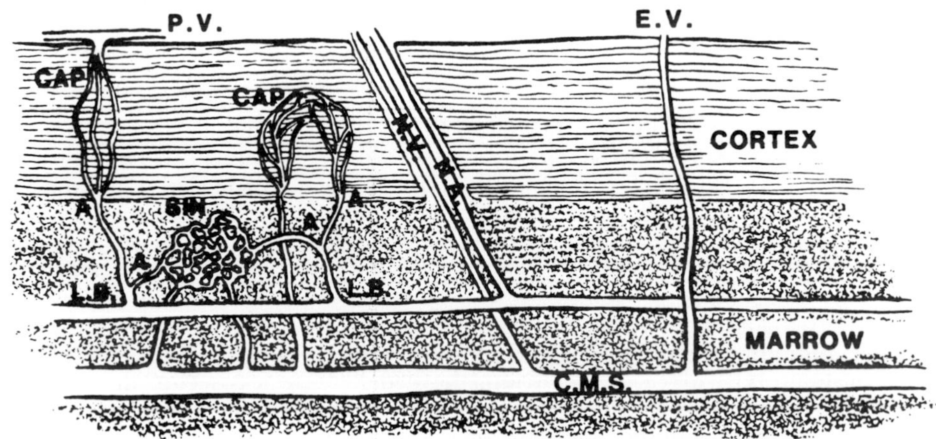

FIG. 6-27. Circulation in the tibial diaphysis. (*N.A.*, nutrient artery; *N.V.*, nutrient vein; *C.M.S.*, central medullary sinus; *A*, arterioles; *SIN*, medullary sinusoids; *L.B.*, lateral branches of nutrient artery; *CAP*, haversian capillaries; *P.V.*, periosteal vein; *E.V.*, emissary vein) (Lopez-Curto JA, Bassingthwaighte JB, Kelly PJ: Anatomy of the microvasculature of the tibial diaphysis of the adult dog. J Bone Joint Surg 62A:1362, 1980)

SELECTIVE IMPAIRMENT OF DIAPHYSEAL BLOOD SUPPLY

If the circulation in bone marrow and periosteum is interrupted, an increase in metaphyseal blood flow occurs.[150] If circulation through nutrient artery and metaphyseal vessels is interrupted, proliferation of the periosteal vessels and increased periosteal blood flow takes place and is often accompanied by periosteal new bone formation.

When blood flow through the nutrient artery is interrupted, approximately two thirds of the cortex becomes ischemic and necrotic, but the outer third remains viable (see Fig. 6-28). On the other hand, when periosteum is stripped and left detached from the cortex, and the nutrient artery is preserved, only the outer third of the cortex becomes ischemic and necrotic. This is often followed by the development of periosteal new bone, which encircles the shaft. When the nutrient artery is suppressed (*e.g.*, by intramedullary nailing), compensatory periosteal vascular proliferation appears to preserve the viability of the cortex to a great extent. When the medullary nutrient blood supply is interrupted and the periosteum is stripped from the bone, the entire thickness of the cortex becomes necrotic.[136]

REVERSAL OF VENOUS BLOOD FLOW

Under certain conditions, blood flow through large peripheral veins of an extremity can be reversed and detoured into alternate routes within the medullary cavity of long bones.[133] When there is interference with venous return through main veins of an extremity, the intramedullary pressures within the regional long bones are increased. In the presence of a significant acute venous obstruction, reversal of blood flow of the larger veins entering the distal femoral metaphysis can be demonstrated, indicating that collateral venous return is taking place through medullary venous channels. This phenomenon may be responsible for the deep, dull bone pain and bone tenderness that is often associated with acute or chronic thrombophlebitis and explains why elevation of the part relieves the pain.

SUMMARY OF CONCEPTS OF NORMAL CIRCULATION IN LONG BONE

The currently accepted concepts regarding the normal blood supply of mature mammalian tubular bone may be summarized as follows:[148]

The nutrient arterial system consists of branches of the nutrient artery and the metaphyseal arteries anastomosing with each other to form the medullary blood supply. This system is largely fed by arterial trunks derived from the large main regional arteries of the systemic circulation.

The periosteal arterial system is derived from and is a component of the larger vascular system that also supplies the muscles that surround the tubular bones.

At least the inner two thirds to three fourths of the compactum are primarily supplied by ramifications of the nutrient (medullary) system.

According to some investigators, the outer third or one fourth of the compactum is primarily supplied by periosteal arterioles. Others believe that the periosteal blood supply is limited to localized areas of compactum that are related to fascial attachments (*e.g.*, the linea aspera of the femur).

The blood flow through the compactum is normally centrifugal, from medulla to periosteum.

Under the abnormal condition of blockade of the nutrient system, the periosteal system is able to reverse the usual centrifugal flow and convey blood supply to the compactum. Those who believe that the periosteal arteries supply a very limited thickness of cortex suggest that these arterioles become more active when the medullary flow is blocked; there is no major reversal in the direction of blood flow.

The most peripheral capillary connections between the nutrient afferent and the periosteal efferent vessels lie in the deep layer of periosteum, in intimate association with the external cortical surface, where the periosteum is attached only loosely to most of the diaphyseal surface.

Larger vascular elements of the periosteal system (arterioles and venules) penetrate the cortical surface in the limited areas where fascial structures are firmly attached to the diaphysis.

EFFECTS OF DIAPHYSEAL FRACTURE

A simple, closed, uncomplicated division of the diaphysis of a long bone, whether the result of fracture or osteotomy, undergoes three types of repair, involving the formation of osseous callus, which, in turn, is dependent on an adequate blood supply.[148] A fracture or osteotomy, when the opposed ends of cortex are not in absolute contact, heals by means of medullary bridging callus, periosteal bridging callus, and intercortical uniting callus.

Medullary bridging callus is the first to effect osseous union. When immobilizaiton is adequate, medullary callus can produce osseous union without the intermediate step of production of cartilage.

Periosteal bridging callus is always interrupted at first by a zone of fibrocartilage that extends outward from, and is directly opposite to, the fracture or osteotomy site. The amount of periosteal callus does not depend on the size of the surrounding hematoma, but it is dependent on the degree of stabilization of the bone fragments. The less secure the fixation, the larger is the mass of reinforcing external callus (*e.g.*, when plate fixation is insecure). Contrariwise, with the greater rigidity afforded by a compression plate, all of the required bridging callus develops within the medulla and little or no periosteal callus need form.

Intercortical uniting callus develops to fill the gap between the bone ends. It grows in from both the medullary and periosteal surfaces, and the amount depends on the size of the gap. When there is no gap, as in compression fixation, little or no intercortical callus forms. Newly formed osteons extend from each bone end and join to bridge the gap and restore bone continuity.

When the diaphysis of a long bone is fractured, especially when the fragments are widely displaced, an area of cortex on either side of the fracture becomes devascularized and necrotic. The extent of the necrotic zone is highly variable, depending on the cause and the degree of interruption of the blood supply. An oscillating saw used to create an osteotomy will produce an area of thermal necrosis of 0.7 mm to 2 mm in depth. A severely displaced fracture will disrupt the main nutrient arteries and produce a wide area of necrosis. Consequently, the repair of a fracture must of necessity be accompanied by the repair processes to restore viable bone (revascularization of haversian canals, bone resorption and widening of haversian canals producing the roentgenographic finding of osteoporosis, and bone deposition).

In the early repair of fractures, bridging periosteal external callus forms early, stabilizing the fracture. An extraosseous arterial supply from the surrounding soft tissues furnishes the blood for external callus formation. Microangiography at this stage reveals multiple small-caliber vessels arranged perpendicular to the external surface of the bone, an angiographic hallmark of early periosteal callus formation. The callus bridging over from both fragments attempts to meet but is always interrupted by a zone of fibrocartilage that is an outward extension from the fracture defect; it does not provide the first osseous union. The periosteal blood supply recedes to its resting level within a few weeks when the regenerated medullary vessels have penetrated the cortex and reestablished their anastomoses with the surface periosteal vessels. Centrifugal cortical blood flow is restored, and the development of external callus is halted.

These stages of repair after fracture and osteotomy and their relation to the blood supply are fundamental. The orderly sequence of repair applies strictly to *undisplaced* closed fractures. Both medullary and periosteal circulatory beds proliferate greatly, but the medullary arterial system plays a major role in supplying blood to the uniting callus and in revascularizing necrotic cortex at the fracture site.[132] The ascendancy of the medullary blood supply increases as healing progresses.

Under various circumstances that interfere with the blood supply to the cortex, alternate routes of blood flow must be provided to meet the needs for repair. The sequence of repair is altered, a situation that must affect the rate and quality of bony union and the physical characteristics of the necrotic bone. The following are examples.

In displaced diaphyseal fractures, the medullary nutrient vessels are disrupted and attempts to regenerate these vessels are at first blocked by the central hematoma.[134] The periosteal circulation, derived from the surrounding muscles,[135] is therefore the chief source of blood supplying the external callus that attempts to bridge the fracture gap. However, periosteal callus never produces primary osseous union, and it always contains an early intermediate zone of fibrocartilage. The disrupted medullary circulation also proliferates at once and mediates the production of endosteal osseous callus.

When reduction of the fragments is stable, continuity of the main medullary nutrient arteries across the level of the fracture is rapidly restored, generally within 3 weeks; when reduction is unstable, the fibrocartilage within the fracture gap delays penetration of the reparative endosteal capillaries. Nevertheless, the dominance of the endosteal blood supply asserts itself. Small caliber vessels from the medullary cavity penetrate the cortex early, revascularizing the haversian canals, resorbing the interior of the necrotic osteons, and producing increasing porosity of the fragments. After 6 weeks, as demonstrated in the experimental animal, larger caliber arterioles from the medulla extend across the cortex to reach and anastomose with the periosteal circulation, supplying most of the blood to the external callus. The medullary callus is responsible for the earliest osseous union. The periosteal callus remains interrupted by a central radiolucent zone of fibrocartilage until, after a variable period, periosteal capillaries ultimately bridge the fibrocartilage and effect an osseous union.

Cortical necrosis adjacent to a displaced fracture will delay bony bridging across the fracture gap. Later, as the necrotic osteons are revascularized and reconstituted, they approach the fracture gap from each fragment and participate in the osseous union. More often, the fibrocartilage, a prominent feature of a displaced fracture, gradually allows ingrowth of medullary vessels and is converted by endochondral ossification.

With complex fractures, when large bone fragments are avascular and instability causes permanent interruption of medullary vessels, the periosteal circulation remains enhanced for a long time and continues to provide the blood supply to the enlarging masses of callus, which, by its own inherent stability, eventually becomes penetrated by capillaries and is ossified.

Following disruption of the medullary circulation by reaming and passage of an intramedullary nail, the intramedullary nutrient arteries are destroyed. Moreover, intramedullary reaming will greatly increase the intramedullary pressure, which will force the fatty marrow into the intracortical canals, thereby blocking the haversian circulation and increasing the depth of cortical necrosis.[153] If intramedullary reaming pressure can be reduced (*e.g.*, by providing egress distally by fenestration of the bone and insertion of suction), the degree of avascular necrosis is greatly lessened.[155] To compensate for loss of the intramedullary supply, normal periosteal longitudinal channels alongside the nail. Osteoclasts viability of the cortex in limited areas where they enter the bone (*i.e.*, at points of tendinous attachments of muscles such as the linea aspera of the femur). The extraosseous arteries aid in the revascularization of the cortex but do not proliferate sufficiently nor for an extended period for repair of the fracture. A few weeks later, the medullary arteries have regenerated sufficiently and once again supply all areas for cortical repair and fracture healing. The regenerative powers of the medullary circulation are enormous, leading to the formation, when necessary for conveying blood a long distance, of new arteries directed longitudinally through the compact bone.[146,153,154] It should be emphasized that although functioning blood vessels, after destruction of the medullary vessels, can be demonstrated, after 1 week, throughout the entire cortex, practically the entire thickness of the cortex is necrotic[156] and must undergo processes of repair.

In certain anatomical regions, where no muscle attachments exist (*e.g.*, at the lower third of the tibia), an extraosseous vascular response is lacking. This is the most common site for delayed union or nonunion.

Within 4 weeks after intramedullary reaming and nailing, the medullary circulation regenerates and highly vascularized and cellular tissue comes to occupy the longitudinal channels alongside the nail. Osteoclasts resorb the endosteal surface of the cortex (Fig. 6-28) to create room for regeneration of intramedullary bone, which eventually surrounds the nail completely. The nutrient arteries regenerate, and vessels enter the haversian canals to reach the periosteal surface outside the external callus. The new vessels can be seen inside the haversian canals as early as the first week, and by 6 weeks the osteoclasts have resorbed the concentric lamellae so that widespread enlargement of the haversian canals results. This is reflected, clinically, by diminished strength of the bone, and, roentgenographically, by diffuse osteoporosis. This osteoporosis mirroring the initial resorptive stage of repair of necrotic bone appears to involve the entire thickness of the cortex by 12 weeks.

In the event that the medullary nutrient supply is permanently obliterated (*e.g.*, following extensive reaming and insertion of acrylic cement), new arteries arise from surrounding tissues and are able, although belatedly, to penetrate the external callus and furnish sufficient blood for cortical repair. An additional source of blood supply may be derived from longitudinal channels within the adjacent viable cortex. This is an extremely slow process. These facts emphasize the need to retain the intramedullary nail and, in the case of cemented intramedullary devices, to protect the extremity against undue force, until both union and repair of necrotic bone are ensured.

When a metallic bone plate is tightly apposed to the outer surface of the cortex, the entire thickness of cortex at the area of contact becomes avascular despite the fact that the medullary vessels normally supply the inner two thirds to three-fourths of the cortex. This occurs because the flow of blood through the cortex requires the existence of a vascular anastomosis between medullary and periosteal supplies. When the plate becomes loosened or removed, the medulloperiosteal anastomosis is restored and the necrotic bone is resorbed and replaced. This appears to support the concept that the normal flow of blood through the cortex is centrifugal.

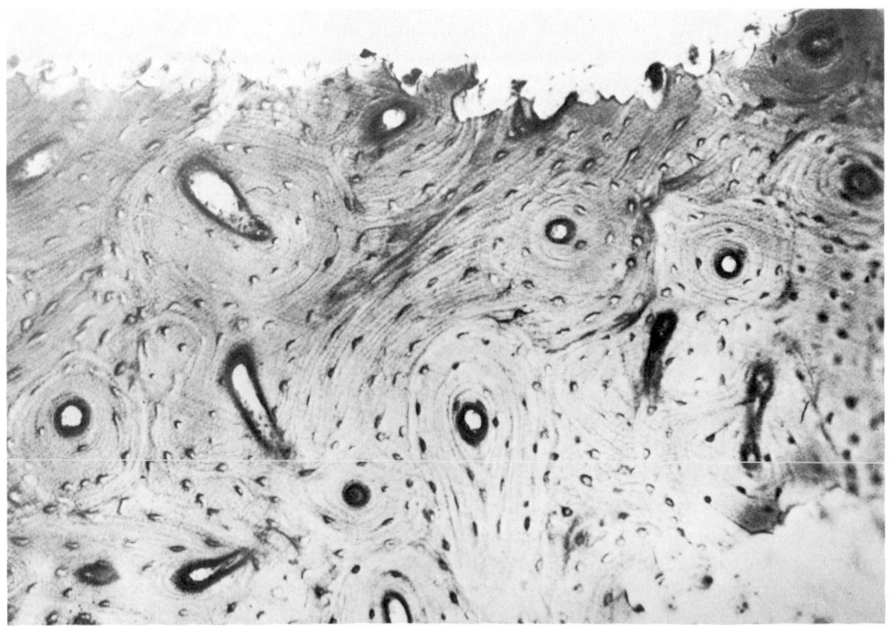

FIG. 6-28. Histopathology of cortex of long bone after intramedullary nail fixation. At 6 weeks the bone is necrotic and avascular. At the upper edge, the endosteal surface is being resorbed by osteoclasts and the process is already beginning to resorb the inner concentric lamellae of osteons near the surface. The deeper haversian canals are empty but soon will be invaded by vascular cellular tissue. (Rhinelander FW: Circulation in bone. In Bourne GH (ed): The Biochemistry and Physiology of Bone, pp 1–78. New York, Academic Press, 1972)

REFERENCES

Biochemistry

1. Clark I: Biochemistry of bone. In Wilson FC (ed): The Musculoskeletal System. Philadelphia, JB Lippincott, 1975
2. Glimcher MJ: Studies of the structure, organization, and reactivity of bone collagen. In Gibson T (ed): Proceedings of the International Symposium on Wound Healing, Rotterdam, 1974, p 253. Montreaux Found. Int. Conf. Med. Science, 1975
3. Neuman WF, Neuman MW: The Chemical Dynamics of Bone Mineral. Chicago, University of Chicago Press, 1958

Basic Physiologic Processes

4. Neumann WF, et al: Cyclic concept in exchange of bone. Calcif Tissue Res 2:262, 1969
5. Talmage RV: Physiological processes in bone. In Wilson FC (ed): The Musculoskeletal System. Philadelphia, JB Lippincott, 1975

Phosphorus

6. Harrison HE, Harrison HC: The interaction of vitamin D and parathyroid hormone on calcium, phosphorus, and magnesium homeostasis in the rat. Metabolism 13:952, 1964

Calcium

7. Avioli LV: Intestinal absorption of calcium. Arch Intern Med 129:345, 1972
8. Faulkner WR, King JW, Damm HC: Handbook of Clinical Laboratory Data, 2nd ed. Cleveland, Chemical Rubber Co, 1968
9. Goldsmith RS: Laboratory aids in the diagnosis of metabolic bone disease. Orthop Clin North Am 3:545, 1972

Fate of Phosphorus and Calcium

10. Arnaud CD, Tsao HS, Littledyke T: Calcium homeostasis, parathyroid hormone, and calcitonin. Mayo Clin Proc 45:125, 1970

Glands of Internal Secretion

11. Adams PH, et al: Effects of hyperthyroidism on bone and mineral metabolism in man. Q J Med 36:1, 1967
12. Adams P, Jowsey J: Bone and mineral metabolism in hyperthyroidism: An experimental study. Endocrinology 81:735, 1967
13. Arnaud CD, Tsao HS, Littledyke T: Radioimmunoassay of human parathyroid hormone in serum. J Clin Invest 50:21, 1971
14. Asling CW, et al: Effects of pituitary factors and of thyroxine on skeletal morphogenesis in the rat. In Reifenstein EC Jr (ed): Transactions of the Third Conference on Metabolic Interrelations, p 125. New York, Macy Foundation, 1951
15. Auerbach GD, Potts JD Jr: Parathyroid hormone. Am J Med 42:1, 1967
16. Bechgaard P: Serum phosphatase in thyrotoxicosis and myxedema. Acta Med Scand 114:293, 1943
17. Bijvoet OLM et al: Effects of prolonged administration of thyrocalcitonin in human senile osteoporosis. In Taylor S, Foster G (eds): Calcitonin. London, Heinemann, 1970
18. Blackburn CM, Power MH: Diagnostic accuracy of protein-bound iodine determination in thyroid disease. J Clin Endocrinol Metab 15:1379, 1955
19. Chase LR, Aurbach GD: Renal adenyl cyclase: Anatomically separate sites for parathyroid hormone and vasopressin. Science 159:545, 1968
20. Chopra LJ, Lam R: Use of 8-anilino-1-napthalene-sulfonic acid (ANS) in radioimmunoassay (RIA) of triiodothyronine (T_3) in unextracted serum. Clin Res 20:216, 1972
21. Cochran M, et al: Renal effects of calcitonin. In Taylor S, Foster GV (eds): Calcitonin 1969. Proceedings of the Second International Symposium, p 523. London, Heinemann, 1969
22. Copp DH, et al: Evidence of calcitonin—a new hormone from the parathyroid that lowers blood calcium. Endocrinology 70:638, 1962
23. Costom BH, et al: Effect of thyrotropin-releasing factor on serum thyroid-stimulating hormone. J Clin Invest 50:2219, 1971
24. DeLuca HF, et al: The interaction of vitamin D, parathyroid hormone and thyrocalcitonin. In Talmage RV, Belanger LF (eds): Parathyroid Hormone and Thyrocalcitonin. Proceedings of the Third Parathyroid Conference. Amsterdam, Excerpta Medica Foundation, 1968
25. Eisenberg E: Effect of varying phosphate intake in primary hyperparathyroidism. J Clin Endocrinol 28:651, 1968
26. Foley TP Jr, et al: Serum thyrotropin responses to synthetic thyrotropin-releasing hormone in normal children. J Clin Invest 51:431, 1972
27. Follis RH Jr: Skeletal changes associated with hyperthyroidism. Bull Johns Hopkins Hosp 92:405, 1953
28. Goldman L, Gordon GS, Roof BS: The parathyroids: Progress, problems, and practice. In Current Problems in Surgery. Chicago, Year Book Medical Publishers, 1971
29. Gordon GS, et al: Clinical endocrinology of parathyroid hormone excess. Recent Progr Horm Res 18:297, 1962
30. Greer MA, et al: Antithyroid compounds. In Pitt-Rivers R, Trotter WR (eds): The Thyroid Gland, vol 1, p 357. London, Butterworth, 1964
31. Habener JR, et al: Parathyroid hormone: Secretion and metabolism *in vivo*. Proc Natl Acad Sci 68:2986, 1971
32. Hershman JM, Pittman JA Jr: Utility of the radioimmunoassay of serum thyrotrophin in man. Ann Intern Med 74:481, 1971
33. Jowsey J: Quantitative microradiography: A new approach in the evaluation of metabolic bone disease. Am J Med 40:485, 1966
34. Kao PC, et al: Development and validation of a new radioimmunoassay for parathyrin (PTH). Clin Chem 28:69, 1982
35. Kao PC: Parathyroid hormone assay. Mayo Clin Proc 57:596, 1982
36. Kinsell LW, et al: Effect of testosterone compounds on nitrogen balance and creatine excretion in patients with thyrotoxicosis. J Clin Invest 23:880, 1944
37. Kivirikko KI, Laitinen O, Lamberg B: Value of serum and urine hydroxyproline in the diagnosis of thyroid disease. J Clin Endocrinol 25:1347, 1965
38. Korenman SG, Granner DK, Sherman BM: Practical Diagnosis: Endocrine Disease, p 166. Boston, Houghton Mifflin, 1978
39. Lamberg BA, Wahlberg P, Forsius PI: The serum protein-bound iodine as a diagnostic aid. Acta Med Scand 154:201, 1956

40. Leboeuf G, Ducharme JR: Thyroiditis in children: Diagnosis and management. Pediatr Clin North Am 13:19, 1966
41. Malkinson FD: Hyperthyroidism, pretibial myxedema, and clubbing. Arch Dermatol 88:303, 1963
42. Martin TJ, Robinson CJ, MacIntyre I: The mode of action of thyrocalcitonin. Lancet 1:900, 1966
43. Mitsuma T, et al: Radioimmunoassay of triiodothyronine in unextracted human serum. J Clin Endocrinol Metab 33:364, 1971
44. Moore EW: Ionized calcium in normal serum ultrafiltrates and whole blood determined by ion-exchange electrodes. J Clin Invest 49:318, 1970
45. Murphy BEP, Pattee CJ: Determination of thyroxine utilizing the property of protein binding metabolism. J Clin Endocrinol 24:187, 1964
46. Nicholas JA, Wilson PD: Adrenocortical response to operative procedures on bones and joints. J Bone Joint Surg 35A:559, 1953
47. Pearse AGE, Carvalheira AF: Cytochemical evidence for an ultimobranchial origin of rodent thyroid "C" cells. Nature 214:929, 1967
48. Pfannenstiel P, et al: Congenital hypothyroidism from intrauterine ^{131}I damage. In Cassano C, Andreali M (eds): Current Topics in Hormone Research, p 749. New York, Academic Press, 1965
49. Potts JT Jr, et al: Parathyroid hormone: Sequence, synthesis, immunoassay studies. Am J Med 50:639, 1971
50. Rasmussen H: Ionic and hormone control of calcium homeostasis. Am J Med 50:567, 1971
51. Rasmussen H, et al: Hormonal control of the renal conversion of 25-hydroxycholecalciferol to 1,25 dihydrocholecalciferol. J Clin Invest 51:2502, 1972
52. Ravel R: Clinical Laboratory Medicine. Chicago, Year Book Medical Publishers, 1973
53. Ray RD, et al: Growth and differentiation of the skeleton in thyroidectomized and hypophysectomized rates treated with thyroxine, growth hormone, and the combination. J Bone Joint Surg 36A:94, 1954
54. Reilly WA, Smyth FS: Cretinoid epiphyseal dysgenesis. J Pediatr 11:786, 1937
55. Reiss E, Canterbury JM: A radioimmunoassay for parathyroid hormone in man. Proc Soc Exp Biol Med 128:501, 1968
56. Reiss E, Canterbury JM: Primary hyperparathyroidism: Application of radioimmunoassay to differentiation of adenoma and hyperplasia and to preoperative localization of hyperfunctioning parathyroid glands. N Engl J Med 280:1381, 1969
57. Riggs BL, et al: Skeletal alterations in hyperparathyroidism: Determination of bone formation, resorption and morphologic changes by microradiography. J Endocrinol 25:777, 1965
58. Riggs BL, et al: Immunologic differentation of primary hyperparathyroidism from hyperparathyroidism due to nonparathyroid cancer. J Clin Invest 50:2079, 1971
59. Shenkman L, et al: Triiodothyronine and thyroid stimulating hormone response to thyrotrophin-releasing hormone. Lancet 1:111, 1972
60. Sherwood LM, et al: Evaluation by immunoassay of factors controlling the secretion of parathyroid hormone. Nature 209:52, 1966
61. Sherwood LM, et al: Parathyroid hormone: Synthesis, storage, secretion. In Talmage RV, Munson PL (eds): Calcium, Parathyroid Hormone and Calcitonin. Amsterdam, Excerpta Medica Foundation, 1972
62. Silberberg M, Silberberg R: Influence of the endocrine glands on growth and aging of the skeleton. Arch Pathol 36:512, 1943
63. Smith DW, Blizzard RM, Wilkins L: The mental prognosis in hypothyroidism of infancy and childhood: A review of 128 cases. Pediatrics 19:1011, 1957
64. Smith R: Total urinary hydroxyproline in primary hyperparathyroidism: An assessment of its clinical significance. Clin Chim Acta 18:47, 1967
65. Stanbury JB, et al: The Metabolic Basis of Inherited Diseases, 2nd ed. New York, McGraw-Hill, 1966
66. Thorn GW, Goldfien A, Nelson DH: The treatment of adrenal dysfunction. Med Clin North Am 40:1261, 1956
67. Walker DC: An assay of skeletongenic effect of levotriiodothyronine and its acetic acid analogue in immature rats. Bull Johns Hopkins Hosp 101:101, 1957
68. Werner SC, Spooner M: A new and simple test for hyperthyroidism employing 1-triiodothyronine and the twenty-four I^{131} uptake method. Bull NY Acad Med 31:137, 1955
69. Wilkins LW: The Diagnosis and Treatment of Endocrine Disorders in Childhood and Adolescence, p 93. Springfield, IL, Charles C Thomas, 1962
70. Wilkins LW: Hormonal influences on skeletal growth. Ann NY Acad Sci 60:763, 1955
71. Wilkins LW: Epiphyseal dysgenesis associated with hypothyroidism. Am J Dis Child 61:13, 1941
72. Wilkins L, et al: Hypothyroidism in childhood. J Clin Endocrinol 1:3, 1941
73. Wilkins L, et al: Developmental goiters in cretins without iodine deficiency: Hypothyroidism due to apparent inability of the thyroid gland to synthesize hormone. Pediatrics 13:235, 1954
74. Winter J, et al: The relationship of juvenile hypothyroidism to chronic lymphocytic thyroiditis. J Pediatr 69:709, 1966

Enzymes

75. Kabat EA, Furth J: Histochemical study of alkaline phosphatase. Am J Pathol 17:303, 1941
76. Lum G, Gambino SR: Serum gammaglutamyl transpeptidase. Clin Chem 18:358, 1972
77. McKelve AM, Mann FC: Role of alkaline phosphatase in osteogenesis after transplantation of bone. Am J Pathol 25:709, 1949

Theories of Mineralization

78. Ali SY, et al: Isolation and characterization of calcifying matrix vesicles from epiphyseal cartilage. Proc Nat Acad Sci 67:1513, 1970
79. Arsenis C: Role of mitochrondria in calcification. Biochem Biophys Res Commun 46:1928, 1972
80. Bader H: Uber das Bindungsvermögen der Lipids für anorganisches Phosphat. Biophysik 1:370, 1964
81. Bernard GW, Pease DC: An electron microscopic study of initial intramembranous osteogenesis. Am J Anat 125:271, 1969
82. Bonucci E: Fine structure and histochemistry of "calcifying globules" in epiphyseal cartilage. Z Zellforsch 103:192, 1970
83. Campo RD, et al: The proteinpolysaccharides of articular, epiphyseal plate, and costal cartilages. Biochem Biophys Acta 177:501, 1969
84. Engstrom GW, DeLuca HF: The nature of Ca^{++} binding by kidney mitochondria. Biochemistry 3:379, 1964

85. Fleisch H: Role of nucleation and inhibition in calcification. Clin Orthop 32:170, 1964
86. Francis MD et al: Diphosphonates inhibit formation of calcium phosphate crystals in vitro and pathological calcification in vivo. Science 165:1264, 1969
87. Glimcher MJ: Specificity of the molecular structure of organic matrices in mineralization. In Sognnaes RF ed: Calcification in Biological Systems, p 421. Washington, DC, Am Assoc Advancement of Science, Pub No. 64, 1960
88. Glimcher MJ: The ultrastructural organization of bone and the mechanism of calcification. *In* Birth Defects, Structural Organization of the Skeleton, Vol 2, p 50. Nat. Found. March of Dimes, 1966
89. Glimcher MJ: The composition, structure and organization of bone and other mineralized tissues and the mechanism of calcification. In Greep RO, Astwood EB (eds): Handbook of Physiology, Endocrinology, Sec 7, Vol VII, cap 3. Washington DC, Am Physiol Soc, 1976
90. Glimcher MJ, Krane SM: The organization and structure of bone, and the mechanism of calcification. In Gould BS, Ramachandran GN (eds): A Treatise on Collagen, Vol II. London, Academic Press, 1968
91. Herring GM: Chemistry of the bone matrix. Clin Orthop 36:169, 1964
92. Howell DS: Current concepts of calcification. J Bone Joint Surg 53A:250, 1971
93. Howell DS et al: Demonstration of macromolecular inhibitors of calcification and nucleation factors in fluid from calcifying sites in cartilage J Clin Invest 48:630, 1969
94. Irving JT: A histological stain for newly calcified tissues. Nature (Lond) 181:704, 1958
95. Irving JT: Theories of mineralization of bone. Clin Orthop 97:225, 1973
96. Irving JT, Wuthier RE: Histochemistry and biochemistry of calcification with special reference to the role of lipids. Clin Orthop 56:237, 1968
97. Irving JT, et al: Effect of condensed phosphates on vitamin D-induced aortic calcification in rats. Proc Soc Exp Biol Med 122:852, 1966
98. McCarty DJ Jr, et al: Studies on pathological calcifications in human cartilage. J Bone Joint Surg 48A:309, March 1966
99. McLean FC: Trends in the theory of calcification. Proc Am Acad Orthop Surg J Bone Joint Surg 50A:826, 1968
100. Martin JH, Matthews JL: Mitochondrial granules in chondrocytes. Calcif Tissue Res 3:184, 1969
101. Matthews JL, et al: Mitochondrial granules in the normal and rachitic rat epiphysis. Calcif Tissue Res 5:91, 1970
102. Neuman WF, Neuman MW: The Chemical Dynamics of Bone Mineral. Chicago, University of Chicago Press, 1958
103. Posner AS: Crystal chemistry of bone mineral. Physiol Rev 49:760, 1969
104. Rolle GK: The distribution of calcium in normal and tetracycline-modified bones of developing chick embryos. Calcif Tissue Res 3:142, 1969
105. Shapiro J, Greenspan JS: Are mitochondria directly involved in biological mineralization? Calcif Tissue Res 3:100, 1969
106. Shuttleworth A, Veis A: The isolation of anionic phosphoproteins from bovine cortical bone via the periodate stabilization of bone collagen. Biochem Biophys Acta 257:414, 1972
107. Solomons CC, Styner J: Osteogenesis imperfecta: Effect of magnesium administration on pyrophosphate metabolism. Calcif Tissue Res 3:318, 1969
108. Spector AR, Glimcher MJ: The extraction and characterization of soluble anionic phosphoproteins from bone. Biochem Biophys Acta 263:593, 1972
109. Urist MR: Recent advances in physiology of calcification. Instr. Course Lect., Am Acad Orthop Surg, J Bone Joint Surg 46A:889, 1964
110. Urist MR: Biologic initiation of calcification. In Zipkin I: Biological Mineralization. New York, John Wiley & Sons, 1970
111. Urist MR, Moss MJ, Adams JM: Calcification of tendon: A triphasic local mechanism. Arch Pathol 77:594, 1964

Bone Formation, Resorption, and Mineralization

112. Bohr H, Ravn HO, Werner H: The osteogenic effect of bone transplants in rabbits. J Bone Joint Surg 50B:866, November 1968
113. Eisenberg E, Gordan GS: Skeletal dynamics in man measured by non-radioactive strontium. J Clin Invest 40:1809, 1961
114. Frost HM: Preparation of thin undecalcified bone sections by rapid manual method. Stain Technol 33:273, 1958
115. Frost HM: Staining of fresh undecalcified thin bone sections. Stain Technol 34:135, 1959
116. Frost HM, Villanueva AR: Observations on osteoid seams. Henry Ford Hosp Med Bull 8:212, 1960
117. Harris WH, Jackson RH, Jowsey J: The in vivo distribution of tetracyclines in canine bone. J Bone Joint Surg 44A:1308, 1962
118. Heaney RP, Whedon GD: Radiocalcium studies of bone formation rate in human metabolic disease. J Clin Endocrinol 18:1246, 1958
119. Jowsey J: Editorial: Quantitative microradiography: A new approach in the evaluation of metabolic bone disease. Am J Med 40:485, 1966
120. Jowsey J, Sissons HA, Vaughn J: The site of deposition of Y^{91} in the bone of rabbits and dogs. J Nucl Energy 2:168, 1956
121. Jowsey J, Kelly PS, Riggs L et al: Quantitative microradiographic studies of normal and osteoporotic bone. J Bone Joint Surg 47A:785, 1965
122. Milch RA, et al: Bone localization of tetracycline. JNCI 19:87, 1957
123. Olerud S, Lorenzi GL: Triple fluorochrome labeling in bone formation and bone resorption. J Bone Joint Surg 52A:274, 1970
124. Prockop DJ, Kivirikko KI: Relationship of hydroxyproline excretion in urine to collagen metabolism. Ann Intern Med 66:1243, 1967
125. Puranen J: Reorganization of fresh and preserved bone transplants. Acta Orthop Scand (Suppl) 92, 1966
126. Riggs BL, et al: Special procedures for assessing metabolic bone disease. Med Clin North Am 54:1061, 1970
127. Sorenson JA, Cameron JR: A reliable in vivo measurement of bone-mineral content. J Bone Joint Surg 49A:481, 1967

The Mature Long Bone

128. Branemark P: Vital microscopy of bone marrow in rabbit. Scand J Clin Invest (Suppl) 38:5, 1959
129. Brookes M, Elkins AC, Harrison RG, Heald CB: A new concept of capillary circulation in bone cortex: Some clinical applications. Lancet 1:1078, 1961
130. Brookes M: The blood supply of bone. In Clark JMP (ed): Modern Trends in Orthopaedics, Vol 4, Science of Fractures, p 91. Washington, DC, Butterworth, 1964

131. Carroll SE: A study of the nutrient foramina of the humeral diaphysis. J Bone Joint Surg 45B:176, 1963
132. Cofield RH, et al: Strontium-85 extraction during trans-capillary passage in tibial bone. J Appl Physiol 39:596, 1975
133. Cuthbertson EM, Siris E, Gilfilian RS: The femoral diaphyseal medullary venous system as a venous collateral channel in the dog. J Bone Joint Surg 47A:965, 1965
134. DeMarneffe R: Recherches morphologiques et expérimentales sur la vascularisation osseuse. Acta Chir Belg 50:469, 568, 681, 1951
135. Ecoiffier J, et al: Etude du réseau veineux dans les os longs du lapin. Rev Chir Orthop 41:29, 1957
136. Foster LN, Kelley RP, Watts WM: Experimental infarction of bone and bone marrow. J Bone Joint Surg 33A:396, 1951
137. Göttman L: Vascular reactions in experimental fractures. Acta Chir Scand (Suppl) 284, 1961
138. Holmdahl DE, Ingelmark BE: The contact between the articular cartilage and the medullary cavities of bone. Acta Anat 12:341, 1951
139. Johnson RW Jr: A physiological study of the blood supply of the diaphysis. J Bone Joint Surg 9:153, 1927
140. Laing PG: The blood supply of the femoral shaft: An anatomical study. J Bone Joint Surg 35B:462, 1953
141. Laing PG: The arterial supply of the adult humerus. J Bone Joint Surg 38A:1105, 1956
142. Larson RL, et al: Suppression of the periosteal and nutrient blood supply of the femora of dogs: A histologic, microangiographic and roentgenologic study. Clin Orthop 21:217, 1961
143. Lopez–Curto JA, Bassingthwaighte JB, Kelly PJ: Anatomy of the microvasculature of the tibial diaphysis of the adult dog. J Bone Joint Surg 62A:1362, 1980
144. Macnab I: The blood supply of tubular and cancellous bone (abstr). J Bone Joint Surg 40A:1433, 1958
145. Nelson GE Jr, Kelly PJ, Peterson LFA, Janes JM: Blood supply of the human tibia. J Bone Joint Surg 42A:625, 1960
146. Rhinelander FW: The normal microcirculation of diaphyseal cortex and its response to fracture. J Bone Joint Surg 50A:784, 1968
147. Rhinelander FW, Phillips RS, Steel WM, Beer JC: Microangiography in bone healing: II. Displaced closed fractures. J Bone Joint Surg 50A:643, 1968
148. Rhinelander FW: Circulation of bone. In Bourne GH (ed): Biochemistry and Physiology of Bone, 2nd ed, p 2. New York, Academic Press, 1972
149. Schulman SS: Observations on the nutrient foramina of the human radius and ulna. Anat Rec 134:685, 1959
150. Trueta J, Cavadias AK: Vascular changes caused by Küntscher type of nailing: An experimental study in the rabbit. J Bone Joint Surg 37B:492, 1955
151. Trueta J: The role of vessels in osteogenesis. J Bone Joint Surg 45B:402, 1963
152. Trueta J, Cavadias AK: A study of the blood supply of the long bones. Surg Gynecol Obstet 118:485, 1964

Effects of Diaphyseal Fracture

153. Danckwardt-Lillieström G: Reaming of the medullary cavity and its effect on diaphyseal bone. Acta Orthop Scand (Suppl) 128, 1969
154. Danckwardt-Lillieström G, Lorenzi GL, Olerud S: Intramedullary nailing after reaming: An investigation on the healing process in osteotomized rabbit. Acta Orthop Scand (Suppl) 134, 1970
155. Danckwardt-Lillieström G, Lorenzi L, Olerud S: Intracortical circulation after intramedullary reaming with reduction of pressure in the medullary cavity. J Bone Joint Surg 52A:1390, 1970
156. Rhinelander FW, Baragry RA: Microangiography in bone healing. I. Undisplaced closed fractures. J Bone Joint Surg 44A:1273, 1962

7

Physiology of Cartilage

CARTILAGE, by its rubberlike resiliency, functions to reduce pressure, and, where it covers the end of a bone, its smooth surface minimizes the friction effect of shearing stresses. Where pressure and shearing stresses are brought to bear at skeletal junctions, cartilage is prone to form. Thus, a rib is joined to the sternum by a segment of cartilage. When movement between osseous structures is small and pressure constitutes the main force, the collagenous component of cartilage is increased (*e.g.*, fibrocartilage of the intervertebral disk). When movement and shearing stresses are maximal, a synovia-lined cleft forms to separate two cartilage-covered surfaces, the diarthrodial joint.

NORMAL ARTICULAR CARTILAGE

Hyaline articular cartilage covers the articulating ends of the component bones. It is a highly specialized form of connective tissue that, during embryonic development, forms independently of the mesenchymal and cartilaginous precursor of the rest of the bone. It possesses unique biochemical and biophysical characteristics well suited to its dual functions as shock absorber and bearing surface in a movable joint.

Articular cartilage is isolated tissue in that in mature animals it is aneural, is alymphatic, and has no direct contact with the vascular system.[2,16] Its nutrition depends on a system by which nutrients must pass through two diffusion barriers to reach the cell. In the mature adult, all nutrients must first diffuse out of the synovial vascular plexus, traverse the synovial membrane to enter the synovial fluid, and pass through the dense hyaline matrix to reach the chondrocyte. In the immature animal, an additional source of nutrients is by diffusion from the vascular structures of the underlying bone.[14]

The permeability of cartilage matrix to nutrients is dictated in large measure by heavy concentrations of polyanionic glycosaminoglycans (GAGs).[22,23] Because of the density of the constituent macromolecules of the matrix, diffusion of substrates is generally related to their molecular size and structure, and a theoretical pore size of 6.8 nm (68A) has been established. Proteins of even low molecular weight and substrates such as glucose diffuse across the matrix very slowly.

In its native state, cartilage consists of approximately 70% water; the remainder is equally divided between ground substance and collagen. Very minor constituents include chondrocytes and enzymes. Half of the dry weight of hyaline cartilage is collagen, whereas the other half is polysaccharide (GAG) together with attached protein.

GROUND SUBSTANCE

Cartilage ground substance is composed of protein-polysaccharides (PPSs, proteoglycans), which are macromolecules consisting of a protein core, the polypeptide chain, whose amino acid composition is variable and extensive, and many chondroitin sulfate and keratan sulfate chains covalently bound to the protein core.[5,31]

The polysaccharides (GAGs) are usually isolated by treatment of the cartilage with a dilute alkali, which releases the polysaccharide from its link with protein. Hyaluronidase will also cleave the link between the polysaccharide chain and the protein backbone.

Chondroitin sulfate consists of alternating units of galactosamine and glucuronic acid. The galactosamine carries an ester sulfate group, so there are two anionic charges per period.

At least three distinct species of GAG have been identified in articular cartilage: chondroitin-6-sulfate, chondroitin-4-sulfate, and keratan sulfate (Fig. 7-1).[25,33] Chondroitin-6-sulfate is the principal GAG, accounting for 45% to 75% of the sugar component of the tissue and approximately 15% of the dry weight.[19] The dimeric sugar unit of this macromolecule consists of glucuronic acid and *N*-acetyl galactosamine linked by a (1-3)-glycoside bond.[25] A sulfate group is located on the sixth carbon atom of the galactosamine. Chondroitin-4-sulfate is identical in structure except for placement of the sulfate group on the fourth carbon atom of the *N*-acetyl galactosamine. This GAG is more prevalent in immature articular cartilage, decreasing in concentration as the animal ages to the adult level of less than 5% of the total.[19]

Keratan sulfate, whose component sugars are galactose and sulfated *N*-acetyl glucosamine, is present in trace amounts in immature cartilage but with advancing age is found in increasing concentrations, with values for adult articular cartilage ranging up to 50%.

The side chains extend at right angles from the protein core (Fig. 7-2). The side chains of the polydimeric sugars of chondroitin sulfate are long, and since the chain

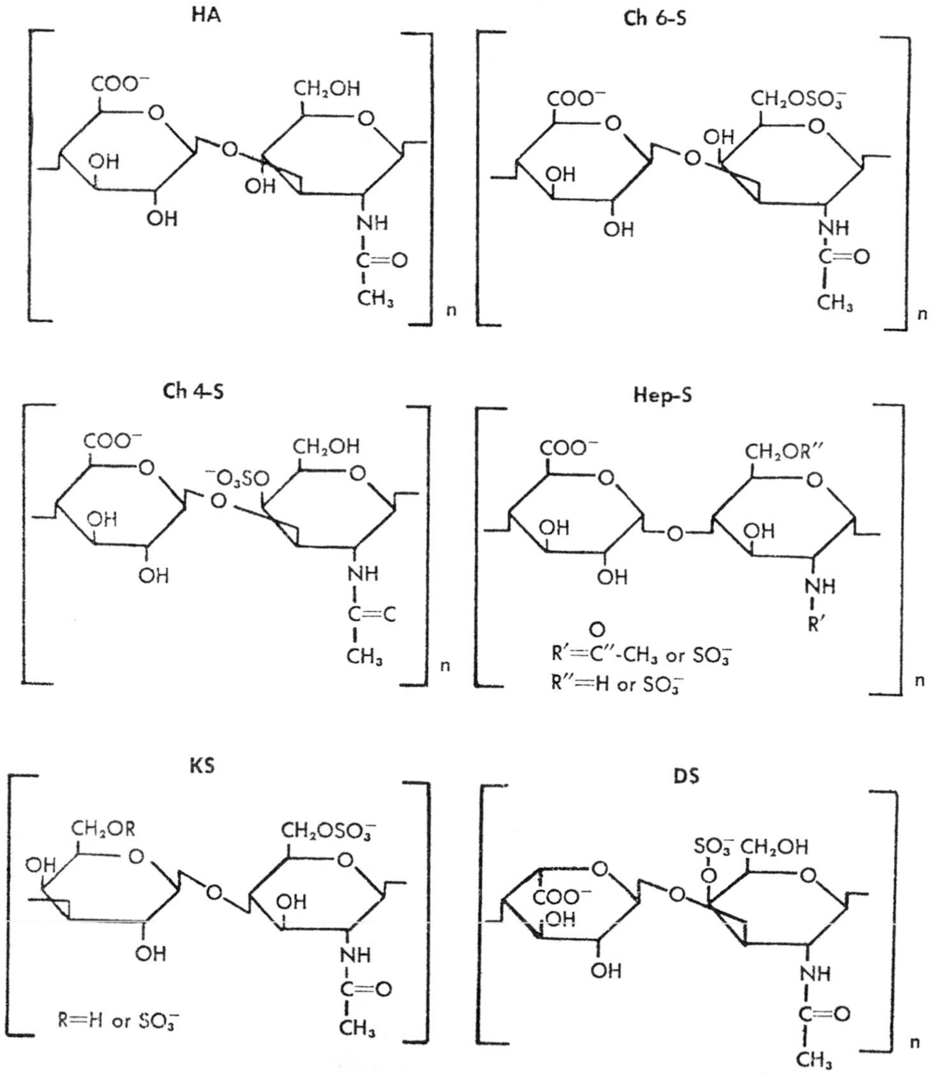

FIG. 7-1. Structure of the repeating subunits of six mucopolysaccharides. (*HA,* hyaluronic acid; *Ch6-S,* chondroitin-6-sulfate—formerly chondroitin sulfate C; *Ch4-S,* chondroitin-4-sulfate—formerly chondroitin sulfate A; *Hep-S,* heparin sulfate—formerly heparitin sulfate; *KS,* keratan sulfate—formerly keratosulfate; *DS,* dermatan sulfate—formerly chondroitin sulfate B) (Meyer K: Am J Med 47:664, 1969)

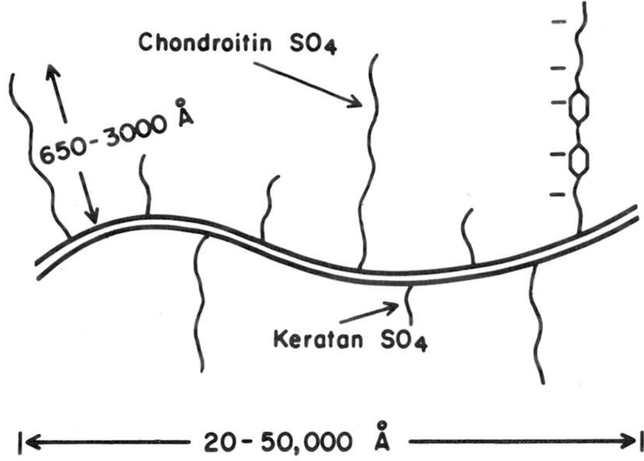

FIG. 7-2. Proteoglycan structure. (Sledge CB: Structure, development and function of joints. Orthop Clin North Am 6B:619, 1975)

weight of chondroitin sulfate is 30,000 to 40,000, there are 50 to 70 disaccharide units per chain. Chondroitin sulfate can be separated from its attachments to protein by treating the cartilage with dilute alkali. The chondroitin sulfate, now free of protein, is easily dissolved in water, but the solution lacks the viscosity of hyaluronate, which is a complete proteoglycan. Chondroitin sulfate can be precipitated from solution as a sodium, potassium, calcium, or barium salt by the addition of ethanol.

The shorter sidechains of proteoglycan consist chiefly of keratan sulfate. Several types of keratan sulfate exist in various tissues, but a species termed skeletal keratan sulfate is the type isolated from cartilage.[24] The repeating dimeric unit consists of galactose and sulfate-carrying *N*-acetyl glucosamine. A keratan sulfate chain is made up of 15 to 30 such dimeric units, so that it is a small polysaccharide. These chains may also contain small amounts of other sugars, such as sialate, fucose, mannose, and galactosamine.

Since the dimeric sugar unit of GAG contains one or two negative charges (COO^- and SO_3^-), these macromolecules produce an enormous negative field.[5,13] The negative charges repel one another, causing the macromolecule to remain stiffly extended in space and establishing an electrostatic field of considerable magnitude.

PROTEINPOLYSACCHARIDES

The proteoglycans are macromolecules consisting of many polysaccharide chains (GAGs) attached to a linear protein core of random coil configuration with a molecular weight of about 200,000 and an average length of about 3400 A (varies in length from 100 nm–400 nm). The proteoglycans are synthesized and sulfated intracellularly on ribosomes and then are secreted into the surrounding matrix for aggregation.[34]

In cartilage, the proteoglycans occupy spaces between a matted network of collagen fibrils, and most of these proteoglycans are noncovalently aggregated to form huge "hypermolecules." Approximately 10 to 30 proteoglycan molecules are linked, through a glycoprotein, with each hyaluronic acid (HA) chain to produce an enormous hypermolecule (Figs. 7-3 and 7-4). The HA chain is a single unbranched chain forming a filamentous backbone, which in individual aggregates varies in length from 400 nm to 4000 nm (average about 2.5μ). Each proteoglycan submit (PGS) is joined at one end by a link glycoprotein to HA to form an aggregate with the nonsulfated HA. The link glycoprotein is noncovalently bound to either HA or PGS but is essential for PGS aggregation to HA. The aggregate has a molecular weight of 30 to 100 × 10^6. The aggregates, because of highly negatively charged chains that repel each other, are spread out over a large domain and are constrained by the relatively rigid network of collagen fibers. Approximately one third of the proteoglycans are tightly bound to the collagen fibrils.

The presently accepted concept is that the ground substance is made up mainly of two distinct macromolecular species that can be isolated by extracting proteoglycans from fresh cartilage. The methods for isolation of proteoglycan aggregate, PGS, link proteins, and HA depend on a fundamental property of the proteoglycan aggregate: Because of the noncovalent bonds between PGS, hyaluronate, and link proteins, the aggregate is reversibly dissociable into these components by concentrated solutions of guanidinium chloride (GuHCl), divalent cations, or lithium bromide, at *p*H 3 to 4, and the crude proteoglycan is then subjected to density gradient centrifugation in cesium chloride.[31] This must be carried out at a low temperature (*e.g.*, 5°C) to avoid degradation of PGS protein by cathepsins. By this method, extraneous matrix proteins and cathepsins are separated into the top of the gradient and a mixture of PGS and proteoglycan aggregate, called proteoglycan complex, is concentrated into the bottom of the gradient. HA is banded in the middle of the dissociative gradient. Two link proteins with molecular weights of approximately 45,000 and 50,000 are concentrated in the top fraction of lowest density.

The basic structural unit of cartilage ground substance is the PGS, the proteoglycan species of lowest molecular weight not further dissociable into smaller units without breaking covalent bonds. Most of the PGS (molecules) is present as aggregates of much higher molecular weight formed by the noncovalent association of subunits with other macromolecular species and linked to the HA chain by a "glycoprotein link," which is a low-molecular-weight non-collagenous protein. Between the aggregates, free PGS exists.

WATER AND ELECTROLYTES

Polysaccharides behave as weak electrolytes, since they contain large numbers of contiguous sulfate and carboxyl

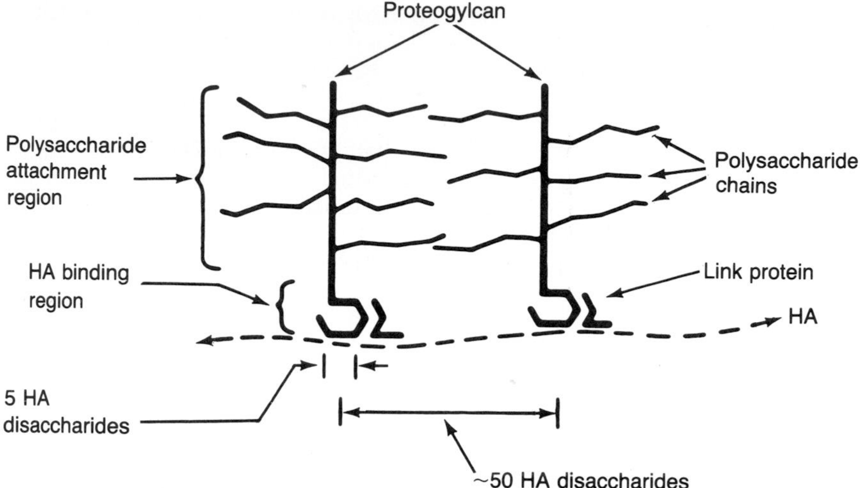

FIG. 7-3. Diagram showing manner of noncovalent linkage of the proteoglycan subunit (PGS) to the filament structure, which is probably hyaluronic acid (HA). This demonstrates that the ground substance of cartilage has a highly ordered structure. The basic structural unit of cartilage ground substance is the PGS, consisting of many chondroitin sulfate and keratan sulfate chains covalently attached mainly to serine and threonine residues of a protein core. PGS units cover a range of molecular weights and composition but cannot be further dissociated into smaller units without breaking covalent bonds. In cartilage ground substance, most of the proteoglycan exists in the form of aggregates of high molecular weight. Approximately 10 to 30 PGS molecules attach by glycoprotein links to each HA chain, producing an enormous hypermolecule. HA is a single unbranched chain about 2.5μ in length. The link proteins are not covalently bound to either HA or PGS but are essential for PGS aggregation to either HA. (Heinegad D, Hascall VC: Aggregation of cartilage proteoglycans. J Biol Chem 249:4250, 1974)

groups (COO^- and SO_3^-) creating a highly negatively charged environment with strong cation- and water-binding properties. A chondroitin sulfate chain carries about 120 negatively charged groups, and each negatively charged group is associated with a cation, usually sodium, and, to a smaller extent, calcium. At the *p*H of this tissue, the protons are scarcely attached at all. Because of the negative charges, the chains are mutually repulsive and tend to assume a widespread configuration over a wide domain.

The strong cation-binding property accounts for the binding of certain cationic dyes, thus altering the absorption spectra of the dye, a property of the dye called metachromasia. Other cations, generally divalent and trivalent cations, by being bound by the polysaccharides, alter the physical properties of the articular cartilage. Water is displaced, elastic recoil is reduced, and the cartilage becomes increasingly deformable. This explains the abnormal cartilage properties observed in certain conditions such as hemophilia, in which the iron ion becomes bound to proteoglycan.

The water content of young articular cartilage is about 85% by weight and gradually lessens to about 70% in adult articular cartilage. Because of the high degree of entanglement of proteoglycan molecules and the large amount of bound or structured water (1,000 to 10,000 times the volume of the proteoglycan molecule), cartilage behaves as a molecular sieve with an effective pore size of about 60 A in diameter. This excludes large molecules, such as the hyaluronate of joint fluid, and retains the chondroitin sulfate and other matrix components. It also excludes immunoglobulins.[34]

SYNTHESIS AND DEGRADATION

The synthesis of proteoglycan occurs intracellularly. First the polypeptide core is manufactured by the ribosomes, and then the carbohydrate chains are added, one sugar at a time, starting with the attachment of xylose to serine. (Chondroitin sulfate is linked to serine. Keratan sulfate is linked to serine and threonine.) Sulfation occurs after the appropriate sugar has been linked to the growing chain. The sugars and the sulfate come from "activated" precursors: sugar nucleotides and phosphoadenosine 5′-phosphosulfate, respectively.[15]

The synthesis of proteoglycan continues throughout

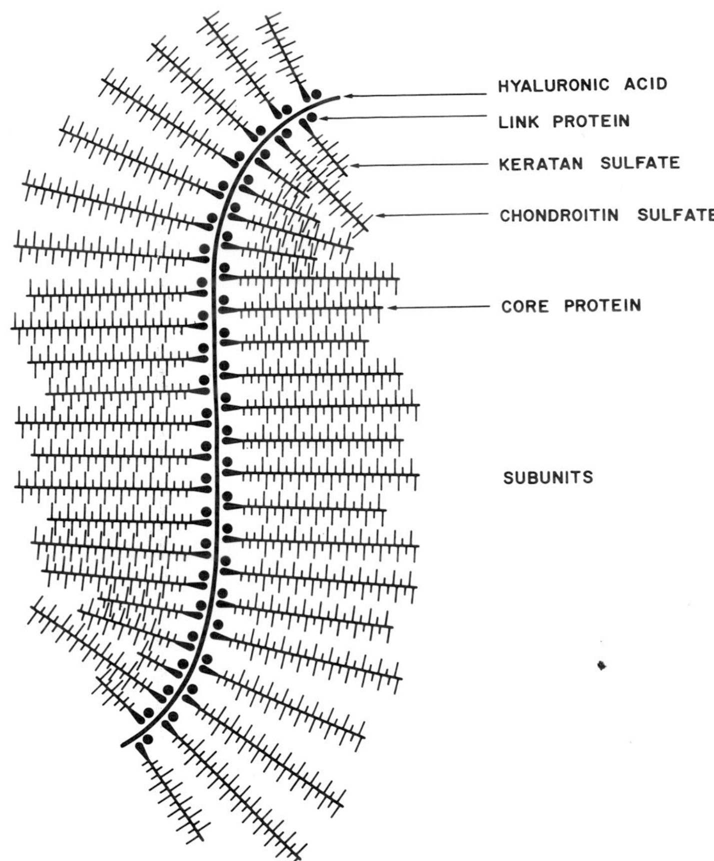

FIG. 7-4. Tentative model of the molecular architecture of the proteoglycan aggregate. The lengths of the HA filament and the PGS (proteoglycan subunit) core proteins and the spacing between the subunits have been drawn to scale, based on measurements of electron micrographs of proteoglycan aggregates from bovine articular cartilage. The lengths of chondroitin sulfate chains have been reduced to about one half to avoid entanglement with neighboring subunits. (Rosenberg L: Structure of cartilage proteoglycans. In Burleigh PMC, Poole AR (eds): Dynamics of Connective Tissue Macromolecules. Amsterdam, North-Holland, 1975)

life. Radioactive sulfate uptake indicates a rapid turnover rate and a half-life of about 8 days.

The degradation of proteoglycan also takes place throughout life and occurs primarily in lysosomes, which contain over 40 known acid hydrolases. It is postulated that the lysosomes release their proteolytic enzyme into the surrounding matrix, and these proteases then depolymerize the proteoglycans by hydrolytic cleavage of the protein backbone (Fig. 7-5). Cathepsin D is the enzyme most likely responsible for this degradative process. However, under experimental conditions, cathepsin D digests proteoglycan compounds at *p*H 5.0 but very little or not at all at *p*H 7.2. Therefore, the action of cathepsin D seen in living cartilage must require various possibilities, including a second enzyme, probably a neutral protease, capable of acting at a neutral *p*H; ingestion of matrix into an intracellular compartment with a low *p*H; and the localized production of an acid milieu outside the cell.[39]

Cathepsin D is elevated severalfold in osteoarthritic cartilage.[1] It appears that this enzyme is the one most likely responsible for the loss of PPS and the resultant cartilage damage.

Chloroquine is a strong inhibitor of cathepsin D. Cortisone and salicylates are not. Antiserums containing antibodies to cathepsin D can be prepared that are capable of inhibiting the autolysis of cartilage.[38] These facts are pertinent to continuing investigations into the pathogenesis and treatment of degenerative arthritis.

METABOLIC ACTIVITY OF THE CHONDROCYTE

Chondrocytes are continuously metabolically very active cells, using both aerobic and anaerobic pathways.[11,17] The chondrocytes from the middle zone of articular cartilage have extensive networks of rough-surfaced endoplasmic reticulum, dilated cisternae, vacuoles, and Golgi apparatus, suggesting that they are actively synthesizing protein, polysaccharides, collagen, and other components of matrix.[36] Metabolic studies using radioisotopes demonstrate that the cell synthesizes the component parts of macromolecules of proteoglycans and collagen, assembles them intracellularly, and rapidly extrudes them into the surrounding matrix.[16,33] Synthesis of proteoglycan is rapid, the proteoglycan having a half-

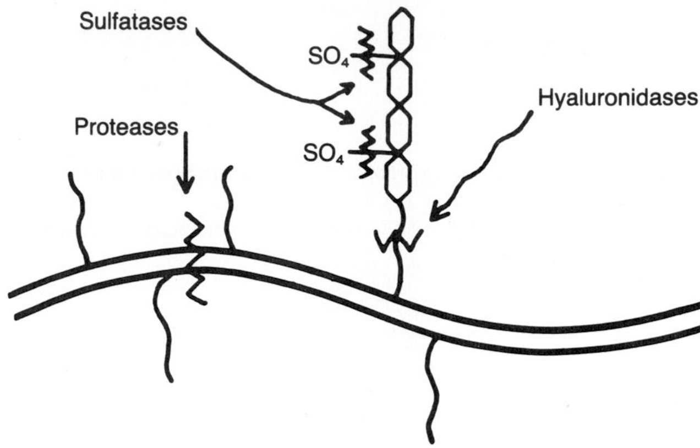

FIG. 7-5. Enzymatic attack on proteoglycans. (Sledge CB: Structure, development and function of joints. Orthop Clin North Am 6B:619, 1975)

life of about 8 days.[18] The turnover rate of collagen is much slower.[29]

Various autolytic enzymes exist both intracellularly and within the matrix. The degradation that normally takes place during tissue turnover is supposedly mediated by lysosomal and extralysosomal enzyme production and release.[32,37]

HISTOCHEMICAL MEASUREMENT OF PROTEOGLYCAN

A quantitative histochemical method can determine the concentration of polysaccharides in ground substance.[30] Safranin-O is a cationic dye that binds stoichiometrically to polyanion, one dye molecule to each negatively charged group of chondroitin sulfate and keratan sulfate. The dye does not bind to collagen (Color Plate 7-1).

When safranin-O is used as a metachromatic dye, keratan sulfate with a less number of anions causes less metachromasia than does chondroitin sulfate. The resulting intensity of color can therefore reflect the amount of mucopolysaccharides and the relative proportions of chondroitin sulfate and keratan sulfate. This constitutes a qualitative measurement. Decreasing metachromasia associated with an increase of keratan sulfate and decrease of chondroitin sulfate, such as occurs with advancing age, is indistinguishable from the lessening metachromasia of degradation.

Treatment of the tissue with ethanol abolishes metachromasia, and safranin-O acts as an orthochromatic dye. One dye molecule combines with one negatively charged group of chondroitin sulfate, or two dye units per uronate-galactosamine repeating unit. In the case of keratan sulfate, one molecule of dye binds to each repeating unit. The absorption spectrum of the dye is proportional to the concentration of the mucopolysaccharide in the tissue section.

COLLAGEN

A review of the synthesis and properties of collagen is essential to understanding the characteristics of normal and diseased cartilage. Collagen is a fibrous protein, often occurring in straight, unbranching bundles that possess high tensile strength and low elasticity. A load of 10 kg to 40 kg is required to break a collagen fiber 1 mm in diameter.[6] Collagen has a characteristic 640 A periodicity by small-angle x-ray diffraction and electron microscopy. It is composed of a high content of glycine (33%) and two unique amino acids, proline and lysine.

Collagen constitutes 50% of the dry weight of cartilage, and its principal function is to provide strength and structural integrity. Cartilage is more resilient to pressure than are other tissues, probably because of the architectural arrangement between collagen and the PPS.

BIOSYNTHESIS

Biosynthesis is initiated in the cytoplasm of the chondroblast or chondrocyte and is carried to completion outside the cell (Fig. 7-6).[27]

First stage. Assembly of amino acids on polyribosomes form procollagen.

Second stage. Enzymatic hydroxylation of some proline and lysine residues takes place.[35] Hydroxylation requires molecular oxygen, ascorbate, ferrous iron, and ketoglutarate.[9] Later, galactose and glucose attach to some hydroxylysine residues.[3]

Third stage. Three α-chains form a rigid, rodlike helical structure, the tropocollagen molecule, which is 3000 A long and only 15 A in diameter. Cartilage contains two types of collagen: identical α-chains and two α1-chains and one α2-chain. Each chain contains about 1000 amino acids, and the three chains are held together by approximately 1000 to 2000 H bonds.

Throughout each polypeptide chain, every third amino acid is glycine (Gly), and collagen can be considered a polymer of tripeptide units, each of which has the formula Gly-X-Y. The amino acid in the X position is frequently proline (Pro), and the third amino acid in the Y position is often hydroxyproline (Hypro). However, lysine (Lys) and hydroxylysine (Hylys) are invariably present, since this amino acid is necessary for cross-linking between tropocollagen molecules. Any amino acid other than proline, hydroxyproline, lysine, and hydroxylysine can occur in the X or Y position.

Fourth stage. Extrusion from the cell. The tropocollagen molecules, probably in solution, are secreted from the cell and proceed at a distance in the ground substance.

Fifth stage. Cleavage of terminal portions of polypep-

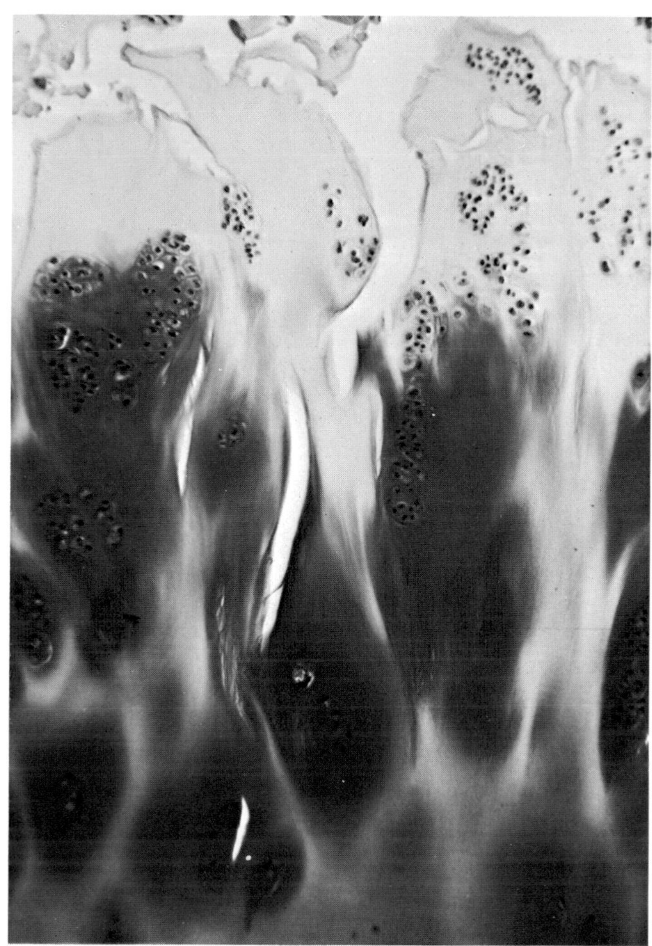

PLATE 7-1. Safranin-O staining of articular cartilage in osteoarthritis. The intense red staining of matrix immediately about the deeply situated multicellular clones reflects their hypermetabolic activity and increased rate of synthesis of glycosaminoglycans (mucopolysaccharides). (Microphotograph courtesy of Dr. Lawrence Rosenberg) (See p. 196.)

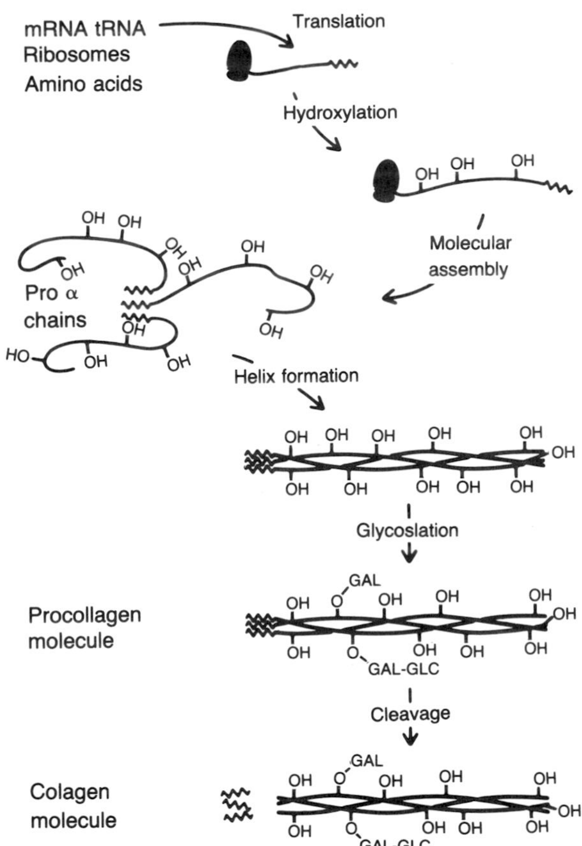

FIG. 7-6. Former concept of the synthesis of collagen. The conversion of procollagen to the collagen molecule supposedly occurs intracellularly by scission of nonhelical polypeptides in the NH_2-terminal region of each constituent pro-α-chain. The modern concept depicted in the following illustration adds the scission of the opposite COOH terminal. The enzyme responsible for this proteolysis is termed procollagen peptidase. (McKusik VA: Heritable Disorders of Connective Tissue. St. Louis, CV Mosby, 1972)

tide chains by proteolytic enzmye results in appropriate length of chains[10] (Fig. 7-7).

Sixth stage. Formation of fibrils. After hydroxylation takes place, tropocollagen molecules are aggregated into fibrils by interaction of charged side groups. This may be initiated within the cell and continues extracellularly.

Experimental model: Water-soluble tropocollagen *in vitro* warmed to 37°C at *p*H 7 spontaneously forms collagen fibrils with typical banding. In this form, the fibrils can be redissolved in neutral salt solution.

Seventh stage. Cross-linking. Microfibrils formed spontaneously by tropocollagen can be seen by the electron microscope in the immediate neighborhood of the chondrocyte. These microfibrils have little tensile strength. For collagen to acquire the tensile strength necessary for functioning tissue such as cartilage, a further phenomenon must occur: the formation of covalent bonds or cross-links between adjacent tropocollagen molecules in the microfibrils.

An amine oxidase enzyme catalyzes a reaction by which the terminal amino groups are removed from several of the lysine or hydroxylysine residues of tropocollagen molecules. The resulting aldehydes on two adjacent α-chains undergo an aldo condensation forming a stable bond. When condensation occurs between an aldehyde of one molecule chain and an amino group of lysine or hydroxylysine in the chain of an adjacent tropocollagen molecule (Schiff-base formation), a less stable cross-link results.

It is very probable that the increasing diameter of collagen fibrils observed in articular cartilage under the electron microscope as one proceeds from the surface to the deeper zones represents progressive cross-linking between adjacent microfibrils.

Collagen synthesis and degradation in adult animals normally is very slow, the estimated half-life of collagen being months or years. Collagen fiber formation is complex, and alteration of any stage of synthesis can be due to many factors and often is genetically determined. For example, genetic deficiency of amine oxidase required to form aldehydes results in an increased amount of uncross-linked tropocollagen. This may produce the skeletal deformities and aortic aneurysms and the increased urinary excretion of hydroxyproline characteristic of Marfan's syndrome.[8] Isotopic studies indicate that uncross-linked tropocollagen is degraded much more rapidly than is cross-linked collagen.[26]

MECHANICAL FUNCTION

The mechanical function of collagen is to resist tensile loads.[7] Any change in fiber density or orientation is reflected in tensile characteristics. Specimens of articular cartilage subjected to tensile tests show the following:

The surface layer is the stiffest. Although these fibers are of small diameter, they are closely aggregated into bundles, with almost no intervening space, and are horizontally disposed. The density of collagen per unit volume is highest at this level.

The deepest layer is the least stiff. Fibrils increase in diameter, are widely spaced, and are oriented haphazardly. The density per unit volume is lowest at this level.

Cartilage resists greater loads when applied in a vertical direction than when applied at 90°. The stiffness and strength of normal articular cartilage therefore depends on surface collagen orientation and density, depth from

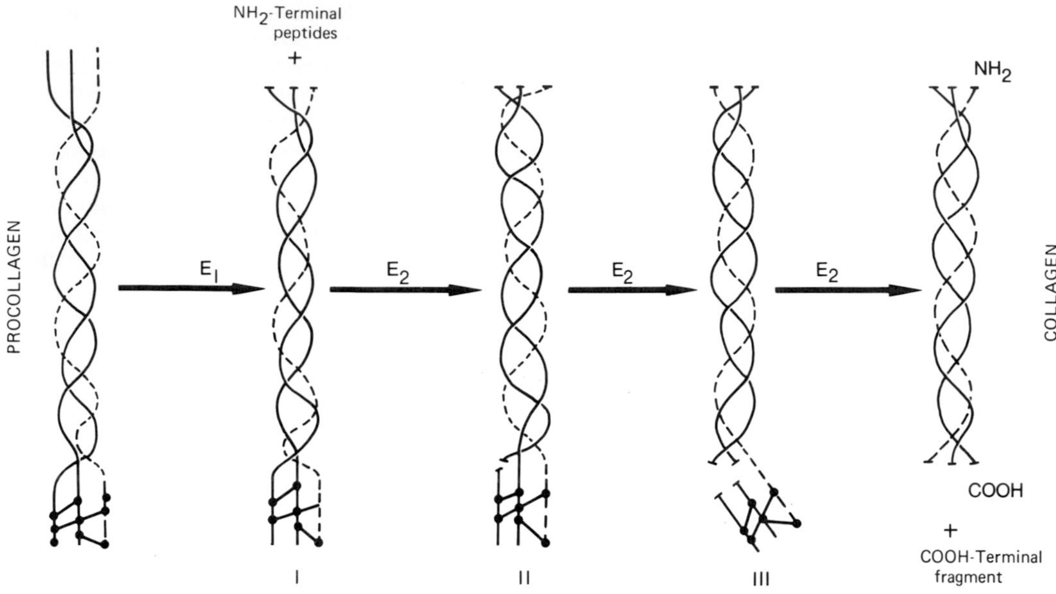

FIG. 7-7. The current proposed model of conversion of procollagen to collagen. The component polypeptide chains are characteristic for the tissue source. Skin and bone collagens consist of two α1(I)-chains and one α2-chain. Collagen from cartilage is composed of three identical chains called α1(II), which are similar in molecular weight to α1(I)-chains but have a different primary structure as well as increased hydroxylation of lysine residues and greater glycosylation of hydroxylysines. The procollagen molecule contains both NH_2- and COOH-terminal nonhelical domains, which are not present in collagen. Both of these regions must therefore be excised during conversion of procollagen to collagen. Intact procollagen with a molecular weight of approximately 450,000 and consisting of two pro-α1-chains (—) and one pro-α2-chain (— — —) contains both NH_2- and COOH-terminal extensions. This molecule is first cleaved by enzyme E_1 to a 390,000-dalton trimer (intermediate I) lacking NH_2-terminal peptides. Sites of cleavage are indicated by bars perpendicular to each chain. Subsequent stepwise scission in a disulfide-bonded COOH-terminal domain by enzyme E_2 produces intermediate II and III and eventually yields a 285,000-dalton collagen molecule with release of a 105,000-dalton disulfide-bonded fragment. This molecule presumes cleavage of a minimum of six peptide bonds per procollagen molecule. Interchain disulfide bonds are indicated as (●—●). (Davidson JM, McEneany LSG, Bornstein P: Intermediates in the limited proteolytic conversion of procollagen to collagen. Biochemistry 14:5188, 1975)

the articular surface, and amount of cartilage degeneration in surrounding areas.

NUTRITION OF CARTILAGE

Cartilage has no blood vessels except for an occasional one passing through to other tissues.

Articular cartilage obtains its nutrition by diffusion from synovial fluid, as evidenced by articular cartilage, which remains viable whereas the underlying bone is avascular (*e.g.*, after a fracture of the femoral neck), and by a cartilaginous fragment, which when separated from the articular surface survives and may increase its dimensions.

Autoradiographic studies demonstrate that the cartilage of the growing immature epiphysis receives nutrients not only from synovial fluid but also from the subchondral vessels.[4,7] After the epiphyseal growth plate has closed, the synovial fluid appears to be the only source of nutrition. Diffusion through the cartilage is enhanced by joint movement.

WATER CONTENT

Most of the 70% of water in articular cartilage is loosely bound in the form of a proteoglycan-collagen gel and is freely exchangeable with the synovial fluid.[21] Theoretically, since cartilage gel is hyperhydrated, the water content is important in maintaining cartilage resiliency and lubrication of the articular surface.[12,28] If a disease state is associated with reduction in water content, these properties may be altered, leading to impaired joint function.

The nature of water binding in cartilage is unknown. The gel-forming property is not exclusively that of the proteoglycan, because the water content of osteoarthritic cartilage, in which the proteoglycan content is reduced, is greater and more firmly bound.[20]

METABOLIC STUDIES OF ARTICULAR CARTILAGE

The metabolism of articular cartilage can be studied by histochemical, biochemical, and radionuclide methods.

HISTOCHEMICAL

The acid mucopolysaccharides are selectively stained by cationic dyes (*e.g.*, safranin-O). The intensity of red color produced by this orthochromatic dye is approximately proportional to the content of acid mucopolysaccharides (GAG) in the matrix.[49]

BIOCHEMICAL

Cartilage can be assayed for deoxyribonucleic acid (DNA), hexosamine, and hydroxyproline (indicator of collagen content).[42,48,50]

RADIONUCLIDES

Slices of cartilage can be incubated with radioisotopes and assayed for radioactivity.[18]

Thymidine-^3H (tritiated thymidine) is a specific indicator of DNA synthesis.[44] The concentration of DNA used in the formation of chromosomes is an index of cell division.

Glycine-^{14}C is a precursor mainly of protein of PPS and of the polypeptide chain of collagen.

Cytidine-^3H is a precursor of both ribonucleic acid (RNA) and DNA, but most of the isotope will enter RNA metabolism. Its incorporation can therefore be equated with nucleic acid synthesis.[46]

$^{35}SO_4$ is a specific tracer of polysaccharide synthesis. It can be traced through the chondrocyte into the matrix.[43]

Labeled proline, after intra-articular injection of ^{3}H-proline, can be recovered from the matrix as labeled hydroxyproline, or it can be identified in autoradiographs. It is an index of the rate of synthesis of collagen.[47]

BASIC PRINCIPLES

From such studies, the following premises have been established;[45]

Chondrocytes from mature articular cartilage do not replicate their DNA or undergo mitotic division, except under conditions of acute or chronic trauma.

The distribution and count of cells are relatively unchanged with aging.

The chemical compositon of the matrix is relatively unchanged, except that the proportion of keratan sulfate to chondroitin sulfate is increased.

The synthesis and breakdown of proteoglycan of articular cartilage take place at a rapid rate throughout life.

As an example of applying these methods to the study of articular cartilage under pathologic conditions, osteoarthritic cartilage shows the following changes:

Significant decrease in polysaccharide content of the matrix without change in collagen

Increase in rate of synthesis of polysaccharide and concomitant increased degradative activity[40,41]

Cell replication proceeding at rates in excess of normal mature articular cartilage. RNA synthesis is unchanged, but DNA synthesis, an indicator of cellular reproduction, is markedly increased.

BIOMECHANICAL FUNCTIONS OF ARTICULAR CARTILAGE

The two main functions of articular cartilage are mechanical load carriage and lubrication. Cartilage experiences compressive stresses normal to the articular surface and tensile stresses mainly parallel to the surface. Until the compressive and tensile properties of cartilage are fully known, the magnitude of these stresses cannot be accurately calculated or the method of load carriage understood. The following discussion of necessity is abbreviated, since the concepts are derived from highly specialized histologic, physiochemical, biomechanical and clinical investigations.

DEFORMATION UNDER LOAD

The stiffness of any area of articular cartilage is highly important to its mechanical functions and can be determined from indentation tests. When load is applied to articular cartilage, an instantaneous deformation develops and is followed by a time-dependent creep phase, in which the indentation increases continuously with time, although a constant load is maintained.[56] During the creep phase, indentation increases rapidly at first and then gradually slows until at 30 minutes the rate of increase is very slow, reaching an equilibrium at 1 hour. When the load is removed, cartilage recovers its original thickness as a result of an initial instantaneous (elastic) recovery followed by a time-dependent recovery phase (reimbibition of water) (Fig. 7-8). The degree of indentation normally varies topographically over a single articular surface. For example, in the femoral head, maximal cartilage stiffness is situated in a banded area over the cephalad area of the femoral head extending around to the anterior and posterior aspects. The band is located diametrically opposite to the similarly contoured acetabular cartilage. The softest cartilage is located about the foveal margin. When the cartilage is fibrillated, or in the softened cartilage area immediately about the fibrillated degenerated cartilage, the degree of indentation is greater than that recorded for normal cartilage.

Cartilage is considered to display an elastic or "spring-like" deformation within 2 seconds after application of a load. Approximately 90% or more of the instantaneous deformation is instantaneously recoverable when the load is quickly removed. During the normal walking cycle, the duration of the applied load is between 0.5 and 1.0 second, and peak loads are applied for less than 0.5 seconds.[53]

The first stage of instantaneous deformation causes a change in contour but not in volume and results from a bulk movement of the matrix and collagen fibers simultaneously rather than from a flow of water through the matrix. During the second stage, cartilage deforms increasingly with passage of time even though the applied pressure is held constant. This is known as "creep" and is related to the flow of water through the matrix. The magnitude of deformation of the cartilage at a given time after application of the compressive load is governed by the magnitude of the applied pressure, elastic stresses in the collagen fiber mesh, permeability of the matrix, and the Donnan osmotic pressure of the proteoglycan gel in the matrix.

The time-dependent compression and recovery of cartilage are closely related to the flow of water through the matrix colloid gel. The expression of water from the cartilage proceeds gradually and continuously with time. Water is expressed from the matrix when the magnitude of the applied load exceeds the osmotic pressure of the matrix colloid. As the load is removed, reimbibition of water is gradual and is governed mainly by the Donnan osmotic pressure.

TENSILE PROPERTIES

Stiffness and strength of articular cartilage, when loaded in tension in planes parallel to the articular surface, are closely related to the extent to which the collagen fibers are orientated parallel to the direction of tension. Collagen fibers are the main tension-resistant elements. Tensile forces are secondary effects of compression and develop parallel to the articular surface. The predominant direction of surface collagen fibers coincides with the maximal surface tensile strains produced by compression of cartilage in a plane perpendicular to its surface.[54]

The tensile stiffness decreases with increasing depth below the articular surface. At the surface zone, the predominant orientation of the collagen fibers follows a direction parallel to the main tensile forces and a definite cleavage pattern. When a sharp awl pierces the articular surface, elongate cracks (instead of round holes) form a systematic pattern over the joint surface. This cleavage pattern indicates the orientation of the collagen fibers in the superficial zone as well as the direction of maximal tensile strains produced by both friction and compression. However, the tensile strains produced by friction are extremely small because of the very low coefficient of friction between cartilaginous articular surfaces.[51] The tensile forces parallel to the articular surface are produced largely as secondary effects of compression.

In areas of visually normal cartilage adjacent to an area of fibrillation, the tensile strength of the surface

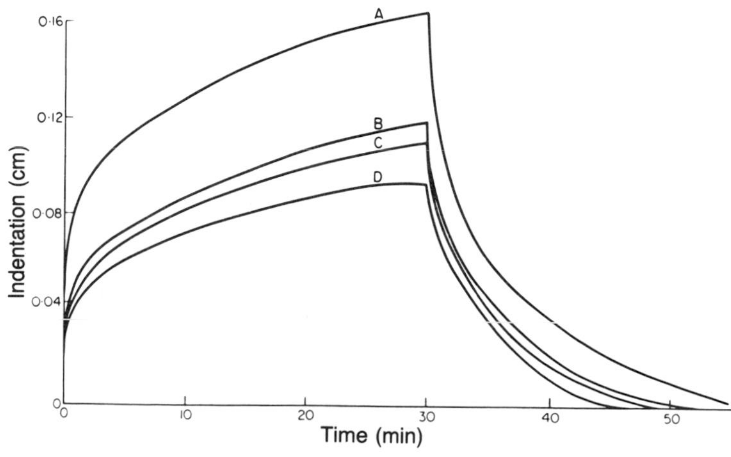

FIG. 7-8. Indentation/time and recovery/time curves for four areas of cartilage on the human femoral head. (Kempson GE, Freeman MA, Swanson SA: Patterns of cartilage stiffness on normal and degenerate human femoral heads. J Biomech 4:239, 1971)

collagen fibers is decreased. Areas remote from such lesions retain their tensile properties.[52]

In normal cartilage, the tensile stiffness depends to a significant extent on the collagen fiber content as well as on the arrangement of the fibers. There is no relationship between tensile stiffness and proteoglycan content.

RESPONSE OF CARTILAGE TO DYNAMIC, CYCLICALLY APPLIED LOADS

In ordinary walking, the articular cartilage in the hip joint is subjected to a load that increases from approximately zero to some five times the body weight at a frequency of approximately 60 times per minute.[55]

Cartilage acts as an energy absorber. The dynamically applied load produces stresses carried partly by mechanical forces in the matrix and partly by liquid pressures. The peak force transmitted by cartilage is at least one-tenth that of cancellous bone. However, cartilage, cancellous bone, and periarticular soft tissues all contribute to force attenuation. Cartilage, because it is so thin, makes a negligible contribution to the reduction of peak forces. Nevertheless, if it were absent, the contact stresses might rise to the point of bone failure stress.

Recovery of deformation when load is removed is greatly expedited by oscillation of the joint. This may be explained by the ability of the temporarily unloaded portion of the cartilage surface to reimbibe fluid and hence to recover.

MECHANICAL FUNCTIONS OF ARTICULAR CARTILAGE

LOAD CARRIAGE

Load carriage is the capacity of cartilage to sustain the loads to which it is subjected without failing mechanically, to compensate for the gross incongruities and small asperities at the subchondral bone surface, and to reduce stresses to the subchondral bone from dynamic loads.[59] Since the bone surfaces do not mate perfectly, stress concentrations are the natural result if the bones make direct contact under load. Cartilage compensates for these bony incongruities by increasing the area of contact in the joint, thereby reducing the contact pressures on the bone (the nominal contact pressure, or stress, on the bone being equal to the load applied to the joint divided by the projected contact area). To compensate for bone incongruities, cartilage must be more deformable than bone and the Poisson's ratio should be such that the lateral expansion under a compressive load should result in a contact area at least as large as that which would result from bone-to-bone contact. If cartilage is to fulfill this function during an activity in which a load is applied and then removed repeatedly, such as normal walking, it is advantageous for cartilage to recover a significant proportion of its deformation during the unloaded phase (*i.e.*, to deform almost elastically so that it retains its thickness throughout a period of repetitive loading).

Most weight-bearing joints are subjected to loads applied rapidly—high loads of short duration. Cartilage protects the bones from these stresses by acting as a shock absorber (*i.e.*, damping and attenuating dynamic loads by deforming a substantial extent in a viscoelastic fashion). Therefore, cartilage should be strong, more deformable than bone, and, from the standpoint of load spreading, elastic. From the standpoint of damping, however, it should be viscoelastic.

Two components contribute to load carriage by cartilage: proteoglycans, by retaining water in the matrix and by regulating its flow, and collagen, by resisting tensile forces within the matrix and by retaining the proteoglycans in place.

The Donnan osmotic pressure generated by the proteoglycans is responsible mainly for the imbibition of water by cartilage, as a result of which the tissue swells and thereby recovers its original volume after a period of prolonged loading. This tendency to swell is limited by the stiffness and strength of the collagen fibers, which are subjected to increasing tensile forces as the swelling increases.[60] The swelling pressure developed mainly by the matrix, as a result of the Donnan osmotic pressure of the proteoglycans, is balanced by the tensile stresses in the collagen fibers when the tissue is not loaded.[65] The net inner osmotic pressure of cartilage has been estimated to be of the order of 1.0 kg/sq (14.5 lb/cm/sq in, 10^5N/sq m).[66]

Articular cartilage is loaded predominantly perpendicular to its surface. The applied compressive load theoretically generates tensile stresses in all directions within the matrix, wherever collagen fibers are distributed.

Since a load applied to cartilage generates a fluid pressure within the matrix, the proteoglycans influence the response of the tissue to the compressive load; the proteoglycans are hydrophilic colloids that bind water and acquire a gellike stiffness in the presence of collagen fibrils.[52] The water is held by the proteoglycans mainly as a result of the Donnan osmotic pressure, and these macromolecules contribute to the low permeability of cartilage, which retards the rate at which water is expressed from the loaded tissue. Therefore, the proteoglycans are a main determinant for the compressive properties of cartilage, because the response of the tissue to compression depends upon the fluid flow in the matrix. Since fluid flow is time dependent, the mechanical behavior of cartilage in compression depends on the length of time for which the load is applied and on whether or not it is applied cyclically.

RESPONSE OF CARTILAGE TO SINGLE APPLICATION OF LOAD OF SHORT DURATION

When a load is applied to cartilage, the fluid pressure within the proteoglycan gel in the matrix must rise immediately and, in the absence of fluid flow, there must be a simultaneous increase in the elastic stresses in the collagen. The net pressure within the cartilage matrix then tends to drive the fluid out of the matrix because it exceeds the osmotic pressure. Water, therefore, tends to be expressed from the matrix. However, the volume of water actually lost within a given period depends on the permeability of cartilage and the length of the flow path. The permeability, which is low even in unloaded cartilage, decreases further as the cartilage is compressed. Loads that are applied for a very short time can therefore be expected to produce negligible fluid flow, even when greater pressures are applied to small, isolated pieces of cartilage. Deformation of cartilage therefore is due to a change in its shape, not in its volume. The larger the loaded area of cartilage, the longer is the time required to express a signficiant quantity of water from it, since, if water is to leave the loaded area, it must flow for substantial distances through the loaded matrix. Thus, the length of the flow path increases with the size of the loaded area. A single step in the walking cycle (in which the articular cartilage of the hip encounters a load of 1000 lbf [4.4 kN, 450 kgf] for only 0.2 sec) causes a loss of only a negligible amount of water, provided the area of contact is large and the pressure is uniformly distributed. However, studies on load distribution within the hip suggest that uniform distribution of pressures is unlikely.

If little water is expressed by loads of brief duration, the cartilage must behave essentially in an elastic fashion during each step of the walking cycle, the applied load causing a rise in the hydrostatic pressure in the proteoglycan gel and a net increase in the tensile stresses in the collagen fibers. On removal of the load, the stressed collagen recoils, causing the matrix to recover its original shape, and the fluid pressure falls to its unloaded value (*i.e.*, the pressure generated by the proteoglycan moiety).

Substanial instantaneous deformation occurs in cartilage when it is loaded due to bulk movement of proteoglycan and water within the loaded region, but without loss of water.

RESPONSE OF CARTILAGE TO SINGLE APPLICATION OF LOAD OF LONG DURATION

When load is applied, instantaneous deformation takes place. As load continues unchanged and pressure within the matrix is maintained, there is a gradual reduction in the volume of the loaded tissue (gradual deformation) as water is driven from the loaded area. As water leaves the matrix, the matrix proteoglycans become more concentrated and thereby increase the osmotic pressure, which tends to draw the water into the matrix. Thus, the rate at which water is expressed from the matrix can be expected to decrease with the elapse of time until the rate finally reaches zero. At this time, no further deformation occurs in the matrix. The new increased fluid pressures in the matrix then balance the applied load plus the new elastic stresses in the collagen.

On removal of the load, the fluid pressure in the previously loaded region of the matrix falls to a value below that in unloaded cartilage. Relieved of tensile stresses, the collagen fibers recover and effect an instantaneous but partial recovery of the total deformation, due to change of shape primarily but not of volume. The osmotic pressure, and possibly the elastic recoil of collagen fibers, causes of gradual imbibition of water until complete hydration and recovery of the original thickness is achieved.

Under a constant load, after instantaneous deformation, the rate of deformation and water loss falls steadily until an equilibrium value is reached. Upon removal of the load, most of the recovery is immediate, but eventually complete recovery is attained.

RESPONSE OF CARTILAGE TO CYCLICAL LOADING

During each cycle, the load is applied briefly and the cartilage behaves elastically. However briefly the load is applied, a small quantity of water is expressed from the matrix, and reimbibition of this water takes a finite time. If a second load is applied before the matrix has fully reimbibed the water lost during the first loading period, incomplete recovery occurs at the end of the first cycle. The unrecovered deformations occurring during consecutive loading cycles summate, and the total unrecovered deformation steadily increases as cyclical loading is continued.

However, at some point the increased concentration of proteoglycans and hence the osmotic pressure increases the tendency of the water to be held in the matrix. The deformation previously unrecoverable is then taken up with an elastically recoverable instantaneous deformation superimposed at each load application.

The theory of additive unrecoverable deformation while load cycling continues unabated is not universally accepted. It has been stated that at normal walking frequencies no permanent residual deformation of cartilage occurs and that the recovery curve is an exact inverted image of the creep curve.[73]

TENSILE STRESSES IN COLLAGEN OF CARTILAGE

Fluid pressures within the matrix generate tensile stresses in collagen fibers. In the superficial zone of cartilage, the fibers are oriented parallel to the surface and provide considerable tensile strength and rigidity on this zone. The four possible ways in which such stresses can be generated are by friction, ploughing, compression, and fluid pressure.

Tensile stresses at the articular surface are mainly parallel to the surface and are chiefly the result of compression where the radius of the area of contact is small compared with the radii of curvature of the two bodies in contact. The Hertz principle applies to two elastic spheres in contact and states that the principal stress (p_2) becomes tensile at a distance equal to the radius of the contact area measured along the curved surface profile. The maximum value of this tensile stress is approximately $0.2 \times p_{max.}$ ($p_{max.} = (3/2) \times p_{mean}$).

The stress distribution in the intermediate and deep zones is different from that in the superficial zone. When the surface of cartilage is loaded, the fluid within the matrix, in attempting to escape laterally, encounters resistance of the collagen network, generating tensile stresses parallel to the articular surface. The magnitude and direction of these forces depend upon the maximum load application and the area of load application. Since the position of the latter varies widely throughout the range of movement of the joint, the magnitude and direction of forces can be expected to vary. Thus, the tensile stresses occur in different directions, hence the need for a random orientation of the collagen network in the intermediate and deep zones.

The deepest zone of collagen fibers shows a tendency toward perpendicular orientation, and it is presumed that this collagen has the additional function of tethering the matrix to the subchondral bone.

RELATIONSHIP OF CARTILAGE-REDUCING STRESSES TO BONE

The absence of articular cartilage leads to a rise in contact stress in the subchondral bone, which in the hip has been calculated as a threefold increase.

The presence of cartilage in the hip joint results in a contact stress between the acetabulum and the femoral head equal to approximately half the ultimate compressive strength of the cancellous bone. In contrast, if, without cartilage, bone-to-bone contact occurred, the contact stress could be nearly twice the ultimate compressive strength of bone. Such stresses can cause fatigue failure in isolated trabeculae in the cancellous bone.

In walking the rate of load application is high because the total cycle time from heel-strike to toe-off is only about 0.5 second. Such rapidly applied loads can cause high transient stresses, which can be reduced by cartilage if the tissues are able to attenuate dynamic loads. Since cartilage behaves almost elastically in the steady state during walking, the force with which it resists deformation is proportional to the force causing the deformation. Moreover, cartilage is more deformable than bone and therefore can be expected to reduce the rate of application of the load more gradually than does bone, or, in other words, attenuate the peak dynamic stresses that can otherwise be encountered in the bone. However, cartilage is so thin that its capacity to reduce peak transient stresses is small compared with the attenuation contributed by the bone. One must conclude that cartilage does not attenuate dynamic loads significantly in a joint during life.

The dampening of a dynamic load, as distinct from its attenuation, depends upon viscous deformation in the loaded material. If little viscous deformation occurs when the cartilage is loaded for a short period, the tissue correspondingly provides little dampening.

EFFECT OF PHYSIOLOGICAL VARIATION

To fulfill its function of reducing contact stresses in a loaded joint, cartilage must possess a stiffness intermediate between zero and a value equal to that of bone. There are variations in topographical stiffness over any single articular surface. Such variations in the stiffness are not expected to affect the ability of the tissue to reduce the contact stresses applied to the bone because these variations are small in relation to the difference in stiffness between cartilage and bone.

EFFECT OF PATHOLOGIC VARIATION

The total absence of cartilage leads to an excessive increase in the contact stresses on the bone. Initially, cartilage becomes softer and thinner while it is gradually and eventually completely lost.

Experimentally, when a hip joint displaying severe cartilage fibrillation and ulceration is subjected to 2000 load cycles, irrecoverable deformation occurs both in cartilage and in subchondral bone. When the cartilage is removed, the bone fails even more extensively.[71]

Softening of the cartilage is equivalent to thinning, since the softer the tissue the thinner it is when loaded. Cartilage thickness must be reduced to at least 25% of normal value before alteration in bone stress is evident. Even after a physiologic loading sequence, fatigue failure in subchondral bone occurs in the presence of total loss or severe fibrillation.

When cartilage fibrillates, it becomes not only thin but also soft, and the softer it is the thinner it becomes when loaded. Thus, loaded, fibrillated cartilage is abnormally thin even though the unloaded tissue is of normal thickness. Clinically, radiologic bone changes may be absent even though the joint space is much diminished, but they appear as soon as it is reduced markedly or lost.

STRENGTH OF NORMAL CARTILAGE

The strength of a material is defined as the minimum stress at which fracture occurs, such stresses including tensile, compressive, or shear stresses, or a combination of these. The strength also depends upon whether a load is applied statically or dynamically. In the case of a dynamic, repeated load, fracture can occur at a load value that is lower than the static load required to cause fracture. In general, the lower the applied load, the larger the number of load cycles required to cause fracture. This kind of behavior is known as fatigue, and fatigue-prone material may be considered as being weaker when it is subjected to a cyclically applied load than when it is subjected to a load that is applied only once. Cartilage may be considered to be fatigue-prone.

MECHANICAL FAILURE IN NORMAL CARTILAGE

Structural failure primarily affects the collagen network that is overstretched in tension. A single load must be of great magnitude (*e.g.*, a violent impact) to produce tensile stresses sufficiently large to fracture the network; in other words, the resulting pressure in the aqueous proteoglycan gel can burst the tissue.

Continuous application of a very high load causes considerable loss of water from the tissue, with consequent large compressive deformation. Such prolonged pressure applied experimentally to a joint causes degeneration of the cartilage and necrosis of chondrocytes.[69] The mechanism of failure of normal articular cartilage in this manner is not yet known.

The collagen network might fracture as a result of a cyclically applied load in tension or in compression. Tensile failure can come about if the "instantaneous" deformations produced in this manner of loading are sufficient to cause fatigue failure. Theoretically, cyclically applied loads of great magnitude, when applied for a long period, can eventually cause the expression of enough water, and hence a sufficiently large deformation, to produce irreversible damages of the cartilage, for the same reasons as those that apply to large, statically applied loads of long duration. This mechanism of failure seems unlikely in life because sufficient water is retained by normal cartilage in such activities as walking.

MECHANICAL FAILURE FROM PROTEOGLYCAN-DEPLETED CARTILAGE

Cartilage that has lost its proteoglycan biologically becomes more deformable than normal. Abnormally large instantaneous deformations probably occur during activities such as walking or by subjecting the collagen network to abnormally large strains. The increase of magnitude of cyclically applied strains can cause fatigue after fewer loading cycles than are necessary to produce fracture in normal cartilage. Moreover, more water is expressed from proteoglycan-depleted cartilage because permeability is increased, with less tendency to reimbibe water because the Donnan osmotic pressure is decreased. The collagen becomes loaded and compressed, and the excessive compressive deformation results in damage to the chondrocytes.

In apparently normal cartilage adjacent to an area of fibrillation, the cartilage is weaker, implying that the collagen fibers may have fractured or that bonds between them have failed. Fibrillation may represent the end result of such progressive tensile failure in the collagen network. The degree of compressive softness and tensile weakness becomes progressively greater across the articular surface as the fibrillated area is approached, until in the fibrillated cartilage itself these changes are extreme.

LUBRICATION

PRINCIPLES OF FRICTION AND LUBRICATION

As one body slides over another, the movement is resisted by a frictional force at the contact surfaces. The ratio of frictional force F to the load or weight W, which presses the two rubbing surfaces together, is called the coefficient of friction μ, that is, $\mu = F/W$. When the joint is at rest, a greater force is usually required to start its movement than to keep it moving at constant velocity. These are referred to as static or sliding frictional forces, respectively.

When two apposing surfaces are unlubricated and slide on each other, friction is the result of interaction of asperities, the minute projections that produce surface roughness. The highest apposing asperities contact each other and are sheared off as surfaces slide on one another. The coefficient of friction of sliding dry surfaces depends on the shear strength of the contact junctions and the extent of the area of contact; as the load is increased, the area of contact increases and friction correspondingly increases. Typical dry coefficients of friction are about 0.1 to 0.3 for plastic on plastic and about 0.3 to 0.8 for metal on metal (Fig. 7-9).

Lubrication reduces frictional resistance and wear of bearing surfaces by interposing a substance that keeps them apart.[28,57]

TYPES OF LUBRICATION

When a fluid is interposed between sliding surfaces, either fluid lubrication or boundary lubrication, or both, takes place.

Fluid

A film of fluid completely separates the opposing bearing surfaces, and resistance to motion arises from the viscosity of the fluid (Fig. 7-10). When the bearing is loaded, the fluid film is supplied by various mechanisms.

Hydrostatic Lubrication. The film of lubricant is maintained under pressure by an external pump. This mechanism is especially suited to oscillating bearings and heavily loaded bearings in low-speed applications.

Squeeze-Film Lubrication. The approaching surfaces generate pressure in the lubricant as they squeeze it out of the area of impending contact between them. The resulting pressure keeps the surfaces apart. In cartilage-on-cartilage bearings, a fluid exudes from the cartilage and forms a film in the transient area of impending contact and may be termed the squeeze film.

Hydrodynamic Lubrication. The relative motion of two bearing surfaces forces lubricant in the form of a wedge between the surfaces, keeping them apart. This mechanism requires uninterrupted motion in the same direction to maintain the integrity of the wedge. It is especially effective in high-speed journal bearings.

Most mechanical bearings are lubricated by oil hydrodynamically. However, it is impossible for animal joints to be lubricated in this manner, because animal joints slide slowly and stop at each reversal of motion, preventing the formation of the wedge.[58]

The coefficient of friction in pure fluid lubrication is very low: 0.001 to 0.01. This is never attained, being limited by factors necessary for maintaining the fluid film.

In cartilage-on-cartilage bearings, the surfaces are elastic enough so that the lubricant pressure, which is generated by motion under a given load, depresses the surfaces a distance greater than the height of their asperities. Consequently, fewer asperities come in contact, and the fluid film is more easily maintained. This is termed elastohydrodynamic lubrication, a form of fluid lubrication. This concept is not universally accepted.

Boundary

Each bearing surface is coated with a thin layer of molecules that slide on the apposing surface more readily than they are sheared off the underlying one (Fig. 7-11). This is very necessary to lowering the frictional effects of cartilage on cartilage. It ceases to function when loads are excessive. The coefficient of friction of boundary lubrication is typically 0.05 to 0.15. The lubrication of most animal joint bearings involves a combination of fluid and boundary lubrication.

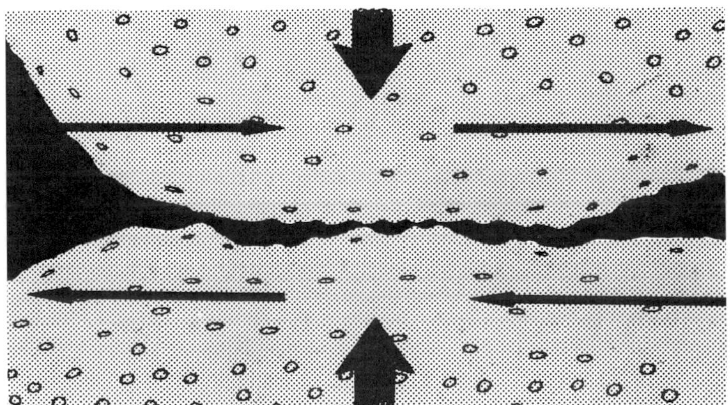

FIG. 7-9. Dry friction. The asperities of the surfaces are in contact and interact. (Radin EL, Paul IL: Response of joints to impact loading. Arthritis Rheum 14:356, 1971)

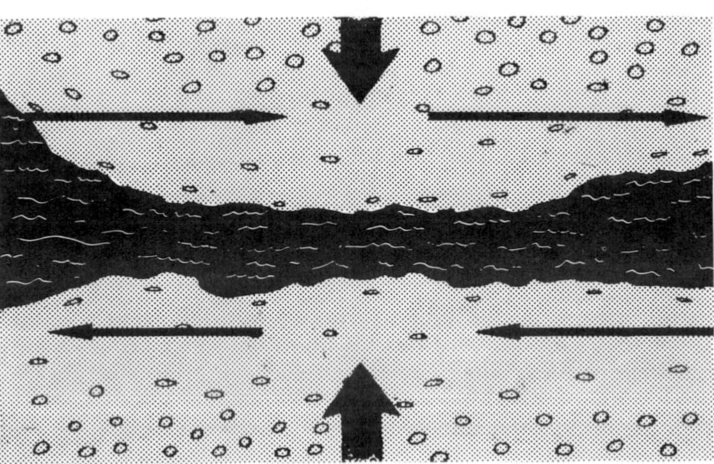

FIG. 7-10. Pure fluid-film lubrication. The fluid film between the surfaces can be maintained by three mechanisms: hydrostatic, squeeze film, or hydrodynamic. (Radin EL, Paul IL: Response of joints to impact loading. Arthritis Rheum 14:356, 1971)

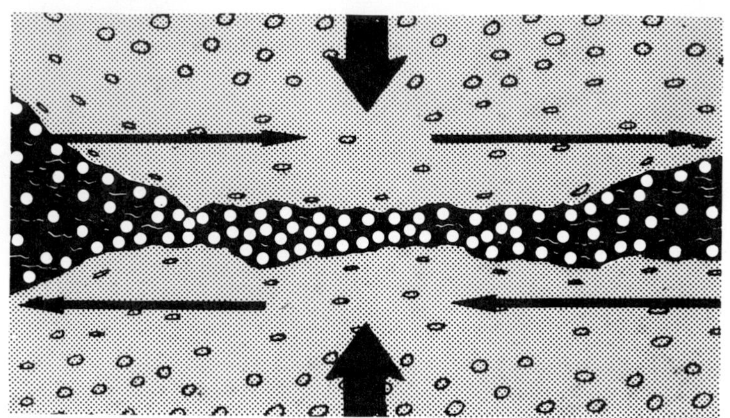

FIG. 7-11. Boundary lubrication. The molecules stick to the surface, keeping them from touching. This acts best in low load situations. Synovial fluid contains a high-molecular-weight glycoprotein that binds to articular cartilage and prevents opposing cartilage surfaces from rubbing against one another. (Radin EL, Paul IL: Response of joints to impact loading. Arthritis Rheum 14:356, 1971)

SYNOVIAL FLUID LUBRICANT PROPERTIES

The component of synovial fluid that provides its viscosity is a hyaluronate, a polysaccharide, sometimes called hyaluronic acid (HA). Viscosity provides the resistance of the fluid itself to shear, so that a less viscous fluid may appear to give a lower coefficient of friction for a given fluid thickness.

Synovial fluid possesses a characteristic property, thixotropy, attributed to its large hyaluronate molecules (*i.e.*, it becomes less viscous as its flow rate, or shear rate, increases). A less viscous fluid will not support as thick a fluid film as will a more viscous fluid. Therefore, hyaluronate molecules, the source of synovial fluid viscosity, are not effective as lubricants for cartilage-on-cartilage bearings. Boundary lubrication is necessary, and this is provided by a hyaluronate-free glycoprotein fraction of synovial fluid. The glycoprotein molecules form a firm coating over the cartilage surfaces and act independent of viscosity or fluid film. When loading pressures become excessive, the glycoprotein molecules are sheared off, boundary lubrication fails, and another mechanism takes over.

RESISTANCE TO MOTION IN JOINTS

Resistance to motion is the result of stretching of soft tissues (ligaments, muscles, tendons) and of soft tissue frictional resistance (synovium on synovium, synovium on cartilage, cartilage on cartilage).

SYNOVIAL TISSUE LUBRICATION

Hyaluronate molecules adhere firmly to synovial surfaces and provide a boundary type of lubrication that keeps synovial surfaces apart.[55] Synovial tissue lubrication does not depend on viscosity, since viscous solutions without hyaluronate do not adequately lubricate synovial surfaces.

CARTILAGE-ON-CARTILAGE LUBRICATION

The two mechanisms involved are the following:

Boundary lubrication. The coefficient of friction may be as low as 0.001.[28] This is not the effect of hyaluronate; digestion by hyaluronidase does not impair the lubrication efficiency of synovial fluid.[68] A glycoprotein fraction is responsible and can only be destroyed by a proteolytic enzyme.

Fluid films. A fluid film forms on the articular surfaces when cartilage is rubbed against cartilage under load in the presence of any lubricant.

In the early phases of loading, fluid is trapped in the existing depressions in the surface of cartilage. The cartilage surface under load, because of its elasticity, undergoes deformation (plowing), creating a depression narrower at its periphery than at its center, trapping the fluid within it so that squeeze-film lubrication occurs.

Compressed articular cartilage weeps fluid, mainly water and small ions, through pores of about 6 nm (60 A).[64] Small pores allow only small molecules to pass, so large molecules of matrix cannot escape or those of synovial fluid enter. This fluid film produces weeping lubrication, a form of hydrostatic lubrication in which the interstitial fluid of hydrated articular cartilage flows out onto its surface when a load is applied to it. The cartilage acts as a self-pressurizing sponge; when the pressure is released, the fluid flows back into the cartilage. Weeping probably occurs beyond the area of impending contact, where counteracting pressure is lower. This mechanism has been termed self-pressurized hydrostatic lubrication (Fig. 7-12).[63]

The hydrostatic pressure built up in the interstitial fluid in cartilage during loading counteracts the pressure in the lubricant, which has been trapped in the area of deformation at the surface. This prevents lubricant from entering the pores in the cartilage. It has been suggested that water from trapped lubricant enters the cartilage, and the hyaluronate molecules left behind become con-

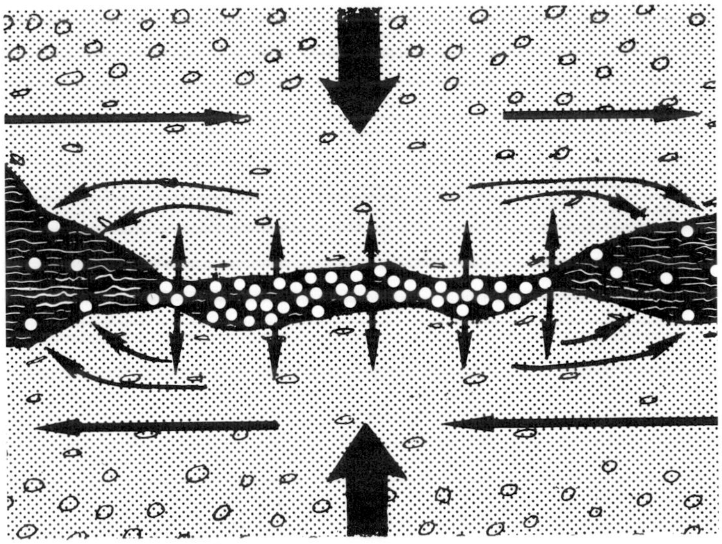

FIG. 7-12. "Weeping" or self-pressurized hydrostatic lubrication. As cartilage is compressed, fluid is forced out in the regions peripheral to the zone of impending contact. Because this fluid flows out only with some difficulty, significant hydrostatic pressures are built up within the cartilage. This pressure traps the fluid caught between the cartilage surfaces; the trapped film keeps the surfaces from touching. The mechanism works best under high load situations. When the load is removed, fluid is resorbed into the cartilage. (Radin EL, Paul IL: Response of joint to impact loading. Arthritis Rheum 14:356, 1971)

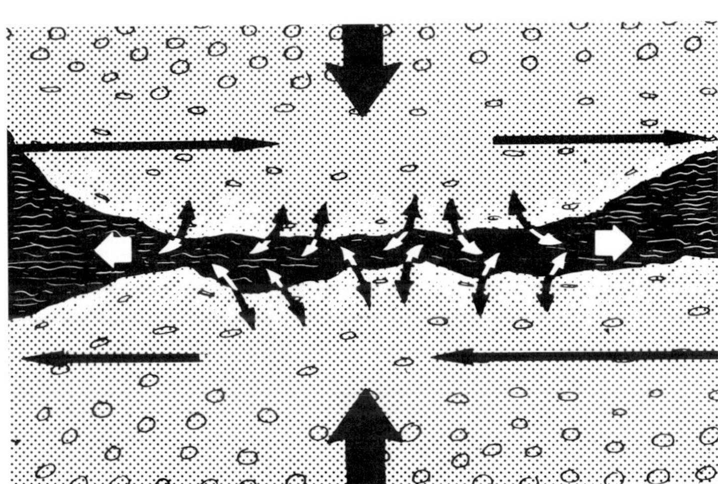

FIG. 7-13. Boosted lubrication. Water from trapped lubricant enters the cartilage, and the hyaluronate and glycoprotein molecules become concentrated and enhance lubrication. (Radin EL, Paul IL: Response of joints to impact loading. Arthritis Rheum 14:356, 1971)

centrated and supposedly enhance lubrication (boosted lubrication).[72]

When cartilage loses its elasticity, weeping is lessened and frictional resistance and wear are increased. In normal animal joints, the coefficient of friction decreases with increasing load. This has been explained by weeping and by boosted lubrication (Fig. 7-13).[61]

FACTORS AFFECTING ARTICULAR CARTILAGE

HYDROCORTISONE ARTHROPATHY

Frequently repeated intra-articular injection of corticosteroids is deleterious to articular cartilage.[77,103,105,106] It causes loss of proteoglycan and as a result the cartilage loses it hyaline luster and becomes soft and fibrillated. Progressive joint degeneration is said to occur, although this may be difficult to establish in an individual instance in which deterioration is already taking place. Further, the question of whether the effects are temporary and cartilage integrity is restored has not been answered. Cystic areas of degeneration within the middle zone of cartilage matrix have been described, but these findings have been questioned as representing vascular spaces.[94]

When the experimental immature animal is given daily corticosteroids, either intra-articular or intramuscular, the following effects are noted:[104]

The surface of the articular cartilage loses its smooth translucent appearance and becomes fibrillated. The loss of matrix exposes unsupported collagen fibers which appear horizontally disposed.

Chondrocytes fail to proliferate and do not mature to become hypertrophic and clustered or arranged in longitudinal columns. As a result, the pattern of subchondral ossification is lost.

Intracytoplasmic metabolic processes are suppressed. The incorporation of glycine-^{3}H into cartilage matrix is decreased, indicating reduced protein synthesis.[98] Uptake[35] of S is suppressed, indicating reduced synthesis of proteoglycan. RNA granules are reduced.

Glycogen and lipids accumulate within the cartilage cells.

Neutral glycoproteins accumulate (are not actively removed).

There is progressive diminution of intracytoplasmic organelles (endoplasmic reticulum, mitochondria, Golgi apparatus).[76]

There is linear decrease of proteoglycan content.

There is an insignificant diminution of collagen content (as indicated by hydroxyproline content) in spite of the reduced production of collagen. This is explained by the long half-life (300 days) of collagen.[76]

Daily systemically administered doses of corticosteroids, such as the large daily doses required in the treatment of lupus erythematosus, cause a progressive decline of matrix synthesis, exposing the collagen fibers that by themselves are unsuited to withstand the normal stresses to which articular cartilage is subjected (Fig. 7-14 and 7-15). A "biochemical lesion" is produced, with consequent breakdown of articular cartilage and eventual denuding of the subchondral bone. The decrease of proteoglycan synthesis takes place only during the period of the effect of the corticosteroid. The biochemical lesion that follows a single intra-articular injection is

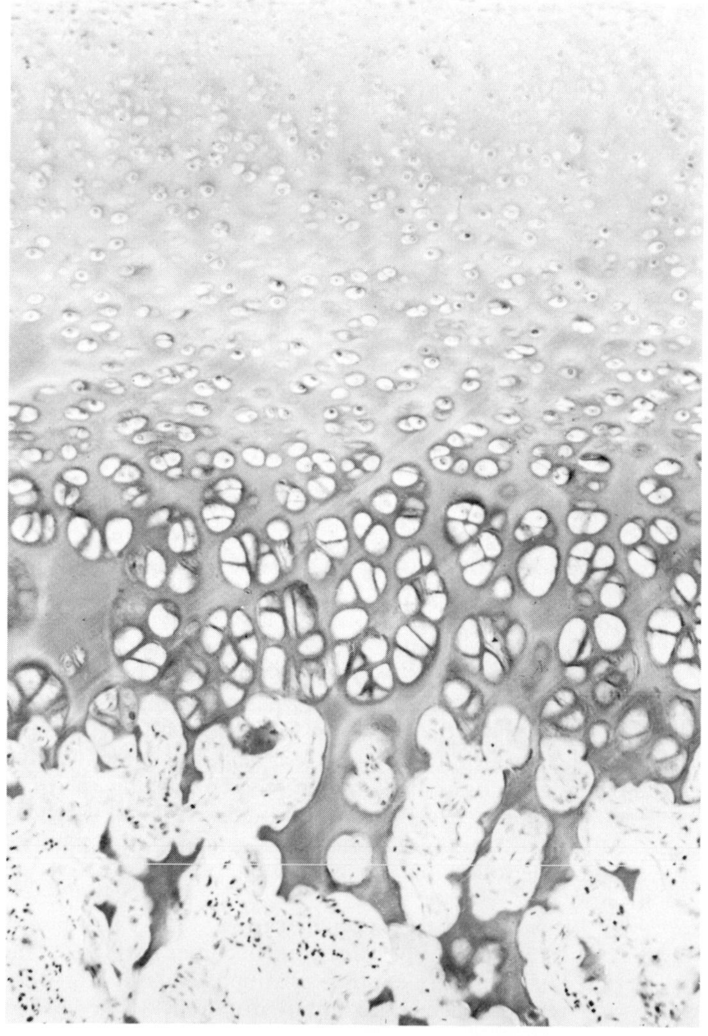

FIG. 7-14. Normal articular cartilage in the experimental animal (rabbit). Alcian blue (*p*H 2.5) stains the acid sulfomucins of the matrix and the calcified matrix between the hypertrophic cells. The calcified matrix is remodeled by osteoclasts, while osteoblasts lay down osteoid and bone to give the typical dentate appearance of subchondral ossification. (× 160) (Shaw NE, Lacey E: The influence of corticosteroids on normal and papain-treated articular cartilage in the rabbit. J Bone Joint Surg 55B:197, 1973)

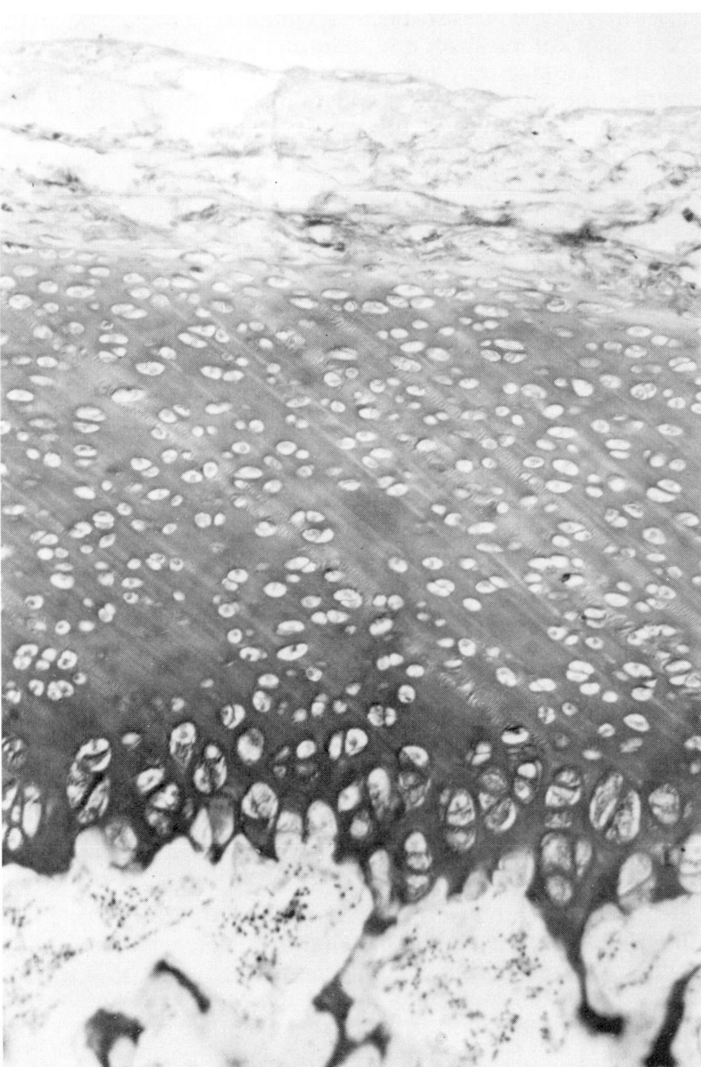

FIG. 7-15. Articular cartilage after 13 daily intramuscular injections of cortisone. Fibrillation is seen at the surface. PPS synthesis is suppressed as indicated by retention of glycogen granules and reduction of RNA within the cells and reduction of ^{35}S uptake. The acid sulfomucins seen in this section represent a residual. Hypertrophic cells are few, and subchondral trabeculae are poorly organized in comparison with the control animal. (Alcian blue *p*H 2.5, × 160) (Shaw NE, Lacey E: The influence of corticosteroids on normal and papain-treated articular cartilage in the rabbit. J Bone Joint Surg 55B:197, 1973)

gradually reversible over a period of 2 weeks.[99] Therefore, when local intra-articular therapy is indicated, an interval of at least 2 weeks should elapse between injections.

ADMINISTRATION OF PAPAIN

After a single intravenous dose of papain (5 mg/kg), the articular cartilage of the experimental animal shows that alcian blue, which stains acid sulfomucins, fails to stain the cartilage matrix, the loss taking place first from the surface and middle zones and last from the deep zone.[104] After injection of papain into a joint, the cartilage becomes fibrillated and the collagen fibers exposed as shown by staining with van Gieson's picrofuchsin. After a papain injection, a 50-fold increase of chondroitin sulfate occurs in the bloodstream.

Recovery then takes place spontaneously and is completed within 3 weeks. The basophilic material reappears first at the superficial and deep zones, where these regions are exposed to synovial fluid and abundant subchondral capillaries, respectively. Repair of papain damage is prevented by the systemic administration of corticosteroids. Autoradiography shows that labeled sulfate is not incorporated into the articular cartilage.

The fact that corticosteroids decrease the incorporation of glycine-^{3}H into cartilage matrix suggests that failure of recovery is due to decreased protein synthesis.[98]

CONTINUOUS COMPRESSION

Continuous compression of cartilage against cartilage, even when transmitted through a fluid-film lubricant, causes irreparable pressure necrosis within a few days.[69,109] Continuing compression and deformation of an area of articular cartilage may prevent nutritive elements from entering the surface pores and diffusing through the interstitial tissue. When this occurs in the immature epiphysis, it may interfere with epiphyseal growth and may produce a surface defect that is a starting point for the development of degenerative arthritis. Simple immobilization of a joint in a forced position causes necrosis within 6 days in the experimental animal. The extent of the lesion varies with the duration of compression. Pressure necrosis of articular cartilage is difficult to detect early because it is painless and occult. The three degrees of damage follow:

Grade I. Superficial necrosis. Gross appearance: loss of normal luster and translucency; cartilage yellowish white and soft. Microscopic appearance: superficial and transitional zones involved; loss of nuclear staining in chrondrocytes

Grade II. Partial thickness loss. Gross appearance: partial loss of cartilage and blister formation in center of lesion. Microscopic appearance: loss of nuclear staining in all layers; disappearance of superficial and transitional zones (liquefaction?); hypertrophy of subchondral bone

Grade III. All layers involved. Gross appearance: full thickness loss of cartilage down to subchondral bone. Microscopic appearance: absence of all cells and matrix; marked hypertrophy of subchrondal bone

Nutrition of cartilage is derived chiefly by diffusion of fluid from the synovial fluid. A solution of proteoglycans, when contained within a collagenous fibrous network so that the macromolecules cannot move, impedes the free flow of water within the tissue when an external force is applied.[101] Although resistance to the flow of interstitial water to a great degree depends upon the concentration, configuration, and entanglement of the proteoglycan molecules, the degree of pressure and the duration of its application are important. Chrondrocytes do not survive deprivation of nutrition as compression continues uninterruptedly over a matter of days. When cartilage is subjected to a physiological compressive load for as little as 12 hours' duration, the open fibrous meshwork of the intermediate zone becomes obliterated, the fibers becoming oriented at right angles to the direction of loading.[96] This appears to impede diffusion of fluid.

TRAUMA AND INFLAMMATION

Many factors are involved in the reaction of a synovial joint to trauma and infection, producing changes in the synovium, synovial fluid, and articular cartilage.

PLASMIN

Synovial fluid may be considered a dialysate of the bloodstream but does not contain macromolecules such as fibrinogen and fibrinolysin unless trauma or inflammation causes increased permeability of synovial blood vessels, which permits these large molecules to enter the joint.[92,93] Fibrinogen disappears quickly from the joint, by proteolytic activity against formed fibrin, resorption by synovial membrane, or both.[88]

Plasmin (fibrinolysin) is a protease resulting from activation of serum plasminogen (profibrinolysin) by diverse means: action of kinases of streptococci and staphylococci; an activator in synovium. Counteracting its proteolytic action is an inhibitor, antiplasmin, contained in synovial fluid. Epsilon aminocaproic acid (EACA) is an effective inhibitor of plasminogen.[95] It is also possible that articular cartilage may contain an inhibitor.

Plasmin acts on cartilage to liberate chondroitin sulfate; the process is stopped by antiplasmin. If sufficient plasminogen is present in the vicinity of cartilage, activation by kinase (*e.g.*, from streptococci and staphylococci) splits off and leaks chondroitin sulfate from the ground substance, with resulting damage to the mechanical properties of cartilage. After intra-articular injection of plasmin, the loss of chondroitin sulfate can be demonstrated within 48 hours.[81] Moreover, chondromucoprotein incubated with human plasmin results in marked reduction of its viscosity.[78] Mack demonstrated that intravenous administration of plasmin or plasminogen causes loss of proteoglycan. Subsequently, however, within a week, the chondrocytes swell and the cartilage is restored to normal.

Leukocytes in synovial fluid are a source of proteolytic enzymes in the vicinity of articular cartilage, particularly during inflammation. The leukocytes contain a protease that acts at neutral *p*H on proteoglycans in the matrix.[91] The degradation of proteoglycans by extracts of cells from rheumatoid synovial fluids is largely due to this enzyme, which may be responsible for initiating the erosion of cartilage in this condition.[111]

SUPPURATIVE INFECTION

Severe cartilaginous destruction is observed in pyogenic nontuberculous arthritis.[81] Both matrix and collagen are broken down on a large scale. Cartilage destruction is most marked at points of maximal contact and pressure.

In vitro studies, using plasmin, demonstrate that the removal of PPS (proteoglycan, chondromucoprotein) by proteolytic enzymes results in no visible alteration of the gross appearance of articular cartilage. Collagen is not disturbed, and this accounts for the preservation of the gross structure, although, because of loss of GAG, the mechanical properties are obviously altered. Collagen loss, therefore, is a necessary requirement for visible structural alteration. *In vivo,* some as yet unknown mechanism is responsible for degradation and removal of collagen, possibly by a combination of enzymatic and mechanical loss.

Collagenase is the only known enzyme capable of degrading undenatured collagen at a neutral *p*H. Presently its properties are being studied from the bone extracts and tissue cultures.[79,83,112] Resorption is induced by vitamin A and inhibited by calcitonin.

Proteolytic enzymes within the lysosomes of chondrocytes and polymorphonuclear leukocytes are no doubt involved in the degradation of collagen but have not been identified.[87]

HEMARTHROSIS

The effect of hemarthrosis on articular cartilage in an otherwise normal synovial joint is controversial. Conflicting reports of experimentally produced hemarthrosis by repeated intra-articular injections of blood continue to appear in the literature. Injections of autologous blood produce a synovial reaction characterized by inflammatory changes (edema, vascular congestion, leukocytic infiltration), deposition of iron, fibroblastic proliferation, and a tendency to pannus formation. Some examples of contradictions with regard to effects on articular cartilage are gross pathologic changes in which cartilage appears yellowish and fibrillated, mainly at points of contact.[89] Surrounding this at areas of least contact, cartilage is overgrown, resulting in an abnormal hypertrophied configuration. Microscopically, fibrillation is observed at areas of contact and pressure. Chondrocytes are rounded, resembling those of the transitional zone, especially adjacent to the area of synovial proliferation. There is clone formation.

However, there may be no pathologic changes.[110] Grossly, the cartilage is smooth, glistening, and translucent. Microscopically, cell morphology and staining of matrix are normal. Metabolic activity is normal as demonstrated by normal incorporation of cytidine-^{3}H (RNA synthesis) and glycine-^{3}H (protein synthesis).

Other studies on immature experimental animals have shown chemical effects by 4 weeks (a reduction of GAG), biomechanical effects by 8 weeks (a reduction of resistance to shear and increased vertical deformation to loading), and gross and microscopic changes by 12 weeks. The intensity of these effects appears to be directly related to the lengthier duration of hemarthrosis and the immaturity of the animal.[80]

The results of numerous investigations on the effect of intrasynovial hemorrhage on articular cartilage in laboratory animals are inconclusive. The studies suggest that a single episode of bleeding into an otherwise healthy joint causes no noteworthy variation in chondrocyte activity or matrix composition. However, repeated hemorrhages may severely compromise chondrocyte function, alter the composition of the matrix, and eventually lead to chondromalacia, osteoarthritis, or destruction of the joint with advancing age.[17] A single episode of intra-articular hemorrhage seems to be of little consequence.

Spontaneous, repeated intrasynovial hemorrhage as seen in bleeding diatheses (*e.g.*, hemophilia) represents a separate category. The combination of repeated hemorrhage, decreased coagulability, chronic trauma, ligamentous laxity, and alteration in the subchondral bone can lead to severe damage to the articular cartilage and subchondral bone structures. The pathogenesis of these changes is obscure.[90,102]

LACERATIVE INJURY

A laceration confined to the substance of the articular cartilage (partial-thickness defect) almost never heals, nor does it lead to osteoarthritis. A full-thickness defect that extends through the underlying bone plate will heal by ingrowth from the underlying marrow spaces of vascular fibroblastic tissue. The fibrous tissue then undergoes progressive chondrification to produce fibrocartilage, firmly welding the wound edges together. At the base of the lesion, new bone forms but stops short of the former cartilage-bone junction.[100]

Immediately following a lacerative injury, an intense biochemical response takes place in the cartilage adjacent to the margins of the defect: increased mitotic activity, increased synthesis of matrix components (as demonstrated by increased uptake of ^{3}H thymidine, $^{35}SO_4$, and ^{3}H glycine).[97] The process is short-lived and ineffectual for healing, and after 1 week the values return to normal.

Enzyme studies show increased levels of cathepsin, β-glucuronidase, hexuronidase, and aryl sulfatase. After 1 week, all values return to normal except aryl sulfatase, which remains transiently increased until about 16 weeks.[108]

The final healed defect is represented by a slightly discolored and roughened pit or a superficial linear defect on an otherwise smooth surface of hyaline cartilage. This implies that osteochondral fractures or surgically induced full-thickness defects will heal, although with fibrocartilage, a mechanically inferior tissue.

IMMOBILIZATION

Under experimental conditions in the immature growing animal, it can be shown that degeneration of the articular cartilage takes place, developing more rapidly in the noncontact areas.[82,85] Initially, at the point of contact between articular surfaces, the cartilage hypertrophies and, simultaneously, degeneration becomes apparent where articular surfaces are unopposed. Before the morphological changes of degeneration become visible, metabolic aberrations are already taking place.[107]

At first, the articular cartilage loses its normal luster, becoming yellowish and soft, and the contact area becomes flattened. The earliest microscopic sign of degeneration appearing in the superficial zone is the loss of an amorphous material that normally lines the surface of articular cartilage (HA).[75] Subsequent changes proceed in a sequential manner from the superficial toward the deep zones. These include loss of chondroitin sulfate (loss of metachromatic staining), loss of surface cells, proliferation, enlargement and clustering of chondrocytes, and, finally, degeneration of cells as evidenced under the electron microscope by complete disintegration of their plasma membranes, mitochondria with distorted cristae, decrease in the amount of cytoplasmic organelles, and many vacuoles. The process moves on to complete destruction of the chondrocytes until the intercellular matrix contains fragments of degenerated nuclei and cytoplasmic organelles. Fissures first appear in the peripheral noncontact areas.

At the contact area, marked proliferation of the fusiform cells is present in the surface layer initially. These appear to be metabolically very active, containing numerous dark-matriced mitochondria, lysosomes, and vacuoles, and some are rich in endoplasmic reticulum. At the same time, the matrix between these cells is decreased and loses its staining qualities. Eventually, here too the chondrocytes become vacuolated and disintegrated, and degeneration takes place, but at a slower pace compared with the peripheral noncontact areas.

Adjacent to noncontact areas, the synovium forms a pannus extending over the cartilage, which becomes thin and irregular.

In some areas, splits in the defective cartilage may be repaired temporarily by vascular fibrous tissue extending from the subchondral bone, but finally denudation in noncontact areas exposes the subchondral bone, which by now has become thick and lamellated instead of soft and woven.

The lack of alternating compression, which causes interstitial fluid to exude from the articular cartilage, and relief of compression, which allows the osmotic potential of cartilage to suck the fluid back, deprives the cartilage of nutrition. Chondrocytes die in the face of absolute immobilization, excessive pressure, or lack of pressure, when each factor operates continuously so that fluid flow is prevented.[105]

COMPLETE RELIEF OF CONTACT

When articular cartilage is completely devoid of contact with an opposing articular cartilaginous surface in a moving articulation where contact is borne elsewhere, it undergoes degeneration.[86] The following sequence of events take place: Early, there is loss of the covering thin amorphous material lining the superficial layer. The fusiform tangentially oriented cells of the superficial layer are lost. These are probably the young chondrocytes, which are the most metabolically active cells in normal articular cartilage. Experimentally, the uptake of radioactive sulfate prior to its incorporation into newly formed chondroitin sulfate occurs maximally in these cells in the superficial and intermediate zones. With early degeneration, the cells of the superficial layer no longer take up $^{35}SO_4$ and disappear prior to degeneration of the matrix.[79] Thus, the metabolic abnormality precedes the morphological changes of degeneration. At a deeper level, after loss of cells from the upper zones, the rounded chondrocytes, instead of forming well-organized and distributed cells, increase in number, clump together (clone formation), enlarge, and exhibit evidence of heightened metabolic activity (*e.g.*, increased organelles, increased uptake of labeled components of matrix elements, and intense staining of the matrix immediately about these cluster formations). The phenomenon suggests a reactive attempt at restoring the matrix. However, at some point, these cells succumb and disintegrate with the surrounding matrix. Small pieces of the noncalcified cartilage sequestrate, and the remaining greater portion of the degenerating cartilage becomes fibrillated by clefts running radially from the surface. As the overlying layers of cartilage are shed, the process of aborted attempts at restoration of matrix is repeated within the deeper zones until all cartilage is lost and the subchondral bone is exposed. In response to loss of its protective cartilage covering, the subchondral bone becomes thicker, and its structure becomes lamellar rather than woven and trabeculated.

After a transarticular amputation, the cartilage covering the end of the bone within the stump undergoes degeneration.[84]

The lack of alternating compression and relief of compression prevents diffusion of interstitial fluid in and out of articular cartilage, and the chondrocytes die for lack of nutrition.[105]

REFERENCES

Normal Articular Cartilage

1. Ali SY, Evan L: Enzymic degradation of cartilage in osteoarthritis. Fed Proc, 32:1494, 1973
2. Barnett CH, Davies DV, MacConnaill MA: Synovial Joints: Their Structure and Mechanics. Springfield, IL, Charles C Thomas, 1961
3. Butler W, Cunningham L: Evidence for the linkage of a disaccharide to hydroxylysine in tropocollagen. J Biol Chem 241:3882, 1966
4. Ekholm R: Nutrition of articular cartilage: A radioautographic study. Acta Anat 24:329, 1955
5. Hamerman D, Rosenberg L, Schubert M: Diarthrodial joints revisited. J Bone Joint Surg 52A:725, 1980
6. Harkness RD: Biological function of collagen. Biol Rev 36:399, 1961
7. Honner R: The nutritional pathways of articular cartilage. J Bone Joint Surg 53A:742, 1971

8. Kivirikko KI: Urinary excretion of hydroxyproline in health and disease. Int Rev Connect Tissue Res 5:93, 1970
9. Kivirikko, KI, Prockop DJ: Purification and partial characterization of enzyme for hydroxylation of proline in protocollagen. Arch Biochem Biophys 118:611, 1967
10. Kohn LD et al: Calf tendon procollagen peptidase. Proc Natl Acad Sci USA 71:40, 1974
11. Krane S, Parsons V, Kunin AJ: Studies of the metabolism of epiphyseal cartilage. In Bassett CAL (ed): Cartilage Degradation and Repair, pp 43–51. Washington, Natl Acad Sci, Natl Research Council, 1967
12. Linn FC, Sokoloff L: Movement and composition of interstitial fluid of cartilage. Arthritis Rheum 8:481, 1965
13. McDevitt CA: Biochemistry of articular cartilage: Nature of proteoglycans and collagen of articular cartilage and their role in aging and in osteoarthrosis. Ann Rheum Dis 32:364, 1973
14. McKibbin B, Holdsworth FW: The nutrition of immature joint cartilage in the lamb. J Bone Joint Surg 48B:793, 1966
15. McKusick VA: Heritable Disorders of Connective Tissue, 4th ed. St. Louis, CV Mosby, 1972
16. Mankin HJ: The articular cartilages: A review. Am Acad Orthop Surg Instr Course Lect vol 19, pp 204–224, St. Louis, CV Mosby, 1970
17. Mankin HJ: The reaction of articular cartilage to injury and osteoarthritis. N Engl J Med 291:1285, 1974
18. Mankin HJ, Lippiello L: The turnover of adult rabbit articular cartilage. J Bone Joint Surg 51A:1591, 1969
19. Mankin HJ, Lippiello L: The glycosaminoglycans of normal and arthritic cartilage. J Clin Invest 50:1712, 1971
20. Mankin HJ, Thrasher AZ: Water content and binding in normal and osteoarthritic human cartilage. J Bone Joint Surg 57A:76, 1975
21. Mankin HJ, et al: Biochemical and metabolic abnormalities in articular cartilage from osteoarthritic human hips: II. Correlation of morphology with biochemical and metabolic data. J Bone Joint Surg, 53A:523, 1971.
22. Maroudas A, Bullough P: Permeability of articular cartilage. Nature 219:1260, 1968
23. Maroudas A et al: The permeability of articular cartilage. J Bone Joint Surg 50B:166, 1968
24. Meyer K, Hoffman D, Linker A: Mucopolysaccharides of costal cartilage. Science 128:896, 1958
25. Muir H: Chemistry and metabolism of connective tissue glycosaminoglycans (mucopolysaccharides). Int Rev Connect Tissue Res 2:101, 1964
26. Prockop DJ: Isotopic studies on cartilage degradation and the urinary excretion of hydroxyproline. J Clin Invest 43:453, 1964
27. Prockop DJ: The biosynthesis of collagen. N Engl J Med 286:194; 242; 291; 1972
28. Radin EL, Paul IL: A consolidated concept of joint lubrication. J Bone Joint Surg 54A:607, 1972
29. Repo RH, Mitchell N: Collagen synthesis in mature articular cartilage of the rabbit. J Bone Joint Surg 53B:541, 1971
30. Rosenberg L: Chemical basis for histological use of safranin O in the study of articular cartilage. J Bone Joint Surg 53A:69, 1971
31. Rosenberg L: Cartilage proteoglycans. Fed Proc 32:1467, 1973
32. Sapolsky AI et al: The action of cathepsin D in human articular cartilage on proteoglycans. J Clin Invest 52:624, 1973
33. Schubert M, Hamerman D: A Primer on Connective Tissue Biochemistry. Philadelphia. Lea & Febiger, 1968
34. Sledge CB: Structure, development and function of joints. Orthop Clin North Am 6:619, 1975
35. Udenfriend S: Formation of hydroxyproline in collagen. Science 152:1335, 1966
36. Weiss C, Rosenberg L, Helfet AJ: An ultrastructural study of normal young adult human articular cartilage. J Bone Joint Surg 50A:663, 1968
37. Weissman, G, Spilberg IL: Breakdown of cartilage protein-polysaccharide by lysosomes. Arthritis Rheum 11:162, 1968
38. Weston PD, Barrett AJ, Dingle JT: Specific inhibition of cartilage breakdown. Nature 222:285, 1969
39. Woessner JF: Cartilage cathepsin D and its action on matrix components. Fed Proc 32:1485, 1973

Metabolic Studies of Articular Cartilage

40. Bollet AJ: Connective tissue polysaccharide metabolism and the pathogenesis of osteoarthritis. Adv Intern Med 13:33, 1967
41. Bollet AJ: An essay on the biology of osteoarthritis. Arthritis Rheum 12:152, 1969
42. Bonting SL, Jones M: Determination of microgram quantities of desoxyribonucleic acid and protein in tissues grown *in vitro*. Arch Biochem Biophys 66:340, 1957
43. Dziewiatkowski DD: Isolation of chondroitin sulfate-S^{35} from articular cartilage of rats. J Biol Chem 237:2831, 1951
44. Mankin HJ: The calcified zone (basal layer) of articular cartilage of rabbits. Anat Rec 145:73, 1963
45. Mankin HJ, Lippiello L: Biochemical and metabolic abnormalities in articular cartilage from osteoarthritic hips. J Bone Joint Surg 52A:424, 1970
46. Mankin HJ, Orlic PA: A method of estimating the health of rabbit articular cartilage by assays of ribonucleic acid and protein synthesis. Lab Invest 13:465, 1965
47. Repo RU, Mitchell N: Collagen synthesis in mature articular cartilage of the rabbit. J Bone Joint Surg 53B:541, 1971
48. Rondle CJM, Morgan WTJ: The determination of glucosamine and galactosamine. Biochem J 61:586, 1955
49. Rosenberg LC: Chemical basis for the histologic use of Safranin-O in the study of articular cartilage. J Bone Joint Surg 53A:69, 1971
50. Woessner JF Jr: The determination of hydroxyproline in tissue and protein samples containing small proportions of this imino acid. Arch Biochem Biophy 93:440, 1961

Biomechanical Functions of Articular Cartilage

51. Fick R: Handbuch der Anatomie und Mechanik der Gelenke. Teil I–III. Fischer, Jena, 1904, 1911
52. Kempson GE et al: Patterns of cartilage stiffness on normal and degenerate human femoral heads. J Biomech 4:597, 1971
53. Murray MP et al: Walking patterns of patients with unilateral hip pain due to osteoarthritis and avascular necrosis. J Bone Joint Surg 53A:259, 1971
54. Pauwels F: Structure of the tangential fibrous layer of the articular cartilage in the scapular glenoid cavity as an example of an unsubstantiated strain field. Z Anat Entwichlungs Gesch 121:188, 1959
55. Radin EL et al: Lubrication of synovial membrane. Am Rheum Dis 30:322, 1971
56. Sokoloff L: Elasticity of ageing cartilage. Fed Proc 25:1089, 1966

Mechanical Functions of Articular Cartilage

57. Bowden FP, Tabor D: Friction and Lubrication. New York, Barnes & Noble, 1967
58. Charnley JW: The lubrication of animal joints. In Symposium of Biomechanics, pp 12–22. London, Institution of Mechanical Engineering, 1959
59. Freeman MAR, Kempson GE: Load Carriage. In Freeman MAR (ed): Adult Articular Cartilage. New York, Grune & Stratton, 1972
60. Harkness RD: Mechanical properties of collagenous tissues. In Gould BS (ed): Treatise on Collagen. Part A. New York, Academic Press, 1968
61. Jones ES: Joint lubrication. Lancet 1:1043, 1936
62. Linn FC: Lubrication of animal joints. J Bone Joint Surg 49A:1079, 1967
63. Linn FC, Radin EL: Lubrication of animal joints: III. The effect of certain chemical alterations of the cartilage and lubricant. Arthritis Rheum 11:674, 1968
64. McCutcheon CW: Mechanism of animal joints. Nature 184:1284, 1959
65. McCutcheon CW: A note upon tensile stresses in the collagen fibers of articular cartilage. Med Electron Biol Eng 3:447, 1965
66. Ogston AG, Wells JD: The osmotic properties of sulphoethyl-sephadex: A model for cartilage. Biochem J 128:685, 1972
67. Paul JP: Bio-engineering studies of the forces transmitted by joints. Part II: Engineering analysis. In Kenedi RM (ed): Biomechanics and Related Bio-engineering Topics, p 369. Oxford, Pergamon Press, 1965
68. Radin EL, Paul IL: Response of joints to impact loading: I. In vitro wear. Arthritis Rheum 14:356, 1971
69. Salter RB, Field P: The effects of continuous compression on living articular cartilage. J Bone Joint Surg 42A:31, 1960
70. Schubert M: Intercellular macromolecules containing polysaccharides. Biophys J 4:119, 1964
71. Swanson SAV et al: Load carriage. In Freeman MAR (ed): Adult Articular Cartilage, p 239. New York, Grune & Stratton, 1972
72. Tanner RI: An alternative mechanism for the lubrication of synovial joints. Phys Med Biol 11:119, 1966
73. Yannas IV: Involvement of articular cartilage in a linear relaxation process during walking. Nature 227:1358, 1970

Factors Affecting Articular Cartilage

74. Aer J, Kivirikko KI: Preliminary characterization of the collagenolytic activity of rat bone. Hoppes-Seylers Z Physiol Chem 350:87, 1965
75. Balazs E et al: Fine structure and glycosaminoglycan content of the surface layer of articular cartilage. Fed Proc 25:1813, 1966
76. Behrens F, Shepard N, Mitchell N: Alteration of rabbit articular cartilage by intra-articular injections of glucocorticoids. J Bone Joint Surg 57A:70, 1975
77. Chandler GH, Wright V: Deleterious effect of intra-articular hydrocortisone. Lancet 2:661, 1958
78. Chrisman OD, Southwick WO, Fessel JM: Plasmin and articular cartilage. Yale J Biol Med 34:524, 1962
79. Collins DH, McElligott TT: Sulphate $^{35}SO_4$ uptake by chondrocytes in relation to histologic changes in osteoarthritic human cartilage. Ann Rheum Dis 19:318, 1960
80. Convery FR et al: Experimental hemarthrosis in the knee of the mature canine. Arthritis Rheum 19:59, 1976
81. Curtiss PH Jr, Klein L: Destruction of articular cartilage in septic arthritis J Bone Joint Surg 45A:797, 1963; 47A:1595, 1965
82. Finsterbush A, Friedman B: Early changes in immobilized rabbit's knee joint: A light and electron microscopic study. Clin Orthop 92:305, 1973
83. Gross J, Lapiere CM: Collagenolytic activity in amphibian tissues. Proc Natl Acad Sci USA 48:1014, 1962
84. Haebler C: Experimentelle Untersuchungen über die Regeneration des Gelenk Knorpels. Beitr Klin Tuberk 134:602, 1925
85. Hall MC: Cartilage changes after experimental immobilization of the knee joint of the young rat. J Bone Joint Surg 45A:36, 1963
86. Hall MC: Cartilage changes after experimental relief of contact in the knee joint of the mature rat. Clin Orthop 64:64, 1969
87. Hamerman D et al: Biochemical events in joint disease. J Chronic Dis 16:835, 1963
88. Harrold AJ: Fibrinogen in synovial joints. J Bone Joint Surg 55B:554, 1971
89. Hoaglund FT: Experimental hemarthrosis. J Bone Joint Surg 49A:285, 1967
90. Jaffe HL: Metabolic, Degenerative and Inflammatory Diseases of Bones and Joints. Philadelphia. Lea & Febiger, 1972
91. Janoff A, Blondin J: Depletion of cartilage matrix by a neutral protease fraction of human leucocyte lysosomes. Proc Soc Exp Biol Med 135:302, 1970
92. Lack CH: Increased vascular permeability, chondrolysis and cortisone. Proc R Soc Med 55:113, 1962
93. Lack CH, Rogers HJ: Action of plasmin on cartilage. Nature 182:945, 1958
94. Levene C: The patterns of cartilage canals. J Anat 98:515, 1964
95. Lewis JH: Effects of epsilon amino caproic acid (EACA) on survival of I^{131} and on fibrinolytic and coagulation factors in dogs. Proc Soc Exp Biol Med 114:777, 1963
96. McCall JG: Load deformation studies of articular cartilage. J Anat 105:212, 1969
97. Mankin HJ, Boyle CJ: The acute effects of lacerative injury on DNA and protein synthesis in articular cartilage. In Bassett CAL (ed): Cartilage Degradation and Repair. Washington, Natl Acad Sci, Natl Research Council, pp. 188–200, 1967
98. Mankin HJ, Conger KA: The acute effects of intra-articular hydrocortisone on articular cartilage in rabbits. J Bone Joint Surg 48A:1383, 1966
99. Mankin HJ et al: The effect of systemic corticosteroids on rabbit articular cartilage. Arthritis Rheum 15:593, 1972
100. Meachim G, Roberts C: Repair of the joint surface from subarticular tissue in the rabbit knee. J Anat 109:317, 1971
101. Muir IHM: Biochemistry. In Freeman MAR (ed): Adult Articular Cartilage. New York, Grune & Stratton, 1972
102. Rodnan GP et al: Postmortem examination of an elderly severe hemophiliac, with observations on the pathologic findings in hemophilic joint disease. Arthritis Rheum 2:152, 1959
103. Salter RB, Gross A, Hall JH: Hydrocortisone arthropathy. Can Med Assoc J 97:374, 1967
104. Shaw NE, Lacey E: The influence of corticosteroids on normal and papain-treated articular cartilage in the rabbit. J Bone Joint Surg 55B:197, 1973
105. Sokoloff L: The Biology of Degenerative Joint Disease. Chicago, University of Chicago Press, 1969
106. Sweetnam DR, Mason RM, Murray RO: Steroid arthropathy of hip. Br Med J 1:1392, 1960

107. Thaxter TH et al: Degeneration of immobilized knee joints in rats. J Bone Joint Surg 47A:567, 1965
108. Thompson RC Jr: An experimental study of surface injury to articular cartilage and enzyme responses within the joints. Clin Orthop 107:239, 1975
109. Trias A: Effect of persistent pressure on articular cartilage. J Bone Joint Surg 43B:376, 1961
110. Wolf CR, Mankin HJ: Effect of hemarthrosis on articular cartilage. J Bone Joint Surg 47A:1203, 1965
111. Wood GC et al: Chondromucoprotein degrading neutral protease activity in rheumatoid synovial fluid. Ann Rheum Dis 30:73, 1971
112. Wood, JF, Nichols G: Collagenolytic activity in rat bone cells. J Cell Biol 26:747, 1965

8

Biophysical Properties of Bone and Cartilage*

ELECTRICAL PROPERTIES OF BONE

Electrical phenomena are integral, although not exclusive, features of biologic processes in all tissues, including bone. Electromechanical interactions are thought to regulate cellular proliferation, differentiation, and function.[2,3] The sources of electrical energy reside intrinsically within the bone (standing potentials); may result from stress applied to the bone, whereby extracellular components of bone, notably collagen, act as transducers to convert mechanical to electrical energy (stress-generated potentials); or are derived from externally applied electricity or time-varying electromagnetic fields. Extensive ongoing investigations are aimed at defining the electrical properties of bone and at defining the mechanisms by which electrical stimuli influence the biologic processes in bone. Although much information is available in both areas, much remains to be accomplished before a detailed, step-by-step understanding of the electrical control of bone cells is forthcoming.[24]

It is now clearly established that extrinsic sources of electrical energy can induce osteogenesis and can be used therapeutically to promote fracture healing and overcome nonunion.[32] Furthermore, inductively coupled electromagnetic fields have been shown to favor bone accretion rates over the rate of bone resorption in the laboratory and to increase blood supply. The preliminary clinical data suggest that they may be of use in osteonecrosis, in bone grafting, and, hypothetically, in osteoporosis. It is therefore essential that the orthopaedic surgeon become informed about the principles of physics and biochemistry as they relate to the electrical properties of bone and the regulation of its cells by electrical means.

BIOELECTRICAL POTENTIALS (NONSTRESS POTENTIALS, STANDING POTENTIALS)

Living bone tissue, like other tissue biologic systems, exhibit steady, resting potentials, recorded in the range of microvolts.[15] These potential differences, thought to exist in all living tissues,[11] are dependent on cell viability and are subject to alteration in polarity and magnitude as a result of changing metabolic processes, mechanical stress, and so forth. In a long bone, when recording electrodes are placed, one in the epiphysis and the other in the metaphysis, the metaphysis is negative with respect to the epiphysis. When a search electrode is placed at successively increasing distances from the epiphysis, the diaphysis exhibits gradually decreasing negative voltage, tending toward isopolarity and even reaching electropositivity in the midshaft.

These standing potentials appear to be derived in part from streaming potentials arising in blood vessels,[3,13] since interruption of arterial flow to the bone causes a

* Drs. C. A. L. Bassett and C. T. Brighton deserve special recognition for offering their expertise in reviewing and editing this chapter.

significant fall in the standing potentials while venous occlusion causes an increase.

In the metaphysis where the large sinusoids are located (just distal to the last transverse septum of the cell columns), there is slow blood flow, low pO_2, electronegativity, and active osteogenesis. Low oxygen tension, which may result from sluggish blood flow, is conducive to osteogenesis.

Despite curtailment of blood supply to bone, the standing potentials, although reduced in degree, are still present for up to 30 minutes after the blood supply has been interrupted. If the bone cells are killed, the standing potentials disappear altogether. This would imply that standing potentials arise, at least in part, from the bone cells.[16]

An opposite view that rapid blood flow is associated with osteogenesis[19] is no longer considered valid.

When the diaphysis is fractured, the entire shaft becomes electronegative, particularly over the fracture site, and the electronegativity of the metaphysis becomes greater. As the fracture heals, the potential differences revert to normal (metaphysis = electronegative, diaphysis = isopolarity or tending toward electropositivity).

It is important to note that electrodes placed on the skin overlying bone, or placed on the periosteum, will give readings corresponding in magnitude and disposition to measurements of direct current (D.C.) potential, to some degree, taken directly from the bone. Consequently, skin readings may be considered a possible index of current potential in underlying bone, if some of the electrical sources of interference and signal coupling can be controlled.

STRESS-GENERATED POTENTIALS

Of various physical forces that act on a bone cell to induce its genetically determined response, only electricity has been extensively studied.[2,3,15] Mechanically stressed bone generates an electrical potential. Areas of compression become electronegative, and areas of tension become electropositive. These stress-generated potentials (SGP) appear to arise by two mechanisms. The currents may represent "piezoelectricity of bone," which probably originates within the collagen fibers (see Piezoelectric Property of Collagen). SGP may also be produced by streaming potentials[13,21] and electrets.[22]

Streaming, or zeta, potentials may be described as follows: As electrically charged bodies, such as ions, cells, and organic molecules in solution are moved, hydrodynamically, through tissues or vessels, an electrostatic repulsion or attraction occurs between the moving charge and the charge in the fixed structures. For example, as a red blood cell with a negatively charged membrane is propelled past negatively charged endothelial cells in the vessel wall, a voltage is produced. Similarly, as cartilage is mechanically deformed, fluid is displaced. The fluid contains ions, and charged molecules, which are forced, hydraulically, through a matrix composed of fixed polyanions (proteoglycans). As a result, a voltage is created, and this is termed a *streaming potential.* Neither of the above-described mechanisms will result in a sustained electric current, since charge separation occurs only while deformation is taking place. As charges are separated within structural components of the tissue, mobile countercharges (*e.g.,* ions) in the extracellular fluids move, electrophoretically, to the charged surfaces, thereby "neutralizing" the charge. The currents are pulsatile, with waveform characteristics reflecting rates and amounts of loading as well as the passive electrical properties (electrical resistance and capacitance) of the tissues in which the generated current is flowing. It should be emphasized that the final current pattern is the result of all electrogenic events, whether local or at a distance (*e.g.,* cardiogenic, neurogenic) and whether in or out of synchrony.[4]

The electrical (ionic) current results in a sequence of biochemical events, depending on the current's characteristics (*e.g.,* D.C. vs. pulsed). These events include changes in ion binding at membranes, changes in enzyme activity (*i.e.,* cyclic adenosine-3',5'-monophosphate [cyclic AMP]), modifications in mitochondrial activity, and alterations in macromolecular synthesis (*e.g.,* collagen, proteoglycan, ribonucleic acid).

When an intact long bone is subjected to a compressive force applied in the direction of its long axis, the periosteum is induced to proliferate and form new bone. It appears that the metabolism of the cambium cells is affected by the mechanical energy, and from an electrophysiological point of view, the biologically hyperactive tissue becomes electronegative.[25] Since force generates electricity equally as well in either viable or nonviable bone, the sequence of biologic events appears to be: force → electricity → modification of bone cell activity. Consequently, chemical, thermal, or mechanical stimuli, which are capable of producing nonfracture callus, have been hypothesized to constitute "environmental conditions which must first be converted to electrical energy which, in turn, acts upon the cells to cause them to proliferate and form callus."[25] By applying the concept of Küntscher,[20] that osteogenesis can be induced, in the absence of fracture, by mechanical, thermal, or chemical means, it may be hypothesized that the ultimate stimulus to osteogenesis may be electrical, and therefore the sequence of events may be: electrical stimulus → change in cellular microenvironmental conditions → callus formation (as one form of cellular response). This postulate, therefore, suggests that when current is passed through bone it will react according to the characteristics of the applied electricity.

RESPONSE OF BONE TO DIRECT CURRENT

A reproducible osteogenic response occurs about a cathode when small amounts of direct current are applied under certain conditions.[7,15,17] The cathode, composed of metal and often of stainless steel, must be placed in a proper osseous milieu (*e.g.*, marrow cavity); 20μamp gives the maximum amount of new bone formation (Fig. 8-1), and higher microamperage tends to cause local tissue necrosis and metal corrosion. The ideal voltage is about 1 V, but because resistance gradually increases at the electrode-tissue interface (due to increasing bone accumulation?), a further increase in voltage is required to keep the amperage at the same optimum level. Osteonecrosis is more likely when the amperage exceeds 30μamp. A P.C. anode inserted within the bone causes local tissue necrosis regardless of the amount of direct current applied.[18]

RESPONSE OF BONE TO ELECTROMAGNETIC FIELDS

Inductively coupled, pulsing electromagnetic fields (PEMFs) produce weak pulsing electrical currents in tissues.[4,8] Because this method does not use implanted electrodes, it does not give rise to polarization, electrolytic by-products, and foreign chemical species theoretically

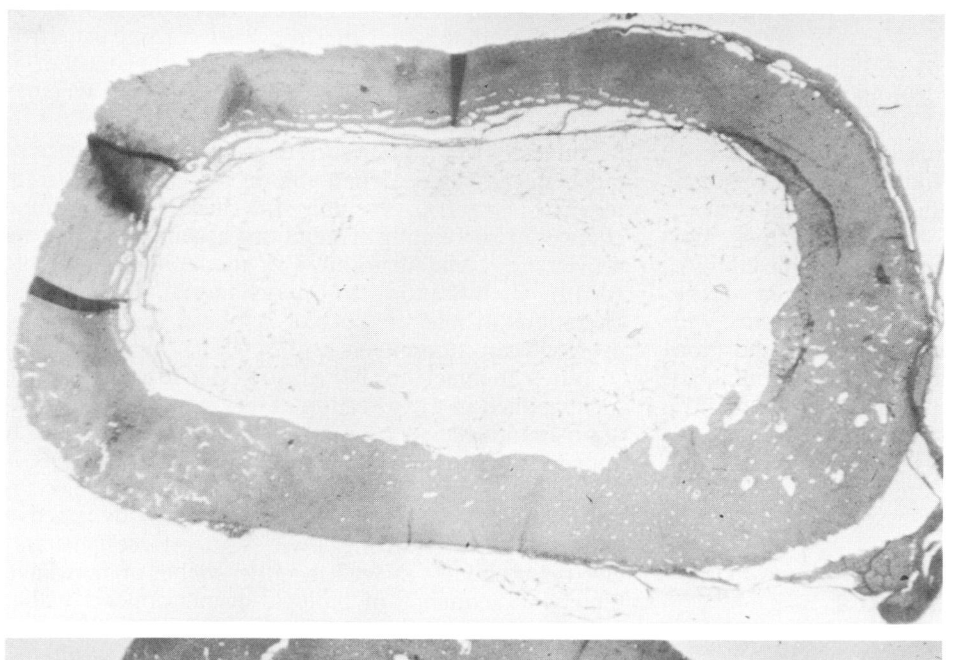

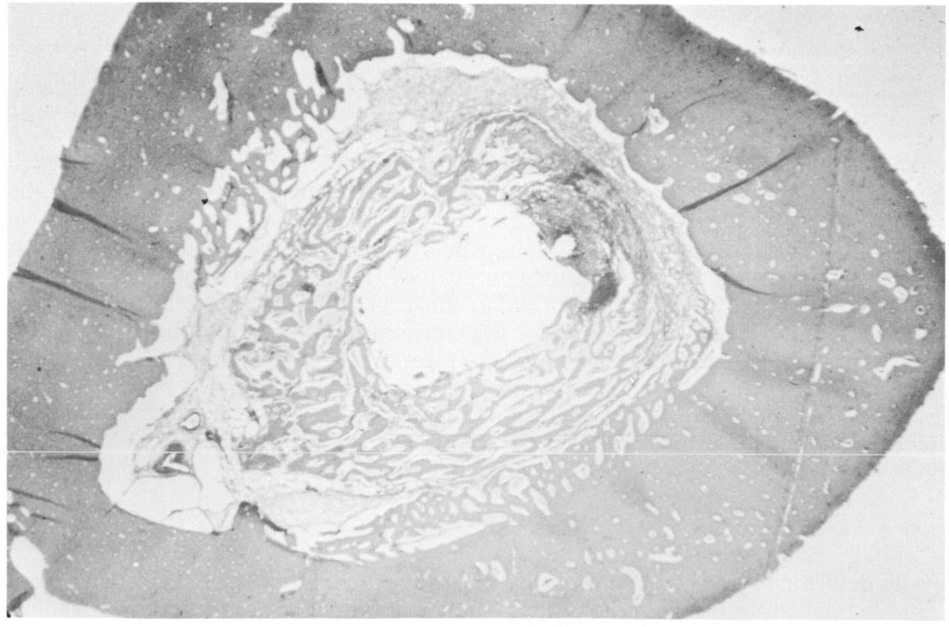

FIG. 8-1. Electrically induced osteogenesis (effect in the experimental animal). (*Top*) Medullary canal in which a dummy electrode existed for 21 days. (*Bottom*) Medullary canal in which an active cathode delivered 20μamp for 21 days. In the latter, a tremendous amount of new bone formation has occurred about the cathode. (Courtesy of Dr. C. T. Brighton)

associated with faradaic (re-dox) action of P.C. electrodes.[26] PEMF-induced currents are not constant and therefore through pulse design may exert a selective influence on ionic species in the cellular environment and may produce resonance effects. Induced pulsing currents will modify cell behavior in bone,[14,23] cartilage,[9,14] and other tissues. Thus by properly programming the electrical events about the mesenchymal cells and their daughter cells, a sequence of histologic changes can be induced. Theoretically, calcification of fibrocartilage within the gap between the un-united bone fragments, regarded as the prelude to ossification (endochondral ossification), is automatically followed by vascular invasion, resorption of the calcified cartilage, and replacement by woven bone, which in turn is replaced by lamellar bone and gap bridging osteons.[9] Periosteal callus does not form.

The possible effects of PEMF-induced currents on fibrocartilage may be explained by the electrical properties of cartilage, its cell membrane surfaces, and the effects on Ca^{2+} flux (probably at the mitochondrial level).

In avascular cartilage, charge-charge interactions may play a role. Because cartilage is rich in proteoglycans, it is largely polyanionic and therefore carries a *net negative charge,* especially when it is dynamically deformed.[6] Endothelium is endowed, as are most cells,[1] with a negatively charged, sialic acid–containing surface coat. A repulsion of negative charges, therefore, may prevent vascular invasion. Until the proteoglycan degradation and provisional calcification take place, vascular invasion and ossification cannot occur. When freed of glycosaminoglycans, collagen fibers, possessing a *net positive charge,* attract cells with a fixed negative charge of their cell surfaces. It is therefore hypothesized that PEMFs act by neutralizing the net negative charge of fibrocartilage, thereby inducing calcification.[2]

Different cellular responses can be evoked by altering pulse characteristics. For example, the calcium content of isolated chondrocytes can be increased or decreased;[9] cyclic AMP, collagen, and proteoglycans can be modified,[14] and deoxyribonucleic acid synthesis can be changed.[23]

It has also been shown that increased resorptive activity and progressive loss of bone secondary to disuse can be minimized by certain pulse characteristics.[10,12]

MECHANISMS OF ELECTRICALLY INDUCED OSTEOGENESIS

The actual mechanisms by which the application of any form of electricity induces osteogenesis is unknown. The evidence elicited by biophysical, biochemical, and clinical studies is largely circumstantial. Much of the data accumulated concerns the use of direct current. For example, around a D.C. cathode, the pO_2 is decreased and the *p*H is increased.[33] Since bone grows best in a hypoxic environment, the low oxygen tension in the vicinity of an active electrode (cathode) may be one of the mechanisms of action of direct current.[34]

In viable, resting, unstressed bone, areas of active growth and repair, as compared with less active areas of bone formation, are electronegative.[15]

Mechanically stressed bone generates an electrical potential. Areas of compressive loading (*i.e.,* the concave side of a long bowed bone) are electronegative and demonstrate increased osteogenesis. Areas of tensile loading of a bowed stressed bone (*i.e.,* the convex side) show electropositivity and reduced osteogenesis.[2,3,15] It has been postulated that such electrical potentials arise from a piezoelectrical effect, presumably derived from mechanical stress applied to collagen,[40,54] and/or streaming potentials[13] and electrets.[22]

At the cellular level, many intracellular metabolic events appear related to biologic processes occurring about the cell membrane. Since it has been demonstrated that the application of direct current will stimulate intracellular activity that can be visualized at ultrastructural levels,[43] and the possibility exists that externally applied PEMFs may exert at least part of their influence on the cell membrane, this cell structure has become the focal point of ongoing investigation.

Many enzymes catalyze intracellular synthesis and the ultimate degradation of biologically important molecules. Hormones control some of these processes, and act by regulating the intracellular level of a small cyclic nucleotide, cyclic AMP.[51] The effect of this small, heat-stable compound is related to the target cell function. For example, cyclic AMP in liver, by increasing formation of active from inactive phosphorylase (PPi), accelerates glycogenolysis. The reaction ATP $\rightarrow$ cyclic AMP + PPi is stimulated by epinephrine. The enzyme, adenyl cyclase, which resides in the cell membrane, catalyzes the reaction.[57]

Adenyl cyclase is a hormone receptor within the membrane and is subject to the influence of various microenvironmental factors (*e.g.,* local ionic concentrations, mechanical pressures that distort the cell membrane), which in turn may affect the electrostatic potential of the plasma membrane. Small changes in a magnitude of a few microvolts may be sufficient to act as a first messenger or signal generator, which acts on the cell membrane to produce adenyl cyclase, which, in turn, increases the level of cyclic AMP, the second messenger.

Many polypeptide hormones carry out their function in specific target tissues by increasing the adenyl cyclase activity, within the chosen cell membrane, and increasing the intracellular level of cyclic AMP.[51] For example, parathyroid hormone acts on the cells of the renal cortex to bring about phosphaturia and calcium reabsorption.[35] In bone cells, parathyroid hormone and calcitonin, by interaction with adenyl cyclase, will modulate the cyclic AMP levels within the bone cells, and thus effect remodeling.[53] The intracellular levels of the cyclic nucleotides cyclic AMP and guanosine 3′,5′-monophosphate (cyclic GMP) also play a role in cytodifferentiation and cell division.[45]

The foregoing facts suggest two messenger hypotheses of hormone action on bone:

1. The hormone is the first messenger; it circulates in the bloodstream, binds to the plasma membrane of the target cell, and activates adenyl cyclase.
2. Cyclic AMP, the second messenger, is generated on the inner surface of the cell membrane, diffuses through the cell, and brings about the appropriate physiological response.

At the intracellular level in bone, cyclic AMP and cyclic GMP are regarded as the mediators of extrinsic factors acting on the cell membrane to induce osteogenesis (*e.g.*, mechanical effects).[52] The cellular membrane–bound enzyme adenyl cyclase catalyzes the formation of cyclic AMP from adenosine triphosphate (ATP) in a reaction that requires magnesium. (Pyrophosphate is the other product of the reaction.)

It has now been amply demonstrated that application or induction of appropriate levels of electrical current through bone will stimulate cellular activity that can be observed at ultrastructural levels, [43] and, in the PEMFs, cyclic AMP activity can be changed[14] as well as the susceptibility of bone cells to parathyroid hormone.[44]

Since it is acknowledged that cell surface activity is a major factor that controls cellular proliferation, differentiation, and function,[37] the electrical characteristics of the membrane and the factors that influence them must be considered.[50,56] Alterations of the cell membrane produced by mechanical, electrical, or chemical perturbation will affect cyclic nucleotide modulation.

The cell membrane of bone cells, like that of other living cells, is composed of a lipid matrix, whose interface with extracellular and intracellular fluids is the site of intense electrical fields that cause both electrostatic and specific interactions between charged species to occur and to whose surface are adsorbed or bound charged, mobile, globular macromolecules (steroids, hormones) and ions, particularly divalent cations.[50] The membrane is excitable and subject to stimulation by various components within the extracellular and intracellular fluids.[36,41] The external membrane surface is known to have a high fixed negative charge. The actual structure of the membrane is unknown, but it is highly potential dependent. Only a few millivolts change results in gross alterations in specifically adsorbed species. Therefore, any perturbation that produces a change in potential across the interface will alter the specific interactions of charged species in the extracellular fluid with, for example, enzymes or steroid hormones, resulting in a modification of cell function.

The principal means by which the membrane interface structure may be influenced are modification of cellular environment, such as tonicity changes, ion substitution, or ion and cell movement (the latter includes electrokinetic effects, such as streaming potential or electrophoresis); mechanical perturbation; and direct input of electrical perturbation.

Changes in local ion concentrations are important.[47,48] Negative electrostatic charges reside in the large macromolecules anchored to the membrane surface, so that changes in local concentrations of ions, particularly divalent cations, are attracted to the membrane surface by the electrostatic potential, resulting in shifts of that potential. The enzyme adenyl cyclase, situated within the membrane, is highly dependent on the divalent cations Ca^{2+} and Mg^{2+}, whose concentration is affected by potential shifts when induced, for example, by pressure, cell contact, and externally applied electrical currents or alterations in an electromagnetic field.

When physiological pressures are applied to cells in cultures, the transmembranous transport of Ca^{2+} is increased and the intracytoplasmic accumulation of this ion depresses the levels of adenyl cyclase, which, in turn, decreases cyclic AMP levels, resulting in marked cellular proliferation.[9,14]

Electrical transmembranous potentials (Em) are involved in affecting ionic-molecular permeabilities. The Em level is significantly lower in actively proliferating cells than in highly polarized nondividing cells and is markedly reduced in proliferating malignant cells.[37,38] Thus a change in the membrane potential can affect the distribution of ions in the immediate cellular environment, control the activity of membrane-bound enzymes and specific ion availability, and indirectly control intracellular metabolism and mitosis.[59]

It must be emphasized that the activity of membrane-bound proteins, particularly adenyl cyclase, is influenced by the concentration of bound divalent cations and hormones,[56] whether by shifts in the potential, increased transmembranous transport, or other means.

When bone cells in tissue culture are subjected to a pressure of physiological magnitude (60 g/sq cm), and electrical current is applied, the levels of cyclic AMP fall and DNA synthesis and cellular division increases.[28] The accompanying voltage must be kept low, preferably at 1 V or less.[52] A decrease in the level of cyclic AMP is an intracellular signal for DNA synthesis and cell division.[49] A subsequent rise in cyclic AMP is a signal for cytodifferentiation.[45,46]

The availability of oxygen in the immediate cellular environment is related to osteogenesis.[55] At low oxygen tension, at about 5%, osteogenesis occurs,* and at higher oxygen tension, measured with oxygen electrodes (*e.g.*, at 35% to 60% of oxygen concentrations), osteoclasia occurs and osteoporosis results.

Electrically induced osteogenesis is maximal about the negative (cathode) electrode, and this phenomenon is associated with very low local oxygen tension and alkalinity.[30,42] Diminished local oxygen concentrations appear to be a necessary requirement for osteogenesis.[29,31,49],* In the case of electrically induced osteogenesis,

* Brighton CT: Personal communication.

when direct current is used, the current should be maintained between 10μ amp and 20μ amp at a potential of less than 1 V.

Experimentally, it has been shown that collagen fibers become oriented in an electrical field.[27] This suggests that the spatial arrangement is a necessary prelude to mineralization.

PIEZOELECTRICAL PROPERTY OF COLLAGEN

Piezoelectricity is defined as electricity resulting from stress on crystals. The phenomenon is described for inorganic crystals that lack a center of symmetry. When the structure is deformed from its unstressed state, the separation in the centers of positive and negative charge produces a net polarization (electric dipole moment per unit volume). Conversely, when an electrical field is applied to the crystal, a change in shape is produced. Piezoelectricity has been observed on various crystalline substances, both inorganic and organic, including the extracellular components of bone,[3,62] particularly collagen.[63,65] Both direct (stress yields polarization) and indirect or converse (electrical field yields strain) effects can be demonstrated in collagen.

The collagen biopolymer is constructed from tropocollagen units. The net charge of this macromolecule is positive, with the head region of the tropocollagen unit being positive with respect to the tail.[60] The tropocollagen units are assembled into fibrils, fibers, and bundles in an orderly array so that the dipole moments are additive.

The two main organic constituents of the extracellular matrix of bone, the macromolecular biopolymers collagen and protein polysaccharide, carry a net charge and are therefore affected by electrical fields occurring in their immediate environment. Both of these macromolecules migrate electrophoretically and assume a preferred orientation in an electric field. It is therefore conceivable that SGP direct the aggregation patterns so that the fibers become oriented in a manner that is conducive to mineralization.[39]

The generation of an electrical potential results from charge separation within a deformed crystalline material. Unmineralized collagen fibrils are positively charged, deformable elements that are close to the negatively charged surfaces of cells for electrostatic interactions to occur. This relationship is ideal for electromechanical regulation of bone cell activity.[40]

The biologic implication of piezoelectricity is that it is a prominent part of the electrical phenomena that regulate the activity of bone-forming cells.[4] The end result of repeated mechanical deformation and muscle contractions is an increase in the pulsing electrical currents in bone through piezoelectric and streaming phenomena. Increased cyclic loading (especially impacting) causes an increase of osseous mass. A reduction of deforming forces (*e.g.*, by bed rest, immobilization, paralysis, buoyancy, or weightlessness) will result in lessening of bone accretion while resorption continues, and a decrease in osseous volume (osteoporosis or osteopenia) will result.[10,61,64]

In the absence of electromechanical factors, it is possible to increase the rate of bone accretion by substituting appropriately configured externally applied electrical currents, such as by invasive, semi-invasive, or noninvasive (electromagnetic fields) methods.

REFERENCES

Electrical Properties of Bone

1. Ambrose EJ: Cell Electrophoresis. London, Churchill, 1965
2. Bassett CAL: Biological significance of piezoelectricity. Calcif Tissue Res 1:252, 1968
3. Bassett CAL: Biophysical principles affecting bone structure. In Bourne GH (ed): Biochemistry and Physiology of Bone, pp. 1–76. New York, Academic Press, 1971
4. Bassett CAL: Pulsing electromagnetic fields: A new approach to surgical problems. In Buchwald H, Varco RL (eds): Metabolic Surgery, pp 255–306. New York, Grune & Stratton, 1978
5. Bassett CAL: Pulsing electromagnetic fields: A new method to modify cell behavior in calcified and non-calcified tissues. Calcif Tissue Int 34:1, 1982
6. Bassett CAL, Pawluk RJ: Electrical behavior of cartilage during loading. Science 178:982, 1972
7. Bassett CAL, Pawluk RJ, Becker RO: Effects of electric currents on bone *in vivo*. Nature 204:652, 1964
8. Bassett CAL, Pawluk RJ, Pilla AA: Acceleration of fracture repair by electromagnetic fields: A surgically non-invasive method. Ann NY Acad Sci 238: 242, 1974
9. Bassett CAL, et al: The effect of pulsing electromagnetic fields on cellular calcium and calcification of non-unions. In Brighton CT, Black J, Pollack SR (eds): Electrical Properties of Bone and Cartilage. New York, Grune & Stratton, 1979
10. Bassett LS, Tzitzikalakis G, Pawluk RJ et al: Prevention of disuse osteoporosis in the rat by means of pulsing electromagnetic fields. In Brighton CT, Black J, Pollack SR (eds): Electrical Properties of Bone and Cartilage. New York, Grune & Stratton, 1979
11. Cater DB, Phillips AF: Measurement of electrode potentials in living and dead tissues. Nature 174:121, 1954
12. Cruess RL, Kan K, Bassett CAL: The effects of electromagnetic fields upon bone formation rates in experimental osteoporosis. Orthop Trans 5:114, 1980
13. Ericksson C: Streaming potentials and other water-dependent effects in mineralized tissues. Ann NY Acad Sci 238:321, 1974
14. Fitton-Jackson S, Bassett CAL: The response of skeletal tissue to pulsed magnetic fields. In Richards RJ, Rajan KT (eds): Culture in Medical Research, vol. II. London, Pergamon Press, 1980
15. Friedenberg ZB, Brighton CT: Bioelectric potentials in bone. J Bone Joint Surg 48A:915, 1966
16. Friedenberg ZB et al: The cellular origin of bioelectric potentials in bone. Calcif Tissue Res 13:58, 1973
17. Friedenberg ZB et al: The response of non-traumatized bone to direct current. J Bone Joint Surg 56A:1023, 1974
18. Friedenberg ZB et al: Bone reaction to varying amounts of direct current. Surg Gynecol Obstet 131:894, 1970
19. Gorham LW, West WT: Circulatory changes in osteolytic and osteoblastic reactions. Arch Pathol 78:673, 1964

20. Küntscher G: Callus ohne Knochenbruch. Zentrabl Chir 68:857, 1941
21. Li ST, Katz EP: Electrostatic properties of reconstituted collagen fibrils. In Brighton CT, Black J, Pollack SR (eds): Electrical Properties of Bone and Cartilage. New York, Grune & Stratton, 1979
22. Mascarenhas S: The electret effect in bone and biopolymers and bound water problems. Ann NY Acad Sci 238:36, 1974
23. Shteyer SJ, Norton LA, Rodan GA: Electromagnetically-induced DNA synthesis in calvaria cells. J Dent Res 59A:362, 1980
24. Spadaro JA: Electrically stimulated bone growth in animals and man: A review of the literature. Clin Orthop 122:125, 1977
25. Yasuda I: Fundamental aspects of fracture treatment. J Kyoto Med Soc 4:395, 1953
26. Zengo AN, Bassett CAL et al: *In vivo* effects of direct current in the mandible. J Dent Res 55:383, 1976

Mechanisms of Electrically Induced Osteogenesis

27. Becker RO, Bassett CAL, Bachman CH: Bioelectric factors controlling bone structure. In Frost HM (ed): Bone Biodynamics, pp 209–232. Boston, Little, Brown & Co, 1964
28. Bourret LA, Bodan GA: The role of calcium in the inhibition of cAMP accumulation in epiphyseal cartilage cells exposed to physiological pressures. J Cell Physiol 88:353, 1976
29. Brighton CT et al: *In vitro* epiphyseal plate growth in various oxygen tensions. J Bone Joint Surg 51A:1383, 1960
30. Brighton CT, Briedenberg ZB: Electrical stimulation and oxygen tension. Ann NY Acad Sci 238:314, 1974
31. Brighton CT, Krebs AG: Oxygen tensions in healing fractures in the rabbit. J Bone Joint Surg 54A:323, 1972
32. Brighton CT et al: Treatment of non-union with constant direct current. Clin Orthop 124:106, 1977
33. Brighton CT et al: Cathodic oxygen consumption and electrically induced osteogenesis. Clin Orthop 107:277, 1975
34. Brighton CT et al: *In vitro* epiphyseal-plate growth in various oxygen tensions. J Bone Joint Surg 51A:1383, 1969
35. Chase LR, Aurbach CD: Parathyroid function and the renal excretion of 3′,5′-adenylic acid. Proc Natl Acad Sci 58:518, 1967
36. Cole KS: Membranes, Ions, and Impulses. Berkeley, University of California Press, 1968
37. Cone CD: The role of surface electrical transmembrane potential in normal and malignant mitogenesis. Ann NY Acad Sci 238:420, 1974
38. Cone CD Jr, Cone CM: Induction of mitosis in mature neurons in the central nervous system by sustained depolarization. Science 192:155, 1976
39. Digby PSB: Mechanism of calcification in mammalian bone. Nature 212:1250, 1966
40. Fukada E, Yasuda I: On the piezoelectric effect of bone. J Physiol Soc Jpn 12:1158, 1957
41. Hodgkin AL, Huxley AF: Currents carried by sodium and potassium ions through the membrane of the giant axon of Loligo. J Physiol 116:449, 1952
42. Howell DS et al: Partition of calcium phosphate and protein in the fluid phase aspirated in calcifying sites of epiphyseal cartilage. J Clin Invest 47:1121, 1968
43. Lavine L et al: Clinical and ultrastructural investigations of electrical enhancement of bone healing. Ann NY Acad Sci 238:552, 1974
44. Luben RA et al: Effects of therapeutic electromagnetically induced current on bone cell responsiveness *in vitro.* J Electrochem Soc (extended abstracts) 80:1130, 1980
45. McMahon D: Chemical messengers in development: A hypothesis. Science 185:1012, 1974
46. Milner AJ: Cyclic AMP and the differentiation of adrenal cortical cells grown in tissue culture. J Endocrinol 55:405, 1972
47. Otten J et al: Regulation of cell growth by cyclic adenosine 3′,5′-monophosphate: Effect of cell density and agents which alter cell growth on cyclic 3′,5′-monophosphate levels in fibroblasts. J Biol Chem 247:7082, 1972
48. Parsegian VA: Possible modulation as reactions on the cell surface by changes in electrostatic potential that accompany cell contact. Ann NY Acad Sci 238:362, 1974
49. Pastan I, Perlman RL: Cyclic AMP and metabolism. Nature 229:15, 1971
50. Pilla AA: Dynamic electrochemical phenomena at living cell membranes. J Electrochem Soc 122:126c, 1975
51. Robison GA et al: Cyclic AMP. Ann Rev Biochem 37:149, 1968
52. Rodan GA et al: Cyclic AMP and cyclic GMP: Mediators of mechanical effects on bone remodeling. Science 189:467, 1975
53. Rodan SB, Rodan GA: The effect of parathyroid hormone and thyrocalcitonin on the accumulation of cyclic adenosine 3′,5′-monophosphate in freshly isolated bone cells. J Clin Invest 53:3068, 1974
54. Shamos MH, Lavine LS, Shamos ML: The piezoelectric effect in bone. Nature 197:81, 1963
55. Shaw JL, Bassett CAL: The effects of varying oxygen concentrations on osteogenesis and embryonic cartilage *in vitro.* J Bone Joint Surg 49A:73, 1967
56. Singer SJ: Structure and function of biological membranes. In Rothfield LI (ed): New York, Academic Press, 1971
57. Sutherland EW, Rall TW: Fractionation and characterization of cyclic adenine ribonucleotide formed by tissue particles. J Biol Chem 232:1077, 1958
58. Vose GP, Smith AW: Effect of water displacement system for gravity counteraction upon skeletal status in the dog. Aerospace Med 39:266, 1968
59. Wolff J, Hope Cook G: Charge effects in the activation of adenyl cyclase. J Biol Chem 250:6897, 1975

Piezoelectrical Property of Collagen

60. Athenstaedt H: Permanent longitudinal electric polarization and pyroelectric behaviour of collagenous structures and nervous tissues in man. Nature 228:830, 1970
61. Birge SJ Jr, Whedon GD: The physiology of inactivity and weightlessness. In Hypodynamics and Hypogravics. New York, Academic Press, 1968
62. Cochrane GVB et al: Electrochemical characteristics of bone under physiologic moisture conditions. Clin Orthrop 58:249, 1968
63. Fukada E, Yasuda I: Piezoelectric effects in collagen. J Appl Physics Jpn 3:117, 1964
64. Johnston RS, Dietlein LE: Biomedical Results from Skylab. Washington, DC, National Aeronautics and Space Administration, 1977
65. Shamos MH, Lavine LS: Piezoelectricity as a fundamental property of biological tissues. Nature 213:267, 1967

Part Two

General Orthopaedic Conditions

9

Metabolic Bone Disease and Related Dysfunction of the Parathyroid Glands

FACTORS AFFECTING CALCIUM METABOLISM

The deposition of calcium is favored by:

- Availability in food
- Alkalinity of serum
- Vitamin D

Resorption from bone is favored by:

- Acidosis
- Hyperparathyroidism
- Hyperthyroidism
- Pregnancy or lactation
- Starvation—acidosis, lack of calcium, phosphorus, vitamin D
- Excessive vitamin D
- Chemical poisoning—strontium, magnesium
- Excessive diuresis
- Local causes—inflammation, vascular congestion
- Inactivity, immobilization—leads to excessive removal of calcium, hypercalciuria, renal stones
- Injury (reflex vasomotor mechanism? Selye adaptation syndrome?)

Absorption from intestine is favored by:

- Acidity of digestate (in distal intestine, alkalinity preciptates the calcium)
- Vitamin D
- Bile salts (to split fats completely and prevent soap formation)
- Parathyroid hormone

Absorption from intestine hindered by:

- Alkalinity—alkalies, achlorhydria
- Excessive phosphates
- Excessive fatty acids—form insoluble calcium soaps
- Excessive carbonates—form insoluble calcium carbonate
- Deficient metabolically active vitamin D (conversion at liver and kidney defective)
- Deficient parathyroid hormone
- Deficient magnesium

Availability from bloodstream depends on its ionization:

- Colloidal calcium is bound to protein and therefore unavailable
- Salt of $Ca_3(PO_4)_2$ in solution exists in equilibrium with ionized calcium

Solution of calcium in serum favored by:

Decreased *p*H
Protein concentration
Lowered serum ionic strength
Magnesium and strontium
Increased parathyroid activity

TABLE 9-1 Normal Values Serum Calcium and Serum Phosphorus

	Infants	Children	Adults
Calcium (mg/dl)	10.5–12.0	10.0–11.5	9.5–10.5
Phosphorus (mg/dl)	4.0–7.0	4.5–5.5	3.2–4.3

PARATHYROID GLANDS

ANATOMY

The parathyroid glands are approximately four very small brownish red structures, about 5 mm × 3 mm × 1 mm that are flattened and ovoid and lie in the posterior aspect of the thyroid gland. Occasionally, the inferior pair may be situated in the mediastinum. As many as 12 glands may be present (Fig. 9-1).

HISTOLOGY

Up to 10 years of age, the gland is composed of a uniform type of cells densely packed as a continuous mass or anastomosing cords; less commonly, they are arranged as follicles with a colloid material at the center. These cells are designated principal or chief cells. They have a large, vesicular, centrally placed nucleus and a faintly staining homogeneous cytoplasm. At about the age of puberty oxyphil cells appear. These cells are larger than the principal cells and have a smaller, darker staining nucleus and a deeply acid-staining cytoplasm.

PHYSIOLOGY

The parathyroid secretes parathyroid hormone (PTH, which has the following functions:

It maintains the serum calcium level (Table 9-1). When the serum calcium level is low, as from dietary lack, the normal level is restored by dissolution and osteoclasis of bone. The low serum calcium causes parathyroid hyperplasia. Conversely, when the serum calcium level is high, parathyroid hypoplasia results; the excess is ex-

FIG. 9-1. (*Left*) Normal parathyroid gland. Note the adipose tissue and vascularity throughout the gland. (*Right*) Adenoma of the parathyroid gland. Note the encapsulation separating the adenoma from the normal gland. Because adenoma causes hypercalcemia, nephrocalcinosis, renal insufficiency, and retention of serum phosphorus, parathyroid hyperplasia takes place in response to hyperphosphatemia. This hyperplasia occurs in all the parathyroid tissue, including that which surrounds the adenoma, as seen in this section.

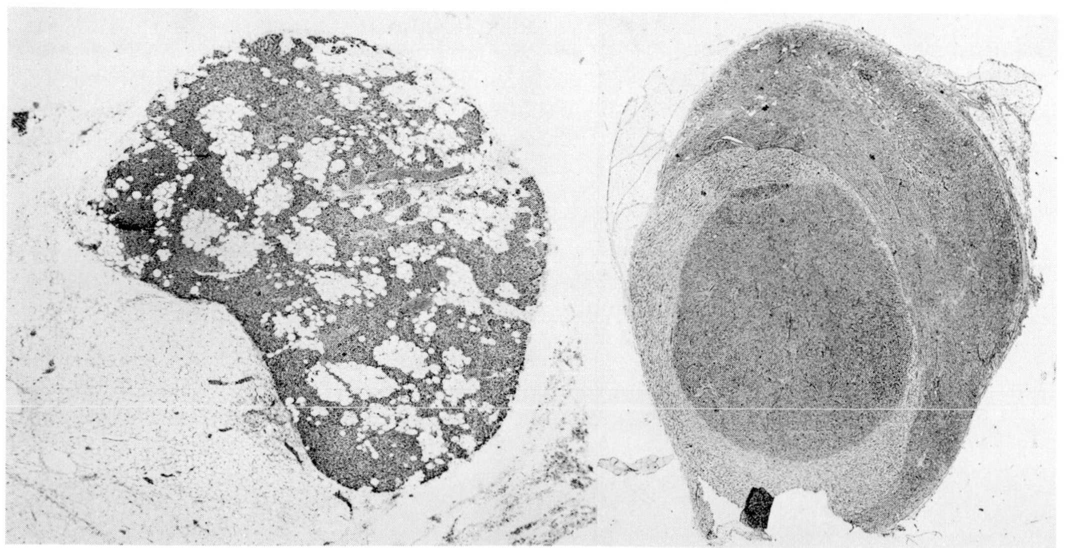

TABLE 9-2 Normal Values for Serum Phosphatase

	Acid (pH 5.0)	Alkaline (pH 8.6–9.3)	
	ADULTS	ADULTS	CHILDREN
Bodansky*	0.0–0.4	1.5–4.0	5.0–12.0
King-Armstrong†		3.7–13.1	15.0–20.0
King-Armstrong† (Gutman's modification)	0.3–3.25		

* Substrate—sodium B–glycerophosphate (unit is based on 1 mg P).
† Substrate—disodium phenylphosphate (unit is based on 1 mg phenol).
(Sunderman FW: Am J Clin Pathol 12:404, 1942)

creted and deposited in bone. Absorption by the gut is reduced.

It lowers the serum phosphorus level. PTH encourages excretion of phosphorus by inhibiting renal tubular resorption. When the serum phosphorus level is high, as in low calcium, high phosphorus rickets, parathyroid hyperplasia develops in an effort to eliminate the excess.

It increases diuresis of phosphorus, mainly by inhibiting tubular resorption.

It promotes tubular resorption of calcium.

It acts with vitamin D to promote intestinal absorption of calcium.

It encourages glomerular filtration of calcium and phosphate ions.

It stimulates osteoclastic resorption of bone.

It will directly effect dissolution of bone. When a gland is placed in direct contact with bone, the latter will absorb, although osteoclasts are not yet apparent.

It inhibits the calcifying effect of vitamin D.

It increases the solubility of calcium and phosphorus, maintaining these substances in ionic form beyond their expected solubilities.

In studying the following metabolic diseases, it is important to determine the part played by the parathyroids. Increased parathyroid secretion can be primary or secondary. Secondary hyperplasia develops as a response to serum calcium and phosphorus levels. An elevation of blood phosphorus increases parathyroid secretion, as does a relative lowering of serum calcium. The PTH will then effect osteoclast formation and osteoclasis and also direct dissolution of bone. When clinical evidence of parathyroid hyperfunction exists, a low serum calcium or high phosphorus level signifies a secondary hyperplasia of the glands, and the cause must be sought, (*e.g.*, diet, renal insufficiency). When the serum calcium level is high and the phosphorus level is low, primary parathyroid adenoma or hyperplasia is the probable cause.

RELATION OF KIDNEY FUNCTION TO SECONDARY HYPERPARATHYROIDISM

Normal kidneys can eliminate phosphorus easily. When nonfunctioning glomeruli form a barrier to passage of phosphorus, the hyperphosphatemia urges the parathyroids to greater activity in an effort to excrete the mineral, resulting in excessive excretion of PTH. A hyperparathyroid state is created. The excess PTH increases the rate of bone absorption with consequent rise of calcium and phosphorus in the bloodstream. Since these elements cannot be eliminated by the kidneys, they are deposited throughout the soft tissues. Deposition in the kidneys themselves forms multiple staghorn calculi. Metastatic pathologic calcification occurs everywhere, including the walls of blood vessels. The large bowel excretes the excess of calcium and phosphorus, although inadequately. All types of kidney diseases and congenital anomalies basically act the same way. The eventual result is renal rickets in the child and renal osteomalacia in the adult. In children the changes are influenced by the presence of actively growing epiphyseal cartilage plates. These plates and the osteoid tissue just beyond become excessively wide and irregular. This is high phosphorus rickets, in contrast to the usual normal or low phosphorus rickets caused by deficiency of vitamin D. The main features include the following:

Marked renal insufficiency of long duration
Phosphate retention with high serum phosphorus
Slight reduction of serum calcium
Marked acidosis
Metastatic calcium deposits near joints
Mönckeberg sclerosis
Osteitis fibrosa generalisata
Enlargement of parathyroid tissue

Treatment consists of lowering the phosphorus intake, of reducing its absorption by aluminum hydroxide, and of directing efforts against the kidney disease. When kidney disease is primarily tubular, loss of calcium is excessive and large quantities of vitamin D and calcium must be administered.

TABLE 9-3 Alkaline Phosphatase Conversion Factors to International Units*

Method	Factor
Bodansky	5.37
Shinowara-Jones-Reinhart	5.37
King-Armstrong	3.53
Kind-King	7.06
Bessey-Lowry-Brock	16.66
AutoAnalyzer (Technicon)	7.06

* IU/liter = μmoles PO_4 released per minute per liter.
(Goldsmith RS: Laboratory aids in the diagnosis of metabolic bone disease. Orthop Clin North Am 3:551, 1972)

PRIMARY HYPERPARATHYROIDISM

In primary hyperparathyroidism (osteitis fibrosa cystica, von Recklinghausen's disease, parathyrotoxicosis), when secretion of PTH becomes excessive it is reflected in bone by a marked increase of osteoclasts, rapid resorption of bone, decrease of osteoblasts, and fibrous replacement of marrow. Both calcium and phosphorus are thrown into the bloodstream; although both are excreted mainly by the kidneys, elimination of phosphorus is accomplished more readily, with the result that the blood calcium level is elevated and the phosphorus level is lowered. The alkaline phosphatase level is elevated, supposedly because of a compensatory effort at restoring the resorbed bone.

PATHOLOGY

Most frequently, an adenoma measuring up to 6 cm in diameter is situated in one of the parathyroid glands.[2] Less often two adenomas or diffuse hyperplasia is the

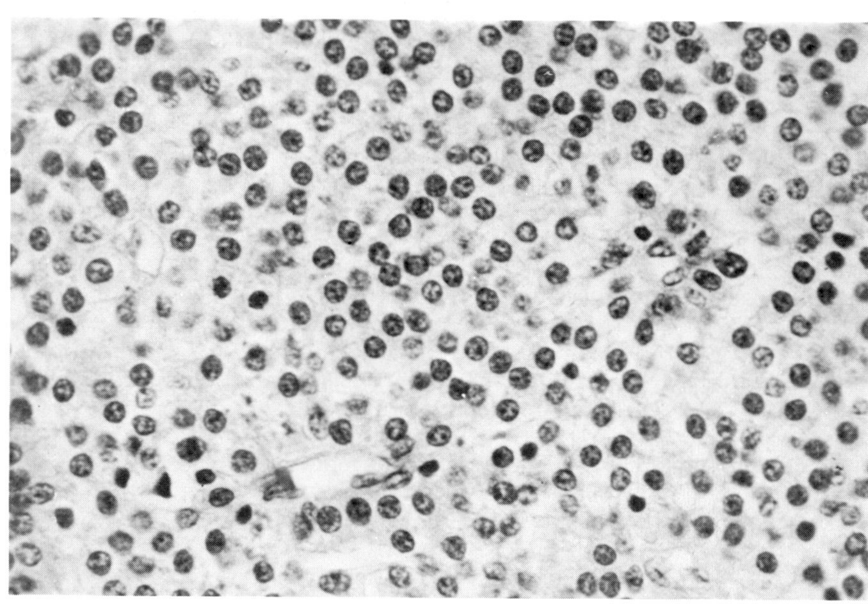

FIG. 9-2. Parathyroid hyperplasia, showing hypercellularity and crowding out of adipose tissue and blood vessels.

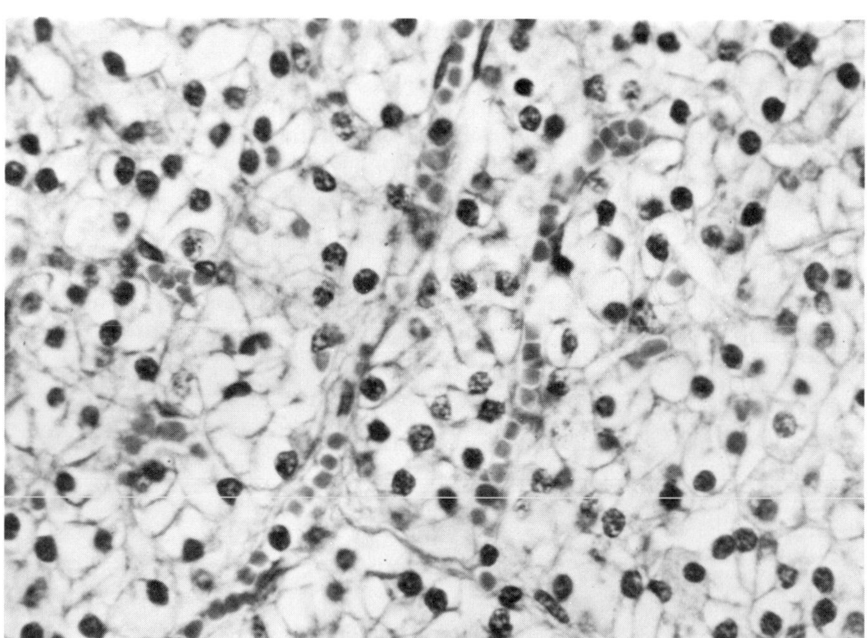

FIG. 9-3. Parathyroid adenoma. Most of the cells are the so-called clear cells or *wasserhelle* cells, which present a vesiculated clear cytoplasm containing glycogen and staining eosinophilic. The cytoplasm of other cells is granular and stains faintly basophilic.

PLATE 9-1. Osteitis fibrosa cystica (hyperparathyroidism). There is active bone resorption by multinucleated giant cell osteoclasts and little or no new bone formation. This same histologic picture may also be observed about the lesions of Paget's disease and fibrous dysplasia and in the wall of a bone cyst during the stage of active local resorption. A generalized distribution of active osteoclastic resorption throughout the skeleton identifies this as hyperparathyroidism. (×108) (See p. 229.)

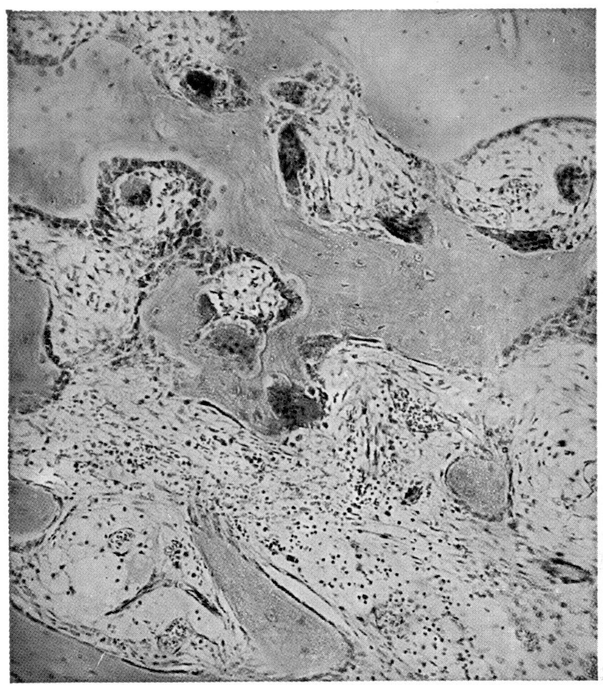

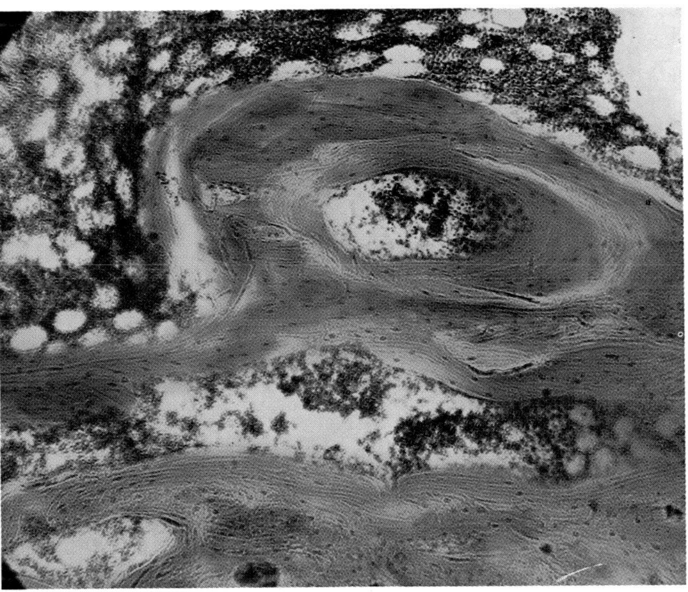

PLATE 9-2. Osteomalacia. The wide pink-staining osteoid seams are deficient in calcium salts. (×70) (See p. 234.)

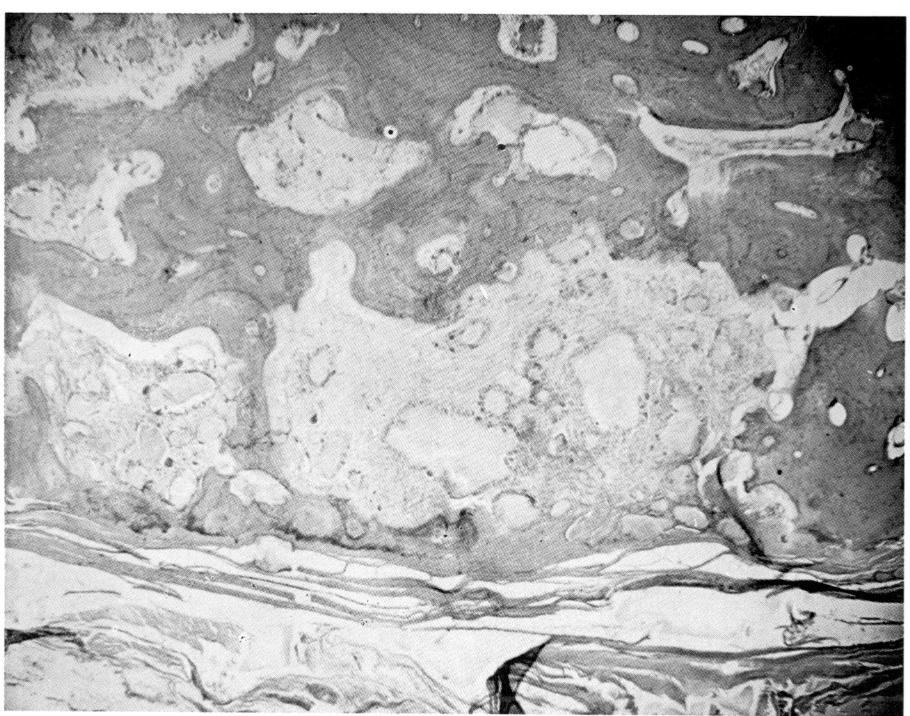

PLATE 9-3. Gout. Microscopic appearance of punched-out bony tophus. (Courtesy of Dr. Edward Rosenberg) (See p. 246.)

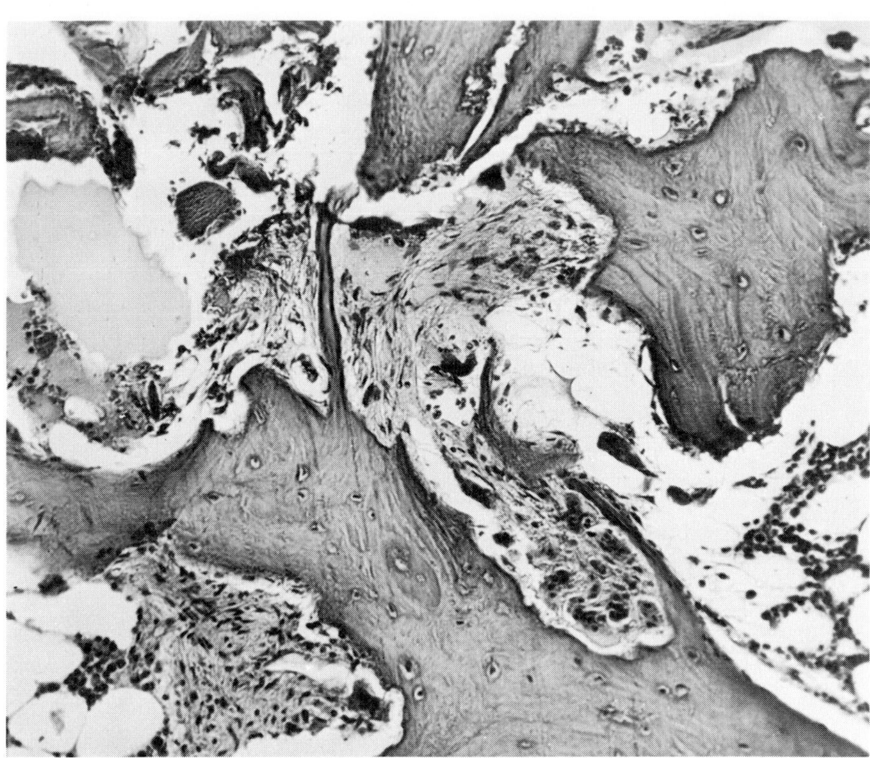

FIG. 9-4. Effect of hyperparathyroidism on bone. Marked osteoclastic resorption of trabeculae. Marrow spaces are filled with vascular fibrous tissue.

cause of excess secretion. The adenoma is composed mainly of the pale, clear, chief or principal cells. Rarely, oxyphils form the main components. The cells tend to form acini, cords, and patternless masses. Normal gland tissue and hyperplasia are characterized by cell uniformity (Figs. 9-2 and 9-3).

Skeletal changes are generalized and include the following:

Diffuse bone resorption. Large numbers of multinucleated osteoclasts are observed in Howship's lacunae, haversian canals are enlarged, and cortices are transformed to paper-thin cancellous bone (Fig. 9-4, Color Plate 9-1).

Deformities. Long bones bend under the stress of weight bearing. Intervertebral disks become ballooned as they indent soft vertebral bodies, forming the "codfish spine."

Pathologic fractures. These fractures occur frequently.

Marrow fibrosis. Replacement of marrow elements may cause anemia.

Brown tumors. These tumors are not actually tumors but are localized accumulations of hemorrhage and blood pigments and reactive masses of osteoclasts in a spindle-cell stroma. The "tumor" is a well-circumscribed dark brown area of soft consistency situated where bone resorption has been thorough. Healing may occur by fibrous tissue replacement, or the center may liquefy, and a bone cyst remains.

Multiple bone cysts. These cysts are unilocular or multilocular; they expand the cortex, leaving a paper-thin covering, and are often the site of pathologic fractures. The walls are composed of dense fibrous tissue, and the contents are serous fluid and fibrin (Fig. 9-5).

Healing. During the active resorptive stage of the disease, an attempt at replacement is observed in thin seams of osteoid apposition. Osteoid formation is especially pronounced at sites of stress, fractures, and bending deformities.

After parathyroidectomy, osteoclasts become sparse and osteoblastic activity becomes pronounced. Cortices thicken. Brown tumors disappear and are replaced by bone or become converted into cysts. The smaller cysts usually disappear, but the larger ones tend to persist. Skeletal deformities generally remain. Fibrous marrow is replaced by lamellar bone, marrow elements are slowly restored, and the blood picture improves.

CLINICAL PICTURE

Both sexes are affected, but the condition occurs most often in middle-aged women. Hyperparathyroidism usually exists for many years in a subclinical state and is

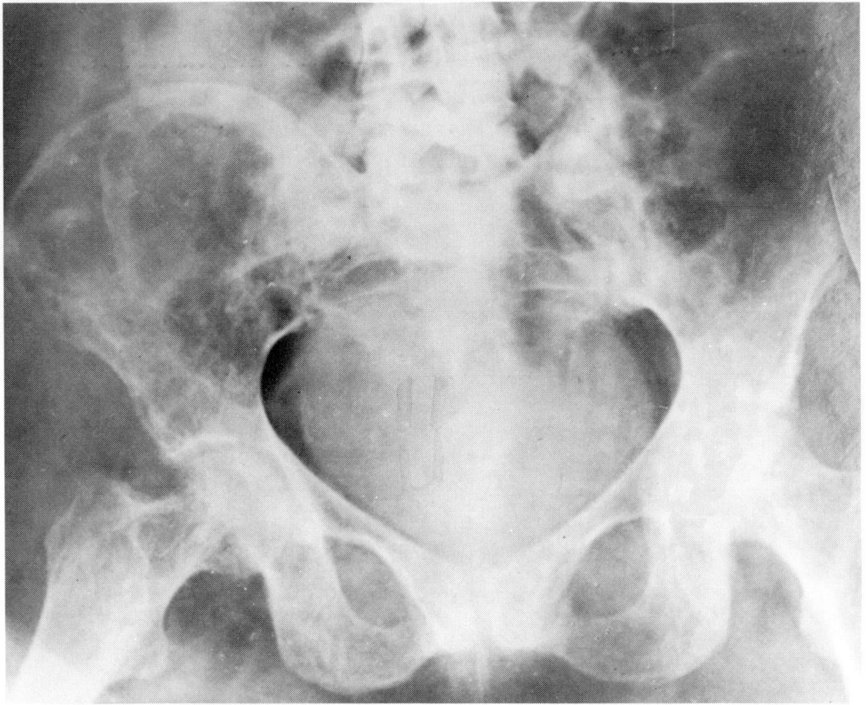

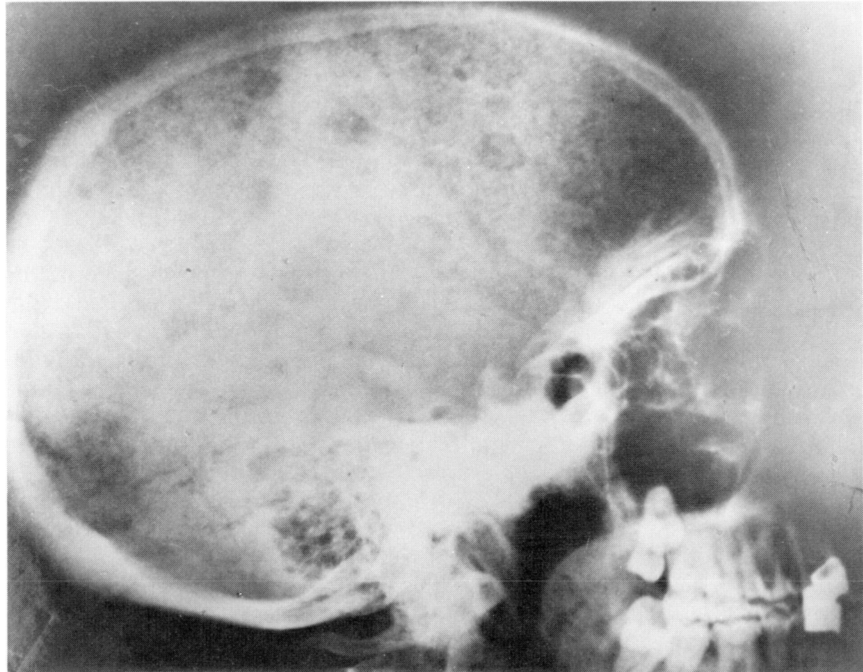

FIG. 9-5. Renal hyperparathyroidism. Multiple areas of cystic bone absorption.

often diagnosed as osteoporosis. Eventually, the following characteristic picture is manifest:

- Severe pain and tenderness in lower limbs and back
- Generalized muscle weakness and hypotonia
- Pathologic fractures and delayed union
- Deformity of limbs and spine
- Polyuria and polydypsia, a consequence of hyperphosphaturia. Sometimes diabetes insipidus is suspected.
- Renal calculi. Calcium salts often deposit as calculi or in the renal parenchyma, producing nephrocalcinosis. Renal colic, urinary infections, and uremia result.

ROENTGENOGRAPHIC FINDINGS

Early findings consist only of generalized deossification. The trabeculae become thinned, transverse trabeculae disappear, and cortices are narrowed. As the disease progresses, cysts appear throughout the skeleton, bending deformities develop, and renal calculi are observed. The skull displays a diffuse osteoporosis described as "pinhead stippling." Vertebrae are porotic and deeply indented by ballooned disks. Collapse of the bodies is frequent. Dental films reveal demineralization of the mandible, disappearance of the lamina dura and epulis tumors.

LABORATORY FINDINGS

Laboratory findings include hypercalcemia, hypophosphatemia, hypercalciuria, hyperphosphaturia, and a high alkaline phosphatase level.

DIFFERENTIAL DIAGNOSIS

Secondary hyperparathyroidism resulting from renal damage produces a high serum phosphorus level, a normal or lowered serum calcium, and often stunted growth. Osteomalacia and senile osteoporosis do not display the extreme degree of marrow fibrosis seen in hyperparathyroidism.

Hypercalcemia is a characteristic feature of sarcoidosis and vitamin D intoxication. Both conditions display excessive absorption of dietary calcium and high renal calcium clearance. These abnormalities are corrected by administration of cortisone. In contrast, cortisone has no effect on the hypercalcemia of hyperparathyroidism. This constitutes the cortisone test, which is particularly useful in differentiating the osteolytic bone lesions of sarcoidosis from those of hyperparathyroidism.[5]

TREATMENT

Experimentally, hyperparathyroidism may be controlled by large amounts of calcium, phosphorus, and vitamin D. However, the danger of calculi and renal destruction is great. The treatment of choice is parathyroidectomy. The neck and the mediastinum should be explored. One fourth of tumors are located in the mediastinum. Preoperative calcium administration is avoided for fear of causing acute parathyroid intoxication. In the presence of normal renal function and a normal alkaline phosphatase level (minimal bone involvement), the tumors should be removed completely. For hyperplasia, three glands and a portion of the fourth are removed. In the presence of an elevated serum phosphatase level and bony lesions, large quantities of calcium and phosphorus leave the bloodstream rapidly after parathyroidectomy. Consequently, the bloodstream is then at a dangerous hypocalcemia tetany level. It is necessary to administer sufficient quantities of these minerals until the gradually lowering alkaline phosphatase level indicates that the bone needs have been satisfied. When the alkaline phosphatase value is high and bone lesions are extensive, probably it is best to remove only a portion of the hyperfunctioning parathyroid tissue. In the presence of kidney damage, surgical resection should be conservative because some of the parathyroid hypertrophy is on a compensatory basis.

SPECIAL DIAGNOSTIC PROCEDURES

The diagnosis of primary hyperparathyroidism is aided by the performance of selected procedures.[1]

Phosphate Excretion Tests

PTH acts directly on the kidney and increases phosphaturia by depressing net phosphorus resorption by the renal tubule. Since the hormone cannot be accurately assayed, urinary excretion of phosphorus constitutes an indirect measurement of tubular resorption and therefore an index of the amount of circulating hormone. Various phosphate excretion tests have been devised. When performed with controlled phosphate intake in a subject with normal renal function and without glycosuria, a phosphate excretion test will delineate a borderline case of hyperparathyroidism.

Phosphorus Loading. Certain cases of hyperparathyroidism show normal phosphorus excretion, but this is usually due to deficient intake or poor absorption of dietary phosphorus. By administering an oral load of phosphorus (2 g to 3 g over 3 days) increased phosphaturia and diminished tubular resorption of phosphorus (TRP) can be brought out. The test is performed when the index of suspicion is high. The normal patient will demonstrate an insignificant fall of the TRP. In contrast, the hyperparathyroid patient will show a precipitous fall to values below 65%.

Dietary Phosphorus and Calcium Deprivation. Restriction of phosphorus and calcium may unmask the biochemical findings in normocalcemic and normophosphatemic patients. Such a dietary insult over a 10-day period will often demonstrate hypophosphatemia, hypercalcemia, and hypercalciuria.

Urinary Hydroxyproline

Hydroxyproline is a nonessential amino acid that occurs almost exclusively in collagen. Urinary hydroxyproline excretion is increased in hyperparathyroidism. This increase is attributed to accelerated bone turnover and collagen degradation. The increased urinary hydroxyproline content occurs usually, but not always, in association with increased alkaline phosphatase levels and roentgenographic manifestations of hyperparathyroidism (*e.g.*, osteitis fibrosa cystica).

Cortisone Suppression

The administration of steroids (*e.g.*, 150 mg cortisone per day for 10 days) will not affect the hypercalcemia of hyperparathyroidism. In contrast the hypercalcemia of sarcoidosis, thyrotoxicosis, multiple myeloma, hypervitaminosis D, and malignant disease is reduced. Exceptions to this rule can occur.

Isotope Studies

^{75}Se selenomethionine parathyroid scan can detect abnormal parathyroid tissue.[3,4]

Limitations of Serum Calcium Determination

Determination of serum calcium without simultaneous protein measurements is misleading, because approximately 0.75 mg calcium is bound to each gram of normal plasma albumin and globulin. In the presence of hypoproteinemia, an elevated serum calcium level may appear "normal" because of an excess of ionized ultrafilterable calcium.

Spontaneous remissions and intermittent hypercalcemia exist in hyperparathyroidism. Therefore, measurements of calcium should be repeated over weeks or months.

Measurement of urinary calcium is of little value because the frequency of hypercalciuria reportedly varies from 30% to 80%. PTH increases tubular resorption of calcium, and renal insufficiency may reduce or even abolish hypercalciuria.

Limitations of Serum Phosphorus Determinations

Of patients with surgically proven hyperparathyroidism and normal renal function 40% to 60% have normal serum phosphorus levels. Serum phosphorus is ordinarily increased in chronic renal disease with its attendant uremia and bone lesions (due to secondary hyperparathyroidism). Since serum phosphorus levels are depressed by estrogens and usually are at the upper limits of normal in postmenopausal females, a relatively low value (less than 3.5 mg/dl) in a postmenopausal woman with recurrent renal calculi should arouse the suspicion of hyperparathyroidism.

Radioimmunoassay

The serum level of PTH can be estimated indirectly by using antibodies prepared against either bovine or porcine PTH.[25] (See Chapter 6.)

HYPOPARATHYROIDISM

Hypoparathyroidism usually results from accidental removal of the parathyroids during thyroidectomy. It is characterized by low serum calcium and high serum phosphorus levels. Clinically, signs of muscle excitability are manifest as twitchings, carpopedal and laryngeal spasms, positive Chvostek and Trousseau signs, and convulsions. Treatment is either by administering expensive PTH or, better, by dihydrotachysterol administered orally 2 ml to 4 ml daily. The dosage of dihydrotachysterol must be regulated daily by the Sulkowitch test, a slightly subnormal serum calcium level being preferred. Calciferol (vitamin D_2) is used occasionally. It is cheaper but not as effective as dihydrotachysterol. The diet must be high in calcium but low in phosphorus. Milk is contraindicated because of its high phosphorus content. Intravenous injections of calcium effectively relieve attacks of tetany.

Parathyroid function is suppressed on diets that are deficient in magnesium. Infusions of magnesium sulfate restore the serum calcium levels to normal.[6] Bone biopsy reveals resumption of the normal histologic pattern.

PSEUDOHYPOPARATHYROIDISM

Pseudohypoparathyroidism is a rare disease first described by Albright that is caused by congenital lack of adenyl cyclase. The production of PTH is adequate, even increased, but the target organs (*i.e.*, kidney, bone) are unable to respond to the hormone. Consequently, the bone architecture is generally unchanged, although certain gross skeletal abnormalities develop and are characteristic, including short stature and shortened ulnar metacarpals. Urinary excretion of cyclic adenosine monophosphate (AMP) is reduced or absent, and urinary phosphorus content is diminished.

DIAGNOSIS

When parathyroid extract is administered, typical clinical and blood chemistry changes fail to develop.

Also, during activation of renal tubular adenyl cyclase by PTH, cyclic AMP is released into the tubular lumen and is secreted in the urine. Measurement of the molecule in the urine evaluates renal responsiveness to PTH. Pseudohypoparathyroidism is characterized by renal unresponsiveness to PTH.

TREATMENT

Therapy with dehydrotachysterol and vitamin D_2 is effective.

LOW-PHOSPHORUS RICKETS AND OSTEOMALACIA

The association of low-phosphorus rickets and osteomalacia is caused by lack of absorption of phosphorus from foodstuffs, due either to dietary insufficiency or vitamin deficiency. The calcium level in the bloodstream is maintained by normal parathyroid activity.

On the other hand, rickets and osteomalacia in which patients show high serum phosphorus and low calcium levels are associated with compensatory parathyroid hyperplasia; the excess phosphorus is excreted, and the calcium level is elevated at the expense of the bone.

These conditions will be described fully under their respective headings.

CALCIUM-DEFICIENCY DISEASES

A physiological level of serum calcium must be maintained or the state of hypocalcemia will result, characterized chiefly by muscle hyperirritability. Calcium is supplied from the diet and from body stores, mainly from bone. Within the bone, processes of new bone formation and old bone resorption are taking place constantly. When calcium absorbed from the gastrointestinal tract is insufficient, the serum level is restored by mobilization from bone. The parathyroids undergo compensatory hyperplasia, and their effect is seen within the bone as ingrowth of vascular fibrous tissue replacing marrow and very active osteoclasis. Bone destruction exceeds bone formation. New protein matrix (pink-staining osteoid) is being laid down in a strong effort at reconstruction. This is reflected in the bloodstream by an increase in the alkaline phosphatase level. However, the osteoid tissue remains uncalcified to a large degree, accumulates in large amounts, and softens the bone (osteomalacia), which in turn yields to stresses and strains.

When this chain of events takes place during infancy and childhood, longitudinal growth is affected. The process of endochondral ossification at the epiphyseal growth plate demands that the cartilage be calcified before it can be resorbed and replaced by osteoid. The latter in turn is meagerly formed at this site and remains uncalcified.

Excessive mobilization of calcium from the skeleton, when not caused by deficient absorption from the intestine, is caused by hyperparathyroidism, which is either primary or secondary to renal disease.

RICKETS

Rickets (rachitis) is defined as a disease of infancy and childhood due to insufficiency of calcium and characterized clinically chiefly by softened and deformed bones. The typical clinical condition to be described is extremely rare except under circumstances of famine. However, the orthopaedic surgeon should bear in mind that, regardless of present-day prophylactic vitamin and nutritional care, a low-grade subclinical type is frequently responsible for certain deformities such as knock-knee and bowleg. Often such a patient, when given additional amounts of vitmin D, will display surprising spontaneous correction. When florid rickets yields only to a very high dosage of vitamin D, the case is classified as vitamin D–resistant rickets. Apparently some unknown factor causes a variable degree of response to the vitamin.

ETIOLOGY

Calcium lack is due to vitamin D deficiency, intestinal diseases, and dietary lack of calcium and phosphorus.

Vitamin D promotes the adsorption of these minerals from the intestine. It is a fat-soluble vitamin, usually associated in foods with vitamin A and found in strongest concentration in fish-liver oils. It is present in lesser amounts in milk, cream, butter, egg yolk, and animal fats. It is prepared commercially by irradiation of ergosterol, a lipid obtained from yeast. The ultraviolet rays of the sun or a mercury quartz lamp convert the sterols of the skin to vitamin D. Dust, window glass, and skin pigmentation will impede penetration of ultraviolet rays.

Intestinal diseases such as steatorrhea, celiac disease, and sprue, as well as the common diarrheas, cause their effect in one of three ways:

1. Fat is inadequately digested and combines with calcium and phosphorus to form soaps, which are eliminated.
2. Vitamin D, being fat soluble, is likewise eliminated.
3. Intestinal irritation reduces absorptive power.

Insufficient calcium and phosphorus implies a diet consisting of foods with minimal amounts of these minerals. Milk, cheese, nuts, and cabbage contain an abundance of calcium phosphate. Rickets is rare during the first 6 months because of ample nutrition derived *in utero*. Prenatal calcium and vitamin lack in the mother (osteomalacia) is the main cause of fetal rickets. Infantile rickets is the most common type, developing between 6 months and 3 years of age. Late rickets, or rachitis tarda, is rare and is observed under conditions of famine or vitamin resistance. An important complication at this age is separation of epiphyses, especially of the upper femoral epiphysis.

The disease occurs mainly in winter and in nontropical regions, which is explained by deficient sunlight. The blacks and the Italians exhibit a marked predisposition. A child who grows rapidly in height is more likely to develop rachitic changes than one whose growth is slow.

Antiepileptic drugs administered to children for prolonged periods of time will induce the formation of hepatic enzymes that interfere with conversion of calciferol to more active forms. About 25% of these children develop rickets, especially in those who are inactive, unexposed to sunlight, and dark skinned. (See Osteomalacia.)

METABOLIC ABNORMALITY

Unavailability of vitamin D or failure of sunlight to produce D_2 and D_3 results in insufficient production of 1,25-dihydroxy vitamin D. The latter substance is the biologically active material that is the end product of metabolic conversion of exogenous and endogenous vitamin D. The result is diminished absorption of calcium through the intestinal wall and decreased transport of calcium in (and out) of bone. Hypocalcemia and hypocalciuria ensue.

Hypocalcemia induces parathyroid hyperplasia. Excess PTH restores blood levels of calcium by mobilization from bone, increasing intestinal absorption of calcium, and increasing renal tubular resorption of calcium. In addition, PTH acts on the renal tubules to reduce resorption of phosphorus, causing phosphaturia and hypophosphatemia. Bone resorption is excessive; nevertheless there are compensatory attempts at bone formation, thus explaining the elevated serum alkaline phosphatase level. A state of negative calcium and phosphorus balance exists; there is insufficient calcium and phosphorus for mineralization of newly formed bone.

PATHOLOGY

The histologic feature of rickets (and osteomalacia) is osteoid tissue, which is the protein base in which the calcium and phosphorus salt has failed to deposit.[2] Rickets and osteomalacia are fundamentally identical disturbances. *Osteomalacia* is the term applied after the epiphyseal plates have disappeared. The process may be divided into active and healing stages.

Active Stage. At the epiphyseal plate, the orderly progression of endochondral ossification is interrupted. Proliferation of cartilage cells, palisade arrangement, and formation of matrix proceeds normally, but calcification of the matrix is deficient. This step is a necessary prerequisite to laying down of new bone about calcified cartilage. Capillary inshoots from the metaphysis invade and destroy the chondrocytes and lay down osteoid about large islands of noncalcified cartilage. The cartilage cell columns proliferate meanwhile to 10 to 20 times the normal depth of cells in a haphazard arrangement. The enormous accumulation of proliferated cartilage and osteoid tissue results in a widened, irregular epiphyseal line of radiolucency extending deeply into the metaphysis.

In the metaphysis and the diaphysis, thick layers of osteoid are laid down about thin old residual fragments of bone and within enlarged haversian canals (Color Plate 9-2). Pink-staining tissue appears everywhere, producing large bizarre-shaped, disorderly arranged trabeculae. A layer of osteoid often develops subperiosteally as an exhuberant growth near the epiphyseal plate. Characteristic globular enlargements are formed in typical situations such as the costochondral junctions of ribs (rachitic rosary). The marrow displays a moderate degree of vascularity and fibrosis.

Healing Stage. Calcium salts are deposited in the zone of preparatory calcification. Capillaries penetrate the columns of proliferated chondrocytes and lay down osteoid about the calcified cartilage. The osteoid promptly becomes calcified and transformed to bone. The thickness of the epiphyseal plate is reduced to normal size. Osteoid trabeculae throughout the metaphysis and the shaft after conversion to bone resume their normal architecture. The fibrotic marrow is replaced by fatty and hematogenous elements. A bowed extremity often corrects itself spontaneously.

CLINICAL PICTURE

A history of dietary deficiency may be obtained. The infant displays increased restlessness at night, profuse diaphoresis, skin pallor, and a disinclination to play. A generalized catarrh of the mucous membranes is manifested by diarrhea and respiratory infection. Occasionally, irritability of the central nervous system (hypocalcemia) results in spasmophilia, convulsions, Chvostek's sign, and opisthotonus. The following features are characteristic:

Head: large bosses over frontal and parietal eminences, flattening of occiput and vertex, causing, enlarged squared appearance (caput quadratum); fontanelles late in closing; bones thin and crackling (craniotabes)
Chest: beading enlargements at costochondral junctions (rachitic rosary); horizontal depression (Harrison's groove) a few inches above lower costal margin caused by pull of diaphragm on softened ribs; chest cage narrowed transversely and elongated anteroposteriorly (pigeon breast)
Abdomen: prominent
Pelvis: compressed transversely by weight bearing, inlet narrowed
Enlarged epiphyses: especially at centers of most rapid growth (knees, wrist)
Delayed dentition
Skin pallor: secondary anemia
Poor tone of muscles: delayed walking
Deformities: lower extremities most often deformed consequent to pressures of weight bearing; knock-knees usually due to deformity at lower end of femurs; bowlegs usually caused by lateral bowing

and internal torsion of tibiae; coxa vara causes waddling gait; ligamentous laxity about deformed joints is typical

Incomplete fractures: frequent and are a result of an insignificant trauma

Growth restriction: lasts only a comparatively short time so that stature is not affected. It is only in nonrecognized rickets that dwarfism is allowed to develop over a long period of time.

ROENTGENOGRAPHIC FINDINGS

In the acute stage, the ossification center in the epiphysis becomes poorly defined and smaller. The epiphyseal border of the metaphysis is cup shaped, ill defined, and frayed. These findings are most pronounced about epiphyseal plates exhibiting the greatest rate of growth (*e.g.*, lower end of femur, upper end of tibia). The metaphyseal cortices flare outward (trumpeting), and the epiphyseometaphyseal junction is widened. There is reduction in the secondary transverse trabeculae; the longitudinal trabeculae persist but are quite thin. The cortices are less sharply defined (because of osteoporosis and osteoid deposition). The bones, especially the long weight-bearing bones, bend, with the cortices thickening on the concave side (Fig. 9-6).

In healing, a dense line appears at the epiphyseometaphyseal junction. This is the newly calcified cartilage. The epiphyseal line becomes narrower and well defined. The epiphyseal ossified nucleus becomes more dense, larger, and well defined. Transverse trabeculations reappear, and cortices resume their density and definition. Bending deformities with continued growth often disappear or subside to a great degree.

LABORATORY FINDINGS

The serum phosphorus level is typically reduced. Often the serum alkaline phosphatase value is high. Compensatory hyperparathyroidism generally maintains a normal serum calcium level but at the same time effects excretion of phosphorus. When this mechanism is defective, the serum calcium level falls and symptoms of neuromuscular irritability ensue.

The urinary calcium level is almost invariably diminished. The urinary output of calcium in a child with rickets may fall considerably below the normal of 5 mg/kg/24 hr. In children on a standard diet, values of 3 mg

FIG. 9-6. Rickets. (*Left*) Thickened and broadened epiphyseal plates. Ossification of the metaphysis is irregular and defective. The metaphysis is wide, its margin pointed, and the central area indented, resulting in a saucer-shaped appearance. The shaft is bowed; the cortex is thin on the convex side and thick on the concave. (*Right*) Broad, saucer-shaped metaphyses, bowing of the diaphyses, and thickening of the cortex on the side of the concavity.

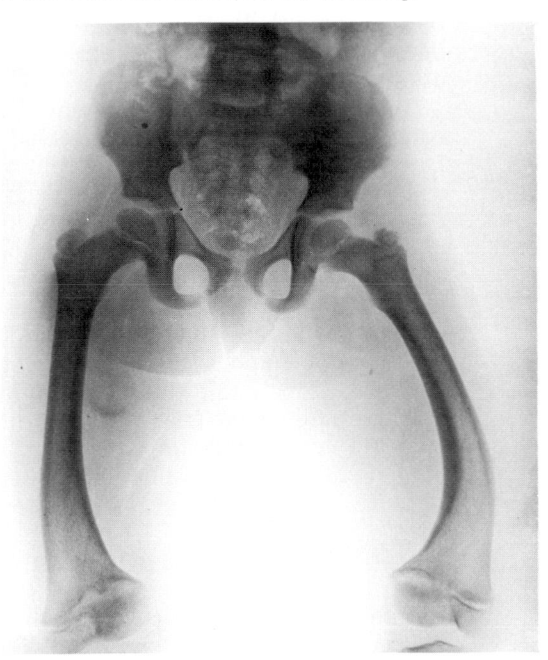

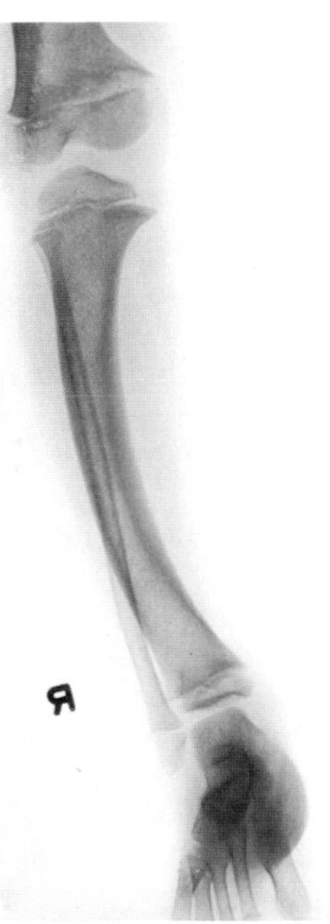

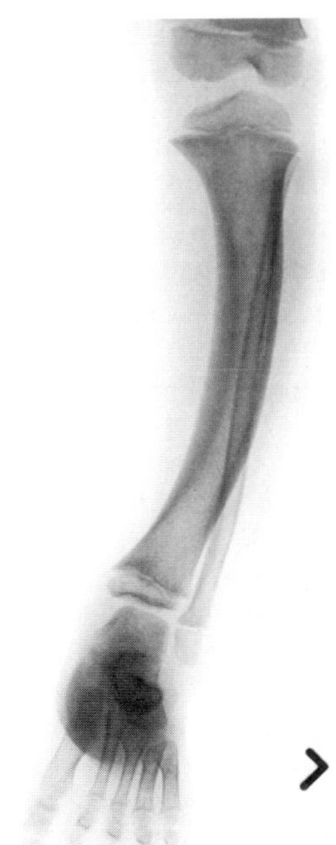

or less/kg/24 hr are considered indicative of a hypocalcemic syndrome.

TREATMENT

Prophylaxis consists chiefly of administration of vitamin D and exposure to sunlight, especially for premature infants and those on artificial milk feedings. Active treatment by vitamin D, calcium preparations, and ultraviolet rays will effect healing, which is demonstrable on roentgenograms within 2 weeks. Deformity of the lower extremities usually spontaneously regresses to a great degree over a period of months. The application of braces or osteotomy to correct deformity is generally unnecessary. Failure of spontaneous correction usually signifies an inadequate dosage of vitamin D. Rarely, when deformity persists, osteotomy is indicated but is best postponed until growth is complete. Knock-knee and bowleg are discussed in detail in Chapter 28.

CELIAC DISEASE

Celiac disease (idiopathic steatorrhea, nontropical sprue, Gee's disease, or Gee-Thaysen disease) is characterized by a malabsorptive defect that allows loss of dietary fat and fat-soluble vitamin D in the stools. It is usually due to a gluten-sensitive enteropathy. An excess of free fatty acids combines with calcium forming precipitates of soap, which are excreted as such in the stool. Parenterally administered vitamin D does not correct the intestinal absorptive defect until gluten is withdrawn from the diet. Rickets sometimes develop in the growing child and osteomalacia in the adult. The finding of excess fat in the stools and positive findings on biopsy of the duodenal mucosa are diagnostic.[19]

CLINICAL PICTURE

The features of celiac disease include the following:

Onset in infancy or early childhood: may persist into adulthood
Diarrhea, anorexia, and irritability: in the infant
Pale, foul, bulky stools: may be absent
Steatorrhea: may be lacking in adult
Retarded growth and development: short stature
Muscle wasting: particularly of proximal groups
Abdominal protuberance: gaseous distention
Iron deficiency anemia
Rickets: may develop in growing child
Osteomalacia: may develop in adult

LABORATORY FINDINGS

The following tests are useful in the laboratory diagnosis:

Duodenal biopsy: peroral method reveals diminished number or total loss of villi
Fecal examination: microscopic fecal smears for fat; quantitative fecal fat (normal up to 5% of ingested fat)
Roentgenographic examination: intestinal dilatation

TREATMENT

A gluten-free diet, high potency vitamin D administered parenterally and calcium lactate injected intramuscularly, and a high protein diet are the modes of treatment.

RENAL CAUSES OF RICKETS AND OSTEOMALACIA

Renal dwarfism, renal pseudorickets, and renal osteitis fibrosa cystica are forms of renal-caused rickets or osteomalacia. Renal insufficiency, whether a result of glomerular or tubular disease, is associated with compensatory parathyroid hyperplasia, which deprives the skeleton of calcium. Typical hyperparathyroid histologic changes in the bone consist of active osteoclastic resorption and fibrosis, with the calcium being mobilized to combat the renal acidosis. Failure of absorption of calcium and vitamin D from the intestine does not occur, so that uncalcified osteoid tissue does not form as extensively as it does in rickets and osteomalacia. However, even the dietary calcium becomes relatively unavailable for bone so that a slight degree of osteoid and bony softening develops. Therefore, weight-bearing deformities are not as pronounced as in rickets.

When the renal factor is present at birth, it is due to congenital cystic disease or congenital hydronephrosis. Later in life chronic glomerulonephritis, chronic interstitial nephritis, and the nephroses due to heavy metal poisoning are etiologic factors. Congenital kidney conditions have an insidious slowly progressive effect throughout childhood, usually becoming clinically manifest at about puberty or adolescence. Typical rachitic changes chronically interfere with endochondral ossification at the epiphyseal plates, thereby restricting longitudinal growth. Shortness of stature and enlarged epiphyses are characteristic. True florid rickets is never seen. The condition is simply low-grade rickets, because of unavailable calcium, superimposed on osteitis fibrosa.

RENAL DISEASE WITH PHOSPHATE RETENTION

The retention of nonprotein nitrogen is almost always associated with retention of phosphorus. The serum calcium level becomes lowered because it adjusts to the high serum phosphorus level, and it is used up as a base to combat the acidosis. The parathyroids hypertrophy to excrete more hormone, which acts either by promoting excretion of serum phosphates or by promoting resorption of bone tissue. Pathologically, one sees a predominance of bone destruction rather than a delay in the calcification of newly formed osteoid.

Clinically, in children before union of the epiphyses, in addition to bony changes of osteitis fibrosa cystica, changes are seen at the epiphyseal line almost identical with those of rickets. Slipping of the upper femoral epiphyses is not uncommon. Retardation of longitudinal growth is a constant finding.

The characteristics of renal osteitis fibrosa generalisata in adults include the following:

- Longstanding and severe renal insufficiency
- Nitrogen and phosphorus retention
- Normal or slightly low serum calcium level
- Severe acidosis with a low CO_2 combining power of serum
- High serum chloride or low serum sodium level
- Mönckeberg type arteriosclerosis (medial arteriosclerosis)
- High serum phosphatase level
- Sometimes calcium deposits around joints
- Generalized skeletal decalcification with a cystic or motheaten appearance seen on roentgenograms.

RENAL DISEASE WITH EXCESSIVE PHOSPHORUS LOSS

Two separate conditions can be distinguished in which tubular function failure results in excessive phosphate excretion.

Failure of Tubules to Form a Base With Which to Excrete Acid in Urine. As demand is made on calcium, which appears in increased amounts in the urine, the low serum calcium level leads to a low serum phosphorus level. Low levels of serum calcium and phosphorus cause failure of mineral deposition in bone. Osteomalacia develops and is less resistant to stresses and strains, osteoblasts are stimulated, and a high serum alkaline phosphatase level results. The low serum phosphorus level delays calcification of newly formed osteoid, so that a greater amount of this tissue is seen.

Hypokalemia is a common complication of renal acidosis. Potassium, like calcium, is used as a base and is excreted in excess in the urine. Symptoms of the low potassium syndrome include pain in the extremities, inability to move the arms and the legs, and electrocardiographic changes.

Nephrocalcinosis and nephrolithiasis frequently accompany this form of renal acidosis. Alkali therapy decreases calcium excretion in the urine and lessens formation of new stones. The etiology of this disorder is obscure.

Fanconi's Syndrome. In Fanconi's syndrome, the renal tubules fail to absorb phosphates, glucose, and many of the amino acids.[22] Consequently, a low serum phosphorus level is associated with glycosuria and aminoaciduria.

Fanconi, in 1936, described the condition as characterized by a hereditary tendency; often a history of consanguinity; retarded growth; rickets; albuminuria; glycosuria; persistently alkaline urine; increase of organic acids, ammonia, phosphorus, and calcium in the urine; marked hypophosphatemia without hypercalcemia; lowering of the blood bicarbonate without azotemia; and degenerative changes in the renal tubular epithelium. Cystine deposits in almost all organs, mainly the reticuloendothelial system, may be associated if the kidney is unable to excrete cystine.

The mechanism of production of late rickets and osteomalacia seems to be an acidosis due to increased urinary excretion of base secondary to increased urinary excretion of organic acids.

Symptoms of this disorder appear early in childhood and become progressively worse.

TREATMENT OF RENAL RICKETS AND OSTEOMALACIA

If properly treated, the relief of skeletal symptoms is often spectacular. Alkaline salts are administered, especially those combinations of the salt of a mineral base with an organic acid (*e.g.*, sodium citrate, sodium lactate, or calcium gluconate). If hypokalemia is a factor, potassium citrate is added. The organic acid is destroyed, leaving the base free to help in the excretion of acid in the urine. Citric acid may be given to increase gastric acidity and aid calcium absorption. To overcome the osteomalacia, a high calcium intake and massive doses of vitamin D will effect a strongly positive calcium balance. Osteomalacia is cured, and normal growth is resumed. Thereafter, loss of calcium can be prevented by alkali therapy alone. Continuation of vitamin D in massive doses is not advisable for fear of causing vitamin D poisoning.

RENAL DIALYSIS PROTOCOL

When the degree of renal insufficiency requires renal dialysis on a regular basis, the following should be incorporated into the regimen.

- *Dialysate Ca^{2+} levels raised* to 6.5 mg/dl (3.25 to 3.5 mEq/l)
- *Oral Ca^{2+}*, only when hypophosphatemia does not exist
- *Dihydrotachysterol,* 0.125 mg to 0.5 mg per day
- *Oral phosphate binders* (*e.g.*, aluminum hydroxide)
- *Dialysate Mg^{2+} level* kept at 1.5 mEq/l

VITAMIN D–RESISTANT RICKETS

Formerly thought to be rare, refractory or vitamin-resistant rickets is known to be quite common and probably is the most frequent cause of dwarfism.[7,24] Compared with the usual form of rickets, refractory rickets is more severe, fails to respond to usual doses, but responds to massive doses of vitamin D. Albright's metabolic studies revealed that vitamin D is absorbed but that the patient does not respond until a threshold level has been exceeded. An adequate response is shown by increased urinary excretion of calcium and decreased fecal excretion of calcium. The serum phosphorus level rises, and the alkaline phosphatase level subsides to normal. Roentgenograms reveal healing at the epiphyseal lines, and growth is resumed at the rate of 1 cm/month.

CLINICAL PICTURE

A marked familial tendency is often observed. The patient is of short stature with all the usual signs of florid rickets. Deformities are severe, particularly in the lower extremities, where bowlegs, knock-knees and a "tackle deformity," consisting of a bowleg on one side and a knock-knee on the other, are seen. Marked ligamentous instability is typical. A waddling gait is due to coxa vara. These deformities are persistent and typically recur after attempted osteotomies. The skull has a characteristic appearance: anteroposterior diameter is increased and transverse diameter is decreased (dolichocephaly); frontal bossing and a marked external occipital protuberance occur. The nose is often saddle shaped.

ROENTGENOGRAPHIC FINDINGS

These findings are the usual findings of rickets. However, the trabeculae are coarser, broader, and more widely spread than usual.

LABORATORY FINDINGS

The serum phosphorus level is generally below 3 mg, the calcium level is normal, and the alkaline phosphatase level is elevated to 20 or more Bodansky units.

Results of the urinary qualitative Sulkowitch test are negative or reveal only a trace of calcium. The urine concentration is normal, and its reaction is acid.

DIFFERENTIAL DIAGNOSIS

Cases that in the past have been wrongly classified as achondroplasia, dyschondroplasia, and chondrodysplasia (and their hopeless prognosis) are now properly identified by blood and urine studies and by response to high dosage of vitamin D.

The condition must also be differentiated from renal rickets and the Fanconi syndrome by its decreased urinary calcium excretion, absence of glucose albumin and amino acids in the urine, and absence of disturbed plasma electrolytes.

In adults the disorder is characterized chiefly by dwarfism. The alkaline phosphatase level is usually normal, but variable phosphorus levels are observed. The roentgenogram displays a coarse architecture of trabeculae, Looser lines, vertebrae typically biconcave with ballooned disks, and degenerative changes at the knees, the hips, and the lumbosacral spine. At the points of attachment of large muscle masses, a bony protuberance suggests the effect of prolonged traction on soft bone. Various bony deformities, especially about the knees, have existed since childhood.

TREATMENT

The aim of treatment is to provide a high dosage of vitamin D and maintain the Sulkowitch test at 1 to 2+ (at this level urinary calcium casts do not appear). First, the threshold level is determined by increasing the dosage until the Sulkowitch test shows that adequate urinary excretion of calcium is occurring. Then the dosage is increased until the serum phosphorus level reaches 5 mg or until toxic symptoms appear, including anorexia, nausea, vomiting, weight loss, occasional hematuria, and rarely oliguria or anuria with nephrocalcinosis. Toxicity is not seen when the serum calcium level is kept below 12 mg and the Sulkowitch result below 3+. Above 12 mg nephrocalcinosis occurs; above 16 mg, general metastatic calcification develops. Blood and urinary changes are noted within a week and roentgenographic changes are observed after 3 to 4 weeks. Vitamin D must be continued until growth is complete to ensure adequate continuance of growth. After cessation of growth, persistence of serum and urinary findings indicates that osteomalacia is present; high vitamin dosage must be continued.

Attempted surgery, especially osteotomies for correction of deformities, are best delayed until the epiphyses have closed. Otherwise, recurrence is almost inevitable. When osteotomy is performed and followed by plaster immobilization, hypercalcemia and hypercalciuria develop, and the extremely high concentration of calcium in the urine may interfere with renal function. Therefore, preoperatively it is advisable to suspend vitamin D administration until 2 weeks postoperatively.

In adults with demineralization and deformity of the spine, especially in a subject of short stature, consideration must be given to the possibility of vitamin D resistance. Appropriate metabolic study may reveal this condition.

DIFFERENTIATING FEATURES OF VITAMIN D–DEFICIENCY RICKETS AND VITAMIN D–RESISTANT RICKETS

Vitamin D–deficient (nutritional) rickets is rapidly reversed by the administration of relatively small amounts of vitamin D, namely, 50μg or less daily (1μg vitamin D_2 = 40 IU).[13]

The term *vitamin D–resistant rickets* may be loosely applied to any condition (*e.g.*, steatorrhea, chronic renal glomerular failure, and renal tubular abnormalities) that requires amounts a thousand times greater (mg rather than μg) to produce healing.

In most civilized countries, renal tubular defects have become the most common cause of rickets today. The most common type of renal tubular rickets, renal tubular hypophosphatemic rickets (phosphate diabetes), is representative of a vitamin D–resistant disorder (Table 9-4).

OSTEOMALACIA

Osteomalacia (mollities ossium) is a condition of adults characterized by softening of the bones because of an accumulation of osteoid tissue, the bone matrix that fails to mineralize. Therefore, it is identical with rickets of infancy and childhood except that longitudinal growth is unaffected.

ETIOLOGY

The process of catabolism (osteoclastic resorption) in bone tissue throughout the body continues normally. On the other hand, the process of anabolism continues normally only as far as laying down of bone matrix (osteoid), but the hardening precipitation of lime salts does not occur.

The most common cause of osteomalacia is vitamin D deficiency. In the Western World, where nutritional needs are met, the most frequent underlying cause is a derangement of vitamin D and phosphate metabolism that is either hereditary or acquired.

PATHOGENESIS

The main theories are those concerned with vitamin D and phosphate metabolism and the effects of chronic systemic acidosis. Less well understood are factors interfering with the synthesis and maturation of collagen fibers that produce a defective osteoid tissue within which mineralization cannot occur.

Vitamin D. The main biologic effects of vitamin D are promotion of calcium absorption by the gut and mobilization of mineral from the bone. Probable effects on bone are bone formation and mineralization; effects on the renal tubule are inhibition of calcium resorption and encouraging phosphate resorption.

The source of dietary (exogenous) vitamin D is irradiated ergosterol, known as calciferol or D_2. Various conditions may interfere with its absorption. Endogenous vitamin D, D_3 or cholecalciferol, is formed from ultraviolet light acting on the precursor substance in the skin. Through a series of conversions, the active principle evolves: 1,25-dihydro vitamin D.

Deficiency of vitamin D, whether dietary lack, malabsorption, or disturbed metabolism, results in failure to mineralize newly formed osteoid tissue (see discussion on vitamin D).

Inorganic Phosphate. Hypophosphatemia impairs bone formation by interfering with the function of osteoblasts (collagen synthesis and mineralization).[17] On the other hand, hyperphosphatemia stimulates bone formation. The level of inorganic phosphate in the body fluids depends on the secretory and resorptive activity of the renal tubules. The main factor governing such function is PTH; it interferes with phosphate resorption, thereby encouraging phosphorus loss and lowering the serum phosphorus level. Therefore, only normal renal tubules can respond to PTH and reject phosphate.

Hypophosphatemia is brought about by renal phosphate "leak," hyperparathyroidism, or phosphate depletion by chronic use of nonabsorbable antacids. The chain of events can be represented as follows:

$$\downarrow \text{P intake} \rightarrow \text{sP} \downarrow \rightarrow \text{sCa} \uparrow \rightarrow \text{PTH} \downarrow \rightarrow \text{TRP} \uparrow \rightarrow \text{uP} \downarrow \rightarrow \text{sP} \uparrow \rightarrow \text{Ca} = \text{N}$$

TABLE 9-4 Differentiating Features of Vitamin D–Deficient Rickets and Vitamin D–Resistant Rickets

Vitamin D–Resistant Rickets	Vitamin D–Deficiency Rickets
Inherited	Acquired
No muscular weakness	Muscular weakness
No hypocalcemic tetany	Hypocalcemic tetany can occur
Serum phosphorus always low before treatment; after treatment, phosphorus rises a little but never returns to normal, even with prolonged treatment with large doses	Serum phosphorus low or normal; if low, returns rapidly to normal with small doses
Growth rate seldom becomes normal with treatment; patient remains dwarfed	Normal growth rate resumed with treatment

Chronic Acidosis. Osteomalacia is often associated with systemic acidosis caused by renal tubular disease and chronic glomerular insufficiency, probably occurring as follows:

Bone mineral buffers hydrogen ions. The increased demand for neutralizing bases uses up the available calcium, which leaves an inadequate supply for mineralization of osteoid.
Acidosis diminishes tubular reabsorption of calcium.
Hypophosphatemia and vitamin D resistance are usually associated with chronic systemic acidosis.

PATHOLOGY

The basic pathologic finding is an excess of persisting osteoid seams, which surround thin, old trabeculae. Here and there a normal degree of osteoclasia is proceeding. Much of the compact bone is transformed into cancellous bone. Osteoblastic activity continues, and layer upon layer of osteoid tissue is formed. The development of osteoid is most pronounced at sites of maximal stress and strain. The marrow appears to be vascular and fibrous, especially in patients with secondary hyperparathyroidism.

Fractures are usually multiple and heal with an abundant callus formation, consisting chiefly of osteoid, so that union is markedly delayed. Grotesque deformities develop as a result of bending with weight-bearing pressures.

CLINICAL PICTURE

Deformities, particularly of weight-bearing structures, constitute the chief findings. The leg and thigh are severely bent. Scoliotic and kyphotic deformities of the spine develop. Pressure of the femoral heads produces coxa vara deformities of the femoral necks and indentation of the acetabulae (protrusio) and the lateral walls of the pelvis.

Generalized skeletal pains and tenderness occur but may be confined to the lower back and lower extremities. An acute onset of localized pain and tenderness may signify an incomplete fracture. Muscle weakness is typical.

Other symptoms are related to the causative dietary, gastrointestinal, or renal factors.

ROENTGENOGRAPHIC FINDINGS

Osteomalacia effects a generalized demineralization with loss of transverse trabeculae, not unlike the appearance of osteoporosis. Laboratory and clinical findings may be necessary to distinguish the two conditions. It is also important to recognize that osteomalacia may be present without roentgenographic evidence.

The two diagnostic findings when bone changes are pronounced are demineralization and persistent transverse Looser zones. The skeleton is diffusely rarefied, and the cortices are thinned. There is no subperiosteal resorption of bone in contrast to hyperparathyroidism. Thus the lamina dura around the teeth is present in osteomalacia and absent in hyperparathyroidism.

Looser lines, or pseudofractures, are frequently found. These transverse, bilaterally symmetrical lines of rarefaction extend incompletely across the bones. Albright believes that these represent incomplete fractures that have healed by callus consisting of osteoid tissue persisting for lack of calcium. A Looser line often occurs in a bone that otherwise may appear to be normal and may be the only evidence of osteomalacia. It occurs repeatedly at characteristic points: the necks of the femurs, the rami of the pubis and ischium, the ribs, and typically in the axillary edge of the scapula immediately below the glenoid. It lasts for months or years without regressing, is bilaterally symmetrical, and occurs only in patients with rickets and osteomalacia. Occasionally, the periosteum overlying these areas may be seen as elevated, with a slight deposit of subperiosteal bone. These osteoid zones invariably heal when the cause of the osteomalacia is identified and appropriate treatment is given.

Similar roentgenographic appearances of fractures in other diseases are really a fibrous and cartilaginous tissue of delayed union. In Paget's disease, polyostotic fibrous dysplasia, and osteogenesis imperfecta, these fractures typically occur at the site of the localized bone pathology and do not respond to measures used to overcome osteomalacia.

As a result of bone softening, bending deformities are seen. In the spine, the vertebral changes are those that are common to demineralized vertebrae of any cause. The nucleus pulposus expands the disks and indents the endplates of the vertebral bodies, which develop a biconcave configuration, resulting in the characteristic "codfish" spine. Compression fractures often occur.

LABORATORY FINDINGS

In typical primary nutritional vitamin D deficiency, the serum calcium level is low or low normal, the phosphorus level is low or normal (most commonly a low normal calcium with a low phosphorus), and the alkaline phosphatase level is moderately elevated.

METABOLIC STUDIES

Before performing metabolic studies, one must inquire whether vitamin D deficiency is the result of inadequate dietary intake, insufficient sunlight, or gastrointestinal dissorders that cause malabsorption.[16]

The following studies should be made:

Investigation for Visceral Disease

Chronic liver disease: inability to convert exogenous D_2 and endogenous D_3 to 25-hydroxy vitamin D, precursor of active principle 1,25-dihydroxy vitamin D which is formed in kidney. In obstructive jaundice, bile salts are unavailable for digestion of fat.

Chronic renal failure: inability to convert precursor to the active principle, 1,25-dihydroxy vitamin D, which is concerned with absorption of calcium by gut; glomerular disease causes phosphate retention and hyperphosphatemia; tubular disease causes failure of resorption of phosphate and hypophosphatemia.

Controlled Low Calcium Diet

A low calcium diet must be started several days prior to laboratory determinations.

Calcium Studies

Fecal calcium: usually increased; almost all of ingested calcium may be in the stools

Serum calcium: pronounced hypocalcemia rarely seen because of compensatory hyperparathyroidism

Urinary calcium: marked decrease in 24-hour output, varying from 80 mg to 150 mg; urinary calcium inversely influenced by dietary phosphorus; therefore, phosphorus-binding substances (*e.g.*, aluminum hydroxide antacids) should be strictly avoided during collection of urine for analysis

Phosphorus Studies

Serum phosphorus: hypophosphatemia usually due to impaired intestinal absorption or to excessive urinary excretion (the exception is chronic glomerular insufficiency, which causes hyperphosphatemia)

Urinary phosphorus: diminished TRP (below 85%, is significant; below 65% is abnormal)[18]

Alkaline Phosphatase

Hyperphosphatasemia is present; values rarely exceed 200 IU to 300 IU. The response to appropriate therapy may be gauged by serum alkaline phosphatase levels.

Serum PTH

Radioimmunoassay can detect an abnormally high value for PTH despite a borderline low value for serum calcium.[25]

Bone Biopsy

Under local anesthesia a bone biopsy specimen is taken from the iliac crest with a trephine to study cancellous bone.[21] The bone should not be decalcified to show the excess of unmineralized bone matrix (*i.e.*, osteoid). More of the bone surfaces than normal are covered with osteoid and an increase in thickness of osteoid is well demonstrated under polarized light. The extent of secondary parathyroid disease can be revealed by an increase of osteoclasts or marrow fibrosis, for example. This is pronounced in renal glomerular disease but is virtually absent in the renal tubular disease.

A large segment of bone taken from an area of radiolucency seen on the roentgenogram (Looser line or umbauzonen, Milkman's pseudofracture) is composed almost entirely of osteoid.

DIFFERENTIAL DIAGNOSIS

Osteoporosis. Osteoporosis is a disturbance of tissue metabolism, not calcium metabolism. Not enough matrix is laid down by the osteoblasts, but whatever is formed is calcified. Therefore, calcium, phosphorus, and alkaline phosphatase levels are normal. Biopsy reveals absence of osteoid tissue.

Osteitis Fibrosa Generalisata. Bone tissue decreases because of increased bone resorption. The compensatory increased activity of osteoblasts leads to a high alkaline phosphatase value. The most common cause is hyperparathyroidism, which causes low serum phosphorus and high serum calcium levels. The lamina dura is absent. Cystic or motheaten changes in the bone are often seen.

TREATMENT

It must be remembered that low-grade degrees of osteomalacia are quite common. The demands of the skeleton may be just barely met until some supervening condition such as pregnancy deprives the body of calcium. Generalized bone pains and tenderness may be the only clue. Muscle weakness is a common complaint; or a compression fracture of a vertebral body or a Looser line may be observed. Blood values may be normal. When a low-grade osteomalacia is suspected, a therapeutic trial is warranted.

Calcium in the form of lactate or gluconate (0.5 g to 3.0 g) is given three times a day. Dicalcium phosphate is also useful.

About 10,000 units of vitamin D is administered daily, and as healing takes place the dosage is reduced to 400 units for children and 800 units for adults. The dosage of vitamin D for treating active rickets and osteomalacia must be adequate but not excessive.

The diet must be high in protein, with the minimum requirement being 3.5 g/kg for infants, down to 1.0 g/kg for adults. Animal protein will supply adequate amounts of phosphorus. Meat, seafood, and dairy products are excellent sources of phosphorus, calcium, and protein.

Gastrointestinal disorders that interfere with absorption of vitamin D and calcium must be corrected. Achlorhydria requires administration of dilute acids with each meal. Bile salts aid digestion and emulsification of fat, which otherwise would combine with and prevent calcium absorption. Other substances that affect absorption of calcium, phosphorus, or vitamin D must be reduced or avoided. For instance, mineral oil prevents vitamin D absorption, phytins decrease calcium available for absorption, oxalic acid combines with calcium and prevents its use even after absorption, and aluminum hydroxide gel binds phosphorus and prevents its absorption.

CLINICAL FORMS OF OSTEOMALACIA

Primary (Nutritional) Vitamin D Deficiency

Primary deficiency of vitamin D is not seen frequently because vitamin D_2 is used to fortify foods. Occasionally it is seen in strict vegetarians who lack exposure to the sun's rays.

Osteomalacia promptly responds to small doses of vitamin D (1,000 IU to 2,000 IU/day). In contrast, osteomalacia associated with intestinal disorders or renal disease responds slowly to large doses (10,000 IU to 50,000 IU/day).

Gastrointestinal Disorders

Postgastrectomy. Steatorrhea, which occurs in one-third of gastrectomized patients, causes negative calcium balance and malabsorption. However, even in the absence of steatorrhea, vitamin D deficiency and osteomalacia may develop.

Small physiological doses of vitamin D supplemented by 1,000 mg calcium may be used both for prophylactic and curative treatment.

Celiac Disease. Steatorrhea causes loss of fat-soluble vitamin D and calcium soaps. There is impaired absorption of vitamin D.[15] Treatment with a gluten-free diet improves vitamin D absorption.

Hepatobiliary and Pancreatic Disease. Loss of bile salts causes steatorrhea and osteomalacia.[9] Absorption of vitamin D is impaired.[26] Cirrhosis of the liver may interfere with the metabolic conversion of vitamin D. Oral doses of vitamin D may prove ineffective and require parenteral administration.

Pseudovitamin D Deficiency (Vitamin D–Dependent Osteomalacia)

This rare disease has all the features of vitamin D deficiency (*e.g.*, muscle weakness, stunted growth, deformities, hypocalcemia, hypophosphatemia) but without demonstrable deficiency of this vitamin or malabsorption. It is inherited as a recessive trait, and it is probably caused by an inborn error of vitamin D metabolism. It is treated by large doses of vitamin D. This is the most severe and deforming type of rickets and osteomalacia.

Drug-Induced Vitamin D–Deficient State

Anticonvulsants (*e.g.*, phenyltoin), tranquilizers, sedatives, muscle relaxants, and oral antidiabetic agents are capable of inducing hepatic microsomal oxidase degradative enzymes that interfere with hydroxylation and conversion of vitamin D to more active metabolites.[10–12,14,20] The result is an inadequate amount of circulating 25-OH calciferol, leading to rickets in children and osteomalacia in adults. Clinically, the condition is rarely overt. Diminished bone mass is not apparent on roentgenograms, since at least 50% of bone mass must be lost before osteopenia is demonstrable.[8] The condition should be suspected in a patient with repeated fractures, delayed union, and bone deformity and with a history of prolonged intake of offending drugs, limited sunlight exposure, and reduced physical activity. A rise in the level of liver alkaline phosphatase isoenzymes should suggest drug-induced osteomalacia or rickets.

Prophylactic treatment for vulnerable people consists of small doses of vitamin D (400 units daily as a dietary supplement). In the child, drug-induced rickets heals rapidly with increased doses of vitamin D above 6,000 IU/day or with 50 units of 25-hydroxycholecalciferol orally. In adult osteomalacia, much larger doses (*e.g.*, 50,000 units once or twice weekly) should be used to overcome the osteomalacia and the tendency to repeated fractures. For overt osteomalacia, treatment may be initiated with the active form of vitamin D, calcitriol or 1,25-dihydroxycholecalciferol, 0.25 μg/day, with appropriate monitoring of serum calcium levels.

Primary Vitamin D–Resistant Familial Hypophosphatemia

Familial hypophosphatemia is inherited as a sex-linked dominant trait. It is expressed first as rickets and later as osteomalacia in the adult. It is characterized by hypophosphatemia, osteomalacia and rickets, retarded longitudinal growth, osteosclerosis, and ligamentous calcification. Hypophosphatemia is present throughout life, but not all patients develop bone disease. Treatment requires large doses of vitamin D (50,000 IU to 80,000 IU/day).

Phosphate Depletion (Secondary Hypophosphatemia)

The prolonged use of phosphate-binding nonabsorbable antacids causes phosphate depletion and osteomalacia. Marked muscle weakness is typically associated with a very low serum phosphorus level. Treatment consists of discontinuing nonabsorbable antacid therapy and administering phosphate supplements.

Renal Tubular Acidosis

Because of impaired tubular transport, the kidney is unable to excrete an excess of hydrogen ion and to acidify the urine. The condition is hereditary or acquired and occasionally is complicated by vitamin D–resistant rickets or osteomalacia. The primary biochemical disturbance is a low plasma phosphorus level with a low renal phosphate threshold. The serum calcium level is normal. Hyperchloremic acidosis, often with hypokalemia due to urinary potassium loss, characterizes the syndrome.[23]

When impaired tubular transport is severe and involves many substances such as glucose, phosphate, and amino acids, the condition is termed the *Fanconi syndrome.*

Treatment requires administration of alkalies ($NaHCO_3$), correction of hypokalemia, and use of phosphate and calcium supplements. Although the bone disease may respond to high doses of vitamin D, this treatment is unnecessary. The response to alkali and phosphate is satisfactory without vitamin D supplements.

Renal Osteodystrophy

Chronic glomerular failure is characterized by marked muscle weakness, progressive deformities (*e.g.*, knock-knees or bowlegs), and loss of height. Inability of the glomeruli to excrete phosphate results in hyperphosphatemia, which in turn causes secondary hyperparathyroidism. Acidosis and an elevated blood urea nitrogen level reflect chronic renal failure.

Osteomalacia is vitamin D resistant, and large initial doses up to 5 mg (300,000 IU) of D_2 are given. Toxicity due to overdose must be controlled by regular serum calcium determinations (see Table 9-1).

Hypophosphatasia

Hypophosphatasia presents clinically as rickets or osteomalacia. It is transmitted as an autosomal recessive and occasionally dominant trait and is characterized by very low plasma alkaline phosphatase and urinary phosphoryl-ethanolamine and pyrophosphate levels.

MALABSORPTION SYNDROME

A malabsorption syndrome refers to the clinical picture produced by a wide variety of conditions that reduce the absorptive ability of the small intestine.[27,28] The main defect appears to be failure to absorb fat and fat-soluble vitamin D, glucose, vitamin A, vitamin B_{12}, and the intrinsic factor.

The dietary calcium combines with fatty acids to form insoluble soaps, which, with the excess of fats and carbohydrates, are excreted in bulky, frothy, foul-smelling stools. In infants and children the condition is called celiac disease and in adults it is designated as idiopathic steatorrhea. Deficiency of vitamin D and calcium is reflected in rickets and osteomalacia.

Deficiency of vitamin B_{12} and the intrinsic factor result in a macrocytic anemia and a beefy red tongue of glossitis. It is similar to pernicious anemia causing paresthesias, but achlorhydria and subacute combined degeneration of the cord is rare. A diffuse brown pigmentation is often observed over the exposed areas of the trunk and the extremities. This disturbance is designated idiopathic sprue when no pathology is demonstrable in the bowel and secondary sprue when specific disease of the small bowel can be identified.

Also included in the malabsorption syndrome are a host of conditions, such as biliary obstruction (bile necessary for emulsification of fat), pancreatitis (absence of lipolytic enzyme), and surgical conditions (gastrectomy, gastrojejunocolic fistula), that effect rapid propulsion of intestinal contents.

CLINICAL PICTURE

The malabsorption syndrome is characterized, in severe cases, by prolonged duration of symptoms, including intermittent diarrhea, marked weakness, weight loss, and glossitis. The patient appears poorly nourished and pale, the abdomen is distended, and often, because of a hypoproteinemia, dependent edema develops.

Osteomalacia, due to lack of vitamin D and calcium, is low grade and manifest by subtle findings such as slight bowing of the extremities and perhaps a Looser line or pseudofracture. In infants, rickets is produced. Osteoporosis is generalized and is a result of protein deficiency. Malnutrition will cause atrophy of the anterior lobe of the pituitary, and likewise the reduced trophic stimulation on sex hormone production will produce osteoporosis. Osteomalacia and osteoporosis frequently coexist in the same patient. "Bone pains" are common complaints, and pathologic fractures occur.

Severe cases of the malabsorption syndrome are uncommon. On the other hand, reduction of intestinal absorption in a subclinical state is very common, particularly after abdominal surgical procedures. One usually does not observe typical diarrhea or a pronounced glossitis. Investigation of the causes of osteomalacia and osteoporosis should include attention to the malabsorption syndrome. The following laboratory procedures are essential to the diagnosis.

LABORATORY FINDINGS

The defect in absorption may affect one or several elements:

Macrocytic anemia
Hypoproteinemia
Hypocalcemia. In low-grade states, the compensatory hyperparathyroidism sustains the serum calcium level, which therefore appears normal. A negative result of a qualitative Sulkowitch test indicates a failure of calcium absorption.
Hypolipidemia, especially serum total and esterified cholesterol
Steatorrhea (may be present without diarrhea). The fecal fat exceeds the normal 20% by dry weight.
A flat glucose tolerance curve when the glucose is administered orally; a normal curve if glucose is administered intravenously
A low oral vitamin A curve ; a normal curve if vitamin A is administered intravenously
Impaired absorption of radioactive vitamin B_{12}
Occasionally, a "typical" appearance of small intestine in roentgenograms

TREATMENT

Intramuscular administration of liver extract, folic acid, and vitamin B_{12} is very effective in inducing a remission. A high-vitamin, high-protein diet that is low in fat is prescribed. Until the absorptive defect is overcome, intramuscular calcium lactate, ultraviolet light, and the sex hormones are necessary for normal bone formation. This treatment must be continued indefinitely in the presence of permanent gastrointestinal pathology.

HYPOPHOSPHATASIA

Hypophosphatasia is a condition clinically resembling rickets but typified by a persistently low serum alkaline phosphatase level.[29,30] It is probably hereditary.

CLINICAL PICTURE

The following findings are characteristic:

Stormy infancy: failure of weight gain, periodic attacks of vomiting, delay in walking, delayed dentition
Stunted growth: shortness of long bones
Rachitic bony changes: such as deformities, thickening about epiphyses and beaded ribs
Liability to fractures, especially at metaphyses; healing takes place in normal fashion
Premature loss of deciduous teeth
Craniostenosis may cause impaired vision; skull peculiarly soft and leatherlike
Gait unsteady, poor tolerance to exercise

LABORATORY FINDINGS

The following findings are typical:

Roentgenograms: generalized demineralization, rachitic irregularities about epiphyseal lines
Low serum alkaline phosphatase level
Excess urinary excretion of phosphoethanolamine
Hypercalcemia and hyperphosphatemia: may be normal

TYPES OF CASES

Severe cases are usually fatal during the first year of infancy, usually attributable to a renal lesion. If the infant survives this period, the outlook for recovery is usually good, the condition remaining stationary or improving and becoming categorized as moderately severe. Mild cases are those in patients without bone changes.

SCURVY

Scurvy (scorbutus) is a nutritional disorder caused by deficiency of vitamin C and characterized clinically by a generalized hemorrhagic tendency. The severe form of the disease is rare, but mild and subclinical types are relatively common. Its main effects are on cells and tissues of mesodermal origin, particularly in the skeletal system.

ETIOLOGY

The disease occurs most frequently in artificially fed infants between 5 and 10 months of age. Since vitamin C is destroyed by heat, exclusive feeding with processed milk that is lacking in this vitamin will result in latent or symptomatic scurvy unless cevitamic acid or orange, lemon, or tomato juice is supplied. An infant fed exclusively on milk to which vitamin D has not been added may also develop rickets. The combination of rickets and scurvy is known as Barton's disease.

Adult scurvy commonly occurs in elderly people who live on a restricted diet. Ordinarily, this vitamin C deficiency is subclinical and manifest by subcutaneous hemorrhages with slight trauma and delay in healing of wounds.

PATHOLOGY

Vitamin C deficiency impairs the cohesive property of the matrix of connective tissue and endothelium.[2] Consequently, capillary hemorrhages occur beneath mucous membranes and other locations of abundant capillary accumulations. Extraskeletal sites include the gums, intestines, conjunctivae, skin, bladder, and kidneys. The most vascular skeletal stiuations are located beneath the periosteum and in the marrow, particularly in the metaphyses and especially adjacent to the most actively growing epiphyses (lower end of femur, upper end of tibia, upper end of humerus).

Subperiosteal hemorrhage is characteristic. The accumulation of blood may be slight or so extensive as to balloon out the periosteum and to resemble a large tumor. The clotted blood is either resorbed or transformed to fibrous tissue. Subsequently, especially when vitamin C is supplied, the organized hematoma becomes ossified with fine periosteal trabeculations. Eventually, with healing, the periosteal bone is resorbed.

Hemorrhages within the metaphysis interfere with ingrowth of osteoblastic tissue. Therefore, endochondral ossification proceeds normally only as far as formation of calcified cartilage (zone of provisory calcification), which accumulates in large amounts. Osteoblasts and osteoclasts are notably deficient or lacking. The broadened layer of calcified cartilage is known as the white line of Fraenkel, which appears as a characteristic transverse line of density on roentgenograms. When scurvy is less severe, a few irregular bone trabeculae may form, within which are contained unresorbed islands of calcified cartilage.

Within the epiphysis itself, a zone of calcified cartilage accumulates about the bony centrum. This encircling dense ring is known as Wimberger's line.

The metaphysis in response to hemorrhage becomes extremely hyperemic. The resultant resorption of bone in addition to failure of laying down of new bone results in extremely deficient ossification, which appears in roentgenograms as a dark zone of radiolucency adjacent to the white line. Lack of bone structure and accumulation of fragile calcified cartilage weakens the epiphyseometaphyseal junction and leads to fractures and epiphyseal separation. The epiphysis and the attached epiphyseal plate may be completely displaced from the shaft. Nevertheless, with vitamin C treatment, although union occurs in the displaced position, continued growth restores normal contour to the bone.

Hemorrhages throughout the marrow result in fibrous organization and replacement of hematopoietic tissue. Secondary anemia results.

Osteogenesis is interfered with, and osteoclasis continues. Trabeculations become thinned and poorly visualized in roentgenograms (ground-glass appearance). Cortices become slender and resemble those seen in osteogenesis imperfecta. Pathologic fractures occur through the metaphysis in infants and the diaphysis in adults.

Porosis of alveolar bone permits loosening of the teeth. Pulp hemorrhages are followed by degeneration and necrosis. Dentine formation ceases, but the enamel is not affected. The gums are swollen and hemorrhagic.

CLINICAL PICTURE

The infant is restless, pale, and febrile. The extremities are held immobile, the muscles are in spasms, and attempts to move them cause the child to cry out with pain. A palpable, excruciating, tender, fixed swelling detected over a bone is the result of subperiosteal hemorrhage. If hemorrhage is recent, the swelling is soft and fluctuant. Later, it is indurated and less tender. Hemorrhages are particularly prone to develop above or below the knee. The voluntary immobilization of the extremities is termed *pseudoparalysis*.

The gums display a bluish, spongy swelling, especially about the upper central incisor teeth. The teeth are loose and brittle. Petechiae or ecchymoses are found in the skin or the mucous membranes. Hematemesis and hematuria may develop. As the disease worsens, there ensue anorexia, weight loss, progressive anemia, hyperpyrexia, pneumonia, and death.

The lower femur, the upper tibia, and the upper humerus are the favored sites for epiphyseal fracture-separations. After treatment is instituted, the fracture heals, and endochondral ossification is reestablished. Although the epiphysis is united in the displaced position, continued longitudinal growth restores the normal contour.

Costochondral separations are typical. The sternum with the cartilaginous portions of the ribs is displaced posteriorly, while the sharp anterior ends of the bony ribs protrude anteriorly. These sharp bony ends form the scorbutic rosary, in contrast to the rounded prominences of the rachitic rosary.

Mild forms of scurvy are seen more commonly. In infants, irritability, restlessness, night cries, pain caused by movement of the extremities, and tenderness over the metaphysis about the knee are the usual symptoms. In adults, pain and tenderness over bony structures are common complaints. A fracture with minimal trauma is suggestive.

LABORATORY FINDINGS

The blood ascorbic acid normal is 1 mg/dl ml; 0.5 mg or less is found in scurvy. A secondary anemia is usual.

ROENTGENOGRAPHIC FINDINGS

The following features are characteristic:[31]

- The white line of Fraenkel, a broadened, irregular radiopaque line caused by calcified cartilage between the epiphyseal line and the metaphysis
- The Pelkan spur, a small bony spur protruding from the lateral, occasionally the medial, border of the metaphysis at its junction with the epiphysis
- The scurvy line, the zone of translucency in the metaphysis adjacent to the white line of Fraenkel

The Wimberger line, the dense line encircling the epiphysis
Ground-glass translucency of the bones
Thin cortices
Subperiosteal hemorrhages, which exhibit a soft tissue shadow or a density of ossification
Epiphyseal fracture-separation
Costochondral and vertebral angulation of the ribs
Subperiosteal fractures

These roentgenographic findings are observed best at the ends of rapidly growing long bones.

DIFFERENTIAL DIAGNOSIS

Poliomyelitis. Paralysis is spotty, appears quickly, and may be transient. Meningeal signs are often present. Bony structure is normal.

Rickets. The metaphyses are deeply cupped. Periosteal bone is minimal. The dense zone of provisory calcification is absent.

Acute Osteomyelitis. Usually only one bone is involved. Local pain and constitutional symptoms are severe. Leukocytosis is high.

Luetic Osteochondritis. This disorder is common before 3 months of age, whereas scurvy occurs later in infancy. The mother's serology is positive, and a history of repeated spontaneous abortions is often elicited.

Osteogenesis Imperfecta. Fractures are diaphyseal rather than metaphyseal, and the liability to fracture lessens with advancing age. Diet is adequate, and blood and urine contain an adequate amount of ascorbic acid.

TREATMENT

Treatment consists of administration of fruit juices or tablets of cevitamic acid. Other vitamins are also prescribed. Processed milk is prohibited. Fractures are immobilized without any attempt at reduction.

GOUT

Gout is a hereditary condition of disturbed uric acid metabolism in which urate salts are deposited in articular, periarticular, and subcutaneous tissues; clinically, it is characterized by recurring attacks of acute arthritis; by intervals of freedom from pain; and, in late stages, by crippling deforming arthritis, nephritis, urinary calculi, and cardiovascular lesions.

ETIOLOGY

The actual cause of gout is unknown. The predisposing causes include the following:

Heredity: occurs in families. Many members of one family may have hyperuricemia without gout; not sex linked.
Sex: males predominantly; rarely, females, usually at the menopause, displaying atypical forms of the disease.
Age: second to fourth decades, usually common at about 40 years of age. Rarely, in children gout is likely to be rapid, severe, polyarticular and crippling.
Adrenal cortex activity: an adequate amount of cortical steroids counteracts the gouty attack. When the cortex is stimulated to overproduction (*e.g.*, by ACTH, surgical trauma), the steroids are depleted and, on withdrawal of the stimulating factor, an acute gouty attack is precipitated.
Vascular changes: an extremity involved by an acute gouty arthritis displays increased blood flow and amplitude, suggesting vascular disturbance as the cause of extreme pain.
Disturbed electrolyte equilibrium: suggested by the marked diuresis that precedes acute attacks of gout.
Decreased urinary 17-ketosteroids: formed from metabolism of adrenocortical and testicular androgens. Reduction below 3 mg/24 h is a constant finding in gout.

PATHOLOGY

Sodium urate is deposited as crystals on the surface of and replacing articular cartilage. The latter is eroded through, and the subchondral bone is replaced in well-circumscribed punched-out areas by the crystalline deposits (Color Plate 9-3). A pannus of granulation tissue grows over the articular surface, invades and replaces the cartilage, and may bridge the joint to the opposite articular surface, producing a fibrous ankylosis. The

FIG. 9-7. Sagittal section of the great toe, removed surgically from a patient 74 years of age, shows urate deposits in and about the joints. (Ciba Clinical Symposia, Vol 2, No. 10, December 1950)

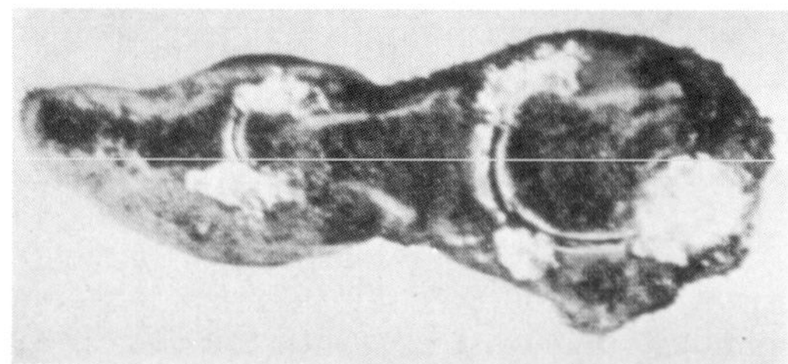

irregularity of the joint surfaces leads to a secondary degenerative arthritis. Urate salts are deposited in the synovial membrane, the periarticular soft tissues, and the subcutaneous tissues (Figs. 9-7 and 9-8).

Microscopically the typical urate crystals are demonstrated by special technique. The deposits are surrounded by an inflammatory reaction, fibrous tissue, and giant cells. The salts are found in articular cartilage, bone marrow, synovial membranes, joint capsules, ligaments, periosteum, tendons, bursae, and subcutaneous and intramuscular tissues. The metatarsophalangeal joint of the big toe is predisposed. Next most affected are the

FIG. 9-8. Gout. (*Top, left*) The white crystalline deposits have invaded the phalanges, the tendon sheath, and the tendon and have penetrated the skin. (*Bottom, left*) Extensive white urate deposits throughout a large joint. (*Top, right*) Microscopic appearance of a gouty nodule. The tissue has been fixed in absolute alcohol, because watery fixatives dissolve out the crystals. Note necrotic amorphous material, bundlelike accumulations of crystals, and reactive inflammatory cells including giant cells. (*Bottom, right*) A silver stain (Galanth's stain) that selectively darkens urate deposits. (Courtesy of Dr. Edward Rosenberg)

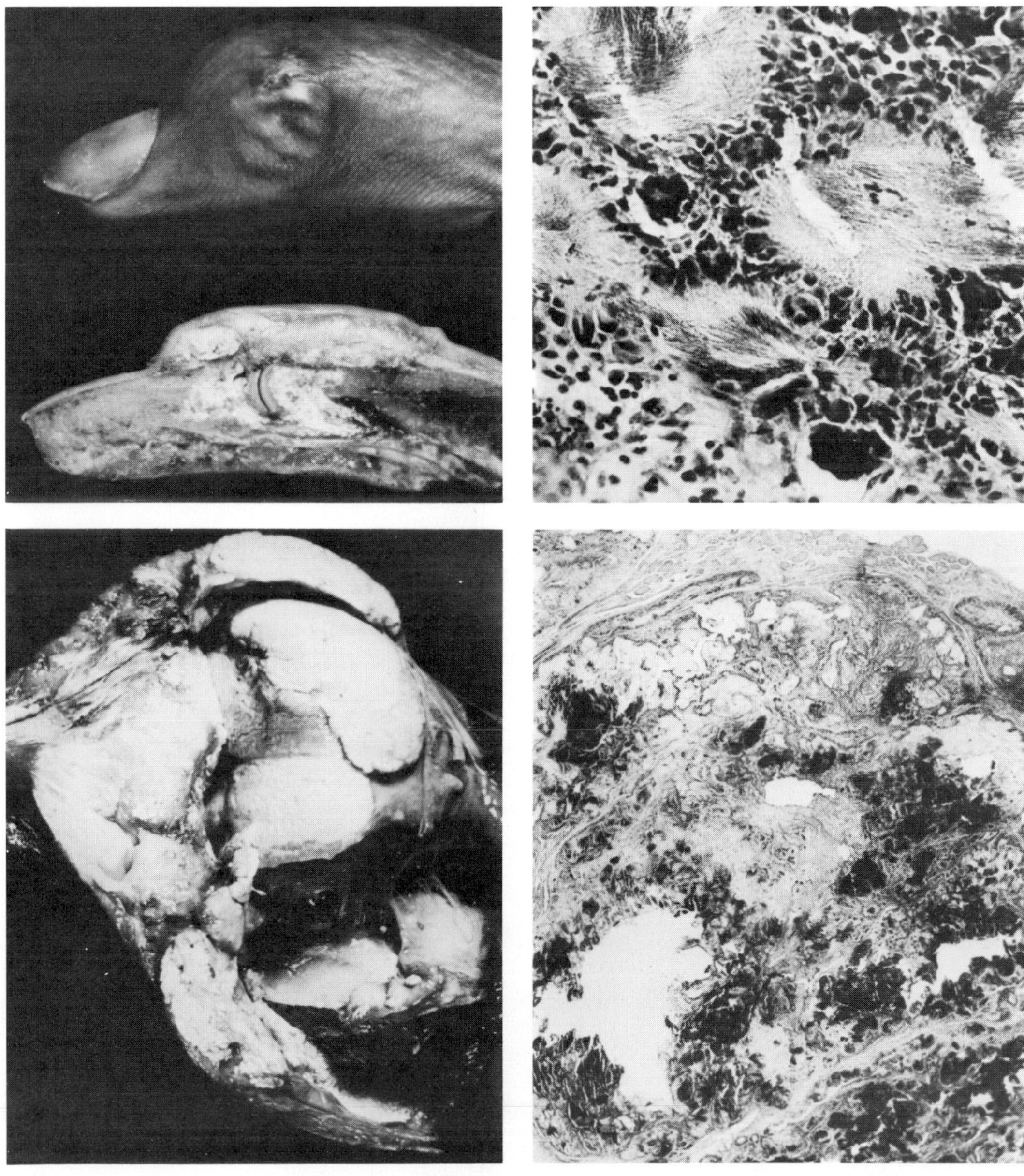

intertarsal joints, the ankles, the fingers, and the wrists. In the kidneys, dots of urate crystals are spread throughout the cortex and linear streaks through the medulla. A glomerular fibrosis is frequent. The cause of death is usually coronary or cerebral vascular disease, or nephrosclerosis with uremia.

CLINICAL PICTURE

The gouty patient definitely has a hyperuricemia for a number of years without symptoms. Measured in terms of urate salt, the serum urate level invariably exceeds 6 mg/dl. The initial acute attack may come without warning and frequently is preceded by a provocative factor such as trauma (long walks), dietary indiscretions (high fat diet), drugs (liver extract), surgical operations, exposure to cold, and withdrawal of ACTH. The patient is usually a man over 30 years of age. The attack has a sudden onset, frequently occurring at night. The joint, often the metatarsophalangeal joint of the great toe, becomes very swollen, red, and tender. The swelling is extreme, simulates a cellulitis, and extends beyond the confines of the joint. A variable amount of increased joint effusion contributes to the swelling (Fig. 9-9). The joint fluid is particularly increased when the knee is the site of the attack. Pain is excruciating. The inflammation may involve a nonarticular urate deposit such as a subcutaneous tophus or in a bursa. Constitutional symptoms include fever, tachycardia, and headaches.

During the acute attack laboratory findings reveal a leukocytosis and an elevated sedimentation rate. The attack may last from a few days to several weeks before it subsides with complete restoration of function of the joint. Desquamation over the involved area is the final stage.

The first interval until the second attack is generally asymptomatic, and its duration is variable. Occasionally, several years may elapse before the next attack appears. Although the intervals vary in length, they tend to become progressively shorter, and the intensity of succeeding attacks become progressively more severe. The later attacks are more likely to be febrile.

Small deposits of urate salts in the subcutaneous tissues are in evidence in the forearm, where they have a pearly white appearance. A characteristic location for these deposits is about the ear. The tophi may increase in size and assume large globular shapes, distending the overlying skin and rupturing to form a chronically draining sinus exuding the chalky white material and discharge of secondary infection. Eventually, with repeated attacks, one or several joints are destroyed by urate deposits, and secondary degenerative changes and a permanent arthritic cripple results.

The main complication is due to deposits of urate salts in the kidneys. Urate calculi are a cause of renal colic and hematuria. Impairment of renal function due to chronic glomerulonephritis and interstitial nephritis leads to uremia and death. Hypertension and arteriosclerosis and consequent coronary and cerebral complications are frequent in these patients. In young patients, attacks are likely to be severe and polyarticular, lasting a long time and becoming crippling. The condition is often misdiagnosed as acute rheumatic fever. In women, gout generally starts at about the time of menopause and is associated with impaired renal function.

DIAGNOSIS

The main diagnostic factors include the following:

Family history of gouty arthritis
Repeated attacks with intervals of freedom from pain
Renal disturbance as urate calculus
Hyperuricemia
Satisfactory response to adequate doses of colchicine

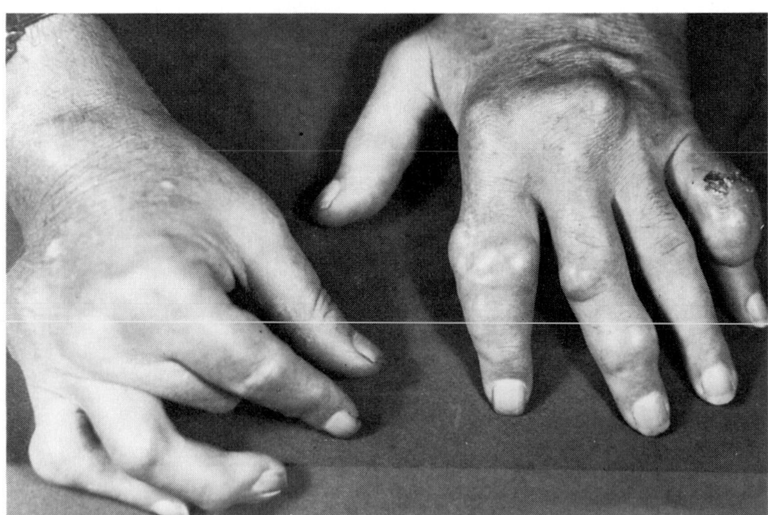

FIG. 9-9. Severe gouty arthritis of the hands.

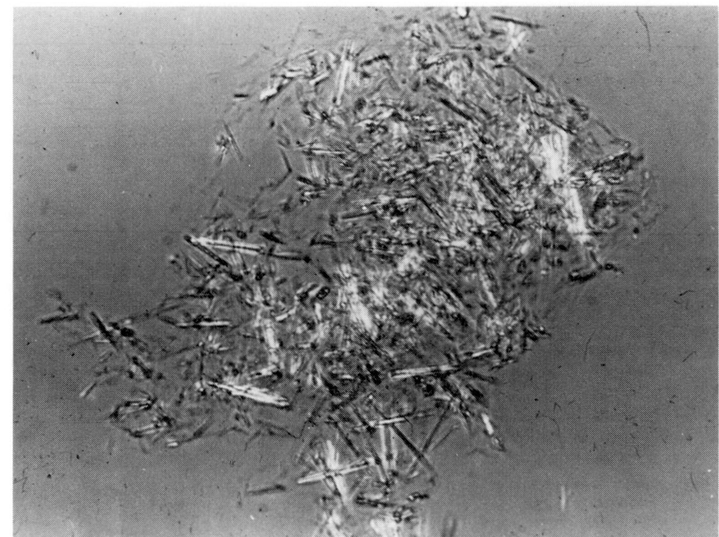

FIG. 9-10. Extracellular monosodium urate crystals as seen in wet preparation of joint fluid under polarized light. (×500) Birefringent needle-shaped crystals are identified under the polariscope by the characteristic flashing color change from blue to yellow and back again as the mechanical stage holding the specimen is rotated. (McCarty DJ, Hollander JL: Identification of urate crystals in gouty synovial fluid. Ann Intern Med 54:452, 1961)

LABORATORY PROCEDURE

Finding an increased concentration of serum urate is necessary for diagnosis. Salicylates and other drugs are uricosuric. They lower the serum level temporarily and must be avoided at the time blood samples are taken. The normal level is less than 5 mg/dl. Nongouty types of arthritis do not respond to colchicine. Therefore, the giving of sufficient amounts of colchicine may be considered as being a therapeutic test. A tophus may be needled or the chalky discharge collected and examined for uric acid crystals.

Microscopic Examination of Joint Fluid

Sodium biurate crystals can sometimes be found in joint aspirates.[34] These rod-shaped, blunt-ended crystals show strong negative birefringence when viewed under the polarizing microscope and are digested by uricase. In contrast, calcium phosphate crystals are rhombic or rod-shaped, show positive but weak birefringence, and are not digested by uricase (Fig. 9-10).

One milliliter of synovial fluid is collected in a tube containing 1 drop of heparin (stock solution of 60 mg heparin in 2 ml distilled water) and centrifuged. The sediment is diluted with a small amount of absolute alcohol as soon as possible, since urate crystals are soluble in water. The sediment is then examined under the polarizing microscope.

Murexide Test

A few drops of nitric acid are added to the suspected substance. The mixture is evaporated to dryness, then moistened with ammonium hydroxide. If uric acid is present, a purple color (due to murexide) results. Thus, the material from a tophus or fluid aspirated from a joint may be tested chemically.

ROENTGENOGRAPHIC FINDINGS

Early, the joint appears normal. Later, replacement of bony structure by urate salts gives the characteristic punched-out appearance. As the cartilage is destroyed, the joint becomes narrowed, and degenerative arthritic changes supervene (Fig. 9-11).

FACTORS INFLUENCING URIC ACID LEVELS

Theories of hyperuricemia vary from increased production to deficient renal excretion and decreased destruction.[36] However, the most logical suggestion is that endogenous uric acid arises from destroyed nuclei, particularly extruded nuclei of normoblasts during the process of maturation of erythrocytes. Therefore, any factor that stimulates the hematopoietic system causes an overproduction of uric acid and can cause attacks of gout. Certain diseases such as polycythemia and drugs such as liver extract can precipitate an acute gouty arthritis. Excretion of urates is effected by cinchophen, high doses of salicylates, caronamide, and probenecid (Benemid). Other agents, such as glycerol, glycine, and glutamic acid, also aid excretion. On the other hand, a high fat diet, sodium bicarbonate, and benzoic acid decrease excretion. Although uric acid is an end product of purine metabolism, foods high in purines (*e.g.*, kidney, liver, brain, pancreas, sardines) appear to have no material effect in elevating the serum urate level. However, the degree of serum urate elevation does not have any relationship to provocation of the acute attack.

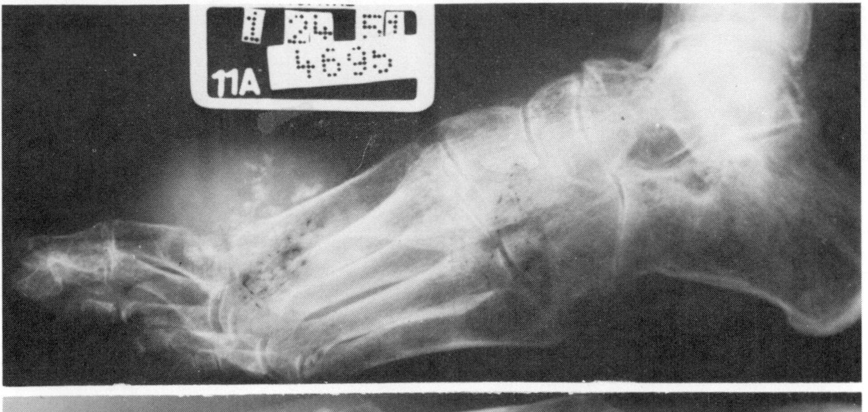

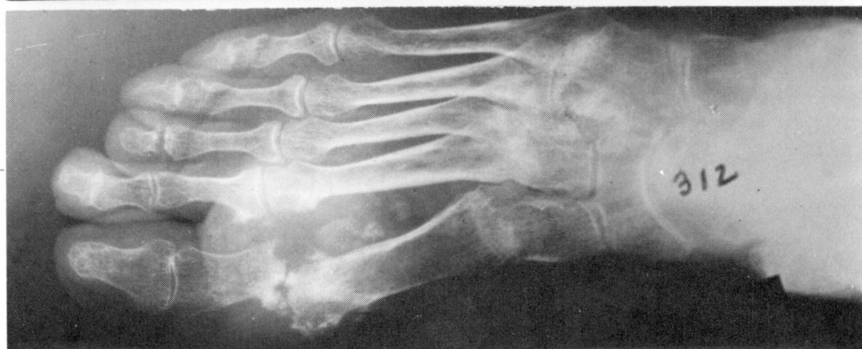

FIG. 9-11. Gouty destruction of first metatarsophalangeal joint.

TREATMENT

Prophylaxis demands avoiding provocative factors.

ACUTE ATTACK

For the acute attack, the patient is placed at absolute bed rest. The affected extremity is immobilized in a soft blanket or pillow splint. An ice pack effectively reduces the pain. A cradle relieves pressure of the bedcovers from the part. Occasionally, moist hot packs are tolerated better than cold. Colchicine is specific for gout; it is both analgesic and diuretic; 1/100- or 1/120-grain tablet is given every hour until pain is relieved or until toxic features, such as nausea, vomiting, and diarrhea, appear. Relief requires 8 to 16 tablets. Medication should be given even through the night if necessary. Joint swelling begins to subside in 12 hours, and complete relief is obtained in 1 or 2 days. The course may be repeated after 3 days. Abundant fluid intake and inclusion of glycine in the diet aid diuresis. Salicylates are also valuable for their uricosuric effect. The diet should be high in carbohydrates. ACTH in dosage of 50 USP units daily is extremely effective, with rapid improvement being noted within the first few hours. Its mechanism of action appears to be by uric acid clearance and a nonspecific antiinflammatory effect. The severe exacerbation of joint distress that follows withdrawal of the hormone is avoided by giving a maintenance dose of colchicine (0.6 mg four times daily) at the same time. Phenylbutazone (Butazolidin) given as enteric coated tablets (200 mg three times daily) or 1.0 g of the sodium salt given intravenously produces complete remission in 48 hours. It is effective in patients resistant to colchicine. However, untoward toxic reactions must be guarded against. Alcohol must be avoided. Compound F injected into the joint produces rapid relief. Oral prednisone or prednisolone, 20 mg to 40 mg/day, is effective.

INTERVAL OR INTERCRITICAL PERIOD

Since hyperuricemia occurs in about 5% of males over 30 years of age, and only one fifth of these eventually develop acute gouty arthritis, aggressive prophylactic drug therapy is not warranted in an asymptomatic patient with mild to moderate hyperuricemia.[35] Periodic examinations, dietary restriction of purine-rich foods, and gradual weight reduction is the appropriate treatment. Weight reduction often leads to a decline in serum urate levels.

When hyperuricemia is pronounced (*i.e.*, greater than 9.0 mg to 10.0 mg/dl) or in the presence of hyperuricosuria (*i.e.*, 1.0 g/24 hr), or both situations exist, preventive drug treatment is rational.

Drug-induced hyperuricemia, which may eventuate in an acute gouty arthritis, is often encountered in the course of treatment of hypertension with thiazides or potent diuretics such as furosemide or when neoplastic disease is treated with cytotoxic drugs. Concurrent control with uricosuric drugs or allopurinol is necessary.

In the interval between acute attacks, colchicine is a safe and effective prophylactic drug that will prevent acute attacks but will not deter the formation of tophaceous deposits. Since colchicine has no uricosuric effect, it should be combined with uricosuric drugs (*e.g.*, probenecid, sulfinpyrazone) or allopurinol. However, when the level of hyperuricosuria threatens stone formation, uricosuric agents are contraindicated. The suggested dose of colchicine is 0.5 mg/day or twice daily.

When allopurinol or uricosuric therapy is initiated, prophylactic doses of colchicine will help prevent an acute attack, which commonly occurs when such treatment is started. During the first 6 months of therapy with uricosuric agents or allopurinol, a dose of 0.5 mg 2 or 3 times a day is adequate. Colchicine is also administered to gouty patients about to undergo surgery for a few days preoperatively and for a similar period postoperatively. Otherwise the surgical trauma may precipitate an acute attack.

Allopurinol (Zyloprim) is an inhibitor of the enzyme xanthine oxidase; it thereby prevents the final step in the production of uric acid.[32] It effectively reduces serum urate levels, and when such levels are maintained at or near normal in tophaceous gout, the size of the urate deposits are consistently reduced and the progression of renal damage is halted.

The principal side-effects of allopurinol therapy are gastrointestinal irritation and dermatitis. Rarely, systemic toxicity may produce fever, blood dyscrasia, and hepatic damage. Therefore, it is essential during such therapy to conduct blood and liver enzyme studies at intervals. In general, the drug is relatively safe and effective for continuous maintenance therapy. By preventing hyperuricemia, the incidence of acute attacks and their severity are markedly reduced. Allopurinol is started at 300 mg/day, and the dosage thereafter is varied to produce the desired effect. Infrequently it is necessary to give as much as 600 mg/day. The maximum permissible dose is 800 mg/day.

SURGICAL PROCEDURES

During an acute attack of gout, immobilization of the affected joint will lessen the degree of joint destruction. In certain situations, excision of the gouty lesion and other surgical measures are necessary. Deposits of urate crystals, whether creamy and semiliquid or chalky and inspissated, may compromise various structures by compression or infiltration and destruction. Nerve tissue is resistant to invasion, but compression of digital nerves causes sensory disturbances. A bursa may become so distended by urate deposits that the overlying skin is thinned and penetrated, resulting in a draining sinus; or the tendon or the bone beneath the bursa may be invaded. Urate crystals within a tendon infiltrate, destroy, and replace tendon fibers. A fusiform, nodular enlargement develops within the tendon, which interferes with tendon motion and may predispose to tendon rupture.

Invasion of a joint destroys articular cartilage and capsular structures. If destruction is mild, a painful degenerative arthritis supervenes. Severe disintegration of joint structure is usually followed by fibrous ankylosis, which is eventually converted into a bony ankylosis. Surgical stabilization of the joint in a functional position is indicated. If a large bony lesion lies adjacent to a joint, removal of the focus may preserve joint function.

Breakdown of skin over a tophus produces a characteristic indolent ulcer with a base of urate crystals and little surrounding inflammatory reaction. Under medical management, the base eventually granulates, and the area epithelializes over with minimal scarring. The process is slow but may be expedited by removal of the gouty deposit, awaiting appearance of granulations, and applying a skin graft. Secondary infection of the gouty ulcer does not occur, suggesting that urates possess a bacteriostatic property.

Surgery of gouty lesions demands observance of the following principles.[33]

- Avoidance of local anesthesia, which might impair local blood supply
- Incisions parallel with course of blood vessels
- Sharp dissection
- Loose suturing to allow escape of liquefied deposits
- Pressure dressing
- Avoidance of prolonged splinting, which encourages ankylosis

Postoperative acute attacks may be minimized by medical therapy. Colchicine (0.5 mg) is given for 3 days preoperatively and 1 week postoperatively. In addition, probenecid (0.5 g to 3.0 g) is given daily preoperatively and is continued indefinitely after surgery.

Orthopaedic measures consist mainly of prevention of joint destruction by immobilization. Large tophi that interfere with joint and tendon motion may be removed.

OCHRONOTIC ARTHRITIS

Homogentistic acid is an aromatic acid resulting from the incomplete breakdown of the amino acids tyrosine and phenylalanine in the body. It has an affinity for certain tissues, particularly cartilage, which in consequence becomes brittle and disintegrates. A secondary degenerative arthritis ensues.

ETIOLOGY

The condition known as ochronotic arthritis (alkaptonuric arthritis) is rare.[37] It is congenital and inherited as a mendelian recessive trait, often occurring in the offspring of consanguineous parents.

PATHOLOGY

Homogentistic acid is a strong reducing agent that, when oxidized, is converted to a dark pigment. The tissues in which it is deposited, particularly sclerae, ligaments, tendons, and cartilage of the ears, the nose, joints, and intervertebral disks, become darkened with pigment. The cartilage loses its elasticity, becomes brittle, and has poor resistance to mechanical strain. It cracks easily and is worn away by friction and compression. The exposed bony surfaces undergo sclerosis and formation of marginal exostoses, which are changes typical of degenerative arthritis. The intervertebral disks, particularly in the lumbar area, degenerate and calcify. The disk spaces narrow, and opposing surfaces of vertebral bodies become irregular and sclerotic. A picture of severe degenerative arthritis of the spine results.

CLINICAL PICTURE

The onset occurs in infancy and childhood. The urine blackens on standing, and the diapers become stained. Gradually over the years a slate brown or black pigment appears first about the concha and the anthelix of the ears and in the sclerae but produces no symptoms. Later, symptoms of degenerative arthritis appear in the large joints and the spine. The entire thoracic and lumbar spine displays rigidity, increased rounding of the thoracic spine, and flattening of the lumbar spine. Often the patient assumes a posture suggestive of Paget's disease. Perspiration stains the clothing.

ROENTGENOGRAPHIC FINDINGS

Films of the spine are characteristic. The disks appear as elliptical, thin, calcified wafers. The apposing vertebral bodies are sclerotic and spurred, and other evidence of degenerative arthritis is seen. The large joints show only degenerative changes (Figs. 9-12 and 9-13).

LABORATORY FINDINGS

Homogentisic acid is a strong reducing agent that is oxidized on exposure to air and turns the urine black. Heating or the addition of alkalies hastens the reaction. Copper solutions (*e.g.*, Benedict's or Fehling's) are reduced, and an erroneous diagnosis of diabetes may be

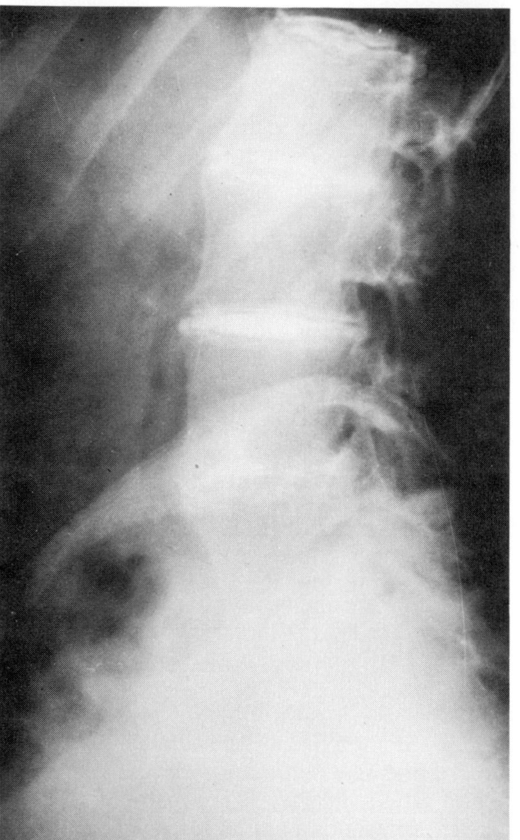

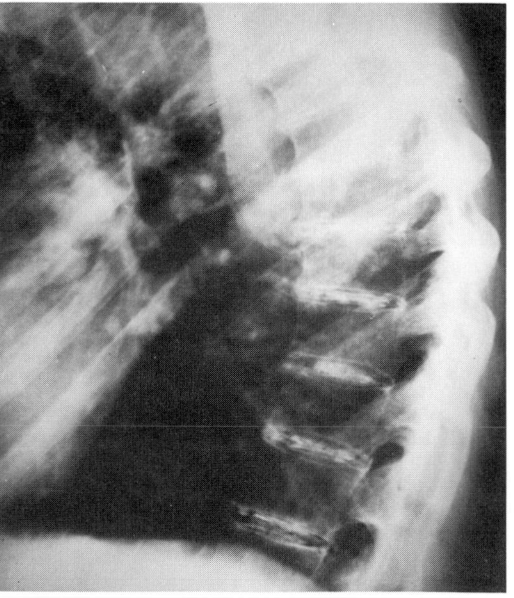

FIG. 9-12. Alkaptonuric (ochronotic) arthritis. The intervertebral disks are narrowed and calcified. (Harrold AJ: Alkaptonuric arthritis. J Bone Joint Surg 38B:532, 1956)

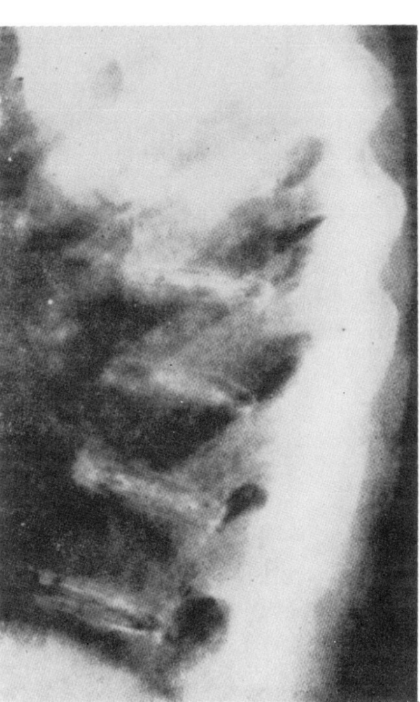

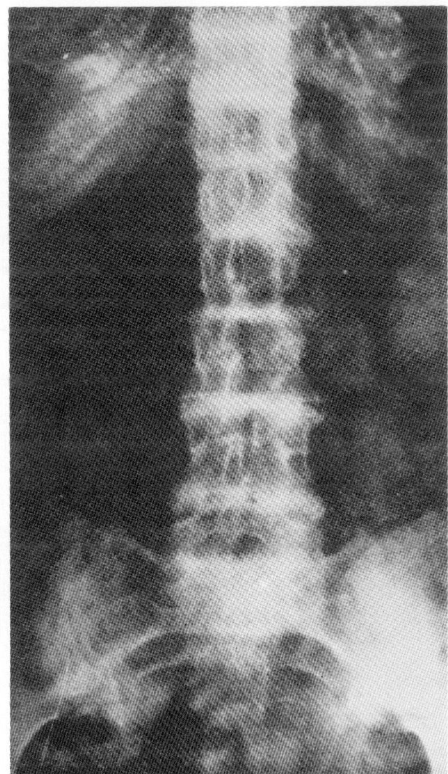

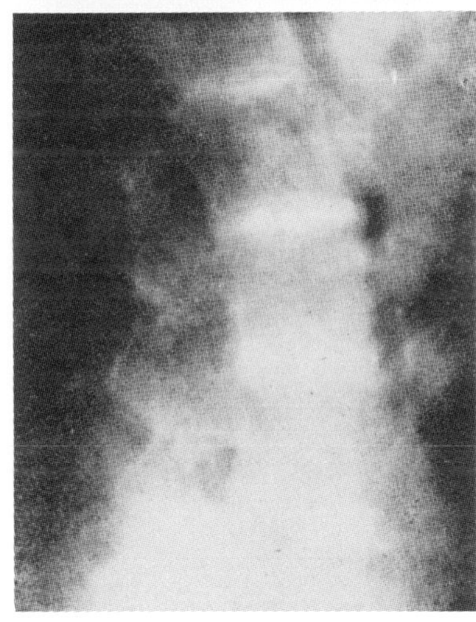

FIG. 9-13. (*Top, left*) Thoracic spine showing narrowed, calcified intervertebral disks. (*Right*) Roentgenograms of lumbar spine. The disks are narrowed and calcified. (Harrold AJ: Alkaptonuric arthritis. J Bone Joint Surg 38B:532, 1956)

made. However, results of fermentation tests are negative and the plane of polarized light is not rotated. A diagnostic reaction is the bluish green coloration produced by the addition of a drop of dilute ferric chloride solution to the urine.

TREATMENT

There is no known treatment for ochronotic arthritis. Reduction of intake of food containing tyrosine and phenylalanine plus administration of a high dosage of vitamin C will reduce excretion of homogentisic acid but have no effect on the progress of the disease. The body will produce the aromatic acid from endogenous sources.

OSTEOPOROSIS

Osteoporosis is a diffuse reduction in bone density that results when the rate of bone resorption exceeds the rate of bone formation. It is most commonly associated with the aging process in which bone formation generally proceeds at the normal rate but bone removal occurs at an increased rate.

Under abnormal conditions, the reduction in bone density may represent the failure of formation of the protein matrix in which the calcium is laid down. Histologically, this is apparent by either diminished osteoblastic activity or excessive osteoclastic activity. Osteoblasts are rare and little or no new bone apposition can be seen. The cortices are reduced in thickness, and cancellous trabeculae become thinned as marrow spaces are widened (Fig. 9-14).

ETIOLOGY

The cause of lack of bone protein varies, and often several etiologic factors are operative in the same patient. Malnutrition causes osteoporosis because insufficient protein is available. At all times there exists a balance of protein anabolism and catabolism in the body. Osseous anabolism cannot be carried on unless protein materials are readily available. In the presence of adequate nutrition, the cause of osteoporosis must be sought in a disturbance of protein metabolism. This can affect all tissues everywhere; it may be limited to the skeletal system as in osteogenesis imperfecta; or it may be confined to one or a few bones within a limited area. Certain bones become porotic more rapidly than others. Cancellous bone becomes porotic more rapidly than compact bone. When osteoporosis is generalized, it tends to be most pronounced in the spine and the pelvis, as for example in postmenopausal osteoporosis.

FIG. 9-14. Osteoporosis, characterized by diffuse demineralization, loss of transverse striations, thinning of longitudinal striations, and decreased width of the cortices. In this case a fracture has occurred in the supracondylar area of the femur as a result of trivial trauma.

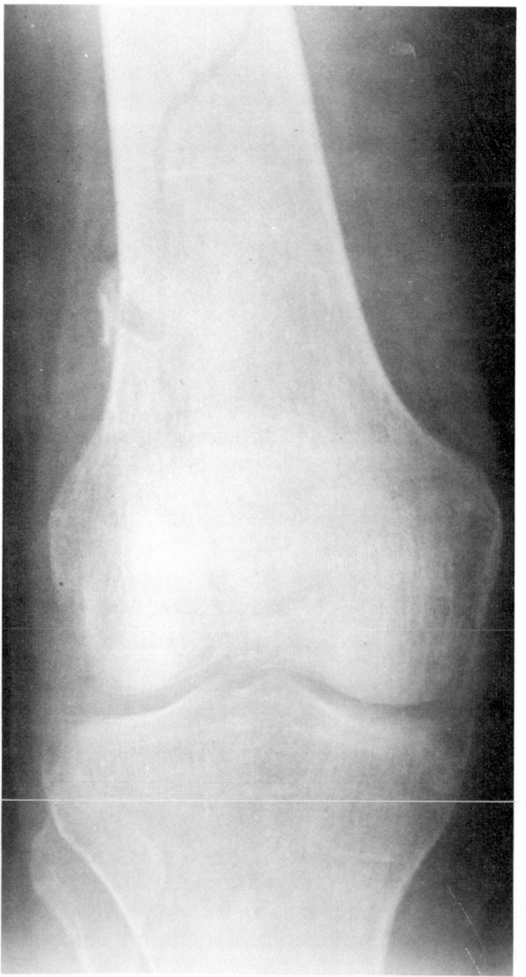

The following conditions produce osteoporosis. When decreased skeletal density is due to disturbance of calcium metabolism, the condition, by definition, is termed *osteomalacia.*

Disuse or Immobilization

The building up of bone exists in balance with the tearing down process. Greater bone production is a response to greater stresses and strains when maintained within physiological limits. When these forces are diminished or absent, the breakdown process exceeds the rate of bone buildup. An immobilized or paralytic limb is a good example of localized porosis of bone. Osteoporosis is generalized when the entire body is inactive. Excessive removal of calcium from bone means that the mineral must be transported elsewhere by the blood stream. As a result, bedridden patients often exhibit extensive deposits of calcium in soft tissues and formation of renal calculi.

Protein Deficiency

Malnutrition at the present time is rare. On the other hand, gastrointestinal disturbances may impair adequate absorption of protein. Conditions that produce loss of protein from the body cause a state of protein deficiency (*e.g.,* extensive third-degree burns, nephrosis, and chronic draining sinuses).

Reflex Dystrophy

Sudeck first described a peculiar mottled osteoporosis of bony structures about an area of trauma. Fractures, sprains, and concussion may initially display a typical picture of local swelling, intense pain, warmth, and the reddish discoloration of vasodilatation. Later, with the onset of vasospasm, the extremity becomes cold, purplish, and edematous, and the skin is glossy and atrophic. Hyperhidrosis is evident. Theoretically, the traumatized area reflexly stimulates the sympathetics. The local vasodilatation and sluggish blood flow, perhaps by an increase of local acidity, are associated with spotty foci of bone resorption. Similarly, vasodilatation in other instances, such as inflammation, vascular tumors, and repair of fractures, produces local osteoporosis.

Hormonal Causes

The formation of protein matrix depends on gonadal hormones. When sex hormones are inadequate, protein anabolism is reduced, while catabolism continues unabated. The condition is more apt to occur in women during the climacteric, especially if the menopause is sudden, as when surgically induced. Less often does it occur in men and then only as a result of total loss of testicular function. Androgen depletion in males is very gradual, inasmuch as the adrenals as well as the testicles produce this steroid hormone. Furthermore, physical activity is greater in men. As a general rule, when osteoporosis is observed in a male, some cause other than hormonal deficiency must be sought.

The sugar or "S" hormone of the adrenal cortex is essential to the process of converting proteins to glycogen. In hyperfunction of the adrenal cortex, whether due to tumor or hyperplasia, an excess of "S" hormone causes excessive breakdown of protein in all tissues, including the skeleton and the musculature. Osteoporosis is, therefore, a feature of Cushing's disease (basophilism of the pituitary) or Cushing's syndrome (primary hyperfunction of the adrenal cortex).

Osteoporosis is part of the hyperthyroid state. Presumably, this develops because an increased catabolism breaks down protein at a faster than normal rate. The result is increased calcium and nitrogen excretion in the urine.

Senility

With advancing age the rate of bone formation is normal or reduced, while bone removal continues at an increased pace. Microscopically, osteoblasts are sparse, trabeculae are thin and vertically disposed, and the marrow is fibrofatty and relatively avascular. The condition appears to be a result of many factors, including inactivity, lessened gonadal hormones, and dietary lack.

OSTEOPOROSIS OF THE SPINE

The spine is often the site of the most profound changes in generalized osteoporosis and will serve as a typical example of the condition. The characteristic pain and pathologic fractures can affect any bone involved by osteoporosis.

ETIOLOGY

The causes include disuse or immobilization, protein deficiency, hormonal causes, and senility. The condition most commonly affects women following the menopause.

PATHOLOGY

As the vertebrae become soft and fragile they undergo typical changes. The vertebral bodies throughout the thoracic spine become wedge shaped as a result of anterior compression forces. Those in the lumbar area are exposed to the expansile force of the intervertebral disks so that superior and inferior surfaces of the bodies become indented. The result is a series of biconcave vertebral bodies and widened disk spaces. Albright likens the appearance to that of the spine of a codfish. The margins of the bodies become radiologically indistinct, and the trabeculations, particularly the transverse ones, disappear. The usual site for a pathologic compression fracture is about the dorsolumbar junction. The occurrence of a fracture elsewhere is cause for suspecting other pathology (Fig. 9-15).

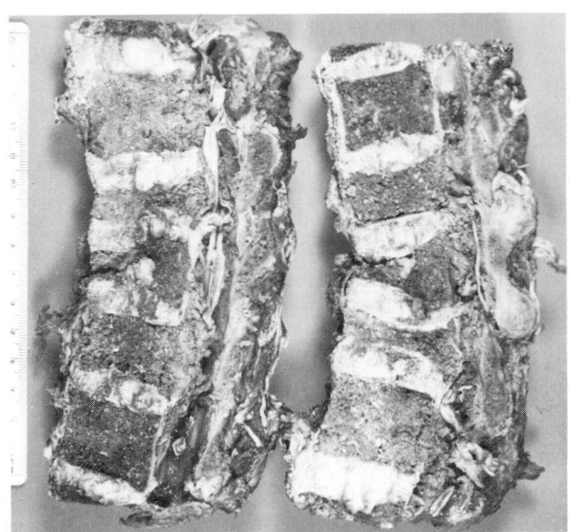

FIG. 9-15. Senile osteoporosis of spine. Ballooning of disks, biconcave vertebral bodies, and pathologic fractures are evident.

CLINICAL PICTURE

Patients with osteoporosis complain of pain in the bones, particularly in the back. The person has a markedly rounded thoracic spine, a stooped habitus, and a shortened stature. Deformities result from spontaneous fractures. A compression fracture may result from a trivial trauma, such as opening a window. Frequent acute attacks of backache suggest minimal fractures that cannot be identified in roentgenograms. The acute onset, the point of tenderness, and relief with recumbency are the chief diagnostic signs.

ROENTGENOGRAPHIC FINDINGS

Diffuse radiolucency is the main feature. The transverse trabeculations have disappeared, and the remaining vertical ones are thinned. Articular cortices are indistinct. Thoracic vertebral bodies are wedge shaped, lumbar bodies are biconcave, and lumbar disks are ballooned. Old or recent compression fracture may be observed.

LABORATORY FINDINGS

Serum calcium, phosphorus, and alkaline phosphatase levels are normal. Urinary excretion of calcium and phosphorus may be slightly greater than the intake; 17-ketosteroid urinary excretion may be increased as a result of adrenal hyperfunction.

DIFFERENTIAL DIAGNOSIS

The main conditions to be differentiated are osteomalacia and osteitis fibrosa generalisata, which likewise cause generalized demineralization of the spine. The former is characterized by low serum phosphorus and normal calcium levels, the latter by a low serum phosphorus level, increased alkaline phosphatase level, hypercalcemia, and hypercalciuria. Biopsy is diagnostic.

Other causes to be considered are osteogenesis imperfecta, blood dyscrasia, multiple myeloma, Gaucher's disease, hyperthyroidism, and Marie-Stümpell disease.

TREATMENT

Estrogen and androgen are given for their protein anabolic effect. Premarin (1.25 mg) is given orally three times a day for 4 weeks, 1 week is skipped, and treatment is repeated. Stoppage of estrogen allows withdrawal bleeding and avoids overstimulation of the breast and the uterus. Estrogenic therapy must be continued for a long time, even years. Androgen may be administered as "linguasorbs" (6 mg) by absorption through the buccal mucous membrane three times a day, or a repository form of both hormones may be injected at bimonthly intervals (Deladumone). These hormones have a sodium retentive effect; a diet low in salt and high in protein is necessary. Estrogenic therapy decreases calcium and phosphorus excretion in all types of osteoporosis except the idiopathic types. Its effects are manifest within 6 days, are maximal in 30 days, and persist for 30 to 50 days after the therapy is stopped. The serum inorganic phosphorus that tends to be high in postmenopausal states falls during estrogenic therapy. Androgen likewise decreases calcium, phosphorus, and nitrogen excretion. These effects persist for a long time after the androgen administration is stopped.[42]

The need for calcium therapy must be determined by calcium balance studies. When a negative calcium balance can be established, calcium and vitamin D should be administered. Over a period of 2 weeks a daily intravenous injection of 10% calcium gluconate is given, limiting the amount to 15 mg/kg body weight. The hypercalcemia produced in this manner is not sustained, with the serum calcium levels returning to normal within 8 hours. The increase in circulating calcium acts to suppress parathyroid function and stimulates the release of thyrocalcitonin, which slows the resorption of bone mineral. Calcium is therefore retained, and often a positive calcium balance is established.[41]

In the absence of a negative calcium balance, the administration of calcium and vitamin D is best avoided, since an excess of calcium may cause hypercalciuria and lead to renal calculi. One must be particularly cautious when administering calcium to a patient taking digitalis, since this may induce cardiac irregularities.

If a malabsorptive defect can be defined, gastrointestinal pathology should be corrected if possible, and medical treatment includes a high vitamin, high protein, and low fat diet and intramuscular injections of liver extract, vitamin B_{12}, and calcium lactate.

Fluoride will cause new bone matrix to be deposited about the thinned trabeculae.[38] The mechanism by which this is brought about is obscure. When calcium intake is inadequate, or when a negative calcium balance exists, as is common in osteoporosis, the new fluoride-induced matrix is not mineralized and microscopically appears as osteoid seams suggestive of osteomalacia. In the presence of an adequate calcium intake, the new bone is well mineralized. This new bone that is laid down about the old trabeculae does not appear to be as well organized as the old bone. Such bone has a higher crystallinity of the hydroxyapatite and is less soluble than normal bone. Fluoride will cause increased nitrogen and calcium retention and often will effect a positive calcium balance.[40,43]

The administration of sodium fluoride is often effective in eliminating bone pain and reducing the tendency to fracture in osteoporosis. This is accomplished even though the roentgenographic appearance of the bone is unchanged. Before undertaking fluoride treatment of osteoporosis, the toxic symptoms of fluoridosis must be recognized.[37] Chronic intake of fluorides can produce neurologic disturbances, renal damage, and increasing calcification of the abdominal aorta. Joint and epigastric pain are common. Gastrointestinal irritation may be avoided by administering the fluoride as gelatin-coated capsules.

The prescribed regimen consists of giving sodium fluoride (0.15 mg/kg/day), calcium, and vitamin D. The effectiveness of treatment can be determined by noting disappearance of bone pain and reduced tendency to fractures and by bone biopsy. Microscopically, although the amount of osteoid about the trabeculae appears to be within normal limits, tetracycline labeling will reveal an increased uptake over bone surfaces, thus establishing increased bone formation.

Excessive immobilization is avoided to deter atrophy of disuse. Back extensor exercises are valuable even for elderly patients. They provide activity necessary for new bone formation and reduce compression forces on the vetebral bodies. The exercises may be instituted as soon as the pain of the fracture has subsided, and the patient is quickly ambulated with the aid of a light hyperextension brace.

REFERENCES

Primary Hyperparathyroidism

1. Avioli LV: The diagnosis of primary hyperparathyroidism. Med Clin North Am 52:451, 1968
2. Luck JV: Bone and Joint Diseases. Springfield, IL, Charles C Thomas, 1950
3. Potchen EJ, et al: External parathyroid scanning with Se^{75} selenomethionine. Ann Surg 162:492, 1965
4. Potchen, EJ, et al: Parathyroid scintiscanning. Radiol Clin North Am 5:267, 1967
5. Schulman LE, Schoenrich EH, Harvey AM: Effects of ACTH and cortisone on sarcoidosis. Bull Johns Hopkins Hosp 91:371, 1952

Hypoparathyroidism

6. Bodell S, et al: Altered response to intravenous magnesium sulfate in magnesium deficiency. Proceedings of the Orthopaedic Research Society, New Orleans, January 28–30, 1976

Calcium-Deficiency Diseases

7. Albright F, Butler AM, Bloomberg E: Rickets resistant to vitamin D therapy. Am J Dis Child 54:629, 1937
8. Ardran GM: Bone destruction not demonstrable by radiography. Br J Radiol 24:107, 1951
9. Atkinson M, et al: Malabsorption and bone disease in prolonged obstructive jaundice. Q J Med 25:299, 1956
10. Avioli LV, Haddad JG: Drug-induced vitamin D deficient state. Metabolism 22:507, 1973
11. Borgstedt AD, et al: Long-term administration of antiepileptic drugs and the development of rickets. J Pediatr 81:9, 1972
12. Conney AH: Prophylactic implications of microsomal enzyme induction. Pharmacol Rev 19:317, 1967
13. Dent CE, Friedman M, Watson L: Hereditary pseudovitamin D deficiency rickets. J Bone Joint Surg 50B:708, 1968
14. Dent CE, et al: Osteomalacia with long term anticonvulsant therapy in epilepsy. Br Med J 4:69, 1970
15. Eddy RL: Metabolic bone disease after gastrectomy. Am J Med 50:442, 1971
16. Fourman P, Royer P: Calcium Metabolism and the Bone, 2nd ed. Philadelphia, FA Davis, 1968
17. Frost HM: The Bone Dynamics in Osteoporosis and Osteomalacia. Springfield, IL, Charles C Thomas, 1966
18. Goldsmith RS: Laboratory aids in the diagnosis of metabolic bone disease. Orthop Clin North Am 3:545, 1972
19. Hamilton JR, Lynch MJ, Reilly BJ: Active coeliac disease in childhood. Q Med J 38:135, 1969
20. Hahn TJ, et al: Serum 25-hydroxycalciferol levels and bone mass in children on chronic anticonvulsant therapy. N Engl J Med 292:550, 1975
21. Jaworski ZFG: Pathophysiology, diagnosis and treatment of osteomalacia. Orthop Clin North Am 3:623, 1972
22. McCune DJ, Mason HH, Clarke HT: Intractable hypophosphatemic rickets with renal glycosuria and acidosis (the Fanconi syndrome). Am J Dis Child 65:81, 1943
23. Morris RC Jr: Renal tubular acidosis: Mechanism, classification and implications. N Engl J Med 281:1405, 1969
24. Pederson HE, McCarroll HH: Vitamin resistant rickets. J Bone Joint Surg 33A:203, 1951
25. Reiss E, Canterbury JM: A radioimmunoassay for parathyroid hormone in man. Proc Soc Exp Biol Med 128:501, 1968
26. Thompson GR, et al: Plasma vitamin D-like activity and vitamin D absorption in man. In L'Ostéomalacie. Paris, Masson, 1967

Malabsorption Syndrome

27. Bossak ET, Wang CI, Adlersberg D: Clinical aspects of the malabsorption syndrome. J Mt Sinai Hosp 24:286, 1957
28. Hartley J: Osseous changes and fractures in the malabsorption syndrome. J Mt Sinai Hosp 24:346, 1957

Hypophosphatasia

29. Dickson W, Harrocks RH: Hypophosphatasia. J Bone Joint Surg 40B:64, 1958
30. Rathbun, JC: Hypophosphatasia. Am J Dis Child 75:822, 1948

Scurvy

31. Kato K: A critique of the roentgen signs of infantile scurvy. Radiology 18:1096, 1932

Gout

32. Hollander JL: The Arthritis Handbook. West Point, PA, Merck Sharp & Dohme, 1974
33. Larmon WA, Kurtz JF: Surgical management of chronic tophaceous gout. J Bone Joint Surg 40A:743, 1958
34. McCarty DJ, Hollander JL: Identification of urate crystals in gouty synovial fluid. Ann Intern Med 54:452, 1961
35. Gutman AB: Pathogenesis and management of primary gout: a review. J Bone Joint Surg 54A:357, 1972
36. Quick AJ: The relationship between chemical structure and physiological response. J Biol Chem 101:475, 1933

Ochronotic Arthritis

37. Harrold AJ: Alkaptonuric arthritis. J Bone Joint Surg 38:532, 1956

Osteoporosis

38. Adams PH, Jowsey J: Sodium fluoride in the treatment of osteoporosis and other bone diseases. Ann Intern Med 63:1151, 1965
39. Jowsey J, Kelly PJ: Effect of fluoride treatment in a patient with osteoporosis. Mayo Clin Proc 43:435, 1968
40. Lukert BP, Bolinger RE: The positive effect of fluoride and methenolone enanthate on nitrogen and calcium balance in osteoporosis (abstr). Clin Res 13:328, 1965
41. Pak CYC: Paper presented to Third International Congress of Endocrinology, Mexico City, 1968
42. Reifenstein EC Jr: Metabolic disorders of bone. In Harrison TR (ed): Textbook of Internal Medicine, Sec 3, p 651. Philadelphia, Blakiston, 1950
43. Rich C, Ensinck J, Ivanovich P: The effect of sodium fluoride on calcium metabolism of subjects with metabolic bone disease. J Clin Invest 43:545, 1964

10

Bone Infections

THE term *osteomyelitis,* taken literally, implies inflammation of bone and its marrow regardless of whether it is due to pyogenic organisms, tuberculosis, syphilis, a specific virus, or the presence of a foreign body such as shrapnel. However, universal acceptance of the term is applied only to infection by pyogenic bacteria, less commonly to the granulomatous inflammation of tuberculosis and syphilis. The infection involves the marrow spaces, the haversian canals, and the subperiosteal space. The bone is involved secondarily. It is destroyed by proteolytic enzymes, necrosed by obliteration of blood supply, decalcified by inactivity and hyperemia, actively resorbed by osteoclasts, and actively reconstructed by osteoblasts.

ACUTE OSTEOMYELITIS

Acute osteomyelitis is a rapidly destructive pyogenic infection, usually hematogenous in origin, occurring most frequently in infants and children; it starts in a metaphysis of an actively growing long bone and runs a fulminating septic course that may terminate fatally.

ETIOLOGY

Predisposing causes are the following:

Age. Infancy and childhood, rarely at other ages
Sex. Males predominate 4:1
Trauma. History of a direct blow frequently elicited
Location. Metaphysis of a long bone; the most actively growing end of the bone (*e.g.,* upper end of tibia, lower end of femur)
Poor nutrition, unhygienic surroundings
Antecedent focus of infection (*e.g.,* boil, tonsillitis)

Exciting causes are *hemolytic Staphylococcus aureus* (most common), *Streptococcus* (less common), *Hemophilus influenzae,* and other organisms (*Escherichia coli, Clostridium perfringens* introduced from septic wounds, pneumococcus, typhoid).

PATHOGENESIS

Although acute osteomyelitis may be initiated by introduction of bacteria from the outside through a wound or continuity from a neighboring soft tissue infection, hematogenous spread from a preexisting focus is by far the most common route of infection.[4] A septicemia or bacteremia is invariably present. An infective embolus enters the nutrient artery and is trapped in a vessel of small caliber. Most of the small end-arteries and capillaries are located in the metaphysis adjacent to the epiphyseal plate (Fig. 10-1). This satisfactorily explains the predilection of the metaphysis to infection. Phemister

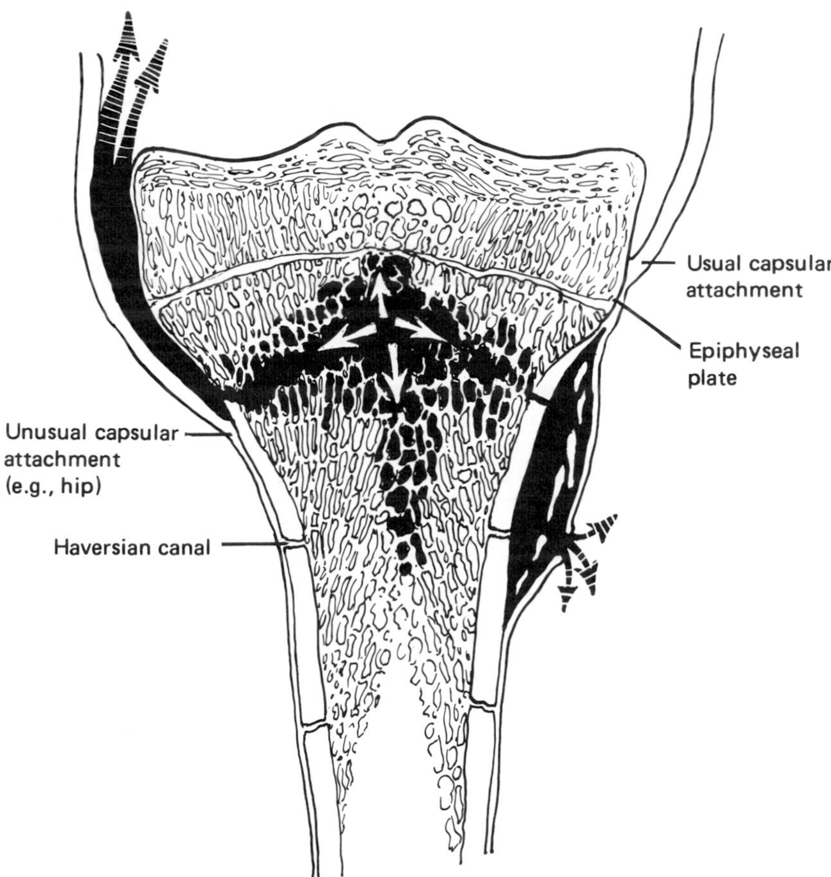

FIG. 10-1. Spread of exudate in acute hematogenous osteomyelitis. Infection occurs in the metaphysis. The cartilaginous epiphyseal growth plate constitutes a barrier to spread toward the epiphysis. The central area of destruction is surrounded by trabeculations rendered atrophic by hyperemia and destruction by proteolytic enzymes. The exudate follows the path of least resistance downward along the medullary spaces and laterally through haversian and Volkmann's canals into the subperiosteal space. The attachment of the capsule about the periphery of the epiphyseal plate blocks spread into the joint. An exception, as in the case of the hip joint, occurs when the capsule attaches beyond the metaphysis. Elevation of periosteum by exudate causes a reactive periosteal osteogenesis in an effort to wall off infection. The exudate reenters the bone through haversian channels, or the periosteum is perforated with spread into the surrounding soft tissues.

showed that the predisposition to infection in the metaphysis of a long bone is in direct proportion to the rate of growth at that area and to the size of the bone. The longer and larger the bone, the more susceptible it is to acute osteomyelitis, particularly at its more rapidly growing end. Thus, the upper metaphysis of the tibia is more likely to become infected than the lower. Other theories offered for involvement of the metaphysis rather than other areas of the long bone include the relative lack of phagocytosis in the metaphysis as compared with the diaphysis and hemorrhage following trauma, which causes locus minoris resistentiae and provides an excellent culture medium.

The infective embolus, which contains virulent organisms in large numbers, blocks a small vessel, and a small area of bone becomes necrotic. An active hyperemia develops in the vicinity, and serum and polymorphonuclear leukocytes are poured out as an exudate to combat the invaders. The hyperemia and enforced immobilization occasioned by pain effect decalcification of the surrounding bone. Proteolytic ferments formed by leukocytes destroy bacteria, necrotic bone, and medullary elements. The debris and the exudate increase in amount and effect pressure within the rigid unyielding walls of bone. Other blood vessels are compressed, and further bone necrosis ensues. The exudate follows paths of least resistance, mainly through the haversian and the cortical Volkmann canals to enter the subperiosteal space. Here an accumulation of exudate gradually strips the periosteum as a subperiosteal abscess. The periosteum in turn attempts to wall off the infection by forming new trabeculae of bone. The underlying cortex, deprived of its periosteal blood supply, becomes necrotic. Perforation of the periosteum permits spread of the infection in the soft tissues along fascial planes.

The exudate may spread down the medullary canal, destroying marrow elements and the blood supply to the cancellous bone and inner aspect of the cortex. In an advanced stage, the cortex may be surrounded externally and internally by pus and deprived of its blood supply, the entire diaphysis sequestrating. It is possible for a small accumulation of pus, by compromising the nutrient artery, to endanger large areas of the diaphysis. The importance of early decompression and adequate drainage is readily apparent.

Dead bone is absorbed by granulation tissue and osteoclastic activity about its surface. When the dead bone is large, it is gradually separated from living bone and is slowly destroyed. Because it has no blood supply, the sequestrum appears to be dense in comparison with surrounding decalcified bone. Spongy bone is absorbed rapidly.

Spread of infection directly into an adjacent joint rarely occurs because the epiphyseal plate forms a barrier. The pus first must penetrate the periosteum, spread along the soft tissues, and penetrate the capsule to cause a suppurative arthritis. The hip is an exception. The metaphysis lies within the confines of the capsule, and the joint is directly involved (see Fig. 10-1).

Healing may take place at any stage because of natural resistance or under the influence of antibiotics. At the earliest stage of minimal destruction, the exudate is resorbed, and new bony trabeculae are formed. Organisms of lesser virulence and inadequate resistance may result in the formation of a persisting abscess that is surrounded by a fibrous membrane and walled off by a ring of dense bone. This is known as Brodie's abscess. The infection may be reactivated at any time, or the organisms are destroyed and a cavity containing sterile pus, serous fluid, or fibrous tissue will remain indefinitely.

Necrotic bone becomes absorbed slowly over its surface, is surrounded by granulation tissue, separates from surrounding living bone, and persists until slowly resorbed or extruded. Until this happens, exudate is formed continually and may drain externally. Walled-off areas of infection may undergo recrudescence of activity at any time in later years. This is the stage of chronic osteomyelitis.

CLINICAL PICTURE

An antecedent infection is usually present. With the onset of osteomyelitis, symptoms of a severely acute illness appear. The child is irritable and restless and complains of headache. Vomiting, convulsions, and chills occur. Fever is high, the pulse is rapid, and leukocytosis is as high as 30,000. The extremity is held in semiflexion, surrounding muscles are in spasm, and passive movement is resisted because of pain. Pain quickly becomes excruciating and occasions fits of screaming and crying. At first no swelling is evident, but within a few days the soft tissues about the affected site become edematous and red, indicating subperiosteal abscess formation. Before periosteal involvement, a localized point of tenderness is found over the affected metaphysis. After inflammatory signs appear, tenderness is quite pronounced. Fluctuation is not elicited until pus has escaped outside the periosteum. An increased effusion in the adjacent joint proves in most cases to be a sympathetic synovitis with sterile clear fluid. If infection and septicemia proceed unabated, the child may become apathetic and unconscious and continue to a fatal termination.

LABORATORY FINDINGS

Films are negative within the first week or 10 days. Thereafter, a localized area of bone destruction is observed in the metaphysis surrounded by a wide zone of decalcified bone. Later, within the next few weeks, the periosteal shadow is elevated at the same level, and multiple laminations of bone deposition parallel with the shaft are seen. Eventually, more spongy trabeculae are destroyed, giving a moth-eaten appearance that extends for a varying distance in the medulla toward the diaphysis. The external or internal surface of the cortex may display multiple scalloped erosions. If a segment of necrotic bone is present, it retains its original architecture and appears denser than the surrounding decalcified bone. When healing takes place in the earliest stage, the bony architecture is quickly restored.

Aspiration of subperiosteal pus reveals by culture the infecting organism and its sensitivity to antibiotics.

Blood culture demonstrates the presence of bacteremia.

Blood count reveals a polymorphonuclear leukocytosis.

COMPLICATIONS

Spread to surrounding soft tissues may cause suppurative tenosynovitis, suppurative arthritis, and thrombophlebitis.

DIFFERENTIAL DIAGNOSIS

The following conditions must be ruled out:

Rheumatic fever. The onset is more gradual, and general constitutional symptoms are less acute. Pain and tenderness are less intense and are confined to the joint. Involvement is polyarticular. Response to salicylates and adrenocorticotropic hormone (ACTH) is dramatic. Antibiotics have no effect.

Ewing's tumor. This, too, causes fever, leukocytosis, and subperiosteal "onion-peel" bone deposition. However, destruction usually is confined to the diaphysis and is more diffuse. The tumor responds rapidly to x-ray irradiation. Constitutional symptoms are less intense. Biopsy demonstrates tumor cells.

Acute suppurative arthritis. Fluid accumulation in the joint occurs earlier, pain and tenderness are definitely limited to the joint, joint movement is greatly restricted, muscle spasm is intense, and aspiration reveals purulent synovial fluid.

PROGNOSIS

The 20% mortality rate of past years has been greatly reduced to the point of rarity with the introduction of antibiotics. Rapid cure of infection in the early stage before bone destruction is evident apparently occurs frequently. It is almost impossible to determine the presence of the disease at this stage. It has become uncommon to observe a case after severe bone destruction has occurred. Small areas of necrotic and sequestrated bone may be resorbed and normal bony architecture restored, especially in children. However, a large sequestrum surrounded by a wall of dense bone may retain infective material within its cavity and cause exacerbations of infection and draining sinuses over many years in spite of treatment with antibiotics. Chronic osteomyelitis continues until the sequestrum is resorbed or extruded.

TREATMENT

Even before the diagnosis can be definitely established, an antibiotic is given immediately in large dosage and continued indefinitely. Penicillin, cephalosporin, and tetracycline are preferred until the organism can be obtained, cultured, and tested for sensitivity. As in any infection in a closed space, immediate provision for drainage is of paramount importance. This must be done at the earliest possible opportunity, even before signs of subperiosteal infection are evident. To wait is to invite disaster. Pressure exerted by pus enclosed within a rigid compartment is tremendous, the circulation to the bone is jeopardized, and extensive necrosis of bone is inevitable. Upon the mere suspicion of acute bone infection, no harm is done by removing the cortex and providing free access to the outside. A waiting period of 24 to 48 hours is permissible if general supportive treatment by transfusions and fluid is necessary to transform a severely ill child into a better surgical risk and if symptoms are not too severe and antibiotics alone offer a chance of cure.

Drainage Technique

The periosteum is incised longitudinally over the point of maximum tenderness. It is stripped laterally for a half inch on either side. Extensive stripping will jeopardize periosteal blood supply to the cortex. If pus is subperiosteal, the site of bone infection is evidenced by pitting and points of exudation through the cortex. Before the stage of subperiosteal abscess formation, the cortex appears normal. Drill holes are made in various directions until the intraosseous exudate is localized. Then an adequate rectangle of cortex is outlined by multiple drill holes, and removal is completed with the osteotome. Curetting of the spongiosa is avoided for fear of disseminating the infection. The cavity is loosely packed with plain gauze to provide a drain and to keep the wound open. A catheter is introduced into the cavity for local instillation of antibiotics. A cast is applied, and the extremity is placed in a position to provide dependent drainage.

Usually pain is relieved immediately, the temperature falls, and the acutely ill patient is transformed dramatically to a well person. The wound should be allowed to heal by secondary intention. If destruction is extensive, immobilization by a cast is continued to prevent a pathologic fracture until new bone formation is sufficient.

CLOSED IRRIGATION AND SUCTION

Instead of allowing the wound to remain open and heal in secondarily, it is closed to obtain primary healing and good skin coverage. Before closure, two plastic tubes are inserted for continuous irrigation, with the appropriate antibiotic and a detergent. The procedure is described under Chronic Osteomyelitis.

CONSERVATIVE APPROACH

If the offending organism and appropriate antibiotic can be determined from blood culture within a reasonable period, vigorous antibiotic treatment without surgical drainage may be sufficient to effect a cure.[2,5] Such a course of therapy is acceptable only when the patient's condition will permit surgical delay and treatment is started early. While awaiting the results of blood culture, intensive antimicrobial treatment is initiated and aimed at the most common offending organism, *Staphylococcus aureus*. For example, the adult will require 10 million units penicillin G or 8 g oxacillin (penicillinase-resistant) per day. Later, the selected appropriate antibiotic is substituted.

In children, because of increased bacterial resistance to various penicillins, the combination of a chemotherapeutic drug with an antibiotic may be used. Fusidic acid and erythromycin are both potent antistaphylococcal drugs unaffected by β-lactamase.[1,3] Further, erythromycin broadens the spectrum to include the next most common organisms, *Streptococcus pyogenes* and *Hemophilus influenzae*. The recommended dosage is aqueous suspension fusidic acid, 5 ml tid (1–5 years) or 10 ml bid (6–12 years), plus erythromycin stearate, 30 mg/kg daily in divided doses.

Surgery is indicated if a definite abscess is present regardless of the clinical course. It is indicated where there has been no response to vigorous antibiotic treatment after 48 to 72 hours.[6]

CHRONIC OSTEOMYELITIS

When the original acute bone infection has subsided, it may persist as a low-grade infection subject to repeated recrudescences of the acute process over many months or years. Hematogenous infection with an organism of low virulence may be chronic from the onset. Infection introduced through an external wound usually causes a chronic osteomyelitis.

PATHOLOGY

In any infection of bone, there is an attempt at repair that, if incomplete, results in chronic persistence of infection. This repair is accomplished by hyperemia of the surrounding tissue, which effects decalcification of the bone. Granulation tissue forms and carries in osteoclasts and osteoblasts. Necrotic cancellous bone is readily absorbed and replaced by new bone. Dead cortex is gradually absorbed about its surface and is detached from living bone to form a sequestrum. The erosive process is brought about by osteoclasis and the action of proteolytic enzymes and causes a jagged irregular surface appearance (Fig. 10-2). Because of loss of blood supply, the sequestrum is not decalcified and appears more dense than the surrounding living bone. Separation of dead bone from living may require several months. Rarely, when infection has been completely eradicated, the necrotic bone does not separate and instead is gradually replaced over many months by the process of creeping substitution. After complete sequestration, so that the dead fragment lies free within a cavity, it is less readily attacked by granulation tissue and is absorbed more slowly. This is especially the case when infective exudate fills the cavity. The surrounding living bone attempts to wall off the infection by forming a thick, dense wall, the involucrum. When neighboring tissue is destroyed, the surface of the sequestrum remains uneroded. Externally, the periosteum lays down new bone to form an involucrum. Rarely, the entire shaft will sequestrate and be enveloped by a new periosteal bone casing that gradually increases in density and thickness. An involucrum usually has multiple openings, the cloacae, through which exudate, bone debris, and sequestra find exit and pass through sinus tracts to the surface. Constant destruction of neighboring soft tissues leads to cicatrix formation, and the skin is thin, distorted, and easily traumatized, the skin epithelium growing inward to line the sinus tracts. Persistence of drainage irritation may cause an epithelioma of a sinus tract.

After a sequestrum has been discharged or removed, the sinus usually closes, and the cavity may fill with new bone. This is more likely in children. In adults, the cavity may persist and harbor organisms that may reactivate the infection at any time.

In chronic osteomyelitis of long standing, multiple cavities and sequestra exist throughout the bone. The shaft becomes thickened, irregular, and deformed.[13]

CLINICAL PICTURE

During the period of inactivity, no symptoms are present. The bone is misshapen, and the skin is dusky, thin, scarred, and poorly nourished. A break in the skin causes

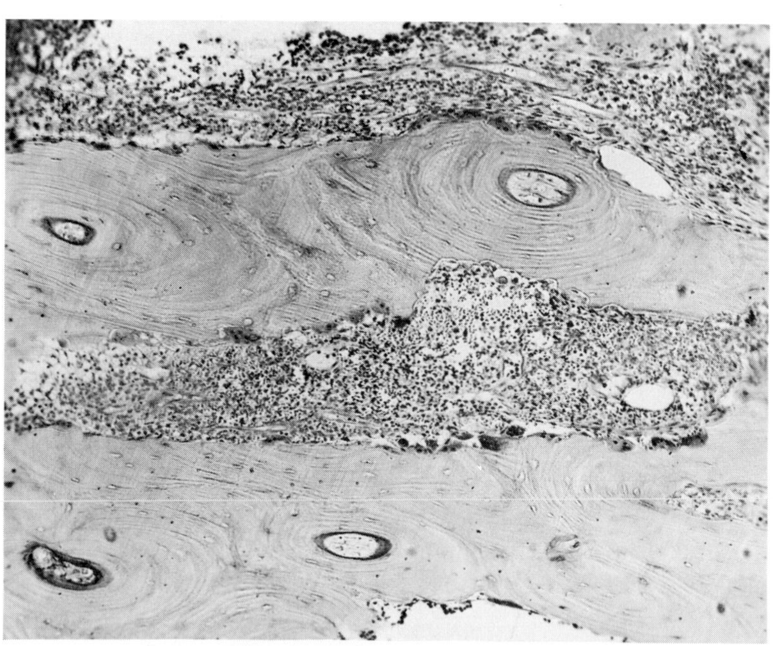

FIG. 10-2. Chronic osteomyelitis. The marrow spaces are occupied by inflammatory exudate (whose cells are composed chiefly of round cells) and detritus. The bone is dead, as evidenced by empty lacunae, and is being actively resorbed by osteoclasts.

an ulceration that is slow to heal. Muscles are scarred and cause contractures of adjacent joints. A lighting up of infection is manifest by aching pain that is worse at night. The overlying soft tissues become swollen, edematous, warm, reddened, and tender. The temperature may be elevated a degree of two. As the infection progresses, a sinus may open and drain indefinitely, extruding small sequestra at intervals. Spontaneous closure of the sinus and subsidence of infection ofter occur following expulsion of a large fragment.

These recurrent acute flare-ups occur at indefinite intervals over months and years. A sinus may drain continuously. On the other hand, an interval of many years between flare–ups is not unusual. Relapse is often the result of poor bodily condition and lowered resistance. Recurrent toxemia over a long period will eventually cause debilitating and sometimes fatal amyloidosis.

COMPLICATIONS

Complications of chronic osteomyelitis include a reduced rate of growth, pathologic fracture, bone lengthening, muscle contracture, epithelioma, and amyloidosis.

BACTERIOLOGY

Staphylococcus aureus, whether penicillinase producing or non-penicillinase producing, is the most common infecting organism.[18] Only about half the cultures grown from the first episode of acute osteomyelitis are susceptible to penicillin. When isolated from recurrent osteomyelitis, the organisms are almost uniformly resistant to penicillin. Certain synthetic penicillins resist destruction by the enzyme penicillinase (β-lactamase). These include dicloxacillin. Instead of penicillin, cephalosporins can be used. Although there is supposed to be a cross-allergenicity between penicillin and cephalosporin, the latter produces a much lower incidence of allergic phenomena. Cefazolin has been shown to produce high levels of the antibiotic in bone.[8]

Most infections are due to more than one organism and require multiple antibiotics. These bacteria most often include group A streptococci, streptococci that are not group A, *Pseudomonas aeruginosa, Proteus, Escherichia coli, Klebsiella, Aerobacter, Staphylococcus epidermidis,* and *Bacteroides.*

Within recent years, the incidence of gram-negative bacteria causing osteomyelitis has increased. Of all the gram-negative organisms, *Klebsiella* causes the most extensive bone destruction.

Hemophilus influenzae is a common cause of bone and joint infections in patients under 2 years of age. It is sensitive to erythromycin.

Proteus species can produce progressive, unrelenting, destructive lesions of bone. Four types are involved. *Proteus mirabilis* is the most common type and is susceptible to penicillin and cephalothin. For the other three species, gentamicin is effective.

Pseudomonas infection of bone is exceedingly rare and generally occurs as a secondary invader. It is treated with gentamicin or tobramycin, which should be used with caution because of potential nephrotoxicity and ototoxicity. Carbenicillin is effective. The combination of gentamicin and carbenicillin may be considered for organisms relatively resistant to either antibiotic.[16]

Osteomyelitis caused by salmonella occurs in association with sickle-cell disease or other disorders of hemoglobin. It is characterized by multiple bone involvement and is susceptible to chloramphenicol.

Bacteroides is the most important of the gram-negative anaerobic bacteria and generally occurs in a mixed infection. It produces foul-smelling, widespread tissue necrosis. *Bacteroides* septicemia is present in more than one half of patients and is uniformly fatal unless recognized early and treated vigorously by appropriate antibiotics, preferably lincomycin (Lincocin), and open wound drainage, permitting the wound to fill in secondarily. Most *Bacteroides* species are susceptible to the tetracyclines.[9,15]

For *Aerobacter aerogenes,* kanamycin and neomycin are the agents of choice.

Brucella causes bone infection in about 10% of patients with brucellosis. The vertebrae are most frequently involved. A combination of tetracycline and streptomycin is effective.

ROENTGENOGRAPHIC FINDINGS

In the early stages, the bone appears moth-eaten and osteoporotic, and areas of sclerosis develop. The periosteum is elevated by subperiosteal laminations of new bone, which become progressively thicker and dense (Fig. 10-3). Sharply delineated areas of density, the necrotic bone, are accentuated by surrounding decalcification. Gradually, each necrotic dense area becomes surrounded by a white ring representing reactive new bone formation, the involucrum. There then develops a narrow zone of diminished density between necrotic and living bone, signifying absorption about the surface of the sequestrum and separation from living bone. If this narrow zone of bone resorption does not appear, infection is probably not present, and the central density represents an area of aseptic necrosis that will be replaced by creeping substitution. Many areas of increased and decreased density may occur throughout the bone, the shaft becoming enlarged and misshapen (Fig. 10-4). A sequestrum may not be visible because of overlying dense bone, unless x-ray exposures are made with varying intensities and from various projections (Figs. 10-5 and 10-6).

TREATMENT

Defense mechanisms of bone constantly strive to absorb or extrude the sequestrum. Exudate is constantly formed under pressure, which further compromises the circulation and spreads the infection. In addition, the hard sclerotic wall, which likewise is infected, prevents obliteration of the cavity in which organisms can reside indefinitely. The wall acts as a barrier, preventing access of antibiotics to the cavity. It is obvious that cure of infection requires removal of the sequestrum and excision of infected granulation tissue, scar, and thick involucrum. By providing a residual bed of normal, bleeding, cancellous bone, bone regeneration and healing are rapid. Removal of bone should not be extensive for fear of inducing a pathologic fracture. If the parent bone is involved diffusely and severely, a conservative approach is best. Only the offending sequestrum is removed. When infection is extensive and uncontrollable, amyloid disease is a definite danger. Amputation is best. The following technique may be applied to chronic osteomyelitis regardless of whether it is caused by penetrating wounds or compound fractures or follows an acute bone infection.

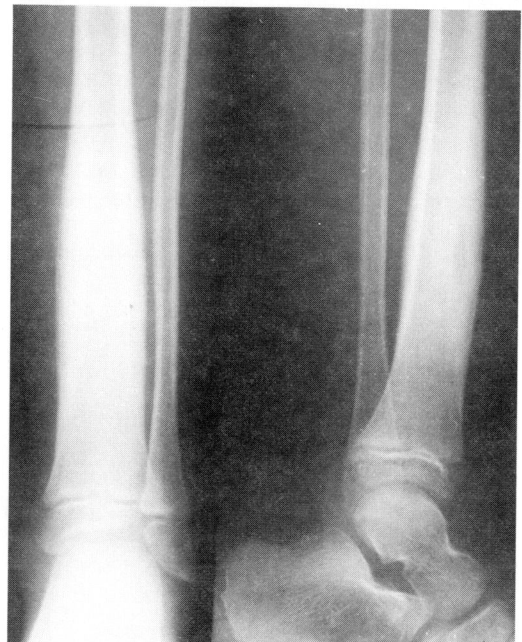

FIG. 10-3. Subacute osteomyelitis. Reactive periosteal new bone completely envelops the shaft. The destructive lesion lies anteriorly.

Technique. Preoperatively, the patient's condition is improved by multiple blood transfusions and a high-protein diet. The exudate is cultured, and the organisms are tested for sensitivity to various antibiotics. The offending organism is usually the *Staphylococcus,* but saprophytes and secondary invaders are also present. These are of importance, since they produce penicillinase, which destroys the antibiotic and allows the *Staphylococcus* organism to survive. These contaminants most commonly include *Escherichia coli* and *Pseudomonas aeruginosa.* Often these can be eliminated by local application of streptomycin. Most strains of *Pseudomonas aeruginosa* are sensitive to aminoglycosides (*e.g.,* tobramycin). Otherwise, the main infecting bacteria is combated by the indicated antibiotic.

A sufficient section of cortex is removed to permit free drainage, and the edges are saucerized. All sequestra, scar tissue, and surrounding dense bone are excised until a bed of raw, bleeding cancellous bone remains. Any tissue causing the mere suspicion of infection or creating doubt as to viability should be removed. The wound is loosely packed open with petrolatum gauze, and a catheter is inserted for local application of antibiotics. A

FIG. 10-4. Chronic osteomyelitis of the upper femur.

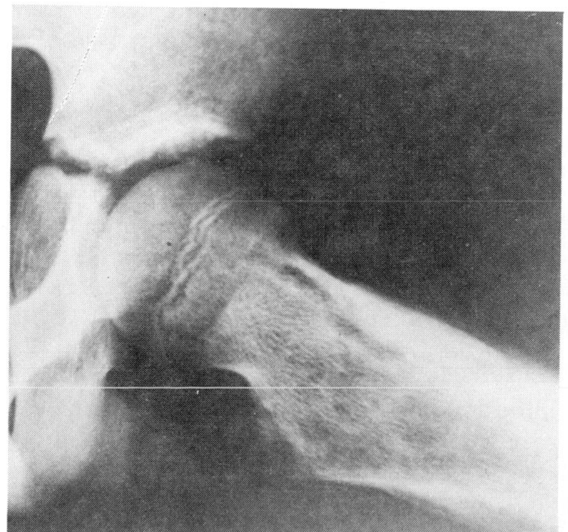

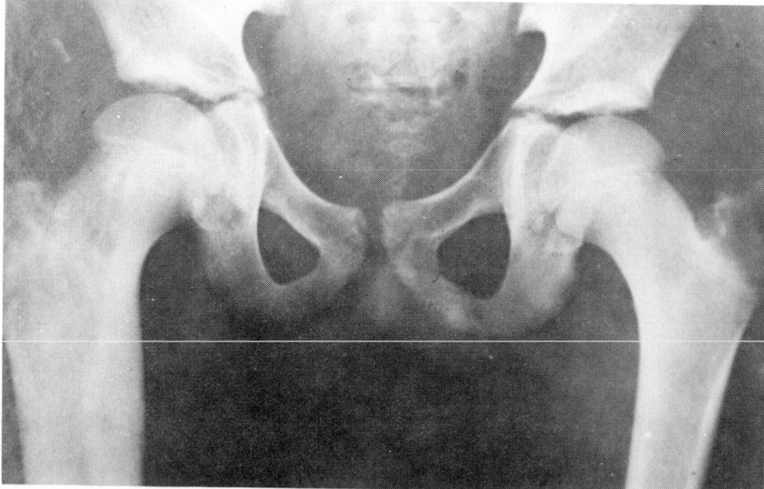

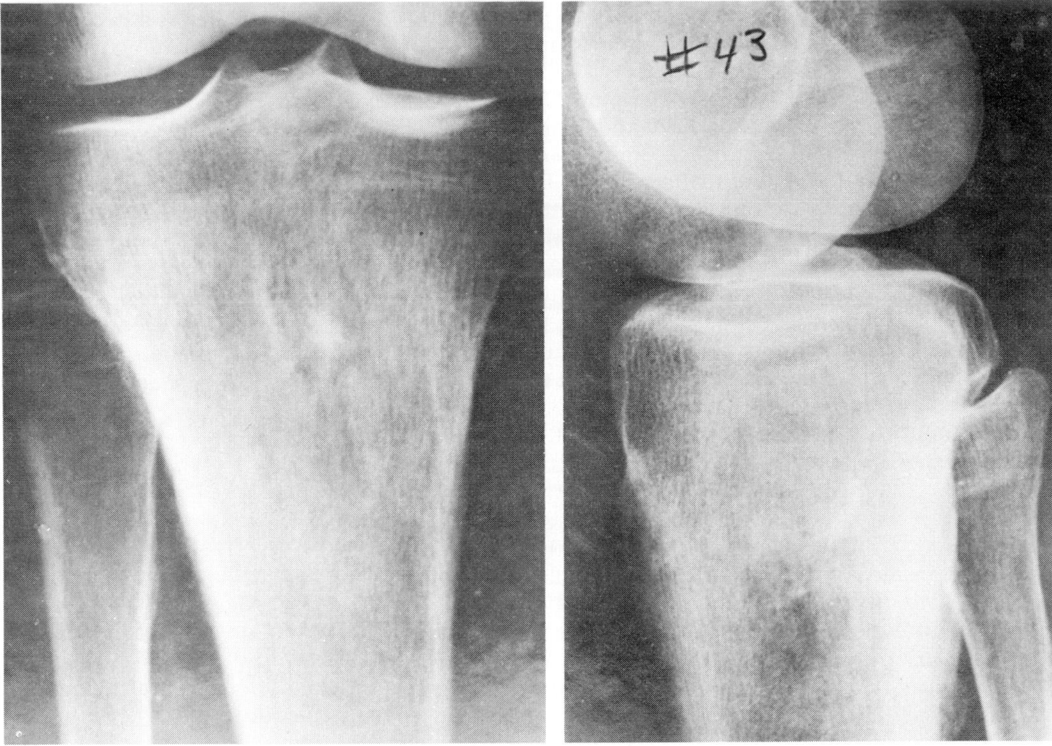

FIG. 10-5. Localized osteomyelitis of the tibia with sequestrum formation.

cast is applied.[12,17] The wound is inspected every week or 10 days until the defect is filled with granulation tissue. Next, a split-thickness skin graft (about 0.012 inch thick) is placed over the granulations, and a pressure dressing is applied. After the take, the area is observed over a period of months to ascertain whether or not the infection is quiescent. Finally, if the bony defect is large, it must be obliterated by cancellous bone chips. Adequate skin covering with thick subcutaneous tissue is necessary for success of a bone-grafting procedure. It is preferable to create a pedicle flap and transfer it gradually until it becomes very viable and well nourished before using it to replace the split-skin covering. After several months, the thick graft will have good circulation and will heal readily following the bone-grafting procedure. Finally, the bone defect is approached, if possible, through normal skin. All scar tissue is excised, and the walls of the cavity are curetted until cancellous, bleeding bone is exposed. Multiple small pieces of iliac cancellous bone are packed into the defect, and the skin is closed. A cast is applied.

Closed Irrigation and Suction. For resistant focal infections, the topical instillation of a solution containing a mild detergent (*e.g.*, Alevaire) and one or more antibiotics seems to be effective. The detergent inhibits or prevents the formation of penicillinase, so that penicillin used with the detergent becomes effective against resistant bacterial strains. Because the detergent is a mucolytic wetting agent, it breaks up pus, mucus, and necrotic

FIG. 10-6. Chronic osteomyelitis. A large sequestrum is enclosed within the cavity.

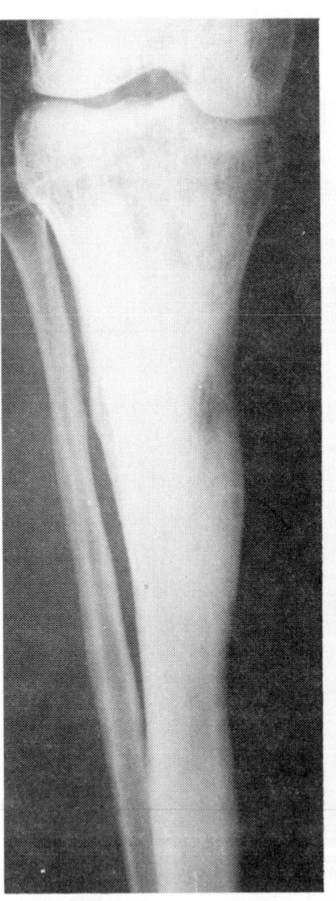

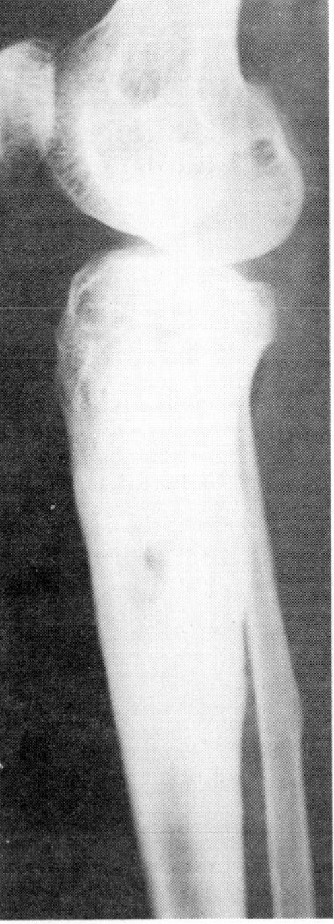

tissue, permitting antibiotics to reach bacteria that might otherwise be inaccessible. The detergent is mildly bacteriostatic.

Technique. Each liter of solution contains 200 ml Alevaire, 800 ml normal saline solution, and 5 million units aqueous penicillin or 2 g of an appropriate broad-spectrum antibiotic, or both. Bacterial cultures and sensitivities eventually determine the most effective antibiotic, which must also be given systemically to supplement the closed irrigation.

All sinuses, sequestra, necrotic tissue, and involucrum are removed. The multiperforated portions of the plastic tubes are laid in the wound. The nonperforated portion of each tube is brought out through normal tissue and anchored to the skin with fine wire suture. The wound is closed tightly with stainless steel sutures. If it cannot be closed, the open wound beneath the dressings may be lavaged.

The inlet tube is connected to the bottle containing the prepared antibiotic-detergent solution. The outlet tube is connected to a suction machine. Instillation drip should deliver 80 ml/hour, or 2000 ml/24 hours. The suction operates at 30 mm Hg to 60 mm Hg. It is stopped every 3 hours during the day to permit the wound to fill with solution. If pressure within the wound causes increasing discomfort, the inlet tube is clamped for 30 minutes. Then the clamp is removed from the tube and the suction pump started.[7,10,11,14]

The material coming through the suction tube is cultured every day. When three successive negative cultures are obtained, the antibiotic-detergent solution is discontinued. It should be emphasized that local and systemic antibiotic treatment is no substitute for thorough surgical excision.

Primary closure plus suction-irrigation is not indicated for anaerobic infections. Instead the wound must be left open for adequate drainage and allowed to fill in secondarily with clean granulation tissue.

SCLEROSING OSTEOMYELITIS OF GARRÉ

Sclerosing osteomyelitis of Garré, also known as idiopathic cortical sclerosis, consists of the gradual development of a spindle-shaped sclerotic thickening of the cortex of a long bone usually confined to one side of the shaft. Infants and children are affected most frequently, and the tibia is the usual site. Pain is constant, dull, boring, and worse at night. A history of trauma is often elicited. Clinically, one finds a diffuse bony enlargement that is only slightly tender. The overlying soft tissues appear normal or occasionally may be slightly warm and reddened. Constitutional symptoms are absent, and the blood picture is normal.

The roentgenologic picture shows a gradual thickening and increased density of the cortex. Within the sclerotic area, a minute focus of decreased density may be observed, particularly when films are taken in various planes and with varying intensities of exposure.

Microscopic examination in most cases fails to reveal evidence of inflammation. The occasional finding of an osteoid osteoma type of lesion suggests this as the causative lesion. Failure to remove the nidus may explain persistence of symptoms. Before excising a section of cortical bone, an attempt should be made to identify and localize a nidus. If symptoms persist, roentgenographic study is repeated, and further bone resection is attempted. Antibiotics are valueless.

The term *osteomyelitis* should be discarded. In the absence of a discoverable etiologic lesion, the general all-inclusive label *idiopathic cortical sclerosis* is suggested.

TUBERCULOSIS OF BONES AND JOINTS

Tuberculosis is a chronic infectious disease caused by the tubercle bacillus. Involvement of bones and joints is secondary to lesions elsewhere (Color Plate 10-1). Therefore, reduction in the incidence of tuberculosis by health measures and lessening of the severity of the disease, particularly by antibiotics and chemotherapeutic agents, has made tuberculosis of bones and joints an uncommon condition.

ETIOLOGY

The exciting factor is the tubercle bacillus. Predisposing factors include the following:

Constitutional. Inadequate diet, fatigue, poor sanitation
Race. Dark-skinned races (*i.e.*, blacks, Mexicans, Orientals, American Indians)
Trauma. Direct violence to a bone or a joint preceding infection suggesting formation of a locus minoris resistentiae.
Age. Infants under 2 years of age, poor tolerance of infection; between 2 and 15 years, infection usually relatively benign; beyond 15, disease severe and may be fatal
Disease. Measles and chickenpox
Puberty and pregnancy. Can reactivate tuberculosis.

PATHOLOGY

Infection in bone and synovial tissue invokes the same response as in the lung except for variations due to the character of the tissue.[20] The initial infection occurs in the lung (human type) or the intestine (bovine type), usually in children under 2 years of age. A natural immunity develops and heals the tubercle at the site of invasion and regional lymph nodes (primary complex). However, allergy to future infection has developed.

Therefore, at the second infection, which may occur years later, the allergic response is an acute inflammatory one, prompt in appearance and marked by outpouring of polymorphonuclear leukocytes and plasma and by massive necrosis. The fresh adult infection provokes an immunological response of the host in whom a sensitized state has been induced by the first lesion.

TUBERCLE

The initial response, especially in reinfection (allergic inflammation of an already tuberculous animal), is polymorphonuclears; these are rapidly replaced by mononuclears (macrophages and monocytes), which are highly phagocytic members of the reticuloendothelial system. After phagocytosing the bacilli, the latter break down, and the lipid is dispersed throughout the cytoplasm, the mononuclear being transformed into the epithelioid cell. This cell, characteristic of the tuberculous reaction, is large and pale with a large vesicular nucleus, abundant cytoplasm, indistinct margins, and processes that seem to pass between the cells, forming an epithelioid reticulum. The characteristic Langhans' giant cells, with their peripherally placed nuclei, are probably formed by fusion of a number of epithelioid cells. They are not formed until caseation necrosis has occurred; often they contain tubercle bacilli. Their function is to digest and remove dead tissue. They occur in other chronic inflammations (syphilis, actinomycosis). After a week, lymphocytes appear and form a ring about the periphery of the lesion. These are one of the sources of gamma globulin, the immune bodies. This mass of newly formed cells constitutes the translucent nodule known as the tubercle (Color Plate 10-2). Several small tubercles may fuse to form a larger one. Caseation necrosis, which is a coagulation necrosis formed by liberation of the protein fraction of bacilli, begins at the second week. The homogeneous center stains red with eosin, surrounded by pale epithelioid cells with one or more giant cells and ringed by a zone of dark blue lymphocytes. The caseous material softens and liquefies.

The future course of the tubercle varies:

- It may resolve completely.
- Fibrous tissue may encircle the lesion, and lime salts may be deposited in the central caseous substance.
- There may develop a low-grade inflammation characterized by many tubercles without proceeding to caseation and encircled by granulation tissue. This fibrosing hyperplastic form is most common in synovial membrane.
- Infection may spread throughout the tissue with formation of many more tubercles.
- When infection is virulent or massive, there may develop an acute inflammatory reaction, an exudative outpouring of polymorphs and serofibrinous fluid. This is seen most commonly in reinfections.

SKELETAL AND ARTICULAR INVOLVEMENT

Skeletal and articular involvement occur during a second infection, the period of allergy. Dissemination takes place through the bloodstream and affects almost all the bones, the immunity apparently healing most of the lesions. On the other hand, the allergic exudative response may be extreme, overcoming the immunity, and a fatal miliary tuberculosis may ensue. Most commonly, the defense is sufficient to overcome all but a few sites. Implantations occur both in bone and synovial membrane. If only bone or synovium is infected alone, the one generally infects the other in a short time. Typically, an active focus is set up in a metaphysis (in a child) or in an epiphysis (in an adult), where the acute exudative reaction may cause local necrosis until caseation occurs. The intense hyperemia causes marked decalcification locally, a characteristic well seen in roentgenograms. Granulation tissue about the site constitutes the fibroblastic healing response. It brings in tremendous numbers of mononuclears and attempts to delimit the process by fibrosis. If unsuccessful, the destruction extends up and down the shaft and peripherally to reach the subperiosteal space. The periosteum may react to a superficial cortical lesion by producing new periosteal bone. The exudate may penetrate outward through the soft tissue to exit through the skin as a fistula chronically draining caseous material, particles of bone, and partially liquefied, thick, grayish yellow substance. Before this abscess erupts, it distends the skin, which appears thinned and slightly darkened, but without acute inflammation (cold abscess). Secondary infection of the sinus tract is frequently superimposed. The prolonged drainage causes amyloidosis and death.

Cartilage is resistant to tuberculous destruction (Color Plate 10-3). Therefore, the epiphyseal plate is not destroyed. However, the granulation tissue may invade the area of calcified cartilage and interfere with longitudinal growth. Asymmetrical impairment of this growth process leads to deformity. Metaphyseal infection reaches the joint through the subperiosteal space, from which it penetrates the capsular attachment about the joint. In the adult, after complete ossification of the epiphysis, the infection spreads in the subchondral area to the periphery where the synovium joins the cartilage; then it enters the joint (see Color Plate 10-3). Destruction of subchondral bone loosens the attachments of the articular cartilage, which may become displaced into the joint cavity (Fig. 10-7).

The synovium may be originally infected and the bone secondarily infected by a reverse process of the one just described. The most common type of synovial infection is one that is low grade. The membrane is swollen and congested with granulation tissue (Fig. 10-8). The articular surface is studded with many translucent tubercles, and deposits of fibrin cover many areas. The joint fluid usually is moderately increased and clear. It contains rice bodies, which are small accumulations of fibrin, and pieces of articular cartilage. Caseation necrosis

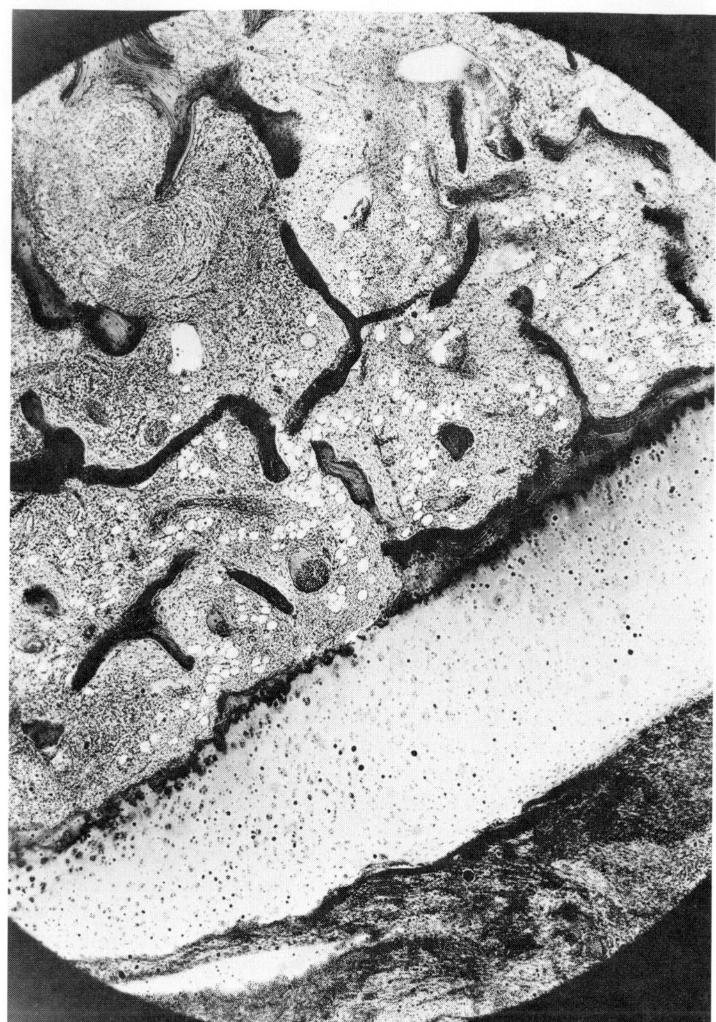

FIG. 10-7. Tuberculosis at the end of a long bone and involving the joint. Between the thin trabeculae, some of which are necrotic, are seen tubercles, granulation tissue, and cellular infiltrate, all of which extend to, but do not directly invade, the articular cartilage. Similarly, the heavily cellular tuberculous tissue overlying the articular cartilage does not seem to affect the latter. (×35)

of the synovium and the capsule is rare. The hydrarthrosis may also occur without the synovium's actually being infected. In this case the inflammatory synovitis and the increased joint fluid is a nonspecific reaction to an adjacent infection in the neighboring bone. Therefore, a negative synovial biopsy does not necessarily rule out tuberculosis. Tuberculosis of the synovium generally heals by fibrosis and marked thickening of the membrane. The granulation tissue extends from the synovium over the articular cartilage at the periphery, where as a pannus it seems to erode the cartilage. When a destructive caseating lesion of bone penetrates the joint, destruction seems to involve the synovium too rather than the usual low-grade fibrosing process. A chronically draining sinus with secondary infection of the joint and generalized amyloidosis may constitute a terminal condition. If the defense reaction overcomes the joint infection, granulation tissue bridges the joint cavity and a fibrous ankylosis results.

A focus of caseation necrosis may be walled off effectively and a clinical cure achieved. However, viable tubercle bacilli remain indefinitely—a potential source of exacerbated activity and reinfection at a later date. As in other types of necrosis, calcium salts frequently are deposited in the caseous material. In roentgenograms this gives the appearance of a sequestrum.

When the lesion in bone is chiefly exudative, the allergic reaction is present; the acute hyperemia causes decalcification in a localized area, revealed in roentgenograms as an osteolytic lesion. If healing occurs rapidly with absorption of exudate, recalcification takes place with restoration of bony architecture.

When caseation is present, the process is less acute; the coagulation necrosis and peripheral fibrosis imply a reaction of immunity. The central osteolytic area seen in roentgenograms is replaced by an increased density as healing and calcification are taking place. During the early necrosing stage, the surrounding bone undergoes

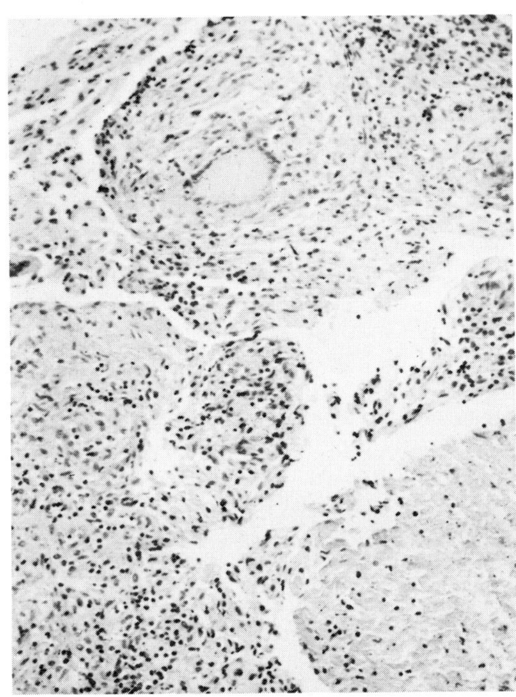

FIG. 10-8. Synovial tuberculosis.

hyperemia and decalcification, but not as severe as in the central area. Occasionally, with healing the perifocal bone may undergo hypertrophy similar to the involucrum in chronic osteomyelitis.

Abscesses in the soft tissues have a tendency to migrate along fascial planes and erupt at a distance from the original focus. This is seen best in the spine, where the infective material may enter the fascia enveloping the psoas muscle and erupt at the groin.

The areas of predilection occur in the following order of frequency: spine, hip, knee, ankle, tarsus, shoulder, and elbow.

CLINICAL PICTURE

Tuberculosis of a bone or a joint is a low-grade slowly progressing infection. The degree of local and general reaction depends on the intensity of infection and the defensive response.

CHARACTERISTICS OF THE DISEASE

Characteristics of the disease are as follows:

An insidious onset
Monoarticular or mono-osseous involvement
Other visceral lesions (*e.g.*, pulmonary, intestinal, renal)
Possible tuberculosis of other family members
Trauma to involved region often preceding onset
Local symptoms and findings: doughy swelling (caused by synovial inflammatory swelling), slight pain and tenderness, muscle spasm, night cries in children (due to relaxation of muscle spasm which allows painful motion), stiffness early, later actual limitation of active and passive motion due to fibrous ankylosis, slight warmth about involved site, increased joint fluid (due to tuberculous synovitis or nonspecific reaction to neighboring bone infection), limp, muscle atrophy that may be quite marked and occurs early
Constitutional symptoms: low-grade fever, especially in the afternoon, anorexia, weight loss, night sweats, tachycardia, anemia

TYPES OF THE DISEASE

For purposes of description, two clinical types are identified: the granular, mild, nondestructive, fibrosing; and the caseous and exudative, destructive, abscess forming. Actually, both types occur together, one predominating over the other.

Osseous

Osseous Granular. In the granular osseous type, bone involvement, usually at the metaphysis or the epiphysis, often follows trauma. The onset is insidious, with limp, vague mild pains, and fatigue. Hydrarthrosis of the adjacent joint is nonspecific and appears late in the day after activity. The periosteum may be palpably thickened and the overlying soft parts slightly warm and tender. Joint movement may be restricted because of hydrarthrosis. Muscle atrophy rapidly appears. Constitutional symptoms are rare. Infrequently, a fluctuant swelling indicates abscess formation.

Osseous Exudative or Caseous. In the caseous and exudative osseous form, the onset is less insidious and is associated with such marked constitutional symptoms as fever, night sweats, weight loss, and anorexia. Pain is more intense and particularly severe at night. Muscle spasm is marked. The overlying soft tissues are warm, swollen, indurated, and quite tender. The tendency to abscess formation is greater. Its appearance is preceded by redness, increased heat, and distention of skin, which becomes thin and shiny. Rupture of the abscess produces a fistula, which drains pus, caseous material, and sequestra for many months. Secondary infection perpetuates the drainage. When the caseous material penetrates the joint, a severely destructive arthritis ensues.

Synovial

Synovial Granular. Granular synovitis is usual when the joint is predominantly involved, particularly in children. Frequently recurring mild hydrarthroses with little or no pain characterize the insidious onset. Constitutional symptoms are mild. Recurrences become more frequent and persistent. Muscle atrophy gradually appears. In time, the joint fluid lessens and the synovial membrane thickens. Motion becomes limited, particularly at the extremes. The synovitis may last for years without involving the bone. Rarely, it may be converted into the caseous form with increase in local and constitutional symptoms. Eventually, contracture and subluxation occur.

Synovial Exudative. The onset of exudative synovitis may be acute, with intense inflammatory signs and general symptoms. The temperature reaches 101°F, and the general condition is poor. Movements are very painful. The regional lymph glands are swollen. The soft tissues about the joint are diffusely swollen and very tender. The condition changes rapidly to exudative caseous involvement of soft tissues and bone, the acuteness subsides, and the tendency is to ankylosis. An abscess usually ruptures externally, and necrotic cartilage is lost. The draining fistula invites secondary infection, which over the years leads to amyloidosis.

LABORATORY FINDINGS

The following laboratory methods are used most commonly:

Tuberculin reaction. This depends on an allergic inflammatory response to an antigen. The intradermal method (Mantoux) is best. A positive reaction indicates only that tuberculosis has been present in the past. Therefore, its value lies in a negative reaction in a known previously negative individual is diagnostic.

Guinea pig inoculation. Guinea pigs have no natural immunity to tuberculosis and rapidly succumb. The pus is injected intraperitoneally, and examination discloses tubercles 5 to 8 weeks later.

Culture. This requires from 5 to 30 days. It should be remembered that the serous exudate of a joint may be a nonspecific inflammatory response to neighboring infection and therefore may not contain bacilli.

Biopsy. Microscopic tissue examination reveals typical tubercles. A regional lymph node should be removed for examination.

Blood. A leukocytosis may be present, particularly in the more intense inflammatory types with constitutional symptoms. A relative lymphocytosis is often found.

Sedimentation rate. This is more likely to be normal in mild granular types of infection. The acutely inflammatory exudative infection gives the highest values.

ROENTGENOGRAPHIC FINDINGS

Osteoporosis is the first sign of active infection. It may also occur as a nonspecific response to an adjacent infection of the joint. The reactive hyperemia, which is most intense in exudative infections, causes decalcification that may be severe enough to stimulate osteolysis. The outline of the articular cortex is lost. When one tarsal or carpal bone is infected, the remaining tarsals and carpals rapidly decalcify, suggesting on x-ray examination that the infection is generalized. In synovitis, decalcification is first noted in the epiphyseal and metaphyseal zones. Its rapid spread indicates an intense exudative reaction. Conversely, recalcification means reduction of activity of the disease.

Swelling of the synovial shadow indicates a hydrarthrosis. This results from primary synovial infection or from a nonspecific inflammatory reaction to a neighboring bony focus that may not yet be visible in roentgenograms.

Small zones of clearly defined subnormal density in bone indicates granular foci. These osteolytic areas are surrounded by diffuse osteoporosis. As caseation takes place, the osteolytic focus is very evident. When healing comes into play, the perifocal bone becomes thickened as a heavy overcalcified ring. If the central decalcified area is merely exudative, healing results in reossification, and once again the trabeculae are apparent. More commonly, a central caseation exists in which calcium is deposited and gives the dense image of a sequestrum. This is surrounded by an osteolytic ring representing the fibrous wall, and beyond this the bone is osteoporotic, normal, or dense, depending on the defense reaction. The final picture may resemble osteomyelitis.

In destructive arthritis, necrosis and separation of articular cartilage cause joint space narrowing. The articular cortices become ragged and osteoporotic. Vague irregular densities in the surrounding soft tissue define abscess formation. The most common is the paravertebral shadow about the spine in the thoracic area and widening of the psoas shadow in the lumbar area. Sinuses are traced by injection of a radiopaque substance.

A synovitis increases the osteogenic activity of the epiphysis, so that premature appearance and enlargement of the ossific nuclei are usual. Similarly, a focus adjacent to the epiphyseal growth plate may stimulate longitudinal growth. If it encroaches on the area of endochondral ossification, growth is irregularly retarded and deformity results. When the focus is superficial, periosteal ossification is seen. This is most apparent in the small long bones of the hand and the foot where the new bone may encircle and enlarge the entire diaphysis.

COURSE AND PROGNOSIS

The newer forms of antibiotics and chemotherapeutic agents have greatly improved the outlook in tuberculosis of bones and joints. In the mild granular infections, healing can often be accomplished without residual joint scarring and ankylosis. These substances permit aggressive resection of larger caseous destructive foci from which later infections may originate. The fatal types of meningitis and miliary tuberculosis are now rare.

The tendency is toward healing by fibrosis. Mild granular types heal slowly. Exudative caseous lesions heal less readily. An epiphyseal caseous lesion may spread into the joint and widely infect the synovium. This type of infection is often associated with similar caseated cavities in other organs and constitutes the most common source of fatal dissemination. Fibrous encirclement of a cavity may effect a clinical cure, but living bacilli in the central area may reactivate the infection at any time. The only final form of healing is recalcification of bone and, in the case of a joint, bony ankylosis. The highest mortality occurs in the young. Meningitis occurs exclusively in caseous forms. Miliary tuberculosis occurs in all forms. The causes of death are meningitis, miliary tuberculosis, pulmonary tuberculosis, and amyloidosis.

TREATMENT

General Care

Absolute bed rest is prescribed. A high caloric and high vitamin diet should be wholesome and appetizing to combat the impaired appetite. Fresh air and a warm dry climate are preferred. Heliotherapy is given daily. General medical management includes good hygienic and nursing care.

The bone lesion is always secondary to a tuberculous focus elsewhere. Therefore, eradication of other active foci is necessary to aid the general bodily resistance in overcoming infection of bone. For example, lobectomy and other surgical measures, as pneumothorax, phrenicotomy, and thoracoplasty, can be carried out concurrently. If possible, surgical treatment should await the building up of the patient's general resistance. The recommended antibiotic and therapeutic drugs are started immediately and continued after the surgical procedure. The most favorable time for operation can be determined by the lymphocyte-monocyte ratio.[21] When this is greater than five, a state of good resistance is indicated. On the other hand, a low lymphocyte count and a high monocyte count indicate a dangerous state of hypergy, which favors development of serious complications.

A trial of conservative treatment is justified in cases of low-grade infection. Recalcification and restoration of bone architecture indicate that healing is taking place. When a bone contains an obviously encircled area of caseation, particularly when abscess formation threatens the integrity of neighboring structures, and when continued drainage is progressively debilitating the patient, removal of the infected focus is indicated. The following procedures are employed: excision of the focus, excision of the entire bone (*e.g.*, a tarsal bone), arthrodesis to put the part at rest, drainage and curettage of the abscess, and amputation when destruction is extensive.

Chemotherapy and Antibiotics

The most effective drugs currently used are isonicotinic acid hydrazide para-aminosalicylic acid or ethambutol, streptomycin, and rifampin.[24] Iproniazid phosphate (INPH) is seldom used. The chemotherapeutic and antibiotic drugs are thoroughly discussed elsewhere in this volume, under the section on treatment of tuberculosis of the spine. The following are their dosages, toxic reactions, and drug resistance.

Para-aminosalicylic Acid. This compound, also known as PAS, has a limited range of usefulness and is inadequate when used alone. Resistance develops after its use for 6 months. Its most useful effect is to prevent the emergence of streptomycin-resistant strains, and it is used in conjunction with streptomycin in a dosage of 10 g to 20 g/day. Its toxic reactions are frequent but mild, including anorexia, nausea, and gastric upset.

Ethambutol. Ethambutol has replaced PAS because it has fewer toxic reactions and is well tolerated. The dose is 25 mg/kg for 60 days and 15 mg/kg thereafter in a single daily dose.

Streptomycin. The sulfate is less painful than the calcium salt when given intramuscularly. It acts best at a *p*H around 9.0 and therefore should be accompanied by a buffered alkaline solution when injected intrasynovially. A single daily intramuscular dose is as effective as divided doses; 2 g/day, though more effective than 1 g, is too toxic for long-continued use. When given with PAS, its dose may be reduced effectively to 1 g twice a week. The permanent toxic effects are related to the eighth nerve and include deafness and vertigo. Vitamin B–deficiency symptoms can occur and respond to large doses of vitamin B. Daily streptomycin, when used alone, results in drug resistance, which is progressive and significant at the 3-month period (75%).

Isonicotinic Acid Hydrazide. Isonicotinic acid hydrazide, known as isoniazid, is given in a dose of 3 mg to 8 mg/kg/day. Toxic effects include rashes, fever, vitamin B–deficiency symptoms and neurologic effects upon reflexes and bladder function. Resistance develops in 11% after treatment for 1 month and increases to 70% in 3 months. It is relatively ineffective when administered alone and should be used in conjunction with PAS and streptomycin to get the maximum prevention of emergence of resistance strains and gain a high bactericidal effect. Isoniazid has the ability to penetrate the cell within which may be contained the tubercle bacillus. Streptomycin and isoniazid together double the rate of killing by either drug alone and will actually sterilize a culture, which neither drug will do alone.

Resistant bacilli tend to die out, and sensitive strains become predominant slowly after a drug is discontinued. Therefore, streptomycin may again become effective at a later date.

Iproniazid Phosphate. Iproniazid is approximately 20 times as effective as isoniazid for tuberculosis of bone and soft tissue.[19] It has certain important toxic side-effects that usually can be avoided or greatly reduced if precautions are taken.

The recommended dosage is 4 mg/kg/day for the first 2 to 4 days. Then it is reduced to 2 mg/kg/day. Osseous lesions require 2 to 3 years of treatment. Soft tissue lesions, such as tendon sheath infections, require 6 months to a year of treatment.

The main side-effects of iproniazid are the following:

Psychosis. Psychosis develops in about 10% of patients when the larger dose is continued, but it is reversible as the drug dosage is reduced.

Jaundice. Liver damage may be caused but is extremely rare when the smaller dosage is used. Periodic liver function tests are recommended. The drug is contraindicated in patients with a history of liver disease.

Cumulative Effect. In patients with impaired kidney function, the drug should be used cautiously to prevent cumulative effects.

Potentiation of Drugs. Iproniazid increases the action of certain drugs such as barbiturates, Demerol, alcohol, and ether. The prescribing of new medications should be watched with care.

Postural Hypotension. This occurs particularly with high dosages.

The side-effects are reversible or greatly lessened by reducing the dosage or discontinuing the drug temporarily. Vitamin B complex administered in conjunction with iproniazid seems to reduce its toxicity.

Antibiotics and Secondary Infection

The proper antibiotic should be carefully selected to cure the staphylococcal secondary infection. An antibiotic may act antagonistically against another antibiotic or chemical when one is bactericidal and the other is bacteriostatic. The former (penicillin, streptomycin, isoniazid, bacitracin, neomycin) affect actively dividing organisms but may be opposed by the latter (chlortetracycline, chloramphenicol, oxytetracycline, PAS, sulfonamides), which act by inhibiting cell division. Thus, for example, oxytetracycline will diminish the effect of isoniazid against tuberculosis. The bactericidal drugs only should be used, but in doubtful instances sensitivity tests should be run.

Streptomycin is very effective against miliary forms of tuberculosis and tuberculous sinuses.[26] The danger of secondary septic infection of tuberculous joints is diminished by the use of sulfonamides and penicillin. Therefore, these complications no longer are an obstacle to surgery of the tuberculous lesion. Streptomycin is unable to penetrate a fibrous wall, so it seems logical to remove the barrier.

Factors Determining Improvement in Joint Disease

Osteoporosis as seen roentgenographically results from acute inflammation, bone destruction, and immobilization. Reossification is manifest by restoration of the bony outlines and the trabecular pattern as the disease becomes quiescent. Restoration of joint motion is the other sign of improvement. After a course of streptomycin, reossification occurs earlier, and return of motion is greater than without the drug, all points of conservative treatment being equal. The duration of treatment is materially reduced. A 3-month course of 0.5 g to 1 g daily is very beneficial in conservative treatment of joint tuberculosis in children. One must remember that because the course of the disease is slow, roentgenologic evidence of increased or decreased involvement generally lags behind the actual stage of pathology.

Sinuses

Sinuses arise from a deep-seated lesion containing sequestra and caseous masses. The latter should be evacuated surgically if necessary by curetting and excising the sinus fibrous wall. Then the open cavitation and the exposed normal-appearing tissues are packed with iodoform gauze for 2 days; this is followed by application of azochloramide dressings and daily irrigation and, finally, in 7 to 10 days by secondary closure. Daily streptomycin, PAS, and isoniazid are given. Firm healing is usual in about 6 weeks. An alternative procedure is to administer antibiotics and chemotherapeutic agents and to withhold surgical intervention until the possibility of spontaneous healing can be determined. Roentgenographic evidence of gross destructive lesions and the presence of sequestra justify immediate surgery.

Abscesses

Accumulations of tuberculous destroyed and liquefied material, whether secondarily infected or not, may be evacuated and heal by primary intention when covered by the combination of streptomycin, PAS, and isoniazid.[23] Before the advent of these agents, open drainage was contraindicated for fear of secondarily infecting the abscess and converting a low-grade infection to one of great virulence. Removal of infected tissue not only prevents spread to the neighboring tissues but also eliminates a potential source of future infections.

Sacroiliac abscesses may be drained and bone grafts immediately inserted to effect an arthrodesis. Paravertebral abscesses can be opened and necrotic bone curetted out of the vertebral body.[25] Streptomycin and penicillin are instilled in the cavity and are also administered systemically. It is not necessary to await quiescence of the disease.[22] Abscesses may be dealt with and an arthrodesis performed at the same time. Occasionally, the juxta-articular lesion may be resected and joint motion preserved. Early drainage is certainly indicated in a thoracic paravertebral abscess, particularly in children in whom multiple vertebral bodies are destroyed. Decompression may often prevent or overcome a paraplegia.

SYPHILIS OF BONES AND JOINTS

The bone, the bone marrow, and the periosteum are favored sites of involvement in syphilis. However, with the advent of antibiotics and supervised prenatal care, luetic lesions have become rarities. The spirochete *Treponema pallidum* is highly susceptible to penicillin, so syphilis of the newborn and tertiary lesions of the adult are becoming extinct. However, an occasional condition requires identification and differentiation from other diseases.

The basic pathology in the skeleton is similar to that of other tissues. The spirochete is blood borne and lodges within the medulla at the site of vessels of smaller caliber, particularly at the metaphysis. Its presence calls forth a low-grade inflammatory response consisting of vasodilatation and a local outpouring of serum and mononuclear cells (lymphocytes and plasma cells). The cells characteristically congregate about blood vessels. If defenses are adequate, the bacteria may be destroyed and the exudate resorbed, the tissues returning to normal, or granulation tissue invades, trabeculae are destroyed, and healing takes place by fibrosis. This granulation tissue and infiltrating cells give a characteristic yellow color to the medulla. If the defenses are inadequate to cope with the virulence of the organism, the tissues locally are destroyed, the necrosis producing a typical yellowish gray gummatous detritus, the gumma. The central necrotic focus is surrounded by small round cells outside of which granulaton tissue and fibrous tissue are seen. Beyond the lesion, reactive new bone forms. The osteoblastic reaction is extensive. The medullary infective material extends through the haversian systems to the subperiosteal space, where elevation of the periosteum results in successive deposits of laminated bone. If the infection infiltrates the periosteum without elevating it, the reactive bone assumes a lacelike appearance. Periosteal bone becomes incorporated within and thickens the cortical bone. Therefore, periosteal ossification is a natural consequence of elevation of periosteum by exudate or granulation tissue or of thickening of the periosteum by granulation tissue that organizes into fibrous tissue and subsequently undergoes osseous transformation. Granulation tissue, fibrosis, and ossification imply that the infection is low-grade and defenses are adequate.

When the infection is virulent and defenses are inadequate, necrosis, destruction, and gummatous formation of the periosteum and the subperiosteal space predominate, new bone formation being held to a minimum. the destruction erodes the cortex and may invade the medullary cavity. In the skull, both cortices may be penetrated and the central nervous system infected, or the infective material may burrow and erupt externally, forming a sinus discharging viscous, sticky material. Later, as a result of secondary infection, the discharge becomes purulent.

The joints are rarely primarily involved. The synovitis causing large painless effusions in late congenital syphilis or occasionally in acquired tertiary syphilis is due presumably to mild synovial infection, but this has never been proved. The synovitis is often bilateral, and the fluid is clear and sterile.

Gummatous osseous destruction of long bones is rare, but when it does occur it usually involves the epiphyseal areas. The infection may then extend into the adjacent joint and cause destruction of cartilage and other soft tissues. Sinus formation is followed by secondary purulent joint infection. Healing takes place by fibrosis, but bony ankylosis does not occur.

EARLY CONGENITAL SYPHILIS

In early syphilis (Parrot's pseudoparalysis) the medulla is always infected in the syphilitic newborn. Because capillary blood supply is richest in the metaphysis adjacent to the epiphyseal plate, this is the site of maximal involvement. Endochondral ossification is interfered with. The infection, round cells, and granulation tissue invade the zone of calcified cartilage, which therefore fails to resorb and accumulates in large amounts. The infected granulation tissue interferes with the laying down of osteoid tissue; therefore, the trabeculae when formed are sparse and irregular. The proliferating cartilage piles up at the epiphyseal plate. These events explain the roentgenographic appearance of a widened translucency of cartilaginous epiphysis and plate, a widened zone of increased density (calcified cartilage) and an irregular saw-toothed contour of the proximal border of the metaphysis, and osteoporosis just beyond the dense zone. The junction between the epiphyseal plate and calcified cartilage is fragile, and fracture with epiphyseal separation often occurs.

Mild metaphyseal infection may stimulate endochondral ossification, and therefore the extremity often displays rapid growth. On the other hand, virulent destructive infection may destroy the growth plate sufficiently to interfere with growth.

In the adjacent periosteum, periosteal involvement results in reactive new bone formation. The long bones, skull, and nasal bones are favored sites of involvement.

If the infant survives the early days after birth, the condition shows a tendency toward healing within a few months. The bone infection clears up, and endochondral ossification is resumed. This suggests that the metaphyses are apparently resistant to infection.

CLINICAL PICTURE

Shortly after birth, the limb displays a large tender swelling about a joint. The child is irritable and restless and cries often. The limb is held immobile as though paralyzed. Other evidence of syphilis may be apparent, such as snuffles, keratitis, skin lesions, mucous patches, and positive serology.

ROENTGENOGRAPHIC FINDINGS

The metaphysis is widened, osteoporotic, or moth-eaten in appearance, and indented. The ossification center has not yet appeared, and it is difficult to ascertain the increased thickness or fracture displacements of the epiphysis. Surrounding the metaphysis and extending toward the diaphysis, the laminations of periosteal ossification are seen (Fig. 10-9).

DIFFERENTIAL DIAGNOSIS

Rickets and scurvy are the main conditions to be differentiated.

Rickets

Syphilis occurs before 6 months of age, whereas rickets does not appear until after 6 months. In rickets, the provisory zone of calcification is demineralized and not apparent on roentgenographic examination. Instead, the epiphyseal plate appears to be widened. Periosteal ossi-

FIG. 10-9. Congenital syphilis. Note the moth-eaten appearance of the metaphyses whose epiphyseal borders are dense and saw-toothed and the periosteal ossification of shafts.

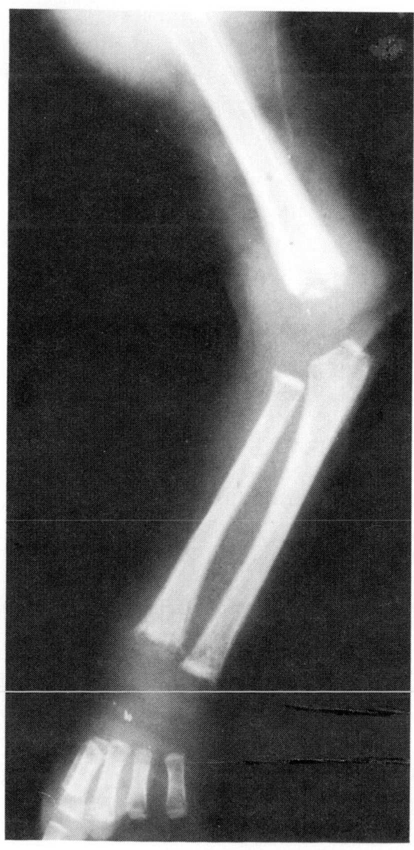

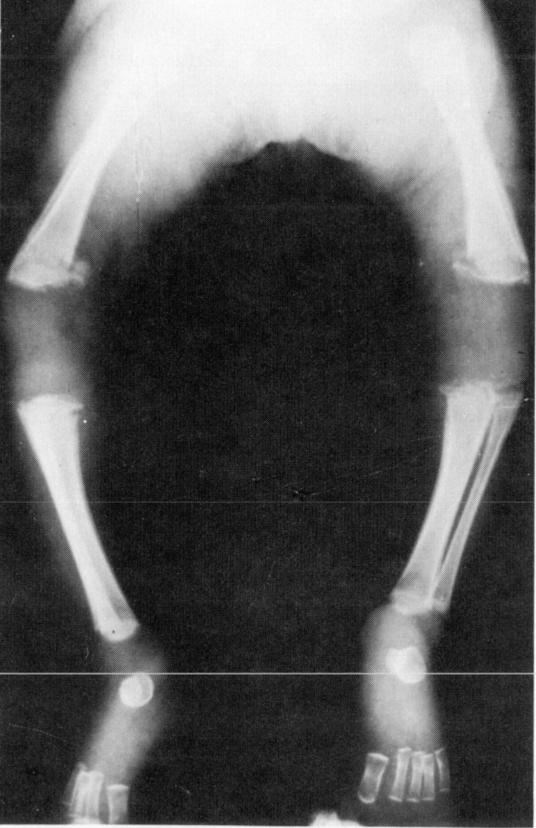

fication in rickets develops on the concave aspect of the long bone in response to static stresses, and deformity results from actual bowing of the bone. In lues, periosteal apposition of new bone has no relation to the concave aspect of the bone and is the actual cause of deformity, not bowing.

Scurvy

The epiphyseal plate is of normal width, but the bony structure of the metaphysis presents a ground-glass appearance. The main changes occur about the circumference of the shaft. Vague densities represent subperiosteal hemorrhage that eventually becomes ossified. The dense white line of Fraenkel in the metaphysis and Wimberger's line of density encircling the epiphysis are characteristic.

TREATMENT

If syphilitic infection of the newborn is not extensive and the infant survives, the osseous involvement is self-limited and heals within several months. Nevertheless, antiluetic therapy brings about a rapid recovery, and interference with subsequent longitudinal growth is less likely.

LATE CONGENITAL SYPHILIS

Late congenital syphilis is usually regarded as the tertiary stage of congenital syphilis, occurring after the second or the third year. Osteoblastic changes characterize the lesions found mainly in the tibia, the femur, and the skull. Periosteal bone formation occurs typically over the anterior aspect of the tibia, causing a bony prominence (saber shin). No actual bowing of the shaft takes place. In the skull, nodular thickenings over the outer table produce deformity. Unless adequate antibiotic therapy is instituted, the periosteal bone is incorporated into the cortex as a permanent deformity. A more virulent subperiosteal infection may erode the cortex from without, or gummatous destruction of the cortex may arise from within the medulla. This destructive osteomyelitis is rare in congenital syphilis. The radiograph, whether destructive or not, displays the increased densities of osteoblastic changes.

Associated evidence of syphilis includes interstitial keratitis, eighth nerve deafness, and deformed incisor teeth (Hutchinson's triad). At least one fourth of syphilitic children have involvement of the central nervous system.

CLUTTON'S JOINTS

Large, bilateral, painless effusions of the knees, occurring in late congenital syphilis in patients between 8 and 18 years of age, are designated Clutton's joints (symmetrical synovitis in congenital syphilis). The condition arises spontaneously and intermittently without apparent cause and disappears as mysteriously. No local inflammatory or constitutional signs are present, and the many recurrences cause no damage to the joints. If the synovial fluid is aspirated, it rapidly reaccumulates. Microscopic examination of the fluid reveals a high content of mononuclears. Radiographic examination is negative.

SYPHILITIC DACTYLITIS

The phalanges and the metacarpals are prone to enlargement and deformity by osteoblastic changes, creating the markedly increased density seen in roentgenograms. The contour of the shaft is spindle shaped, and the surface may display bone erosion. When multiple areas of gummatous destruction are present within the enlarged bulbous bone, the radiograph may be confused with that of tuberculous dactylitis. Clinically, the finger displays a large, spindle-shaped, boggy, painless swelling. Bilateral lesions are not uncommon.

ADULT SYPHILIS

Bone and joint lesions occur in the tertiary stage years after the primary stage. At least 50% of luetics have bone involvement, although a smaller number are manifest clinically and roentgenographically. The infection may be mild and resolve without apparent alteration of bony architecture. A slightly more virulent infection, assuming that the defenses are adequate, stimulates an osteoblastic reaction, the cortex becoming dense and thick and encroaching upon the medullary cavity. On the other hand, a more virulent infection, although continuing to stimulate surrounding osteoblastic reaction, is destructive. The resultant lesion is the gumma. The products of necrosis produce a yellowish gumlike material. The infective material may spread through the haversian canals to the subperiosteal space, where further gummatous necrosis occurs, or the medullary infection may progressively destroy the cortex, the periosteum, and the soft tissues, finally erupting as a chronically draining sinus. Secondary infection is usual. Sequestra are rare. Involvement is greatest at the ends of the long bones, where the joint may be invaded, and a gummatous arthritis may result.

Periostitis is the most common lesion, occurring in both skull and long bones. The periosteum becomes edematous and infiltrated with round cells and granulation tissue. The granulation tissue is converted to fibrous tissue, which in turn is ossified by a lacelike deposition of new bone.

In the skull the outer table is chiefly involved, but gummatous destruction may erode through the inner table and produce a luetic meningitis.

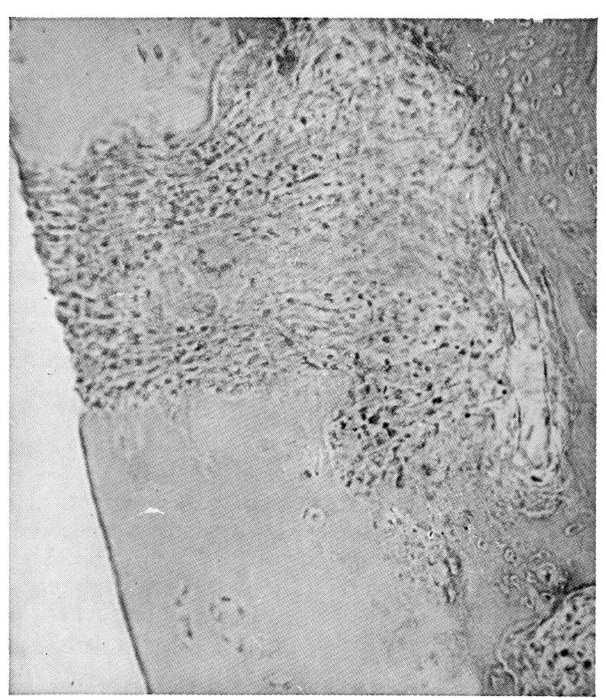

PLATE 10-3. Tuberculosis. The tuberculous granulation tissue is seen undermining and separating the articular cartilage from the bone. It does not directly destroy cartilage but instead enters the joint through a split in the cartilage. Several typical Langhans' giant cells are present. (×210) (See p. 267.)

respiratory infection has subsided, within several weeks or months the patient begins to have a low-grade fever and loses weight and strength. A skin ulcer or a subcutaneous abscess is often the first symptom suggesting fungous infection. A subcutaneous nodule may break down, discharge a sanguinopurulent material, and heal with a dense depressed scar, or it may persist as a chronic ulcer.

The bone lesions of blastomycosis and coccidioidomycosis are identical. The lesions arise in cancellous bone and are predominantly destructive with little periostitis, bone production, or marginal reaction. A well-defined area of osteolytic destruction is seen in roentgenograms.

PATHOLOGY

The lesion is a granuloma.[38] The tubercle may liquefy and form a chronic abscess and a sinus. Healing occurs by fibrosis and occasionally by bone reconstruction. Dissemination is by lymphatics and the bloodstream.

Microscopically, the appearance is granulomatous. the cells include histiocytes, epithelioid cells, polymorphonuclear leukocytes, and lymphocytes. A fibroblastic reaction is present. Giant cells are present in moderate numbers. The small spherical bodies with double contoured capsules lie free in the tissues and within giant cells. They contain central clumps of basophilic material. *Blastomyces* show small single buds being extruded externally. *Coccidioides* show central multiple spores resembling cocci. No new bone formation is seen.

DIAGNOSIS

Predominantly pulmonary or cutaneous mycotic infection can present concomitant involvement of bones and joints in up to 50% of patients.[28,29] When pulmonary abscesses and osteolytic lesions occur together, the diagnosis of tuberculosis is suggested. Rarely, coccidioidomycosis and blastomycosis may present as an osteomyelitis that defies recognition and treatment. All cases of chronic osteomyelitis should be studied for fungus.

Culture

Pus and sputum are first examined microscopically as wet preparations without potassium hydroxide. The material is then cultured on Sabouraud's glucose agar at room temperature for 10 to 40 days. The culture colonies are placed in 10% potassium hydroxide, which dissolves everything but the spores.

Tissue Stains

Biopsy specimens of bone and skin lesions are prepared by special stains such as periodic acid—Schiff or silver methenamine.[35] The granulomatous reaction and organisms are observed.

Skin Testing

Skin tests are performed with blastomycin or coccidioidomycosis antigen. It is important to recognize that the skin test is often negative. Further, patients with blastomycosis tend to have positive responses at times to histoplasmin. Therefore, if a positive histoplasmin test is obtained in the presence of a negative blastomycin test, further investigation is suggested.

Complement Fixation Test

A complement fixation test is of value only when positive. Although external manifestations of the disease may be minimal, the true extent of visceral dissemination and activity of the infection is revealed by the titer. Titers above 1:32 are considered indicative of active disease. Surgery is best attempted during a period of low titer.[31]

TREATMENT

Amphotericin B is effective in the treatment of blastomycosis and coccidioidomycosis; 2-hydroxystilbamidine is nearly as effective and is much less toxic.[40,42] Both drugs are given intravenously over a period of weeks until a total dose of 2 g to 3 g amphotericin B or 8 g to 12 g 2-hydroxystilbamidine is given.

Amphotericin B is preferred in the acutely ill patient with severe or rapidly progressive disease. It is given in an initial dose of 1 mg intravenously over several hours. On subsequent days the dose is increased until a maintenance dose of 0.5 mg to 1.0 mg/kg is achieved. Alternate-day therapy seems to diminish toxicity without reducing effectiveness.

The following are side-effects of amphotericin B:

Constitutional. Anorexia, nausea, vomiting, fever, chills (during infusion, infrequent and controllable)
Hematopoietic. Anemia (reversible on withdrawing drug)
Nephrotoxic. Azotemia, mild proteinuria, isosthenuria, hypokalemia, inability to acidify

Nephrotoxicity is the most important side-effect and is due to three factors: renal artery constriction, direct tubular damage, and fluid-electrolyte imbalance. The blood urea nitrogen and creatinine clearance must be repeatedly checked for the duration of therapy. If abnormal, the dosage must be adjusted accordingly. In addition, the fluid-electrolyte imbalance must be corrected (*e.g.*, by sodium bicarbonate supplements and oral potassium).

The osteomyelitic lesion should be excised down to normal-appearing bone.[32] Additional bacteriologic studies should identify secondary invaders and the appropriate antibiotics. Amphotericin B may be infused directly through a catheter and removed by suction. A continuous infusion of 20 mg/day is given for several weeks. If the wound cannot be closed primarily, it may be skin grafted later.

Ketoconazole (Nizoral) is an imidazole compound similar in antifungal activity to amphotericin B, but it has the advantages of being orally administered and lacking nephrotoxicity. It requires acidity for dissolution and therefore should not be given concomitantly with antacids, anticholinergics, and H_2 blockers. In adults, the recommended starting dose of ketoconazole is a single 200-mg tablet daily; in serious infections, the dose may be increased to 400 mg once a day. The minimal course of treatment for systemic mycoses is 6 months.

In the disseminated type of disease, the outlook is poor. On the other hand, when a single focus exists, such as in a bone, cure is quite possible. Resection of the osseous lesion is often followed by complete bony replacement. Extensive involvement of a part may justify amputation.

MADUROMYCOSIS

Maduromycosis (madurellamycosis, Madura foot) is an uncommon mycotic infection involving bone and occurring in tropical and subtropical zones and in the southermost points of the United States, especially Texas. It is characterized by progressive local necrosis and abscess formation, intermittent discharge of a peculiar fluid through fistulous tracts, and replacement by granulation and fibrous tissue.[33,36,37,39,41]

ETIOLOGY

People between 20 and 40 years of age are affected. The mycelia are coarse and contain numerous round and oval bodies, the chlamydospores. They form grains or granules that vary in color but often are jet black. The mycelial threads are often arranged in clusters of radially arranged eosinophilic clubs. The mode of transmission is unknown, but patients usually are agricultural workers giving a history of suffering from thorn wound.

PATHOLOGY

Microscopically, the dark grains are composed of coarse, dark mycelial elements, pigments, and debris. A typical granulomatous reaction surrounds the abscess cavity (*i.e.*, granulation tissue, round cells, giant cells, and extensive scarring).

CLINICAL PICTURE

Maduromycosis predominantly affects the foot. The earliest stages of infection are rarely observed. The condition starts with multiple, hard, deep-seated and fixed papules or nodules that soften at their centers and form abscesses. The abscesses rupture and produce persistently draining fistulas. The progress of extension is very slow, the infection spreading and deeply involving tendons, muscle, and bone and spreading proximally toward the ankle and up the leg. Pain is minimal, and inflammatory signs are absent, so the individual continues walking and furthering destruction. The big toe is often affected first. Involvement of bone invariably occurs with gross destruction and disorganization of all bones of the foot. The foot becomes swollen, indurated, misshapen, and punctured with sinuses draining exudate containing varicolored granules but mainly black grains resembling caviar. Systemic reaction is absent, and the blood picture is normal. Infection and destruction are slowly progressive and persistent. The offending mycelia may be identified by culture and hanging-drop examination.

ROENTGENOGRAPHIC FINDINGS

Roentgenographic findings are extremely variable. The disease is most often observed at an advanced stage that exhibits extensive destruction of all bones of the foot (Fig. 10-10). Rarely, a single lesion may be seen in the tibia where the picture is identical with chronic osteomyelitis.

DIFFERENTIAL DIAGNOSIS

Leprosy, syphilis, tuberculosis, malignant neoplasm, and other mycotic infection must be ruled out.

TREATMENT

Early bone lesions heal readily under the influence of sulfonamides and antibiotics. Severe destructive lesions with draining sinuses require amputation.

SPOROTRICHOSIS

Sporotrichosis is a fungus infection producing granulomatous lesions usually involving skin and subcutaneous tissue; uncommonly, it is disseminated systemically, involving various tissues and viscera. When bone is infected, the slow destructive and exudative process resembles chronic osteomyelitis or tuberculosis.[30,34] The condition is being recognized with increasing frequency.

ETIOLOGY

The causative organism is *Sporotrichum schenckii*. It is almost never identified in secretions from the lesions or in biopsy material but is seen best in a suspension of a culture. It appears as tangled, filamentous threads with short side branches on which lie clusters of small oval

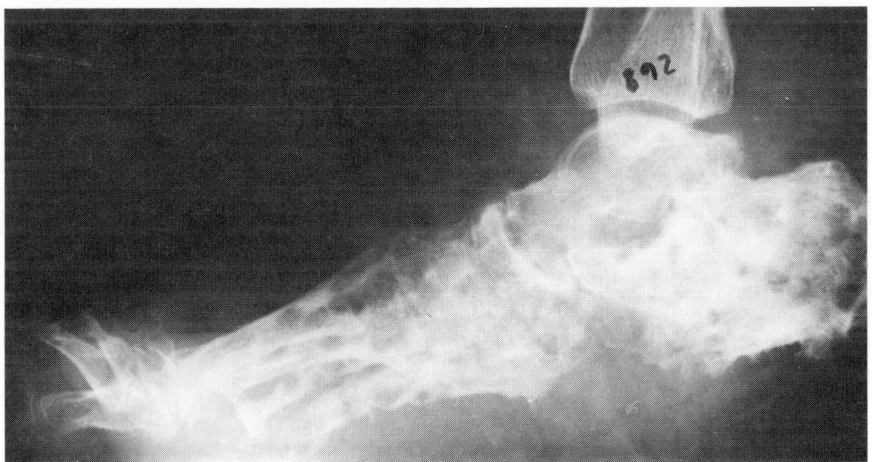

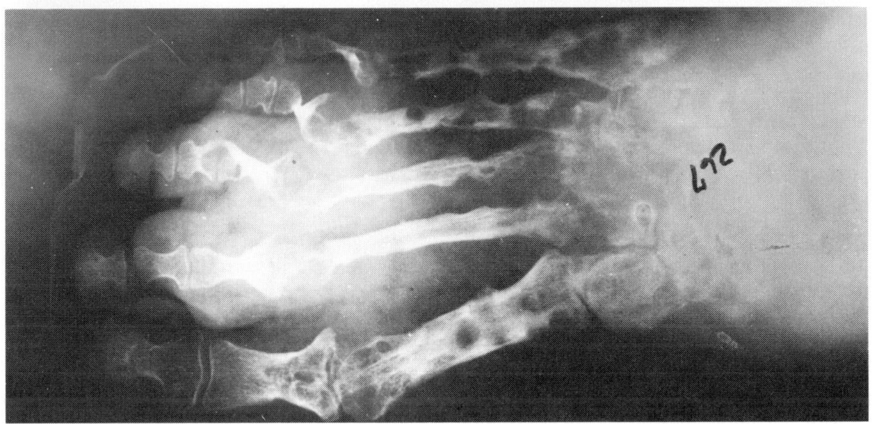

FIG. 10-10. Madura foot.

bodies called conidia. The fungus exists in nature as a saprophyte of plants, flowers, and trees, particularly in an environment of high humidity. Consequently, farmers, horticulturists, fruit pickers, and the like are favored victims of this occupational disease. The usual mode of infection is through a trivial wound in the skin (*e.g.*, a thorn prick), but the disease can be transmitted by an animal bite or by the handling of dressings of patients.

PATHOLOGY

The lesion is a granulomatous reaction with central area of necrosis surrounded by epithelioid cells, chronic inflammatory cells, and an occasional giant cell. Activity varies from destruction and exudation at one extreme to healing by resorption of exudate and fibrosis at the other. The granulomatous lesions in bones and joints are comparable with an extremely low-grade form of tuberculosis (Fig. 10-11.)

CLINICAL PICTURE

The initial lesion most often involves the upper extremity, usually the hand. A history is often elicited of a specific trauma (*e.g.*, pricking the finger on a rose thorn a number of days or weeks previously). At this site an indurated, nontender, freely movable nodule develops and is covered with reddened skin. Later, the color becomes violaceous, the nodule becomes adherent to the deep tissues and the skin and then softens and becomes fluctuant, and the overlying skin breaks down to form an indolent, granulomatous ulcer, which repeatedly bleeds and crusts and which heals very slowly over weeks to months. Within a few days to a week after appearance of the initial lesion, infection spreads through and thickens lymphatic channels in the forearm, and these are palpable as thick cords (see Fig. 10-11). Along a prominent cord, a chain of nodules characteristically forms, and these too break down, forming ulcers that discharge a watery exudate and persist for months or years. The general health is usually unaffected in this lymphatic form.

Uncommonly, systemic involvement occurs, with or without a recognizable antecedent lesion on the extremity. Granulomatous lesions can involve any tissue, supposedly by hematogenous spread, but pulmonary and central nervous system involvement are rare. Bone infection may appear as an osteomyelitis or periostitis, and synovial infection is not unusual. In addition to widely spread subcutaneous nodules, a generalized lymph gland

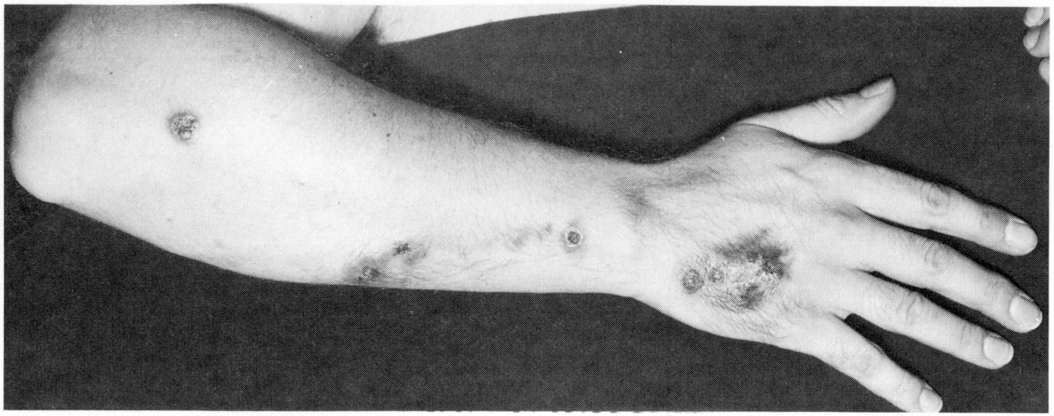

FIG. 10-11. Sporotrichosis. Shown are characteristics to be sought in identifying this cause of chronic granulomatous osteomyelitis, periostitis, or synovitis. (*Top*) Typical primary lesion on dorsum of hand with multiple nodular and ulcerative secondary lesions arranged in linear fashion along a thickened lymphatic cord. (*Center*) *Sporotrichum schenckii* from culture showing tangled filamentous threads with short side branches upon which lie clusters of piriform conidia. (*Bottom, left*) Tubercle formation. (*Bottom, right*) Infiltration of histiocytes and giant cells without necrosis. (Duran RJ, Coventry MB, Weed LA et al: Sporotrichosis. J Bone Joint Surg 39A:1330, 1957)

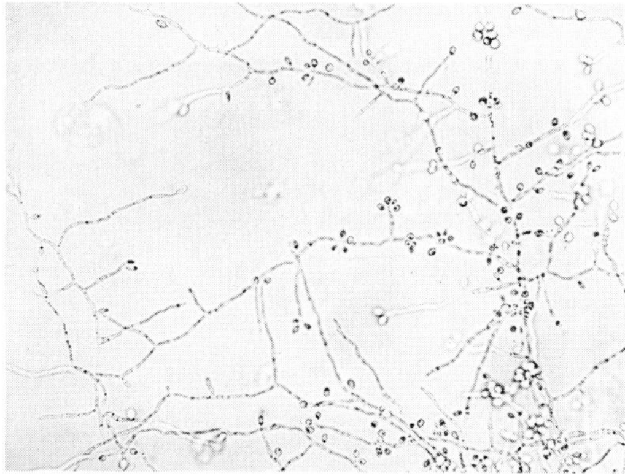

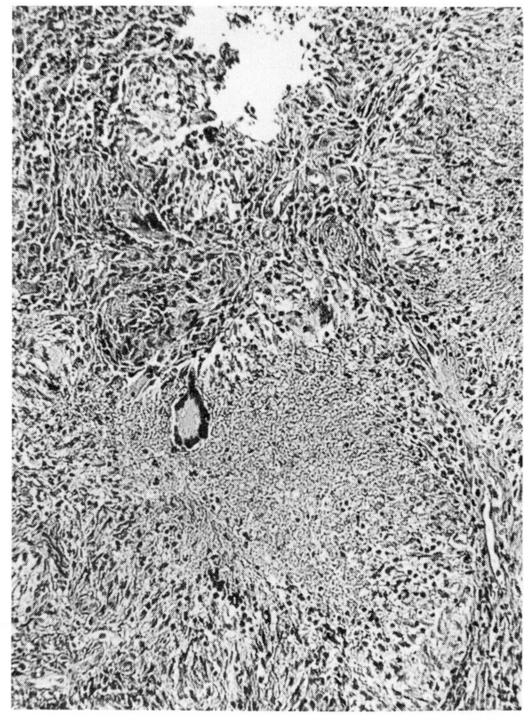

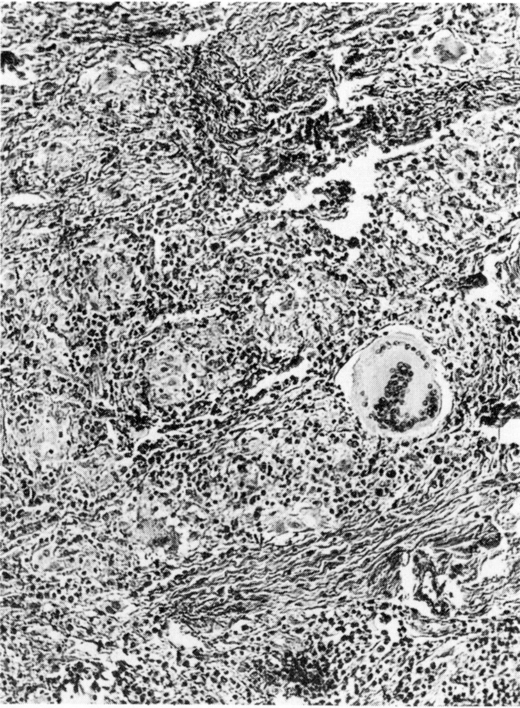

enlargement is often apparent. A low-grade fever and slight leukocytosis with eosinophilia are often associated. Systemic sporotrichosis is a chronic, progressive illness with a grave outlook.

DIAGNOSIS

The fungus cannot be identified in secretions or biopsy material. Instead, the biopsy tissue is ground up and cultured, and typical colonies are produced. A suspension of the growth reveals the fungus. Complement fixation tests, agglutination tests, and skin tests are not specific.

If an externally draining ulceration is found to communicate with subjacent infected and destroyed bone, secondary infection by bacterial contaminants makes this unsuitable for culture. Instead, a nodule or an enlarged lymph gland should be used.

Sporotrichosis must be differentiated from tuberculosis, syphilis, pyogenic infection, tularemia, coccidioidomycosis, blastomycosis, histoplasmosis, squamous cell epithelioma, and granulomas caused by drugs.

TREATMENT

Potassium iodide is the drug of choice, especially for the localized lymphatic form. The dosage is gradually increased up to 50 mg/day. The skin lesions readily heal, but treatment must be continued another 6 weeks to preclude recurrence.

For systemic sporotrichosis, 2-hydroxystilbamidine is given slowly intravenously in daily 225-mg doses. Dangerous toxic drug reactions are frequent.

The problems of handling bone and joint involvement are similar to those of tuberculosis.

SALMONELLA OSTEOMYELITIS

Salmonella organisms, which most commonly cause food poisoning, will rarely produce acute and chronic osteomyelitis. The genus *Salmonella*, of which more than 960 types are known, are gram-negative bacilli, possessing motility by means of flagella. Three kinds of infection are identified in humans: gastroenteritis, occasionally severe enough to be fatal; salmonella fever, similar to typhoid fever; and a septicemia characterized by multiple metastatic abscesses.

Salmonella infections are a relatively common complication of sickle cell anemia. Only three of the innumerable serotypes of *Salmonella* are usually found in association with sickle cell anemia: *Salmonella choleraesuis, Salmonella paratyphi B*, and *Salmonella typhimurium*. These serotypes are responsible for about two thirds of the cases of osteomyelitis associated with sickle cell anemia. Once *Salmonella* bacteremia develops in patients with sickle cell anemia, it is almost invariably associated with localization in bone.

Other hemoglobinopathies have been shown to be associated with *Salmonella* infections. In hemoglobinopathies, *Salmonella* exceeds by almost ten times other pyogenic organisms as the etiologic agent in osteomyelitis.

CLINICAL PICTURE

The clinical picture is similar to other types of acute osteomyelitis. Intestinal symptoms are usually absent. The acute infection shows a tendency to subside and persist as a chronic infection. The ends of the long bones and the lumbar spine are usually involved, but infections of small bones and sternoclavicular joints can occur.[43–45] An infective destructive process affecting several bones at the same time is characteristic.

DIAGNOSIS

The causative organisms may be cultured from the bloodstream, the lesion, and, rarely, the stool. The clinical picture of *Salmonella* osteomyelitis may closely resemble that of intraosseous sickling. Therefore, blood cultures should always be drawn during an acute sickling crisis.

Agglutination tests are diagnostic. The organism may be traced to, or isolated from, certain foods.

TREATMENT

The organism is susceptible to chloramphenicol (3 g–4 g/day in the adult). High doses of ampicillin or penicillin may be used.

A complete wound toilet is important. Pus and necrotic tissue are removed, and dependent drainage is established. Sinus tracts, scar tissue, and devitalized soft tissue and bone are excised. The wound may be closed tightly and continuous closed suction and irrigation instituted.

BRUCELLAR SPONDYLITIS

Osteomyelitis caused by the organisms of undulant fever peculiarly seem to favor the spine (see Chapter 30).

REFERENCES

Acute Osteomyelitis

1. Blockey NJ, McAllister TA: Antibiotics in acute osteomyelitis in children. J Bone Joint Surg 54B:299, 1972
2. Harris NH: Some problems in the diagnosis and treatment of acute osteomyelitis. J Bone Joint Surg 42B:535, 1960
3. Jensen K, Lassen HCA: Combined treatment with antibacterial chemotherapeutic agents in staphylococcal infections. Q J Med 38:91, 1969

4. Luck JV: Bone and Joint Diseases. Springfield, IL, Charles C Thomas, 1950
5. Waldvogel FA, Medoff G, Swartz MN: Osteomyelitis: A review of clinical features, therapeutic considerations and unusual aspects. N Engl J Med 282:198–206, 260–266, 316–322, 1970
6. Winter FE: The surgical treatment of pyogenic osteomyelitis. Clin Orthop 51:139, 1967.

Chronic Osteomyelitis

7. Compere EL, Metzger WI, Mitra RN: The treatment of pyogenic bone and joint infections by closed irrigation (circulation) with a non-toxic detergent and one or more antibiotics. J Bone Joint Surg 49A:614, 1967
8. Cunha BA et al: The penetration characteristics of cefazolin, cephalothin, and cephradine into bone in patients undergoing total hip replacement. J Bone Joint Surg 59A:856, 1977
9. Finegold SM et al: Antibiotic susceptibility patterns as aids in classification and characterization of gram-negative anaerobic bacilli. J Bacteriol 94:1443, 1967
10. Grace EJ, Bryson V: Topical use of concentrated penicillin in surface active solution. Arch Surg 50:219, 1945
11. Grace EJ, Bryson V: Chronic osteomyelitis in war wounded: A report of two veterans discharged with intractable osteomyelitis and successfully treated with local penicillin-detergent therapy. NY State J Med 47:2204, 1947
12. Hazlett JW: Treatment of osteomyelitic defect by cancellous bone grafts. J Bone Joint Surg 36B:584, 1954
13. Hodges PC, Phemister DB, Brunschwig A: Diseases of Bones and Joints. New York, Nelson, 1938
14. McElvenny RT: The use of closed circulation and suction in the treatment of chronically infected, acutely infected, and potentially infected wounds. Am J Orthop 3:86–87; 154–160, 1961
15. Nettles JL et al: Musculoskeletal infections due to *Bacteroides*. J Bone Joint Surg 51A:230, 1969
16. Smith CB et al: In-vitro activity of carbenicillin and results of treatment of infections due to *Pseudomonas*. J Infect Dis 122 (Suppl):514, 1970
17. Speed JS, Smith H: Miscellaneous affections of bone. In: Campbell's Operative Orthopedics, 2nd ed, p 1147. St. Louis, CV Mosby, 1949
18. Symposium, Proceedings, American Academy of Orthopaedic Surgeons. J Bone Joint Surg 51A:1022, 1969

Tuberculosis of Bones and Joints

19. Bosworth DM: Treatment of tuberculosis of bone and joint. Bull NY Acad Med 35:167, March 1959
20. Boyd W: Textbook of Pathology. Philadelphia, Lea & Febiger, 1953
21. Campos OP: Bone and joint tuberculosis: Treatment. J Bone Surg 37A:937, 1955
22. Evans ET: Tuberculosis of bones and joints: Reference to streptomycin and special surgical techniques. J Bone Joint Surg 34A:267, 1952
23. Ostman P: Combined surgical and chemotherapy of abscesses in bone and joint tuberculosis: Early results. Acta Orthop Scand 21:204, 1951
24. Stevenson, FH: The chemotherapy of orthopedic tuberculosis (the Robert Jones Prize Essay, 1952). J Bone Surg 36B:5, 1954
25. Wilkinson MC: Curettage of tuberculous vertebral disease in treatment of spinal caries. Proc R Soc Med 43:114, 1950
26. Wilkinson MC: Chemotherapy of tuberculosis of bones and joints. J Bone Joint Surg 36B:23, 1954

Mycotic Infections

27. Alfred KS, Harbin M: Blastomycosis of bone. J Bone Joint Surg 32A:887, 1950
28. Busey JF et al: Blastomycosis: A review of 198 cases. Am J Respir Dis 89:659, 1964
29. Cherniss EI, Waisbren BA: North American blastomycosis: A clinical study of 40 cases. Ann Intern Med 44:105, 1956
30. Conant NF, Smith DT, Baker RD et al: Manual of Clinical Mycology, 2nd ed, p 222. Philadelphia, WB Saunders, 1954
31. Conaty JP, Biddle M, McKeever FH: Osseous coccidioidal granuloma. J Bone Joint Surg 41A:1109, 1959
32. Cushard WG Jr, Kohanim M, Lantis LR: Blastomycosis of bone. J Bone Joint Surg 51A:704, 1969
33. Downing JG, Conant NF: Medical progress: Mycotic infections. N Engl J Med 233:153, 1945
34. Duran RJ, Coventry MB, Weed LA et al: Sporotrichosis. J Bone Joint Surg 39A:1330, 1957
35. Emmons CW, Binford CH, Utz JP: Medical Mycology. Philadelphia, Lea & Febiger, 1963
36. Gammel JA: Etiology of maduromycosis. Arch Dermatol Syph 15:241, 1927
37. Gammel JA: Correction. Arch Dermatol Syph 15:477, 1927
38. Hall, RH, Mendeloff J: Blastomycotic osteomyelitis. J Bone Joint Surg 34A:977, 1952
39. Kulowski J, Stovall S: Maduromycosis. JAMA 135:429, 1947
40. Sen BL et al: Pulmonary blastomycosis in eastern North Carolina. NC Med J 28:264, 1967
41. Thompson HL: Present status of mycetoma. Arch Surg 16:774, 1928
42. Witorsch P et al: The polypeptide antifungal agent (X-50790): Further studies in 39 patients. Am Rev Respir Dis 93:876, 1966

Salmonella Osteomyelitis

43. Hook EW: Salmonellosis: Certain factors influencing the interaction of *Salmonella* and the host. Bull NY Acad Med 37:499, 1961
44. Ralston EL: Osteomyelitis of the spine due to *Salmonella choleraesuis*. J Bone Joint Surg 37A:580, 1955
45. Widen AL, Cardon L: *Salmonella typhimurium* osteomyelitis with sickle-cell-hemoglobin C disease: A review and case report. Ann Intern Med 54:510, 1961

11

Congenital Deformities

Section I
Etiology

The actual cause of a deformity found at birth is theoretical. However, the two known factors are genetic and embryonic trauma.

GENETIC FACTOR

The genes in the chromosomes of the ovum and the sperm transmit the specific anomalous characteristic. Transmission follows Mendel's law. When the genetic factors are dominant, the anomaly will develop in a large number of offspring. When the factors are recessive, the anomaly occurs infrequently. For example, osteogenesis imperfecta follows a pattern similar to hemophilia in that the disease occurs almost exclusively in the male but is transmitted by the female, as a mendelian recessive.

FACTOR OF EMBRYONIC TRAUMA

Experimental and clinical evidence has shown that many things can injure the developing embryo. In the early weeks of differentiation of the embryonic tissues into specific tissues and component parts of the fetus, the embryo is most susceptible to extraneous factors. Each component part rapidly differentiates at a specific time when it is most sensitive to trauma. Also, each injurious factor seems to have an affinity for a particular area or tissue. Therefore, the type of deformity might be determined theoretically by the traumatic agent and the time at which it exerts its deleterious influence.

TERATOGENESIS

The experimental production of congenital anomalies is teratogenesis.[1] The following are known teratogenic factors:

Metabolic. Hypoglycemia is due to various disorders, including hyperinsulinism.

Hormonal. When hormones, particularly adrenal corticosteroids or adrenocorticotropic hormone (ACTH), are administered, whether to experimental animals or to humans, during the early embryonic stages, congenital anomalies may develop. Clubfoot deformity is common following such treatment during pregnancy.

Nutritional deficiency. Lack of riboflavin in particular is a factor of nutritional deficiency. It is interesting to note that experimental production of deformities by insulin can be largely prevented by injecting nicotinamide and riboflavin at the same time as the insulin.

Chemical. Lead nitrate, for example, can induce hydrocephalus, meningoencephaloceles, and meningomyeloceles in chick embryos.

X-radiation. A cleft palate can be produced experimentally.

Infection. The frequent association of cataracts and cardiac septal defects with maternal intercurrent infection of rubella during the early months of pregnancy strongly suggests the cause and the effect.

Mechanical. Injury by direct mechanical trauma to the embryo in the early weeks of pregnancy must be considered in the light of experimental evidence. For example, "rumplessness" can be produced in chickens by shaking of the eggs.

Thermal. The earliest postconceptional phase is the most susceptible time in experimental animals.

Anoxia. Anencephaly, spina bifida, and other defects produced in laboratory animals suggest an important clinical application in pregnancy maternal hypoxia of anemia.

Maternal Rh isoimmunization. Antigens present in the blood of the fetus (inherited from the father), though lacking in the mother's blood, produce maternal Rh isoimmunization, which may interfere with normal fetal development and result in extensive abnormalities of the central nervous system. the following are the features: severe mental deficiency; asymmetrical hypertonicity and weakness of the extremities, the neck, and the back; and choreoathetosis. In almost all cases it is possible to obtain a neonatal history compatible with erythroblastosis fetalis and an Rh setup in the mother and the child compatible with the diagnosis.[2]

Duraiswami, after his classic experiments in experimental production of skeletal defects, made the following summarizing hypothesis:

> The development of an embryo, which is presumably guided by a series of organizing processes, may be interfered with during critical periods by genetic or environmental teratogenic factors. Such disturbances caused to the organizer system may, in their turn, produce metabolic, biochemical, and other changes through the intervention of hormones and enzyme systems and thus interfere with the normal development of the embryo. The resulting abnormalities in development would not occur in a random assortment, but tend to fall into certain categories corresponding to the critical stages of development of susceptible tissues and the quality and intensity of the noxious agent. Developmental malformations may result not only from arrest of growth and differentiation of the embryo as a whole, or some of its parts, but also from degeneration in tissues which had developed normally up to a certain stage, as has clearly been demonstrated in the case of insulin-induced deformities and rubella-induced lenticular lesions. It is possible to demarcate in the life of the human embryo certain critical periods which are peculiarly associated with catastrophic changes in the development of the skeleton. The fourth and fifth weeks of intrauterine life are definitely associated with the development of the cartilage skeleton. The seventh and ninth weeks present widespread calcification of the cartilage of the long bones as the main feature. The last two weeks of fetal life are marked by the rapid growth in length of the long bones, as distinct from the increase in size of the epiphyses. The orderly progression from the mesenchymatous condensation to cartilage, and then through calcified cartilage to bone may be disturbed by genetic or environmental teratogenic factors and a variety of skeletal deformities result.[1]

The following sections describe conditions more commonly seen and treated in orthopaedic practice.

CONGENITAL SKELETAL LIMB DEFICIENCIES

Congenital anomalies characterized by absence of skeletal components are of two types: the so-called true amputation (limb-bud arrest) and the gross limb abnormality. To properly analyze these anomalies, it is essential to review the early development of the limbs in the human embryo.

The upper and lower limbs appear first as small buds of tissue on the lateral body wall at 4 postovulatory weeks. These buds grow and differentiate rapidly in the ensuing 3 weeks, and the various regions of the limbs develop in a proximodistal sequence. The arm and forearm, for example, appear before the hand, and the thigh and leg appear before the foot.

The skeletal elements of the limbs are found first as condensations of mesenchyme within the limb buds. These condensations soon chondrify in a definite order, and ossification follows. Initial bone formation is found in the clavicle at 5 postovulatory weeks, in the humerus, radius, ulna, distal phalanges of the hand, femur, and tibia at 7 postovulatory weeks, and in the scapula and fibula at 7 weeks.

Endochondral ossification in the shaft of a bone occurs generally from 1 to 5 weeks after initial bone-collar formation has taken place. By 7 weeks, all the skeletal elements of the limbs (with the exception of the clavicle, which has a different mode of development) are present as cartilaginous models, some of which have collars of bone in their shafts. By 7 weeks, the skeleton is a replica in miniature of that in postnatal life.

Anomalies in which the number of skeletal elements are increased (*e.g.*, polydactylia) must arise during the first 7 weeks of embryonic life. Further, failure of a skeletal element to develop during this time results in a decrease of skeletal parts (*e.g.*, radial hemimelia).

The classification of congenital skeletal limb deficiencies proposed by Frantz and O'Rahilly is presented in Table 11-1.[3] The defects are either terminal (T), where there are no unaffected parts distal to, and in a line with, the deficient portion or intercalary (I), where the middle portion of a proximodistal series of limb components is deficient but the proximal and distal portions are present. Each of these two main groups may be either transverse,

TABLE 11-1 Classification of Congenital Skeletal Limb Deficiencies

Terminal (T)	
TRANSVERSE (−)	LONGITUDINAL (/)
1. *Amelia* (absence of limb)	1. *Complete paraxial hemimelia* (complete absence of one of the forearm or leg elements and of the corresponding portion of the hand or foot)—R, U, TI, or FI*
2. *Hemimelia* (absence of forearm and hand or leg and foot)	2. *Incomplete paraxial hemimelia* (similar to above but part of defective element is present)—r, u, ti, or fi*
3. *Partial hemimelia* (part of forearm or leg is present)	3. *Partial adactylia* (absence of one to four digits and their metacarpals or metatarsals): 1, 2, 3, 4, or 5
4. *Acheiria or apodia* (absence of hand or foot)	4. *Partial aphalangia* (absence of one or more phalanges from one to four digits): 1, 2, 3, 4, or 5
5. *Complete adactylia* (absence of all five digits and their metacarpals or metatarsals)	
6. *Complete aphalangia* (absence of one or more phalanges from all five digits)	
Intercalary (I)	
TRANSVERSE (−)	LONGITUDINAL (/)
1. *Complete phocomelia* (hand or foot attached directly to trunk)	1. *Complete paraxial hemimelia* (similar to corresponding terminal defect but hand or foot is more or less complete)—R, U, TI, or FI*
2. *Proximal phocomelia* (hand and forearm, or foot and leg, attached directly to trunk)	2. *Incomplete paraxial hemimelia* (similar to corresponding terminal defect but hand or foot is more or less complete)—r, u, ti, or fi*
3. *Distal phocomelia* (hand or foot attached directly to arm or thigh)	3. *Partial adactylia* (absence of all or part of a metacarpal or metatarsal): 1 or 5
	4. *Partial aphalangia* (absence of proximal or middle phalanx or both from one or more digits): 1, 2, 3, 4, or 5

A line below a numeral denotes upper-limb involvement, for example, T-$\underline{2}$ represents terminal transverse hemimelia of the upper limb. A line above a numeral denotes lower-limb involvement, for example, I-$\overline{1}$ represents intercalary transverse complete phocomelia of the lower limb.

* In capital letters when the paraxial hemimelia is complete, in small letters when the defect is incomplete.

(*1, 2, 3, 4,* or *5,* digital ray involved; *FI* or *fi,* fibular; *R* or *r,* radial; *TI* or *ti,* tibial; *U* or *u,* ulnar)

(Frantz CH, O'Rahilly R: Congenital skeletal limb deficiencies. J Bone Joint Surg 43A:1202, 1961)

denoted by a hyphen (-), where the defect extends transversely across the entire width of the limb, or longitudinal, denoted by a vertical line (/), where only the preaxial or postaxial portion is absent and hence the deficiency is longitudinal (Fig. 11-1).

Section II
Upper Extremity

CONGENITAL HIGH SCAPULA

Congenital high scapula (Sprengel's deformity, undescended scapula, elevated scapula) consists of a permanent elevation of the shoulder girdle.

ETIOLOGY

Like other congenital deformities, the unknown causative factor is operative during early embryonic life, but most particularly at the time of development of the cervical spine and the upper limb buds and the subsequent descent of the latter. This explains the frequent association of deformities of the occiput and the base of the skull, the cervical and the upper thoracic spine, and the ribs and the surrounding muscle tissues. Before the third month, the mesenchymal tissues take form as the cervical spine and, at the same level, the upper limb buds. The limb buds then descend to the level of the thorax. The failure of descent results in a permanently high shoulder girdle and imperfect development of the surrounding tissues, described as incomplete segmentation and the failure of fusion of bony elements.

PATHOLOGY

The scapula is smaller in its vertical diameter and appears broad. The suprascapular portion arches forward where it fits over the superior thoracic cage in its elevated position. Looking at it from the posterior aspect, it is rotated counterclockwise so that its inferior angle is approximated to the spine. The enveloping muscles

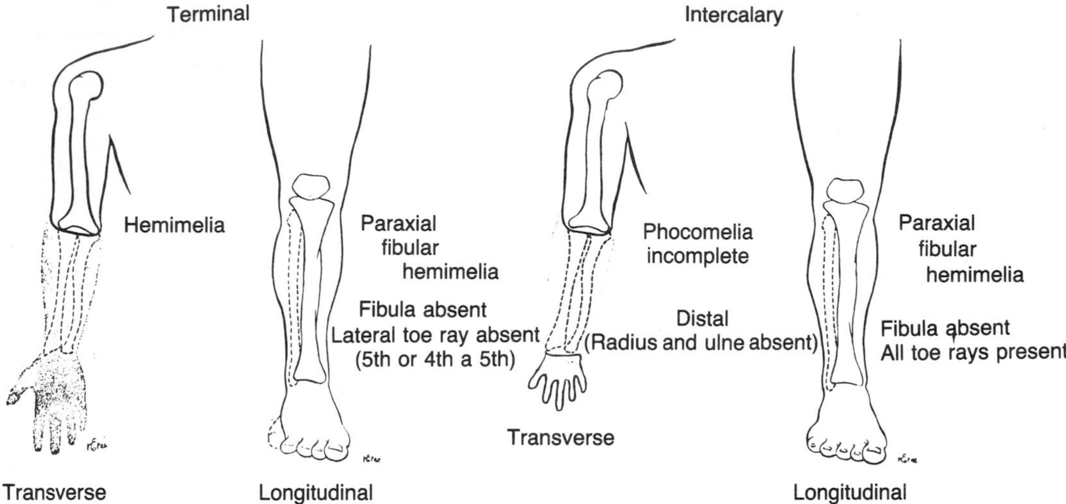

FIG. 11-1. Diagrams illustrate the typical congenital skeletal limb deficiencies and their nomenclature. (Frantz CH, O'Rahilly R: Congenital skeletal limb deficiencies. J Bone Joint Surg 43A:1202, 1961)

(supraspinatus, infraspinatus, subscapularis) and those that attach to the scapular spine and the vertebral border (trapezius, levator scapulae, rhomboids, serratus anterior) are composed of normal muscle tissue, or imperfectly developed muscle fibers having the appearance of myoblasts, or wholly of fibrous tissue. From the superior angle, a sheet or bandlike structure composed of fibrous tissue, cartilage, or bone extends upward to attach to the transverse processes of several cervical vertebrae. Occasionally, it reaches the base of the occiput of the skull. This structure probably represents the levator scapulae. Associated errors in segmentation are represented by wedged and fused cervical and thoracic vertebrae, hemivertebrae, and fused ribs, all of which are responsible for the frequently associated scoliosis. Congenital failure of fusion is displayed by the spina bifida in the cervical spine and the separation of the occipital bones extending upward from the foramen magnum.

CLINICAL PICTURE

As viewed from the rear, the shoulder and the scapula are higher than on the opposite side (Fig. 11-2). When the condition is bilateral, the upward displacement of both shoulders gives the neck a shortened appearance (Fig. 11-3). The scapula is rotated counterclockwise, the inferior angle displacing toward the spine. At the upper angle of the scapula, the band that extends up toward the cervical spine or even the base of the skull may be apparent as an elevated ridge. On attempted abduction of the arm, the lower angle of the scapula does not rotate outward as it should in normal scapulohumeral rhythm. The amount of restriction of shoulder movement is variable and generally proportionate to the pathologic replacement of periscapular muscle tissue and the presence of the superior restricting band. Very often the range of motion and strength is surprisingly excellent. Cervicothoracic scoliosis and torticollis are frequently associated features. Pain is absent.

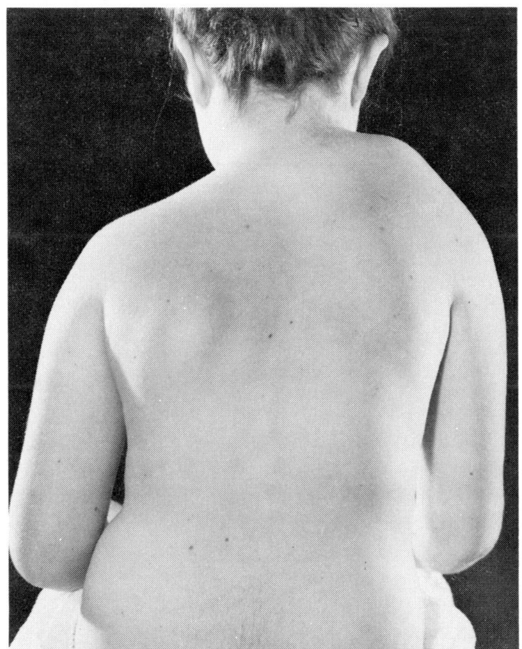

FIG. 11-2. Sprengel's deformity, or congenital elevation of the scapula.

TREATMENT

Treatment is undertaken for cosmetic reasons only. There is no other justification for undergoing the extensive surgery necessary for correction. When function at the

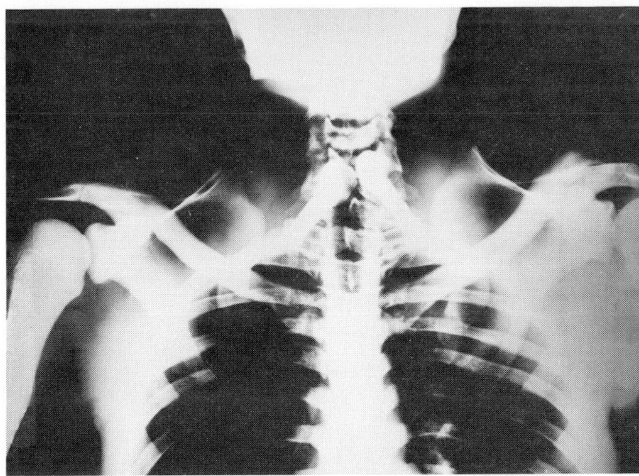
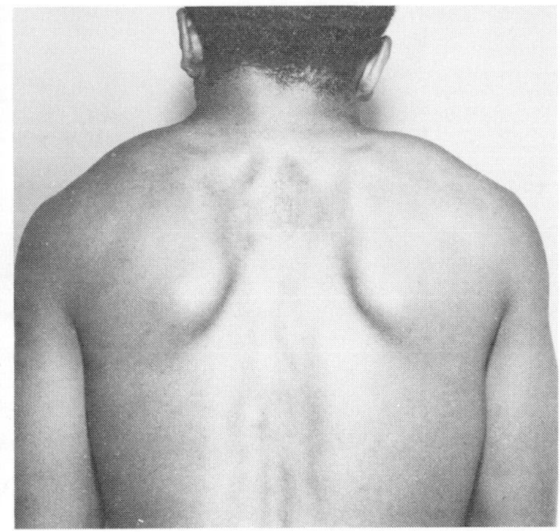

FIG. 11-3. Bilateral undescended scapulae. The roentgenogram reveals persistence of the embryonic connection with the cervical spine, the omovertebral bone, on each side. Clinically, the omovertebral bones form prominences extending from the cervical spine to the superior angle of the scapulae. (U.S. Army photograph. Blair JD, Wells PO: Bilateral undescended scapula associated with omovertebral bone. J Bone Joint Surg 39A:201, 1957)

shoulder is restricted, restoration of position to the scapula does not improve function. Correction should be undertaken in childhood. The downward displacement may cause traction on the brachial plexus, and the nerve trunks may be compressed by lowering the clavicle, which thereby narrows the costoclavicular space.

A longitudinal incision is made along the vertebral border of the scapula. The attachments of the muscles to the vertebral edge are incised. The rhomboids are reflected toward the spine, the supraspinatus and the infraspinatus are elevated laterally, the trapezius is cut from its attachment to the spine of the scapula, the subscapularis is freed from the undersurface, the serratus magnus is removed from the medial border, and the fibrous or chondrous or osseous band is cut from the upper angle and removed. In exposing the band, the posterior scapular artery should be sought and ligated. The suprascapular nerve and artery are identified and protected at the suprascapular notch. The completely denuded scapula is now freed for displacement except for the clavicle, which prevents descent. A Z-plastic osteotomy of the clavicle permits lengthening of the bone and downward movement.

An alternative is removal of the outer end of the clavicle, including the conoid and the trapezoid ligaments, which attach to the coracoid process of the scapula. A wire suture is inserted through two drill holes in the scapula and directed downward to emerge through the skin distally. This wire will be fixed to a body spica cast under tension to maintain the lower position of the scapula. A number of muscle fibers may be freed from the erector spinae from below and attached to the inferior angle; supposedly, this aids in maintaining the new position. Fixation of the lower angle to a rib is not recommended, since this may restrict scapular motion. The wire is removed when the clavicle has united.

CLEIDOCRANIAL DYSOSTOSIS

Cleidocranial dysostosis is a congenital developmental condition in which membranous bones fail to ossify sufficiently, particularly in the calvarium and the clavicles, where fibrous tissue replaces the bone.[4,5] Characteristically, the pubic bone also participates in the pathologic process, but the replacing tissue gives rigidity and strength to the pelvis which therefore does not feel deficient to the examining finger. Muscle deficiencies occur at the shoulder.

CLINICAL PICTURE

Clinically, the characteristics are as follows:

The slender build, large head with small shrunken face, long neck, drooping shoulders, and narrow chest are typical.

The skull shows well-marked bosses over the frontal, the parietal, and the occipital areas. A median groove separates the frontal prominences. The anterior fontanelle is large and may never close completely. A mild degree of hydrocephalus may be present. The maxilla is small, and the relatively large mandible may appear prognathous. Delayed or deficient dentition is common.

Clavicles may have a defect at the inner, middle, or outer third or may be altogether devoid of bone. The remaining bone segment, particularly at the outer third, may compress the underlying nerves of the brachial plexus. The shoulders droop and can be approximated voluntarily (Fig. 11-4). The bone defect is usually bilateral. Absence of the clavicular portion of the trapezius and the anterior fibers of

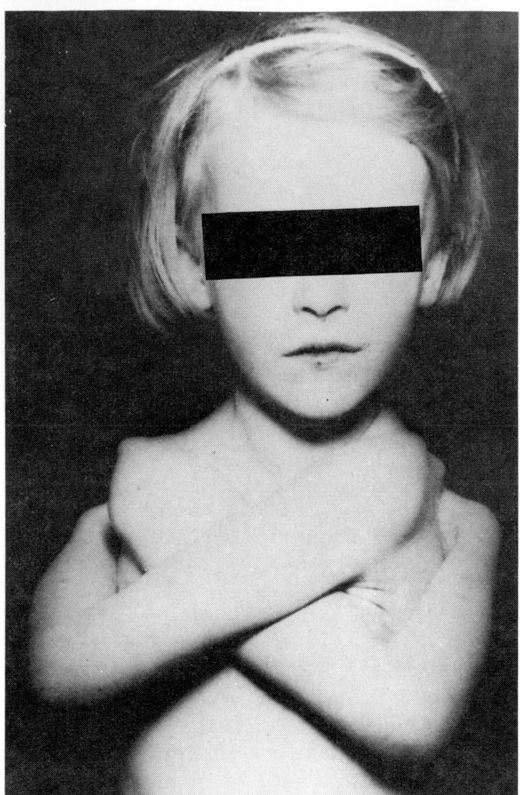

FIG. 11-4. Cleidocranial dysostosis.

the deltoid may occur occasionally. However, impairment of shoulder function is unusual. The scapulae may be small, deformed, and winged.

Widespread spina bifida occulta is common.

Deficient ossification of the pubic bones causes no clinical impairment.

ROENTGENOGRAPHIC FINDINGS

Roentgenographic findings include the following:

- Membranous calvarium imperfectly ossified (Fig. 11-5)
- Base of skull normally ossified
- Sutures that often fail to close normally
- Anterior fontanelle large, may never close
- Wormian bones in occipital and posterior parietal regions

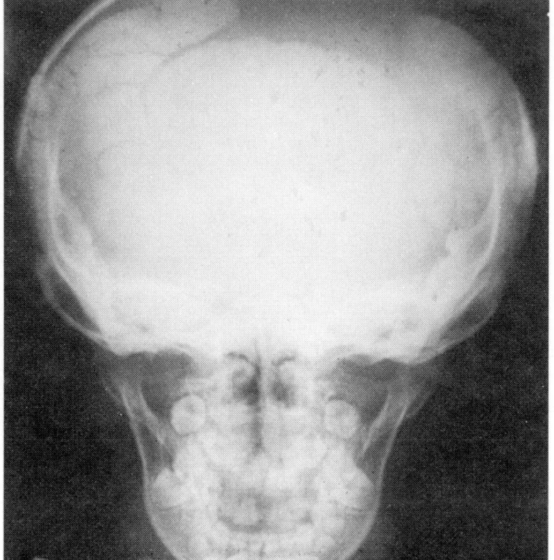

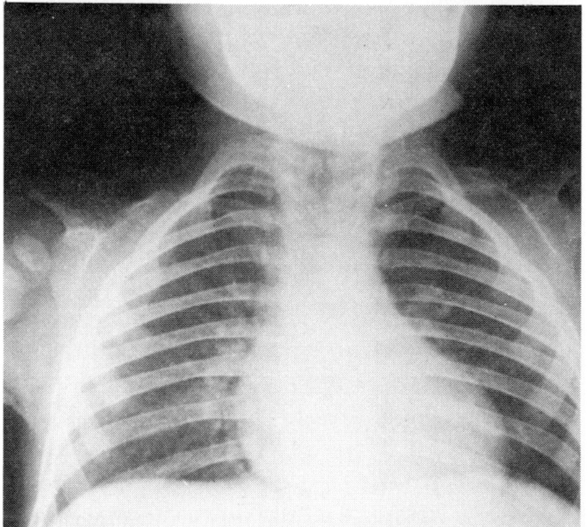

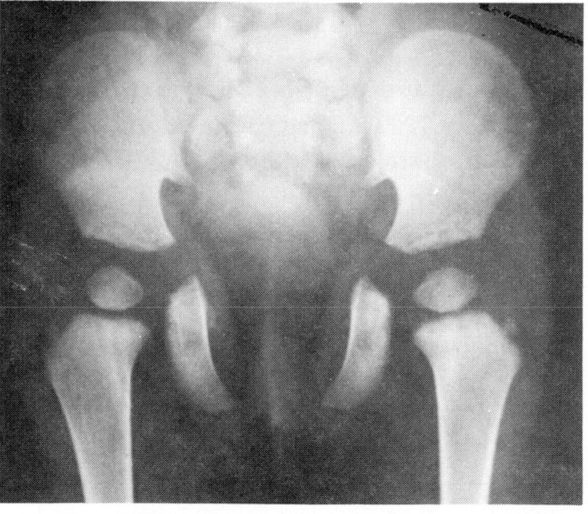

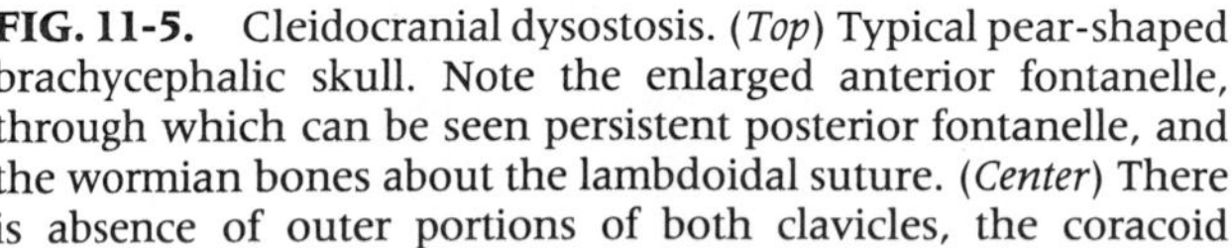

FIG. 11-5. Cleidocranial dysostosis. (*Top*) Typical pear-shaped brachycephalic skull. Note the enlarged anterior fontanelle, through which can be seen persistent posterior fontanelle, and the wormian bones about the lambdoidal suture. (*Center*) There is absence of outer portions of both clavicles, the coracoid processes, and the supraspinous fossae of both scapulae. (*Bottom*) Note the wide separation of symphysis and acetabulum and the irregular ossification of the capital femoral epiphyses and acetabula. (Eisen D: Cleidocranial dysostosis. Radiology 61:21, 1953)

Maxilla hypoplastic; mandible of normal size
Partial or complete defect of clavicles
Bilateral deficient ossification of pubic bones
Congenital coxa vara frequently associated
Failure of fusion of neural arches common
Epiphyses found at both ends of metacarpals and metatarsals

TREATMENT

No treatment is necessary, since no disability is present. These patients live normal, useful lives and have a normal life expectancy.

CONGENITAL ANOMALIES OF THE HAND

The accepted etiologic theories are those of maldevelopment or mutations that are subsequently inherited.[6] A mutation is defined as a permanent transmissible change in the character of an offspring from that of his parents.

SYNDACTYLISM

Syndactylism is defined as joined fingers (Fig. 11-6). It is the most common deformity of the hand and is most frequent between the middle and ring fingers and between the second and third toes It is often associated with polydactylism. Occasionally, hypodactylism and deficiencies of the long bones are accompanying anomalies. Experimentally, a diet deficient in riboflavin produces shortened or absent bones and syndactylism. The degree of syndactylism varies from two otherwise normal fingers being joined by skin (webbing) to the similar webbing between all the fingers (mitten hand). The webbing may be shallow or involve the entire length of the digits. The extreme degree involves fusing between the bones and joining of tendons and nerves. Therefore, it is essential that adequate preoperative roentgenographic study be made and careful deliberate dissection at surgery be enforced.

Treatment. Treatment is surgical. The skin of the web is rarely sufficient for covering defects when the fingers are separated. A free full-thickness graft is usually necessary. The generally accepted surgical procedures follow:

Flap operation (Didot procedure). At the area corresponding to the web, a triangular flap of skin with the base proximal is cut. It is routed through an opening cut on the volar aspect and is sutured to the palmar skin. The tunnel is kept open during healing by a wax stent or a glass rod. Later, an incision is made longitudinally over the dorsal aspect of one finger and the volar aspect of the other, and the flaps are brought over to cover the defects. Rarely are the flaps of sufficient length, and the resulting scar-tissue formation jeopardizes any future surgery.

Free full-thickness graft. This procedure is the most successful. The web is split, and a free graft, including skin to cover the commissure, is placed. A pressure bandage and splint are applied. If more than two fingers are involved, only one side of a finger is operated on at a time to avoid bilateral compression of the finger, which might compromise the circulation. If only one common tendon is found, it is detached from the less developed finger and left attached to the better developed one. Later a tendon may be transferred.

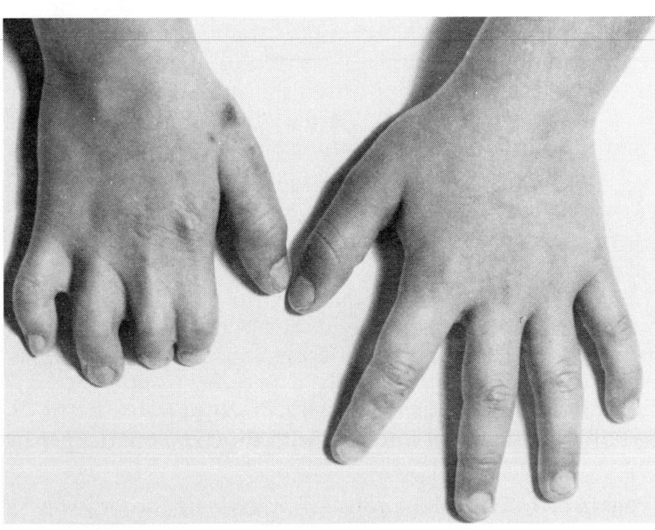

FIG. 11-6. Syndactylism. The skin bridge between the index and middle fingers is complete and that between the other fingers is incomplete.

SYMPHALANGISM

Symphalangism is fusion of interphalangeal joints, usually the middle with the proximal or distal phalanx. It occasionally accompanies syndactylism. Treatment is by arthrodesing in the functional position of partial flexion. However, if the symphalangism involves only the proximal joint and the distal one is moved by an adequately functioning profundus tendon, arthroplasty may be attempted.

POLYDACTYLISM

Reduplication of fingers varies from a completely developed finger to the doubling of a single phalanx. There is a tendency for the accessory digit to be located on the radial or ulnar margin of the hand. The types of polydactylism include an extra fleshy mass that is not adherent to the skeleton and is devoid of bones, cartilage, or tendons; duplication of a digit that is composed of normal components and articulates with an enlarged or bifid metacarpal; and a digit with its own metacarpal, which is rare.

Treatment. Treatment consists in removal. One must ascertain whether the remaining digits have functioning tendons, because it may be necessary to transfer the tendon of the accessory digit, for example, to the thumb. Reduplication of the distal phalanx is most common in the thumb (bifid thumb). If one segment is well developed, the other may be removed. Usually, it is better to excise a central wedge from each tip and join the remaining segments (Bilhaut-Cloquet operation).

BRACHYDACTYLISM

Shortening of the fingers as a result of decreased length or number of phalanges or shortened metacarpals is a hereditary condition transmitted as a simple mendelian dominant. Frequently, it is associated with webbed fingers or polydactylism. The fingers may have good profundus tendons and function well. On the other hand, the tendon is absent, and the distal joint is flail or is a fused nonfunctioning joint. A flail distal joint should be fused to improve the function of pinch and grasp.

ANNULAR GROOVES AND CONGENITAL AMPUTATIONS

Congenital constricting bands vary from a shallow groove in the skin or the subcutaneous tissue in one finger to a deep groove almost to the bone with a small distal segment of finger attached by a pedicle. Usually, it is associated with syndactylism and brachydactylism. The shallow ring does not interfere with function, but deeper rings cause distal edema.

Treatment. Treatment consists in excising the grooves down to normal structures, approximating the subcutaneous tissue, and closing the skin by a Z-plasty to avoid a constricting annular scar. Only one half the circumference of the finger should be operated on at a time. Complete congenital amputation of fingers or hand is regarded as the extreme degree of congenital constricting ring.

CLEFT HAND OR LOBSTER-CLAW HAND

Cleft hand is extremely rare. A defect exists in the central portion of the hand. A V-shaped cleft tapering proximally may divide the hand into two parts, each part consisting of webbed fingers; the middle finger and the metacarpal are missing, and no true thumb is present. Grasping is accomplished by approximating the claws. In another type, the middle finger is absent but the metacarpal is present and the cleft is shallow. The third type consists of a radial digit or thumb and an ulnar digit, the other fingers and the metacarpals being absent.

Treatment. In attempting to treat this condition, one should remember that any procedure that eliminates the cleft probably will reduce the function. The ability to grasp is accomplished by approximating the claws over an object held in the cleft. On the other hand, deepening a shallow cleft will improve function. When one considers amputation for unsightliness, the factor of excellent function of the lobster-claw hand as compared with the artificial hand should countermand the procedure.

THUMB-CLUTCHED HAND

Thumb-clutched hand, a rare deformity, has been described as congenital absence of the extensor pollicis longus, pollex varus, congenital clasped thumb, and flexion-adduction deformity of the hand.[7,8] It is a result of developmental deficiency of the extensor mechanism of the thumb so that only rudimentary musculotendinous structures exist. Sometimes the anomalous development is associated with similar involvement of adjacent digits or with clubfoot. No familial incidence has been noted.

The condition must be differentiated from spastic thumb-clutched deformity of cerebral palsy, which is due to spasticity of the adductor pollicis. The latter condition discloses diminution of deformity by passively flexing the wrist and intact thumb extensors evidenced by electromyographic studies.

Arthrogryposis multiplex must also be ruled out. This condition involves multiple joints and severe crippling deformities resistant to treatment.

Treatment. At first the volar contractures which have been secondarily developed must be released by adductor tenotomy, full-thickness skin grafts, Z-plasty, splinting, and exercise. Satisfactory passive extension may require several years and must be accomplished before tendon transfer is attempted. Arthrodesis of the metacarpophalangeal joint may be necessary. Superficial flexor tendons are appropriate for transfer and are passed about the radial aspect of the wrist and fastened to the extensor hood over the proximal phalanx of the thumb. At the same time, a similar procedure may be used for other digits if involved.

MEGALODACTYLISM OR MACRODACTYLISM

True congenital hypertrophy of the digits or hand is rare. The second or the third finger is usually involved. If unsightly, and particularly if unnecessary to hand function, it may be amputated. More frequently an enlarged finger is due to a local process, such as a neurofibroma, an angioma, and another type of tumor, which when removed improves appearance.

CONGENITAL ABSENCE OF THE RADIUS

The common congenital anomaly of absence of the radius is usually associated with a clubhand that is deviated radially (Fig. 11-7). The bone may be completely absent, or a portion, usually at its upper end, may remain. The hand lacking the support of the radius at the wrist deviates radially until it lies at right angles to the long axis of the forearm. The ulna gradually bows in following the hand with the concavity on the radial side. It is usually short and thickened. The radial carpal bones are absent or fused. A contracture exists on the radial side of the forearm in the form of muscles that are shortened, fibrotic, fused to each other, or absent. These muscles are the brachioradialis and the muscles to the radial side of the wrist, the thumb, and the index finger.

Treatment. The contracture must be released. In mild deformity, this can be accomplished by stretching and splinting. In the severe type, surgical release is necessary. The tendons are lengthened or, when their absolute lack of function can be determined, are severed. The fascia is cut transversely; the deformity is not straightened immediately for fear of cutting off the circulation through the radial artery. Gradual stretching and splinting secure the correction, if necessary by an osteotomy of the ulna. Finally, the wrist is arthrodesed in the position of function.

CONGENITAL RADIOULNAR SYNOSTOSIS

The term *primary radioulnar synostosis* is applied to the congenital condition, in contrast to the *secondary* or

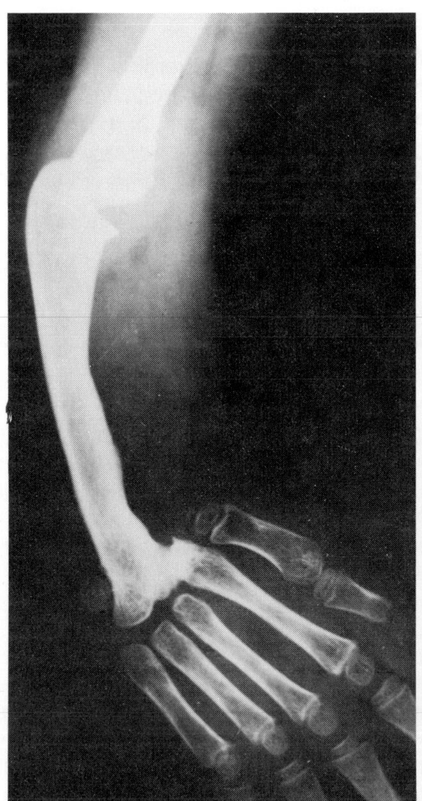
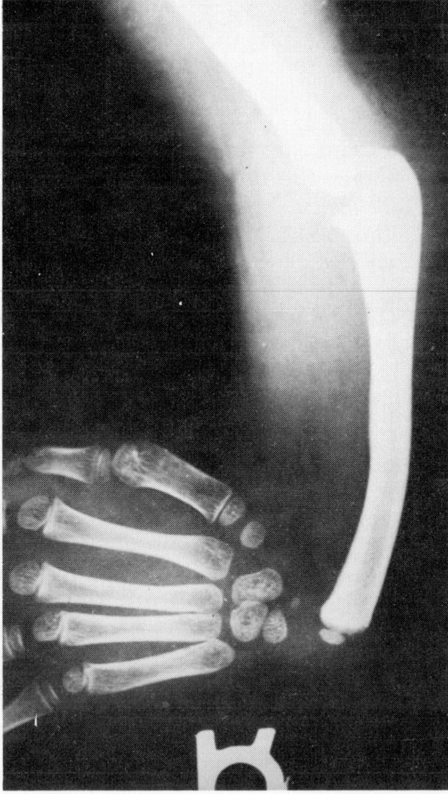

FIG. 11-7. Congenital absence of the radius. The deformity was corrected by ulnarmetacarpal arthrodesis. (Courtesy of D. Miller)

traumatic type. Primary synostosis is usually bilateral and at the upper third of the forearm, although the junction can occur anywhere. The marrow cavity of the synostosis may be continuous with that of both bones. The upper end of the radius may or may not be perfectly formed, and anterior or posterior dislocation at the elbow is not unusual. The supinator brevis is absent and may be replaced by bone. Other muscles concerned with rotation of the forearm, such as the pronator teres and the quadratus, are imperfectly formed or absent. The shaft of the radius crosses over the ulna in close relationship to the latter so that a fixed pronation of the forearm and a tightened, narrow interosseous membrane result.

TREATMENT

Treatment is limited to osteotomy to place the forearm in the midposition for better function. Attempts to overcome the synostosis and give rotatory function to the forearm are doomed to failure because of lack of properly functioning muscles. Freeing of the radius requires extensive surgery, which is not justified by results. Briefly, the procedures that have been attempted are the following:

- Resecting the synostosis
- Resecting the head of the radius, covering the stump with fascia lata
- Looping of fascia lata about the shaft of the radius and attaching to a drill hole in the ulna to keep the radius from displacing
- Severing the interosseous membrane along much of its length
- Osteotomizing the radius and rotating to midsupination or full supination
- Transferring tendon to the radius to effect active supination

CONGENITAL HUMERORADIAL SYNOSTOSIS

Like radioulnar synostosis, this is an error in segmentation in embryonic life. Therefore, very commonly it is associated with other synostoses throughout the forearm and the hand. When a joint is nonexistent, the muscles that would ordinarily move that joint are absent or imperfect. Therefore, it is unwise to attempt an arthroplasty unless adequate muscle for transfer is available. In this condition, if the arm-forearm angle is nonfunctional, the position should be corrected by an osteotomy. The lack of epiphyses at the lower humerus and the upper radius may cause some reduction in longitudinal growth, whereas the ulna would continue at its normal rate, resulting in a bowing deformity. This can be corrected by osteotomy. Fortunately, most of the longitudinal growth in the upper extremity takes place at the upper humerus and the lower radius and ulna so that eventual length is not reduced seriously.

Section III *Lower Extremity*

CONGENITAL DISLOCATION OF THE HIP

If displacement of the femoral head from its normal position within the acetabulum is found at birth, it is regarded as a congenital dislocation of the hip. This must be distinguished from dislocations due to trauma, paralysis, or infection occurring after birth.

ETIOLOGY

The actual cause is unknown. The hereditary factor is pronounced, and involvement of several members of one family is not unusual. Females are more commonly affected, by a ratio of 9:1. The condition is prevalent in Mediterranean countries, notably Italy, where whole clinics may be devoted to the care of such cases.

PATHOLOGIC ANATOMY

Anatomical studies of the human fetus have demonstrated that at 10 weeks the femoral head, the acetabulum, and the capsule are well developed and proportionate as in the adult.[16] The pathology develops before the tenth week in the anlage of the hip. At birth, the acetabulum and the femoral head are entirely cartilaginous; the anteroinferior acetabulum is shallow, and the cartilage is thin; the labrum glenoidale and the acetabular rim are well developed; anteversion of the femoral neck is 20° to 40°; inclination of the femoral neck is 110° to 120°; and extension at the hip is limited to 160°, the range of motion improving when the child starts walking. Deviations from this basic picture are associated with displacement of the femoral head.

The femoral head may be partially displaced upward (subluxated) or completely dislocated out of the acetabulum (Fig. 11-8). The clinical picture and the treatment as well as the pathology vary with the two situations.

SUBLUXATION

The acetabular fossa is shallow and small, and the roof or superior portion is oblique, even vertical, offering no resistance to the upward glide of the head by muscle pull or weight bearing. The superior acetabular pole is grooved and irregular due to constant friction, and at

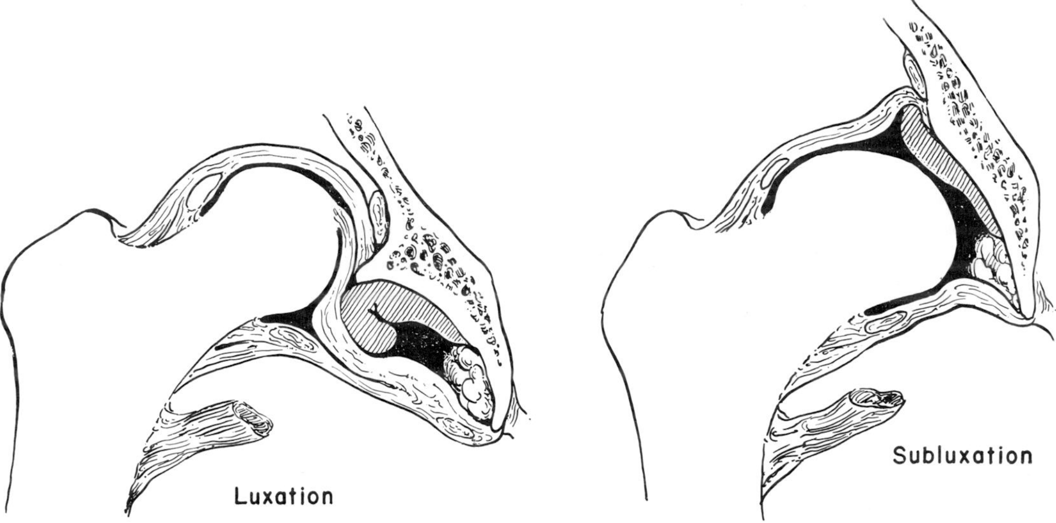

FIG. 11-8. (*Left*) Luxation or complete dislocation. The acetabulum is well formed, and the head is of normal size and contour. Note that the hypertrophied labrum, ligamentum teres, and haversian gland obstruct replacement. (*Right*) Subluxation or incomplete dislocation. The head is enlarged and oblique, the acetabulum is shallow, and the roof is inadequate. The labrum and haversian gland are thin.

this point the labrum and the reflected tendon of the rectus femoris are pushed against the ilium and attenuated. The acetabular fossa assumes an oval or triangular shape. In comparison with the small size of the cavity, the femoral head is enlarged and cannot be adapted to the inadequate socket. The capsule is thickened, and its cavity is enlarged to accommodate the movement of its contents. The ligamentum teres may be elongated, hypertrophied, degenerate, attenuated, or absent. The anteversion of the femoral neck may be increased. The inferior and central portion of the acetabular fossa may be filled with fibrofatty tissue. The picture suggests atrophy of the socket due to lack of normal pressure by the head of the femur. When the head is replaced, especially early while the structures are mainly cartilaginous, the cavity will re-form.

COMPLETE DISLOCATION

The femoral head is completely displaced out of the acetabulum and comes to rest against the lateral wall of the ilium (Fig. 11-9). Howorth states that most commonly it lies anteriorly adjacent to the anterior-inferior iliac spine and secondarily comes to lie in the posterior area near the sciatic foramen. The pressure of the head against the ilium causes the former to be somewhat flattened posteriorly and the femoral neck to increase its anteversion. The capsule is greatly hypertrophied and increased in extent, and frequently this laxity of the capsule has been blamed for the dislocation. However, it is well known that a joint capsule will stretch from abnormal pressures within it and conversely will contract adaptively

FIG. 11-9. Complete dislocation of the hip. (*Top*) The anteroposterior view demonstrates an apparently foreshortened neck which is in reality a forward-pointing bone. The acetabulum is somewhat inadequate. (*Bottom*) The anteversion is readily demonstrable in the lateral view.

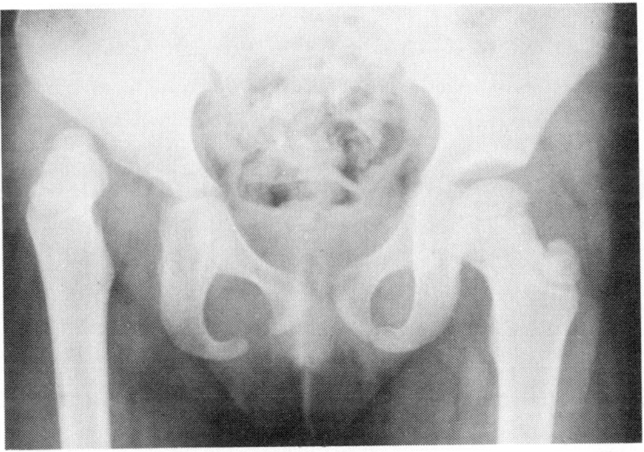

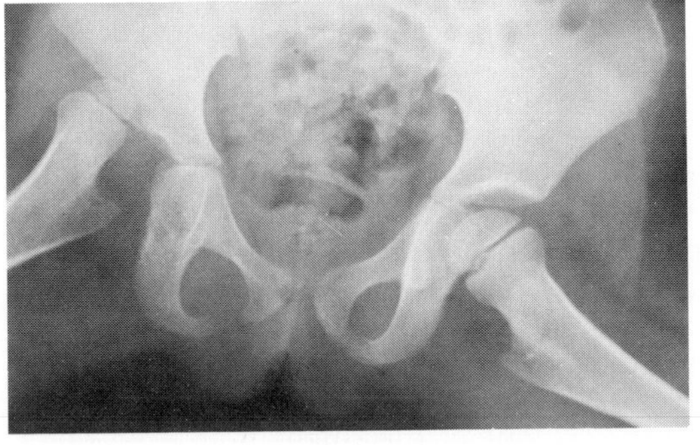

when intracapsular pressures are absent. As the capsule is pulled upward, it drags up the transverse ligament, and both capsule and ligament become adherent to the floor of the fossa and obstruct replacement. The femoral head pushes the capsule above the superior acetabular lip, and the capsule becomes adherent to the ilium. Pressure of the head against the ilium at the supra-acetabular area causes the capsule and the periosteum to differentiate into a fibrocartilaginous tissue lining a depression in the bone, thus forming a secondary socket or false acetabulum. Below this, the reflected rectus tendon and the labrum glenoidale obstruct replacement. The ligamentum teres may be elongated and markedly hypertrophied and in itself may interfere with reduction. However, it may also be attenuated or absent. The haversian gland and a thick labrum glenoidale fill the socket, which, however, is deep and well developed. The iliopsoas tendon crosses the capsule and gives the latter an hourglass appearance. The muscles that originate on the pelvis and insert distally as well as the fascia lata are adaptively shortened and prevent distal replacement of the femur.

CLINICAL PICTURE

The normal infant displays symmetrical folds in the groins, below the buttocks, and several along the thighs. In hip subluxation and dislocation these folds are asymmetrical. As the infant lies on the examining table, the pelvis and the limb on the affected side are pulled proximally by muscle action as though the ipsilateral abdominal and spinal muscles were overactive, as well as the hip adductors. Indeed, this factor should be considered in the etiology. The proximal displacement of the limb causes an apparent shortening, which is never as pronounced by actual measurement, except in actual dislocation.

In the subluxated hip, when applying traction or testing abduction, a palpable or audible click is discernible as the head slips back and forth over the acetabular rim, and abduction is limited (Ortolani's sign). When the hips of the normal infant are flexed to 90° and the thighs are abducted, the latter will nearly reach the table. In subluxation or dislocation, the abduction is restricted.

In a complete dislocation, the findings are more prominent. The femoral head may be palpable below the anterior-superior iliac spine or posteriorly at the sciatic notch. The shortening of the extremity is definite by actual measurement. The limb can be displaced by pushing and pulling, the femoral head being palpated as it moves to and fro. This is known as telescoping. The trochanter is prominent on the affected side.

When both hips are involved, the prominent trochanters give a widened appearance to the pelvis, and the lateral displacement of the thighs from each other causes a widened perineum. The child is late in walking.

In unilateral dislocation, the typical gluteus medius gait is apparent. Because the femoral head floats freely, the gluteus medius has lost its fulcrum and cannot perform its function of elevating the opposite side of the pelvis as the opposite extremity is lifted off the ground. Compensation is obtained by swaying the body toward the affected side so that the center of gravity is thrust over the femur. This gait is found also in other conditions with gluteus medius deficiency (*e.g.*, poliomyelitis). When both hips are dislocated, the swaying from side to side produces the characteristic "duck-waddle" gait. The Trendelenburg sign tests the efficiency of the gluteus medius. Normally, when the lower extremity is lifted from the ground, the pelvis on that side rises owing to contraction of the contralateral gluteus medius. If the pelvis sags downward, the sign is positive and the muscle is regarded as inadequate. Looking at the patient from the side, the lumbar spine is extremely lordotic, and the abdomen is protuberant as the pelvis tilts forward when a bilateral dislocation exists and the femoral heads lie posteriorly. When the dislocations are anterior, the converse is true (*i.e.*, the pelvis is horizontal, and the lumbar spine is flattened). A unilateral dislocation can be demonstrated by the Allis sign. With the infant lying on his back, the knees are flexed and the feet are resting on the table. The knee of the affected limb will lie at a lower level (Fig. 11-10).

Normally, walking starts at 11 or 12 months. In this condition, however, walking is late. Older children will complain of pain, weakness, and fatigability. Occasionally, the condition surprisingly occasions little complaint. In cases of subluxation, osteoarthritic symptoms eventually appear. Therefore, it is extremely important to recognize the earliest signs, particularly limitation of hip joint abduction (due particularly to contracture of adductor muscles), asymmetry of thigh folds, and slight or apparent shortening. Roentgenographic studies are invaluable in concluding the diagnosis.[14]

FIG. 11-10. The Allis or Galeazzi sign. The knee is lower on the dislocated side.

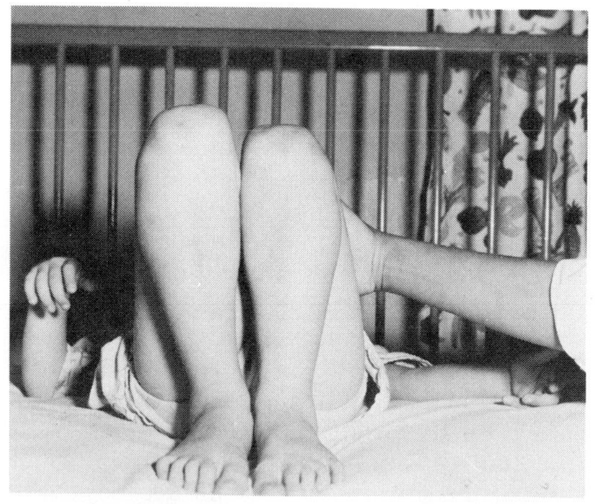

ROENTGENOGRAPHIC FINDINGS

At birth, the acetabulum and the upper femoral epiphysis are cartilaginous and therefore not visualized in roentgenograms. Complete dislocations are easily detected, but displacement of the femoral head outward and upward to a minimal degree, constituting a subluxation, is more difficult to recognize. Yet it is most important to diagnose a subluxation at this early date, for it is then that replacement results in an excellent anatomical and functional result.

With the newborn supine and both lower extremities held parallel, an anteroposterior view of the hips is taken while traction is exerted on the suspected limb. The procedure is repeated while the extremity is pushed proximally. This "push-pull" film may demonstrate instability of the femoral head. Slight displacements may be detected by the following procedure. A transverse line is drawn on the film through the clear area of acetabulum, which represents the triradiate cartilage. From this a perpendicular is erected that passes through the edge of the acetabular roof. Four quadrants are formed where the two lines cross. By following the ossified femoral neck upward, the approximate location of the cartilaginous head is ascertained. This head should lie in the inferomedial quadrant. Displacement into the outer inferior quadrant constitutes subluxation, and a position in the outer upper quadrant reveals a frank dislocation. The following characteristic findings are shown in Figure 11-11:

- The femoral head is in the upper outer quadrant.
- The neck appears foreshortened (in reality it is anteverted).
- The acetabulofemoral space is widened.
- The underborder of the femoral neck lies above Shenton's line, whereas normally it is continuous with the upper border of the obturator foramen.
- The acetabulum is shallow.
- The acetabular roof is oblique, almost vertical.

Ossification of the femoral head is delayed on the abnormal side. Next, the infant's hips are flexed, the thighs are abducted (frog position), and the next exposure made. This reveals the lateral view of the femoral neck, which normally forms an angle of 20° to 40° with the shaft. The angulation forward may be increased to as much as 90°, an excessive amount of anteversion. The neck may be shorter than on the opposite side.

In children, the head is ossified and so the findings are more definite. The widening of the joint space, the change of position in push-pull films, the obliquity of the roof, change in contour of the head, and anteversion are easily ascertained.

The following sections pertain to refinements in roentgenographic diagnosis that are not absolutely necessary to diagnosis.

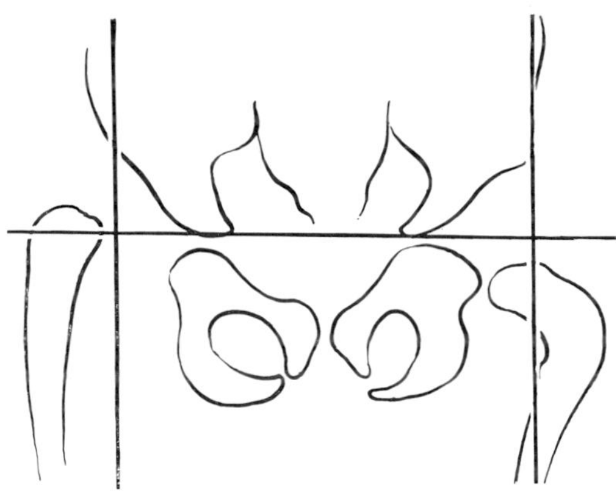

FIG. 11-11. Identification of dislocation before femoral head ossification. The approximate position of the head is above and medial to the ossified neck. A transverse line is drawn through the top of both triradiate cartilages. This intersects a line dropped from the edge of the acetabular roof, forming four quadrants. Normally, the head lies in the lower inner quadrant. The displaced head lies in either of the outer quadrants.

ARTHROGRAPHY

A radiopaque solution such as 17.5% Diodrast or 30% Tenebryl is injected into the joint. The needle is usually inserted anteriorly at a point below Poupart's ligament and lateral to the femoral artery. Information is obtained (*e.g.*, the contour and the position of the cartilaginous head, the depth of the acetabulum, and the extent and constriction of the capsule). The procedure seems to be superfluous inasmuch as failure to obtain reduction by a closed method leads to operative exposure at which time all pathology can be observed and dealt with. The radiopaque solution is completely absorbed within the hour.

CE ANGLE OF WIBERG

The CE angle of Wiberg is used after the age of 3 to 4 years, when the femoral head is fully ossified and its relationship to the acetabulum is fully established.[26] By this method, the femoral head-acetabular relationship can be expressed by a single figure.

In Figure 11-12, note: Since the normal head subtends a perfect circle, the central point of the circle denotes the center of rotation of the head, which maintains a constant relationship with any point on the acetabulum, irrespective of the position of the femoral head. The edge of the superior acetabular roof is designated E. The angle formed by a line passing through E and the center of the femoral head and intersecting a vertical line (B) dropped from the edge of the roof is the CE angle. The average CE angle is 36°, the normal range varying from 20° to 46°. The center of rotation of the head lies at a

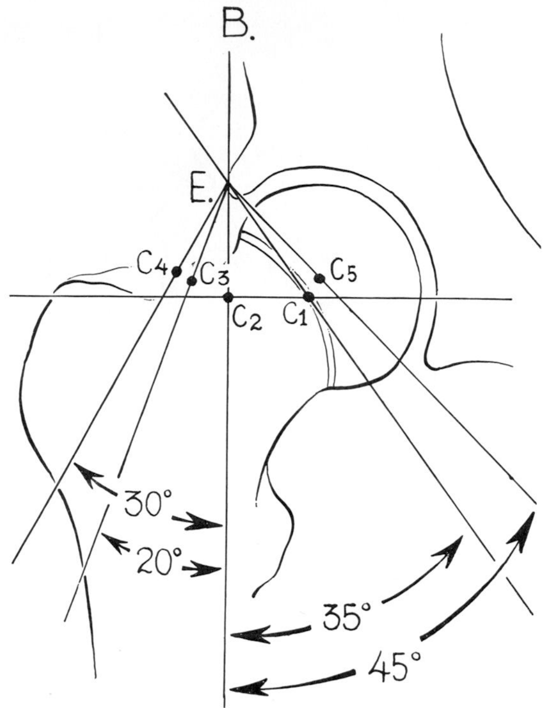

FIG. 11-12. The CE angle of Wiberg. Variations in the CE angle are seen when the center of rotation of the head is altered.

point equidistant from the two poles of the epiphyseal line and just proximal to the metaphyseal border (C1). The displacement of this center of rotation causes the following variations in the CE angle:

C1: normal
C2, C3, C4: varying degrees of subluxation
C2: coxa magna
C5: coxa plana (center displaced inward)

ACETABULAR INDEX

A horizontal line is drawn through the triradiate cartilage. Another is drawn along the roof of the acetabulum and intersects the horizontal line, forming an angle, the acetabular index. This indicates the obliquity of the roof. The normal in the newborn is 27.5°, and in children at 2 years of age it is 20°. As the angle approaches 30°, instability of the head becomes manifest.

DETERMINATION OF THE AMOUNT OF ANTEVERSION OF THE FEMORAL NECK

Generally, it is necessary only to rotate the femur internally during closed or open reduction until the head is firmly fixed within the socket and the full extent of the femoral neck is revealed in outline (Fig. 11-13).[13] The amount of internal rotation of the extremity denotes the degree of anteversion and the necessary derotation when corrective osteotomy is done. To determine the amount of anterior torsion accurately, the patient is placed supine on the x-ray table, and his hip is flexed 90°. The thigh is abducted 10°, and the x-ray tube is directed over the hip so that the central ray is perpendicular to the plane of the film. A radiopaque bar is placed lateral to the greater trochanter at right angles to the transcondylar axis or frontal plane of the femur. The lateral roentgenogram of the hip thus obtained will exhibit this bar as a reference line that is at right angles to the shaft. A line is drawn through the central axis of the neck of the femur and is projected to meet the shadow of the reference bar. At this point a perpendicular line is erected to the reference line. The amount of torsion is the angle formed by this perpendicular line and the line of the central axis of the neck. The normal amount of anteversion is 30° in the infant, which is gradually reduced to 8° in the adult. In congenital dislocation of the hip, the anteversion may increase to 85° or more.

TREATMENT

CONSERVATIVE

As is true of other congenital deformities, the earlier treatment is instituted, the more likely is a successful result to be realized. Within the first few months, redevelopment of the acetabulum is the normal response of pressure of the femoral head within it. The parts are still mainly cartilaginous and plastic and are easily molded by restoring normal anatomical and physiological conditions.

FIG. 11-13. Anteversion of the femoral neck. (*Left*) The limb is in neutral rotation. The neck points forward and appears foreshortened. The epiphyseal ossification center appears small and rounded. The lesser trochanter is prominent. (*Right*) The extremity is rotated internally. The neck in full profile is longer. The ossification center is ovoid and larger. The lesser trochanter is rotated backward and is barely visible.

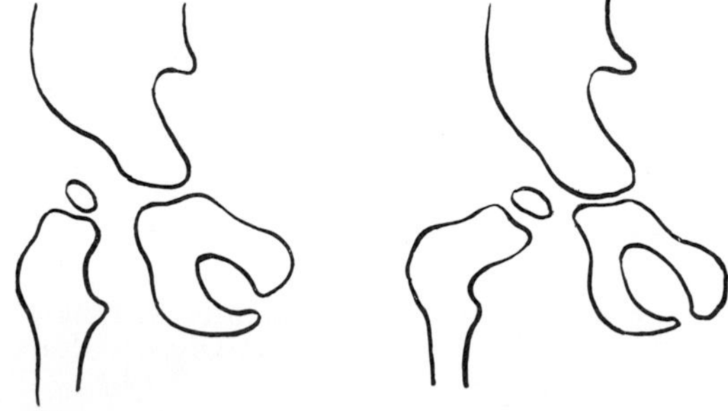

Basic Principles

Normal acetabular development depends on a normally placed femoral head. The usual presenting situation at birth is a dysplastic acetabulum that is shallow and is more vertical than normal, with the roof deficient anteriorly and laterally, permitting the femoral head to slip out of its socket when the hip is extended and adducted. The dysplasia becomes worse and the femoral head and neck become progressively misshapen as long as the abnormal acetabular-femoral head relationship is permitted to exist. Conversely, restoration of the femoral head to its normal position will reverse the process, and the earlier this is accomplished the more normal will be the final result. Normal or nearly normal hips will result if the hip dislocation is reduced in infancy when the acetabular dysplasia is not severe.[19] If the dysplastic undislocated hip is left untreated, it may develop normally, but a few persist into adult life as subluxations, or subluxation may eventuate as a complete dislocation during early childhood.

The reduction should be gentle, and the joint should not be positioned under strain. Continuous forcible compression of the articular surfaces must be avoided to prevent ischemic necrosis of the femoral head and irreparable damage to the articular cartilage. Tight adductors should be released by subcutaneous tenotomy. After reduction, full extension and adduction at the hip will encourage the head to slip out at the shallow anterior and lateral edge of the acetabulum, so the flexed and abducted position is mandatory. Further, maintaining the hip in internal rotation for prolonged periods will increase the degree of anteversion of the femoral neck, so only the least amount of internal rotation necessary to secure stable reduction is permissible.[21] The most desirable initial position is that of Lorenz: 90° to 100° flexion and 70° abduction. This position appears to reduce the tendency toward anteversion and may eliminate the need for derotation osteotomy.

Closed reduction of high dislocation, especially if delayed, requires observance of the principles of preliminary traction, routine subcutaneous adductor tenotomy at the time of reduction, and avoiding abducting the thighs too much, for only in this manner can one reduce the incidence of ischemic necrosis of the femoral head. This sequela develops more commonly in children treated from 8 to 20 months of age and is rare when treatment is initiated before the age of 4 months. The first roentgenographic evidence of this condition is irregular fragmented ossification of the femoral head. Although a normal head may yet develop, more often a flattened femoral head will result.

By forcing the femoral head into an extreme position of abduction and internal rotation even for a short period, the femoral head may be deprived of its blood supply and ischemic necrosis may ensue.[15] In the newborn, both the lateral and the medial circumflex femoral artery supply the developing femoral head (Fig. 11-14). At about 5 or 6 months of age, as the femoral head develops and elongates, the epiphyseal contribution from the lateral circumflex artery regresses, and the principal source of blood is from the medial circumflex femoral artery, which sends ascending vessels along the posterior aspect of the neck and then sends a prominent vessel through the notch between the greater trochanter and the head and enters the lateral aspect of the head as the lateral epiphyseal artery.

When the hip of an infant over 5 months of age is placed into maximal abduction, the superior acetabular rim may impinge against the notch between the greater trochanter and the epiphysis. If, in addition, the hip is rotated inward, the medial circumflex femoral artery may be compressed between the iliopsoas and pectineus muscles as it passes backward after its origin from the femoral or profunda femoral. In this site, the medial circumflex is especially vulnerable when these muscles are contracted.[17]

Arteriographic studies on infant cadavers demonstrate that arterial blood flow is reduced by marked abduction and internal rotation and is increased by adductor tenotomy. Consequently, the incidence of avascular necrosis can be substantially reduced (to less than 5%) by avoiding the extremes of abduction and internal rotation, particularly if preceded by traction and adductor tenotomy. The tissues about the hip must be loose to permit gentle, nonforceful reduction.

The Human Position

The preferred position for immobilization is more than 90° of flexion and 30° to 60° of abduction, because this results in the lowest incidence of avascular necrosis.[21a]

During the First Year

Most commonly, only a moderate incomplete displacement or subluxation is found. Merely abducting the limb causes the femoral head to descend toward the center of the acetabulum, where pressure forces cause the socket to deepen and a roof to form. Whether the condition is unilateral or bilateral, both hips are maintained in abduction continuously for a number of months. This can be accomplished by various devices that maintain flexion and abduction (Fig. 11-15). Only when roentgenograms demonstrate that the femoral epiphysis lies well within the acetabulum in the inferomedial quadrant and an adequate roof has formed can the splinting be discontinued. This may require anywhere from 3 months to a year.

When a complete dislocation is present, it is usual to find an acetabulum of adequate depth. Reduction is accomplished as follows: The infant is recumbent on the table, and an assistant holds the pelvis and the opposite extremity firmly fixed. The dislocated hip is flexed to relax the capsule and adducted to relieve the pull of the

(Text continues on page 300.)

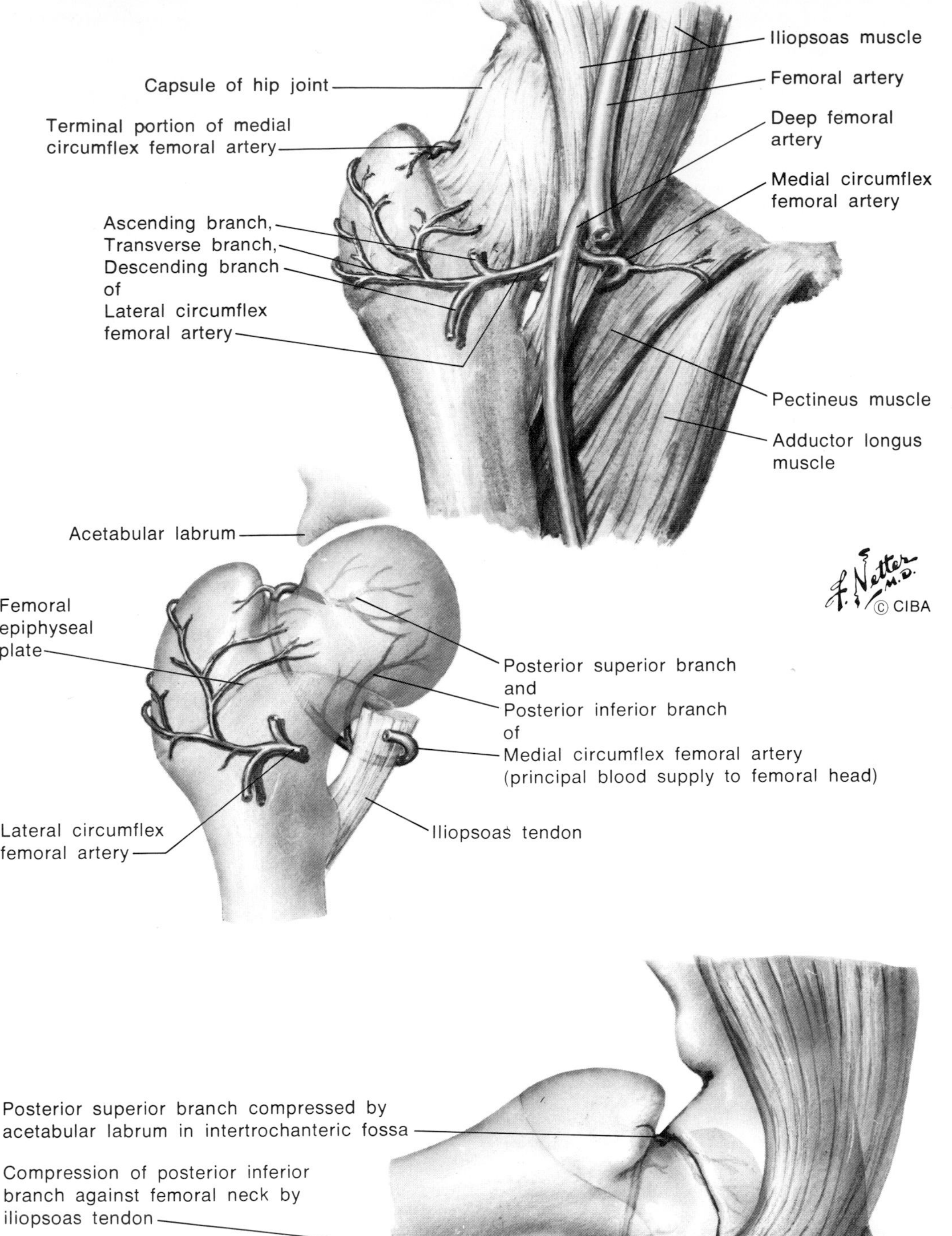

FIG. 11-14. Blood supply to the femoral head in infancy (after Ogden). (*Top*) Extracapsular course of medial and lateral circumflex femoral arteries. (*Center*) Distribution of medial and lateral circumflex arteries to the head and neck of femur. (*Bottom*) Compression of medial circumflex femoral artery in extreme abduction, internal rotation, and flexion. (Hensinger RN: Congenital dislocation of the hip. Ciba Clin Symp 31:3, 1979)

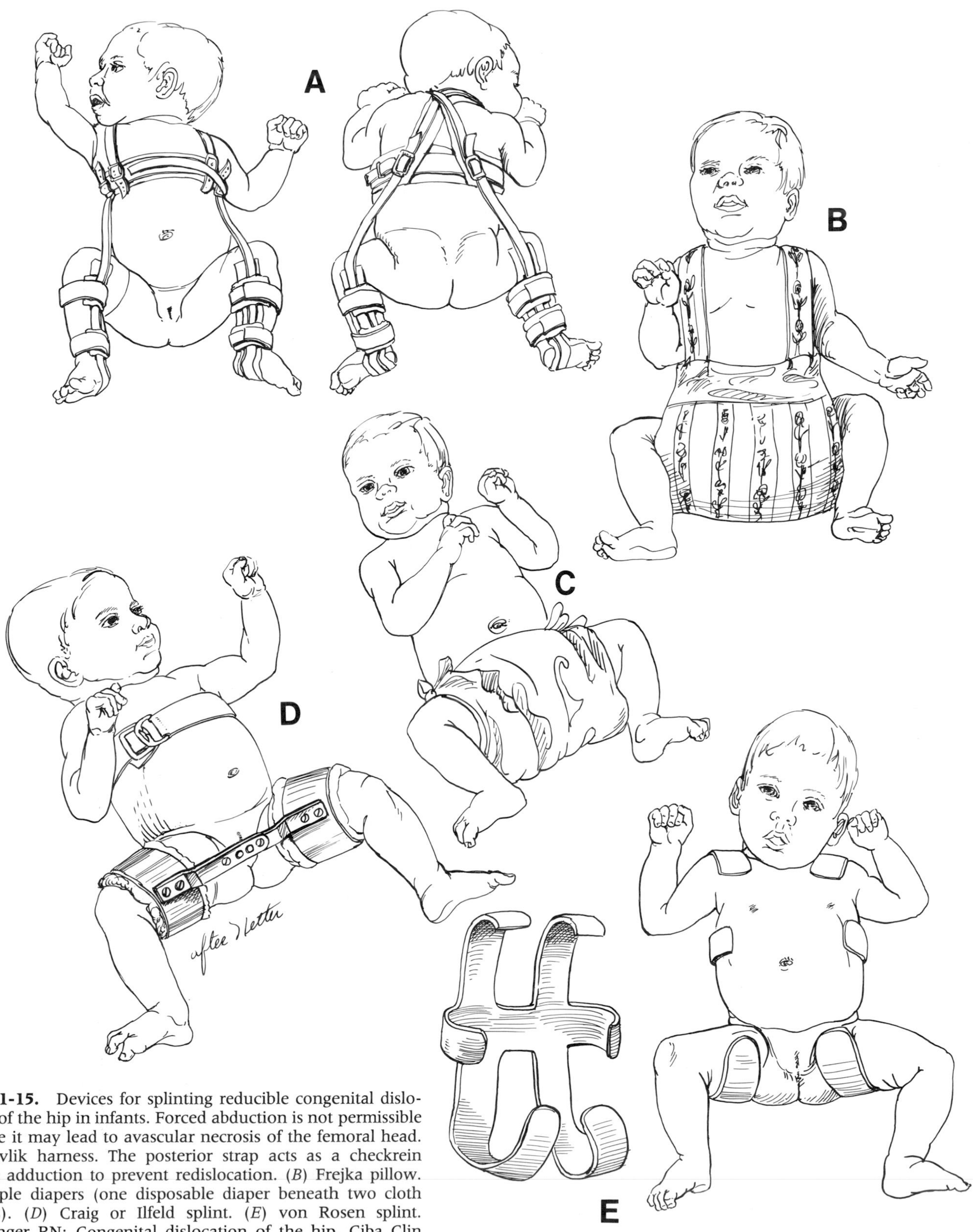

FIG. 11-15. Devices for splinting reducible congenital dislocation of the hip in infants. Forced abduction is not permissible because it may lead to avascular necrosis of the femoral head. (*A*) Pavlik harness. The posterior strap acts as a checkrein against adduction to prevent redislocation. (*B*) Frejka pillow. (*C*) Triple diapers (one disposable diaper beneath two cloth diapers). (*D*) Craig or Ilfeld splint. (*E*) von Rosen splint. (Hensinger RN: Congenital dislocation of the hip. Ciba Clin Symp 31:3, 1979)

adductors. Then the hip is fully flexed, bringing the femoral head around the acetabulum to its shallow posteroinferior aspect. At this point, while the thigh is abducted, the other hand holds the trochanter posteriorly and pushes and guides the head into the socket. Usually, there is an audible snap or a palpable click as the head passes over the acetabular rim. After reduction, the hamstrings are taut and prevent the knee from being fully extended. One can test stability of reduction by push-pull maneuvers, and roentgenograms confirm the reduction. Bilateral dislocations can be reduced at the same sitting. If the reduction is stable, it may be necessary only to maintain the limbs in wide abduction for several months (see Fig. 11-15). However, it is safer to immobilize both extremities in a plaster cast with both hips flexed and abducted, the so-called frog-leg position (Fig. 11-16 *Left*). Both patellae face outward. If excessive anteversion of the neck is suspected, only minimal internal rotation of the thighs is permissible but not advisable (Fig. 11-16 *Right*). Immobilization is maintained for 3 months, and another cast is applied with the abduction and the rotation partially reduced. Subsequent casts gradually obtain the fully extended and neutral position of the limbs. Manipulation should be done gently to avoid traumatizing the hip. Forceful handling and immediately fully abducting and internally rotating the hip (which stretches the capsule and wrings out the blood vessels) have been blamed for subsequent development of degenerative changes in the femoral head that suggest aseptic necrosis (coxa plana). The length of time of immobilization and changes of casts are left to the discretion of the individual operator.

From 1 to 3 Years

Normal development of the acetabulum and femoral head depends on reestablishing a normal acetabulofemoral relationship that is sufficiently stable to permit early motion. Because the potential for remodeling after the first year has markedly diminished, it is essential to secure a complete reduction and to remove all factors that encourage redisplacement. Although, generally speaking, the need for surgical intervention increases with advancing age, there are so many variations that each case must be planned to adapt to the individual situation while adhering to certain basic principles of treatment.

First, the anatomical features of each dislocation or subluxation must be defined. One may predict a situation in which closed reduction may fail. The acetabular roof may be inadequate (acetabular index). The arthrogram may reveal soft tissue interposition. Anteversion may be extreme.

Second, closed reduction is preferable, but excessive force should be avoided because this may lead to osteochondrosis, growth disturbance, and a stiff hip. The incidence of these sequelae is greatly reduced if reduction is accomplished gradually by traction and abduction.[22]

Third, after reduction is supposedly accomplished, the femoral head should nestle deeply and concentrically within its socket. If soft tissue interposition is suspected, an arthrogram will usually define the nature of the obstruction, which in most cases is found to be the limbus.[24] One may elect to remove the limbus immediately, or traction and abduction may be continued for several weeks, during which time the femoral head, in most instances, will sink deeper as the interposing tissue thins out.[23] If this does not occur within a reasonable period, the obstruction should be removed.

In a borderline situation, the factor of instability may not be ascertained until conservative treatment over a period of several months has proved unsuccessful. The acetabulum should be redirected by the innominate osteotomy of Salter or the pericapsular osteotomy of

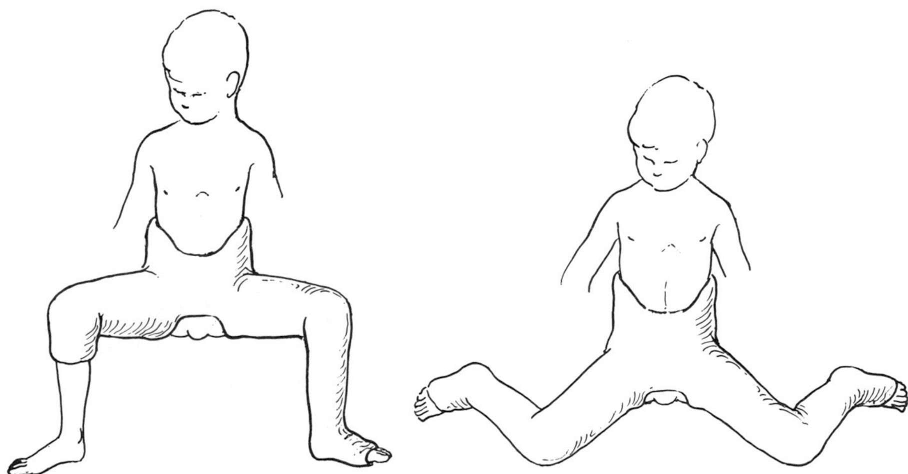

FIG. 11-16. Retentive casts after reduction of the congenital dislocated hip. (*Left*) Frogleg position: flexion-abduction-external rotation. The preferred position for immobilization is the "human position" (more than 90° flexion, 30° to 60° abduction) which is associated with the lowest incidence of avascular necrosis. (*Right*) Reversed position: flexion-abduction-internal rotation. Originally used for excessive anteversion of the femoral neck, it is no longer acceptable because it increases the incidence of avascular necrosis.

Pemberton. Marked anteversion of the femoral neck is corrected by rotation osteotomy.

The question of whether to continue conservative treatment by traction and immobilization or to intervene surgically will depend on signs of normal development of the acetabulum. Normally, three small ossification centers—the ossa acetabuli anterior, superior, and posterior—appear in the developing rim after 11 years of age. However, after the reduction of a dislocation, even at 2 to 3 years of age, an ossification center appears at the upper acetabular rim. This is probably an attempt at reconstitution of the roof. The appearance of these centers after reduction of a dislocation is of value in giving a good prognosis for the acetabulum.[27] Plaster immobilization is continued until stability is assured. An open reduction must be done if closed reduction fails, and redirection of the acetabulum or reconstruction of the acetabular roof must be strongly considered if a tendency to subluxation is noted.

By the 18th month, the acetabulum is ossified and no longer soft and yielding to the pressure of the femoral head. After this age most patients will require surgical procedures.

The following plan of treatment may be modified and

FIG. 11-17. (*A*) The Wingfield frame (in use at Nuffield Orthopaedic Centre) used for gradual reduction of congenital dislocation of the hip. (*B*) Note the sling about the upper thigh pulling the femoral head caudally as the limb is abducted. (Courtesy of E. W. Somerville)

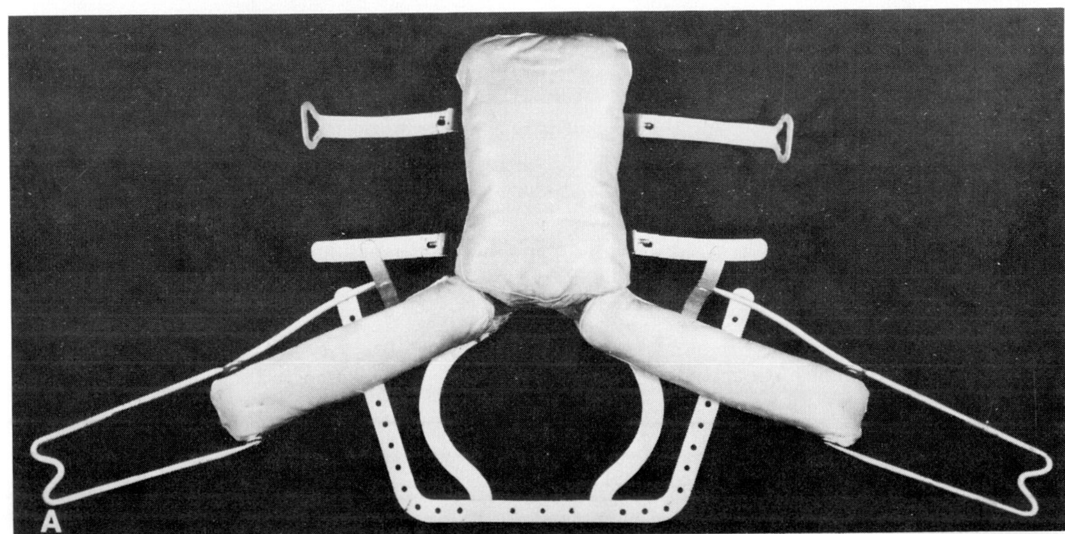

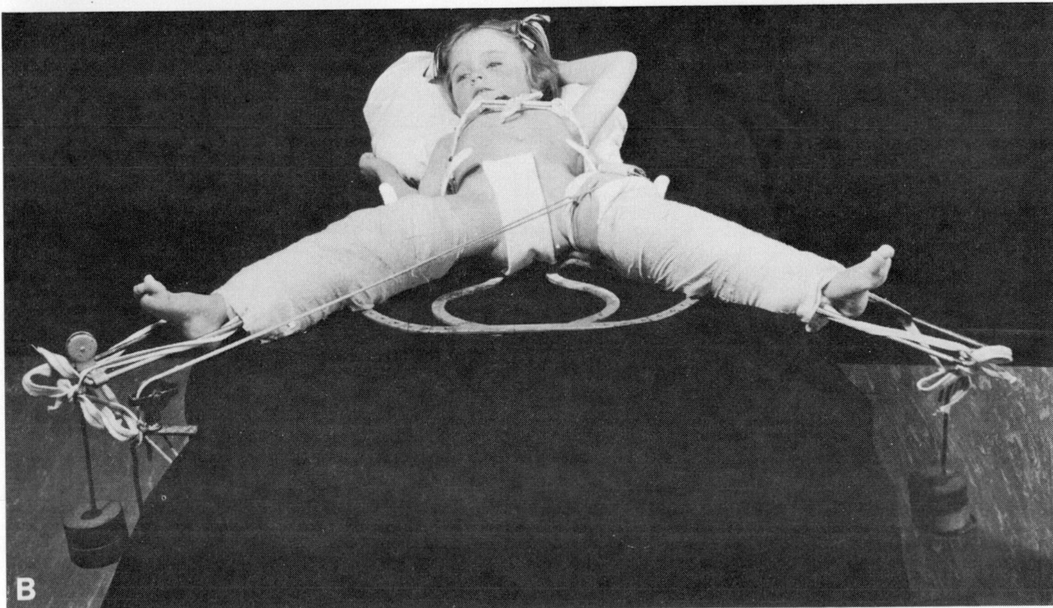

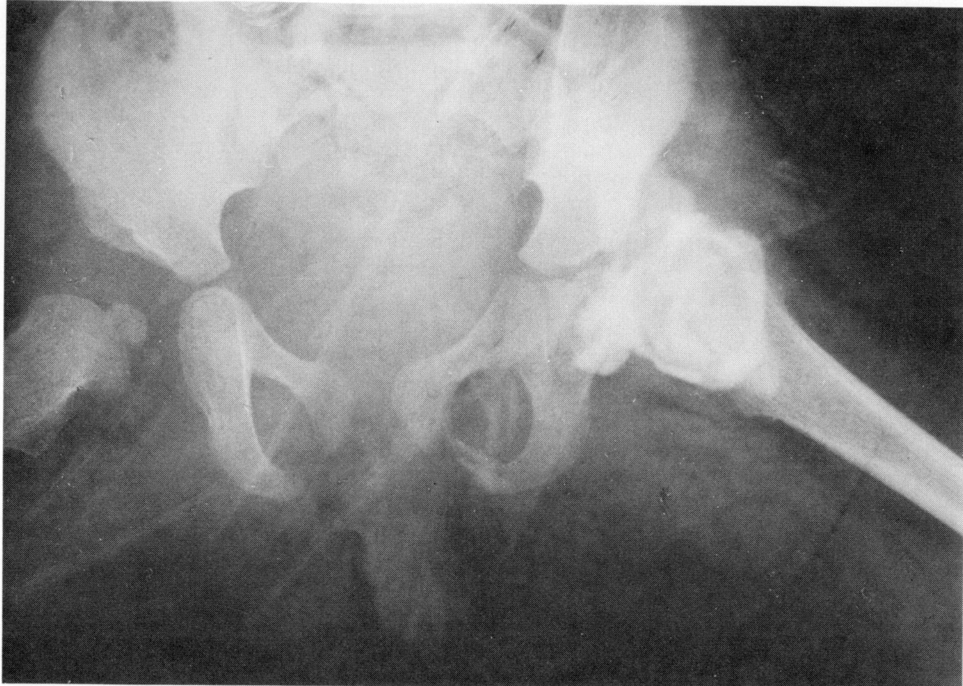

FIG. 11-18. The dislocated hip is reduced on a frame, but the femoral head is held out by the inverted limbus. (Courtesy of E. W. Somerville)

FIG. 11-19. Arthrogram in congenital dislocation of the hip shows the inverted limbus. (Courtesy of E. W. Somerville)

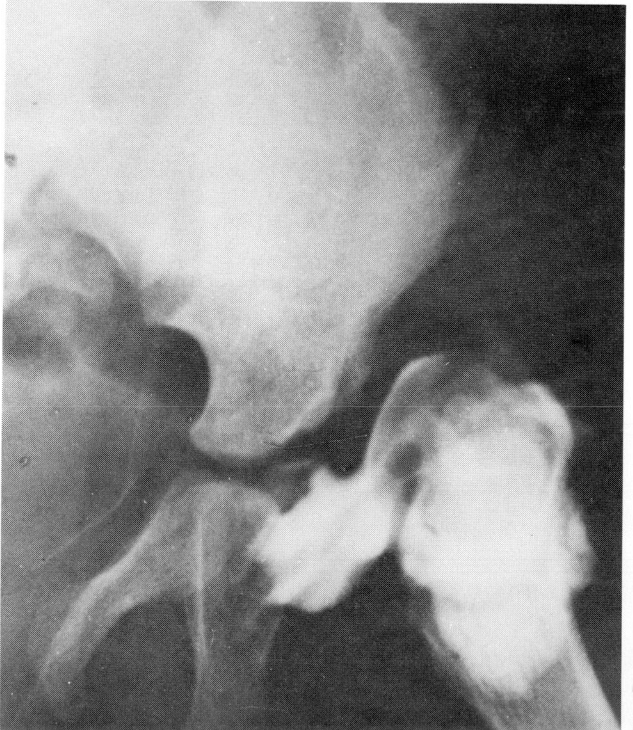

FIG. 11-20. Arthrogram of subluxation. Note the absence of an interposed limbus. (Courtesy of E. W. Somerville)

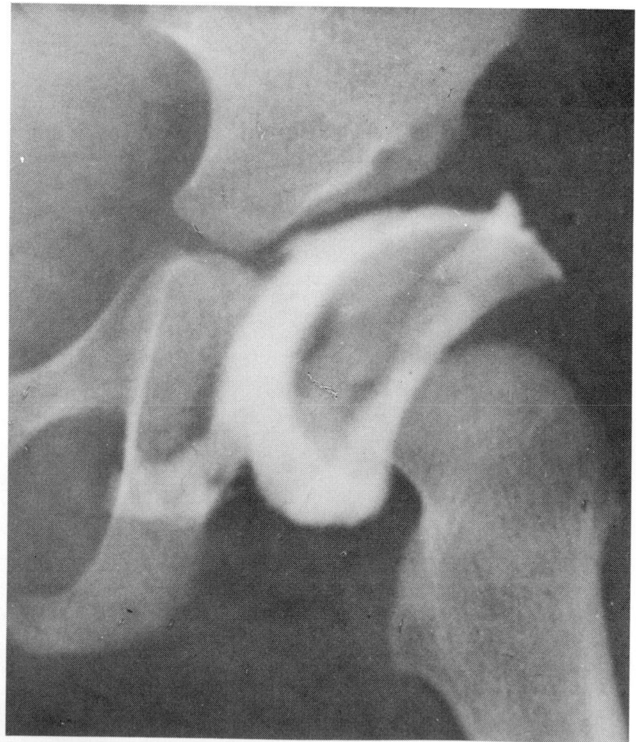

adapted to the individual case requirements. The hip is first slowly reduced by traction and abduction on a suitable frame (*e.g.*, Wingfield frame, Putti divaricator) until the head is opposite the acetabulum (Fig. 11-17). The principle is gradual reduction without the use of force. Longitudinal pull should not exceed 2 or 3 pounds, and the legs are abducted at a rate of 5° per day until 60° of abduction is reached. At this point, a cross pull will aid in achieving the reduction. If, after 4 or 5 weeks, plain radiography shows the femoral head standing out in an eccentric position, an arthrogram may reveal interposed tissue, usually the limbus, and the contrast medium collecting abnormally within the depths of the acetabulum (Figs. 11-18 through 11-20). At this point one may elect to remove the limbus, or conservative treatment may be continued and serial roentgenograms will demonstrate that the femoral head gradually sinks deeper to a more concentric position as the interposed tissue atrophies.

FIG. 11-21. Operation to correct anteversion of the femoral neck. The entire extremity is rotated internally so that the femoral neck lies in the proper plane. The degree of internal rotation is determined by preoperative roentgenographic study. A threaded pin inserted into the subtrochanteric area of the femur maintains this position. A threaded pin is inserted into the condylar area of the femur. A supracondylar osteotomy is performed, and the distal fragment is rotated externally until the knee faces forward. The pins are incorporated into the cast.

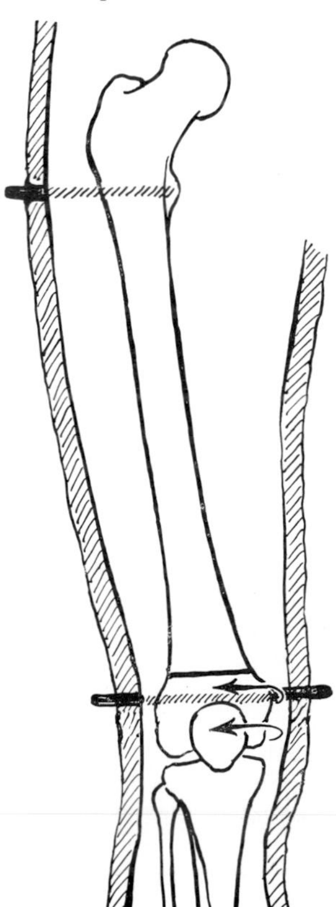

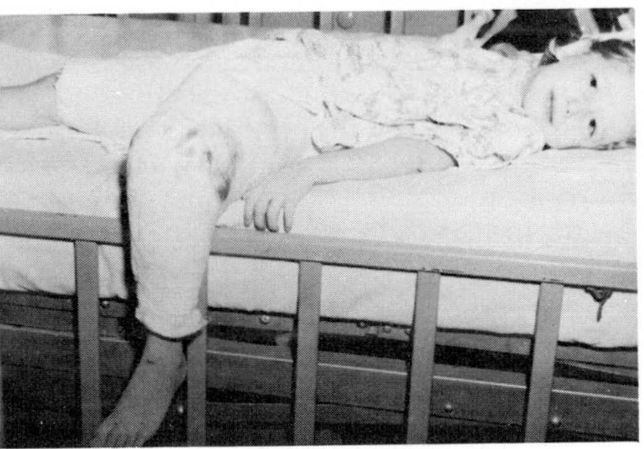

FIG. 11-22. A second cast after supracondylar osteotomy to correct anteversion. The distal fragment and leg have been rotated clockwise 90° from the internal rotated position.

Nonsurgical treatment is generally effective in about two thirds of cases, traction, abduction, and medial rotation being continued for about 2 months. The remainder require some type of surgical procedure to provide stability. Excessive anteversion requires a rotation osteotomy (Figs. 11-21 and 11-22). If an abnormal degree of obliquity of the acetabular roof will not permit retention of the femoral head after several weeks of treatment on the frame, an innominate osteotomy should be done. Removal of interposed tissue may be sufficient to effect an immediate stable reduction.

After the Age of 3

The lack of function leads to shallowness of the acetabulum. The cavity is filled with fibrofatty tissue and adherent capsule. The shortened muscles and fascia keep the femoral head riding high. Marked anteversion is very probable. Attempting reduction at this stage is very traumatizing, and its success is highly improbable. A high percentage of painful stiff hips or redislocations result from nonsurgical treatment. This is especially true in later childhood. After 8 years of age, the shortening is too severe to allow reduction of the head into the original acetabulum even by surgical means. Any attempt to restore the head to the normal position should be done before this time. In general, surgical correction is the treatment of choice beyond 3 years of age but may be undertaken before this time if closed reduction fails.

SURGICAL

Selection of the appropriate operation depends on the pathology.

Preliminary Traction. The soft tissue structures strongly resist the reduction of the femoral head to the level of the acetabulum. This varies with different people and increases with age. A hip that is reduced with the soft tissues tense will be subjected to enormous pressure on the articular surfaces with resultant degenerative changes and possible recurrence of dislocation. Reduction is facilitated if traction is applied preliminary to operation for several days to weeks. Roentgenograms will reveal the descent of the head to the acetabular level. Sometimes it is necessary to perform adductor tenotomies and even a preliminary operation by which the capsule with the gluteal muscles is stripped from the ilium before skeletal traction is applied. The simpler methods are first tried. Bryant's traction is used for the younger child, and sliding skin traction with a Thomas splint is used for the older child (Fig. 11-23). Adequate descent of the head is absolutely necessary before operating.

Open Reduction. The anterior iliofemoral or Smith-Petersen incision is used. This skirts along the anterior half of the iliac crest, then extends distally between the sartorius and the tensor fascia femoris. The lateral femoral cutaneous nerve is avoided. The gluteus medius and minimus are elevated subperiosteally from the ilium, and the dissection is continued deeply between sartorius and tensor. The reflected head of the rectus femoris above the acetabulum is divided, and the large, elongated, sometimes constricted capsule is exposed and freed where it is adherent to the ilium; the upper edge of the acetabulum is encountered. Here the capsule is incised transversely near and parallel with the rim, and the femoral head is exposed. The acetabulum is cleared of the fibrocartilage of the thickened labrum and the fibro-fatty haversian gland as well as adherent capsule until the normal articular cartilage is exposed. The depth of the socket can now be ascertained. Some surgeons practice gouging out the cartilage to deepen the socket, and they quote excellent results, but degenerative changes probably would seem to be invited by this procedure. While the acetabulum is mainly cartilaginous, ordinary pressure of the reduced head will effect adequate restoration of the socket.

FIG. 11-23. Preliminary traction. Bryant's traction is sufficient in this case. A more resistant hip requires skeletal balanced traction.

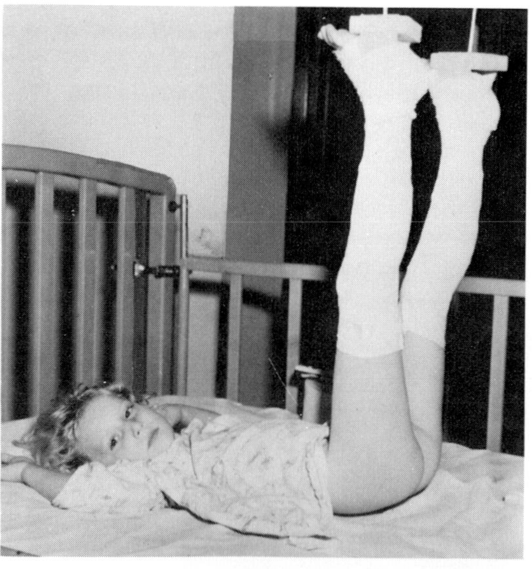

Before 5 years of age, some degree of remodeling may be expected, although this potential is markedly reduced after 18 months. The tendency to regain normal anatomical features is improved by providing stability. This can be accomplished by redirecting the acetabulum to face more lateral and anterior by the Salter procedure. Where the acetabulum is very shallow and large, the Pemberton procedure may be applicable.

After 4 or 5 years of age, reconstruction of the acetabular roof is mandatory. This can be accomplished by a shelving procedure by which a bone buttress is extended outward over the femoral head or by displacing the acetabulum inward so that the remaining overhanging ilium creates a new roof (Chiari procedure).

After the required soft tissue and bone procedures have been completed, the femoral head is reduced and stability is noted. The best position of abduction and the amount of internal rotation required to secure apposition are ascertained and held until the operation is completed and the cast applied. The degree of internal rotation denotes the amount of anteversion to be corrected by osteotomy at a subsequent procedure in 3 or 4 weeks. The ligamentum teres is excised. It may be necessary to elongate the rectus femoris and the sartorius before the head can be adequately replaced. The capsule is also partially excised and shortened and sewed firmly to aid in stabilizing the head. Postoperatively, the cast extends from the nipples to the toes and to the thigh on the opposite side.

Removal of the Limbus (Somerville). If the case is first seen between the ages of 1 and 3 years, a high percentage of successful results can be obtained by the following program:[25]

1. Gradual reduction by traction and abduction on a frame
2. Arthrography to determine the nature of soft tissue interposition (see Figs. 11-18 through 11-20)
   a. Subluxation (limbus not turned in)
   b. Dislocation (limbus inverted)
3. Excision of the limbus in cases of dislocation
4. Derotation osteotomy

Removal of the limbus is a quick, simple procedure that usually will effect an immediate stable reduction.[24] If the question of soft tissue interposition cannot be resolved by arthrography, the frame reduction may be continued for a few weeks, but if the head remains in an eccentric position, removal of the interposing tissue is indicated. If on rare occasions the reduction cannot be accomplished by removal of the limbus, the surgical exposure can be extended.

The patient is removed from the frame and the legs are allowed to adduct. The incision is made along the anterior half of the iliac crest, the abductor muscles are reflected subperiosteally, and the capsule is exposed. The reflected head of the rectus is exposed, its edge defined, separated from the capsule, and retracted. A small transverse incision is made in the capsule close to the acetabular lip, creating an opening through which the white shining cartilage of the femoral head is exposed. The incision is carried forward beneath the rectus. Traction is applied to the leg, and a gap is produced within the joint. Sometimes the infolded limbus can be seen, but usually it is not obvious, and the acetabulum may appear to be deep and well formed. A blunt hook is slipped into the joint and over the edge of the limbus. The tip of the hook can then be forced through the base of the fold where a small incision identifies the periphery of the fold. The knife is then carried forward along the acetabular edge to the anterior end of the limbus, which is then freed. The free segment of limbus is then grasped with a Kocher forceps and separation of the posterior portion is completed with scissors. After the limbus is removed, the extremity is rotated medially and abducted about 30° as the head sinks deeply into the acetabulum. The position is held while the wound is closed and a hip spica applied. It is unnecessary to close the capsule. Immobilization is continued about 3 months; a rotation osteotomy is then done, and a cast is applied for an additional 6 weeks before mobilization is permitted.

Correction of Anteversion. Inasmuch as anteversion increases with age and persistence of the abnormal position of the head, correction is indicated more frequently after 3 years of age. A section of the cast is removed from the lower third of the thigh, and the lateral aspect of the femur is exposed. A threaded pin is drilled into the bone and extends out of the operative wound to be held in the plaster for fixation of the upper fragment. While the pin is held firmly, the bone is osteotomized, and the distal fragment is rotated until the patella points forward. After closure of the wound, the two sections of the cast are joined. The pin is removed when union is observed on roentgenograms.

Innominate Osteotomy (Salter). In congenital dislocation or subluxation of the hip, the acetabulum is shallow and insufficiently inclined so as to encourage redisplacement. The reduced hip may be stable in the position of flexion, abduction, and varying degrees of rotation, but redislocation occurs when the limb is brought down to the functional position of extension and adduction. In this position, the dysplastic acetabulum is deficient where it covers the femoral head laterally and anteriorly. By changing the inclination of the ace-

FIG. 11-24. Technique of innominate osteotomy. (1–4) Diagram of principle involved. (Salter RB: Innominate osteotomy in the treatment of congenital dislocation and subluxation of the hip. J Bone Joint Surg 43B:518, 1961) (*Figure continues on pages 306–308.*)

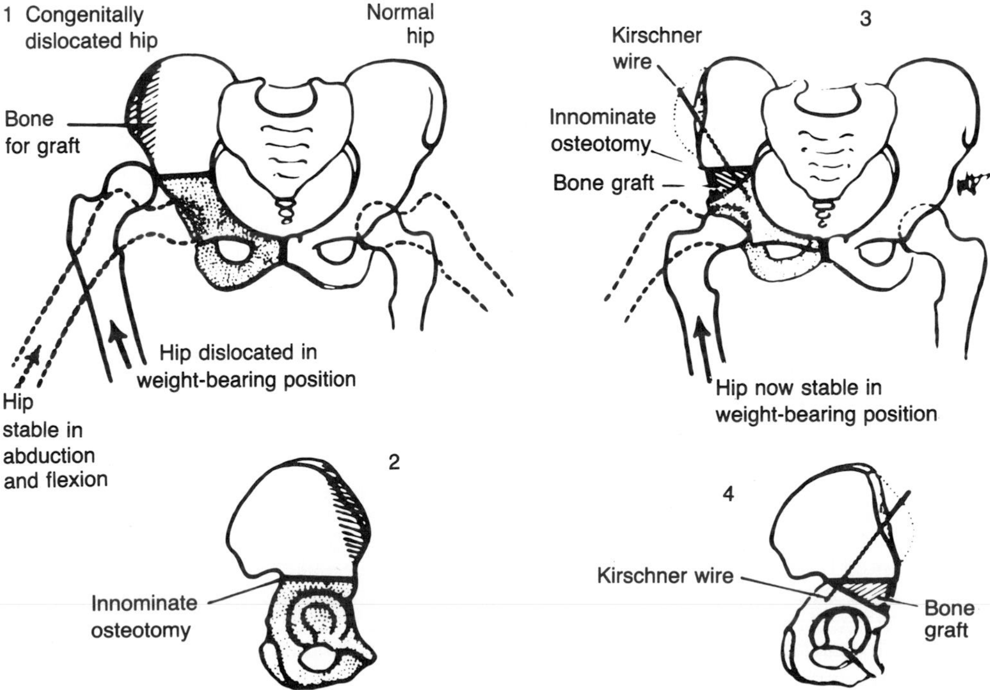

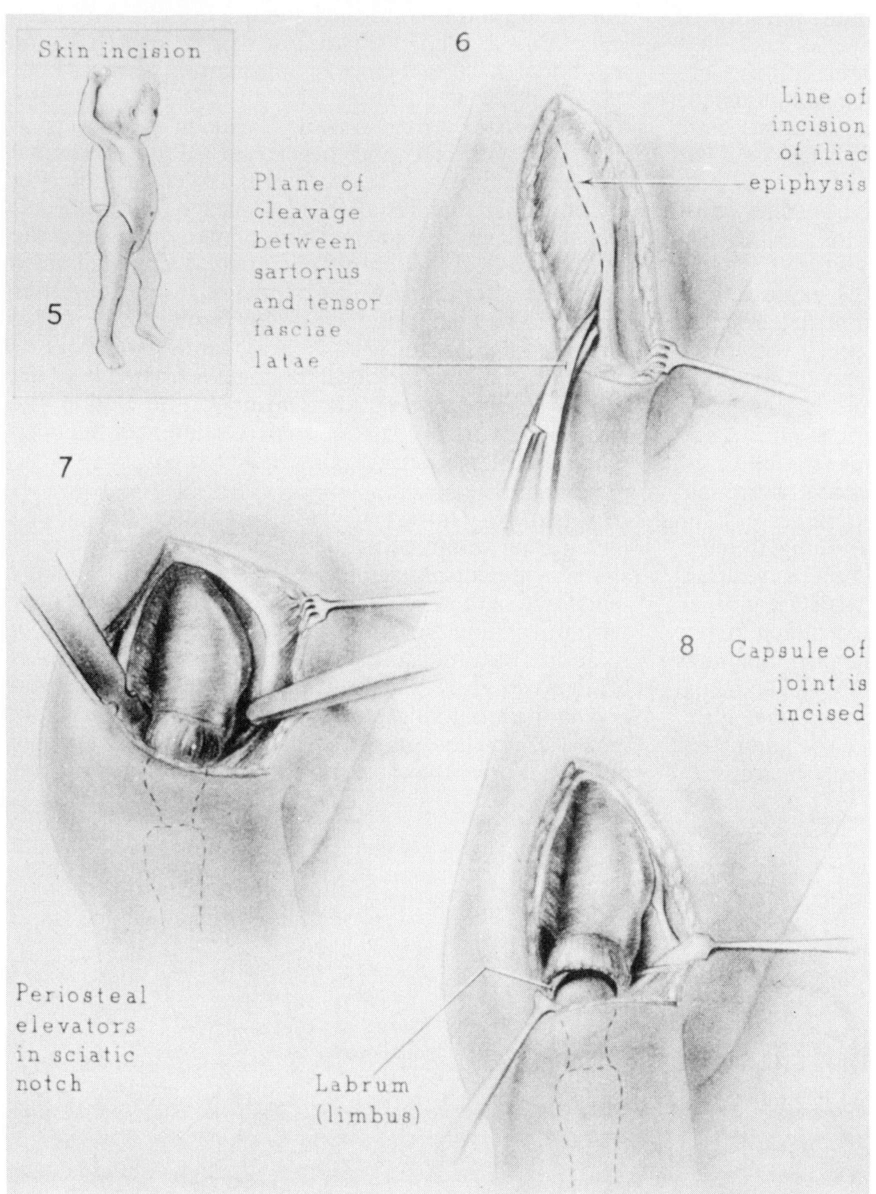

FIG. 11-24. (*Continued*). (5–8) Technique of innominate osteotomy.

tabulum, stability can be provided and early hip motion attained. This is accomplished by completely dividing the innominate bone just above the acetabulum. The distal half of the innominate bone containing the acetabulum is rotated, and the newly directed position is secured by bone graft and pins (Fig. 11-24). Salter believes that the procedure is applicable to congenital dislocation in children from 18 months to 6 years of age and to congenital subluxation up to early adult life. Complete reduction of the hip is an essential prerequisite.

The hip is exposed through a Smith-Petersen incision modified by carrying the incision along the iliac crest beyond the anterior-superior iliac spine to the midpoint of the inguinal ligament (see Fig. 11-24).[20] An incision is made in the iliac apophysis down to the bone along the iliac crest from its midpoint to the anterior-superior spine and then distally to the anterior-inferior spine. The lateral part of the apophysis with the periosteum of the lateral surface of the ilium is then stripped in a continuous sheet inferiorly to the lateral edge of the acetabulum and posteriorly to the greater sciatic notch, and this space is packed. If the fibrous capsule of the hip has become adherent to the lateral aspect of the ilium above the acetabulum by being stretched upward by the intracapsular dislocation, it is freed by a periosteal elevator. Blunt dissection between the capsule and the abductor muscles

FIG. 11-24. (*continued*). (9–12) Technique of innominate osteotomy.

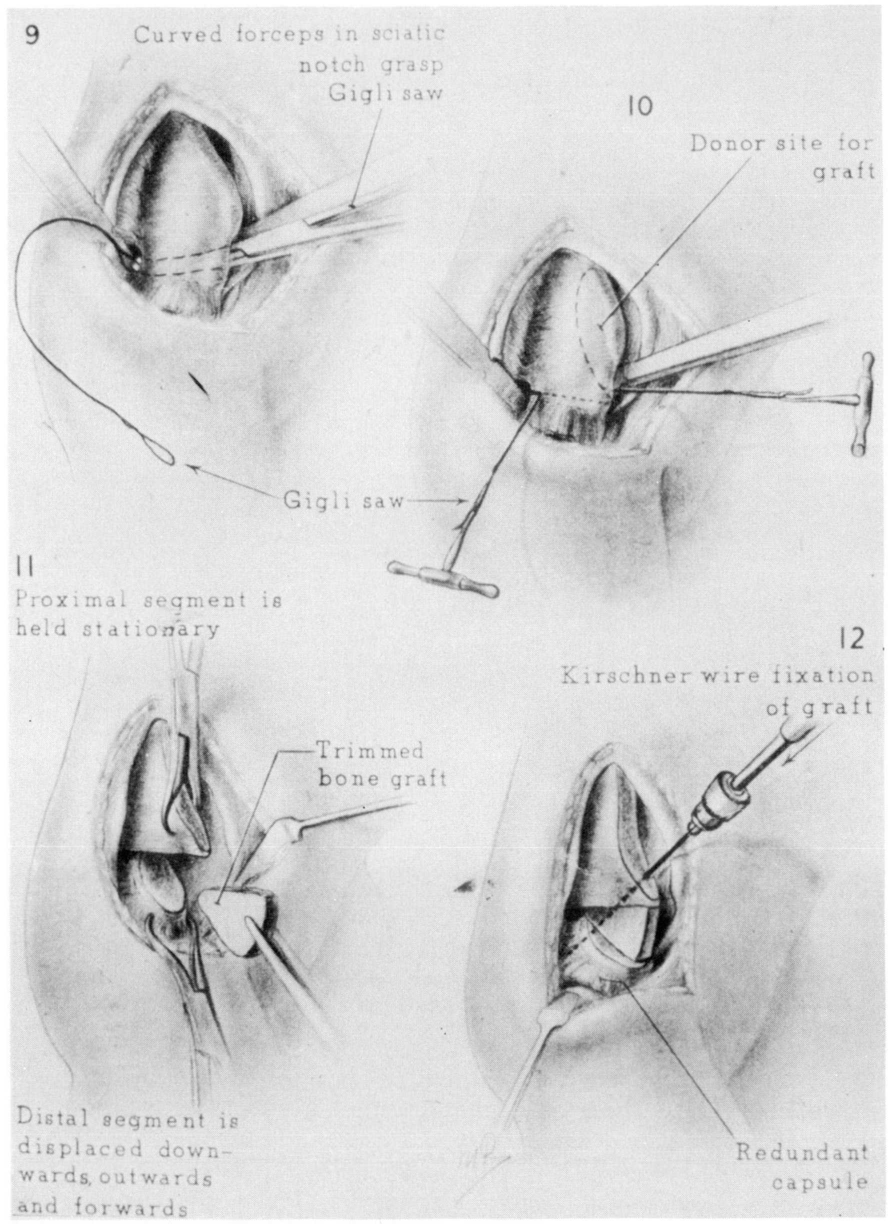

provides excellent exposure of the lateral and anterior aspects of the capsule.

The capsule is widely opened close to the superior and anterior margins of the acetabulum. Excessive fibrofatty tissue is removed from the acetabulum, but the ligamentum teres is left undisturbed unless it is hypertrophied and prevents reduction. If the limbus is inverted and interferes with the reduction, it should be removed. Otherwise it is retained, since it adds to the depth and stability of the acetabulum. The femoral head is reduced under direct vision. If the ilipsoas is tight, renders reduction difficult, and limits abduction and internal rotation, its tendinous portion should be divided. Stability is then assessed. Redisplacement is found when the adduction causes the femoral head to slip laterally and when extension or external rotation causes it to slip anteriorly.

The remaining portion of the cartilaginous iliac apophysis is displaced medially from the anterior half of the crest with an elevator, and the periosteum of the inner surface of the ilium is stripped off in a continuous sheet to expose the sciatic notch. Care is taken to remain in the subperiosteal plane throughout, but particularly behind the sciatic notch because of the proximity of the

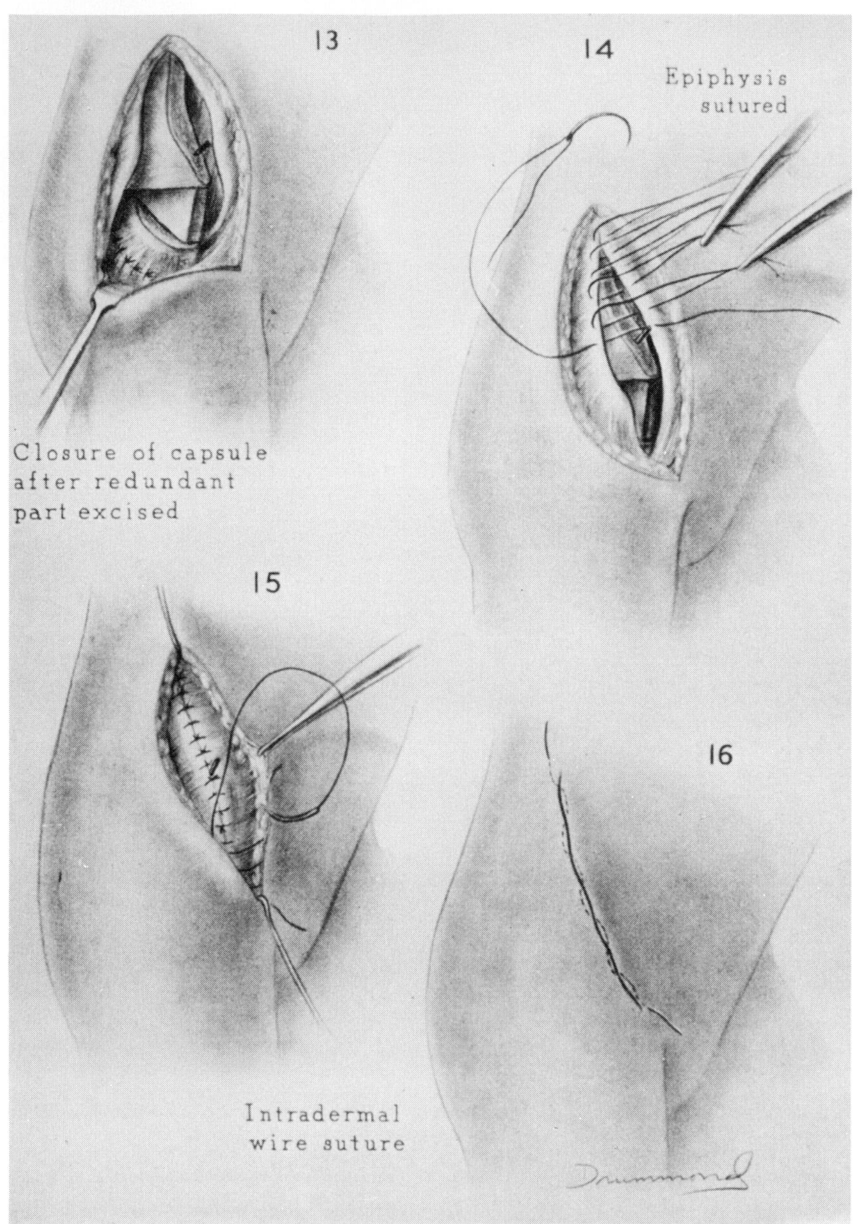

FIG. 11-24. (*Continued*). (13–16) Technique of innominate osteotomy.

sciatic nerve and the superior gluteal artery. The tip of a curved forceps is passed subperiosteally behind the notch from the medial side in order to grasp one end of the Gigli saw. The osteotomy extends in a straight line from the sciatic notch to the anterior-inferior spine and is at right angles to the vertical line of the ilium. A generous full-thickness bone graft is removed from the anterior part of the iliac crest and is trimmed to the shape of a wedge, the base of which should correspond to the distance between the anterior-superior and anterior-inferior spines. One stout towel forceps is used to steady the proximal segment of the innominate bone, and a second is used to grasp the distal segment posterior to the anterior-inferior spine. By means of a curved elevator in the sciatic notch and traction on the distal towel forceps, the distal segment of the innominate bone containing the entire acetabulum is shifted forward, downward, and outward so that the osteotomy site is opened anterolaterally. The best displacement of the distal fragment is obtained by allowing the femoral head to remain in the dislocated position. It is most important to avoid any backward or inward displacement of the distal segment.

The wedge-shaped bone graft is then inserted on its

edge into the osteotomy site, and when traction is released the graft will be found to be held firmly between the two segments of the innominate bone. A stout Kirschner wire is then inserted from the proximal segment through the graft and into the distal segment posterior to the acetabulum. The femoral head is then reduced, and if the displacement of the acetabulum is correct the reduction will be stable even with the hip in the functional position of walking. Throughout the remainder of the procedure an assistant holds the lower extremity with the hip in a position of slight abduction, slight flexion, and slight medial rotation. The knee is kept flexed to overcome the relative shortening of the hamstring muscles.

The residual pocket of joint capsule, formerly occupied by the dislocated femoral head, is obliterated by appropriate excision of redundant capsule followed by careful suturing of the edges. The halves of the iliac apophysis are then sutured together over the iliac crest. The Kirschner wire is cut so that its end lies in the subcutaneous fat. After skin closure, a unilateral hip spica is applied with the hip in the same position of slight abduction, slight flexion, and slight internal rotation; the knee is fixed in flexion to diminish hamstring tension.

Postoperatively, the hip spica is removed after 6 weeks. It is replaced by toe-to-groin plaster casts with an abduction bar for 4 weeks more. After removal of the abduction casts, the child is permitted to walk.

Pericapsular Osteotomy of the Ilium (Pemberton). The upper portion of the acetabulum is rotated forward and laterally to cover the femoral head.[18] Pemberton pointed out the importance of the anterior defect of the acetabular rim, which is not apparent in the usual radiographic view and permits the femoral head to displace when the hip is extended. After osteotomy, the superior acetabular component rotates through an axis corresponding with the horizontal limb of the triradiate cartilage, which extends across the acetabulum. Flexibility of the triradiate cartilage at an early age permits the superior portion of the acetabulum to be brought laterally and forward so that it is literally wrapped around the femoral head. Obviously the capacity of the acetabulum is reduced. Therefore, the procedure is applicable to situations in which the femoral head is disproportionately small in relation to the acetabulum, particularly the relatively large acetabulum of the subluxated hip. If the operation is done early, while remodeling potential is great, incongruity between femoral head and acetabulum corrects spontaneously. Consequently, the operation should be done before 4 years of age and preferably at 1 year. Exceptionally it can be done up to 12 years of age in girls and 14 in boys, but disproportionate articular surfaces at this age usually eventuate in later degenerative change. When it is done for a dislocated hip that is difficult to reduce, coxa plana may develop but eventually disappears.

The hip joint is exposed through the Smith-Petersen approach. The superior part of the incision is made well below the iliac crest. The glutei and tensor fasciae latae are stripped subperiosteally down to the hip joint and posteriorly until the greater sciatic notch is seen. The iliac apophysis, with its attached muscles, is then separated from the anterior third of the iliac crest using a sharp elevator; the muscles are stripped subperiosteally from the inner aspect of the ilium until the sciatic notch is reached on the inside of the pelvis. The rectus femoris attachment is not sectioned. In a subluxating hip joint in a patient under 6 or 7 years of age, it is usually not necessary to open the hip capsule; in a high dislocation, in which replacement of the head may be difficult, or in children above 7 years of age, the capsule should be opened to check the reduction.

Two flat-blade retractors are inserted into the sciatic notch, one from the inner side and the other from the outer, thus exposing the entire anterior third of the ilium. The retractors should be inserted in such a manner as to protect the sciatic nerve and superior gluteal vessels. The osteotomy is then done separately through each table of the ilium (Fig. 11-25). With a narrow curved osteotome, a cut is first made through the outer table of the ilium, starting just above the anterior-inferior iliac spine and extending backward parallel to, and about a quarter of an inch above, the attachment of the joint capsule. The osteotome is driven backward under direct vision until it can be seen to be well in front of the retractor. At this point the blade of the osteotome will be in such a position that when it is driven further it will disappear from sight, since the overlying tissue cannot be retracted beyond the sciatic notch. It is important that the tip of the instrument be directed so that it will not enter the sciatic notch but will reach the ilioischial limb of the triradiate cartilage at its midportion about halfway between the anterior margin of the sciatic notch and the center of the posterior rim of the acetabulum. After making certain that the curved osteotome is properly directed, it is driven the final half inch to complete the cut of the outer table.

A corresponding cut is then made through the inner table of the ilium. The osteotome is started anteriorly at the previous point of entrance above the anterior-inferior iliac spine. It is directed backward parallel to and on a level with the cut in the outer table. Again the cutting edge will disappear from sight in front of the sciatic notch as it is driven the last half inch to reach the triradiate cartilage. By varying the relative position of the posterior portion of this second cut, the direction of displacement of the acetabular roof can be controlled. If the acetabular defect is chiefly anterior and the roof must be displaced directly downward to cover the anterior portion of the head, the osteotomy of the inner table should conform exactly to the one in the outer table. If it is necessary to cover the head more laterally, the posterior portion of the osteotomy in the inner table is shifted forward in relation to the cut in the outer table, and the acetabular roof will tilt laterally as it is displaced.

After cutting through both cortices, the cancellous

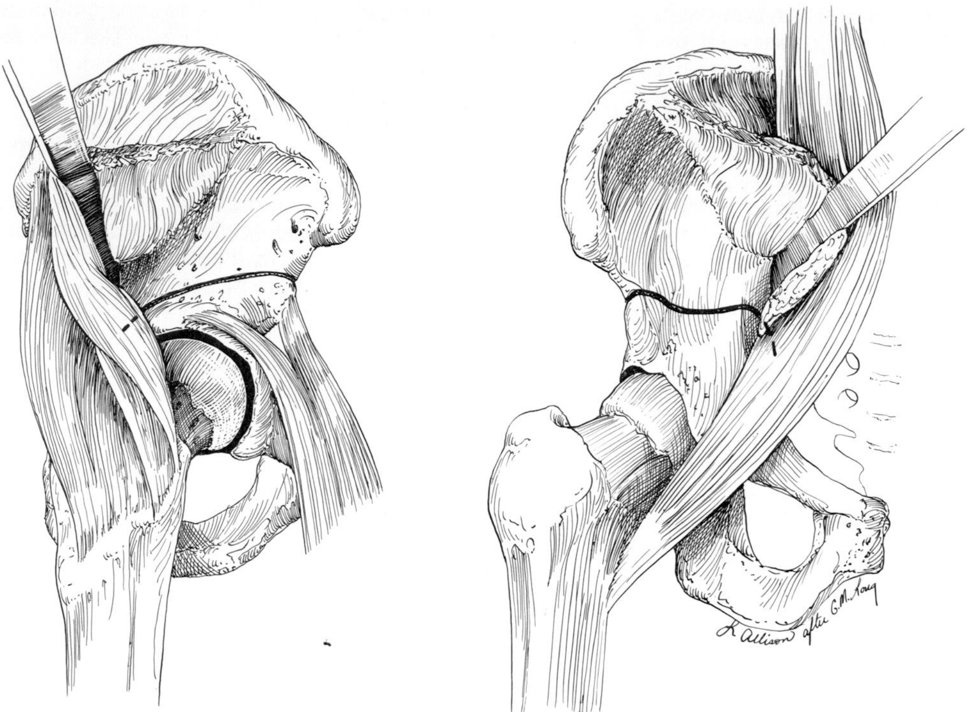

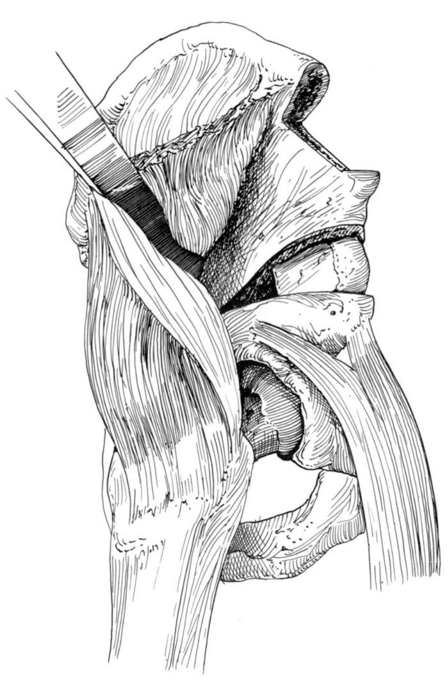

FIG. 11-25. Technique of pericapsular osteotomy of Pemberton. (*Top right*) Osteotomy through the outer table of the ilium extending backward from just above the anterior-inferior iliac spine parallel to the capsular attachment as far as the triradiate cartilage. (*Top left*) Osteotomy through the inner table of the ilium curving backward from the same starting point as that shown in the top right diagram and also reaching the triradiate cartilage. (*Bottom*) The acetabular roof is turned down and held by a wedge of bone inserted into grooves cut on both surfaces of the osteotomy. (Pemberton P: Pericapsular osteotomy of the ilium for treatment of congenital subluxation and dislocation of the hip. J Bone Joint Surg 47A:65, 1965)

bone between them is divided by inserting a wide curved osteotome. After this osteotome is inserted, it is levered downward so that the anterolateral rim of the acetabulum is lowered to close the existing anatomical defect.

While the surfaces of the osteotomy are held apart, a groove is cut into each surface with a narrow gouge. A wedge of bone is then removed from the anterior portion of the wing of the ilium, including the anterior-superior iliac spine. After the dislocation is reduced and the acetabular roof is turned down, the wedge of bone is inserted into the grooves, locking the acetabular roof firmly in place (see Fig. 11-25). It is important to lower the detached portion of ilium as much as possible, which means separation of the anterior edges of the osteotomy an inch to an inch and a quarter. The iliac apophysis is then sutured into place over the remaining ilium, and the wound is closed. A spica cast is applied with the hip slightly abducted and internally rotated.

Shelf Operation. The older the patient when reduction is effected, the less likely is the deepening of the acetabulum and the greater is the subsequent disability and inevitable symptoms of pain, stiffness, and fatigue. The roof can be re-formed at the same time as the reduction. However, it is best to do it after 5 years of age, when the ossification within and about the acetabulum is sufficient to ensure success of this bone plastic procedure. Preliminary traction for several weeks to overcome the muscle pull is necessary to lessen the danger of the femoral head's being pulled proximally against the newly formed buttress and compromising the result. At operation all soft tissue structures that may similarly interfere are dealt with. Then a cortical flap of bone, starting immediately above the upper acetabular rim and extending inward and downward, skirting the articular aspect, is turned downward over the head and is maintained by insertion of bone blocks and chips (Fig. 11-26). Traction must be continued postoperatively until bony consolidation is complete.

In irreducible dislocations, a shelf operation is necessary when instability causes symptoms. The lumbar lordosis resulting from posterior position of the femur may cause low back pain. At operation, the femoral head is brought forward to a point just above the acetabulum, and the shelf is constructed. The pelvic tilt and lordosis are reduced, and stability is effected. This procedure is likely to be successful when performed in patients over 10 years of age.

Acetabular Deepening Procedures. Acetabulum deepening is indicated when the acetabulum is shallow (acetabular dysplasia) and the enlarged femoral head (coxa magna) subluxates. By displacing the socket medially, an adequate covering for the femoral head is created and stability provided. The lateral abductor muscle moment is lengthened, and the medial weight-bearing moment is decreased; reducing the load and distributing it over a greater surface area lessens the likelihood of later degenerative change. The abductor muscle efficiency is improved by the reduced load and by increasing the resting muscle length. The Trendelenburg gait, pain, and fatigue are eliminated. The procedure is done after 4 or 5 years of age and is indicated for the dysplastic subluxating hip. Intra-articular procedures (*e.g.*, capsular arthroplasty of Colonna) are inadvisable because they are prone to cause stiffness.[11]

The Chiari operation is entirely extra-articular and is the preferred procedure.[9,10] An innominate osteotomy is done immediately adjacent to the upper acetabular rim without entering the joint. The distal fragment containing the acetabulum is displaced medially so that the exposed raw bony surface of the proximal fragment forms an extension of the roof and is separated from the femoral head by the capsule. Intracapsular exposure must be avoided because this results in a stiff hip (Figs. 11-27 and 11-28).

Through a Smith-Petersen anterolateral incision, the abductor muscles are elevated subperiosteally and retracted backward to expose the greater sciatic notch.[12] The anterior two thirds of the iliac crest bearing the attachments of the abdominal muscles are detached. A malleable retractor is passed to enter the greater sciatic notch. The inner surface of the ilium is freed subperiostally as far back as the sciatic notch, and a second retractor is then passed to the medial side of the innominate bone and into the notch to make contact with the first retractor. The retractors protect the sciatic nerve and the internal iliac vessels from injury.

The level for the osteotomy is immediately above the attachment of the joint capsule to the ilium, between the capsule and the reflected head of the rectus femoris. Frequently, the interval between the capsule and the reflected head may be difficult to define, because the capsule may adhere proximally to the outer surface of the ilium and may misdirect the osteotomy at too high a level. The problem may be obviated by locating the proper level with a guide pin under radiographic control. Then the guide pin is inserted at 10° upward and inward, preferably under image amplifier control. The osteotomy follows the guide pin.

One must guard against inadvertently allowing the

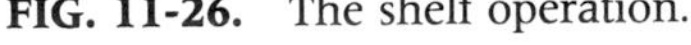
FIG. 11-26. The shelf operation.

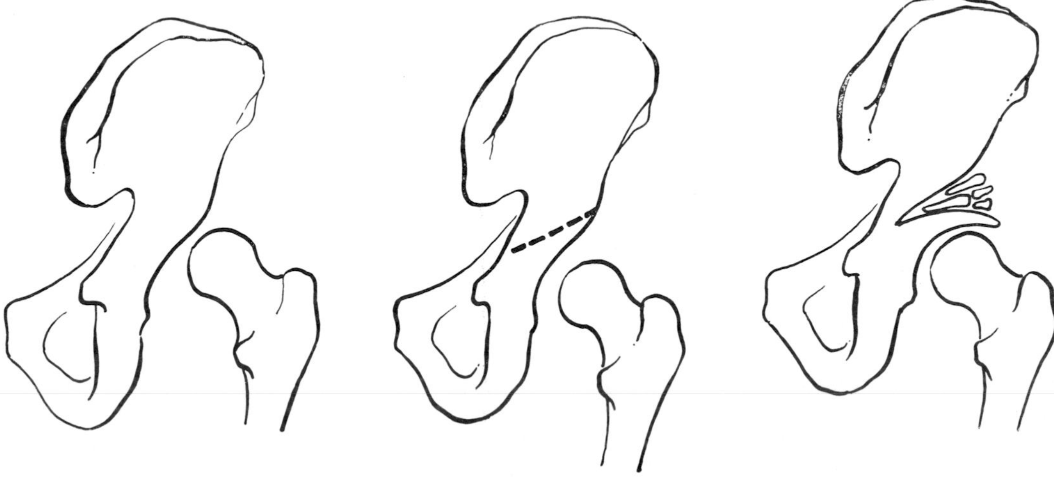

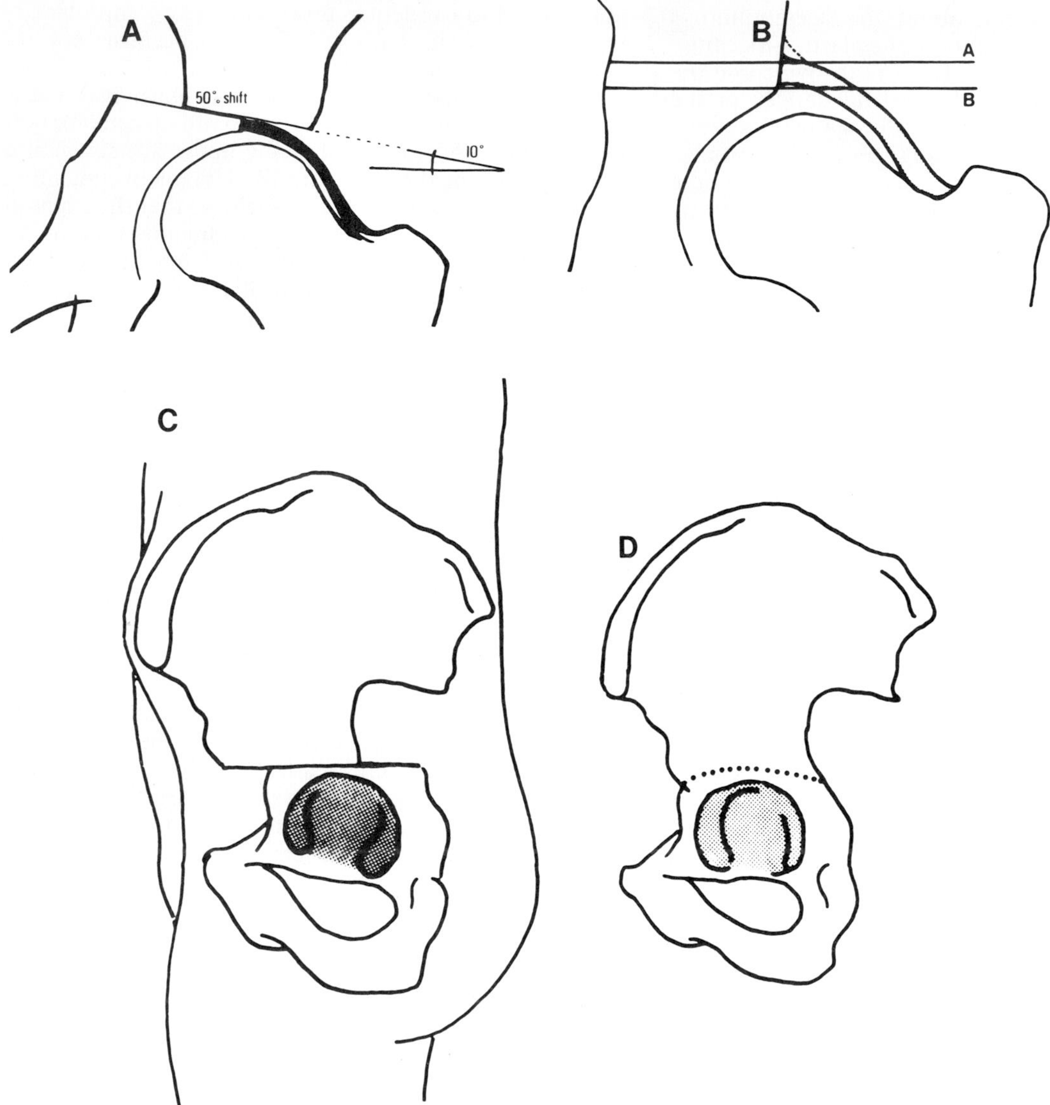

FIG. 11-27. The Chiari osteotomy. (*A*) The ideal osteotomy is sited immediately above the capsular attachment, directed inward and upward at an angle of 10°, and displaced inward 50%. (*B*) Level at *A* is ideal for osteotomy. Level at *B* is too low and damages the capsule. The short dotted line shows how capsular adhesion to the ilium can invite too high a level for the osteotomy. (*C*) The lateral view shows how the posterior slip causes prominence of the anterior-superior iliac spine and (*D*) how the osteotomy is curved to prevent posterior slip. (Colton CL: Chiari osteotomy for acetabular dipplasia in young subjects. J Bone Joint Surg 54B:578, 1972)

distal fragament to settle posteriorly; this displacement can produce an ugly prominence of the anterior-superior iliac spine and a flexion deformity of the hip. This can be avoided by slightly curving the osteotomy. Multiple drill holes first outline the osteotomy before it is completed with osteotomes. The osteotomy of the pelvis extends anteriorly, then posteriorly to the greater sciatic notch, dividing the innominate bone. The leg is then abducted gradually, and gentle inward pressure is exerted against the distal fragment, causing it to displace medially. About 50% displacement is desirable. The displacement must not be excessive so that the raw surfaces lose contact. If the fragments appear to be unstable, a lag screw can be inserted for fixation from proximal fragment directed distally and medially into the distal fragment.

A spica cast is applied to the toes on the affected side and to the knee on the opposite side and extended proximally to the nipple line. It is removed after 4 to 6 weeks and weight bearing is permitted thereafter.

The capsule must not be opened because it forms a

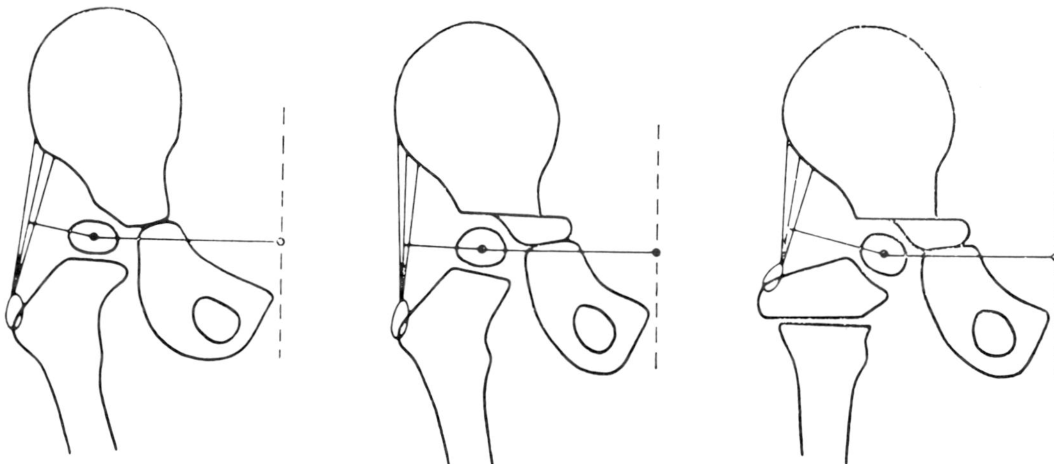

FIG. 11-28. Diagrams showing how the Chiari osteotomy improves the biomechanics of the hip joint. (*Left*) Original short lateral abductor lever, long medial lever. (*Center*) The ratio of the medial lever to the lateral lever is reduced. (*Right*) The position after adding varus osteotomy to correct coxa valga. The ratio is even further reduced. (After Burch: In Beckenosteotomie. Stuttgart, Georg Thieme, 1965)

lining for the new roof where it is converted to fibrocartilage. If the capsule is damaged, a stiff hip results.

Before undertaking this procedure, the potential for relocating the femoral head must first be established. A preliminary operation to achieve correction of valgus by a varus osteotomy and to overcome anteversion by a derotation osteotomy may be necessary.

Stabilizing Osteotomies. At a late age, stabilizing osteotomies are the procedures of choice to eliminate pain at the site of the false acetabulum on the wing of the ilium. A bony support on the femur is formed. Two main types are used—the Lorenz and the Schanz.

Lorenz Bifurcation Osteotomy. A long oblique osteotomy in the subtrochanteric area is made so that the proximal end of the distal fragment lies at the level of the acetabulum. The plane of the osteotome is directed from the distal end at the posterolateral aspect toward the proximal end at the anteromedial aspect of the bone. Then the limb is abducted and extended so that the proximal end of the distal fragment is directed medially and anteriorly into the acetabulum (Fig. 11-29). Such large raw surfaces of the osteotomized bones are apposed to each other that union in the angulated position takes place readily. A cast is applied for about 3 months or until union is demonstrated by radiographic examination.

Schanz Osteotomy. The femur is sectioned transversely at the lower border of the pelvis, and the upper fragment is angled inward until it rests against the side wall of the pelvis (Fig. 11-30). Thus, the body weight gains a bony support, and stability is demonstrated by improvement of the Trendelenburg sign. The adduction of the proximal fragment lengthens the distance of the gluteus medius and provides a fulcrum so that adequate leverage of the muscle is obtained. Preliminary to operation, an anteroposterior roentgenogram is taken with the lower extremity completely adducted. A measuring stick with radiopaque markers is placed alongside the limb, and the level of osteotomy and the degree of angulation are ascertained. A Vitallium plate is prepared and angulated sufficiently, not only to deviate the upper fragment medially against the pelvic wall but also anteriorly to overcome the posterior displacement of the upper femur. At operation the bone is sectioned transversely, and the plate is attached to the upper fragment. Then the distal shaft is abducted and extended and approximated to the distal half of the plate, which is then attached. The cast is generally necessary for about 3 months. This procedure is contraindicated before 15 years of age because loss of angulation is common during the growth period.

Old Subluxation of the Hip. A persistently subluxating hip will ultimately develop progressively painful osteoarthritis. In the young active adult, cup arthroplasty or hip resurfacing procedures will provide stability and relief of pain. At a later age, total hip replacement is the procedure of choice. The development of these procedures has largely obviated the need for stabilizing osteotomies. This is discussed more fully in the section on the hip (Fig. 11-31).

CONGENITAL CLUBFOOT

DEFINITION

Congenital clubfoot (talipes) is a gross deformity of the foot present at birth. The direction of deformity of the individual components of the foot is described in the following terms:

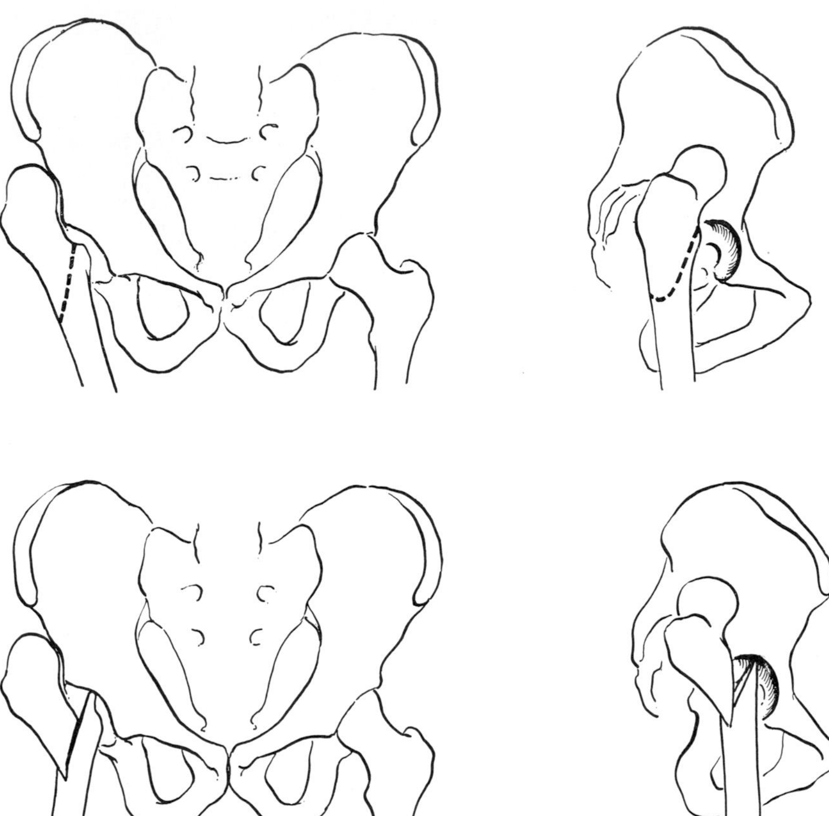

FIG. 11-29. Lorenz bifurcation osteotomy. (*Top*) Direction and level of section. (*Bottom*) Position after displacement of distal fragment into the acetabulum.

Equinus. The forefoot is plantar flexed (at ankle and midtarsal areas).
Calcaneus. The forefoot is dorsal flexed. The calcaneus forms the plantar prominence.
Varus. The heel and forefoot are inverted. The plantar surface faces medially.
Valgus. The heel and forefoot are everted. The plantar surface faces laterally.

For example, talipes equinovarus, the most common type (95%), describes the foot that is plantar flexed and inverted. Talipes calcaneovalgus, calcaneovarus, and equinovalgus are the other less common types.

ETIOLOGY

The causative factor is unknown, but the theories are intrauterine compression; arrest in fetal development, explaining frequently associated anomalies; dysplasia of muscles, causing muscle imbalance; and abnormal tendon insertion, particularly anterior tibial.[31]

Deformities of feet that are due to obvious causes are not usually included in this discussion of clubfoot, because the exciting cause demands primary consideration in treatment. These conditions are discussed under the appropriate headings and include central nervous system diseases (spina bifida, poliomyelitis, Friedreich's ataxia), imperfect muscle development (arthrogryposis), lymphatic stasis (congenital constriction band), and absent bony structures (*e.g.*, tibia).

Brief mention should be made of spina bifida, which is not always clinically evident, but roentgenographic investigation for it always should be conducted in cases of clubfoot deformity. When the spinal defect is large and associated with extrusion of spinal contents, muscle imbalance, sphincter paralysis, and sensory loss accompany a severe foot deformity (Fig. 11-32).

PATHOLOGY

In talipes equinovarus the leg muscles are smaller than in the normal leg and microscopically may show signs of possible degeneration. The tendo Achillis passes downward and medially toward the calcaneus, thereby helping to maintain the bone in inversion. The ligaments between the calcaneus, the talus, and the navicular are thickened and contracted. The navicular is displaced downward and medially and is maintained by the shortened posterior tibial tendon and the contracted ligaments, including the deltoid ligament. The anterior end of the calcaneus

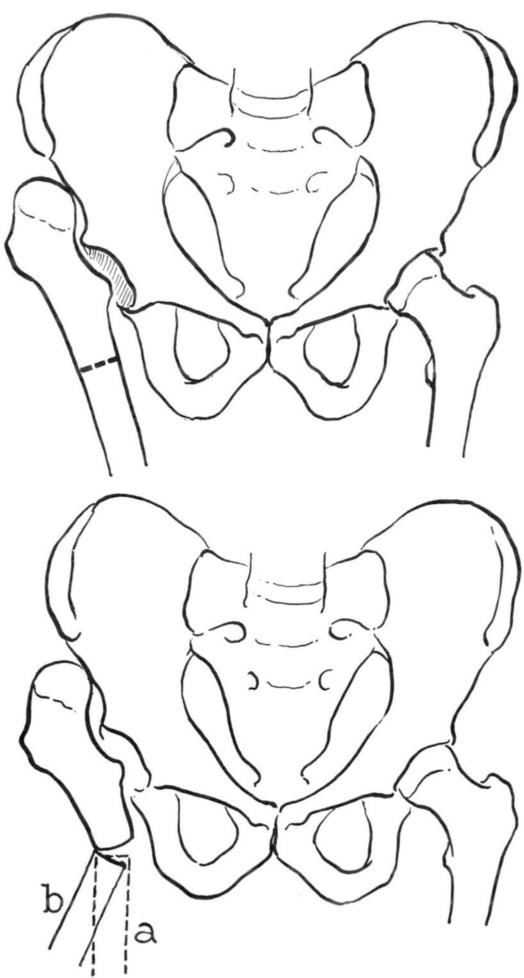

FIG. 11-30. Shanz osteotomy. (*Top*) Preoperatively. A film taken with the limb completely adducted will indicate the angle of correction. The level of section is well shown. (*Bottom*) Position after osteotomy. The usually accepted positioning is at *a;* hyperabduction is indicated for extreme shortening and instability, *b*.

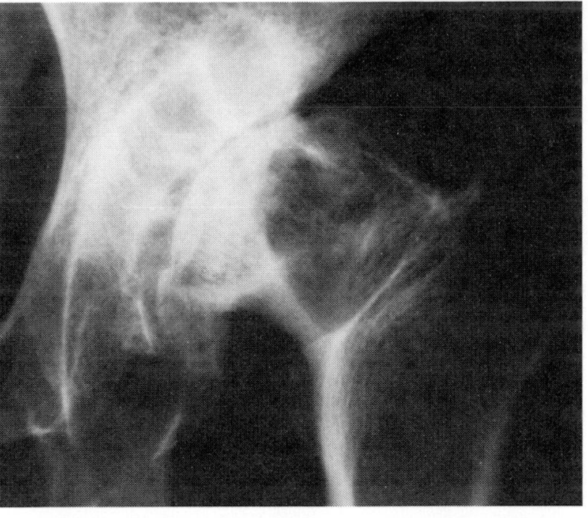

FIG. 11-31. Old subluxation of the hip. Originally, this was a complete dislocation that was adequately reduced during infancy, but sufficient deepening of the acetabulum did not take place. Instability has caused erosion of the acetabular roof and degenerative changes throughout the joint. This demonstrates the necessity for prolonged immobilization after reduction of the congenitally dislocated hip.

is displaced medially beneath the head of the astragalus. The plantar aponeurosis is thickened and contracted along with the short plantar muscles, so a high-arch deformity (cavus) is created, and the forefoot is held in equinus. The forefoot is adducted and inverted by the combined action of the tight anterior and posterior tibial muscles.

At first the bony structures are normal. Later they become deformed as an adaptation to their persistently abnormal position. The top of the talus becomes flattened. The talar head enlarges. The calcaneus angulates medially. All metatarsals are curved medially. The cuneiforms and the cuboid become wedge shaped with the bases disposed dorsolaterally. Internal torsion of the tibia is a frequently associated deformity.

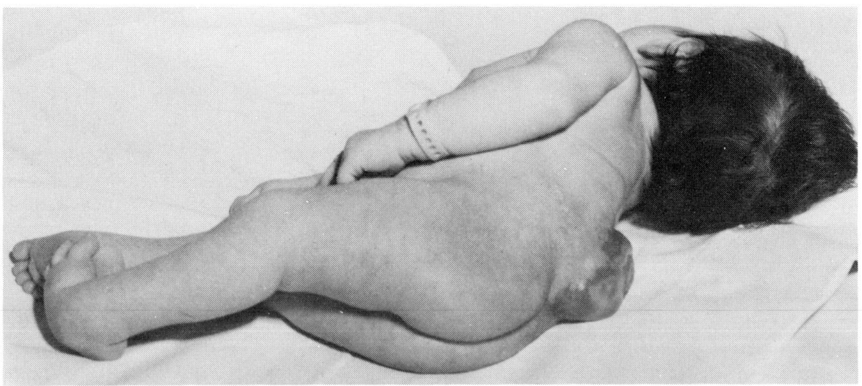

FIG. 11-32. Spina bifida. The associated clubfoot deformity is severe.

In talipes calcanovalgus, which constitutes the major part of the remaining clubfoot types, no definite pathology can be ascertained, because the deformity usually corrects spontaneously or with a minimum of treatment. However, should the deformity persist, the scaphoid displaces laterally with the forefoot structures, the head of the talus points medially and inferiorly, and the longitudinal arch is flattened. All ligamentous structures are lax and elongated.

CLINICAL PICTURE

The deformity is divisible into the following three main components:

Equinus. The forefoot is dropped plantarward. At the ankle, heel cord tight; at the midtarsal area, plantar structures tight.
Varus of heel. The tight medially inserted heel cord and medially contracted ligaments resist correction.
Adduction and varus of forefoot. The anterior and posterior tibial muscles pull the first metatarsal and the scaphoid into inversion.

In addition, the contracted plantar aponeurosis and muscles create a cavus deformity. The anterior end of the talus forms a dorsal and lateral bony prominence. The tibia is twisted inwardly. The deficient musculature causes an atrophic appearance of the leg. Flexibility of the foot is lost to a varying degree, depending on the severity and the age of the deformity (Fig. 11-33).

ROENTGENOGRAPHIC FINDINGS

Normally, the talus, the scaphoid, the inner cuneiform, and the first metatarsal form a straight line. In clubfoot, the scaphoid is displaced medially and inferiorly to the head of the talus, carrying the cuneiform and the metatarsal with it. The center of ossification for the scaphoid normally does not appear before the third or the fourth year, but the position of the cuneiform and the metatarsal indicates displacement of the scaphoid. The shadows of the talus and the calcaneus normally overlap except at the anterior end, where the calcaneus is displaced laterally, the axis of the calcaneus in line with the fourth and fifth metatarsals. In talipes equinovarus the anterior end of the calcaneus is displaced medially and overlaps the talar head. Correction demands that the medial and lateral axes be restored.

When the deformity has persisted for several years, the metatarsals become curved medially, the scaphoid becomes deformed and enlarged medially, and the talar head is asymmetrical and enlarged laterally and forms an obstacle to reduction. An anteroposterior view of the calcaneus reveals a varus deformity of the bone. The body of the talus is in equinus; only its posterior portion articulates with the tibia and is flattened and sclerotic.

In calcaneovalgus, radiographs are normal at first, but as time passes the scaphoid comes to lie lateral to the talar head, which in turn presents medially and plantarward. A lateral weight-bearing view reveals flattening of the longitudinal arch, evidence of ligamentous inadequacy.

FIG. 11-33. Talipes equinovarus deformity. Note the internal tibial torsion.

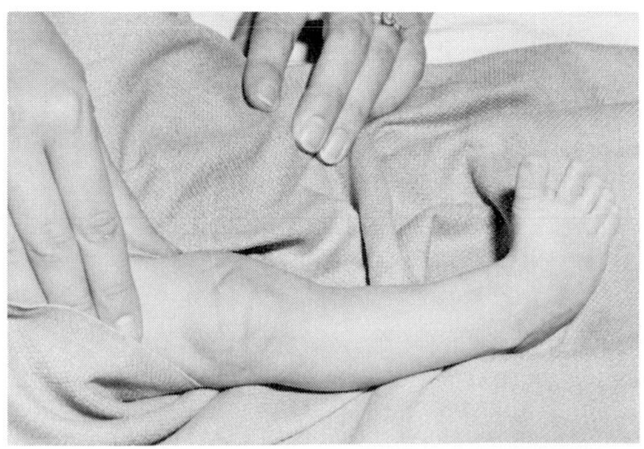

DIAGNOSIS

Assuming that no primary causative factors can be discovered, the deformity must be regarded as the typical primarily occurring clubfoot. The condition must be differentiated from the "Z" foot, which consists of metatarsus adductus and a relaxed valgus of the rear foot. This is a special entity in which the scaphoid lies lateral to the talus and therefore treatment by the usual method will displace the scaphoid further and produce a severe flatfoot.

TREATMENT

Conservative treatment consists in gradual manipulative reduction of the deformity and maintenance by retentive apparatus. This treatment is applicable to cases seen early, within the first year or two.

Surgical intervention is reserved for the clubfoot that resists conservative treatment or is seen at a late date, after the deformity has become fixed by the changing contour of the bony structures. The longer conservative treatment is delayed, the more resistant will be the deformity and the greater will be the need for surgical correction.

CONSERVATIVE

Manipulation is directed to stretching the contracted tissues gradually and repeated over a period of time—

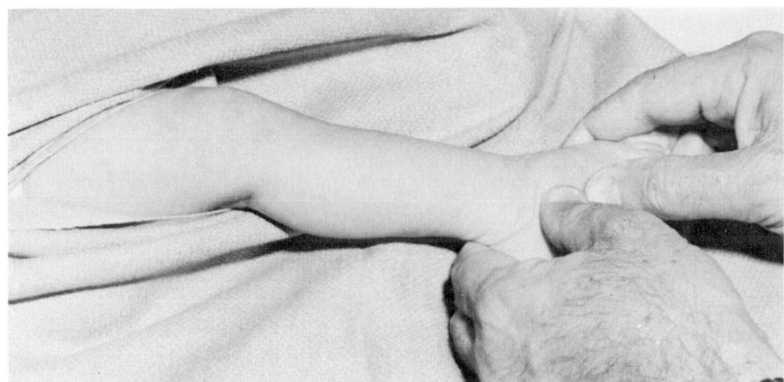

FIG. 11-34. Manipulation of talipes equinovarus. The tips of the thumbs form the fulcrum against which the fingers of the left hand evert the heel and the fingers of the right hand abduct and evert the metatarsals. Pressure is gentle, maintained a few seconds, and repeated.

weeks to months. No anesthesia is necessary. Gentleness and deliberateness are the essence of treatment. The adduction and varus components are corrected first. The foot is grasped by both hands so that the thumb tips press over the lateral bony prominence formed by the cuboid and the base of the fifth metatarsal. This acts as the fulcrum while fingers about the heel and the metatarsals pull these structures into abduction and eversion (Fig. 11-34). This is done gently and repeatedly. Forceful manipulation tears the contracted tissue medially, resulting in cicatrix; the joints will be damaged and eventually will become ankylosed. A stiff, permanently deformed foot would result.

When the deformity can be partially corrected with a minimum of pressure, a cast is applied, maintaining a position just short of the obtained correction. An assistant holds the limb with the knee flexed to a right angle while another assistant holds the foot in the corrected position. A few layers of protective sheet wadding are applied, and the cast bandage is rolled on smoothly from toes to upper thigh (Fig. 11-35). While the plaster is setting, the surgeon holds the foot in the corrected position. Attempts to obtain correction after applying the plaster will cause points of pressure necrosis and constriction of the foot and the leg. The parents are alerted to watch for danger signs over the ensuing hours. Cyanosis and swelling of the toes and continued irritability and crying by the infant are sufficient indication for removal of the cast and relief of pressure. At 2-week intervals the cast is removed and the procedure is repeated, a little more correction being secured at each visit. When varus and adduction have been overcome (as denoted by radiographic realignment of the axes), correction of the equinus is initiated. If this is started while the scaphoid is still displaced medially, recurrence of the deformity is the rule, because with weight bearing the talus will push on one side of the scaphoid and redisplace it. The foot should not be brought up before proper axial alignment has been obtained. Manipulation by stretching the calf muscles and the posterior capsule of the ankle is accomplished by direct upward pressure on the anterior end of the calcaneus. Pressure distal to the midtarsal joints causes the small tarsal bones to move dorsalward, resulting in a rocker-bottom foot. Repeated stretchings and castings are done until adequate dorsiflexion has been obtained.

FIG. 11-35. The finished cast. Note the equinus position during correction of the adduction and the varus. The cast extends above the knee, which is in the flexed position to prevent rotation of the limb within the cast, and relaxes the calf muscles.

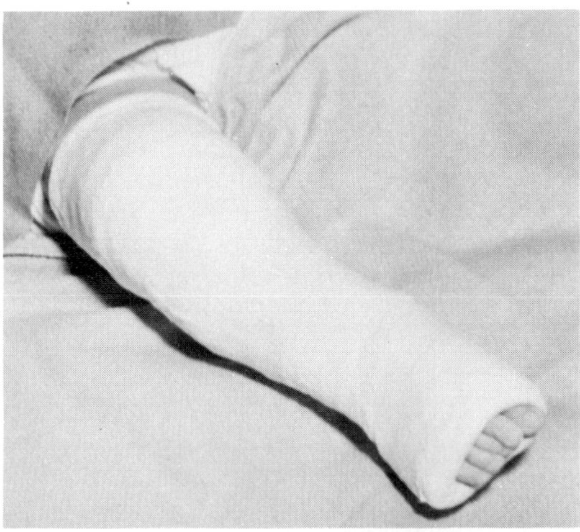

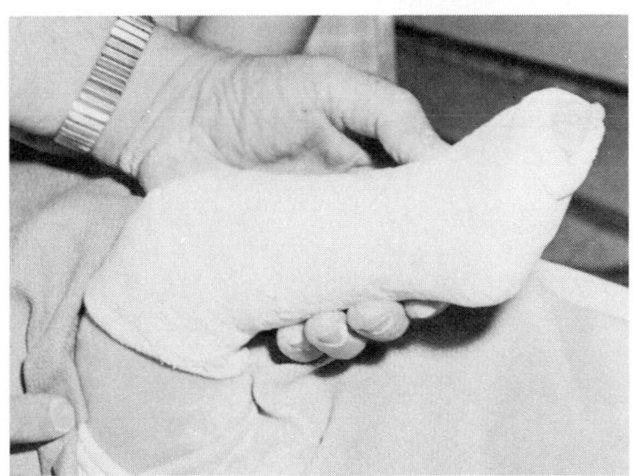

The tendency to recurrence is strong. Therefore, overcorrection to some degree toward the opposite deformity is advised by some authorities. However, Kite states that overcorrection of the scaphoid displacement leads to another disabling deformity, a flatfoot in which the scaphoid lies lateral and dorsal while the talar head protrudes medially and plantarward.[33] Nevertheless, persistence is necessary until complete anatomical restoration is attained. The correction is maintained by daily, continued, repeated manipulations and stretchings by the parents. The infant wears a "prewalker" shoe to aid in holding the correction until he can stand and walk (Fig. 11-36). This is a high-top shoe with an outflare last, a steel sole plate, a rigid extended counter, and a strap across the anterior aspect of the ankle to hold the foot snugly in the shoe.

The Denis Browne splint is also used to preserve correction. This consists of a metal bar with a sole plate at either end to which the feet are attached by adhesive bandaging. On the treated side, the plate is bent outward so that the foot is kept tilted in eversion, abduction, and external rotation. Theoretically, the child's kicking motions aid the correction. The Fillauer splint is a modification using clamps to hold shoes at the outer ends of the splint, which simplifies its application (Fig. 11-37). The parents need only insert the infant's feet in the shoes, which are already fixed in the appropriate position. The method does not eliminate the need for manipulations, particularly heel cord stretchings. By maintaining the feet continuously in external rotation, the internal tibial torsion may gradually be overcome.

Recurrence of deformity demands return to the original cast procedure. Resistant deformity should be overcome surgically.

SURGICAL

More than 50% of all clubfeet treated from birth by conservative methods have incomplete corrections and recurrent deformities requiring surgical measures. Operations are confined to the soft tissues when done before the age of 8 or 9 years. Before this time bony fusion is not feasible, because the bone structures are not sufficiently ossified. The surgical objective is to provide lasting correction and a flexible, plantigrade foot. Surgery is preferably done at an early age, as early as 1 or 2 years.

Soft Tissue Operation

The soft tissue procedure is based on the original Brockman operation under the premise that congenital atresia of the socket for the head of the talus was the cause of the deformity. The aim was to lengthen the shortened muscles acting upon the navicular and enlarging the socket.[28] Recurrences following this procedure were frequent.

Recent studies on biomechanics and pathologic anatomy have led to modifications of the original technique and improved the rate of success. Knowledge of the pathologic anatomy and of the mechanics of the articulations about the talus (talocalcaneonavicular joint) is essential to intelligent surgical planning.

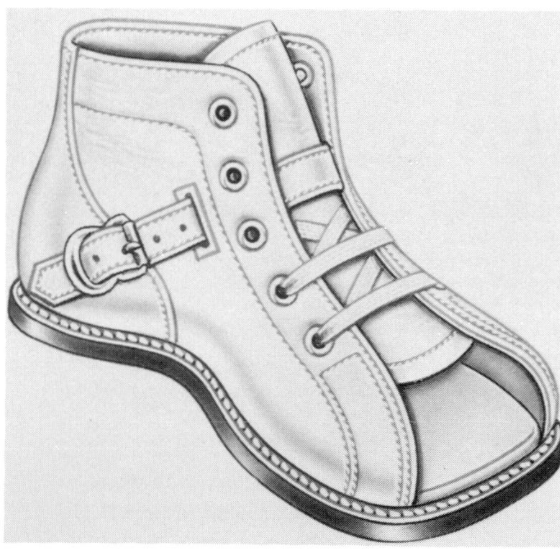

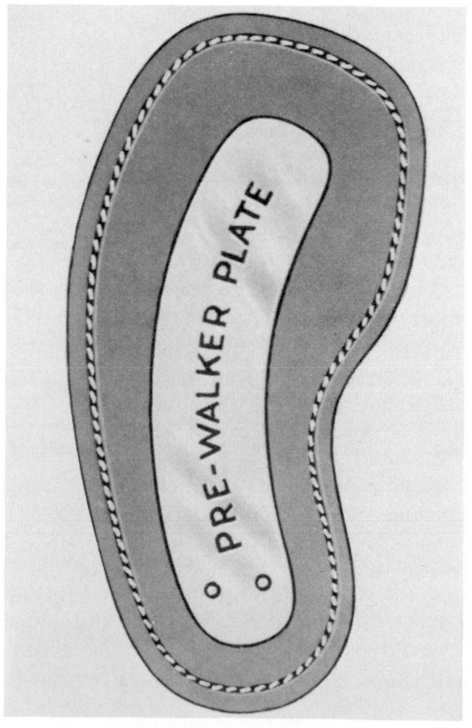

FIG. 11-36. The prewalker clubfoot shoe is used to maintain correction obtained by other means. It has no corrective function. Note the pronounced outflare of the forepart of the shoe, the retentive strap and buckle across the ankle, and the flat steel plate over the sole. (Courtesy of I. Sabel Company, Philadelphia)

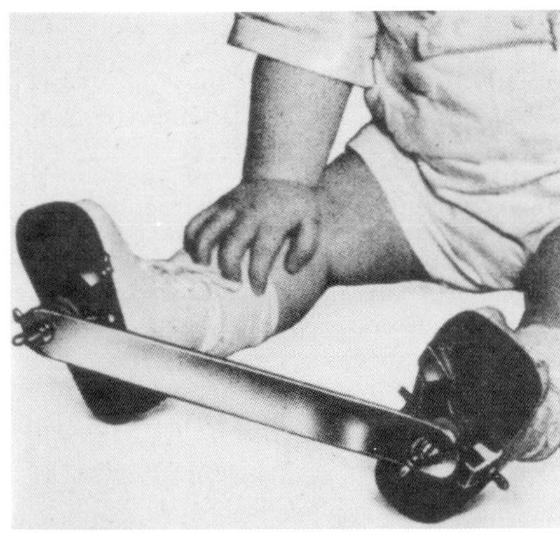

FIG. 11-37. Fillauer splint. The removable splint is useful for treating clubfoot and rotational deformities of the lower extremity. The shoe clamps may be rotated internally and externally. The flat intervening bar may be bent to hold the feet in inversion or eversion. An oversized bar will maintain wide abduction useful in treating dysplasia of the hip or after reduction of a dislocated hip. (Courtesy of The Fillauer Company, Chattanooga, Tenn.)

The talocalcaneonavicular joint complex comprises the midtarsal and subtalar articulations, excepting the calcaneocuboid joint.[32,38] The complex includes the talonavicular joint, the anterior and middle talocalcaneal articulations, and the plantar calcaneonavicular (spring) ligament. It is a ball-and-socket joint with a common synovial cavity separate from the posterior subtalar articulation. The head of the talus is contained in a socket that is formed anteriorly by the navicular; dorsomedially by the deltoid ligament, talonavicular joint capsule, and posterior tibial tendon; and laterally by the bifurcated (Y) ligament. The floor supporting the head of the talus is formed by the middle and anterior subtalar articular surfaces of the calcaneus and the spring ligament.

In contrast to the usual ball-and-socket articulation, the socket moves about the ball and expands and contracts, because it is composed in part of fibroelastic ligaments. The calcaneus and navicular do not articulate with each other, but together they move as a unit because of strong ligamentous attachments between them.

During dorsiflexion and plantar flexion of the foot, there is motion not only of the tibiotalar joint but also of the talocalcaneonavicular joint. As dorsiflexion occurs, the forefoot pronates and the calcaneus everts. The anterior end of the calcaneus moves laterally with the navicular while the posterior tuberosity moves downward. The talocalcaneonavicular socket deepens in dorsiflexion and covers more of the head of the talus.

During plantar flexion, the forefoot supinates and the calcaneus inverts, its anterior end moving downward and medially beneath the talus, while the posterior end moves upward and laterally. At the same time, the navicular moves medially on the head of the talus and the capacity of the socket becomes smaller, exposing more of the talar head laterally. Most of the varus and valgus motion takes place at the middle and anterior subtalar articulations and in the talonavicular joint. Very little motion takes place at the calcaneocuboid and posterior subtalar articulations.

Dorsiflexion of the foot takes place by two mechanisms, which occur simultaneously and which are interdependent. At the ankle joint, rotation of the talus requires relaxation of the calcaneal tendon. At the subtalar joint, around which the remainder of the foot rotates, the posterior tibial tendon must release to allow the naviculocalcaneal unit to shift outward. Shortening of either or both of these tendons will prevent full normal dorsiflexion. If both are tethered, the heel remains in equinus. If one is involved, dorsiflexion will occur but will be incomplete.[37]

Equinus of the calcaneus is associated with posterior displacement of the lateral malleolus. As the calcaneus everts and moves toward dorsiflexion, the lateral malleolus assumes its normal position. Therefore, when presistent equinus deformity of the calcaneus and posterior displacement of the lateral malleolus are noted on the roentgenogram, reduction of the clubfoot is regarded as incomplete.

Clubfoot is regarded as an exaggerated equinus and varus displacement of the talocalcaneonavicular joint, which is fixed by thickening and contractures of the soft tissues. In planning surgical correction, it is essential to recognize the mechanics and the pathologic contractures preventing reduction. Interference with the mobility at the talocalcaneonavicular socket will limit both vertical and horizontal motions of the foot. Restricted mobility of the navicular on the talus will limit subtalar motion.

The following three types of contractures are found:

Posterior. Posterior capsule, Achilles tendon, posterior talofibular and calcaneofibular ligaments

Medial. Deltoid and spring ligaments, talonavicular capsule, the tendon of the posterior tibial, and, to a lesser degree, tendons of the flexor digitorum longus and flexor hallucis longus

Subtalar. Anterior interosseous ligament, bifurcated ligament

Correction of the equinus position of the talus is resisted by the underlying calcaneus and posterior capsule, including the posterior talofibular ligament. With the talus in equinus, the posterior tuberosity of the calcaneus is displaced upward and laterally by the pathologic contractures of the posterior talocalcaneal capsule, the heel cord, and the calcaneofibular ligament. The anterior end of the calcaneus is displaced in the opposite direction downward, medially, and beneath the head of the talus. Correction of the anterior part of the deformity is resisted by contractures of the deltoid and spring ligaments, the posterior tibial tendon, and the subtalar interosseous ligament. The navicular is displaced medial to the head of the talus.

The result of the medial contractures is that the navicular, sustentaculum tali, and medial malleolus are pulled together by the contracted posterior tibial tendon, deltoid and spring ligaments, and talonavicular capsule. At surgery these structures are usually fused together into a dense mass of scar tissue that obscures the joint lines and the neck of the talus.

In older children, marked cavus deformity is added and is due to contracture of the plantar fascia and muscles that derive their origin from the calcaneus.

Posterior Release. For equinus deformity of the hindfoot, Achilles tendon lengthening is necessary. When deformity is minimal, subcutaneous tenotomy is sufficient. For severe deformity, lengthening under direct vision must be done. The tendon must be divided longitudinally in the transverse plane so that, after separation of the tendon segments, the distal exposed raw tendon surface lies anteriorly and the proximal exposed raw surface lies posteriorly, well protected by overlying thick subcutaneous tissue. If inadequate dorsiflexion is gained by tenotomy, posterior capsulotomy is added. The tibiotalar and talocalcaneal capsule and the calcaneofibular ligament are severed transversely, and the posterior talofibular ligament is severed vertically. After complete posterior release, a lateral roentgenogram is made in the operating room while the foot is dorsiflexed. If dorsiflexion of the calcaneus is inadequate and the lateral malleolus remains displaced posteriorly, medial release is necessary.

Sufficient strength of calf muscles is a necessary prerequisite for posterior release. Structural alteration of the talus that prevents its engaging in the ankle mortise is a contraindication.

A longitudinal incision, 8 cm to 10 cm, is made medial to the heel cord.[34] The tendon is divided longitudinally in a transverse plane. The posterior half remains attached to the calcaneus below, and the anterior half remains attached to the muscle belly above. The anterior half should remain anchored and not be freed from its peritendinous attachments in its proximal two thirds.

In most cases complete transection of the posterior ankle joint capsule with the posterior talotibial and talofibular ligaments is necessary. This requires ample exposure with retraction of the overlying tendons, nerve, and blood vessels. A dorsiflexing stretching force against the sole is maintained. The Achilles tendon is resutured in its elongated relationship and the wound closed. A cast is applied from the toes to the knee, and the knee is allowed to gradually straighten over several days. The need for wedging of the foot into increased dorsiflexion will depend on the initial amount of correction and the tension of the wound.

Medial Release. When equinus and varus deformity coexist, both must be overcome, either separately or at the same time. Posterior release alone will not correct hindfoot equinus, because the anterior end of the calcaneus is locked beneath the talus. Both ends of the calcaneus and the navicular must be freed so that the anterior end moves outward and upward with the navicular as the posterior tuberosity of the calcaneus moves downward. Varus and adduction displacement cannot be corrected without overcoming the equinus deformity.

Many techniques have been described. With minor variations, all embrace the principles of posterior, medial, and subtalar release, and all agree on eliminating the deforming force of the posterior tibial muscle. The following technique is representative of the basic principles (Fig. 11-38).

The medial incision begins at the base of the first metatarsal and extends backward, curving beneath the medial malleolus to end at the Achilles tendon.[38] The tendon of the abductor hallucis is secured distally and traced backward to the muscle, which is folded plantarward exposing the tendons and neurovascular structures. The posterior tibial tendon is exposed first and its sheath incised. In the clubfoot it lies more anterior and vertical than in the normal foot. The flexor digitorum longus is next exposed just below the posterior tibial tendon and freed from its sheath. Just behind this lies the neurovascular bundle in a common sheath; it is mobilized and retracted posteriorly. Then the flexor hallucis longus is identified under the sustentaculum tali and freed from its sheath. When the bundle is retracted anteriorly, the Achilles tendon is exposed. Finally, the exposure is completed by dividing the master knot of Henry. This fibrocartilaginous structure is attached to the undersurface of the navicular and envelops the flexor digitorum longus and flexor hallucis longus where they cross. It is necessary to excise the master knot of Henry to mobilize the navicular.

The Achilles tendon is lengthened by Z-plasty, detaching the medial calcaneal insertion. After the Achilles tendon is divided, anterior retraction of the neurovascular bundle and flexor hallucis longus brings the posterior aspect of the ankle into view. The posterior margin of the tibia is identified, and posterior capsulotomy of the tibiotalar joint is done. By extending the capsulotomy laterally, the posterior talofibular ligament is severed. Next the posterior capsule of the subtalar joint and the calcaneofibular ligament are divided.

Finally, the neurovascular bundle is retracted posteriorly. The posterior portion of the deltoid ligament is incised by extending the posterior subtalar capsulotomy medially.

Medial release is next accomplished. The tendons and neurovascular bundle are retracted, exposing a mass of scar tissue composed of the posterior tibial tendon, the superficial deltoid ligament, the capsule of the talonavicular joint, and the spring ligament. The mass obscures the joint lines and the neck of the talus.

The navicular is displaced medial to the head of the

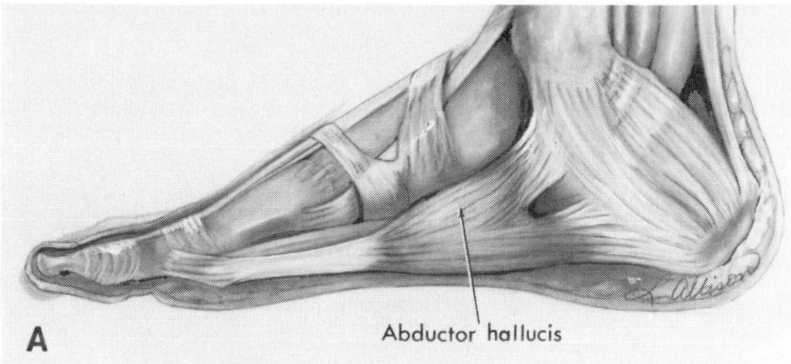

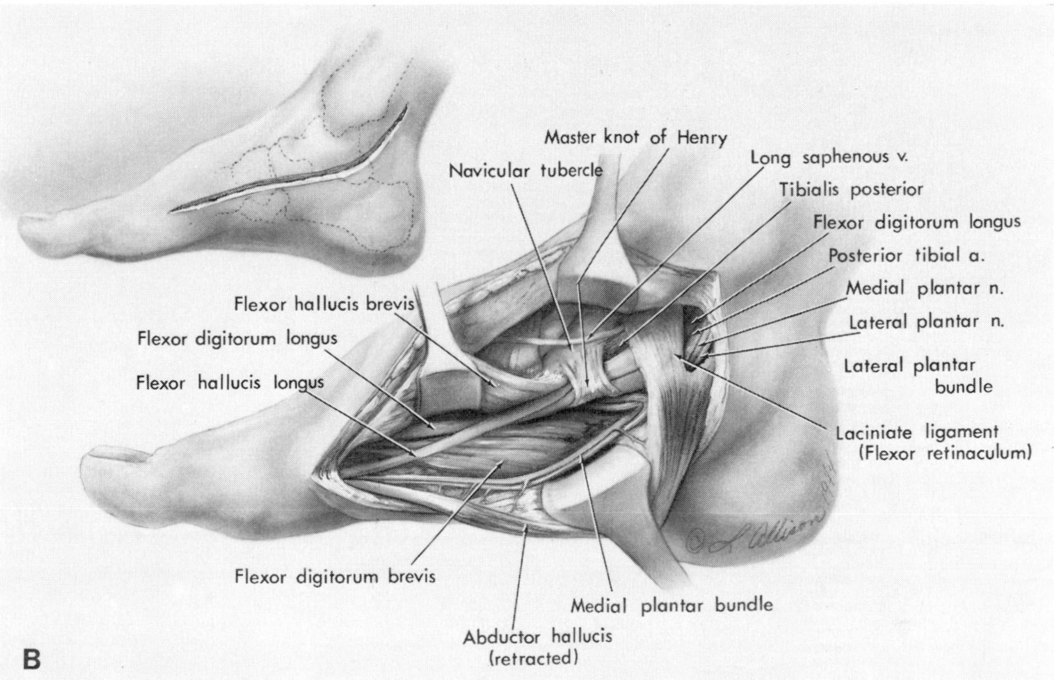

FIG. 11-38. Surgical correction of resistant talipes equinovarus. (*A*) The abductor hallucis muscle is the key to the medial approach. By freeing its anterior border and its posterior attachment to the laciniate ligament, it can be folded outward as a hinge exposing the medial structures. Adjoining the abductor hallucis on its inner aspect is the flexor hallucis brevis; the two muscles can be reflected together exposing the capsuloligamentous structures on the plantar aspect of the foot. (*B*) Exposure of medial aspect of the foot. The direction and length of the incision may be varied depending on whether posterior release is done at the same time. The abductor hallucis is retracted exposing the master knot of Henry. A mass of fibrous tissue may envelop all structures making identification difficult, but the posterior tibial tendon can be secured proximally and traced distally to its insertion at the navicular tubercle. (*Figure continues on pages 322–323.*)

talus. Mobilization of the navicular is begun by cutting the posterior tibial tendon just above the medial malleolus. The proximal end of the tendon is allowed to retract. The mass of scar tissue is excised. Traction on the distal stump of the posterior tibial tendon opens the talonavicular joint and permits excision of the deltoid ligament insertion on the navicular and the talonavicular capsule. The posterior tibial attachments to both the sustentaculum tali and the spring ligament are incised, and the spring ligament is detached from the sustentaculum tali. Mobilization of the navicular now exposes the false articular facet on the proximal and medial aspect of the head of the talus. The talar head usually faces slightly more medially toward the medially displaced navicular than it normally does.

The medial release is completed by returning to the posterior capsulotomy and everting the foot. The subtalar joint is thereby exposed, permitting release of the superficial layer of the deltoid ligament from the calcaneus. The deep portion of the deltoid ligament, which inserts

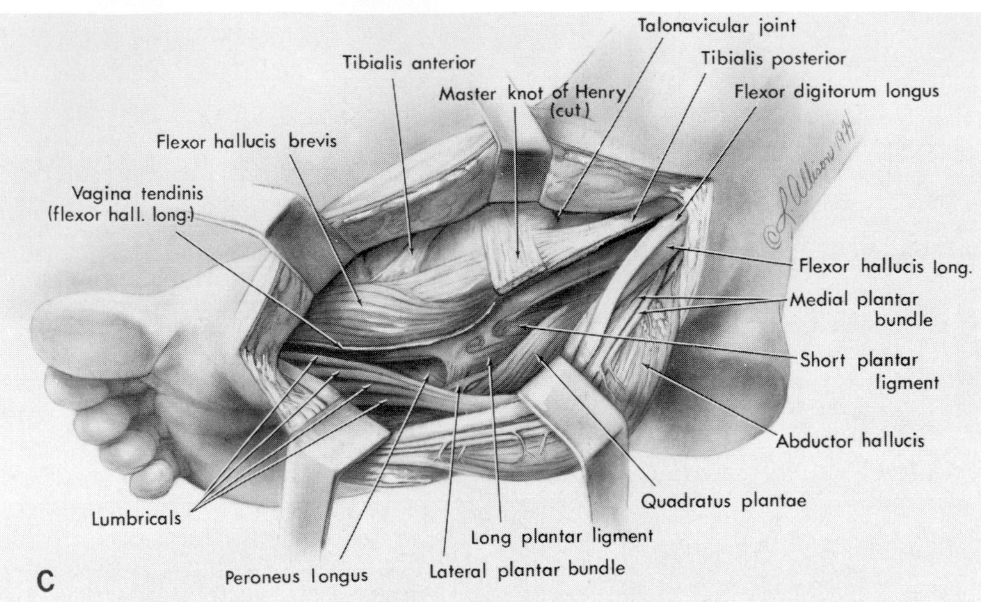

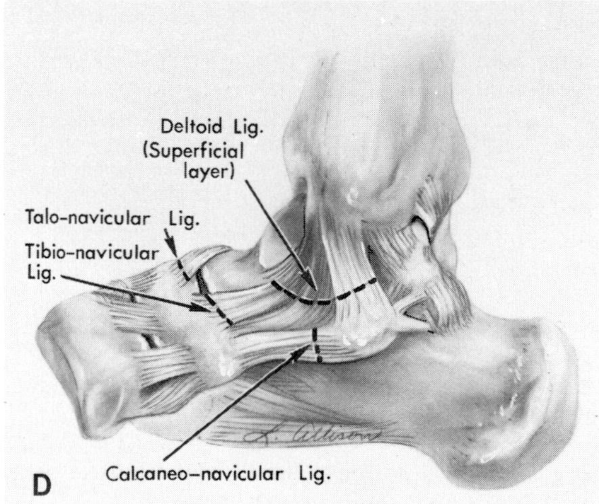

FIG. 11-38 (*continued*). (*C*) Medial approach at a deeper level. The master knot of Henry has been cut; the approach to the plantar aspect is made between the abductor hallucis and flexor hallucis brevis, and the plantar ligaments are exposed. The tibialis posterior must be divided at its insertion and allowed to retract, or it may be divided proximally for lengthening later and retracted posteriorly with the tendons of the flexor digitorum longus and flexor hallucis longus and the neurovascular bundle, exposing the sustentaculum tali and deltoid ligament. Later, these tendons and neurovascular bundle may be retracted anteriorly while exposing the posterior capsule. (*D*) Medial release. Division of the deltoid ligament must be limited to the superficial layer. The plantar ligaments originating from the calcaneus need not be divided unless cavus deformity is associated. Adduction and plantar flexion deformity of the first ray, usually seen in late cases, may require division of the naviculocuneiform capsule.

into the body of the talus, must be preserved. If this is divided, a flatfoot deformity with tilting of the talus may develop,

Subtalar release completes the mobilization of the anterior end of the calcaneus and the navicular. The talocalcaneal interosseous ligament is exposed by everting the foot and is transected. Mobilization of the navicular is completed by cutting the bifurcated ligament. This ligament extends from the calcaneus to the lateral border of the cuboid. The distal remnant of the posterior tibial tendon is cut from the navicular.

The deformity can now be reduced without force, replacing the navicular in front of the head of the talus. The anterior end of the calcaneus moves laterally and

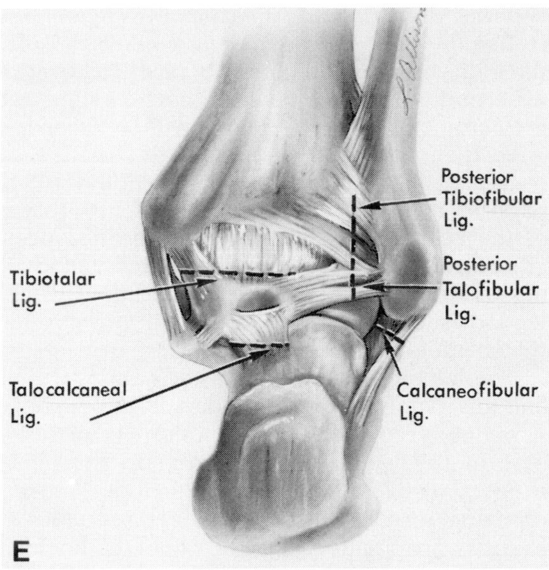

FIG. 11-38 (*continued*). (*E*) Posterior release is indicated when Achilles tendon lengthening does not correct equinus deformity sufficiently. Usually only division of the tibiotalar and talocalcaneal ligaments is necessary; the posterior talofibular and calcaneofibular ligaments may be added. This will correct most of the equinus, but complete correction must await medial release.

everts while its posterior end moves downward and away from the ankle joint. Overcorrection must be avoided, since this will result in flatfoot and eventual metatarsus adductus. The talonavicular joint is transfixed with a Kirschner wire. The Achilles tendon is repaired with interrupted chromic sutures. After closure, the protruding wire is bent outside the skin but is not incorporated in the cast.

After 3 weeks the cast is changed under general anesthesia and a new above-the-knee cast is applied. The cast is changed at 6 weeks when the Kirschner wire and sutures are removed. Immobilization continues over a 4-month period. Then the foot is protected with a Denis Browne splint with everting crossbar.

Technique in Older Child With Cavus Deformity. Children 3 to 5 years old have an associated severe cavus deformity with plantar flexion of the first metatarsal. A Steindler stripping must be added. The origin of the plantar fascia is excised, and the abductor hallucis, intrinsic toe flexors, and abductor digiti quinti muscles are stripped subperiosteally from the calcaneus. The navicular often presents an enlarged tuberosity that must be excised. If the forefoot is adducted, the capsule between the navicular and cuneiform is incised and multiple capsulotomies of the tarsometatarsal joints may be necessary.

Tendon Transfer. True congenital equinovarus shows no evidence of muscle imbalance. The anterior tibial and the peronei may be weakened by stretching but are not truly paralyzed and are capable of regaining their strength once the deformity is corrected. The posterior tibial acts as an adducting and inverting deforming force because its insertion is often found to consist of a thick, hard fibrous mass from which radiate thick strands of fibrous tissue extending over and engulfing structures on the dorsal, the medial, and the plantar aspects of the foot.[30] Posterior tibial action is reduced by tendon lengthening or entirely eliminated by tendon resection. Rarely, when deformity is severe and recurrence is probable, the posterior tibial tendon may be transferred by way of the interosseous route to the dorsal aspect of the foot.

Deformity in paralytic equinovarus in the growing child is extremely prone to recurrence even when tarsal arthrodesing procedures have been done. Transfer of the posterior tibial tendon, if available, is essential. Tibialis anterior transfer is much less effective.[36] In any equinovarus deformity in which muscle imbalance is suspected, electromyographic studies should be done to determine whether tendon transfer should be considered. Tendon transfer is best done when the child is old enough to cooperate in muscle re-education.

Technique. First, the deformity is corrected by manipulation and casts. At surgery, the entire posterior tibial tendon and its fibrous prolongations are freed and detached. Achilles tenotomy and posterior capsulotomy of the ankle are done. The posterior tibial muscle is freed well proximally with care to preserve its innervation. Then the tendon and muscle are passed through a large opening in the interosseous membrane to emerge between the bellies of the extensor hallucis longus and the extensor digitorum longus. The free tendon is passed down the sheath of the extensor digitorum longus and fixed in a hole drilled in a dorsoplantar direction in the third cuneiform. Postoperatively, cast immobilization of 6 weeks is followed by a night splint for an additional 3 months.

Combined Soft Tissue and Bone Operation. When deformity remains uncorrected beyond the age of 3 years, adaptive bone architecture changes take place. The bone structures at the outer border of the foot become elongate and are arranged in a convex manner. The cuboid assumes a wedged configuration, its proximal and distal articular surfaces diverging outward. The calcaneus gradually assumes a varus shape. The metatarsals deviate medially at the tarsometatarsal joints. Soft tissue release no longer suffices to overcome the deformity. Bone procedures must be added.

At an early stage of resistant clubfoot, in addition to medial, posterior, and subtalar release, the outer column must be shortened. Between 3 and 6 years of age, the calcaneocuboid and cuboid metatarsal joints must not be violated to avoid interfering with growth. Instead, decancellation of the interior of the cuboid is accomplished by curetting through a small opening. Then, as the deformity is overcome by forcible wrenching, the cuboid is compressed to a fraction of its former size.

Beyond 6 years of age, tarsal distortion is greater and the deformity is more resistant to correction. A dorsolateral wedge is removed from the calcaneocuboid joint. The opening thus created is extended medially to communicate with the talonavicular joint, forming one continuous articulation (Chopart's joint). The forefoot with the distal tarsals is then moved outward and upward, closing the calcaneocuboid interval, which is then fixed with a staple.

Severe varus deformity of the calcaneus can be corrected later by a Dwyer osteotomy. Metatarsal adduction requires multiple capsulotomies of the tarsometatarsal joints or multiple osteotomies at the base of the metatarsals.

Rarely, it may be advisable to transfer the posterior tibial through the interosseous membrane to the third cuneiform.[35] The tibialis anterior should not be used. Removal of this tendon from its normal position results in dropping of the forefoot, depression of the first metatarsal head, and a cocked-up hallux.

The following technique embodies the principles but may be modified to suit the individual case.

Technique. Preliminary manipulations and corrective casts reduce the deformity as much as possible.[29]

The medial incision starts just in front of the tubercle of the navicular bone and runs backward along the line of the tendon of the tibialis posterior, beneath the medial malleolus and up the leg along the anterior border of the tendo calcaneus for a distance of 2 or 3 inches. The tight plantar structures are divided with a tenotome (or Steindler stripping may be done). The tendon of the tibialis posterior is exposed throughout its length from the medial malleolus to its insertion into the navicular. In some feet it will be found to be a well-differentiated tendon; in others it may be poorly differentiated in its distal half inch and may even merge with a small mass of fibrocartilaginous tissue that may occupy the space between the medial surface of the head of the talus and the medially subluxated navicular bone. The tendon must be dissected free from this slab of tissue and the tissue mass excised to expose the talonavicular joint. Then the tendon is lengthened by Z-plasty, taking care to allow for a substantial increase in length, and the capsule of the talonavicular joint is divided on its superior, medial, and inferior surfaces, thereby allowing free lateral movement of the navicular on the talus. (However, this may not be possible until further medial release is accomplished by sectioning the superficial layer of the deltoid ligament and the subtalar interosseous ligament.) Next, the proximal half of the incision is deepened to expose the tendo calcaneus, which is isolated and lengthened by Z-plasty.

This will only occasionally allow correction of equinus; in most cases it is also necessary to divide the posterior capsule of the ankle and any tight strands of fibrous tissue that may be running parallel with the tendon; in some cases the tendon will be poorly differentiated, and very free dissection and division of tissue will be needed to free the back of the ankle and allow dorsiflexion of the joint. In a small minority of older feet even this free dissection will not permit correction to a right angle, and the extra leverage of a wrench will be needed, but this wrench should not be used strongly, and it should not be used at all unless every strand of contracted soft tissue has been divided. (It is particularly essential that eversion of the calcaneus is possible after medial and subtalar release.) It is essential to correct equinus before proceeding to the next part of the operation. The elongated tendons should not be sutured until the second part of the operation has been completed.

The lateral incision crosses the calcaneocuboid joint and runs parallel with the tendon of the peroneus brevis. A wedge is removed from the calcaneocuboid joint, the base of the wedge corresponding to the direction of maximal convexity. Then the forefoot is rotated in a pronatory direction, the cuboid rotating on the calcaneus in such a way as to bring the head of the first metatarsal to the ground. At the same time the navicular bone moves laterally on the head of the talus. The calcaneal and cuboid raw bone surfaces are apposed and held with two staples.

The elongated tendons are sutured, and the wounds are closed. The foot is immobilized in plaster until the joint is arthrodesed, usually after about 5 months. Roentgenologic evidence of fusion is not seen in the young child. Walking in a plaster cast is permitted after 6 weeks.

The procedure may be modified by freeing the posterior tibial tendon and muscle proximally, routing the tendon through an adequate opening in the interosseous membrane and fixing it to the dorsolateral aspect of the foot.

Roentgenographic Evidence of Satisfactory Correction

The A-P (anteroposterior) view shows adequate divergence of the axes of the talus and the calcaneus (Kite's angle). This in itself is not certain evidence that the calcaneus and navicular have been repositioned correctly. A lateral roentgenogram must be made with the foot held in maximum dorsiflexion. In the uncorrected clubfoot, this view shows inadequate dorsal movement of the anterior end of the calcaneus, parallelism of the talus and calcaneus, and absence of the normal overlap of the anterior end of the talus and calcaneus. Failure of the calcaneus to dorsiflex is evidence of incomplete subtalar correction regardless of the apparent normal appearance on the A-P roentgenogram. When full dorsiflexion of the calcaneus can be demonstrated repeatedly over several months, recurrence is unlikely.

LATE DEFORMITY

The calcaneus and all tarsals become adaptively contoured to a deformity that is allowed to persist throughout

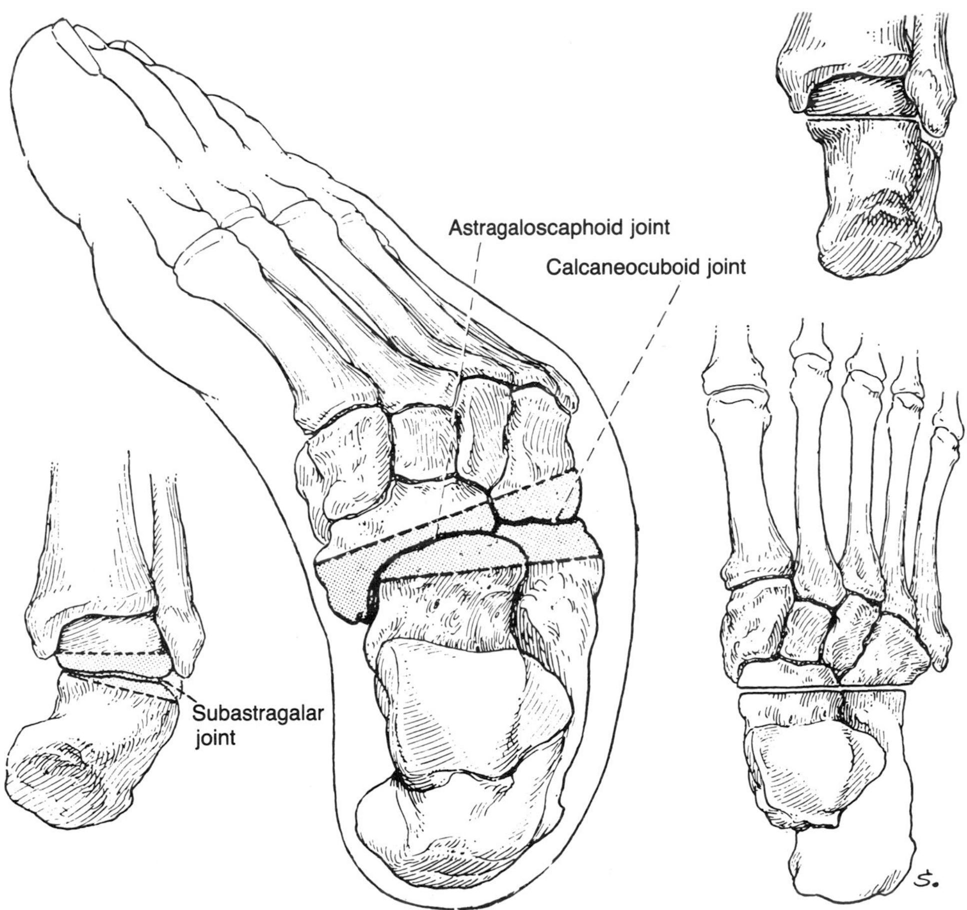

FIG. 11-39. Bony reconstruction for neglected equinovarus deformity. The wedges are removed from the midtarsal and the astragalocalcaneal joints with their bases directed toward the direction of convexity. (Speed JS, Knight RA: Campbell's Operative Orthopaedics. St. Louis, CV Mosby, 1971)

the growth period. Except for posterior release, soft tissue operations are useless. The deformity must be corrected by ample bone resections, preferably after 10 years of age. Triple arthrodesis requires removal of wedges of bone with the bases directed laterally from the midtarsal joint and from the subtalar joint (Fig.11-39).

CONGENITAL METATARSUS ADDUCTOVARUS

Congenital metatarsus adductovarus (congenital metatarsus varus, metatarsus adductus, pes adductus, skewfoot) appears to be increasing in frequency or recognized more often and consists of medial displacement of the distal shafts of the metatarsals (adduction), inversion of the forepart of the foot (supination), eversion and lateral displacement of the navicular and calcaneus (pronation), and often the development of a cavus arch.[40–42]

At birth, in contrast with clubfoot, the deformity is mild and often overlooked. However, within the first few weeks, the big toe and first metatarsal are pulled medially by strong contractions of the abductor hallucis. The deformity becomes more evident by gently stroking the inner aspect of the foot. The deformity appears to be adversely influenced by the infant's sleeping prone posture with the lower extremities flexed and tucked in beneath the buttocks. As the deformity increases, the forefoot becomes inverted (varus) and pulled upward and inward by the anterior tibial. This muscle has an anomalous insertion wrapping extensively about the medial side of the first metatarsal and passing to the inferomedial aspect of the foot. This action eventually elevates the longitudinal arch into a cavus. Meanwhile, the navicular displaces toward the outer aspect of the talar head as the calcaneus everts. This component of the deformity becomes more evident at a later age, when the infant stands. The outer border of the foot becomes convex, and a palpable prominence develops, representing the cuboid and base of the fifth metatarsal.

Initially, in most cases, the deformity is passively correctable and, if untreated, will spontaneously correct, resulting in a normal foot or at the most a minimal deformity.

Approximately 10% of cases are progressive. The adductocavovarus and calcaneonavicular eversion deformities become increasingly rigid and resistant to passive correction, all metatarsals being drawn medially and inverted. When weight is borne on this foot, in order that the medial border of the foot make contact with the floor, the foot rotates (pronates) on its longitudinal axis so that the hind foot, or calcaneonavicular unit, is thrown into eversion or valgus. Finally, a rigid severe deformity results in the adult: All metatarsals, especially the first, are adducted and supinated; the adducted first metatarsal forms a bunion, and the big toe deviates outward (hallux valgus) in response to shoe pressure. Thus, what appears to have been a mild deformity consisting of intoeing of the big toe may have serious long-term implications. With advancing age, the "serpentine or Z-foot" deformity develops, consisting of adduction and varus of the metatarsals, hallux valgus, valgus of the calcaneus, and cavus. Although disability may not be extreme, gait is ungainly, the shoes wear out quickly over its outer border, and intermittent pressure annoyances (*e.g.*, bursitis, calluses, bunion) are common.

EARLY RECOGNITION

If treatment is to be successful, the condition must be recognized before deformity is severe and fixed. An overacting abductor hallucis can be demonstrated by stroking the inner aspect of the foot, whereupon the big toe moves medially and the first metatarsal deviates away from the second. Normally, during infancy the longitudinal arch is filled with a fat pad and therefore is not apparent. However, by making an imprint of the sole, early cavus deformity may be detected. At first the tarsal area and the metatarsals appear quite mobile and remain so in most cases, but serial examinations will eventually disclose the occasional case that will not spontaneously correct. Passive correctability becomes increasingly difficult. Early development of rigidity causes the first metatarsal to become persistently adducted. The heel now is rigidly everted. A bony prominence over the outer border of the foot consists of the cuboid and base of the fifth metatarsal. Equinus deformity is never observed. Medial tibial torsion is usually associated.

ROENTGENOGRAPHIC FINDINGS

The A-P x-ray exposure is made with the infant's foot placed firmly against the cassette (Fig. 11-40). As the deformity develops, the findings are characteristic and are most pronounced by the second year. The metatarsals become sharply and medially angulated at the tarsometatarsal joints. The base of the first metatarsal articulates with the medial aspect of the first cuneiform, which is irregular in shape. The ossification centers for the first and second cuneiforms and the navicular are normally not evident before the second year, and their appearance may be delayed. By tracing proximally the direction of the first metatarsal as it points toward the lateral aspect of the talar head, this defines the location of the navicular. The first and second metatarsals are widely separated. When varus or inversion is present, the metatarsals are rotated about their axes so that their dorsal convexities are visible in the A-P view, producing spurious medial curving of the shafts. Valgus of the heel is evidenced by an extraordinary wide divergence of the longitudinal axes of talus and calcaneus.

TREATMENT

CONSERVATIVE

Mild, passively correctable deformities require no treatment, because they tend to correct spontaneously. Nevertheless, every deformity, however mild, should be observed repeatedly within the first year, since an occasional case with progressive deformity and increasing rigidity will be disclosed at the earliest moment, when conservative treatment (manipulations and corrective casts) is most effective. Improperly carried out manipulations, particularly when entrusted to the novice who may be misled into attempting to correct the deformity by forcefully pronating the foot, will increase valgus deformity of the heel and result in a severe flatfoot and a disability worse than the original. Manipulations should not be delegated to the parents. Swungout shoes and an abduction bar (Denis Browne splint) are ineffectual and encourage eversion of the heel.

Manipulation is gentle and carried out without anesthesia. The deformity of the hindfoot is corrected by supinating the calcaneus underneath the talus. The anterior aspect of the calcaneus must be brought beneath the head of the talus. Since the plane of the subtalar joint rises slightly in a lateral and backward direction, medial displacement of the anterior process of the calcaneus requires slight plantar flexion of the heel before the heel can be inverted. When the heel is adducted and inverted, it is accompanied by medial displacement and inversion of the scaphoid and cuboid bones together with the cuneiforms. The bases of the metatarsals are now in proper alignment with the talus and calcaneus. Next, adduction of the metatarsals is corrected by simply abducting them while counterpressure is applied over the cuboid. The forefoot is not pronated.

Application of the cast is done while an assistant holds the toes between the thumb and index finger of one hand while holding the knee at a right angle with the other hand. The heel is held in a few degrees of equinus and in complete inversion. Since no effort is made at this time to correct the medial tibial torsion, the foot will point medially. One layer of sheet wadding is applied,

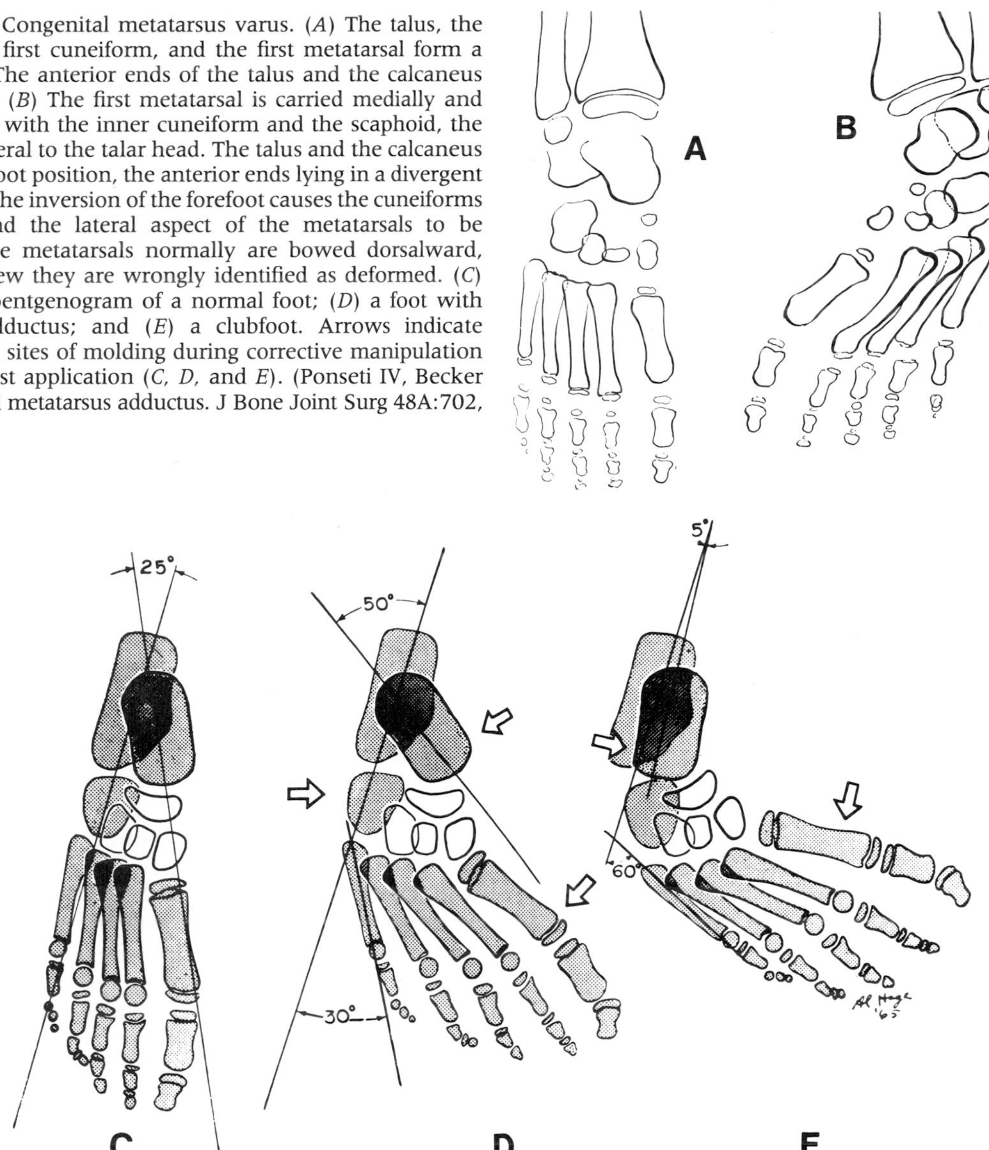

FIG. 11-40. Congenital metatarsus varus. (*A*) The talus, the scaphoid, the first cuneiform, and the first metatarsal form a straight line. The anterior ends of the talus and the calcaneus are separated. (*B*) The first metatarsal is carried medially and is in line only with the inner cuneiform and the scaphoid, the latter lying lateral to the talar head. The talus and the calcaneus are in the flatfoot position, the anterior ends lying in a divergent relationship. The inversion of the forefoot causes the cuneiforms to overlap and the lateral aspect of the metatarsals to be visualized. The metatarsals normally are bowed dorsalward, and in this view they are wrongly identified as deformed. (*C*) Diagram of roentgenogram of a normal foot; (*D*) a foot with metatarsus adductus; and (*E*) a clubfoot. Arrows indicate directions and sites of molding during corrective manipulation and plaster-cast application (*C, D,* and *E*). (Ponseti IV, Becker JH: Congenital metatarsus adductus. J Bone Joint Surg 48A:702, 1966)

with an additional layer about the head of the fibula. Then a 3-inch plaster bandage is applied. The first section of the plaster cast extends from the toes, covering the assistant's fingers, to just below the knee. The plaster is closely wrapped about the foot and ankle and less snugly about the leg. Corrective molding is accomplished as follows: The hindfoot is inverted and slightly plantar flexed to correct the valgus deformity of the heel, while counterpressure is applied over the cuboid and the anterior part of the foot is abducted with slight pressure applied to the head and neck of the first metatatsal. To avoid a cavus deformity, the anterior part of the foot must not be pronated. The longitudinal and transverse arches and the heel are well molded. After the first section of the cast hardens, the foot and leg are externally rotated to correct the medial tibial torsion and a 4-inch plaster roll is applied to the knee and thigh. Manipulations and casts are repeated at 10-day to 2-week intervals. A slightly overcorrected position should be sought.

SURGICAL

If the deformity is initially seen at an advanced stage and is rigid and unresponsive to conservative treatment, surgical correction is indicated.

Early Deformity

Within the first few years, soft tissue release is sufficient. The abductor hallucis may be severed, and the distal portion of the anterior tibial insertion may be severed. Capsulotomies of the tarsometatarsal joints require that both the capsules and the intermetatarsal ligaments be completely severed to facilitate outward angulation. The lateral portion of the capsule of the fifth metatarsocuboid joint must be preserved to provide a stabilizing hinge, which will prevent lateral displacement of the base of the fifth metatarsal. At this site, the insertion of the peroneus brevis must be preserved.

Capsulotomy of the first metatarsocuneiform joint may be sufficient. The growth plate of the first metatarsal is situated near the base and must be protected.

Usually capsulotomies of all tarsometatarsal joints are necessary.[39] When the calcaneonavicular unit is fixed in eversion, the Grice procedure may be added. Although limiting operations to soft tissue procedures at an early age is designed to preclude interference with bone growth, the foot often remains slightly undersized.

Late Deformity

Bone procedures are reserved for severe deformities after adequate growth has been attained. If deformity is moderate and the child is more than 8 years of age, osteotomies at the bases of the metatarsals will allow correction of the metatarsus adductus. The Grice procedure must be added. Any bone procedure adjacent to the growth plate at the base of the first metatarsal may compromise further growth and is a distinct hazard.

After full growth is attained, severe adaptive bone changes can be overcome only by wedge resections and a triple arthrodesis. Since late deformity is mainly disfiguring, disability for the activities of daily living is generally not severe enough to warrant such extensive surgery. Under exceptional circumstances (*e.g.*, an occupation requiring prolonged standing and walking), a bone reconstruction procedure may be indicated.

CONGENITAL HALLUX VARUS

Congenital hallux varus is a deformity found at birth, consisting of medial angulation of the large toe at the metatarsophalangeal joint. One or more of the following conditions are present:[43]

First metatarsal bone usually short and thick
Accessory bone and toes often associated
Varus deformity of one or more of the other metatarsal bones
Firm fibrous band extends from inner side of large toe to base of first metatarsal. Over the medial aspect of the first metatarsal, an articulation with a small accessory bone represents a vestigial accessory toe. This may be the incompletely developed medial segment of a primary double hallux.

Other causes of hallux varus include overcorrection of a bunion operation, paralysis of the adductor hallucis, infection about the metatarsophalangeal joint, and malunion of fractures about the joint.

TREATMENT

The correction is surgical. Through a dorsal longitudinal incision, the interspace between the first two metatarsal heads is developed, and bone is excised from the lateral aspect of the head of the first metatarsal. The capsule is freed from about the dorsal, medial, and plantar aspects of the metatarsal head. Next, the accessory bone, the fibrous band, and the medial sesamoid are removed from the medial side of the metatarsal. Then freeing of the capsule from the metatarsal is completed. At this stage the toe can easily be displaced laterally. The extensor hallucis brevis tendon is severed at its junction with the muscle, and while the toe is held laterally in the corrected position the tendon is routed through a drill hole in the metatarsal neck. The lateral capsule is imbricated to maintain the new position. Postoperatively, firm bandaging to the other toes is all that is necessary.

CONGENITAL OVERLAPPING LITTLE TOE

In congenital overlapping little toe, which is usually bilateral, the small toe is dorsiflexed, rotated so that its dorsal surface faces laterally, and adducted over the fourth toe. By passively flexing the toe, the taut extensor tendon stands out prominently as the main factor preventing reduction of the deformity. Little or no disability arises, although occasionally pain from shoe pressure and formation of corns are sources of annoyance. Therefore, surgical correction is rarely indicated (Fig. 11-41).

TREATMENT

When the deformity is mild, passive stretching into flexion and abduction may suffice.

For pronounced deformity, correction requires surgery. Since the problem is mainly cosmetic rather than disabling, surgery is rarely necessary.

The principal deforming factors that must be overcome are a taut long extensor tendon, relative shortening of the dorsal skin, dorsal capsular contracture, and, frequently, capsular adherence to the volar aspect of the fifth metatarsal head.

The multiplicity of procedures that has been devised attests to their drawbacks: incomplete reduction, recurrence rate, and complications such as circulatory impairment with possible loss of the toe, delayed wound healing, and marked scarring. It is highly inadvisable to invite such risks for what is basically a cosmetic defect.

I use the following procedure, which appears to pose the least risk or rate of recurrence: extensor tenotomy,

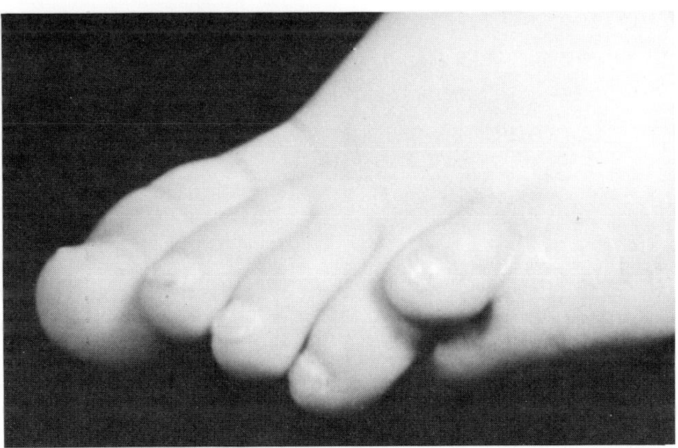

FIG. 11-41. Overlapping little toe. The toe is short, dorsiflexed, rotated, and adducted.

capsulotomy, partial phalangectomy, artificial syndactylism.

1. The toes are held widely apart, exposing the web space. A horizontal incision is made across the web extending along the side of each toe as a paradigital incision as far distally as the level of the base of the nail.
2. A dorsal longitudinal incision is made bisecting the dorsal edge of the horizontal incision and exposing the long extensor tendon; the latter is severed.
3. Dorsal, medial, and lateral portions of the capsule are severed. This allows the toe to drop down. Plantar flexion may be limited by adherence of the volar plate to the undersurface of the metatarsal head, which must be freed by blunt dissection.
4. The base of the proximal phalanx is excised. During the growth period, the proximal portion of the phalanx must be preserved and the distal portion removed.
5. A V-shaped segment of skin is removed from the plantar flap.
6. The toes are apposed, and the dorsal and plantar wound edges are sutured together, effecting an artificial syndactylism.
7. The toes are strapped for several weeks to maintain the correction.

The simplest, most expeditious procedure is amputation of the little toe. However, this exposes the head of the fifth metatarsal to excessive weight-bearing pressures, which may produce an adventitious bursitis.

CONGENITAL DISLOCATION OF THE KNEE

One or both knees may be found at birth in a position of hyperextension (congenital genu recurvatum), and in extreme cases it may be possible to approximate the leg to the anterior surface of the thigh (Fig. 11-42). The proximal end of the tibia is displaced anteriorly and laterally on the femur. The quadriceps tendon and the iliotibial band are shortened. The patella is small or absent but begins forming after correction of the deformity. The anterior half of the capsule is contracted, but the posterior portion and the anterior cruciate ligament are elongated and lax.

Two types are recognized. The traumatic developmental type is due to malposition *in utero* or fibrofatty degeneration of the quadriceps. The second type is a primary embryonic defect, as indicated by such accompanying defects as harelip and clubfoot. The first type is far more common.

TREATMENT

Conservative treatment consists in repeated manipulations and castings to permit gradual flexion. Subcutaneous tenotomy of the iliotibial band is often necessary, and braces may be required to maintain reduction.

For severe resistant cases, surgical correction involves lengthening or sectioning the quadriceps tendon, the iliotibial band, the anterior capsule, and the posterior cruciate ligament. The posterior capsule and the anterior cruciate ligament are reefed. A maldisplaced gastrocnemius should have its proximal ends anchored to the femoral condyles.[44]

CONGENITAL COXA VARA

Normally, the infantile femoral neck forms an angle with the shaft of 120° to 140°. Reduction to a more acute angle constitutes a coxa vara deformity and is due to a variety of causes, including congenital, infection, trauma, tumor, and slipped upper femoral epiphysis. Congenital coxa vara (infantile coxa vara, developmental coxa vara) is that type found at birth or shortly thereafter.[45,46,48] Pathologically, it consists of a progressively increasing acuteness of the neck-shaft angle, shortness of the neck, a vertical direction of the epiphyseal plate, an oblique defect in the neck which extends from the proximal medial to the distal lateral borders of the neck and is composed of cartilage and osteoid tissue, a greater trochanter extending upward toward the ilium as a beak, a shortened femur, and secondary degenerative changes in the acetabulum due to malapposition. Histologically, the head of the femur is normal.

CLINICAL PICTURE

Clinically, a painless limp is the usual complaint. On examination, one finds a shortened lower extremity and a positive Trendelenburg test, the latter because the shortened distance from origin to insertion has weakened the gluteus medius. The greater trochanter lies above

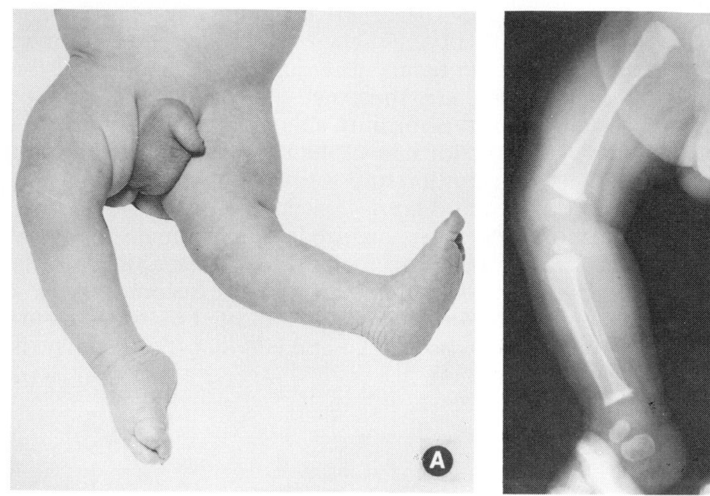

FIG. 11-42. Congenital dislocation of the knee. (Clayburgh BJ: Congenital dislocation of the knee. Proc Staff Meet Mayo Clin 30:396, 1955)

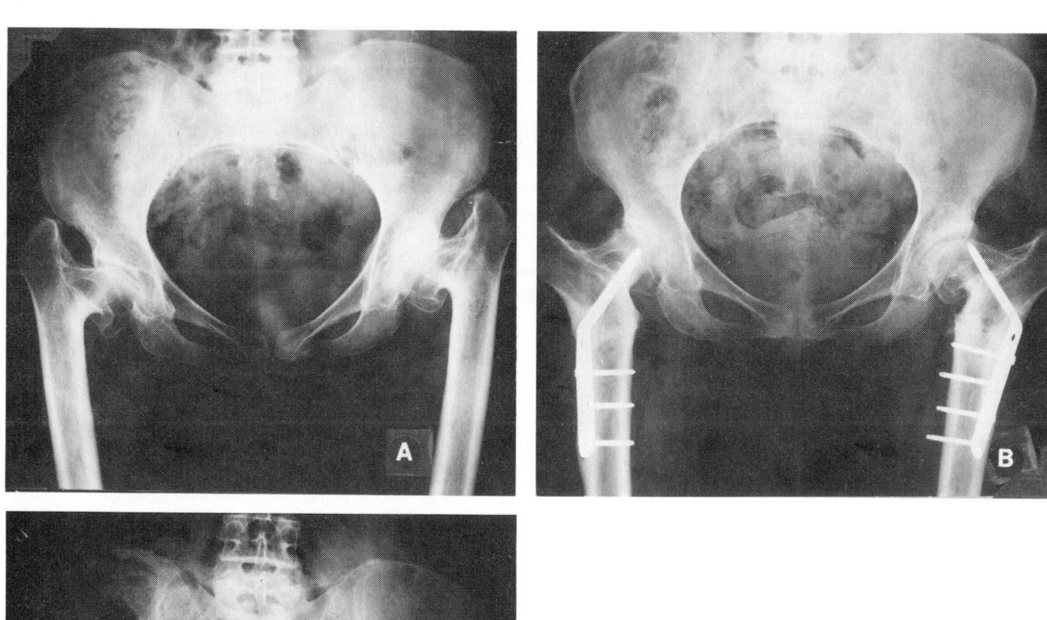

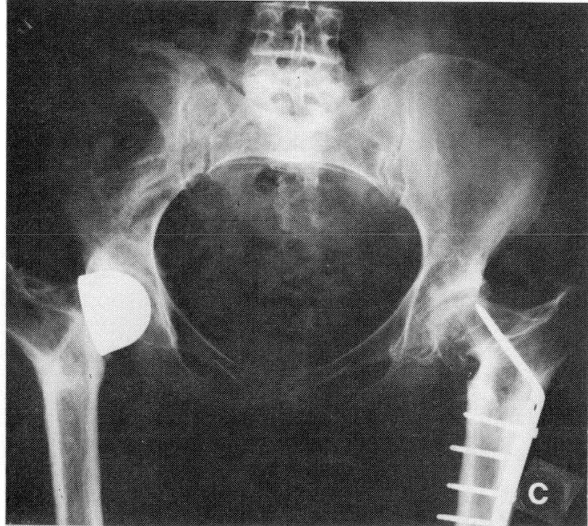

FIG. 11-43. Congenital coxa vara. (*A*) Typical decrease of neck-shaft angle, defect in neck, greater trochanter rides high. (*B*) Valgus osteotomies and fixation with blade plate. The weight-bearing surfaces of the femoral head have been changed; the efficiency of the gluteus medius muscle has been increased by lowering the greater trochanter. (*C*) Vitallium mold arthroplasty was done on the left because of degenerative changes. (Coventry MB: Proc Staff Meet Mayo Clin 29:48, 1954)

Nélaton's line. When the condition is bilateral, the bilaterally weakened hip abductors cause a waddling gait, and the increased lumbar lordosis suggests dislocated hips, but no telescoping is demonstrable. The neglected case in adult life has degenerative arthritic symptoms superimposed, such as pain, stiffness, and weakness. A progressive limitation of abduction and internal rotation is noted.

ROENTGENOGRAPHIC FINDINGS

Roentgenographic findings are typical (Fig. 11-43). The oblique defect in the femoral neck extending upward toward the proximal portion of the vertically disposed epiphyseal plate forms with the latter an inverted V or Y. This defect has the appearance of a nonunion. The triangular fragment may be irregular and fragmented. The neck is short, and the greater trochanter is beaked. The head is large and somewhat translucent. One unit, consisting of the head, epiphyseal cartilage, and triangular fragment, appears to be slipping downward.

TREATMENT

Treatment is aimed at obliterating the neck defect and thereby halting progression of the deformity and at correcting the already existing deformity. A subtrochanteric osteotomy and widely abducting the distal fragment will convert the oblique almost vertical defect, which is perpetuated by shearing stresses, into a horizontally displaced defect, which will fuse or unite by exposure to compression forces. A bone graft placed through the neck will aid in completely ossifying the neck. The operation is described briefly below.

Through a lateral incision, the femur is exposed subperiosteally below the greater trochanter. A transverse osteotomy is performed, and the shaft is widely abducted so as to form a wide obtuse angle with the upper fragment. The position is held by a Smith-Petersen nail inserted in the head and the neck and attached at its outer end to a plate that has been affixed to the shaft (see Fig. 11-43). Instead of using a nail and a plate, a one-piece metallic unit, such as a Moore or a Blount plate, consisting of a neck section and a shaft section, may be prepared preoperatively and bent to the appropriate angle and inserted at surgery. Postoperatively, a cast is unnecessary. Reossification almost inevitably occurs. The operation lengthens and thereby strengthens the hip abductors, and the Trendelenburg test becomes negative. Also, the femur is lengthened, and some of the limp due to shortening is overcome. However, the prognosis should be guarded inasmuch as recurrence can occur slowly regardless of any method, but most particularly during the growth period and when bone grafts alone are used.[47]

As an alternative method, a Y-shaped osteotomy will obtain a valgus position. By this method the static forces

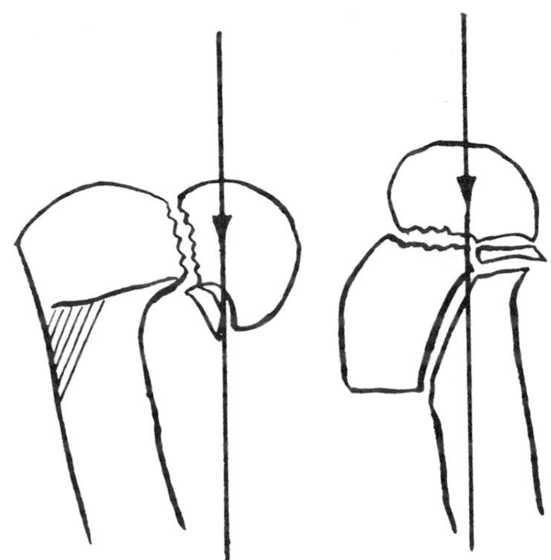

FIG. 11-44. The Y-shaped osteotomy of Pauwels. (Pauwels, F: Osteoplastic operations on the lower extremity. Rev Chir Orthop 47:125, 1961)

are converted from shearing to impacting forces, rapid union takes place, and recurrence is less likely. The procedure is represented by Figure 11-44.

CONGENITAL PSEUDARTHROSIS OF THE TIBIA

Congenital pseudarthrosis of the tibia is a congenital condition of unknown origin in which discontinuity of the bone at the junction of the middle and distal thirds or beyond is present at birth or develops thereafter during the growth period, permitting persisting abnormal mobility and creating the illusion of a false joint (Fig. 11-45). The upper and lower portions of the bone are joined by a mass of fibrous tissue that may contain fibrocartilage and, rarely, a synovial-lined cleft. It may develop as a result of a pathologic fracture or an ill-advised osteotomy through the dysplastic region of the bone.

ETIOLOGY

The cause is unknown. Approximately 40% of patients present with lesions typical of neurofibromatosis, or von Recklinghausen's disease (*e.g.*, café au lait spots, cutaneous fibromas), which is inherited as an autosomal dominant trait with variable penetrance and a high rate of mutation.[56–58,61] A possible relationship of neurofibromatosis, fibrous dysplasia, and congenital pseudarthrosis has been suggested.[49] Whatever the cause of the tibial defect that leads to fracture and nonunion, mechanical forces accentuate the problem.[55]

Congenital pseudarthrosis is also rarely encountered in the clavicle and very rarely in the humerus, femur, ulna, and first rib.

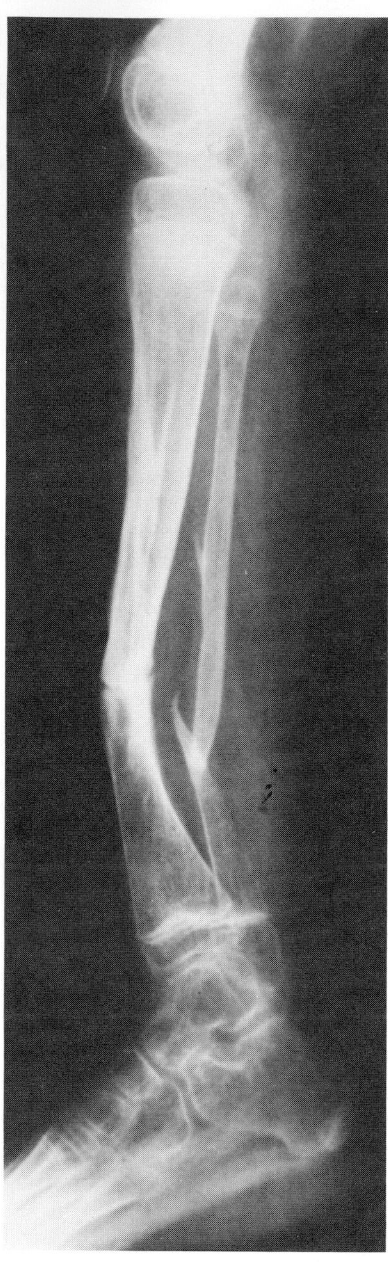

FIG. 11-45. Congenital pseudarthrosis of the tibia. Several unsuccessful attempts have been made to obtain union by bone grafting.

PATHOLOGY

Three types of lesions are described:[52,59]

A complete defect in the bone is the typical pseudarthrosis found at birth. The upper and lower segments represent variable portions of the tibial diaphysis, ranging from a proximal segment representing two thirds to three fourths, rarely as much as seven eighths, of the bone and a shorter distal segment ranging from one third to a very small portion of the bone. The upper and lower epiphyseometaphyseal components of the long bone have a normal structural appearance, but as each portion of the diaphysis approaches the defect, which is most often located at the junction of the middle and distal thirds, they become progressively tapered, their ends sclerotic and their medullary canal obliterated. The configuration of the bone ends in juxtaposition to the pseudarthrosis varies. At one extreme, the diaphyseal segments may be only slightly tapered and sclerosed; their ends are transversely disposed and are well apposed to one another with little malalignment, and the pseudarthrotic interval is narrow. This situation is usually the presenting appearance following a pathologic fracture through a congenitally bowed tibia.

At the other extreme, the diaphyseal fragments approaching the pseudarthrosis are markedly tapered, sclerosed, and foreshortened, and the interfragment interval is wide. The distal portion of the tibia, consisting of the lower epiphysis, the physis, and a variable amount of diaphysis, is often angulated backward, carrying the foot into equinus, and the Achilles tendon is contracted.

Occupying the interval between and surrounding the bone ends is a very cellular fibrous tissue. This tissue extends outward and seems to be continuous with what appears to be a thickened periosteum. When the fibers are arranged in whorls and contain an occasional fine-bone trabeculum, it resembles the histologic picture of fibrous dysplasia. Rarely, one observes poorly formed fibrocartilage and slits likened to synovia-lined spaces.[52]

A congenital bone cyst occurs in the lower third of the tibia, the microscopic picture of which closely resembles that seen in fibrous dysplasia. Although the diameter of the tibia is neither narrowed nor appreciably expanded, fracture invariably takes place through the weakened shaft, and conditions identical with an established pseudarthrosis follow.

Congenital bowing of the tibia, complicated by a fracture, will result in a pseudarthrosis. Anterolateral bowing is usually predisposed to this complication. Posteromedial bowing rarely undergoes a pathologic fracture. Congenital bowing and congenital cysts of the tibia are properly called prepseudarthrotic lesions.

ROENTGENOGRAPHIC FINDINGS

Roentgenograms of a typical pseudarthrosis demonstrate a lack of bone formation in the tibia, usually at the junction of the middle and distal thirds but possibly situated more distally. The portions of the diaphysis approaching the pseudarthrotic interval may assume varying degrees of tapering, sclerosis, and obliteration of the medullary canal. At a distance from the false joint, the bones assume a normal shape and structure, including preservation of the epiphyses and growth plates. As a general rule, the fibula is unaffected and is more often bowed, although it may display a pseudarthrosis at the same level. The distal tibial segment is usually angulated backward, resulting in equinus of the foot. Longitudinal growth of the bone is slightly to moderately retarded.

Prepseudarthrosis lesions may present as a cystic well-defined translucency that closely resembles that seen in fibrous dysplasia. The adjacent cortices may be thinned, but the diameter of the bone is usually neither narrow nor enlarged. These lesions may also present as anterior bowing of the tibia with variable degrees of local narrowing, sclerosis, and obliteration of the medullary cavity.

TREATMENT

Treatment may be categorized as prophylactic, directed toward the prepseudarthrosis lesions, and active, directed toward the fully developed congenital pseudarthrosis (or congenital nonunion) of the tibia.

PROPHYLACTIC

Patients with anterolateral bowing of the tibia at the junction of the middle and distal thirds of the diaphysis or beyond, particularly when accompanied by narrowing and sclerosis and loss of definition of the medullary canal, are considered at high risk for developing pathologic fracture and nonunion. The extremity must be protected by an orthosis and the child guarded against activity excesses. As longitudinal growth and remodeling take place, there is a tendency toward spontaneous, although slow, correction of the deformity and restoration of normal architecture. This may require years. The threat of fracture is ever present until skeletal maturity is reached. Corrective osteotomy is absolutely prohibited.

If fracture and resultant pseudarthrosis appear imminent, particularly when the bone structure is inadequate, and especially in the presence of a cyst, and the child's activity cannot be controlled, prophylactic reinforcement with bone transplants, preferably autogenous or homogenous cortical bone struts, is indicated.[60,62] The weakened region of the tibia is bypassed by a cortical or rib transplant (see Congenital Angulation of the Tibia) (Fig. 11-46.)

Since a congenital cyst in this region invariably fractures, it may similarly be treated by the bypass procedure. Afterward it may be necessary to curet the defect, fill it with bone transplants, and immobilize the leg in a cast until the defect is obliterated and a tibia of adequate size is obtained.

ACTIVE

Whatever the cause of the dysplastic process, the pseudarthrosis is perpetuated by detrimental stresses: bending, shearing, torsion. For an established pseudarthrosis, surgical treatment is necessary. As a general rule, the older the patient when surgical treatment is done, the more likely the success of union, so that the age of puberty would seem to be appropriate. However, by this time, the leg is underdeveloped, deformed, and short, and amputation is frequently preferable. Therefore, aggressive surgical intervention is better undertaken early in childhood because sufficient time remains for growth factors to operate so that when skeletal maturity is reached, a well-developed, even normal, extremity results. Moreover, if the initial surgery should fail, the procedure may be repeated. Repeated surgical procedures in the past reflect the difficulties of achieving a solid bony union, and the success rate of all patients, whether a single procedure or repeated procedures are done, was approximately 40%. With the advent of electrically induced osteogenesis, with or without surgical stabilization and bone transplants, the rate of success has increased to 70%. The chances of overcoming the pseudarthrosis appears to be correlated with adequate structural development of the bone ends adjoining the pseudarthrosis. The markedly tapered, narrowed, and highly sclerotic diaphyseal segments adjoining a wide defect has the lowest rate of achieving a bony union.

Surgery can be attempted as early as 4 years of age. If surgery must be postponed for any reason, further deformity should be prevented by an orthosis.

The principles of treatment are as follows:

1. Stabilization
   a. Dual onlay bone grafts (Boyd).[51] Provides both stability and induction of osteogenesis. Tapered slender bones will not permit its use.
   b. Intramedullary rod (Charnley).[54] Disadvantage: permits rotatory forces, which, however, can be controlled with a thigh-length cast with the knee flexed at 45°. Advantage: permits osteogenesis-inducing axial compressive forces; controls a small distal fragment by transtarsal insertion of the rod
   c. External skeletal fixation (fixateur externe).[66] Useful for maintaining length, when the bone structure about the defect is inadequate, and when poor soft tissue about the pseudarthrosis will not permit local fixation device
2. Stimulation of osteogenesis
   a. Bone transplants. Autogenous cancellous bone is preferred.
   b. Electrical stimulation. Used alone or as an adjunctive measure with stabilization and bone transplants. This will increase the rate of bony union.
3. Maintenance of cast immobilization. This is accomplished until bony bridging is adequate and the structure and size of the tibia are sufficient to with-

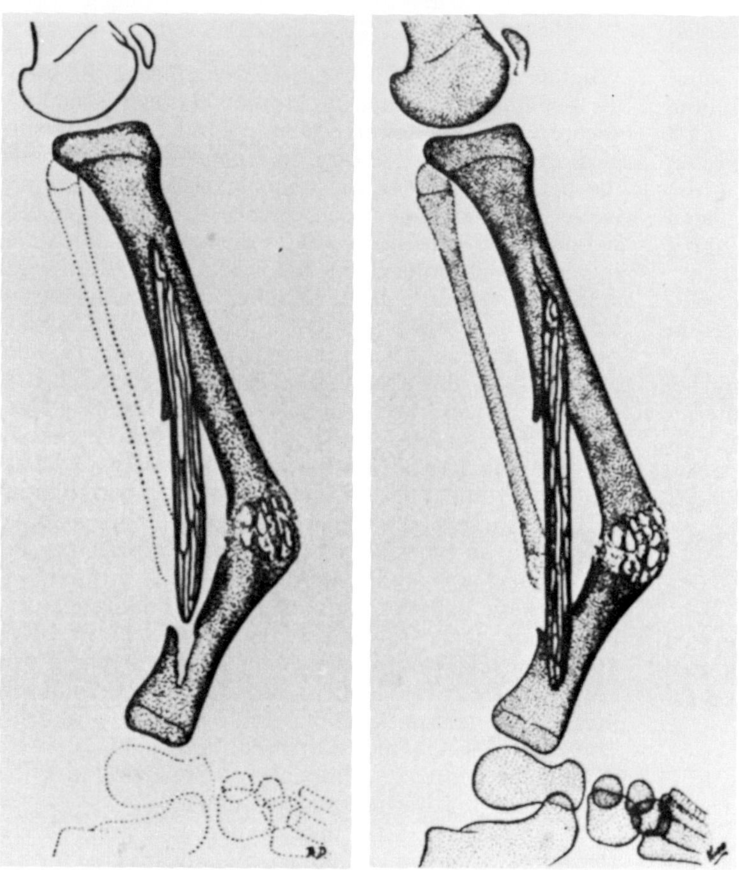

FIG. 11-46. The bypass operation for prophylactic treatment of an imminent fracture and pseudarthrosis in congenital angulation of the tibia. Except at the upper and lower sites of implantation, the transplant is entirely extraperiosteal. The operation is also used preliminary to curettage and bone grafting of a congenital cyst, a pre-pseudarthrotic lesion. (McFarland B: Pseudarthrosis of the tibia in childhood. J Bone Joint Surg 33B:36, 1951)

stand the possiblity of a pathologic fracture. The cast must be applied to the upper thigh, and the knee must be kept flexed at 45° to prevent gravity-induced tensile forces.

4. Compression versus noncompression stresses. Proponents of intramedullary rodding advocate immediate weight bearing to encourage compression stresses that induce osteogenesis. Advocates of electrical stimulation advise early avoidance of weight bearing until roentgenograms show early ossific bridging; then cyclic axial loading is initiated.

Dual Onlay Bone-Grafting Operation (Boyd). Two tibial cortical grafts and a supply of cancellous bone chips are removed from a donor or obtained from a bone bank.[51] The pseudarthrosis is exposed, and the fibrous tissue, which may surprisingly extend into the surrounding soft tissue, is completely excised. The eburnated bone is removed from the bone ends, and the medullary canal is opened up by drilling. To correct bowing and the equinus deformity, an Achilles tenotomy and a fibular osteotomy are required. If possible, the fibula should be preserved to aid postoperative immobilization. The lateral surfaces of the tibia above and below are shaved down flat, and the tibial cortical transplants are affixed, one medially and the other laterally. A space is left between the ends of the tibial fragments into which are packed the cancellous bone chips (Fig. 11-47). Only skin and subcutaneous tissue are closed. A cast is applied, and immobilization is continued until union is apparent. Fracture and nonunion are postoperative complications, and protection of the leg by a leather lacer brace or plastic orthosis until skeletal maturity is mandatory.

Intramedullary Nailing (Charnley). Fixation by an intramedullary rod eliminates angulatory strain while permitting beneficial axial compressive forces.[54,65] Despite the criticism that it still allows rotational stresses, rodding of the tibia by the transtarsal approach is the most commonly used method of fixation.[50] It can be used alone with external plaster support, but generally autogenous cancellous bone or osteoperiosteal bone transplants are added. Fixation in the tarsus will prevent the nail from cutting out of the short distal segment of tibia. Before introducing the nail, an Achilles tenotomy will overcome the bowstring action that prevents correction of the deformity.

Previously, the method used for osteogenesis imperfecta (*i.e.*, fragmentation, reversal of fragments, and realignment—Sofield procedure) has been practiced, but now this is known to afford no advantage.[64]

Intramedullary nailing, with or without bone transplants, has about a 40% rate of success of achieving a union, and the procedure may need to be repeated before this can be achieved. With the addition of electrically induced osteogenesis, the rate of success has risen to 70%.[50]

Electrical Stimulation. Osteogenesis within the pseudarthrotic defect can be enhanced by induction of electrical currents within the defect. This therapeutic modality consists of direct current of small magnitude (*e.g.*, 20 microamperes) administered continuously by a totally implanted apparatus (power pack and electrodes); or by a semi-invasive method by percutaneous insertion of electrodes, the power pack remaining external; or by inductive coupling, which is noninvasive and produces pulsing electromagnetic fields.[50,53,63]

The most favorable types of lesion for ultimate healing of the defect by electrically induced osteogenesis, with or without surgical stabilization and bone transplants, are a pseudarthrosis following a spontaneous fracture or an osteotomy of a bowed tibia and a fracture through a cystic lesion of the lower tibia. It is desirable for electrical stimulation to be augmented by cancellous bone transplants and, if possible, by internal fixation by an intramedullary rod or double cortical transplants. When the bone ends are markedly tapered and a gap exists of more than 5 mm, the outlook for repair is unfavorable and only about 20% will succeed.

CONGENITAL ABSENCE OF THE FIBULA

Congenital absence of the fibula (paraxial fibular hemimelia) is the most common congenital absence of long bone, followed in frequency by the radius, femur, tibia, ulna, and humerus. Failure of the entire bone to appear is rather rare. Partial absence usually involves the prox-

FIG. 11-47. Boyd dual graft for congenital pseudarthrosis. (*A*) The first graft is held in position temporarily by two short screws. (*B*) Subsequently, both grafts are fixed in position by screws that pass through both grafts and intervening bone. Temporary screws have been removed and replaced by permanent screws, and the trough has been filled with cancellous bone. (*C* and *D*) Union and incorporation of the grafts. (Boyd HB: Congenital pseudarthrosis: Treatment by dual bone grafts. J Bone Joint Surg 23:497, 1941)

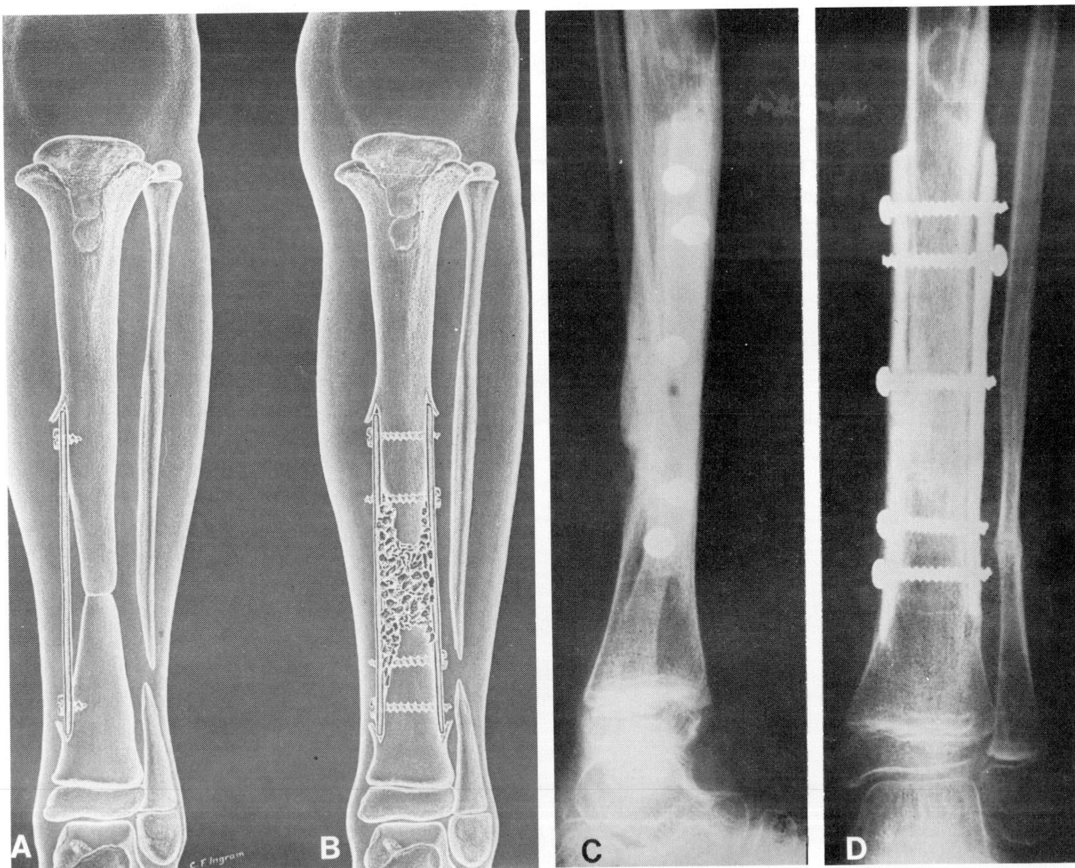

imal portion of the bone, preserving the lateral malleolus at the ankle and an essentially normal clinical appearance. Consequently, partial congenital absence of the fibula is often overlooked, and its incidence may be greater than is generally appreciated. A genetic factor has never been established. Experimental reproduction of the defect has been achieved by metabolic, nutritional, and physical means before limb-bud formation (between 6 and 8 weeks' gestation in the human).[1,72,76]

The deformity may be minimal, consisting of partial unilateral absence of the fibula and slight limb shortening, with no associated anomalies elsewhere. A typical complete unilateral absence of the fibula is but one component of an extensive dysplasia of the entire extremity that may also include congenital shortening of the femur, shortening of the tibia (frequently with anteromedial bowing and hypoplastic deformed epiphyses), equinovalgus deformity of the foot, tarsal anomalies (coalition, absent tarsal), metatarsal anomalies, and, often, absence of the fourth and fifth rays, a skin dimple over (but not adherent to) the bowed tibia, and a fibrocartilaginous tight band, which probably represents the remnant of the fibular anlage, running from the proximal end of the tibia to the calcaneus (Fig. 11-48). More than 3 inches overall shortening of the extremity develops during childhood, and the discrepancy may reach as much as 5 inches in the adult. The deformity may be bilateral and often is associated with other congenital anomalies in the contralateral limb and upper limbs. Hypoplasia of the corresponding femur is frequent.

CLASSIFICATION

The following classification is useful for prognosticating the outcome:[73]

Type I. Partial unilateral absence of the fibula with minimal gross deformity except for shortening.

Type II. Classic form, with absence of most or all of the fibula, anterior bowing of the tibia, and equinovalgus deformity of the foot. The outlook for overcoming the deformity is poor.

Type III. Congenital absence of one fibula, associated with one or more congenital deformities elsewhere, or bilateral congenital absence of the entire fibula. Again the outlook is poor, especially when many congenital anomalies are present.

DIFFERENTIAL DIAGNOSIS

In the infant, difficulty arises in interpreting the roentgenograms to rule out the following conditions:

Congenital absence of the tibia. Differentiation is important because this entity invariably requires a high amputation. In contrast, congenital absence of the fibula requires an early amputation only in the severe classic types (II and III), and then a modified Syme's type of amputation.

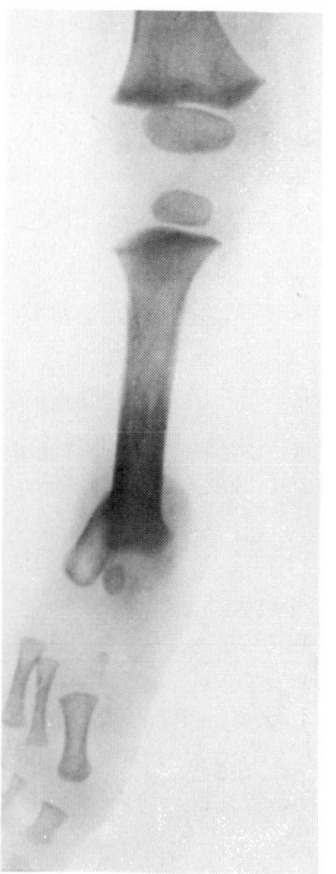
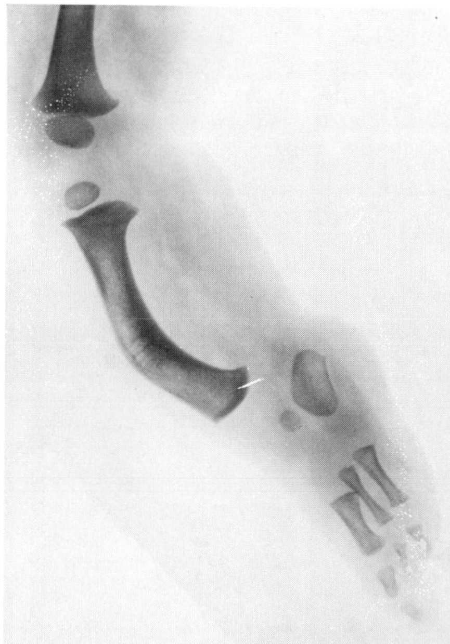
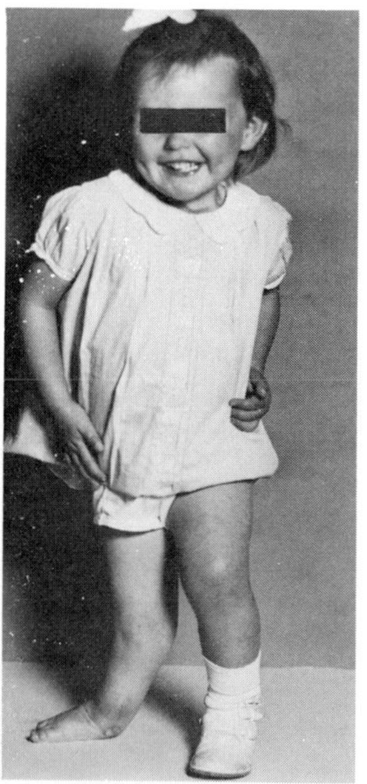

FIG. 11-48. Congenital absence of the fibula. The lateral displacement of the foot at the ankle, anterior angulation of the tibia, equinus, and frequently associated absence of digital rays are well shown. The patient displays the typical deformity of shortening of the leg and equinovalgus. (Coventry MB, Johnson EW Jr: Congenital absence of the fibula. J Bone Joint Surg 34A:941, 1952)

In congenital absence of the tibia, the foot and ankle are in a varus position, not valgus, and the medial malleolus is missing; there is no anterior bowing of the tibia, and there is dislocation at the knee where the fibula rides laterally and upward.

Congenital pseudarthrosis of the tibia. In this condition, the appearance of the leg is somewhat similar to that of congenital absence of the fibula. In congenital absence of the fibula, an osteotomy to correct tibial bowing is followed by rapid union; in congenital pseudarthrosis, osteotomy is dangerous.

In congenital pseudarthrosis, roentgenograms demonstrate that the tibia and fibula are thickened and may be angulated or fractured. The fibula is always present except at the site of pseudarthrosis. In congenital absence of the fibula, the fibula, or a portion of it, is absent and the tibia is not markedly sclerotic or thickened.

TREATMENT

The principal aims of surgery are obtaining a plantigrade foot and a functional ankle with no deformity and equal limb lengths.[77]

MILD DEFORMITY

When no apparent deformity other than slight shortening is present (type I), a heel lift on the affected side may be sufficient. For greater limb discrepancy, epiphyseal arrest on the opposite side may be necessary.

Somewhat greater degrees of dysplasia, usually with a portion of the fibula absent, slight tibial bowing, preservation of at least four rays of the foot, an ankle that can be passively aligned, and mild growth inhibition, can sometimes be remedied by soft tissue release procedures (Achilles tendon lengthening, capsulotomy, peroneal tenotomies), a bone procedure (*e.g.*, reconstructing the lateral malleolus), and leg equalization operations. Resection of the deforming fibrocartilaginous band should be considered. Osteotomy to overcome tibial bowing is seldom necessary; as a rule, diaphyseal bowing improves spontaneously. In patients with partial absence of the fibula and an intact foot (incomplete intercalary fibular paraxial hemimelia), leg-length discrepancy at skeletal maturity is usually less than 3 inches, and no other deformity is apparent. Leg equalization procedures are generally sufficient.

The growth inhibition pattern can be studied based on scanogram measurements or, in children less than 1 year old, on teleoroentgenograms. The percentage of growth inhibition remains relatively constant throughout the growth period.[69,70,77] By using tables of the lengths of the femur and tibia, one can estimate the ultimate leg-length discrepancy.[71,74]

SEVERE DEFORMITY

The classical case displays a severe deformity at an early age.[67,77] The two major problems, severe shortening of the extremity and equinovalgus deformity of the ankle and foot, are generally irremediable by reconstructive procedures. An extreme leg-length discrepancy, which can be predicted to occur at maturity, generally 7.5 cm or more, is not amenable by leg-lengthening procedures or suitable for epiphyseal arrest on the contralateral limb.

A modifed Syme's amputation done at an early age will provide nearly normal function of the limb and a prosthesis of excellent appearance.[69,70,75,77] The gait pattern is essentially normal, the stump does not become bulbous as in the adult, bony overgrowth does not occur, and the child becomes active and proficient at sports.[68]

In the modified Syme's amputation, an ankle disarticulation is performed without disturbing the distal tibial epiphysis, cutting across the distal end of the tibia and its malleolus to make a flat surface and covering this with a heel pad.[78] Posterior migration of the heel pad may occur, but the normal skin will hypertrophy to permit weight bearing. The prosthesis is end bearing with a flexible inner wall and is patellar tendon bearing. It is essential to preserve intact the specialized subcutaneous tissue of the heel flap.

CONGENITAL ABSENCE OF THE TIBIA

Part or all of the tibia may be absent at birth (congenital tibial hemimelia). The affected extremity is shorter not only because the fibula is short but also because the fibula is displaced upward and lies alongside the lateral femoral condyle. The lower fibula lies lateral to the astragalus and the calcaneus. The lack of tibial support allows the foot to swing medially into severe equinovarus. The entire leg deviates medially in relation to the longitudinal axis of the femur, and the fibula is bowed (Fig. 11-49).

TREATMENT

The aim of treatment is to restore osseous continuity between the thigh and the foot. Surgery should be done as early as possible. The upper fibula is mobilized by cutting away the attachment of the biceps (after the common peroneal nerve is isolated and protected). Then it is placed in the intercondylar notch and held with sutures. It is immaterial whether a synostosis or a freely movable joint develops. At first the tight soft tissue structures will not allow the knee to be fully extended. However, extension can be accomplished by successive casts. Finally, a leather lacer corset is fitted to the leg and holds the foot in extreme equinus, thereby overcoming the shortening and allowing the child to walk. Constant walking exercise prevents atrophy and en-

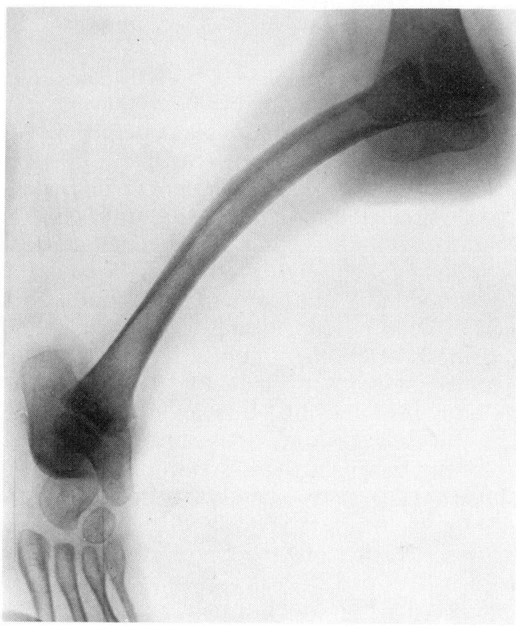

FIG. 11-49. Congenital absence of the tibia. The fibula is hypertrophied and dislocated at the knee. (Coventry MB, Johnson EW Jr: Congenital absence of the fibula. J Bone Joint Surg 34A:941, 1952)

courages bony and muscular development. Within a few years, when the lower end of the fibula and the astragalus and the calcaneus are more ossified, the distal fibula is arthrodesed to the astragalus or, in its absence, to the calcaneus, with the latter in extreme equinus. Weight bearing in walking is on the toes. Over the years, the fibula will hypertrophy to several times its original size. The only alternative to this procedure is amputation.

A severe foot deformity may dictate the need for an ankle disarticulation with a Syme flap. A below-knee prosthesis requires a thigh corset with knee joints, because the patient never develops sufficient mediolateral stability for a patellar tendon bearing (PTB) prosthesis.

If reconstructive procedures distal to the knee are not possible, a knee disarticulation may be done and the patient fitted with a knee disarticulation type of prosthesis. Such surgical conversion is necessary to equalize leg lengths, correct malrotation, and provide stability.[67]

CONGENITAL TORSION IN THE LOWER EXTREMITY

Torsion of a bone is defined as twisting or rotation on its longitudinal axis. The condition is found most commonly in the lower extremities in the tibia or the femur. It is congenital or acquired. When present at birth, spontaneous correction occurs to a variable degree in the first few years in response to the stresses of walking and weight bearing. The deformity that persists is compensated for by additional deformities at the hip, the knee, and the foot, which permit forward progression of the foot in walking.

TIBIAL TORSION

The angle that the median sagittal plane of the tibia forms with the coronal plane is known as the angle of torsion. When the sagittal plane is directly anteroposterior, both of the malleoli of the ankle should lie in the coronal plane, the talus facing forward and the foot itself pointing directly in front of the body. This angle is considered as 0°. Normally, a small amount of external rotation is present and ranges from 0° to 40°, the foot pointing outward and the malleolus displacing backward. When the distal tibia is twisted outward more than this amount in relation to the proximal tibia, it is considered an abnormal amount of external tibial torsion.[79] When the distal tibia is twisted inward so that the foot points medial to the median plane, internal tibial torsion exists. Measurement of the angle is determined by placing the patient in the sitting position, flexing his knee to a right angle, pointing his patella forward (which positions the proximal tibia), and placing his foot on the floor. The angle is estimated by noting the deviation of the foot from the midposition (Fig. 11-50).

INTERNAL

When the congenital type is present, it is detected by the ease with which the extremity can be rotated passively

FIG. 11-50. Internal tibial torsion. To test, the knees are flexed and the ankle is held at a right angle. The relation of the foot to the sagittal plane measures the angle of torsion.

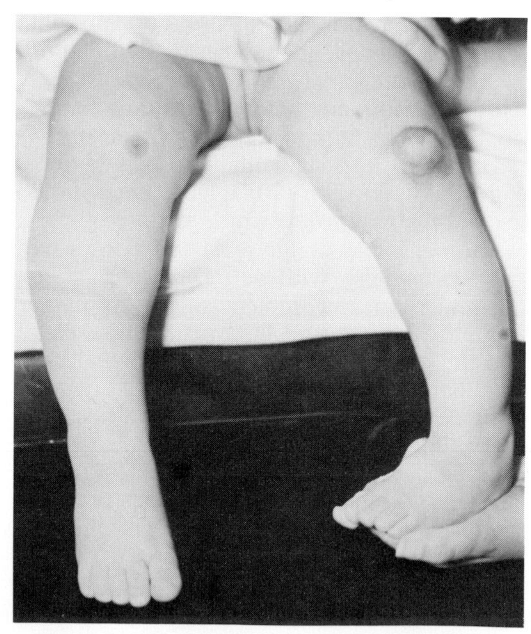

externally and internally to the normal range, as noted by the patella rolling out and in, respectively. The amount of angulation is chiefly at the distal end of the bone. When the child stands, in order that the feet be placed pointing forward, the patellae and the knees are rolled outward, giving a semilateral view of the knees. This simulates bowing of the knees. The pseudobowlegs are identified as such by facing the patellae forward, which automatically eliminates the deformity. Frequently, the mother's complaint may be bowlegs rather than pigeon toes. Occasionally, actual bowing may develop eventually. In such a case, the test of forward-pointed patellae fails to eliminate the deformity. Without treatment, the prognosis is poor. Spontaneous improvement rarely occurs. Treatment consists of holding the feet rotated continuously and externally by means of a Denis Browne or a Fillauer splint, derotation taking place gradually over several months. The older the child, the less likely is the correction by conservative means. This is particularly true after 6 or 7 years of age. If in such cases the deformity is extreme and disabling so that stumbling and falling is frequent, surgical correction by osteotomy is justified.

The acquired type of internal tibial torsion results from abnormal sleeping and sitting positions. The infant generally sleeps on his stomach in the knee-chest position with the toes turned in. On examination, the range of motion externally is limited (*i.e.*, the patellae cannot be rolled out sufficiently). After sleeping habits are corrected, spontaneous derotation is usual. However, return to normal is expedited by bracing in the externally rotated position.

EXTERNAL

The anatomical outward twisting of the bone should not be confused with the outward rotation of the leg secondary to spastic paralysis or poliomyelitis. An overacting biceps femoris or a tight iliotibial band attached to the upper outer aspect of the leg will turn the leg outward, but actual torsion of the tibia is not present. External torsion of the bone results from faulty sleeping and sitting habits. The infant sleeps on its abdomen or its back in the frog or spread-eagle position. The limbs can be passively turned inward until the patellae face straight forward but not much farther. Rotation outward is excessive. Later, during the standing period, the feet turn outward and are usually flat. If the child turns the feet in order to point them forward, the patellae are rotated inward, affording a semilateral view of the knees which thus appear in valgus. The pseudo-knock-knee condition is exposed by bringing the patellae to the forward position, which automatically eliminates the deformity. The mother's complaint, as a matter of fact, may be knock knees rather than flatfeet or an abnormal external rotation or "Charlie Chaplin" gait. Occasionally, actual knock knees may exist. These secondary deformities should always be sought and evaluated prior to treatment. Treatment consists in breaking faulty sleeping habits and continuously maintaining the feet in the inward position by bracing. Derotation is gradual over several months, but, as in acquired internal torsion, is limited by age of the patient. Persistent disabling deformity may require osteotomy.

CORRECTION BY SURGERY

When torsion is associated with genu valgus or varus, a transverse osteotomy of the tibia is done just below the tibial condyles, where union is most probable and displacement of the fragments less likely. The tibia and the fibula are sectioned, the distal tibia is rotated, and angulation is corrected at the same time as a cast is applied.

The controlled rotation osteotomy is used when no varus or valgus correction is necessary (Fig. 11-51).[80] A Z-osteotomy is made through the upper third of the tibia. The distal horizontal limb of the Z-step-cut is always made on the side of the direction of correction. The proximal limb extends in the opposite direction. Between the two transverse cuts, a wedge-shaped section of bone is removed from the anteromedial aspect of the tibia. The bone is osteotomized longitudinally on its posterior aspect, thereby freeing the two segments of tibia. The rotation is corrected by turning the distal fragment inward or outward, as the case may be, thereby approximating the edges anteriorly. Fixation of fragments is by sutures or transfixion screws.

FEMORAL TORSION

Internal torsion of the shaft of the femur occurs in congenital dislocation of the hip and constitutes a compensatory phenomenon secondary to femoral neck anteversion. In order that the person may walk with the patella directed forward, the entire femur must be turned outward carrying the neck and head of the femur forward. Forward placement of the excessively anteverted femoral neck makes it difficult to retain the femoral head within the acetabulum. The femoral torsion, and therefore the femoral neck anteversion, must be corrected by a derotation osteotomy. This is described in the section on congenital dislocation of the hip.

CONGENITAL DISLOCATION OF THE PATELLA

The patella may be small and imperfectly developed at birth.[82] It lies permanently in a laterally displaced position over the lateral or anterolateral aspect of the lateral femoral condyle. It is anchored in this position by the shortened fibers of the capsule and the vastus lateralis.

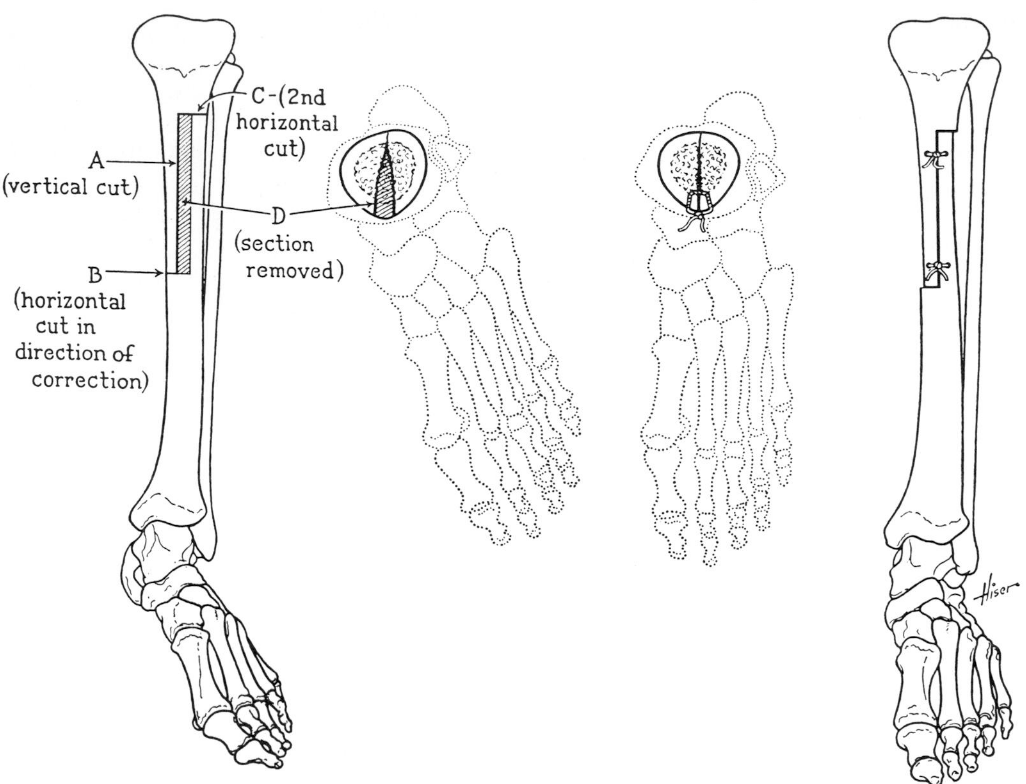

FIG. 11-51. Controlled rotation osteotomy of the tibia (method of O'Donoghue). (O'Donoghue DH: Controlled rotation osteotomy of the tibia. South Med J 33:1145, 1940)

The vastus medialis and the medial capsule are stretched. The anterior portion of the lateral femoral condyle is flattened, but this may be a secondary change. Usually, the tibia is rotated externally, and genu valgus may or may not be present. The abnormal lateral position of the patella causes pain and instability, which in early childhood may be mild and cause no concern. However, with advancing age, the pain comes on with lesser forms of activity and the weakness becomes so pronounced that the patient falls easily and eventually crutches are required. The imperfect mechanical situation causes flakes of cartilage to be sheared off into the joint, where they develop into multiple loose osteocartilaginous bodies. Severe degenerative arthritis with narrowing of the joint space is the final result with passage of years.

The condition must be differentiated from the common recurrent dislocations of the patella occurring later and apparently without the hereditary factor.

TREATMENT

Treatment procedures generally used in recurrent dislocation have not been entirely successful for the congenital condition. Conn's operation gives satisfactory results.[81] First, the external rotation and the valgus of the tibia are corrected by casts (only in the infant). In older people, the valgus and rotation need correction by a supracondylar osteotomy. Next, the knee capsule is exposed through a U-shaped incision that is deepened to include the synovium. The tendinous attachments of the vastus lateralis and the vastus medialis of the quadriceps mass are freed from the quadriceps tendon itself. The patella is pushed into its normal position in the midline, which leaves a diamond-shaped gap in the line of the lateral incision. A piece of similar shape (which conforms to a piece of aluminum placed over this gap) is then cut from the redundant capsule on the inner aspect of the joint, which includes the capsule and the synovial membrane. This piece is transferred to and sutured to the margins of the opening in the lateral aspect. The medial opening is closed with sutures. The elongated fibers of the vastus medialis are shortened and sutured to the quadriceps and the upper border of the patella. The already short vastus lateralis is sutured to the quadriceps tendon. Weight bearing is permitted in 3 weeks.

At a later age, removal of the patella and, if necessary, a knee "housecleaning" is done.

MULTIPARTITE PATELLA

The ossification center of the patella usually makes its appearance between the third and fifth years and gradually enlarges. Occasionally two, rarely more, centers are present and fuse to form the parent bone. When these centers fail to fuse and remain as discrete components of the composite bone, a bipartite, or a tripartite or a multipartite, patella results. The importance of this condition lies in the fact that often it is confused with, or misrepresented as, a fracture, since it is usually discovered on the roentgenogram taken following an injury.[83]

ROENTGENOGRAPHIC FINDINGS

The most common anomaly consists of two segments, the so-called bipartite patella, in which the patella is composed of a main large bone, occupying most of the patella, and a small bone usually situated at the upper outer quadrant (Fig. 11-52). The two segments fit accurately together to form a normally contoured parent patella. The features that distinguish this condition from a fracture are that it is frequently bilateral, although not invariably so; there is a line of demarcation running downward and laterally; and opposing margins are smooth and dense and can be seen to be composed of bone cortices.[84]

SYMPTOMS

The condition is generally asymptomatic. Occasionally, when axial views of the patella demonstrate that the articular surfaces of both segments do not form a continuous smooth line, one must consider disruption of the line of junction as a possible cause of knee pain. Removal of the smaller fragment may effect complete relief of symptoms.

CONGENITAL FLATFOOT

The normal newborn foot lacks a longitudinal arch because a fat pad fills the plantar concavity. This should never be interpreted as a flatfoot. Within the first year or two, the pad disappears and the true extent of the arch is revealed. In the normal foot, the talus, the navicular, the first cuneiform, and the first metatarsal form a straight line as visualized from the A-P and lateral aspects. The true criteria of a flatfoot include a break in the line of the first ray so that the head of the talus points medially and downward, with or without the navicular; in the A-P view, the head of the talus points medially and the navicular is displaced laterally in relation to the talar head; the heel is everted (valgus) so that in order for the metatarsal heads to be placed equally on the ground the forefoot must be inverted (supinated). In the non-weight-bearing state, the deformity is less and no deformity may be evident. The true extent of the displacement and flattening of the longitudinal arch is revealed on weight bearing. The examiner can restore the longitudinal arch to its normal appearance by plantar flexing the forefoot, inverting the heel, and everting the forefoot.

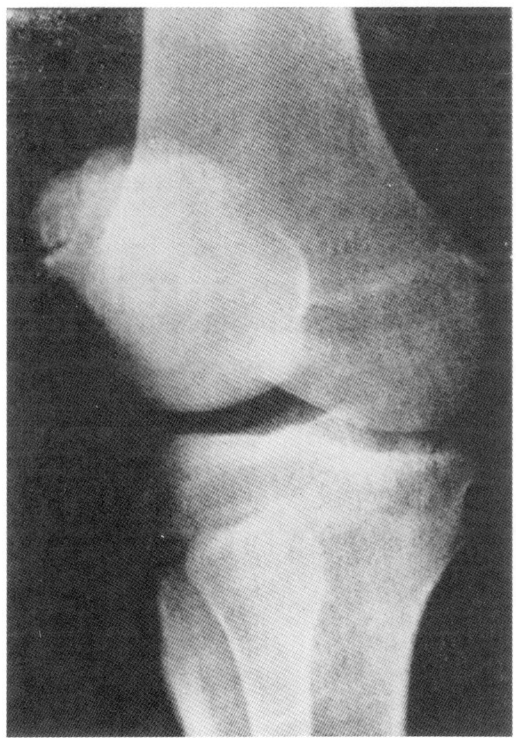

FIG. 11-52. Bipartite patella. Note features that distinguish this from a fracture: situated at upper and outer quadrant; well-defined line of separation runs in an undulating curve downward and outward; opposing margins consist of unmistakable cortices; roentgenogram of opposite knee often exhibits identical findings.

Roentgenographic studies are important in establishing the presence of congenital flatfoot. Normally, the talus, navicular, inner cuneiform, and first metatarsal comprise an unbroken line seen in the A-P and lateral projections. In the A-P view, the axes of the talus and calcaneus form a slightly divergent angle, the calcaneus pointing outward. In the hypermobile flatfoot in the resting position, normal roentgenographic findings are usual. It is essential to take roentgenograms while the foot is weight bearing. Before 2 years of age, the navicular is unossified, but its position can be established by following the line of the first metatarsal and inner cuneiform and noting its relationship to the axis of the talus. If the two lines form an angle medially and plantarward, the diagnosis of flatfoot is certain. In extreme degrees of ligamentous hyperlaxity, the talus may be angulated downward and medially even in the non-weight-bearing position, but continuity of the inner ray is easily restored by plantar flexing the forefoot and inverting the heel.

When normal anatomical restoration of the inner ray cannot be passively secured by placing the foot in equinus and inverting the heel, a rigid flatfoot is said to exist. In such a situation, either one of two conditions is responsible and must be clearly defined. Congenital vertical talus when treated early in infancy is often amenable to serial manipulations and casts followed by surgery. Tarsal coalition likewise restricts tarsal motion. This condition cannot be positively identified on roentgenograms until sufficient ossification of the tarsals has taken place. (Flatfoot is further discussed in Chapter 29.)

CONGENITAL VERTICAL TALUS

Congenital vertical talus (congenital rocker-bottom foot or convex pes valgus) is a rare condition found at birth in which the navicular is displaced dorsal to the neck of the talus and the talus is disposed vertically so that its head forms the most prominent part of the sole. The contour of the foot is such that the sole is convex and the heel is in equino-valgus (rocker-bottom foot) (Fig. 11-53). The forefoot is deviated outward and dorsally. It is important to define and treat this condition early because failure to do so results in a rigid flatfoot. Congenital vertical talus is often overlooked early, since its appearance is quite similar to talipes calcaneovalgus, a benign condition from which it must be differentiated.[87,89]

ETIOLOGY

The condition develops in the embryo stage almost invariably associated with other congenital deformities. It is often found in arthrogryposis multiplex congenita (arthrogryposis) and is sometimes associated with spina bifida. Anomalies of the central nervous system can produce the deformity by muscle imbalance (*i.e.*, weak posterior tibial and strong peroneals).[86] It may be one of many anomalies associated with autosomal trisomy.[93,94]

PATHOLOGY

The talus points downward and medially, and the navicular is displaced dorsally and laterally, where it is often lodged firmly against the neck of the talus, preventing reduction (Figs. 11-54 and 11-55). The calcaneus is rotated outward and held in eversion by the contracted interosseous ligament and the calcaneofibular ligament; it is held fixed in equinus by the contracted posterior capsule and Achilles tendon. Occasionally, a dorsolateral dislocation or extreme subluxation of the calcaneocuboid joints occurs. The dorsal capsules of the talonavicular and calcaneocuboid joints and the tibionavicular ligament (anterior portion of the deltoid ligament) are markedly contracted and constitute a formidable obstacle to reduction. The break in the midtarsal joints allows the forefoot to displace outward and dorsally. As a result, the course and insertion of the peroneus longus tendon comes to lie dorsal to the axis of the talus, bowstringing across the ankle joint and acting as a strong dorsiflexor and evertor. In addition, the forefoot dorsiflexors (anterior tibial, extensor hallucis longus, extensor digitorum longus) are contracted.

On the medial side, the calcaneonavicular ligament (spring ligament) is elongated and attenuated. The posterior tibial tendon splays out and becomes attenuated as it passes over the medial and plantar surface of the displaced talar head. It divides into a larger medial half, which inserts on the plantar aspect of the navicular, and a lateral segment, which attaches distally into the base of the second, third, and fourth metatarsals.

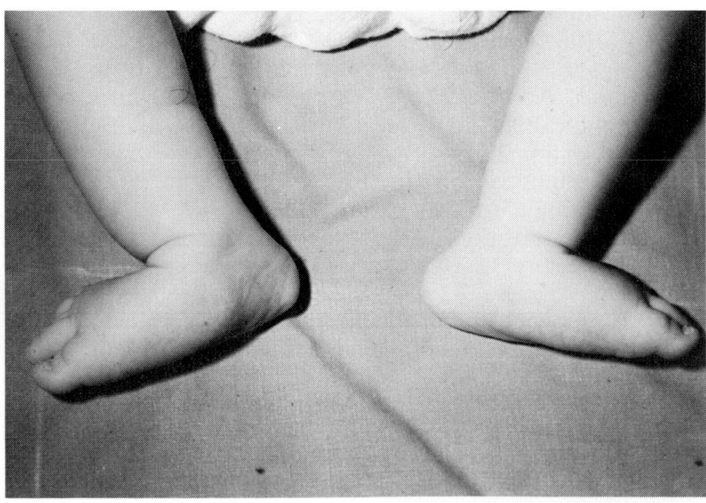

FIG. 11-53. Congenital rocker-bottom foot (congenital convex pes valgus, congenital vertical talus). The heel is in valgus and equinus. The forefoot is abducted. The sole is convex. The head of the talus is prominent on the medial aspect of the tarsus. The foot is rigid, and passive correction of the deformity is not possible. (Patterson WB, Fitz DA, Smith WS: The pathologic anatomy of congenital convex pes valgus. J Bone Joint Surg 50A:458, 1968)

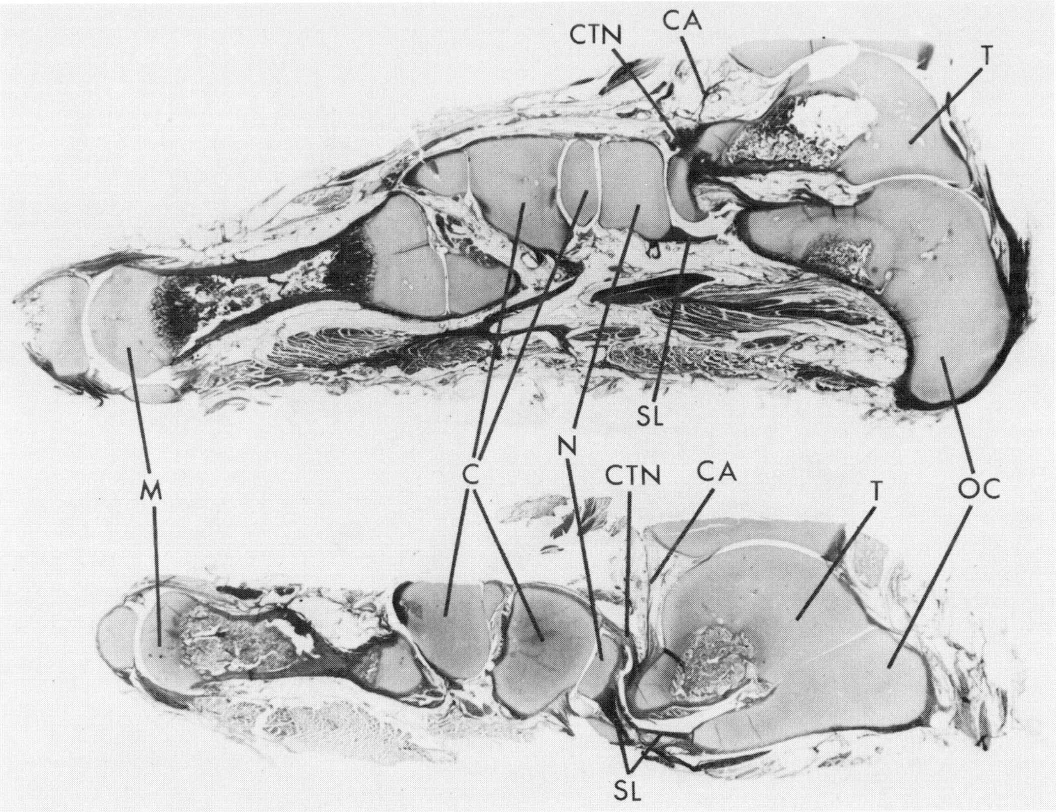

FIG. 11-54. Pathology of congenital convex pes valgus. Sagittal section through first ray of normal foot (*above*) and convex valgus foot (*below*). The spring ligament, capsule of the ankle joint, and capsule of the talonavicular joint are elongated compared with those of the normal foot. The talonavicular articulation is covered by a dense connective tissue. Note the difference between this articulation and the smooth contiguous cartilaginous surfaces of this joint in the normal foot. The equinus position of the talus and calcaneus is evident in the abnormal foot. The pointed appearance of the head of the talus is demonstrated. (*OC,* calcaneus; *T,* talus; *SL,* spring ligament; *N,* navicular; *CA,* capsule of ankle joint; *CTN,* capsule of talonavicular joint; *C,* cuneiforms; *M,* first metatarsal) (Patterson WR, Fitz DA, Smith WS: The pathologic anatomy of congenital convex pes valgus. J Bone Joint Surg 50A:458, 1968)

If the deformity persists into late childhood and adolescence, the talus becomes altered to assume an hourglass configuration, and often the calcaneus becomes curved dorsally at its anterior end, becoming beak shaped. Changes in the articulating facets between the talus and calcaneus take place, which encourage redisplacement even after surgical correction.

CLINICAL PICTURE

At birth, the foot resembles and is often misdiagnosed as talipes calcaneovalgus. However, the sole of the foot is characteristically convex, the dorsolateral fold is deep and situated at the midtarsal area, and the head of the talus is prominent over the plantar and medial aspects. The deformity from the outset is rigid; therefore, passive attempts to plantar flex and invert the foot are restricted.

Later in childhood, the flatfoot deformity is quite characteristic. The sole is so convex and the heel cord so tight that on weight bearing the posterior portion of the heel fails to touch the ground. The forefoot is abducted and dorsiflexed, the heel is in valgus, and the deformity persists even in the resting state. The foot is rigid, and attempts to passively correct the deformity are rarely successful. The gait is awkward and resembles a waddle. The shoes are rapidly worn out over the inner sides. Pain may develop late in childhood and adolescence.

Associated congenital deformities are common, especially arthrogryposis and spina bifida.

ROENTGENOGRAPHIC FINDINGS

The important roentgenographic characteristics of the infant include the following:

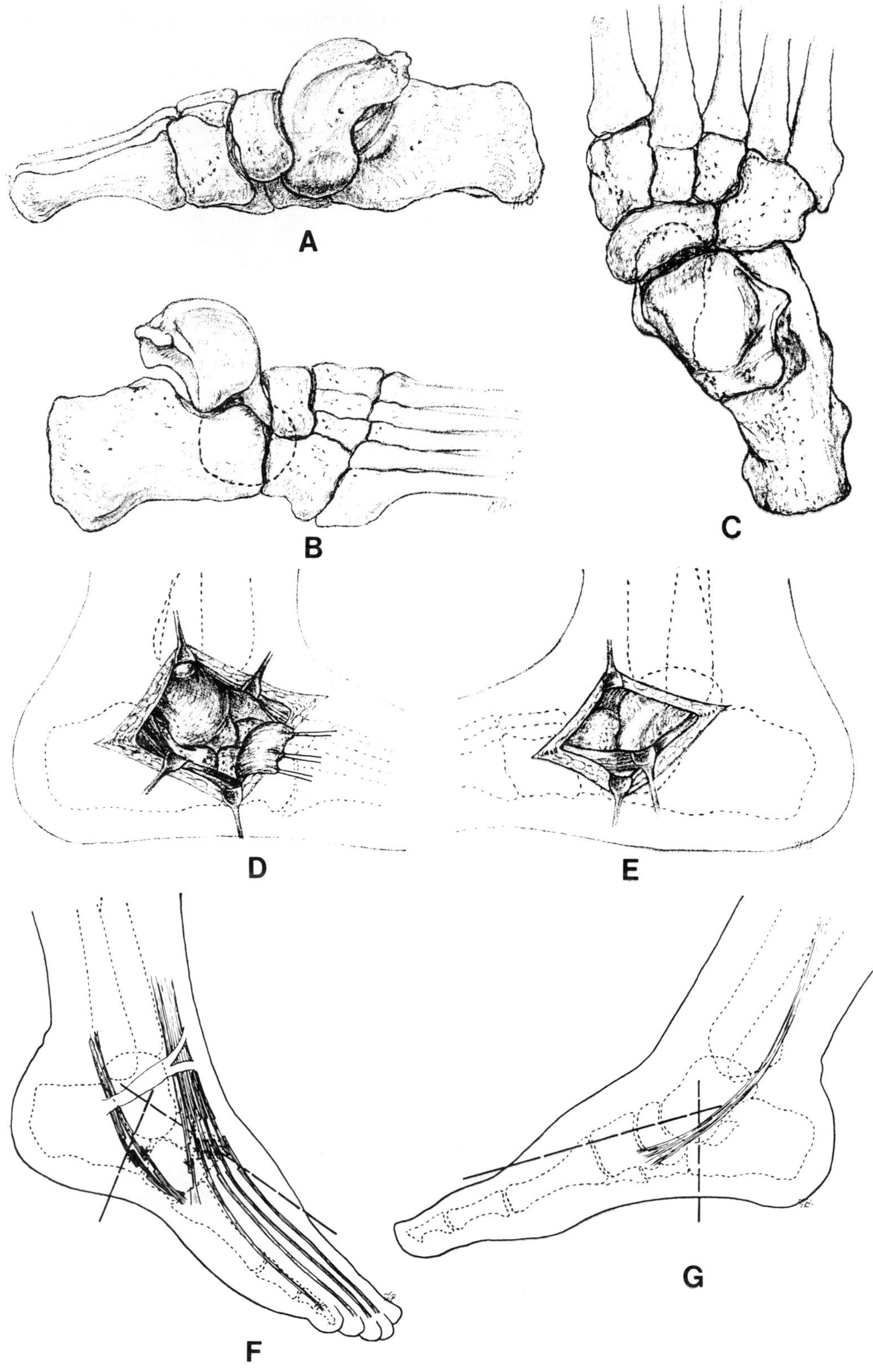

FIG. 11-55. (*Caption on facing page.*)

FIG. 11-55. The pathologic anatomy of congenital convex pes valgus. The bone relationships in a foot with congenital convex pes valgus as seen from (*A*) the medial aspect, (*B*) the lateral aspect, and (*C*) the dorsal aspect. Note the downward rotation of the talus into a vertical position; the subluxation of the navicular, which articulates with the dorsal aspect of the neck of the talus, locking it in a plantar flexed position; the relative posterior displacement and lateral rotation of the calcaneus on the talus; the abduction of the forepart of the foot; and the mild equinus of the calcaneus. (*D*) Bone relationships seen through a lateral incision. The peroneal tendons are retracted downward, the short extensor of the toes has been dissected free and retracted distalward, the long extensor tendons of the toes are retracted medially, and the sinus tarsi has been cleaned. Note the posterior position of the calcaneocuboid joint; the navicular articulates with the dorsal aspect of the neck of the talus. (*E*) Bone relationships seen through the medial incision. The posterior tibial tendon is retracted downward. Note subluxation of the navicular. (*F*) Lateral view of foot after talonavicular and subtalar ligamentous and capsular structures have been divided, contracted tendons have been lengthened, deformity has been reduced, and Kirschner wires have been inserted to maintain reduction. Only those tendons that are contracted to the extent that they prevent reduction are lengthened. Because of the equinus of the calcaneus and the tight heel cord, reduction is in equinus, which is corrected at a second-stage procedure by heel cord lengthening and posterior capsulotomy. (*G*) Medial view of the foot described in (*F*). (Herndon CH, Heyman CH: Problems in the recognition and treatment of congenital convex pes valgus. J Bone Joint Surg 45A:413, 1963)

The vertical talus is almost perpendicular.

The navicular on the head or neck of the talus is dorsally displaced. The navicular is not ossified within the first year or two, but its position is established by following the alignment of the inner ray; the continuity of the inner ray cannot be reestablished by plantar flexing the large toe. After 2 years of age, the navicular has ossified and the abnormal talonavicular relationship is readily identified.

There is equinus of the heel.

Characteristically, the abnormal relationship of the talus to the calcaneus in lateral views remains constant as the foot is dorsiflexed or plantar flexed. In contradistinction, the other forms of convex pes planovalgus, which are flexible and also have a vertically disposed talus, will reveal restoration of a more normal relationship of the tarsal bones as the foot is plantar flexed. This is a valuable means of differentiating congenital vertical talus from less resistant congenital flatfoot.

Bone deformities developing as a result of the abnormal displacement include hourglass constriction of the talus, beaking of the calcaneus, wedging of the navicular, and dorsolateral subluxation of the calcaneocuboid joint.

DIFFERENTIAL DIAGNOSIS

The differential diagnosis includes the following:[90]

Idiopathic flatfoot. There is no deformity in the non-weight-bearing state. On weight bearing, the foot is flat but the heel remains on the ground. The foot is flexible, and the deformity can be passively reduced in infancy and childhood, becoming rigid in later years. In the lateral roentgenographic view, the inner ray can be restored by plantar flexing the foot. In the standing position, the talus displaces toward the sole but never becomes perpendicular, and the talonavicular displacement is never complete. Secondary changes in the navicular, talus, and calcaneus never occur. When the heel cord is tight, the calcaneus may be horizontal but is never in equinus.

Paralytic flatfoot. Usually caused by poliomyelitis or spina bifida, paralytic flatfoot produces weakness of the invertors. The foot is mobile, and roentgenographic findings are similar to those of idiopathic flatfoot.

Spurious correction of clubfoot. Roentgenographic findings are similar, the talus and calcaneus being in equinus, but the distinction is made by history.

Talipes calcaneovalgus. The calcaneus is dorsiflexed, and the deformity can be readily corrected.

Tarsal coalition. Although this deformity is also rigid, both in the resting and in the standing position, the navicular is never dislocated, the talus does not assume a perpendicular position, and the heel is never in equinus. Bony bridges become apparent after tarsal ossification is completed.

TREATMENT

CONSERVATIVE

The deformity is rarely amenable to manipulation. However, one may attempt correction by closed methods in early infancy when the deformity is not severe and some degree of flexibility remains.[88,91] The objective is to restore a competent medial ray by replacing the navicular in front of the head of the talus. This is achieved by repeated manipulation of the forefoot into plantar flexion, forcing the head of the talus upward and inverting the heel, and holding the correction in closely fitting plaster. If this does not succeed within a few weeks, it should be abandoned in favor of surgery.

SURGICAL

The basic principles that should be emphasized are that conservative measures usually fail, the talonavicular joint must be reduced and the reduction maintained, a posterior release must nearly always be done, and the bone structures primarily involved must be held in the corrected position until they are stable, or recurrence is the rule.[85]

Although nonoperative manipulation nearly always fails, preliminary serial manipulations and casts bringing the foot into equinus are helpful to stretch the extensor tendons and the skin. This may obviate the need for tendon lengthening and reduce the skin tension that occurs when reduction is achieved at surgery.

Operative Technique. The procedure is performed in two stages, preceded by 4 to 6 weeks of plantar flexing casts (see Fig. 11-55*D* through *G*). The first stage attacks the midtarsal deformity. A generous oblique incision is made over the sinus tarsi. The tendons of the extensor digitorum longus, extensor hallucis longus, and anterior tibial are lengthened. A complete talonavicular and calcaneocuboid capsulotomy is done, which usually permits reduction of the talonavicular joint. However, it is often necessary to sever the talocalcaneal interosseous ligament before the calcaneus can be moved medially beneath the talus and the talus pulled upward while the navicular is reduced to its normal position in front of the head of the talus. With the forefoot in the appropriate degree of plantar flexion, the reduced talonavicular joint is transfixed with percutaneous Kirschner wire. Another wire directed vertically through the sole transfixes the calcaneus to the talus, preventing recurrence of eversion of the hindfoot.

Plantar flexion of the forefoot restores foot alignment, because the hindfoot is in equinus. Lengthening of the peroneus longus tendon should be avoided if possible so as not to weaken balanced dynamic forefoot flexion.

In the older child over 3 years of age, a talocalcaneal extra-articular bone block (Grice procedure) may be necessary to help effect and stabilize reduction.

The lengthened tendons are sutured, and the wound is closed. A long cast is applied with the knee bent and the foot in equinus. In 6 to 8 weeks the Kirschner wire is removed and the second stage is done when the skin is healed and there is evidence of union of the subtalar bone block.

The second stage consists of heel cord lengthening, posterior capsulotomy, and advancement of the posterior tibial tendon to the plantar surface of the navicular. The calcaneonavicular (spring) ligament is shortened. The cast is removed after 6 weeks and the patient wears a spring-loaded dropfoot brace for several months.

When surgery is delayed until adaptive bone changes have taken place, correction of deformity and relief of pain are accomplished by a triple arthrodesis.

Complications of surgery include aseptic necrosis of the navicular or talus, which may be averted by limiting the amount of dissection.

Alternative Technique. Removal of the navicular bone will reduce tension on the soft tissues medially and allow easier reduction.[92] This procedure consists of peritalar soft tissue release, excision of the navicular bone, implantation of the tibialis anterior into the talar neck, and posterior release of the hindfoot. A Kirschner wire transfixes the talus, medial cuneiform, and first metatarsal. Occasionally, multiple dorsal tendon lengthenings are added.

CONGENITAL ANGULATION OF THE TIBIA

Congenital angulation of the tibia is also called congenital bowing of the tibia and congenital kyphoscoliotic tibia. The tibia and the fibula may be bowed anteriorly or posteriorly and twisted internally or externally (Fig. 11-56). This occurs at the junction of the middle and the lower third, at the site of origin of the primary ossification center and the usual area of predilection for pseudarthrosis. The degree of involvement varies from mild bowing of a well-developed tibial shaft to severe bowing and torsion in a tibia in which the bony architecture is deficient, thinned, and even cystic about the apex of the angulation. the cortex is thickest over the concave side of the curve. The remainder of the shaft and the epiphyses

FIG. 11-56. Congenital angulation of the tibia and fibula.

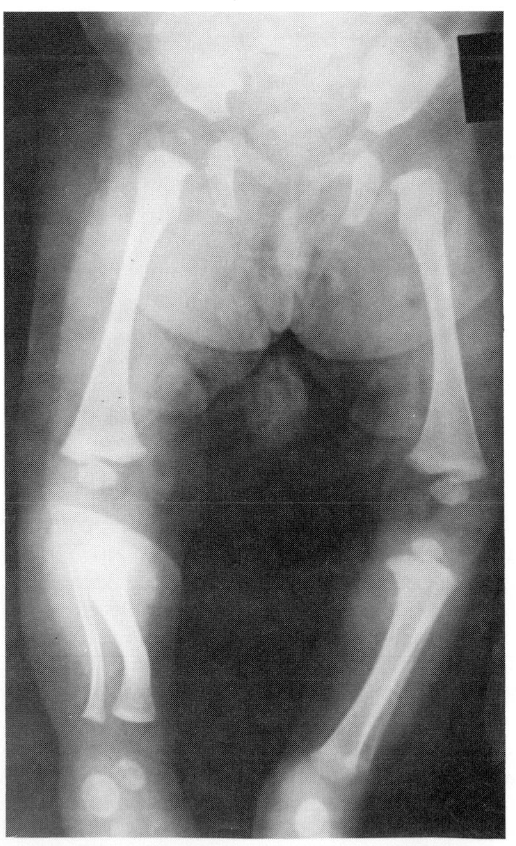

are normal. The skin is dimpled or retracted over the apex. A tendency to spontaneous fracture and subsequent pseudarthrosis exists. Occasionally, the growth in length of the limb is slightly retarded, although the epiphyseal plates seem to behave normally in appearance and time of fusion. When the bowing is anterior, talipes equinus is an associated deformity. The resistance of the clubfoot to treatment seems to parallel the severity of the bowing and its tendency to fracture and pseudarthrosis. Posterior and medial bowing is associated with severe talipes calcaneus. In this condition there is a tendency to shortness of the extremity and weakness of the calf muscles. However, there is no detectable abnormality of bony structure, no unusual tendency to fracture, and an excellent chance for spontaneous correction.[97,99]

When angulation of the tibia is part of a generalized disorder in which a number of long bones in the upper and the lower extremities are bowed, the underlying cause is usually rickets. If rickets can be excluded, hypophosphatasia is usually the cause, especially when the skin overlying the tibial angulation is retracted or dimpled.[96] A rare cause of bowing of the long bones in infants and children is Fanconi's anemia, hypoplastic pancytopenic anemia.[100]

CHARACTERISTICS

The main characteristics of this condition are the following:[95]

- Congenital anterior or posterior bowing, with rotation of the tibia
- Location in the distal portion of the middle third
- Site corresponding to the site of origin of the primary ossification center
- Thick ossification of cortex on the concave side of the curve; trabeculations arranged radially from apex of curve
- Normal bone growth from epiphyseal ends
- Tendency to spontaneous correction
- Potential danger of pathologic fracture and nonunion; pseudarthrosis more apt to develop in cases with anterior bowing
- Associated deformities: hypoplasia (failure of development of a part; fibula may be absent), hyperplasia (partial gigantism, as enlarged thumb), syndactylism of the hands or feet, neurofibromatosis with café au lait spots, dimpling of skin at apex of curved tibia

TREATMENT

Cautious and conservative treatment should be used even though the bony structure seems to be adequate and in spite of the angulation being posterior where the danger is supposedly slight. All cases should be regarded with respect. The infant should be constantly protected from injury until spontaneous correction of the curve and restoration of the bony architecture have occurred and the tendency to pseudarthrosis has lessened. This may require years. The temptation to osteotomize the tibia should be resisted. It is permissible to fit a long-length brace and apply a soft leather cuff over the apex which can be gradually tightened. Clubfoot deformities are treated with gentleness, avoiding a strain thrown above on the tibia during correction of equinus or calcaneus.

Posteromedial bowing of the tibia resolves spontaneously, usually over a period of about 3 years. The calcaneovalgus deformity found at birth resolves rapidly. Although serially applied corrective casts followed by bracing have been used, such treatment appears to be superfluous. The main problem concerns the leg-length inequality that may reach sufficient proportions, often as much as 5 cm, to require epiphysiodesis at an appropriate time.[98] The parents should be alerted and scanograms carried out at intervals. The affected foot usually remains one or two sizes smaller than the opposite foot.

When fracture and development of a pseudarthrosis apear imminent in anterolateral angulation of the tibia, particularly when the bone structure appears inadequate and the child's activity is uncontrollable, prophylactic reinforcement with autogenous bone grafts may be justified (see Fig. 11-46).[60,62,101] Through a longitudinal incision, the periosteum is elevated over half the circumference on the concave side of the tibia, extending as far as the metaphyses, and bone grafts of ribs are applied beneath the periosteum. Protective casts are worn for several months after which full activity is permitted.

Since the affected segment of tibia is often involved by fibrous dysplasia or neurofibromatosis, the bone graft may need to be placed extraperiosteally to bypass the abnormal area (Fig. 11-57). This is effective both as a preventative measure and as definitive treatment for pseudarthrosis.

PROXIMAL FEMORAL FOCAL DEFICIENCY

Proximal femoral focal deficiency is an uncommon congenital deformity characterized by defective morphogenesis (dysgenesis) of the proximal portion of the femur.[102] The femoral head, neck, and trochanters are formed in cartilage and joined to the ossifying diaphysis through a pseudarthrosis, remaining so for long periods. The orderly sequence of endochondral ossification is impaired, resulting in delayed appearance of ossification centers and retarded longitudinal growth of the femur. The proximal femoral components remain persistently cartilaginous and unable to withstand the stresses of weight bearing and muscle forces, especially at the site of pseudarthrosis, resulting in severe coxa vara deformity. The ultimate shortening of the femur at maturity may

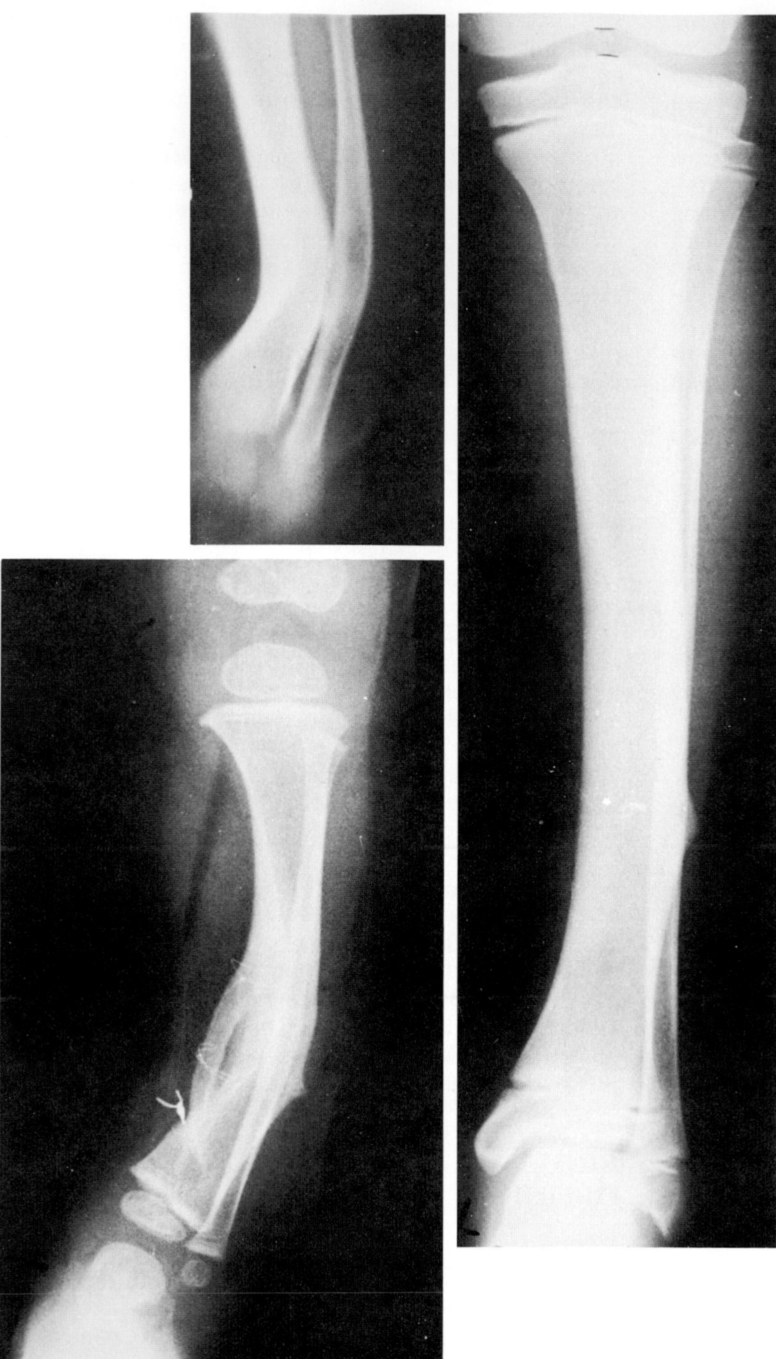

FIG. 11-57. Prophylactic surgical procedure for congenital angulation of the tibia. (*Top, left*) Preoperative roentgenogram. (*Bottom, left*) Postoperative roentgenogram of the leg at 1 year of age demonstrates placement of autogenous bone grafts. (*Right*) Roentgenogram at 12 years of age shows excellent straightening, development of bone architecture, and unimpaired longitudinal growth. (Courtesy of Dr. Panu Vilkki)

be severe, the discrepancy often exceeding 12 inches in severe cases.

Extreme forms of this anomaly are those in which the proximal components of the femur fail to develop at all. The mild forms include those with minimal shortening and coxa vara deformity. Because other congenital anomalies are often associated, a teratologic factor acting upon the developing embryo during the stage of active limb-bud formation appears to be the most plausible cause of this condition.

Proximal femoral focal deficiency must be differentiated from congenital coxa vara. The latter condition, more appropriately called developmental coxa vara, is characterized by the lack of a hereditary or teratologic factor, absence of associated anomalies, relatively normal diaphyseal development, minimal shortening (rarely exceeding 2 inches), bilateral involvement in about one third of patients, and minimal symptoms, so the diagnosis is frequently delayed (see Congenital Coxa Vara).

EMBRYOLOGY

In the developing human embryo, the first evidence of limb buds appears at the 5-mm crown-rump stage (32 days), with rapid and progressive development thereafter. The mesoderm of the limb is laid down in a proximodistal fashion, becoming complete at the 12-mm stage 10 days later.[106] During the fifth week the individual muscles begin to differentiate, and after mesenchymal condensation and chondrification, ossification of the bones is first observed at the seventh week. Differentiation of the primitive limb bud is self-determined, and transplantation at this stage before nerve ingrowth will be followed by normal development.

Orderly progression and development from mesenchymal condensation to cartilage, and through calcified cartilage to bone, may be disturbed by some teratologic factor, especially when that agent is operative during the period of active limb-bud formation and differentiation, usually from 4 to 6 weeks after conception.[1] This is the time when the noxious agent produces its greatest effect, and major limb deformities are produced.

The elements of the ilium and proximal femur develop from a common cartilaginous anlage, with subsequent cleft formation to produce a joint cavity.[108] Although movement may be essential to the development of a normal joint space and to sculpturing of the articular cartilage of femur and acetabulum, all components of the adjacent bones develop fully and are of normal size and contour in the absence of movement.[105] Consequently, if an acetabulum is seen on the roentgenogram within the first year of life, a femoral head and neck will also be present even if not visualized on the film.

At birth, ossification of the diaphysis extends to the metaphysis, whereas the femoral head and greater trochanter are entirely cartilaginous, their distal ends constituting the growth plates by which they contribute approximately 30% of longitudinal growth to the femur. The ossification center for the femoral head appears within the first year of life, but ossification of the greater trochanter is delayed until the fourth year. Thus, there are two separate areas of growth; the relative amount of growth in these two areas determines to a great extent the neck-shaft angle and the length of the proximal diaphysis.[104]

Furthermore, certain physiological forces tend to force the femoral neck into varus or valgus. The major factors encouraging varus are body weight and the longitudinally acting muscles about the hip: abductors, rectus femoris, longitudinally directed adductors, and hamstrings. The opposing valgus forces are the horizontally directed external rotators and adductors.

The differential epiphyseal growth and interrelated physiological forces combine under normal conditions to decrease the neck-shaft valgus during growth and development. At 1 year, the angle is approximately 150°, and the angle decreases thereafter, even after maturity, reaching an angle of about 120° in the aged.[112]

The mean anteversion angle of the newborn is approximately 31°. This decreases during growth to an adult average of about 12°, but the latter is highly variable.[115] Therefore, to accurately measure the true neck-shaft valgus or varus angle on the roentgenogram, it is necessary to position the extremity to correct for the amount of anteversion or retroversion.

TYPES OF DEFORMITY

Partial deficiency of the proximal femur can be graded from the mildest deformity, simple femoral hypoplasia, to the severest, femoral aplasia (Fig. 11-58).[111] Since simple femoral shortening often presents problems similar to those when greater deficiency is present, this group is included as the mildest form of this condition.

Type 1. Congenital short femur with bowing, coxa vara, and a normal acetabulum. Although ossification of the femoral capital epiphysis may be delayed, a normal hip ultimately results. Sclerosis of the medial femoral diaphyseal cortex is associated with bowing, conditions uniquely similar to those observed in milder forms of tibial pseudarthrosis.

Type 2. Short femur with subtrochanteric pseudarthrosis, progressive coxa vara, and a normal acetabulum. Ossification of the pseudarthrosis will follow in most cases, but significant residual coxa vara is the rule.

Type 3. Short femur with bulbous proximal end and delayed appearance of the femoral capital epiphysis. The acetabulum is present and mildly dysplastic. There is a tendency for the pseudarthrosis to ossify but less readily than for type 2, and the resultant varus may be extreme.

Type 4. Short femoral segment tapering sharply to a point at the proximal end. There is progressive proximal migration of the tapered sclerotic femoral shaft, with little evidence of spontaneous ossification. The femoral capital epiphysis will ultimately appear but is often delayed for several years and seldom develops fully. The acetabulum is present and becomes progressively more dysplastic.

Type 5. Small bony segment representing the distal femoral shaft, with no evidence of the proximal femoral components and no acetabulum. There is a tendency for the femoral segment to elongate, but a hip joint does not develop.

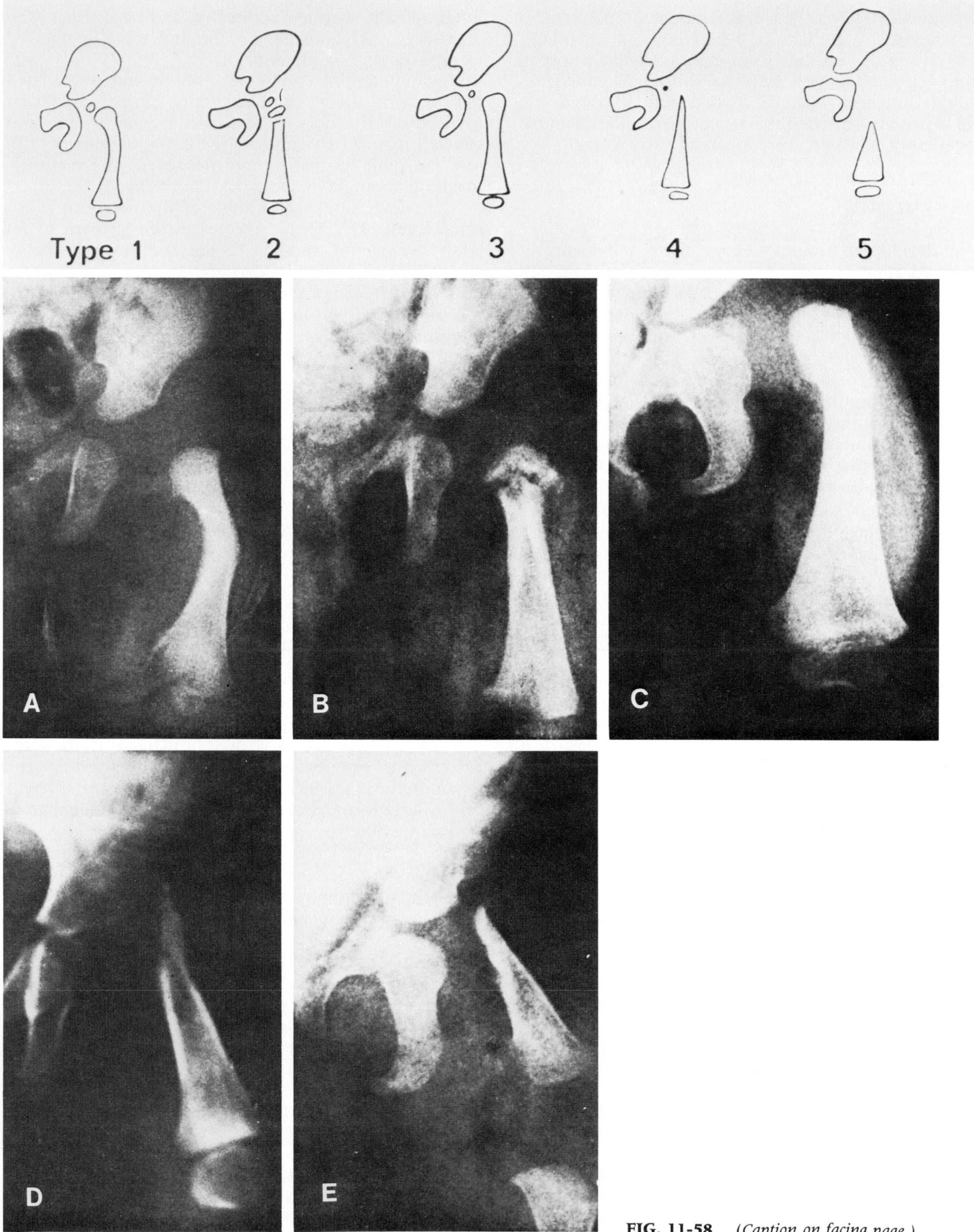

FIG. 11-58. *(Caption on facing page.)*

FIG. 11-58. Types of proximal femoral focal deficiency are shown by the line drawings at the top of the illustration. Types 1 to 5 correspond respectively to roentgenograms *A* to *E*. Type 1: short bowed femur with coxa vara; acetabulum normal. Type 2: short femur with subtrochanteric pseudarthrosis and progressive coxa vara; acetabulum normal. Type 3: short femur with bulbous proximal end; acetabulum slightly dysplastic. Type 4: short femur tapering sharply to a point; acetabulum dysplastic. Type 5: short femoral segment; no acetabulum. (Panting AL, Williams PF: Proximal femoral focal deficiency. J Bone Joint Surg 60B:46, 1978)

TREATMENT

Proximal femoral focal deficiency presents multiple problems of management, depending on the degree of the various elements of the deformity, including instability of the hip, malrotation, inadequate proximal musculature, and inequality of leg lengths. Each of these factors should be evaluated in formulating a regimen.

INSTABILITY OF THE HIP

Instability is related to iliofemoral maldevelopment and muscle inadequacy. In milder forms of deficiency, coxa vara leads to proximal displacement of the greater trochanter, which in turn causes relative abductor insufficiency and a lurching gait. In moderate types of deficiency, a persisting pseudarthrosis adds to the instability, and in the severe type of deficiency, failure of joint formation permits the imperfectly formed femoral head to slip proximally. When the proximal portion of the femur fails to develop at all, extreme instability is the natural consequence.

As a general rule, when an acetabulum can be identified on the roentgenogram of the infant, a cartilaginous head and neck, although not yet visible, are already present. One may elect to allow spontaneous ossification of the head and neck, and bony bridging across the site of pseudarthrosis, to take place.[110,116] On the other hand, in an effort at encouraging these processes and reducing the degree of coxa vara deformity, bone grafts can be placed across the pseudarthrosis extending into the femoral head and neck.[109] Before this is attempted, the presence of the proximal elements of the femur should be confirmed by arthrography. This surgical procedure is generally not accepted inasmuch as it may compromise the already insufficient contribution to longitudinal growth of the femur. Moreover, spontaneous ossification, although delayed, generally takes place, and the coxa vara deformity can be dealt with later.

In type 1 or 2 deformity, the coxa vara is corrected and held with a fixation device. This should be done at an early age and repeated when the deformity recurs.

In type 3, the pseudarthrosis usually remains unossified and the cartilaginous proximal components are joined through the bulbous pseudarthrosis to the diaphysis. The pseudarthrosis should be excised, the varus corrected, and a single-unit fixation device inserted. Alternatively, it may be preferable to encourage ossification of the proximal femur and healing of the pseudarthrosis by inserting a bone graft (*e.g.*, fibula) from the base of the greater trochanter into the neck and head and implanting its distal end, together with cancellous grafts, into the diaphysis. The coxa vara deformity can be corrected at a second operation.

In type 4, a hypoplastic head is widely separated from the tapered sclerotic femoral shaft. Nothing is gained by attempting to achieve union; such efforts are unrewarding, and even were they successful the functional result would be poor because of associated muscular hypoplasia.

In type 5, reconstruction is impossible because the acetabulum is absent. One might remove the vestigial elements of the proximal femur, place the proximal end of the shaft into a reconstructed acetabulum, and attempt to arthrodese the femur to the pelvis.[116] Some additional stability may be gained by improving muscular development by active exercises.

MALROTATION AND INADEQUATE PROXIMAL MUSCULATURE

The hip usually has a fixed flexion and external rotation contracture, sometimes associated with an abduction contracture. However, the range of preserved motion, generally flexion to 90° and abduction to 30°, is functionally useful. The gluteal muscles are usually good, whereas the quadriceps is hypoplastic. On attempted active flexion of the hip, a bulky, strongly contracting sartorius can be demonstrated. Its action is to draw the limb into the "sitting tailor's" position. Consequently, despite the hip flexion contracture, function is good and treatment for this is not required. When the femoral and tibial components are converted into a single lever by arthrodesis of the knee, this usually results in reduction of the fixed flexion at the hip.

LEG-LENGTH INEQUALITY

All femora show hypoplasia and shortening to a variable degree, ranging from mild in type 1 to severe in type 5. In general the femur is 20% to 40% of normal length. The proportional difference remains constant during growth, except for proximal migration at the pseudarthrosis.[103,113]

When lower-limb inequality is mild, it can be managed by epiphysiodesis or leg-lengthening procedures. Usually the femoral shortening is severe and progressive, and the discrepancy may exceed 12 inches at maturity; therefore, the foot of the affected leg will come to lie at approximately the same level as the normal knee. This temporally related progressive deformity should be handled in the following manner (Fig. 11-59):

Patten. In the young child, while the shortening is not yet severe, a shoe elevation is sufficient.

Extension prosthesis. Within the prosthesis, the foot is placed on a platform in full equinus. As the shortening increases, both the knee and the foot are placed within the socket of the extension prosthesis with the hinge immediately distal. These prostheses are cosmetically unacceptable.

FIG. 11-59. Methods of treating proximal femoral focal deficiency. (*A*) A patten or elevated shoe of appropriate height to maintain leg length equality. (*B*) Foot placed in equinus in a below-knee extension prosthesis. (*C*) An above-knee prosthesis with the foot in equinus. (*D*) Rotation-plasty (van Nes) allowing ankle to function as the knee with an extension prosthesis. (*E*) Conventional above-knee prosthesis after a Syme's amputation and fusion of the knee. (Panting AL, Williams PF: Proximal femoral focal deficiency. J Bone Joint Surg 60B:46, 1978)

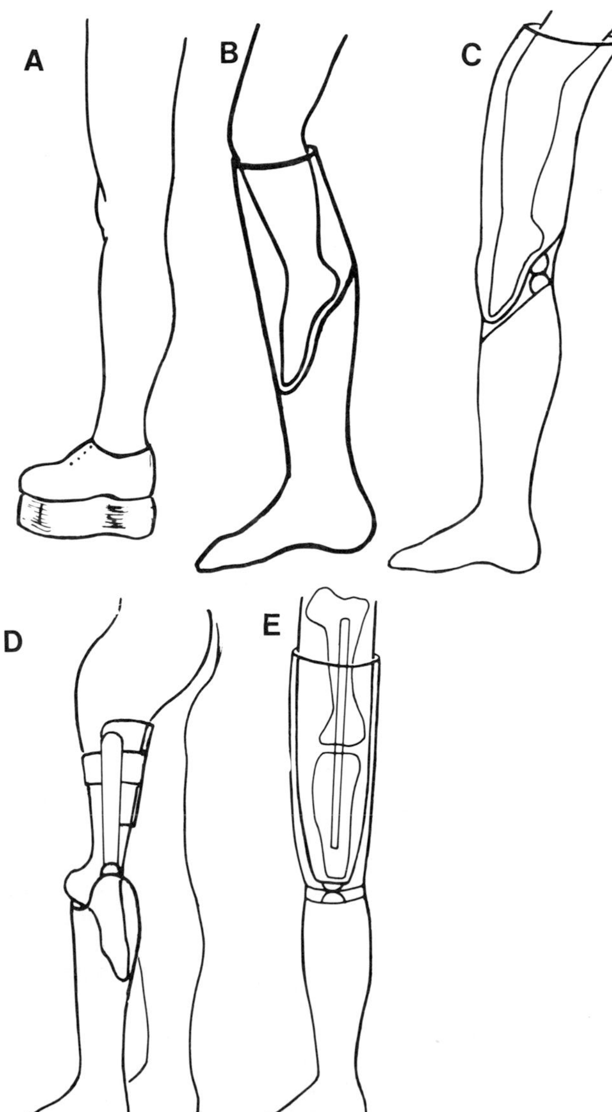

van Nes rotation-plasty.[114] Arthrodesis of the knee and rotation of the distal portion of the limb through 180° brings the ankle into a position where it functions as a knee, with the calf muscles acting as a quadriceps. However, gradual derotation usually takes place with growth and causes considerable difficulty with fitting a functional prosthesis.

Currently, because of the development of improved prostheses, the need for a substitute knee becomes less important, so there are few indications for this operation.

Syme's amputation.[67,111] This provides an excellent end-bearing stump allowing ready fitting of a prosthesis at an early age when the child quickly adapts to the prosthesis. The amputation should be done as soon as the foot can no longer reach the ground in the child in whom a severe discrepancy is expected.

Arthrodesis of the knee.[107] This provides a single skeletal lever so that available muscles can act more efficiently across the hip joint, particularly when done in conjunction with a Syme's amputation.

The procedure of choice is an early Syme's amputation as soon as walking is established and an end-bearing prosthesis. With further growth, as thigh-to-leg disproportion increases, arthrodesis of the knee is done. By removing a minimal amount of bone and inserting a smooth rod across the knee joint, continued epiphyseal growth is preserved.

It is impossible to predict the ultimate length of the stump at maturity, because many factors are involved. Therefore, all epiphyses should be preserved initially; later, epiphysiodesis should be carried out to produce a stump 3 inches to 4 inches above the level of the normal knee. In this manner a mature limb is created that is cosmetically and functionally comparable to other above-knee amputees.

Section IV
The Spine

CONGENITAL TORTICOLLIS

Torticollis (congenital wryneck) is the deformity of tilting of the head toward one side and rotation toward the opposite side. It is generally caused by muscle contraction or shortened soft tissue structures on one side of the neck, but other less common causes include paralysis of muscles on one side with resultant overaction of the muscles on the other side; congenital deformities of cervical vertebrae; subluxation of a cervical vertebra, usually spontaneous and occurring in children; cervical adenitis secondary to upper respiratory tract infection; destructive cervical spine lesions; Sprengel's deformity; unilateral soft tissue infection; neck tumors; myositis; and a central nervous system disorder, particularly diseases of the basal ganglia. In any torticollis at any age, these causes must be considered in the differential diagnosis.

ETIOLOGY

The cause is unknown. The theories of causation include intrauterine malposition (compression of vascular supply leads to ischemia and fibrosis of the sternocleidomastoid), clotting in terminal veins to the muscle during labor, and tumor formation in the sternocleidomastoid.

PATHOLOGY

At birth or within the first 2 weeks, a hard, fusiform swelling within the sternocleidomastoid muscle is found to consist of immature fibrous tissue, well demarcated from the surrounding normal-appearing muscle tissue. The "tumor" may occupy the entire thickness of the muscle, usually in the lower third. No evidence of hemorrhage or hemosiderin is found, so a remote possibility of trauma certainly cannot be substantiated. The fibrous mass subsides spontaneously, and the sternocleidomastoid becomes shortened and contracted, the process taking place over several months. Microscopically, the muscle throughout is deficient in muscle fibers, which are separated by mature fibrous tissue. The fibrous, unyielding shortening of the muscle permits neighboring structures to become contracted likewise (*i.e.*, the deep cervical fascia and the scaleni muscles). The face becomes asymmetrical and the head deformed secondary to the continued altered position over the years. The eyes eventually are situated at unequal levels. The cervical vertebrae over the growth years become deformed and adapted to the position. Thus it can readily be understood why the deformity becomes progressively fixed with passage of time.

CLINICAL PICTURE

At birth or soon thereafter the infant's head gradually tilts to one side and rotates to the opposite side (Fig. 11-60). The sternocleidomastoid muscle on the tilted side becomes taut, prominent, and shortened. This is easily demonstrated on attempting passive correction of the rotation and the tilt. An elongated, indurated, nontender swelling appears in the lower third of the muscle in many cases. Occasionally, the circumscribed tumor is absent, but the muscle has a rigid, nonelastic feel to palpation. The deformity becomes progressively worse in degree and rigidity as the other soft tissue structures and the cervical spine undergo adaptive changes. The head and the face eventually assume an asymmetrical shape, and a fixed scoliosis of the cervical spine results. In the adult, the deformity is practically uncorrectable.

TREATMENT

When treatment is instituted early and the deformity is mild and readily overcome by passive movement, con-

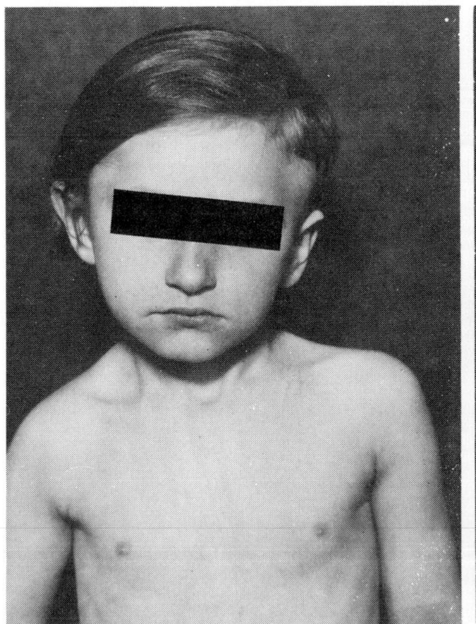

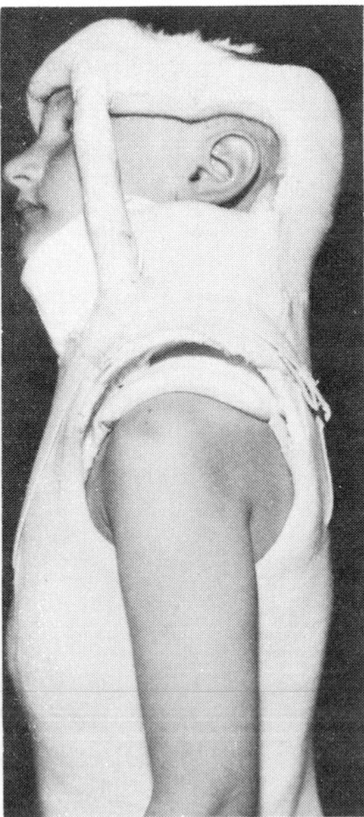

FIG. 11-60. Congenital torticollis. (*Left*) Clinical appearance. Note the facial asymmetry and prominent sternocleidomastoids, particularly on the left side. (*Right*) Postoperative cast.

servatism is adequate. The head is manipulated repeatedly toward the opposite position so that the sternocleidomastoid muscle is stretched. The daily stretchings are done by a parent with utmost gentleness. The child is placed in the crib in a strategic position of being forced to look and lift the head toward the direction of correction. For example, if the deformity is a right torticollis, the infant is positioned with its toys on the left side of the crib and the entrance to the room at the left so that he is forced to gaze toward the left at the person entering the room.

The severe and progressive cases should be determined early, before rigidity and deformity of the face and the head set in. Surgery can be performed on infants as early as 3 months of age. Through a transverse incision just above the clavicle, the platysma muscle is split and the sternocleidomastoid muscle is exposed. The sheath of the muscle is slit, and the tendinous insertions are cut at the medial end of the clavicle and the manubrium sterni. The muscle is allowed to retract. Chandler and Altenberg recommend removal of the fibrous tumor.[117] This can be shelled out and the muscle freed from underlying structures. It is questionable whether this step is necessary, inasmuch as the mass invariably recedes in a few months and does not seem to compromise the result. The clavicular attachment of the platysma and the deep fascia may also be severed. Some surgeons cut the tendinous origin of the sternocleidomastoid at the mastoid process, but this endangers the spinal accessory nerve. When this nerve traverses near the operative field, it should be identified and isolated and kept out of harm's way. Release of the soft tissue structures should permit ample correction immediately. Postoperatively, manipulative stretchings are encouraged, and head traction is applied for several weeks. This maintains correction and strengthens the antagonist muscles. An alternative is to overcorrect the deformity at the conclusion of surgery and to apply a cast about the head and the chest (Calot jacket). The cast is removed several weeks later, and manipulations and exercises are instituted.

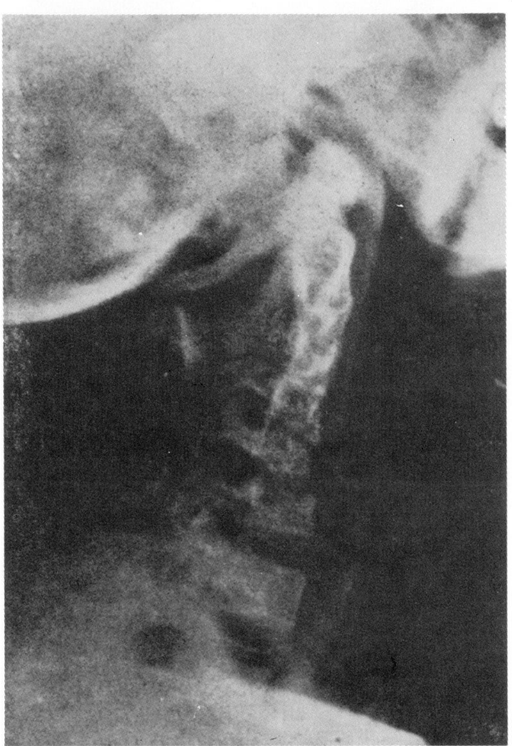

FIG. 11-61. Klippel-Feil syndrome. Lateral view of the cervical spine. The first cervical vertebra is elongated and tilted. The second to the sixth cervical vertebrae are anomalous and fused. The normal cervical lordosis is completely absent. (Shoul MI, Ritvo M: Clinical and roentgenographical manifestations of Klippel-Feil syndrome. Am J Roentgenol 68:369, 1952)

KLIPPEL-FEIL SYNDROME

Klippel-Feil syndrome (congenital fusion of cervical vertebrae, brevicollis) is a condition of congenitally fused and deformed cervical vertebrae that results in restricted neck motion and neurologic phenomena (Figs. 11-61 and 11-62).

PATHOLOGY

Typically, several vertebrae are fused, usually in pairs, and the number of vertebrae is reduced, thereby shortening the spine in the cervical region. The two vertebrae are joined by one continuous spinous process, and the bodies, if not joined by bony fusion, may be separated by a vestigial disk. The articulating processes are nonexistent, and the intervertebral foramina are narrowed and may encroach on the nerve roots. Deformities of the cervical vertebrae, mainly of the bodies, result in scoliosis, kyphosis, and torticollis, which secondarily cause nerve root pressure and pheripheral nerve symptoms. Spina bifida, particularly of the lowermost cervical vertebrae extending into the upper thoracic area, is frequent. Platybasia may be associated.

CLINICAL PICTURE

The main clinical characteristics follow:

Short neck. The trapezei may be unduly prominent laterally and give a webbed appearance—webbed neck (Fig. 11-63).

Limited neck motion. This particularly involves lateral bending and rotation.

Lowered hairline

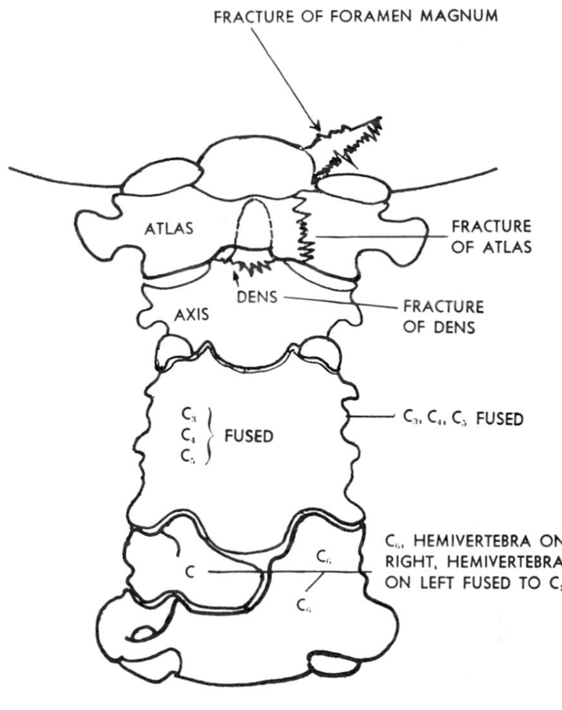

FIG. 11-62. Klippel-Feil syndrome. This diagram represents findings in cervical vertebrae at postmortem examination following accidental death. There are fractures of the foramen magnum, the atlas, and the dens. The third, fourth, and fifth cervical vertebrae are fused. The sixth cervical vertebra is in the form of two hermivertebrae, that on the left being fused to the seventh cervical vertebra. (Shoul ML, Ritvo M: Clinical and roentgenographical manifestations of Klippel-Feil syndrome. Am J Roentgenol 68:369, 1952)

Neurologic signs and symptoms. These are variable, depending on the degree of pathology.[119] The nerve roots may be compressed by osseous malformation, scoliois, kyphosis, and torticollis, leading to signs of peripheral nerve irritation, such as pain, burning sensations, and cramps, or signs of actual nerve compression, such as hypoesthesia or anesthesia, weakness or paralysis, fibrillations, and reduced deep reflexes. When the spinal cord itself is involved, the lower extremities present signs of the upper motor lesion.

ROENTGENOGRAPHIC FINDINGS

Two or more vertebrae are found to be fused, particularly at their spinous processes, and are deformed. Oblique views demonstrate absence of articulations and the inadequacy of neural foramina. The pathology found varies from only two vertebrae, discovered on routine examination, which are asymptomatic, to involvement of all cervical vertebrae, severe malformations, curvatures, reduced number of vertebrae, and spina bifida.

IMPORTANCE OF CONDITION

The importance lies mainly in distinguishing Klippel-Feil syndrome from Pott's disease and congenital torticollis, which require other forms of treatment. Deformity and rigidity of the cervical spine make it susceptible to fracture from insignificant trauma such as whiplash injury. Compression of nerve roots and the spinal cord itself is common following such trauma, even in the absence of definitely discernible fracture.

FIG. 11-63. Klippel-Feil syndrome. Note the short neck and low hairline. (Shoul MI, Ritvo M: Clinical and roentgenographical manifestations of Klippel-Feil syndrome. Am J Roentgenol 68:369, 1952)

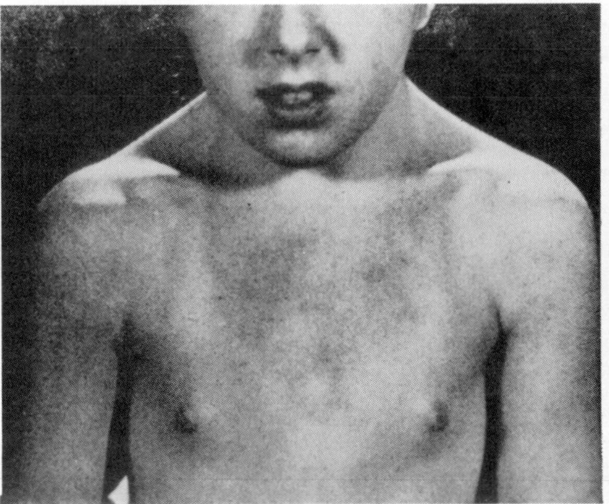

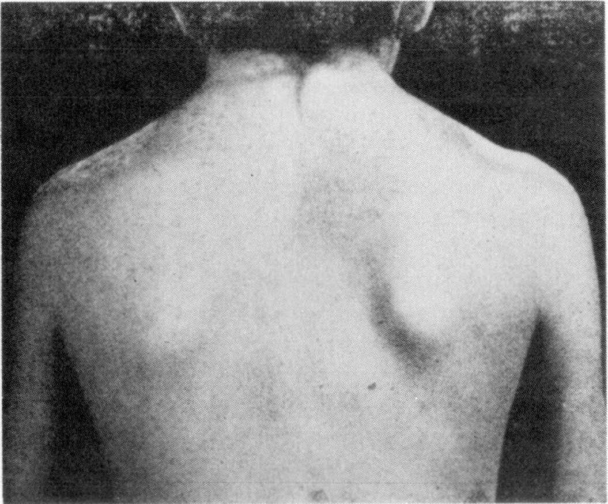

TREATMENT

Symptoms and findings of nerve root irritation, particularly when mild and of short duration, can frequently be relieved by traction and immobilization by a cast or a collar. However, neurologic phenomena that are resistant to conservative treatment and are disabling will require decompression of spinal cord and nerve roots. When one segment of the cervical spine is rigid, the segment immediately above suffers severe flexion strains, and disk rupture is probable. Removal of the disk may be indicated. Loss of the disk will eventuate in localized degenerative arthritic changes and spur formation that encroaches on the nerve root at the foramen. Decompression of this root is sufficient. Many cases are asymptomatic and require no treatment.

The shortening of the neck may be due to actual diminution in size or number of cervical vertebrae; large cervical ribs and congenital elevation of the scapulae are often associated, accounting for an apparent shortening. The cervical ribs and first three thoracic ribs may be removed.[118] Not only will this produce apparent lengthening of the neck but also, when freed of their attachments, the upper thoracic vertebrae become more mobile, act more as cervical vertebrae, and provide added flexor-extensor movement to the cervical spine. The scapulae are lowered surgically. Occasionally, one encounters prominent folds of skin on each side of the neck (pterygium colli) associated with the Klippel-Feil syndrome, particularly in females. This is corrected by resection of fascia and part of muscle, when necessary, and a double Z-plasty in the skin.

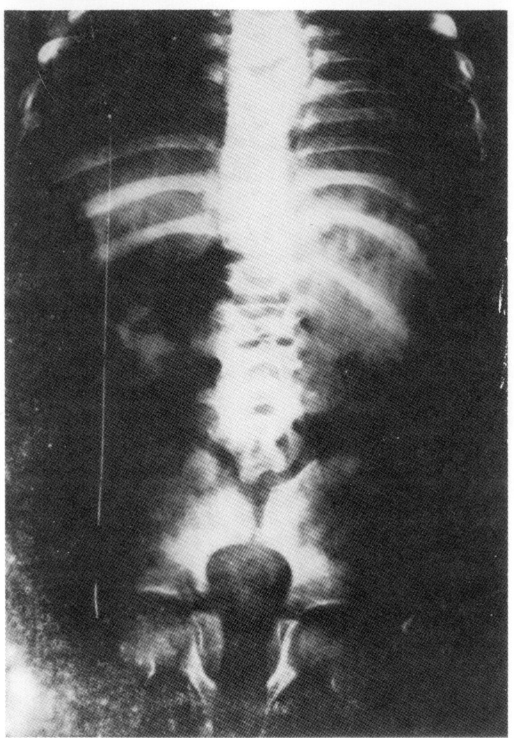

FIG. 11-64. Roentgenogram demonstrating congenital absence of the sacrum and the coccyx. (Katz JF: Congenital absence of the sacrum and coccyx. J Bone Joint Surg 35A:398, 1953)

CONGENITAL ABSENCE OF SPINAL SEGMENTS

Agenesis of segments of the spinal column is rare and usually occurs in its terminal portions.[120,121] Failure of development varies from the mere absence of the lower coccygeal segment to the complete nonexistence of vertebrae below the 10th thoracic segment. The extreme degrees of involvement are incompatible with life. Survival is possible only with absence of the sacrum or lesser degrees of the anomaly. The condition probably is due to some deleterious factor operative during the early weeks of fetal existence.

When the sacrum is not present and the iliac bones meet posteriorly in the midline, the buttocks are flattened, the intergluteal fold is shortened, the sacrococcygeal prominence is lacking, and the transverse diameter of the pelvis is diminished. Neurologic involvement is prominent. There are atrophy and diminution of muscle power in the lower extremities and urinary and fecal incontinence. A characteristic cone-shaped appearance of the lower half of the body is apparent. The feet are deformed (Figs. 11-64 and 11-65).

Section V
General Defects

POLYDACTYLISM

Extra appendages may be present in the hand or the foot at birth. The appendage may vary in degree of development from a small skin tag to a completely formed finger or toe with phalanges and a metacarpal or a metatarsal (Fig. 11-66). Usually, it consists of a small but recognizable digit containing phalanges and protruding from the lateral border of the hand or the foot and articulating with the distal end of the metatarsal or the metacarpal of the fifth toe or finger, respectively. It should be removed by disarticulation and cutting away the excess bone about the joint. When a fully developed digit is present, it is necessary to remove in addition the corresponding metacarpal or metatarsal. When doubt arises as to which of the digits is the accessory one, the digit with the least function is removed.

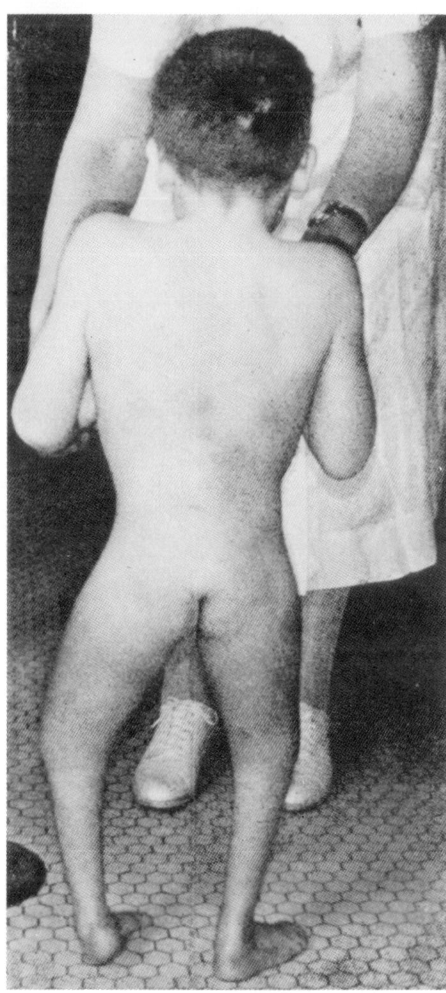

FIG. 11-65. Congenital absence of the sacrum and the coccyx. (Katz JF: Congenital absence of the sacrum and coccyx. J Bone Joint Surg 35A:398, 1953)

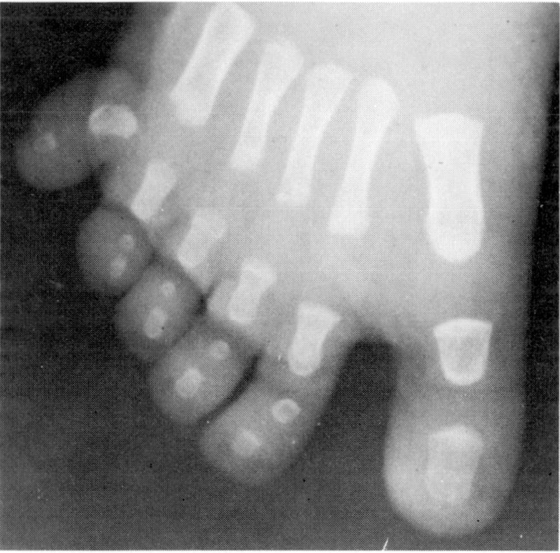

FIG. 11-66. Polydactylism. The proximal phalanx of the sixth or supernumerary toe articulates with the head of the fifth metatarsal.

AMYOPLASIA CONGENITA

A rare congenital condition, amyoplasia congenita (arthrogryposis multiplex congenita, myodystrophia fetalis) displays a marked hereditary tendency. The muscles of the extremities are aplastic, the muscle fibers being replaced by fibrofatty tissue. As a result, the joints on which they act are very rigid. Clinically, these joints display limitation of both active and passive motion and usually are fixed in a position of flexion, adduction, and inversion. In the foot the deformity is one of equinovarus that is extreme and unyielding, and a comparable deformity is found in the hand. The knees and the elbows present a fusiform appearance because of the muscle atrophy above and below. The muscles have a peculiar firm or rubbery feel, and the overlying skin is tense and glossy. The condition is painless. The spine and the back are practically never involved. The prognosis for overcoming the deformity is poor, but the life expectancy is not altered. Correction by conservative measures is valueless, because the factor of recurrence is strong. Improvement by operations on the bony structures (*e.g.*, osteotomy or arthrodesis) should be done only if the patient's mental condition warrants it.

The importance of this condition lies in its recognition. An innocent-looking clubfoot may prove to be impossible to cure because of an aplastic musculature. The typical signs of resistance to active and passive motion in all directions, symmetry of involvement, atrophic muscles, glossy skin, and mental retardation should be sought in all cases of clubfoot and the unfortunate outlook made known (see Chapter 17.)

CONGENITAL CONSTRICTING BANDS

Well-defined transverse indentations of the skin and the underlying soft tissues completely encircling the extremity at one or several levels have the appearance of a band of tissue constricting the limb. The constriction varies in degree from a slight depression to a deep one simulating an embryonic attempt at amputation (Fig. 11-67). Indeed, the disorder is frequently associated with absent parts of the extremities (*e.g.*, fingers and toes). Other congenital anomalies such as clubfoot are also found.

The lower third of the leg is the most common site for the band, where anterior or posterior bowing of the tibia may be present. The fibrous band extends down to the deep fascia but not beyond, so the deep nerve and

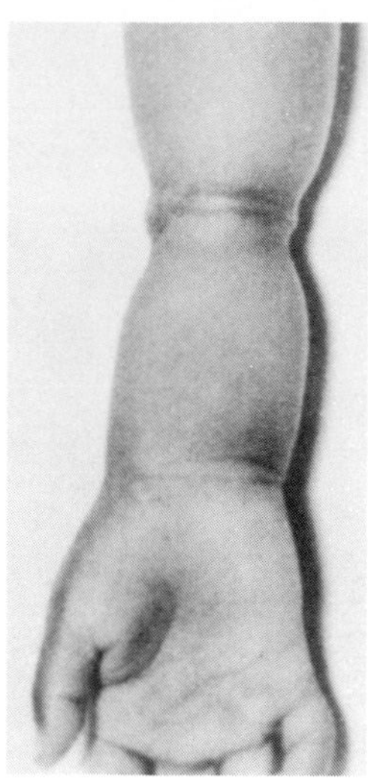
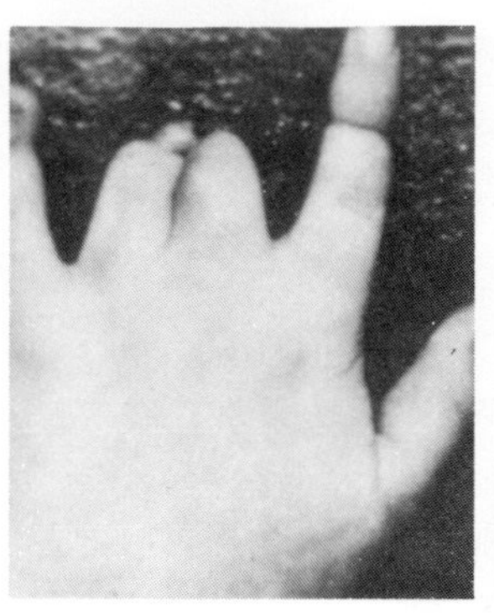
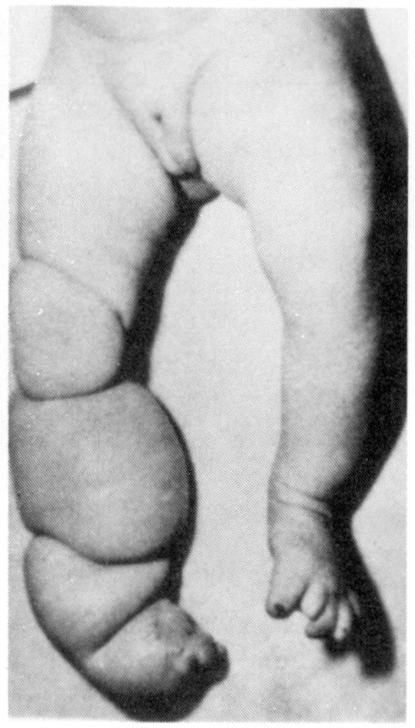

FIG. 11-67. Congenital constricting bands. These are attempts at segmentation. Swelling peripheral to the bands is due to lymphatic obstruction and will subside after removal of the constriction. (Blackfield HM, Hause DP: Plast Reconstr Surg 8:101, 1951)

vascular structures are spared. However, the superficial lymphatics may be obstructed, resulting in marked swelling of the foot distally. This swelling is globular in appearance, so completely enveloping the toes that the latter appear to be absent. When the obstruction is overcome, the swelling subsides and a more normal-looking foot is apparent.

Treatment is surgical. The band and the overlying skin are removed by a Z-plasty excision and suture of the skin, preferably in two stages, the anterior and posterior halves being done at separate times. If resection is extensive, skin grafting is necessary.

AINHUM

Ainhum affects the fifth toe, less commonly the fourth, characterized by the formation of a constriction band appearing first on the plantar surface of the base of the toe and finally producing complete encirclement. Collagenic degeneration of the soft tissues and rarefying osteitis of bone develop distal to the point of constriction. It is most common in blacks in tropical countries. Its congenital origin is controversial.

CONGENITAL HYPERLAXITY OF JOINTS

Congenital hyperlaxity of joints (arthrochalasis multiplex congenita) is characterized by diminished resistance and elongation of fibrous and elastic tissue, on a heredofamilial basis, with consequent hypermobility of joints.

PATHOLOGY

The muscles are small and elongated; ligaments, tendons, and aponeuroses are poorly developed and elongated. The joints are hypermobile, subluxations and dislocations occurring particularly about the hips and the knees.

It is entirely possible that this may be a lesser form of the Ehlers-Danlos syndrome, consisting not only of hyperlaxity of joints but also of hyperelasticity of skin, fragility of skin, and development of pseudotumors beneath the skin following trauma.

CLINICAL PICTURE

The excessive joint motion is first noted in early childhood. Many joints are involved symmetrically, especially the hips, the knees and the metacarpophalangeal joints. The degree of involvement varies from excessive range of motion to severe flaccidity, subluxation, and complete dislocation. A pronounced characteristic is the ability to hyperextend the finger joints. Hypermobility of the spine produces scoliosis; the patient stands with the knees hyperextended; and excessive hyperlaxity in the foot is manifest by a severe flatfoot deformity. The muscles are atrophic, but muscle power is only slightly diminished. Other congenital anomalies are often associated.[122,123]

REFERENCES

Teratogenesis

1. Duraiswami PK: Experimental causation of congenital skeletal defects and its significance in orthopaedic surgery. J Bone Joint Surg 34B:646, 1952
2. Yannet H: Mental deficiency due to prenatally determined factors. Pediatrics 5:328, 1950

Congenital Skeletal Limb Deficiencies

3. Frantz CH, O'Rahilly R: Congenital skeletal limb deficiencies. J Bone Joint Surg 43A:1202, 1961

Cleidocranial Dysostosis

4. Fairbank HA: Atlas of General Affections of the Skeleton. Baltimore, Williams & Wilkins, 1951
5. Marie PS, Sainton P: Observation d'Hydrocephalie Hereditaire (Pere et Fils) Pare Vice de Developpement du Crane et du Cerveau. Bull Mem Soc Med Hop Paris 14:706, 1897

Congenital Anomalies of the Hand

6. Barsky AJ: Congenital anomalies of the hand. J Bone Joint Surg 33A:35, 1951
7. Crawford HH, Horton CE, Adamson JE: Congenital aplasia or hypoplasia of the thumb and finger extensor tendons. J Bone Joint Surg 48A:82, 1966
8. White JW, Jensen WE: The thumb-clutched hand. J Bone Joint Surg 34A:680, 1952

Congenital Dislocation of the Hip

9. Chiari K: Ergebnisse mit der Beckenosteotomie als Pfannendachplastick. Z Orthop 87:14, 1955
10. Chiari K: From proceedings of the British Orthopaedic Association. J Bone Joint Surg 52B:174, 1970
11. Colonna PC: Capsular arthroplasty for congenital dislocation of the hip: A two stage procedure. J Bone Joint Surg 35A:179, 1953
12. Colton CL: Chiari osteotomy for acetabular dysplasia in young subjects. J Bone Joint Surg 54B:578, 1972
13. Dunlap K et al: A new method for determination of torsion of the femur. J Bone Joint Surg 35A:289, 1953
14. Hart VL: Congenital dislocation of the hip: Early recognition and treatment during first six months of life. Minn Med 32:749, 1949
15. Hensinger RN: Congenital Dislocation of the Hip. Clinical Symposia, vol 31, No. 1. Summit, NJ, Ciba-Geigy, 1979
16. Howorth MB: Congenital dislocation of the hip. Ann Surg 125:216, 1947
17. Ogden JA, Moss HL: Pathologic anatomy of congenital hip disease. In Weill UH (ed): Progress in Orthopaedic Surgery, Vol 2, Acetabular Dysplasia—Skeletal Dysplasia in Childhood. New York, Springer-Verlag, 1978
18. Pemberton P: Pericapsular osteotomy of the ilium for treatment of congenital subluxation and dislocation of the hip. J Bone Joint Surg 47A:65, 1965
19. Ponseti IV, Frigerio ER: Results of treatment of congenital dislocation of the hip. J Bone Joint Surg 41A:823, 1959
20. Salter RB: Innominate osteotomy in the treatment of congenital dislocation and subluxation of the hip. J Bone Joint Surg 43B:518, 1961
21. Salter RB: Role of innominate osteotomy in the treatment of congenital dislocation and subluxation of the hip in the older child. J Bone Joint Surg 48A:1413, 1966

21a. Salter RB, Kostiuk J, Dallas S: Avascular necrosis of the femoral head as a complication of treatment for congenital dislocation of the hip in young children. A clinical and experimental investigation. Canad J Surg 12:44, 1969

22. Scott JC: Frame reduction in congenital dislocation of the hip. J Bone Joint Surg 35B:372, 1953
23. Severin E: Congenital dislocation of the hip: Development of the joint after closed reduction. J Bone Joint Surg 32A:507, 1950
24. Somerville EW: Open reduction in congenital dislocation of the hip. J Bone Joint Surg 35B:363, 1953
25. Somerville EW: Results of treatment of 100 congenitally dislocated hips. J Bone Joint Surg 49B:258, 1967
26. Wiberg G: Studies on dysplastic acetabula and congenital subluxation of the hip joint. Acta Chir Scand (Suppl) 83:58, 1939
27. Wiberg G: Shelf operation in dislocation of the hip. J Bone Joint Surg 35A:65, 1953

Congenital Clubfoot

28. Brockman EP: Congenital Clubfoot. London, Wright, 1930
29. Evans D: Relapsed clubfoot. J Bone Joint Surg 43B:722, 1961
30. Fried A: Recurrent congenital clubfoot. J Bone Joint Surg 41A:243, 1959
31. Garceau GJ: Talipes equinovarus. Am Acad Orthop Surg Instructional Course Lectures 7:119, 1950
32. Grant JCB: Atlas of Anatomy. Baltimore, Williams & Wilkins, 1962
33. Kite JH: Theories on the increase in the occurrence of congenital metatarsus varus deformity. Am Acad Orthop Surg Instructional Course Lectures 7:116, 1950
34. McCauley JC: Surgical treatment of clubfoot. Surg Clin North Am 31:561, 1951
35. Singer M: Tibialis posterior transfer in congenital clubfoot. J Bone Joint Surg 43B:717, 1961
36. Singer M, Fripp AT: Tibialis anterior transfer in congenital clubfoot. J Bone Joint Surg 40B:252, 1958
37. Swann M, Lloyd-Roberts GC, Catterall A: The anatomy of uncorrected clubfoot. J Bone Joint Surg 51B:263, 1969
38. Turco VJ: Surgical correction of resistant clubfoot. J Bone Joint Surg 53A:477, 1971

Congenital Metatarsus Adductovarus

39. Heyman CH, Herndon CH, Strong JM: Mobilization of the tarsometatarsal and intermetatarsal joints for the correction of resistant adduction of the forepart of the foot in congenital clubfoot or congenital metatarsus varus. J Bone Joint Surg 40A:299, 1958
40. Kite JH: Congenital metatarsus varus. J Bone Joint Surg 32A:500, 1950
41. McCormick DW, Blount WP: Metatarsus adductovarus. JAMA 141:449, 1949
42. Ponseti IV, Becker JH: Congenital metatarsus adductus. J Bone Joint Surg 48A:702, 1966

Congenital Hallux Varus

43. McElvenny RT: Hallux varus. Q Bull Northwestern Univ Med School 15:277, 1941

Congenital Dislocation of the Knee

44. Clayburgh BJ: Congenital dislocation of the knee. Proc Staff Meet Mayo Clin 30:396, 1955

Congenital Coxa Vara

45. Babb FS, Ghormley RK, Chatterton CC: Congenital coxa vara. J Bone Joint Surg 31A:115, 1949
46. LeMesurier AB: Developmental coxa vara. J Bone Joint Surg 30B:595, 1948

47. LeMesurier AB: Letter to the Editor. J Bone Joint Surg 33B:428, 1951
48. Zadek I: Congenital coxa vara. Arch Surg 30:62, 1935

Congenital Pseudarthrosis of the Tibia

49. Aegerter EE: The possible relationship of neurofibromatosis, congenital pseudarthrosis and fibrous dysplasia. J Bone Joint Surg 32A:618, 1950
50. Bassett CAL, Caulo N, Kort J: Congenital "pseudarthrosis" of the tibia: Treatment with pulsing electromagnetic fields. Clin Orthop 154:136, 1981
51. Boyd HB: Congenital pseudarthrosis: Treatment by dual bone grafts. J Bone Joint Surg 23:497, 1941
52. Boyd HB, Sage FP: Congenital pseudarthrosis of the tibia. J Bone Joint Surg 40A:1245, 1958
53. Brighton CT et al: Direct-current stimulation of non-union and congenital pseudarthrosis. J Bone Joint Surg 57A:368, 1975
54. Charnley J: Congenital pseudarthrosis of the tibia treated by the intramedullary nail. J Bone Joint Surg 38A:283, 1956
55. Commurati M: Le pseudartrosi congenite della tibia. Chir Organi Mov 15:1, 1930
56. Ducroquet R: A propos des pseudarthrosis et inflexions congénitales du tibia. Mem Acad Chir 63:863, 1937
57. Fienman NL, Yacovaks WC: Neurofibromatosis in childhood. J Pediatr 76:339, 1970
58. Green WT, Rudo N: Pseudarthrosis and neurofibromatosis. Arch Surg 46:639, 1943
59. Inglis K: The pathology of congenital pseudarthrosis of the tibia. J Coll Surg Aust 1:194, 1928
60. Lloyd-Roberts GC, Shaw NE: The prevention of pseudarthrosis in congenital kyphosis of the tibia. J Bone Joint Surg 51B:100, 1969
61. McCarroll HR: Clinical manifestations of congenital neurofibromatosis. J Bone Joint Surg 32A:618, 1950
62. McFarland B: Pseudarthrosis of the tibia in childhood. J Bone Joint Surg 33B:36, 1951
63. Paterson DC, Lewis GN, Cass CA: Treatment of congenital pseudarthrosis of the tibia with direct current stimulation. Clin Orthop 148:129, 1980
64. Sofield HA, Millar EA: Reversal of shaft and intramedullary-rod fixation in the treatment of congenital pseudarthrosis of the tibia: A ten-year appraisal. J Bone Joint Surg 46A:1370, 1964
65. van Nes CP: Congenital pseudarthrosis of the leg. J Bone Joint Surg 48A:1467, 1966
66. Weber BG, Čech O: Pseudarthrosis. Bern, Hans Huber, 1976

Congenital Absence of the Fibula

67. Aitken GT: Amputation as a treatment for certain lower-extremity congenital anomalies. J Bone Joint Surg 41A:1267, 1959
68. Aitken GT: The child amputee. Orthop Clin North Am 3:447, 1972
69. Aitken GT: Congenital short femur with fibular hemimelia. J Bone Joint Surg 56A:1306, 1974
70. Amstutz H: Natural history and treatment of congenital absence of the fibula. J Bone Joint Surg 54A:1349, 1972
71. Anderson M, Messner MB, Green WT: Distribution of lengths of the normal femur and tibia in children from one to 18 years of age. J Bone Joint Surg 46A:1197, 1964
72. Bagg NJ: Disturbance in mammalian development produced by radium emanation. Am J Anat 30:133, 1922
73. Coventry MB, Johnson EW Jr: Congenital absence of the fibula. J Bone Joint Surg 34A:941, 1952
74. Green WT, Anderson M: Skeletal age and the control of bone growth. Am Acad Orthop Surg Instructional Course Lectures Vol. 17:199, 1960
75. Kruger IM, Talbott RD: Amputation and prosthesis as definitive treatment in congenital absence of the fibula. J Bone Joint Surg 43A:625, 1961
76. Warkany J, Nelson RC, Schraffenberger E: Congenital malformations induced in rats by maternal nutrition deficiency: III. The malformations of the extremities. J Bone Joint Surg 25:261, 1943
77. Westin GW, Sakai DN, Wood WL: Congenital longitudinal deficiency of the fibula. J Bone Joint Surg 58A:492, 1976
78. Wood WL, Zlotsky N, Westin GW: Congenital absence of the fibula: Treatment by Syme amputation: Indications and technique. J Bone Joint Surg 47A:1159, 1965

Congenital Torsion in the Lower Extremity

79. Kite JH: Tibial torsion. J Bone Joint Surg, 36A:511, 1954
80. O'Donoghue DH: Controlled rotation osteotomy of the tibia. South Med J 33:1145, 1940

Congenital Dislocation of the Patella

81. Conn HR: A new method of operative reduction for congenital luxation of the patella. Boston Med Surg J 150:169, 1904
82. Mumford EB: Congenital dislocation of the patella. J Bone Joint Surg 29:1083, 1947

Multipartite Patella

83. Adams JD, Leonard RD: A developmental anomaly of the patella diagnosed as a fracture. Surg Gynecol Obstet 41:601, 1925
84. Smillie IS: Injuries of the Knee Joint. Edinburg, E&S Livingston, 1946

Congenital Vertical Talus

85. Coleman S, Stelling FH, Jarrett J: Pathomechanics and treatment of congenital vertical talus. Clin Orthop 70:62, 1970
86. Drennan JC, Sharrad WJW: The pathologic anatomy convex pes valgus. J Bone Joint Surg 53B:455, 1971
87. Hark FW: Rocker foot due to congenital subluxation of the talus. J Bone Joint Surg, 32A:344, 1950
88. Herndon CH, Heyman CH: Problems in the recognition and treatment of congenital convex pes valgus. J Bone Joint Surg 45A:413, 1963
89. Lamy L, Weissman L: Congenital convex pes valgus. J Bone Joint Surg 21:79, 1939
90. Lloyd-Roberts GC, Spence AJ: Congenital vertical talus. J Bone Joint Surg 40B:33, 1958
91. Silk FF, Wainwright D: The recognition and treatment of congenital flatfoot in infancy. J Bone Joint Surg 49B:628, 1967
92. Stone KH (for Lloyd-Roberts GC): Congenital vertical talus: A new operation. Proc R Soc Med 56:12, 1963
93. Towns PI et al: Trisomy 13–15 in a male infant. J Pediatr 60:528, 1962

94. Uchida IA et al: A case of double trisomy no. 18 and triple X. J Pediatr 60:498, 1962

Congenital Angulation of the Tibia

95. Badgley CE et al: Congenital kyphoscoliotic tibia. J Bone Joint Surg 34A:349, 1952
96. Bain AD, Barrett HS: Congenital bowing of long bones. Arch Dis Child 34:516, 1959
97. Heyman CH, Herndon CH: Congenital posterior angulation of the tibia. J Bone Joint Surg 31A:571, 1949
98. Hofmann A, Wenger DR: Posteromedial bowing of the tibia: Progression of discrepancy of leg lengths. J Bone Joint Surg 63A:384, 1981
99. Miller BF: Congenital posterior bowing of the tibia with talipes calcaneovalgus. J Bone Joint Surg 31B:50, 1951
100. Silverman FN: Systemic diseases of childhood with local manifestations. Am Acad Orthop Surg Institutional Course Lectures 14:249, 1957
101. Vilkki P: Preventative treatment of congenital pseudarthrosis of tibia. J Pediatr Surg 12:91, 1977

Proximal Femoral Focal Deficiency

102. Aitken GT: Proximal femoral focal deficiency: Definition, classification and management. In Aitken GT (ed): Proximal Femoral Focal Deficiency: A Congenital Anomaly, pp 50–76. Washington, DC, National Academy of Sciences, 1968
103. Amstutz HC: The morphology, natural history and treatment of proximal femoral focal deficiencies. In Aitken GT (ed): Proximal Femoral Focal Deficiency: A Congenital Anomaly, pp 50–76. Washington, DC, National Academy of Sciences, 1968
104. Compere EL, Garrison M, Fahey JJ: Deformities of the femur resulting from arrestment of growth of the capital and greater trochanteric epiphyses. J Bone Joint Surg 22:909, 1940
105. Drachman DB, Sokoloff L: The role of movement in embryonic joint development. Dev Biol 14:401, 1966
106. Hamilton WJ, Mossman HW: Hamilton, Boyd and Mossman's Human Embryology, 4th ed, pp 541–547. Cambridge, W. Heffer and Sons, 1972
107. King RE: Providing a Single Skeletal Lever in Proximal Femoral Focal Deficiency. Inter Clinic Information Bulletin, vol 6, No. 2:23. New York, Committee on Prosthetics Research and Development, 1966
108. Laurenson RD: Development of the acetabular roof in the fetal hip. J Bone Joint Surg 47A:975, 1965
109. Lloyd-Roberts GTC, Stone KH: Congenital hypoplasia of the upper femur. J Bone Joint Surg 45B:557, 1963
110. Meyer LM, Friddle D, Pratt RW: Problems of treating and fitting the patient with proximal femoral focal deficiency. Inter Clinic Information Bulletin, vol 10, No. 2, pp 1–4. New York, Committee on Prosthetics Research and Development, 1971
111. Panting AL, Williams PF: Proximal femoral focal deficiency. J Bone Joint Surg 60B:46, 1978
112. Pick JW, Stack JK, Anson BJ: Measurements on the human femur: Lengths, diameters and angles. Q Bull Northwestern Univ Med School 15:281, 1941
113. Ring PA: Congenital short femur. J Bone Joint Surg 41B:73, 1959
114. van Nes CP: Rotation plasty for congenital defects of the femur. J Bone Joint Surg 32B:12, 1950
115. von Lanz T, Mayet A: Die Gelenkkörper des menschlichen Hüftgelenkes in der progredienten Phase ihrere umwegigen Ausformung. Z Anat 117:317, 1953
116. Westin GW, Gunderson FO: Proximal femoral focal deficiency: A review of treatment experiences. In Aitken GT (ed): Proximal Femoral Focal Deficiency: A Congenital Anomaly, pp 100–110. Washington, DC, National Academy of Sciences, 1968

Congenital Torticollis

117. Chandler FA, Altenberg A: "Congenital" muscular torticollis. JAMA 125:476, 1944

Klippel-Feil Syndrome

118. Bonola A: Surgical treatment of the Klippel-Feil syndrome. J Bone Joint Surg 38B:440, 1956
119. Mosberg WH Jr: Klippel-Feil syndrome: Etiology and treatment of neurological signs. J Nerv Ment Dis 117:479, 1953

Congenital Absence of Spinal Segments

120. Freedman B: Congenital absence of the sacrum and coccyx: Report of a case and review of the literature. Br J Surg 37:299, 1950
121. Katz JF: Congenital absence of the sacrum and coccyx. J Bone Joint Surg 35A:398, 1953

Congenital Hyperlaxity of Joints

122. Hass J, Hass R: Arthrochalasis multiplex congenita. J Bone Joint Surg 40A:663, 1958
123. Key JA: Hypermobility of joints a sex-linked hereditary characteristic. JAMA 88:1710, 1927

12

Developmental Conditions

OSTEOGENESIS IMPERFECTA

Osteogenesis imperfecta (fragilitas ossium, idiopathic osteopsathyrosis, periosteal dysplasia) is a hereditary condition characterized by fragility of bone, deafness, blue sclerae, laxity of joints, and a tendency to improvement with age.[1–3,6,7]

ETIOLOGY

The factor of heredity is demonstrable in many cases. Many prenatal cases are inherited as a mendelian recessive; the postnatal cases are inherited as a dominant. One or several of the characteristics of the condition may be present in other members of the family. The presence of blue sclerae is said to be associated with hereditary types only.

PATHOGENESIS AND PATHOLOGY

The primary defect is the failure of formation of osteoblasts. At the epiphyseal plate endochondral ossification proceeds normally as far as the stage of provisional calcification of cartilage. Very few osteoblasts appear, and osteoid formation is minimal. Some of the calcified cartilage may undergo direct metaplasia to bone. The formation of bone by periosteum is likewise deficient. The periosteum is thick, but the cambium layer is thin and relatively acellular. Occasionally, cartilage cells are formed at this site, perhaps representing persistence of the fetal histogenesis. In the skull small scattered foci of bone formation and delayed closure of the fontanelles are characteristic.

Grossly, the bones are shorter and thinner. The epiphyses in contrast to the shaft appear bulbous. Trabeculae are sparse, delicate, and longitudinally disposed. No transverse trabeculae are seen. The cortex is very thin. Medullary contents are fatty or fibrous and rarely lymphoid. Deformity results from fractures and bending. The fracture often is subperiosteal and seems to heal mainly by periosteal bone formation. Callus is abundant except in severe cases.

Associated deformities include vertebral bodies that are translucent, shallow, and biconcave as a result of disk indentation. Scoliosis is frequent. The skull is thin and globular. It may be crushed in severe cases at birth. The pelvis may be compressed from side to side.

CLINICAL PICTURE

The condition may vary from mild to severe. The onset occurs at any time from before birth to late adolescence, rarely in adults.

Classification of Cases

Three forms are noted:

1. *Fetal or prenatal form.* Usually this form is severe, with many fractures throughout the body being present at birth. The skull feels like a membranous bag of bones. The infant may be stillborn or die at birth or within a few weeks.
2. *Infantile form.* This form is less severe; multiple fractures occur; the skull is thin and globular and may resemble that of a hydrocephalic. If the child survives the first few years, the chance for lessening of the tendency to fracture and continued survival is good.
3. *Adolescent form or osteogenesis imperfecta tarda.* In this type the child is normal at birth, and fractures as a result of trivial trauma become manifest later in childhood. Later, the tendency to fracture is lost.

Characteristics

The characteristics, one or all of which may be present in the patient and other members of his family, include the following:

Fractures. The number of fractures varies. In severe cases they may be spontaneous. Pain is slight or absent. Healing readily occurs, usually with deformity that tends to lessen with continued longitudinal growth. The tendency to fracture lessens with advancing age.
Blue sclerae. A fairly deep indigo color, not merely the light blue seen in normal infants, is noted.
Deafness. Hearing is reduced in many patients by the third decade of life. Otosclerosis is frequently the cause.
Laxity of joints. The susceptibility to strain and dislocation is common in families of the patients.
Feeble musculature
Dwarfing. This is caused by deformities of lower limbs and spine.
Broad skull. Parietal and occipital bones are prominent (*crâne à rebord*).
Poorly calcified deciduous teeth. Permanent teeth are normal.
Normal blood chemistry

ROENTGENOGRAPHIC FINDINGS

The skeleton is osteoporotic, and the long bones appear elongate and thin, with thinned cortices and bulbous ends (Figs. 12-1 through 12-3). The skull is thin, and wormian bones may be present. Vertebral bodies are translucent, shallow, and biconcave, with the disks being biconvex. Severe prenatal cases exhibit numerous fractures, particularly in the ribs, and the major long bones may be short, broad, and thick.

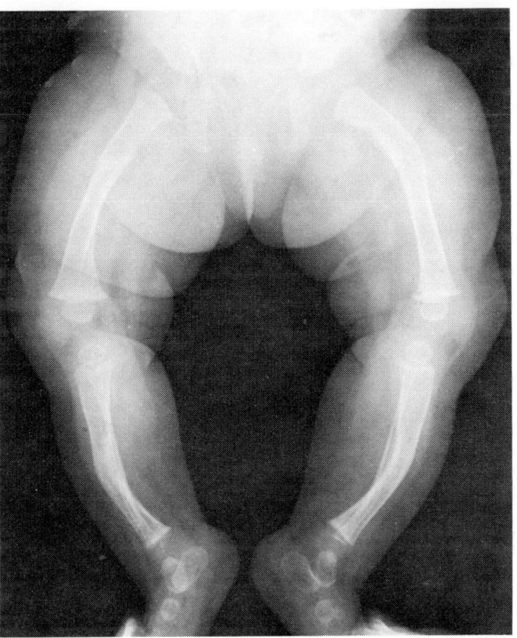

FIG. 12-1. Osteogenesis imperfecta. There is marked osteoporosis. Note loss of transverse trabeculations. Longitudinal trabeculations are poorly defined, cortices are thinned, and deformities occur at sites of healed fractures.

PRENATAL DIAGNOSIS

Prenatal determination of the probability of the presence of osteogenesis imperfecta in the fetus can be achieved by amniocentesis and measurement of inorganic pyrophosphate.[5] This compound is consistently elevated at 3.4 to 3.7 times the normal value for the gestational age. Rarely, such alterations can occur in normal fetuses. The normal values of pyrophosphate are listed below:

0–14 weeks = 6μg/dl
15–24 weeks = 18μg/dl
25 weeks to term = 13μg/dl

TREATMENT

Treatment consists essentially of protection of the child until the tendency to fracture has lessened. Adequate vitamin intake for bone deposition is necessary, but one must guard against excessive vitamin D medication by overzealous parents, which would contribute to decalcification. The administration of estrogens and androgens may have a beneficial effect.

Severe deformity of a long bone may be corrected by multiple osteotomies through the metaphyses and through the shaft of the bone and threading the fragments on an intramedullary rod.[4] Union occurs rapidly, and the rod may be left in as a precaution against recurrence of

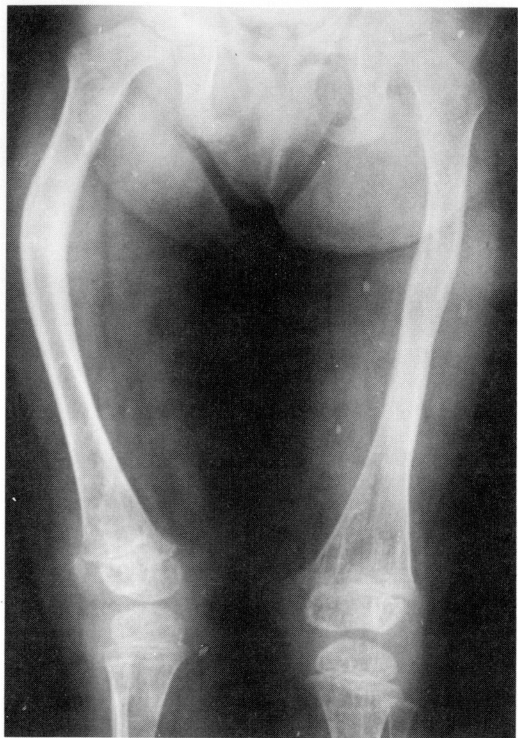

FIG. 12-2. Osteogenesis imperfecta. Same case as in Figure 12-1. Trabeculations are better defined, and some transverse trabeculations are present. Cortices are thicker. There is a tendency to straightening of deformities with growth. This demonstrates progressive return to normal bony architecture and lessening tendency to fracture with advancing age.

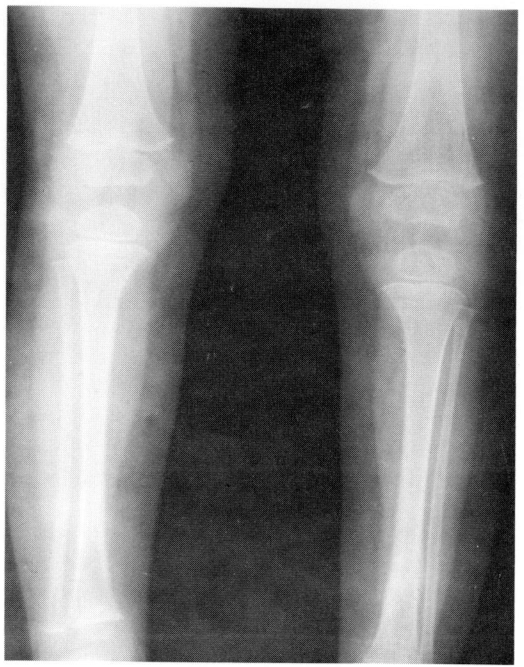

FIG. 12-3. Osteogenesis imperfecta, appearance later in childhood.

fracture and deformity. When the bone is too thin for surgical handling, it may be replaced with homogenous bone (either bank bone or a fibular graft from a relative). The transplanted bone is replaced in time by the imperfect bone characteristic of osteogenesis imperfecta. As a rule, no disturbance of epiphyseal growth occurs. The procedure may also be used for the fracture of a long bone. The technique (Fig. 12-4) is described in the following paragraphs.

The shaft is exposed subperiosteally along its entire length, osteotomized through the proximal and the distal metaphyses, and removed from its bed. The shaft is studied and sectioned into the least number of fragments necessary for straightening, and the fragments are threaded on an intramedullary rod. The rods commonly used are round in cross section and range from $\frac{5}{64}$ to $\frac{1}{4}$ inch in diameter. Since the cross-sectional anatomy of the medullary canal is usually distorted, difficulty may be encountered in attempts to pass the rod through the canal, and a fragment may be split longitudinally. In such a situation, the pieces only need to be fixed about the rod in barrel-stave fashion. Then the straightened shaft is replaced into its bed. The projecting distal end of the rod is inserted into the distal metaphysis so that it extends almost to the distal epiphyseal line, and the proximal end lies either in the medullary canal close to the proximal epiphyseal line, as in the case of the tibia, or projects just above the proximal end of the bone, as in the case of the femur, the ulna, and the humerus, where the rod is inserted in a retrograde manner.

After fixation of the tibia, the rod tends to displace anterior and protrude through the anterior portion of the bone. Therefore, it is essential to maintain an intact anterior cortex. After the distal end of the rod has been secured in the distal metaphysis, a slot, approximately 1 inch in length and the width of the rod, is made with a curet in the posterior cortex of the proximal metaphysis. Next, the proximal portion of the protruding rod is manipulated over the lateral cortex of the proximal metaphysis, through the posterior slot and into the medullary cavity of the metaphysis.

In the femur the proximal end of the rod is driven retrograde up the medullary canal to emerge just medial to the greater trochanter and, after the fragments of the shaft are threaded on the rod, the distal end is driven into the distal metaphysis (Fig. 12-5).

In the humerus the rod is similarly driven in retrograde fashion through the proximal metaphysis, coming out at the lateral margin of the epiphysis. Then it is gradually driven distally, and the fragments are threaded on to it until its distal end is seated in the distal metaphyseal fragment.

Fixation of the ulna after fragmentation and realignment of the shaft is accomplished either by inserting the

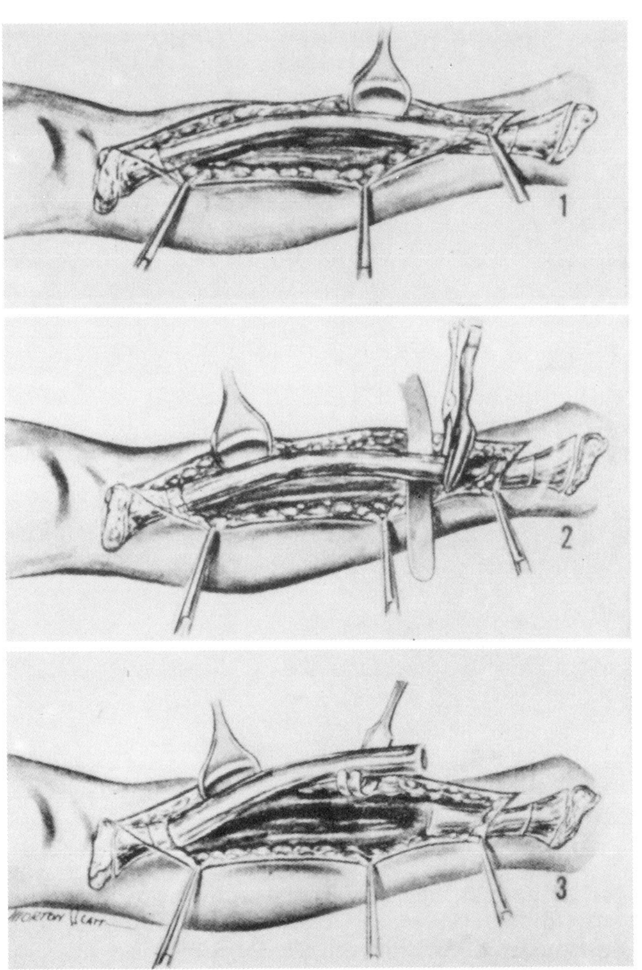

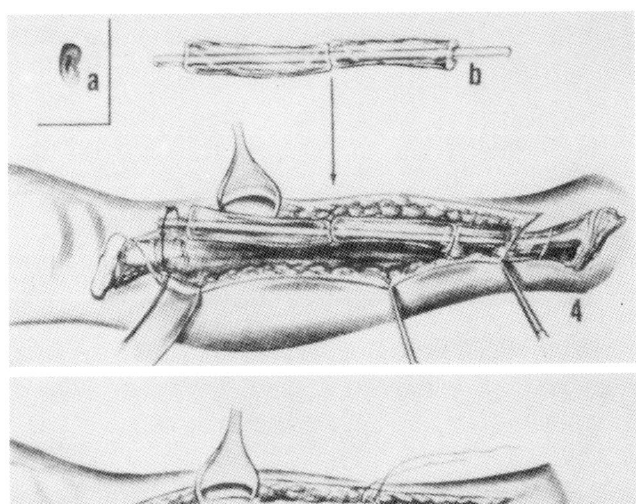

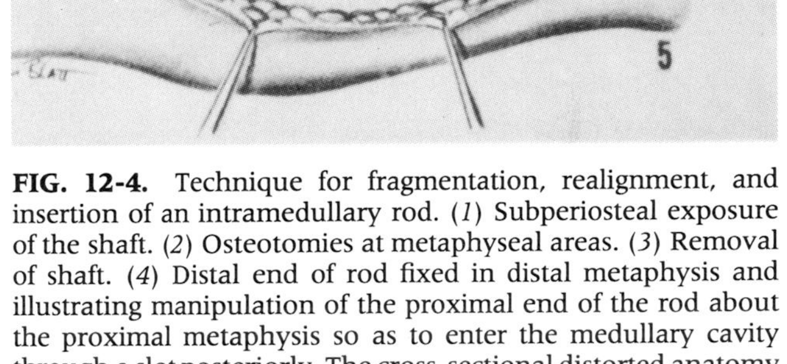

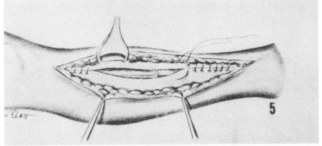

FIG. 12-4. Technique for fragmentation, realignment, and insertion of an intramedullary rod. (*1*) Subperiosteal exposure of the shaft. (*2*) Osteotomies at metaphyseal areas. (*3*) Removal of shaft. (*4*) Distal end of rod fixed in distal metaphysis and illustrating manipulation of the proximal end of the rod about the proximal metaphysis so as to enter the medullary cavity through a slot posteriorly. The cross-sectional distorted anatomy (*a*). Fragments realigned and threaded on rod (*b*). (*5*) Closure of periosteum. (Sofield HA, Millar EA: Fragmentation, realignment, and intramedullary rod fixation of deformities of the long bones in children. J Bone Joint Surg 41A:1371, 1959)

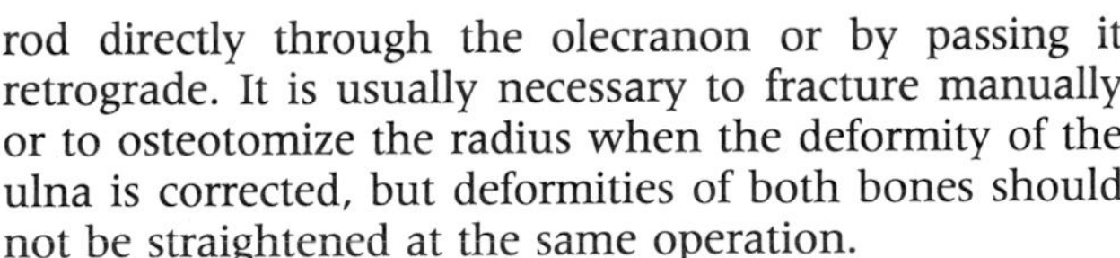

rod directly through the olecranon or by passing it retrograde. It is usually necessary to fracture manually or to osteotomize the radius when the deformity of the ulna is corrected, but deformities of both bones should not be straightened at the same operation.

Once the rod and the attached fragments are in position, the periosteum is closed as much as possible. The remaining soft tissues are sutured over the bone, and the extremity is immobilized in a plaster cast. Tourniquets are used where possible, but they seldom can be used in patients with the severe form of the disease.

CHONDRO-OSTEODYSTROPHY

This rare condition (also called Morquio-Brailsford disease) is characterized by dwarfism; flattening of the vertebral bodies; marked kyphosis; defective ossification of many epiphyses, mainly in the spine and the hips; normal intelligence; and progressive weakness of the musculature.[2,8,9] Familial tendencies are common. An early fatal outcome is usual.

CLINICAL PICTURE

The infant appears to be normal in all respects during the first 3 or 4 years. Gradually, a kyphotic deformity develops about the dorsolumbar junction. The neck appears shortened, failure to gain in height is noted, and the knees assume a valgus angulation. Because of muscle weakness, the child frequently supports himself by placing the hands on the thighs. The typical appearance, as described by Morquio, is a round-backed, knock-kneed, flatfooted child who stands with the hips and the knees flexed in a crouching position. The neck is shortened, and the head is displaced forward and sunk between the shoulders; the gait is waddling. The facial appearance and intelligence are normal. A marked kyphosis is evident at the dorsolumbar junction. The chest is narrowed in the transverse diameter and elongated in the anteroposterior diameter (pectus carinatum). Although dwarfing is general, the spine is chiefly affected. All epiphyses are often enlarged and even bulbous. The joints, particularly the hips, are frequently stiff. Occasionally, ligamentous laxity with hypermobility occurs about the hands and

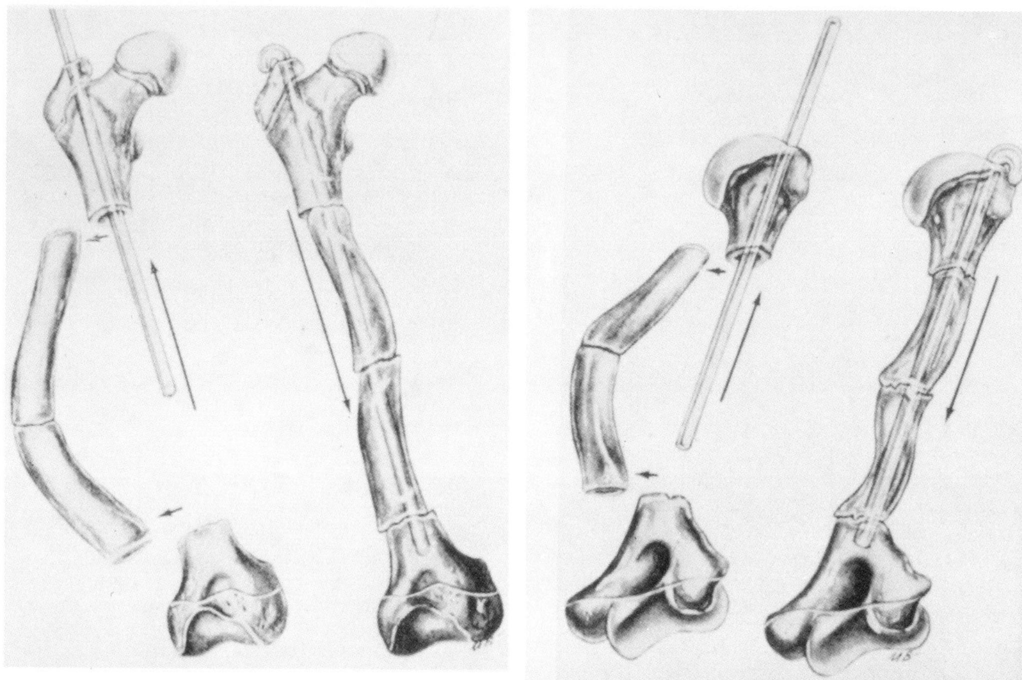

FIG. 12-5. Technique for realignment of fragments and retrograde insertion of the intramedullary rod in the femur (*left*) and the humerus (*right*). In each case, after insertion into the distal fragment, the proximal end of the rod is cut off and bent to form a hook to discourage migration of the rod.

the feet. The fingers are usually broad and blunt. Pain is unusual (Fig. 12-6).

The course is for the dwarfing, the deformities, and the muscle weakness to become progressively more marked. Survival beyond childhood is rare.

ROENTGENOGRAPHIC FINDINGS

Characteristic findings occur in the spine and the hips (Figs. 12-7 and 12-8). The vertebrae are flattened and are elongated anteroposteriorly. The superior and the inferior margins are irregular and ill defined. Anterior wedging is most marked at the cervicodorsal junction, which causes the shortened neck, and at the dorsolumbar junction, which creates a kyphosis. A characteristic tonguelike process extends forward from the anterior aspect of the vertebral bodies. Ossification of the epiphyseal rings is delayed and irregular. The disks are unusually wide.

The upper femoral epiphysis displays delayed ossification with formation of multiple irregular centers. Eventually, the femoral head becomes irregular, flattened, and fragmented. The femoral neck appears short and thick. A coxa vara deformity is common. The acetabulum is quite large and irregular. The joint space appears unusually wide since it is occupied by a large amount of dystrophic cartilage. Occasionally, dislocation is a consequence of extreme muscle flaccidity.

Similar changes are seen in other epiphyses. The result is a large epiphysis, irregularly ossified, and a shortened diaphysis.

DIFFERENTIAL DIAGNOSIS

Rickets. Rickets is simulated by the swollen joints. However, patients with rickets display generalized osteoporosis, mainly in the diaphyses. The epiphysis is ossified from a single central nucleus. Shafts of weight-bearing bones become bent. Genu varum is far more common. In Morquio's disease, knock-knees are typical. Fractures are frequent. Patients with rickets respond to administration of vitamin D.

Achondroplasia. The spine is normal in length, and the limbs, in contrast, are very short. Muscle power is unusually well developed. Gross epiphyseal and articular changes are never seen, because epiphyseal growth takes place from a single nucleus that progresses to maturity.

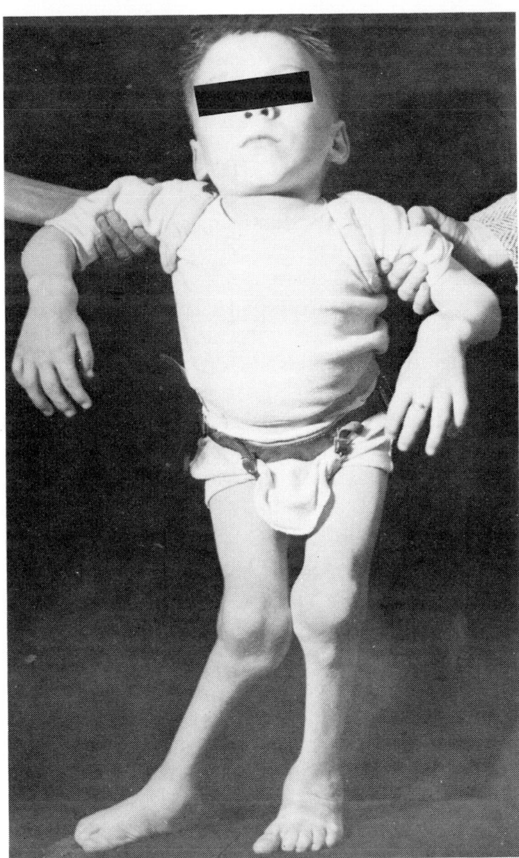

FIG. 12-6. Chondro-osteodystrophy. Note the typical dwarfism, muscular weakness, crouched position, knock-knees, enlarged epiphyses, joint laxity, intelligent facies. (Courtesy of J. F. Brailsford)

Gargoylism. This chondro-osteodystrophy type of dwarf is characterized by mental deficiency, heavy facies, cloudy corneae, and enlargement of the liver and the spleen. The shapes of the vertebral bodies are different.

Hypothyroidism. A generalized delay in ossification is typical. Epiphyseal centers appear late, are multiple, and become deformed with weight bearing. The condition responds to thyroid medication; the multiple nuclei fuse into one well-formed nucleus.

Dysplasia Epiphysialis Multiplex. This simulates Morquio's disease. However, stunting of growth is general and not chiefly caused by the spine. The multiple ossific centers in the epiphysis are mulberrylike; several small centers surround one main center and the epiphysis becomes flattened. Muscle power is normal. Hereditary and familial influences are common. The tendency is toward improvement, and life expectancy is normal. Dwarfing is not as severe as in chondro-osteodystrophy.

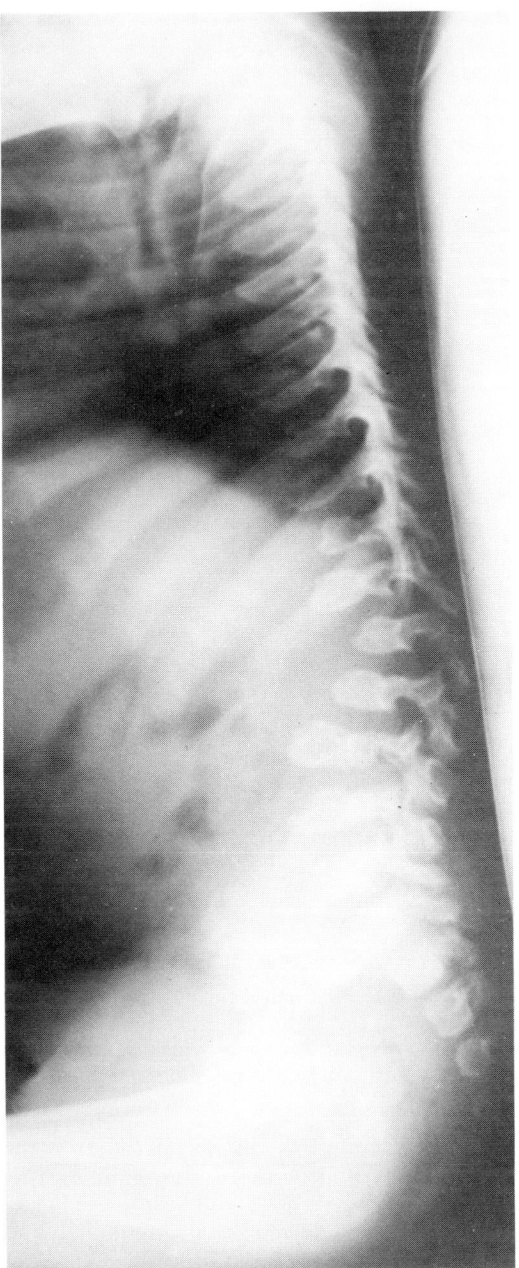

FIG. 12-7. Chondro-osteodystrophy. The vertebrae are flattened and elongated anteroposteriorly. There is kyphosis at the dorsolumbar junction. A characteristic tonguelike process extends forward from the anterior aspect of the vertebral bodies. Ossification of apophyseal rings is delayed.

DYSPLASIA EPIPHYSIALIS MULTIPLEX

Dysplasia epiphysialis multiplex is a rare, often hereditary, developmental defect characterized by abnormal ossification of many epiphyses and stunting of growth,

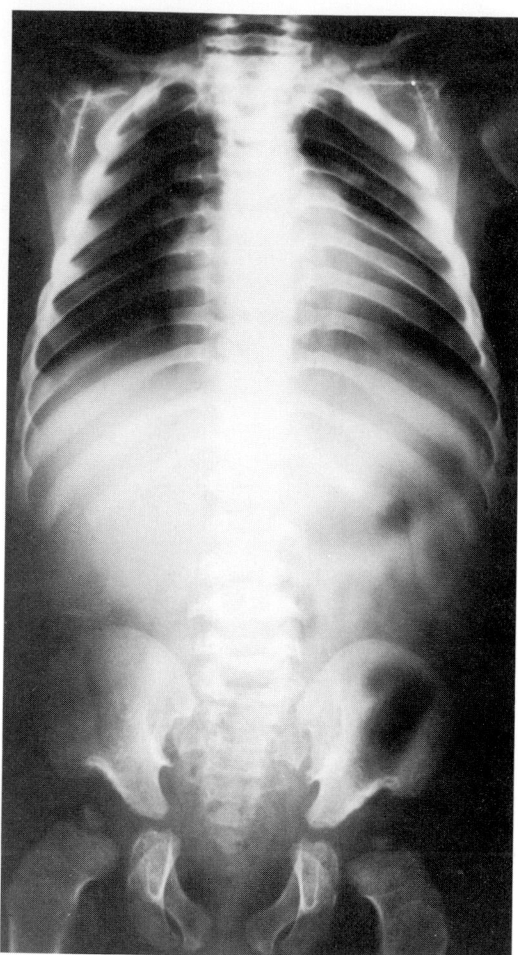

FIG. 12-8. Chondro-osteodystrophy. Delayed ossification of upper femoral epiphyses. The femoral head consists chiefly of a large amount of dystrophic cartilage, which occupies the enlarged acetabulum. The femoral neck is short and thick.

which, contrary to Morquio's disease, is not chiefly caused by restriction of growth of the spine.[10] The tendency is toward improvement, the epiphyses being moderately malformed, and degenerative arthritic changes in the adult are usual. The musculature is unaffected.

CLINICAL PICTURE

Pain and stiffness in the knees and the hips, difficulty in walking, and restriction of motion at the shoulders are early complaints. The hands present short, thick fingers. Most commonly the hips, the shoulders, the knees, and the ankles are involved. The spine may be affected, but kyphosis is unusual. No deformity is apparent other than short stature. In the adult, bilateral symmetrical osteoarthritic changes common in the hips should suggest roentgenographic studies of other joints. Several members of a family may be affected. Life expectancy is normal.

ROENTGENOGRAPHIC FINDINGS

The centers of ossification are late in appearing, are multiple, and are often arranged in a mulberrylike fashion about one main central nucleus. Eventually, the epiphysis becomes normal in density and fusion of the epiphyseal line occurs at the usual time. The epiphysis is smooth in outline but flattened, often with a bony prolongation inferiorly. The joint space becomes narrowed, and degenerative changes supervene in the adult. The glenoid and the acetabulum, at first normal, eventually conform to the shape of the epiphysis (Fig. 12-9).

A characteristic deformity at the ankle consists of the lower tibial epiphysis diminishing in depth from within outward so that the joint surface is oblique. The shafts of the long bones are shorter than normal. Carpal and tarsal bones ossify late.

FIG. 12-9. Dysplasia epiphysialis multiplex, adult appearance. The epiphysis is dense and flattened, with the glenoid conforming to its shape. Note the narrowing and degenerative changes that characteristically and early restrict shoulder motion. Findings are bilateral and symmetrical and occur in large joints, especially hips, shoulders, knees, and ankles.

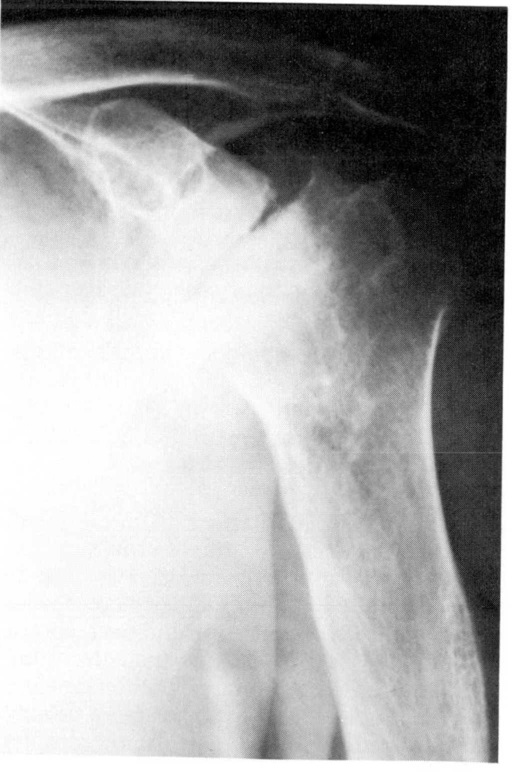

The spine, when involved, shows only delayed ossification and fragmentation of the epiphyseal plates with wedging of the bodies, but the deformity is never as severe as in Morquio's disease.

DYSPLASIA EPIPHYSIALIS PUNCTATA

Dysplasia epiphysialis punctata (also called chondrodystrophia calcificans congenita and stippled epiphyses) is a rare congenital condition characterized mainly by discrete spots of calcification affecting cartilaginous structures. It is not hereditary and is rarely familial.[11-14]

PATHOLOGY

Throughout the entire body multiple focal areas of calcification develop in cartilaginous precursors of bones. Interspersed between calcified foci are patchy areas of mucoid and cystic degeneration. The spots of calcified cartilage are found especially in epiphyses, where they tend to concentrate adjacent to the metaphyses. The long bones are shortened, and the diaphyses are widened at their metaphyseal ends. If the patient survives beyond infancy, the epiphyses become completely calcified and subsequently ossified.

CLINICAL PICTURE

The subject is usually stillborn or seldom survives infancy. The rare patient living beyond childhood develops shortness of the affected extremities. The main characteristics of the disease are listed below:

- Flexion deformities of joints, especially knees and elbows. The cause is probably muscular and capsular fibrosis.
- Bilateral congenital cataracts. These cataracts are found in most patients.
- Dwarfism of short-limb type as in achondroplasia. Femurs and humeri are chiefly involved. A single limb may be affected

ROENTGENOGRAPHIC FINDINGS

Opaque, discrete, or coalescing dots occupy cartilaginous structures such as the epiphyses, carpals, and tarsals; cartilaginous portions of ribs; and iliac apophyses (Fig. 12-10). These dots appear earlier than the usual time of appearance of ossification centers. One or more long bones may be shortened, thickened, and bowed. The metaphyses of the shortened bones are splayed, and their epiphyseal borders are irregular.

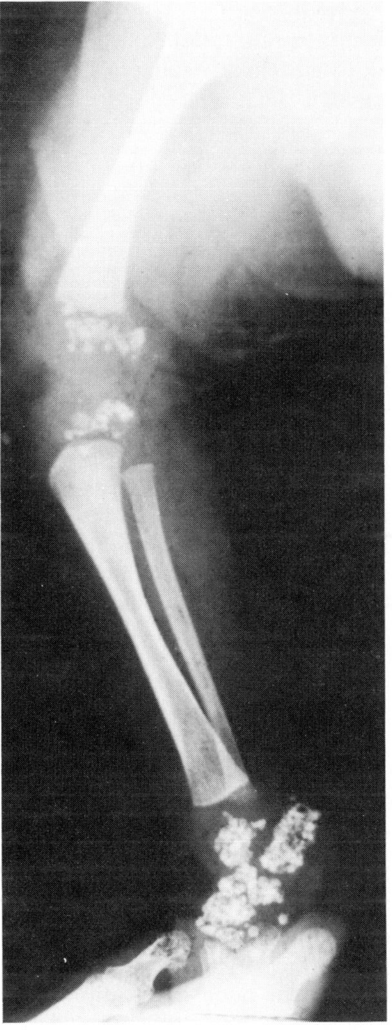

FIG. 12-10. Dysplasia epiphysialis punctata. (Karlen AG, Cameron JAF: Dysplasia epiphysialis punctata. J Bone Joint Surg 39B:293, 1957)

DIFFERENTIAL DIAGNOSIS

Dysplasia epiphysialis punctata must be differentiated from dysplasia epiphysialis multiplex and cretinism.

OSTEOPETROSIS

Osteopetrosis (also called Albers-Schönberg's disease, marble bones, and chalk bones) is a rare developmental abnormality in which the bony structure throughout the body becomes increasingly dense and brittle.[2,15-21] Complications are caused by insufficient development of the bone marrow, which may prove to be fatal, and by bony encroachment on the cranial foramina, which may produce optic atrophy, deafness, and facial paralysis.

The etiology is unknown. Consanguinity of parents may be an underlying genetic factor. The disease appears to be inherited as a simple mendelian recessive, but the severe congenital type may be transmitted as a mendelian dominant trait.

PATHOLOGY

The process appears to be continued deposition of new bone on unresorbed calcified cartilage or primary spongiosa. A failure of remodeling results in marked widening of the metaphyses and a club-shaped appearance of long bones. The condition starts before or at birth and continues uninterruptedly or intermittently until growth stops. The bone grossly is grayish white on section. It may be as hard as marble or have the consistency or brittleness of chalk. The medullary cavity is obliterated. Microscopically, the trabeculae are greatly increased in number and thickness and appear to be disorganized. Haversian canals are rare. Many islets of hypercalcified cartilage persist among the dense bony trabeculae. Marrow spaces are small, infrequent, and fibrotic. Osteoblasts are normal or increased in number. Osteoclasts are normal or absent (Color Plate 12-1).

The typical long bone is very dense and white, is solid on cross section, and possesses club-shaped extremities due to widened metaphyses. If the process is intermittent, transverse bands of dense bone alternate with bands of normal bone throughout the shaft. In the epiphysis, concentric alternating rings of dense and normal bone are often formed. The vertebral body typically forms a transverse band of dense bone at either extremity with an intervening area of normal bone. Skull diploë are fused as one. The air sinuses are often replaced by dense bone or are entirely absent. The pituitary fossa is shallow, and the posterior clinoid processes are clubbed and encroach on the fossa. Bony enlargement narrows the skull foramina and compresses nerve structures, particularly the optic nerve. Peculiarly, the mandible is immune.

CLINICAL PICTURE

Osteoporosis starts during gestation and is progressive until longitudinal growth stops. The intensity of the disorder varies. In a mild type, formation of dense bone occurs slowly, intermittently, and incompletely and the patient survives. The more severe malignant type often occurs when consanguinity of parents exists. All bones early and rapidly become very dense, devoid of architecture, and usually intensely hard or chalky and brittle. Fractures are frequent and heal slowly. The fracture is transverse and sharply abrupt. An anemia develops because of bony or fibrotic replacement of the marrow. Its severity depends on the capacity for extramedullary hematopoietic tissues to undergo compensatory hypertrophy. Optic atrophy, facial or ocular palsy, deafness, and hydrocephalus are complications.

LABORATORY FINDINGS

Serum calcium, phosphorus, and phosphatase levels are normal.

ROENTGENOGRAPHIC FINDINGS

The entire long bone, including the epiphyses, may be uniformly dense and completely devoid of structure. Occasionally, less dense areas of normal bone are interspersed. When the process is active temporarily, a dense band forms in the metaphysis and with continued growth displaces distally along the diaphysis. The metaphyses are chiefly affected, becoming clubbed; the enlargement ends abruptly at its junction with the diaphysis. The ilia often show alternating dense and clear curved bands parallel with the crests. Density of the skull is greatest at the base. The pituitary fossa is small, and the thick clubbed posterior processes close in on the fossa. Air sinuses are absent or dense. The maxilla is affected, but the mandible almost invariably escapes. Each vertebra displays dense bands at either end and a clear band between. An epiphysis may show a central focus of dense or normal bone surrounded by alternating rings of increased or normal density (Fig. 12-11).

PROGNOSIS

The age at onset and the severity of the disease determine the outcome. As a general rule, when the condition appears at birth and its manifestations are pronounced, the outlook is poor and the patient's condition rapidly deteriorates with a fatal termination within 2 years. The severity of the anemia appears to be the determining factor. When the disease develops later during childhood and is mild or moderate and when anemia and intercurrent infections can be controlled until adolescence, especially when roentgenograms show intermittent bands of unremodeled bone between bands of widely spaced normal trabecular bone, the chances for survival are good.

MELORHEOSTOSIS

Melorheostosis (Leri type of osteopetrosis, monomelic flowing hyperostosis) is a rare condition in which dense bone formation in a bone resembles the flow of candle drippings.[2]

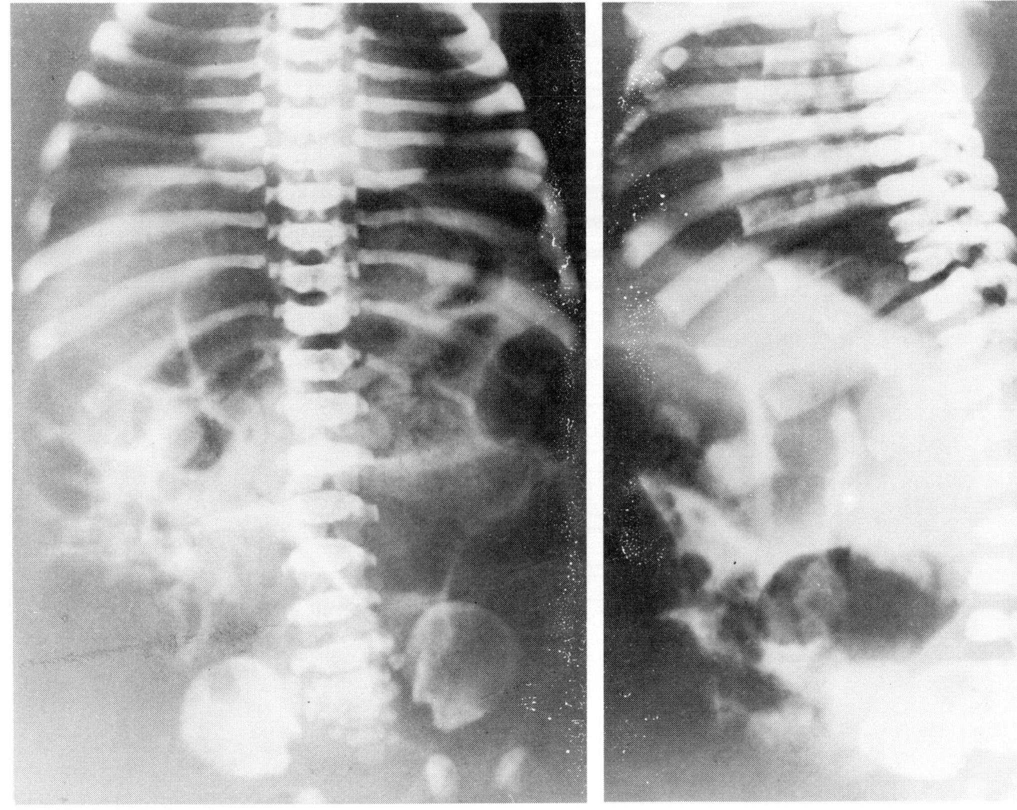

FIG. 12-11. Osteopetrosis. (N. U. Case No. 294)

ETIOLOGY

The cause of melorheostosis is unknown. Heredity plays no part. Suggested theories include ischemia secondary to sympathetic system disturbance and a developmental error.

CLINICAL PICTURE

Age. The disorder begins in childhood.

Area of Predilection. The lower more often than the upper extremity is involved; typically, changes are confined to one limb.

Symptoms and Signs. The characteristics are listed below:

Dull and aching pain is seldom severe and likely in older patients.
Limitation of motion occurs in joints of the affected limb.
Deformity of bone is due to irregular thickening.
Shortening of the limb occurs in some cases.
Swelling, edema, induration, coldness, increased perspiration and skin changes (scleroderma) suggest sympathetic ischemic phenomena. The resulting fibrosis of muscles and other soft tissues is reponsible for stiffness and limitation of motion.

ROENTGENOGRAPHIC FINDINGS

A dense structureless streak or blotch of part of a bone resembles the flow of radiopaque substance. The surface is undulated. The scapular or half pelvis corresponding to the affected limb usually shows dense patches. The skull, the spine, and the ribs invariably escape involvement (Figs. 12-12 through 12-15).

PATHOLOGY

Microscopically, there is a compact overcrowding of lamellae arranged in a bizarre manner and an interlacing of immature and adult bone.

TREATMENT

Sympathectomy may effect relief of pain, appearance of warmth and dryness, and increase of motion. The effect should be tested presurgically by sympathetic block.[22]

DYSCHONDROPLASIA

Dyschondroplasia (Ollier's disease, multiple enchondromas) is a rare developmental condition characterized by large rounded masses or columns of cartilage in the metaphyses of certain bones, particularly the long bones.[2] The cartilage proliferates normally at the epiphyseal plate but fails to become calcified, resorbed, or replaced by newly formed bone. This results in accumulation of large amounts of cartilage in the metaphysis and reduction of longitudinal growth. The cartilaginous masses bulge the metaphysis and may penetrate the cortex with formation of enchondromas. Dense septa of normal bone divide the

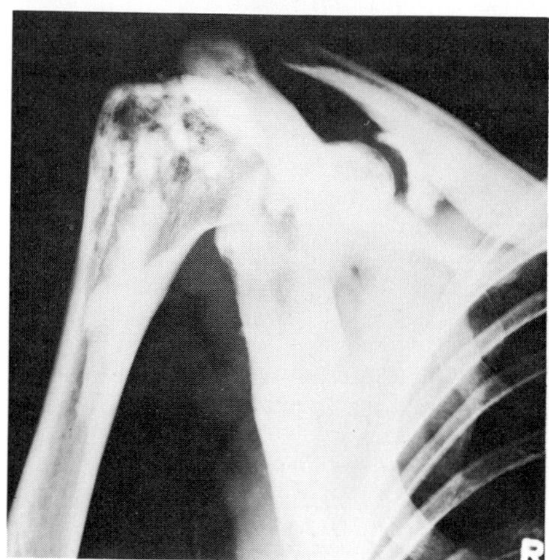

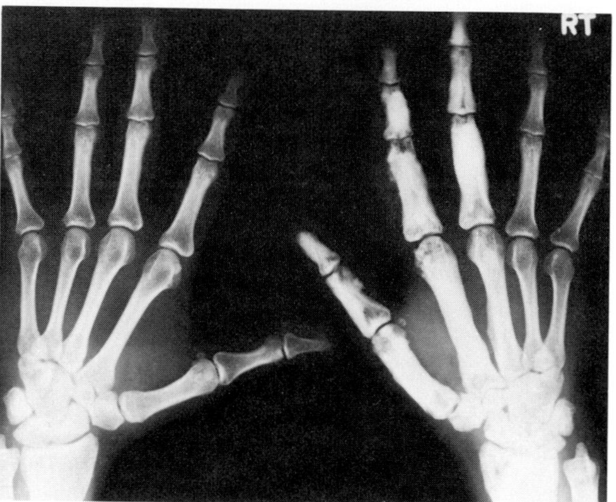

FIG. 12-12. Melorheostosis. The peculiar streaked sclerosis of bone resembling candle drippings is well demonstrated. It is frequently associated with congenital neurofibromatosis. (McCarroll HR: J Bone Joint Surg 32A:601)

FIG. 12-13. Melorheostosis of the tibia. The structureless dense streak that extends beyond the surface in undulating fashion resembles candle drippings.

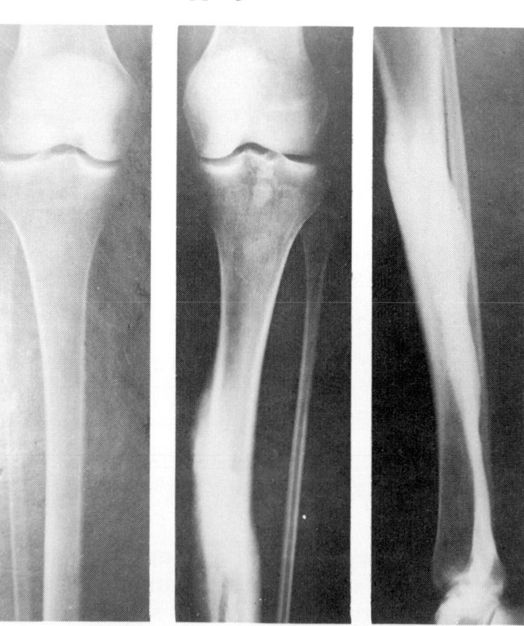

FIG. 12-14. Melorheostosis of the tarsals and metatarsals. The dense blotches are most apparent in the scaphoid and first cuneiform.

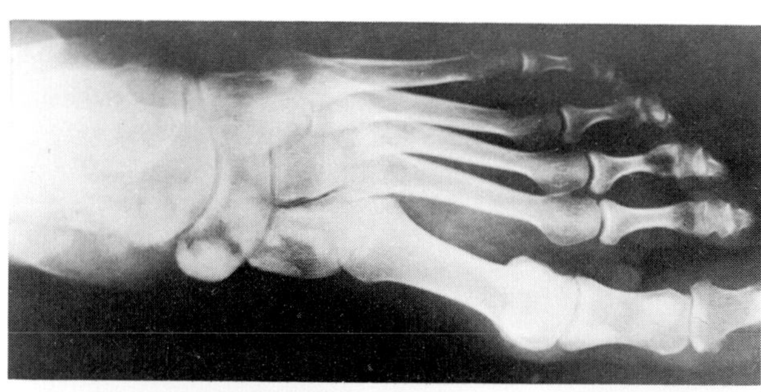

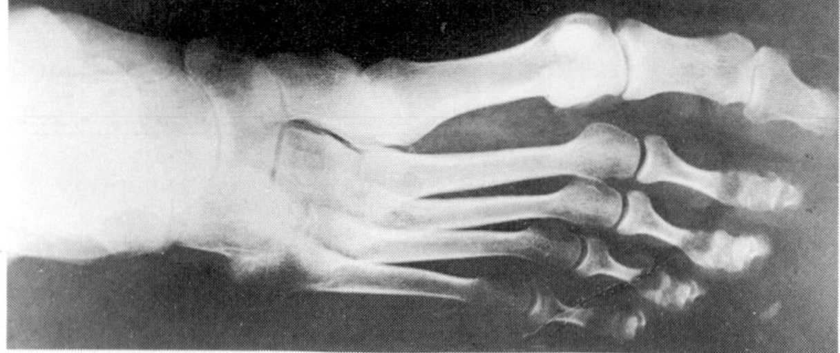

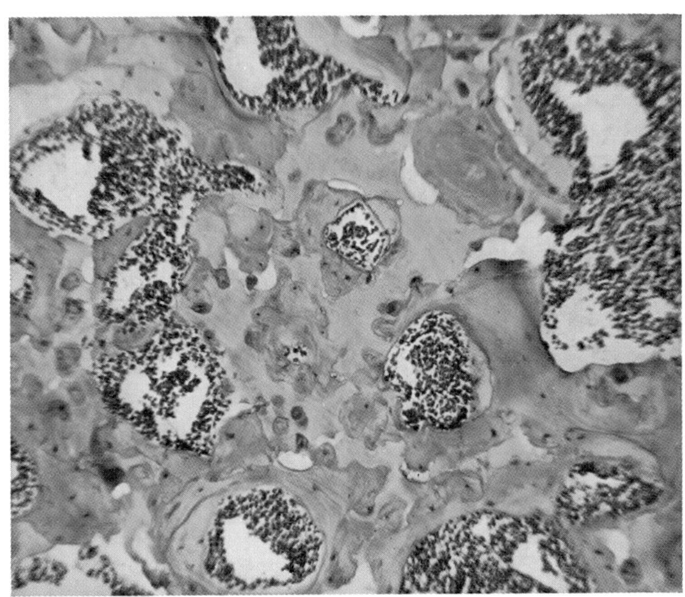

PLATE 12-1. Marble bone. (×85) (See p. 370.)

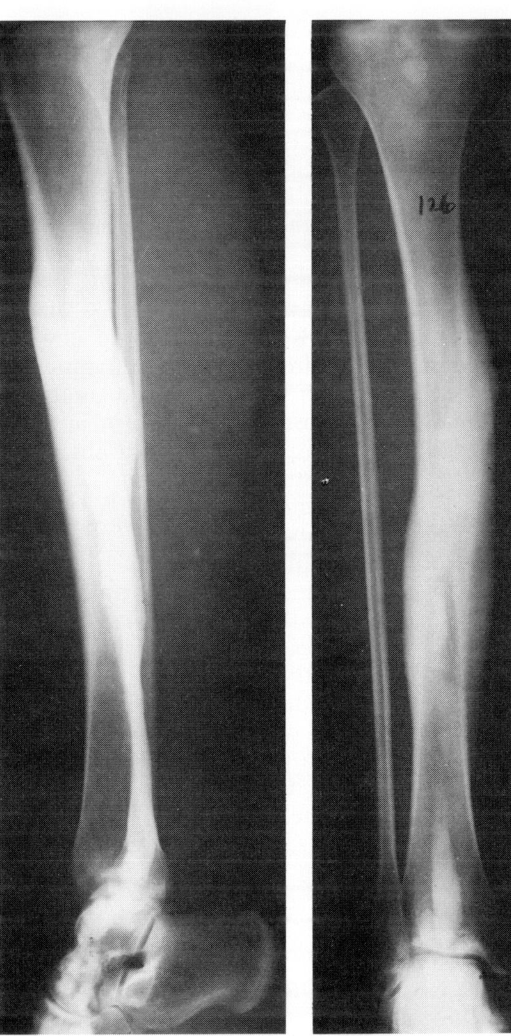

FIG. 12-15. Melorheostosis. Dense, structureless, cortical, and endosteal bone, with flowing hyperostosis resembling candle drippings.

cartilage into lobules. The diaphysis is short and broadened. Chiefly involved are the long bones formed in cartilage, particularly at the more rapidly growing ends (*e.g.*, about the knee and at the distal ends of the radius and the ulna). The condition is predominantly unilateral. In the small long bones of the hands, the enchondromas occupy the entire bone and grow to large size, seriously deforming the hand. Microscopically, the masses consist of hyaline cartilage with cells of varying size irregularly arranged. Some calcification and replacement by ossification is seen in older patients approaching adolescence.

CLINICAL PICTURE

Age. The patient is normal at birth; the condition becomes manifest at any time during the growth period.

Area of Predilection. The main sites are the long bones, especially at actively growing ends; knee; distal ulna and radius; upper end of humerus; long bones of hands and feet, especially the phalanges; and pelvis, particularly the iliac crest.

Symptoms and Signs. The affected extremity is shortened. Valgus or varus deformities result when growth is retarded unequally at the epiphyseal line; the ulna is shortened more than the radius, which in consequence becomes bowed and dislocated at the radial head; large enchondromas of the phalanges cause gross deformity of the hand. Fractures are uncommon except in the hand.

ROENTGENOGRAPHIC FINDINGS

Cartilage-filled clear spaces of varying size and shape appear in the metaphysis and tend toward a columnar arrangement. The columns are separated by septa of increased bony density, which cause a striated or streaky appearance. The metaphysis is irregularly expanded. The diaphysis is short and thick and occasionally curved. The large mass of cartilage may bulge and interrupt the continuity of the cortex. The epiphysis adjacent to an involved metaphysis often displays dense mottling. In the phalanges all semblance of the original bone may be lost. Ilium involvement is characterized by cartilage columns that radiate in a fanlike manner toward the crest. As adolescence approaches, the cartilage columns and spaces become less well defined, with dense spots appearing throughout the metaphysis, suggesting replacement by ossification (Fig. 12-16).

TREATMENT

Occasionally, osteotomy is necessary to correct deformity. The fragments readily unite. Epiphyseal arrest in the opposite extremity combats limb inequality.

MAFUCCI'S SYNDROME

Mafucci's syndrome consists of dyschondroplasia associated with cavernous hemangiomas and phleboliths in the soft tissues.

HEREDITARY MULTIPLE EXOSTOSES

In hereditary multiple exostoses (also called hereditary deforming dyschondroplasia, metaphyseal aclasis), many osteocartilaginous exostoses form at the metaphyses of long bones. Several members of a family are usually affected.

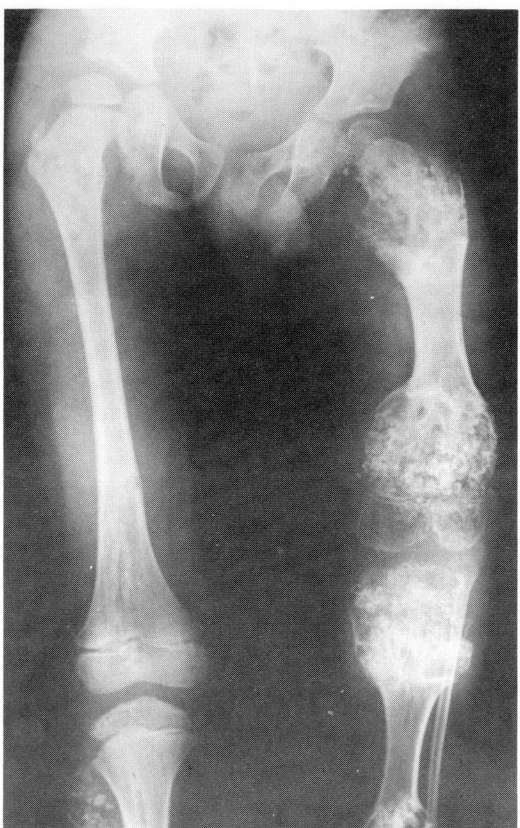

FIG. 12-16. Dyschondroplasia. Note cartilage-filled clear spaces of varying size and shape; columnar arrangement; density of bone between cartilage columns, which is increased; metaphyseal enlargement; thickened shaft; shortening of bone; and mottled epiphyses.

ETIOLOGY

The cause is unknown, but the following theories of pathogenesis have been advanced:

Failure of Development of the Periosteum.[25] The cortex fails to attain full thickness, and the inadequate periosteum cannot restrict the outward growth of bone.

Failure of Osteoclastic Activity.[28] The modeling and shaping process of bone is deficient, which explains the widened trumpet-shaped appearance of the metaphysis. If this theory were correct, the term *metaphyseal aclasis* should be applied to this condition.

Deficient Perichondrium, Permitting Overgrowth of Cartilage.[23] The cartilage becomes transformed into bone. Because all displaced cartilage is prone to malignant change, the occasional malignant degeneration of an exostosis is clear.

PATHOLOGY

Only bone arising in cartilage and eventually enclosed by a sheath, such as subperiosteal bone, is affected. Membranous bone is immune. Therefore, exostoses develop at the growing ends of long bones and especially where such growth is most active (*i.e.*, the distal end of the femur and the radius and upper end of the tibia and the humerus). The metaphysis is uniformly enlarged, has parallel sides, and, on approaching the central part of the shaft, abruptly narrows to the normal diameter, a configuration that Keith calls "trumpeting."[28] Irregular projections extend from the surface and point away from the end of the bone. They may be conical, spiked, or globular. These exostoses first occur near the epiphyseal cartilage and are displaced along the shaft with growth. One can almost estimate their time of appearance by measuring the distance from the epiphyseal line. Growth in length of the bone is interfered with as the cartilage grows outward so that, for example, if the fibula lags behind the tibia, the latter may become curved.

Microscopically, the metaphysis shows poor trabeculations, which are continuous with those within the central portion of the exostosis. Jaffe describes the exostosis as an outpouching of the cortex.[26] The surface is a zone of hyaline cartilage with active endochondral ossification beneath it. When growth stops, the surface has a thin layer of nonproliferating cartilage resting on a thin layer of bone. Underneath is spongy bone with delicate trabeculae, fatty marrow, and islands of calcified cartilage.

CLINICAL PICTURE

The patient may or may not be of shortened stature, depending on the severity of the process. Irregular hard prominences near the ends of long bones may be visible or at least palpable and may be tender. The overlying skin, if subjected to pressure or friction, is tender, reddened, and swollen. Numbness, paresthesias, and muscle weakness may result from nerve pressure. Involvement of adjacent tendons restricts movement. The excrescences may be fractured but unite readily. When an asymptomatic exostosis suddenly without cause becomes enlarged and painful, malignant degeneration should be suspected.

ROENTGENOGRAPHIC FINDINGS

Roentgenograms reveal a trumpetlike metaphysis with very little compact cortical bone that is continuous with that of the exostosis. The paucity of normal trabeculae causes a relatively less dense appearance of the interior of the growth (Fig. 12-17).

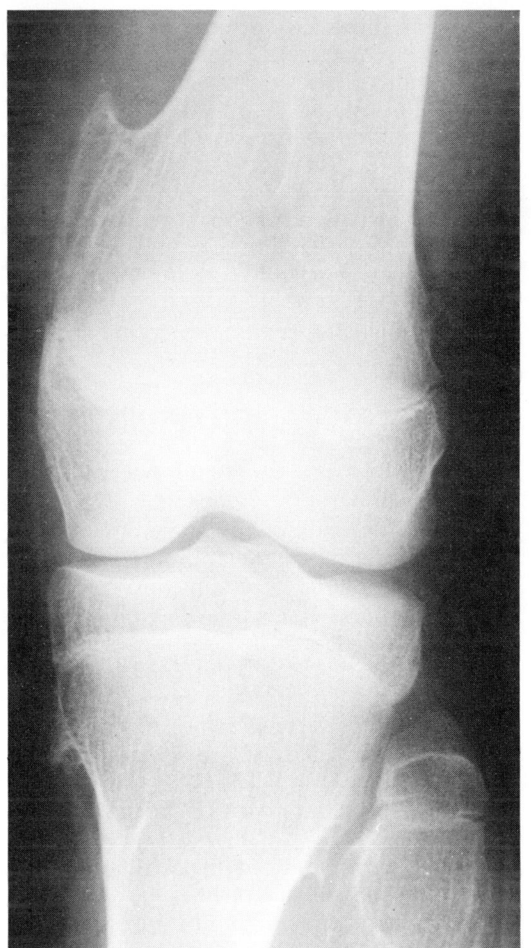

FIG. 12-17. Hereditary multiple exostoses. The metaphyses are trumpet shaped and poorly trabeculated. The exostoses that point away from the ends of the bones are actually much larger than those represented on the roentgenogram because they are capped with thick hyaline cartilage.

COMPLICATIONS

Complications include fracture, overlying bursitis, pressure on tendons and nerves, shortening and bowing of the extremities, and sarcomatous degeneration.

PROGNOSIS

Ordinarily, these are benign growths that cause local problems such as a fracture of its base, adventitious bursitis, and compresion of neighboring structures. Growth of the exostoses is halted when skeletal growth ceases.

When a previously asymptomatic exostosis suddenly becomes painful and produces increasing local swelling and when roentgenograms show irregularity of its cartilaginous cap and osteolytic foci in the subchondral trabeculae, malignant transformation must be suspected. It is generally believed that the risk of developing chondrosarcoma is 1% to 2% for patients with a solitary exostosis and 5% to 25% for patients with multiple osteocartilaginous exostoses.[24,27,29]

TREATMENT

The exostosis is removed when it is constantly subjected to injury, causes deformity, compresses important structures, or is suspected of undergoing malignant transformation.

ACHONDROPLASIA

Achondroplasia (chondrodystrophia fetalis, micromelia) is a congenital developmental condition characterized pathologically by defective endochondral ossification, affecting chiefly the long bones, and clinically by a peculiar dwarfism in which the extremities are shortened, whereas the trunk remains relatively unaffected.

ETIOLOGY

The actual cause is unknown. Hereditary tendencies are occasionally apparent, the condition being manifest in half the children of parents, one of whom is an achondroplastic dwarf. Females are more often affected.

PATHOLOGY

The process of endochondral ossification at the epiphyseal growth plates is disturbed. Instead of orderly proliferation, palisading, and formation of scaffolds of calcified cartilage, the cartilage is degenerate and very vascular. Therefore, ossification for longitudinal growth is greatly retarded. On the other hand, periosteal ossification proceeds normally, and bone diameter is ensured. This form of ossification may even be excessive, particularly at the metaphysis where the cortex flares outward and appears to embrace the epiphysis. Within the epiphysis itself, where palisading and provisional calcification are unaffected, ossification proceeds at a normal pace.

Although all bones dependent on endochondral ossification are involved in the process, the long bones of the limbs are chiefly affected. The base of the skull, which develops in cartilage, is compromised by premature fusion, forming a single mass of bone. Growth is retarded, with the base remaining short while the rest of the skull grows normally.

CLINICAL PICTURE

Dwarfism is often apparent at or soon after birth. Prematurity is frequent; most of the newborns are stillborn or fail to live beyond the first year of life. Those that survive become healthy and robust, and life expectancy is normal.

During childhood, the extremities lag behind in longitudinal growth so that, although the spine is affected to some extent, the limbs appear strikingly short in comparison with the trunk (Fig. 12-18). The hands present a typical "trident" appearance. They are short and broad, and the fingers short, thick, and divergent. Because the humeri and the femora are intensively involved, shortening affects the arms and the thighs more than the forearms and the legs. The fibula is relatively unaffected in contrast with the tibia. As a result, the head of the fibula appears prominent and lies at a high level on the lateral aspect of the knee joint.

The musculature is well developed, and often muscle power is superior, enabling these people to perform feats of strength and acrobatics.

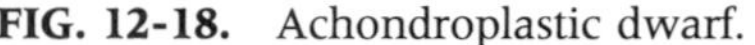

FIG. 12-18. Achondroplastic dwarf.

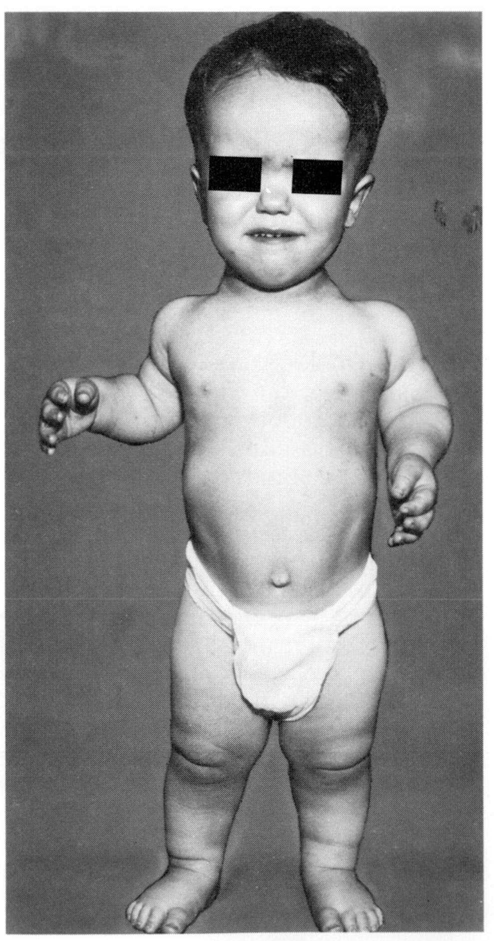

The hip joints lie posterior to the central axis of the pelvis. Consequently, the pelvis tilts forward, the buttocks are prominent, the sacrum lies in a horizontal plane, lumbar lordosis is exaggerated, and a compensatory increase of the thoracic kyphosis develops. The peculiar rolling gait has been attributed to hip displacement and pelvic tilting.

The head is brachycephalic. The forehead is prominent, and the bridge of the nose is depressed.

The chest is small and flat, and the ribs are abnormally short.

Intelligence and sexual development are normal.

ROENTGENOGRAPHIC FINDINGS

The long bones are short and, because of reduction in length, are apparently, rather than actually, increased in diameter. The ends of the shafts are splayed. The epiphyseal border of the metaphysis is often indented at its center. The epiphyseal ossification center, which forms by endochondral ossification, is well developed and well circumscribed. It lies in close apposition to the metaphysis, fitting snugly into the V-shaped indentation. This displacement of the center away from the joint gives the illusion of marked widening of the joint space. The clavicles and the fibulae are less affected by shortening than the other long bones. The ribs are short, and the sternum is broad and thick. The scapula is rectangular and small.

The pelvis is reduced in all dimensions. The ilium presents a characteristic rectangular appearance. The roof of the acetabulum is flat and horizontally disposed. The hip joint lies farther back than usual, and the acetabulum is close to the sacrosciatic notch. The sacrum is narrow and horizontally disposed.

The skull is large. Premature fusion of the basal centers considerably shortens the base of the skull, with the foramen magnum remaining small and funnel shaped. The facial bones are not involved.

In the spine, endochondral ossification seems to be relatively unaffected so that, although the depth of the vertebral bodies is reduced, the total length of the spine is much less diminished than that of the extremities. However, important morphologic changes develop in the posterior arches, consisting of shortening of the pedicles and reduction in the interpedicular distance with consequent narrowing of the spinal canal in both diameters (spinal stenosis).[30] These patients suffer a high incidence of cord and nerve root compression.[31]

OSTEOPOIKILOSIS

Osteopoikilosis (also called osteopathia condensans disseminata) is characterized by the development of multiple dense spots in many bones. These spots appear during the growth period, are asymptomatic, and persist throughout adult life. The affection is rare.

ROENTGENOGRAPHIC FINDINGS

Multiple small, circular or ovoid, dense spots are situated in many bones, with the elongate lesions lying in the long axis of the bone. They occur profusely in epiphyses, in metaphyses, and in the small bones of the carpus and the tarsus. Occasional scarce spots may be found in the skull, the ribs, and the spine. They are particularly numerous in the pelvis. Regions containing cancellous bone seem to be predisposed, whereas the shafts are relatively immune (Fig. 12-19).

PATHOLOGY

The trabeculae of the spongiosa are increased in number and thickness.

DIFFERENTIAL DIAGNOSIS

Melorheostosis must be differentiated because it exhibits, in addition to similar small spots, broad bands of dense bone described as blotches that also occupy the shafts of long bones.

ENGELMANN'S DISEASE

Engelmann's disease (also known as progressive diaphyseal dysplasia and progressive diaphyseal hyperostosis) is characterized by symmetrical fusiform enlargement and sclerosis of the shafts of major long bones associated with similar hypertrophic dense changes in the skull. The etiology is unknown.[2,32–34]

FIG. 12-19. Osteopoikilosis.

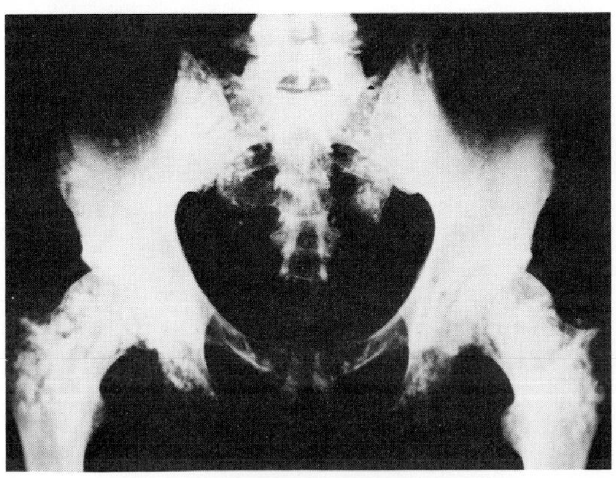

CLINICAL PICTURE

The condition is first observed in early childhood. Both sexes are equally affected. Infants walk late, and dentition is retarded. Often the patient is gaunt and thin, has poor muscle tone, and fatigues easily. The diaphyses of long bones are often palpably thickened. Soon or late, usually before 7 years of age, aching pain in the legs becomes a prominent complaint. A peculiar waddling gait is often noted. With the passage of years, the bony changes extend, weakness becomes pronounced, and pain may become severe. Puberty is late, and the genitalia and secondary sex characteristics are poorly developed.

Results of all laboratory tests are negative.

ROENTGENOGRAPHIC FINDINGS

One, several, or all of the long bones display a fusiform enlargement of the diaphysis, usually ending abruptly at the metaphysis but occasionally extending to involve one or both epiphyses. The widened dense cortex not only increases the external circumference of the bone but also encroaches on the medullary canal (Figs. 12-20 and 12-21).

FIG. 12-20. Engelmann's disease. The cortical thickening involves the diaphyses, ends abruptly at the metaphyses, and encroaches on the medullary canal. (Gillespie JB, Mussey RD: J Pediatr 38:55, 1951)

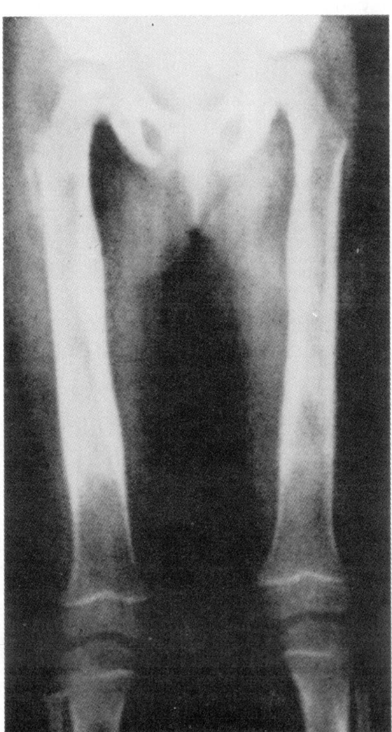

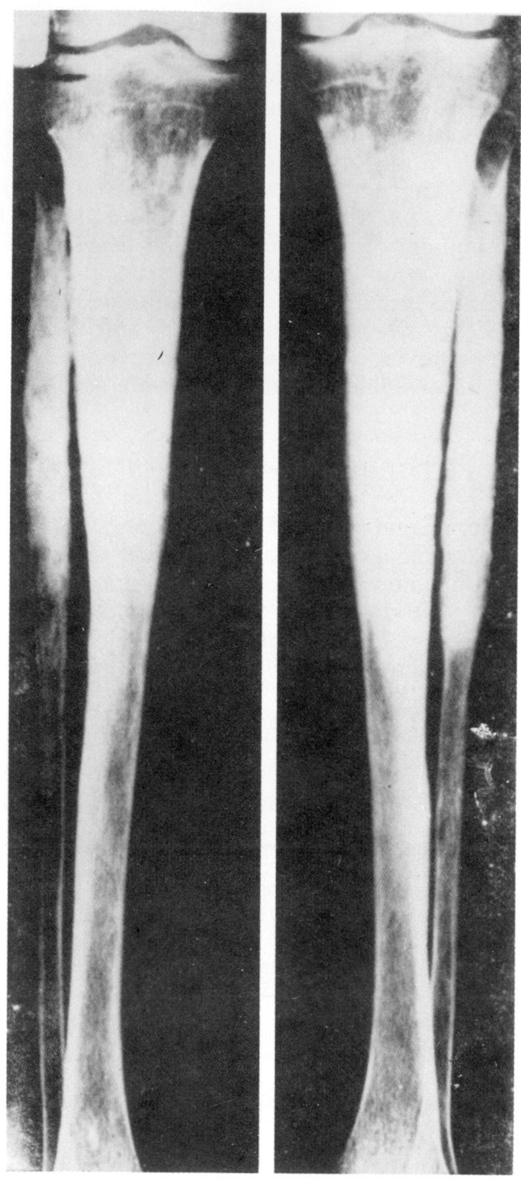

FIG. 12-21. Engelmann's disease. (Griffiths DLL: Engelmann's disease. J Bone Joint Surg 38:312, 1956)

The skull typically is affected by the thickening and sclerosis over the frontal region, the base of the skull at the basiocciput, and the petrous portion of the temporal bone.

DIAGNOSIS

Only Caffey's disease (infantile cortical hyperostosis) must be differentiated. Caffey's disease is observed within the first year, often before 6 months of age, and is invariably accompanied by fever; increased density is often unilateral, the mandible is frequently affected, and the roentgenographic changes disappear with complete recovery.

PATHOLOGY

Nothing unusual is noted. The cortices are thickened by apposition of mature lamellar bone, both on the periosteal and the endosteal aspects (Fig. 12-22).

PYCNODYSOSTOSIS

Pycnodysostosis (Gk. *pycnos* = thick, dense; *dys* = defective; *ostosis* = of bone) is characterized by short stature, dysplasia of skull, obtuse mandibular angle, dysplasia of outer end of clavicles, partial or total aplasia of distal phalanges, and generalized increased density of the skeleton. Repeated fractures resulting from minimal trauma are common. The condition is genetic, inherited

FIG. 12-22. Engelmann's disease, microscopic appearance. (*Top*) Cross section of fibula, displaying cortical thickening and regular lamellar structures of the bone. (*Bottom*) Microscopic section (×40) showing abundant osteoblasts and fibrous marrow structure. Note the absence of mosaic architecture such as occurs in Paget's disease. (Griffiths DLL: Engelmann's disease. J Bone Joint Surg 38B:312, 1956)

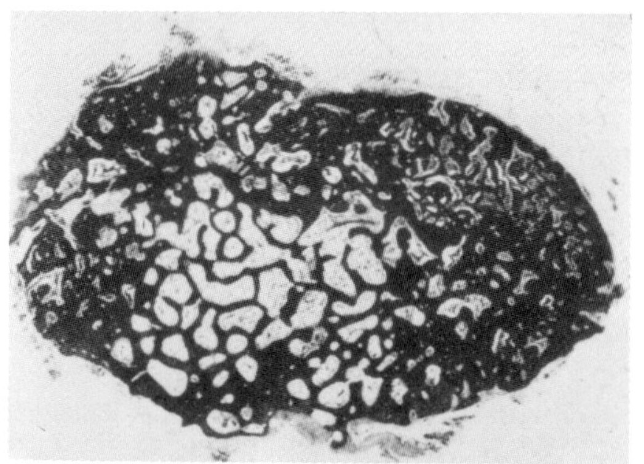

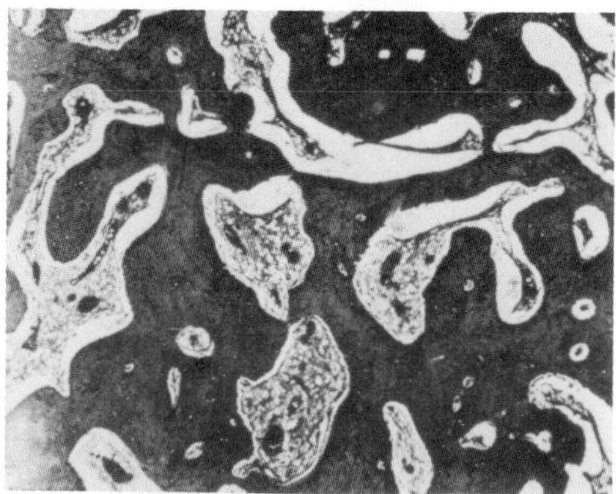

as an autosomal recessive trait, and often the product of a consanguineous union. The disorder resembles cleidocranial dysostosis and is often regarded as a variation of that condition. It must also be differentiated from osteopetrosis, but patients with pycnodysostosis have a longer life expectancy because bone marrow hematopoiesis is preserved. The artist Henri Toulouse-Lautrec supposedly was affected by this condition.[35–38]

PATHOLOGY

The histologic appearance is similar to that seen in osteopetrosis, except for preserved areas of active hematopoietic bone marrow.

CLINICAL PICTURE

Repeated fractures from trivial trauma are common. Fractures of the mandible during tooth extraction may occur. Average adult height is short. The head is disproportionately large with frontal bossing. The anterior fontanelle and cranial sutures remain open until adulthood. The eyes are proptosed, resembling exophthalmos. The face is small as a result of underdeveloped facial bones, and the angle of the mandible is flattened. As in cleidocranial dysostosis, the deciduous teeth persist into adulthood, interfering with the eruption of the permanent teeth and creating a double row of deformed teeth. The acromial ends of the clavicles are aplastic. Various trunk deformities include scoliosis, kyphosis, and spondylolisthesis. The terminal phalanges are short and aplastic, and usually only the tufts are missing. Ambulation is unaffected.

ROENTGENOGRAPHIC FINDINGS

The entire skeleton shows increased density. The skull is large and brachycephalic. The anterior fontanelle and cranial sutures persist as widened defects into adulthood. The wormian bone pattern is apparent in the parietal bone. Facial bones are hypoplastic. Nonpneumatization of sinuses is common. The mandibular angle is typically obtuse, often approaching 180°. Spinal abnormalities are frequently associated, often reflecting failure of segmentation.

Medullary canals of long bones are poorly formed but nevertheless are present, indicating preservation of the bone marrow and hematopoiesis and thus distinguishing this condition from osteopetrosis. Sometimes a widened distal femur (Erlenmeyer flask deformity) similar to that seen in Gaucher's disease is present.

The distal phalanges of hands and feet are tapered, and the tufts are absent. Persistent transverse radiolucent lines (umbauzonen?) are often observed in tubular bones (Fig. 12-23).

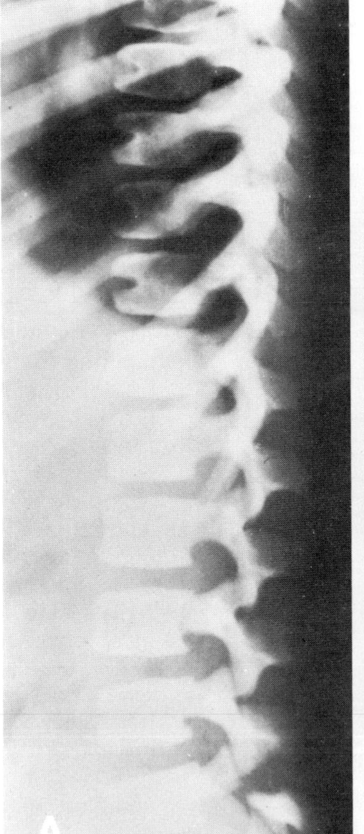

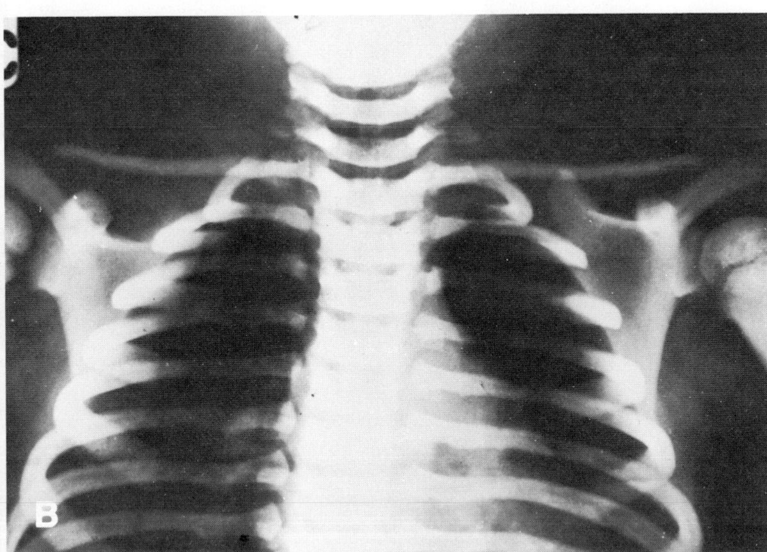

FIG. 12-23. Pycnodysostosis, showing increased bone density and the following distinguishing roentgenographic features: (*A*) Deep anterior clefts in dorsal vertebrae. (*B*) Short and straight clavicles; the acromial ends are aplastic.

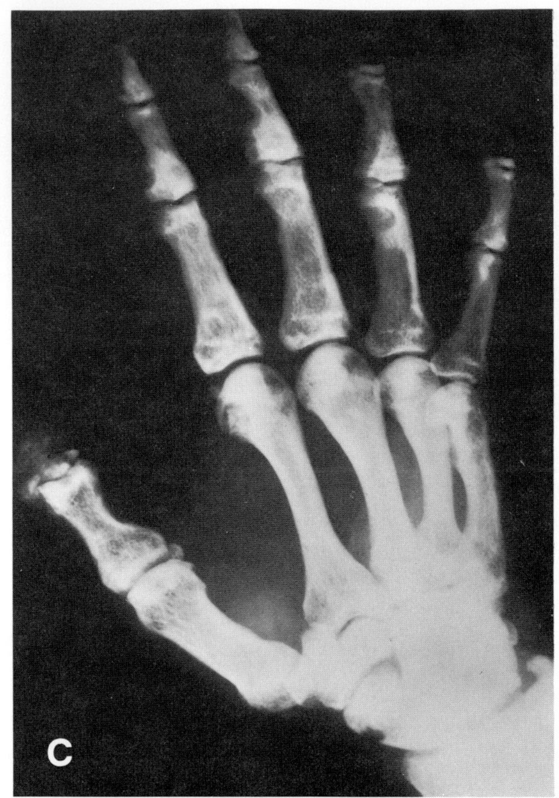

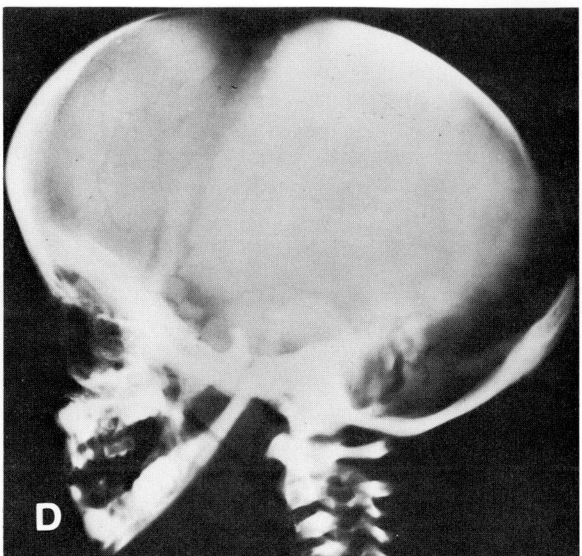

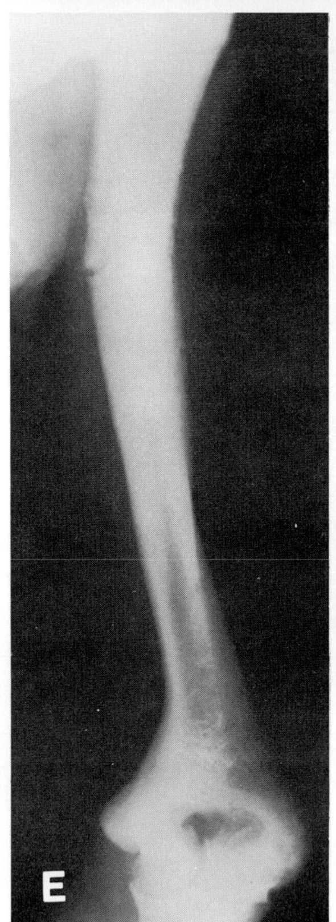

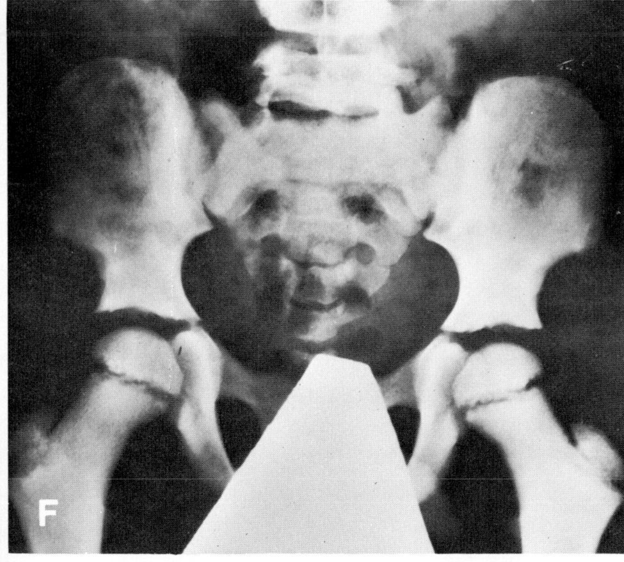

FIG. 12-23. (*continued*) (*C*) Acro-osteolysis, absence of tufts, tapering of distal phalanges. Closure of distal radial and ulnar epiphyseal growth plates is premature. (*D*) Large head with frontal bossing. Open fontanelles, wide persisting sutures, wormian parietal bones, hypoplastic facial bones, straightening, and loss of mandibular angle are evident. (*E*) Dense long bone displaying an incomplete fracture (umbauzonen?); the medullary cavity is preserved. (*F*) Pelvis and hips with horizontal acetabular roofs showing marked generalized osteosclerosis. (Courtesy of Christine Hall and Ruth Wynne-Davies)

REFERENCES

Osteogenesis Imperfecta

1. Brailsford JF: Osteogenesis imperfecta. Br J Radiol 16:129, 1943
2. Fairbank Sir T: An Atlas of General Affections of the Skeleton. Baltimore, Williams & Wilkins, 1952
3. Luck JV: Bone and Joint Diseases. Springfield, IL, Charles C Thomas, 1950
4. Sofield HA, Millar EA: Fragmentation, realignment, and intramedullary rod fixation of deformities of the long bones in children. J Bone Joint Surg 41A:1371, 1959
5. Solomons CR, Armstrong DA: Prenatal testing for osteogenesis imperfecta. Proc Orthop Res Soc New Orleans, January 28–30, 1976
6. Weber M: Osteogenesis imperfecta congenita. Arch Pathol 9:984, 1930
7. Wright PB, Gernstetter SI, Greenblatt RB: Osteogenesis imperfecta: Therapeutic acceleration of bone age. J Bone Joint Surg 33A:939, 1951

Chondro-Osteodystrophy

8. Brailsford JF: Chondro-osteodystrophy. J Bone Joint Surg 34B:53, 1951
9. Morquio L: Sur une forme dystrophie osseuse familiale. Arch de med d enf 32:129, 1929; 38:5, 1931

Dysplasia Epiphysialis Multiplex

10. Fairbank T: Dysplasia epiphysialis multiplex. Br J Surg 34:225, 1947

Dysplasia Epiphysialis Punctata

11. Conradi E: Vorzeitiges Auftreten von Knochen—und eigenartigen Verkalkungskernen bei Chondrodystrophia fotalis hypoplastica. Jahrbuch fur Kinderheilkunde 80:86, 1914
12. Fairbank HAT: General diseases of skeleton. Br J Surg 15:120, 1927
13. Frank WW, Denny MB: Dysplasia epiphysialis punctata. J Bone Joint Surg 36B:118, 1954
14. Karlen AG Cameron JAP: Dysplasia epiphysialis punctata. J Bone Joint Surg 39B:293, 1957

Osteopetrosis

15. Albers-Schönberg H: Röntgenbilder einer seltenen Knockenerkrankung. Munch Med. Wchnschr 51:365, 1904; Fortschr Geb Röntgenstr 11:261, 1907
16. Breck LW, Cornell RC, Emmett JE: Intramedullary fixation of fractures of the femur in a case of osteopetrosis. J Bone Joint Surg 39A:1389, 1957
17. Cohen J: Osteopetrosis: Case report, autopsy findings, and pathological interpretation: Failure of treatment with vitamin A. J Bone Joint Surg 33A:923, 1951
18. Engfeldt B, Engstrom A, Zetterstrom R: Biophysical studies on bone tissue. III. Osteopetrosis (marble bone disease). Acta Paediatr 43:152, 1954
19. Enticknap JB: Albers-Schönberg disease (marble bones): Report of a case with a study of the chemical and physical characteristics of the bone. J Bone Joint Surg 36B:123, 1954
20. Hasenhuttl K: Osteopetrosis: Review of the literature and comparative studies on a case with a twenty-four year follow-up. J Bone Joint Surg 44A:559, 1962
21. Pirie AH: The development of marble bones. Am J Roentgenol 24:147, 1930

Melorheostosis

22. Hess WE, Street DM: Melorheostosis, relief of pain by sympathectomy. J Bone Joint Surg 32A:422, 1950

Hereditary Multiple Exostosis

23. Bennett GE, Berkheimer GA: Malignant degeneration in a case of multiple benign exostoses. Surgery 10:781, 1941
24. Dahlin DC: Bone Tumors, 3rd ed. Springfield, IL, Charles C Thomas, 1978
25. Geschickter CF, Copeland MM: Tumors of Bone, 3rd ed, p 79. Philadelphia, JB Lippincott, 1949
26. Jaffe HL: Hereditary multiple exostosis. Arch Pathol 36:335, 1943
27. Jaffe HL: Tumors and Tumorous Conditions of Bones and Joints. Philadelphia, Lea & Febiger, 1958
28. Keith A: Studies of the anatomical changes which accompany certain growth-disorders of the human body. J Anat 54:101, 1920
29. Lichtenstein L: Bone Tumors, 4th ed, St. Louis, CV Mosby, 1972

Achondroplasia

30. Donath J, Vogel A: Untersuchungen über der chondrodystrophischen Zwerg wuchs. Wien Arch Med Grenzgebiete 10:1, 1925
31. Nelson MA: Spinal stenosis in achondroplasia. Proc R Soc Med 65:1028, 1972

Engelmann's Disease

32. Camurati M: Di un Raro Caso di Osteite Simmetrica Ereditaria degli arti Inferiori. La Chir degli Organi de Movimento 6:662, 1922
33. Engelmann G: Ein Fall von Osteopathia hyperostotica (sclerotisans) multiplex infantilis. Fortsch Geb Rontgenstr 39:1101, 1929
34. Griffiths DL: Engelmann's disease. J Bone Joint Surg 38B:312, 1956

Pycnodysostosis

35. Elmore SM: Pycnodysostosis: A review. J Bone Joint Surg 49A:153, 1967
36. Elmore SM, Nance WB, McGee BJ et al: Pycnodysostosis with a familial chromosome anomaly. Am J Med 40:274, 1966
37. Marateaux P, Lamy M: Deux observations d'une affection osseuse condensante: La pycnodysostose. Arch Fr Pediatr 19:267, 1962
38. Marateaux P, Lamy M: The malady of Toulouse-Lautrec. JAMA 191:715, 1965

13

Diseases of Joints

SYNOVIAL FLUID

CHARACTERISTICS

Normal synovial fluid has the following characteristics:

Gross Appearance. Clear, pale yellow, viscous, does not clot; similar in traumatic arthritis

Amount. From the normal knee, 0.13 ml to 3.5 ml.

Intra-articular Pressure. Minus 8 cm to minus 12 cm H_2O

Sterile.

Contains Immune Antibodies. These are identical with those of blood serum.

Cytology. Average number 65/cu mm, mostly lymphocytes and monocytes. Acute inflammation will evoke a response of polymorphs. Later, as the acute inflammation subsides or becomes chronic, mononuclear phagocytes predominate. An effusion in which the leukocyte count is above 5000/cu mm or the absolute polymorph count is above 55/cu mm is probably not of traumatic origin.

Specific Gravity. This is 1.008 to 1.015; it is somewhat higher in fluids of traumatic or degenerative arthritis.

Protein. This is about 2 g/dl, consisting of mucin, albumin, and globulin. The A-G ratio is about 20:1. The protein concentrations in joint effusions are often two or three times higher. Electrophoretic patterns of synovial fluid show evidence of differential permeability of the synovial membrane. For example, albumin is much higher in synovial fluid than in serum, α_1- and β-globulin are essentially the same in both, and α_2- and γ-globulin are lower in synovial fluid.

When the membrane is inflamed, it becomes easily permeable to proteins, and the difference in the permeability between albumin and globulin ceases to exist. Therefore, the concentrations of albumin and globulin approach that in serum, except that α_2-globulin remains lower in the synovial fluid. The globulin concentration always increases in proportion to the intensity and the duration of the inflammation.

Contains No Fibrinogen. This is also true in effusions of traumatic arthritis. The fluids of specific infections and rheumatoid arthritis coagulate and form large firm clots because they contain fibrinogen.

Mucin. The amount varies. It is responsible for the viscosity, which averages 235 at 38° C but can range from 5.7 to as high as 1160. The mucin content is low under conditions of marked inflammation (high total protein, turbidity, high total leukocyte and polymorph counts, high globulin, low sugar). In traumatic fluids, the mucin content is normal.

Enzymes. Amylase, protease, lipase; extremely low alkaline phosphatase

EXAMINATION

Collection of fluid is done without adding an anticoagulant, except a few milliliters for cytologic study to which is added 2 mg potassium oxalate per milliliter of fluid.[1]

Gross Appearance. Note the color, turbidity, apparent viscosity, and tendency to clot. Blood streaks are caused by needle puncture. The viscosity may be estimated by allowing the fluid to drip from the end of a small syringe. Normally, the viscous fluid falls drop by drop. The thin, nonviscous fluid of inflammation flows freely and uninterruptedly.

Bacteriology. Culture is done at the bedside and should include guinea pig inoculation.

Cytology. For a total cell count, saline is used as a diluent, since routine diluents contain an acid that will precipitate the mucin. Methylene blue is added to the saline to stain the nucleated cells. A standard hemacytometer is used.

The differential count is done on very thin dried smears stained with Wright's stain. The mucinous amorphous deposit stains deeply basophilic.

In traumatic joint disease, the total cell count varies from a normal of 60 to 3000, seldom higher, and consists mainly of mononuclears. In inflammatory joint disease, the total count is above 3000, mainly polymorphs. One must be cautious in interpreting the fluid in mild rheumatoid arthritis, since this may resemble that of traumatic arthritis.

Mucin and Viscosity. Normally, when acetic acid is added to synovial fluid, a tight, ropy clump is formed in a clear solution and does not break up on agitation (Ropes test). In mild inflammation, mucin is precipitated in a clump but is soft and friable, breaking up on agitation. In more severe inflammation, a flocculent precipitate forms in a cloudy solution.

Viscosity indicates the state of the mucin. This may be tested with a Hess viscosimeter or in a fairly satisfactory manner by the syringe-drip test described above.

Sugar. Sugar is measured by the Somogyi-Nelson method (which measures true glucose only). The concentration of sugar in synovial fluid is the same as that in the blood. Values are normal in traumatic arthritis and reduced in rheumatoid and infectious arthritis.

Protein. In traumatic fluid, the total protein does not rise above 5.5 g/dl, and the albumin fraction determined electrophoretically is more than 60% of the total. In rheumatoid arthritis, the total protein may rise above 8 g, with a proportionately higher amount of globulin, so that the albumin concentration is lower, often below 50%.

CLASSIFICATION OF DISEASES AFFECTING JOINTS

Infectional Arthritis
- Acute (*Streptococcus, Staphylococcus,* gonococcus)
- Chronic (tubercle bacillus)

Probably Infectional
- Rheumatic fever
- Rheumatoid arthritis (atrophic arthritis, proliferative arthritis, chronic infectious arthritis)
- Ankylosing spondylitis (Marie-Strümpell disease)
- Psoriatic arthritis

Toxic Arthritis
- Arthritis associated with various infections

Degenerative Arthritis (osteoarthritis, hypertrophic arthritis, osteoarthrosis)
- Generalized
- Localized
  - Secondary to previous trauma
  - Secondary to structural abnormality
  - Secondary to rheumatoid arthritis
  - Cause unknown

Arthritis Associated with Metabolic Diseases
- Gout
- Other metabolic diseases

Neuropathic Joints
- Tabes dorsalis
- Syringomyelia

Neoplasms of Joints (cyst, xanthoma, hemangioma, giant cell tumor, synovioma)

Traumatic Arthritis
- Direct trauma
- Indirect trauma (secondary to postural strain)

Systemic Disease Manifestation
- Serum sickness
- Hemophilia
- Intermittent hydrarthrosis
- Pulmonary osteoarthropathy
- Hysterical joints

Local Joint Disturbances
- Aseptic necrosis
  - Known etiology (fracture, dislocation, air embolism)
  - Unknown etiology (juvenile osteochondritis or Legg-Calvé-Perthes disease, Köhler's disease, Freiberg's disease, Osgood-Schlatter disease)
- Osteochondritis dissecans (aseptic necrosis?)
- Osteochondromatosis
- Pigmented villonodular synovitis

DEGENERATIVE JOINT DISEASE

The terms *osteoarthritis* and *osteoarthrosis* (also chondromalacic arthrosis, degenerative arthritis, hypertrophic arthritis, arthritis deformans) are currently used to define an idiopathic, slowly progressive disease of diarthrodial (synovial) joints, occurring late in life and characterized pathologically by focal degeneration of articular cartilage, subchondral bone thickening (sclerosis), marginal osteochondral outgrowths (osteophytes), and joint deformity; clinically by recurring episodes of pain, synovitis with effusion, stiffness, and progressive limitation of motion; and roentgenographically by narrowing of the joint interval, increased density and thickening of the subchondral bone, subchondral cysts, and marginal bony excrescences. The degenerative process first affects the articular cartilage; it initially appears to affect the surface and progressively extends deeply throughout the entire cartilage thickness. Alterations of the physicochemical characteristics diminish cartilage resistance to compressive and tensile forces, and it develops fibrillations, deep clefts, shredding, and, finally, complete erosion, exposing the subchondral bone. Coincident with the earliest stage of involvement at the surface, the subchondral bone becomes increasingly vascular, and blood vessels invade the deep calcified layer, penetrating the tidemark. As the overlying cartilage is eroded, the subchondral lamellar bone and the adjacent trabeculae become thickened.

The presently accepted view is that osteoarthritis (osteoarthrosis) is a degenerative process of unknown etiology affecting articular cartilage of a previously healthy joint; it is designated in the literature most commonly as primary osteoarthritis. Although the disease occurs mainly in older people, the articular cartilage possesses morphological, chemical, metabolic, and physical characteristics separate and distinct from those of aging cartilage. It is therefore necessary to accurately define the changes that take place with aging in human articular cartilage before describing the parameters of the osteoarthritic process.

The secondary type of osteoarthritis is a degenerative process of articular cartilage that is precipitated by specific factors (*e.g.*, incongruity of joint surfaces).

Although this disease is generally recognized as degenerative rather than inflammatory, the term *osteoarthritis* will be used, since it is the commonly applied reference term in the literature. *Chondromalacic arthrosis* appears to be more descriptive.

ETIOLOGY

The cause of primary osteoarthritis is unknown; however, there are predisposing factors.

PREDISPOSING FACTORS

Age. The process appears to begin in the second decade of life, but degenerative changes are not apparent until middle age, and by 55 to 65 years of age approximately 85% have roentgenologic evidence, to a variable degree, of the disease.[34]

Sex. Men and women are equally affected. Up to 54 years of age, the pattern of involvement is similar in both. Thereafter, the disease is more severe and more generalized in women.

Heredity. An epidemiologic study suggests that osteoarthritis is an articular expression of a generalized constitutional condition resulting from inherited metabolic abnormalities.[25] Heberden's nodes may be inherited as a single autosomal gene, sex influenced to be dominant in females and recessive in males. The age at penetrance is variable. In elderly women, when penetrance is complete, the frequency due to the dominant trait is 30%. In men, as a result of the recessive trait, the frequency is 3%. The exact mode of transmission is unknown.[71,72]

Obesity. The disease is twice as prevalent in the obese and mainly affects the weight-bearing joints. In obese men, the disease often assumes the generalized pattern more typical of women.

Areas of Involvement. There is a variable involvement from person to person and from joint to joint. However, certain patterns appear to emerge from studies of populations. Before 54 years of age, the pattern of joint involvement is similar in men and women. In women, a more generalized involvement is usual, and the distal interphalangeal joints and the first carpometacarpal joints are often affected. In men, the hips are more commonly involved.

Any synovial joint may be affected, but the most severe degeneration occurs in joints subjected to greatest compression. Those affected by weight bearing and compressional forces include the lower spine, hips, and knees. Those affected by strong, repetitive muscle forces include the first metatarsophalangeal and the first carpometacarpal (trapeziometacarpal) joints and the midcervical joints.

Within a single joint, the initial osteoarthritic changes are mainly confined to the nonpressure areas. When Trueta examined the femoral heads of people of various ages, from 14 to 100 years, showing evidence of cartilage degeneration, 71% of femoral heads were shown to exhibit degeneration confined to the nonpressure areas and only 3% to the pressure areas. In the remaining 26%, the cartilage lesion was present in both areas.[76]

INCITING FACTORS

Primary osteoarthritis implies that the cause is unknown. Secondary osteoarthritis arises in a joint that, by definition, is previously healthy, and the cartilage is altered by various conditions. It is entirely possible that the inciting factors, listed below, may increase the rate of progression of an already existent, but not clinically manifest, degenerative process.

Inflammatory Process. In such a process as rheumatoid disease, the periarticular and synovial tissues invade and destroy the articular cartilage.[58]

Metabolic Disorders. For example, gouty deposits of urates, and in alkaptonuric ochronosis deposits of pigments, accumulate in articular cartilage, altering its physical properties and making it susceptible to destruction.[33] Hemochromatosis acts similarly.[13,20]

Biomechanical Factors. Cartilage is fatigue prone (*i.e.*, it will fail when a stress of sufficient magnitude is cyclically applied). Thus, cyclical loading will not only produce fractures of collagen fibers but also produce proteoglycan (PG) depletion at the surface. Such stresses are increased by bone deformity.

Structural abnormality, as a result of articular fracture, dislocation, acetabular dysplasia, slipped epiphysis, and Perthes' disease, will cause increasingly high contact pressures as a result of reduced load-bearing areas. Avascular necrosis, by permitting osseous collapse, similarly deforms the articular surface and leads to dangerously high load-bearing pressures.

Malalignment of a joint (*e.g.*, genu valgum or varum) imposes unequally distributed increased loads on one side of the joint, eventuating in breakdown of cartilage.

Abnormal physical forces may be the result of an internal derangement of the joint.[15] The concept of an instant center pathway is used to determine the velocities and direction of forces acting on the joint. The velocity at any point at the surface is found by connecting the instant center (point of rotation at a given time) to the surface and constructing a perpendicular to it. In the normal instant center pathway, the velocity at the joint contact surface is parallel to the surface (Fig. 13-1*A*). In a patient with a tear of the medial meniscus, the instant center pathway is distorted, so that as the knee is extended, the velocity at the joint line tends to force the femur into the tibia (Fig. 13-1*B*). This high contact force produces wear and subsequent degenerative joint disease.

Compression of opposing articular surfaces interferes with the nutrition of cartilage and results in necrosis of chondrocytes. Matrix PG depletion ensues, the cartilage is unable to withstand compressive and shear stresses as movement is resumed, and degenerative changes take place.[64]

FIG. 13-1. Pathomechanics of an internal derangement of the knee. The instant center of rotation for each successive arc of movement is determined as the knee goes from flexion to extension. The direction of velocity of forces at the contact point of the joint line is determined by drawing a line from the instant center of rotation to the surface and drawing a perpendicular. The direction of velocity force is indicated by the perpendicular. (*Left*) The velocity at the surface of contact is normally parallel to the surface. (*Right*) With a bucket-handle tear of the medial meniscus, the instant center about which the knee rotates for 30° of flexion has been displaced posteriorly from its normal location, and the direction of velocity tends to force the surfaces together, producing excessive wear. (Frankel VH, Burstein AH, Brooks DB: Biomechanics of internal derangement of the knee. J Bone Joint Surg 53A:945, 1971)

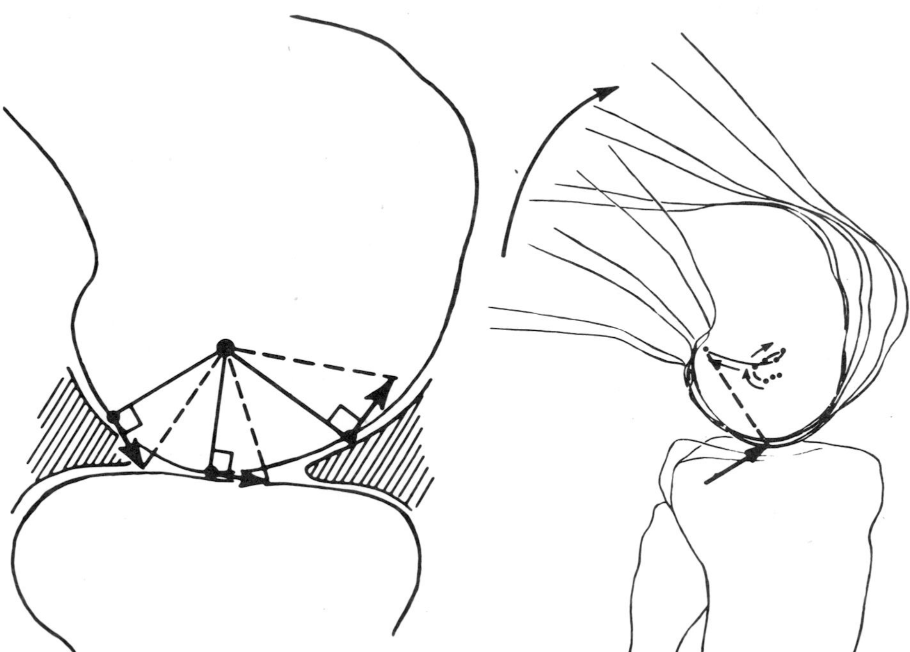

Prolonged immobilization of the experimental animal's knee in forced flexion is followed by adherence between the synovial membrane and the articular cartilage in that part of the joint where the articular surfaces are not in contact. The underlying cartilage undergoes degeneration, presumably as a result of impaired nutrition.

Hormonal Effects. Acromegaly notably affects cartilage.[9,68] Somatotropin stimulates chondrocytes, resulting in acceleration and intensification of metabolic activity. As the animal ages, somatotropin deficiency becomes pronounced and chondrocyte regressive changes and reduced metabolic activity ensue.

Diabetes shows progressive abnormalities of chondrocytes, and diabetics are uniquely susceptible to osteoarthritis.

Chemical Injury. Systemically or locally administered chemical agents affect the viability and metabolic activity of articular cartilage chondrocytes.

Corticosteroids injected into the joint produce substantial depression of synthetic activity lasting from several hours to a week or more.[45] When corticosteroids are administered systemically for many weeks in immunosuppressive doses, a similar reduction of synthetic rates and loss of PG results.[51] The histologic lesion is described as focal chondromalacia or incipient osteoarthritis.[59,65]

Alkylating agents (*e.g.*, nitrogen mustard or thiotepa) injected intra-articularly may be injurious to articular cartilage.[73]

Repeated Intrasynovial Hemorrhage. In patients with defective clotting factors, repeated hemorrhage can lead to severe damage to articular cartilage as well as to subchondral bone structures.[24,62] Iron and pigment in matrix may alter the physical and chemical properties of cartilage, or the chondrocytes engulf large quantities of iron pigment within their cytoplasm, perhaps causing lysosomal release of degradative enzymes. It has been shown that the PG concentration is diminished and synthetic activity of the chondrocyte is depressed.[11]

A single or occasional hemorrhage probably causes no problem.

Changes With Aging. Some observers believe that fibrillation of the surface layer of articular cartilage is age related, asymptomatic, and peculiar to certain locations (hip: inferomedial to fovea and zenith of femoral head; patella: medial facet) and sometimes can lead to osteoarthritis.[12]

Certain changes occur during aging in normal human articular cartilage. These age-related changes take place in immature cartilage, during maturation associated with skeletal development, and during aging in adult life. It is essential to distinguish such alterations from those of disease processes, particularly those of osteoarthritis.

Cellular Changes. In the immature epiphyseal cartilage, the number of cells in proportion to the amount of matrix is higher than in the adult.[11] Mitotic activity is evident in two zones. Near the articular surface, cell replication is responsible for gradual enlargement of the cartilage mass of the epiphysis. In the basilar area, cellular proliferation is a prelude for endochondral ossification, forming a microepiphyseal plate for ossification of the epiphyseal center. As the animal ages, usually after the early months of life, mitotic activity is no longer demonstrable, and a progressive decline in cellularity takes place during the first 2 years of life.[74] In the adult, there is no change in the overall cellularity. It is important to note that the cell count in the superficial zone does not change with advancing age.[56] When visually intact articular cartilage shows a reduction in cellularity in the superficial zone, especially if associated with signs of degeneration of cells, and increased cellularity of the transitional zone, the early onset of osteoarthritis is evident.

Collagen. Aging is associated with increased maturity of collagen fibers. Fibers in all zones are increased in diameter, often appear fragmented, and, in the vicinity of degenerating cells, often contain nuclei of calcification.[80] At birth, except for tangential orientation at the superficial zone, the fibers assume a random arrangement. This pattern persists during normal aging, except for a tendency to vertical orientation in the deepest layer adjacent to the bone.[36] In the superfical zone, the fibers frequently lose their bundle arrangement but remain tangential to the articular surface. The lamina splendens in older tissue is often replaced by an accumulation of amorphous debris.[80]

Protein and Glycosaminoglycan (GAG) Synthesis. In immature animals, the synthesis of protein and other matrix components is quite active but decreases as maturity is approached.[43] The rate of synthesis then remains remarkably constant to balance the normal rate of degradation. PG in the adult rabbit articular cartilage has a short half-life, and a large portion has a half-life of approximately 8 days.[7] Other components, including collagen, have a very slow turnover rate. The constant level of synthesis is altered under pathological conditions and is markedly increased following a lacerative injury and during certain phases of osteoarthritis.[44,48]

Chemical Composition. Chondroitin-6-sulfate forms the principal GAG, accounting for 45% to 75% of the sugar component. In immature cartilage, the remainder of the GAG is mainly chondroitin-4-sulfate and trace amounts of keratan sulfate. As the animal ages, the concentration of chondroitin-4-sulfate steadily decreases to the adult level of less than 5% of the total GAG. On the other hand, the amount of keratan sulfate increases with age, reaching concentrations as high as 50% in the adult. Normally, significant amounts of chondroitin-4-sulfate are found only in immature cartilage. In a reparative response to injury or a disease process (*e.g.*, osteoarthritis) the chondrocyte reverts to its chondroblastic function of synthesizing large amounts of chondroitin-4-sulfate, and appreciable amounts of this GAG are found in this tissue.

Little change occurs in the composition of normal human articular cartilage after the animal becomes skeletally mature. No appreciable change with age occurs in the water, collagen, total hexosamine, chondroitin sulfate, total nitrogen, sulfur, and ash content of the tissue.[2]

In the case of collagen, it is not known whether the fiber morphology alters during aging in humans or whether aging affects the physicochemical properties of human cartilage fibers. Moreover, the effect of aging on the amount of cross-link formation in collagen is unknown.[18]

Physical Alterations. The permeability of articular cartilage decreases with aging, reaching its maximum in the period from 10 to 40 years of age. Then a variable increase in permeability takes place, more marked in the superficial than in the deeper zone.[32,55]

The elastic properties of normal human articular cartilage are unchanged with aging.[69] When a load is applied, deformation is instantaneous, followed by a creep phase. When the load is removed, the cartilage recovers its original thickness as a result of instantaneous recovery followed by a time-dependent recovery phase. Approximately 90% or more of the "instantaneous" deformation is instantaneously recovered when the load is quickly removed. On the other hand, indentations of fibrillated cartilage are much larger and recovery is slow and incomplete.

Tensile stiffness refers to forces parallel to the articular surface produced largely as a secondary effect of compression, and the ability to resist such forces is a function of collagen fibers.The effect of aging on the tensile strength of articular cartilage is unknown and requires further study. In osteoarthritis, articular cartilage is considerably less stiff and weaker, mainly at the surface, and stiffer with increasing depth.

Nutrition of Articular Cartilage. Only during the embryonic period and for a short time thereafter, vascular channels extend from the metaphysis into the basilar portions of the articular cartilage and from the perichondrium directly into the epiphysis.[35,37] The immature articular cartilage with open epiphyseal plates thus derives its nutrition from the underlying vasculature of the metaphysis and by diffusion from the synovial fluid.[14,38] After maturation, as the epiphyseal plate closes, the calcified zone is established, and the tidemark becomes apparent, almost all nutrition is derived by diffusion from synovial fluid.[23] Under pathologic conditions, such as osteoarthritis or a complete cartilage defect that extends through the subchondral plate, the metaphyseal vessels, in an apparent reparative response, once again penetrate the deep calcified zone.

PATHOLOGY

Normal cartilage is smooth, glistening, and bluish white. The synovial membrane is smooth and pale, and at its attachment to the joint margins it merges with the articular cartilage. Normally, a physiological aging process starts in the second decade and increases with advancing age. Such changes in the chemical composition, histologic appearance, synthetic and degradative activity, and physical characteristics have been described in the preceding section and should be distinguished from the changes that occur in osteoarthritis or osteoarthrosis.

Early degeneration of hyaline articular cartilage is a focal process within the individual joint. Grossly, it appears as a dry, dull, yellowish, opaque, soft, and fibrillar surface having a velvety feel. Microscopically, as many as 20 chondrocytes occupy each enlarged lacunar space (Weichselbaum's lacuna), a multicellular aggregation termed a chondron or clone. (Fig. 13-2). Later, the cells degenerate and assume a stellate or amorphous appearance. With movement of the joint, compressive and frictional forces erode and shred the exposed degenerated articular surface cartilage, which becomes shagged and pitted.

The normal matrix consists of closely aggregated collagenous bundles of fibers at the surface, randomly arranged network of fibers at a deeper level, and vertically arranged fibers in the basal layer. Between the collagen fibers are the PGs, the intensely hydrophilic protein polysaccharide (PPS). Both the fibers and the PGs have the same index of refraction, so the fibers are not visible. As the degenerative process advances, the PGs become degraded and removed, and the fibers become visible. The tissue splits into many clefts. The fibrillary and fissured appearance produced as the collagen fibers assume a vertical position between the deepening clefts is highly characteristic of osteoarthritic cartilage (Color Plate 13-1). The superficial tufts of fibers can be observed

FIG. 13-2. Cartilage in degenerative arthritis. Clefts, Weichselbaum's lacunae, fibrillar appearance, and irregular staining qualities are well displayed. (×108)

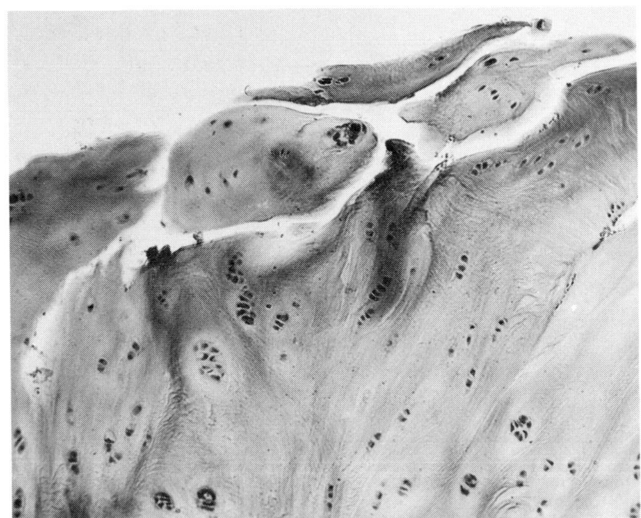

as tiny hairy waving processes when the cartilage is submerged in water and produce a velvety appearance and feel to the surface.

In some areas, the cartilage appears to regenerate and cover denuded areas. This can be traced to the following sequence of events: Complete loss of the overlying articular cartilage exposes the subchondral bone to stresses to which it is not suited, and microfractures occur. Vascular cellular tissue fills the defect and forms fibrocartilaginous tissue. The process is similar to the reparative response to complete defects of articular cartilage, either traumatic or surgically induced.

Degenerated cartilage, particularly as the disease becomes advanced, is often sheared off and lies free within the joint cavity as a "joint mouse."

In the deeper layers, the chondrocytes may appear to line up in columns as they approach the calcified zone where vascular tufts invade from the subchondral bone and marrow, and new layers of lamellar bone thicken the subchondral cortex. This latter process appears to represent a response to increased vertical loads imposed by the loss of the overlying articular cartilage.

In the intermediate (moderately advanced) stages, the soft, degenerated cartilage is worn down and completely resorbed (by lysosomal enzymes?), or is extruded into the joint. The exposed subchondral bone, now exposed to excessive stresses, undergoes an intense osteogenic response associated with a marked degree of vascularity. This phenomenon spreads toward the joint margins, where, unimpeded by compressive forces and perhaps encouraged by traction of capsular attachments, it produces osseous outgrowths that often extend into the capsule (Fig. 13-3).

The synovial membrane undergoes hyperplasia and villous formation and may display hyperemia and infiltration of mononuclear cells. The reactive synovial inflammatory changes seem to be less intense in inactive or non-weight-bearing joints. The synovial membrane may contain foci of cartilage cells that may arise either by metaplasia or by engulfing cartilage fragments from the joint cavity. The nests of cartilage cells may undergo calcification followed by ossification or may be completely resorbed or the cartilaginous and osteocartilaginous bodies may be extruded into the joint.

Fig. 13-3. Osteoarthritis of the distal interphalangeal joint. Note bony outgrowths at the margin of the base of the distal phalanx, clinically termed Heberden's nodes.

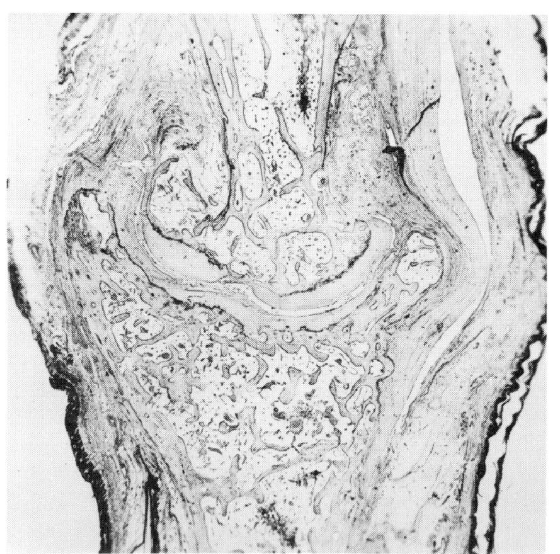

In the advanced stage, the cartilage is completely worn away, and the subchondral cortex becomes extremely thick, smooth, and polished by continuous shearing forces (Fig. 13-4). The subchondral bone is incapable of sustaining vertical loads as before and subchondral fractures occur. Subchondral cysts seem to develop at points of greatest stress. Chondromas and osteochondromas continue to form in the synovial membrane and either remain attached by a pedicle or lie free within the joint. When a joint mouse loses its attachment and therefore its blood supply, its bony core becomes necrotic while its cartilage covering, which derives its nutrients from the synovial fluid, survives and adds additional layers of cartilage. At intervals, the surface layer of cartilage may calcify and then may become covered by an additional layer of cartilage, and the process is repeated over and over again. The sectioned surface of such a joint mouse may, therefore, display multiple alternating layers of calcified and noncalcified cartilage and perhaps a central core of necrotic bone.[8,11]

Vascular Changes. A state of vascular profusion and dilatation in the subchondral area exists.[76] The osteoarthritic process from its inception, when the superficial zone exhibits the earliest changes, shows vessels from the subchondral marrow already penetrating the basal zone of calcified cartilage. The bony architecture of the subchondral trabecular bone becomes rarefied and weakened by the hyperemia. As a result of the loss of the resilient articular cartilage, increased forces are borne by the underlying bone, which is even less suited to dissipate these forces, and trabecular fractures occur. As the bony trabeculae collapse and become compressed, and as the new bone forms, the conglomeration of fractured, partially necrotic, compressed bone with new bone forms a dense-appearing segment.

The increased vascularity represents a response that is responsible for the formation of new bone, in the non-weight-bearing area causing the production of osteophytes and in the weight-bearing area producing dense new bone.

Altered Hemodynamics. Hyperplasia of intraosseous arteries in the subchondral cancellous bone implies an increased arterial inflow.[21] Venous outflow from the epiphysis is impaired.[5] Normally, when a contrast medium is injected into the intraosseous cancellous portion of the epiphysis, the radiopaque shadow quickly outlines

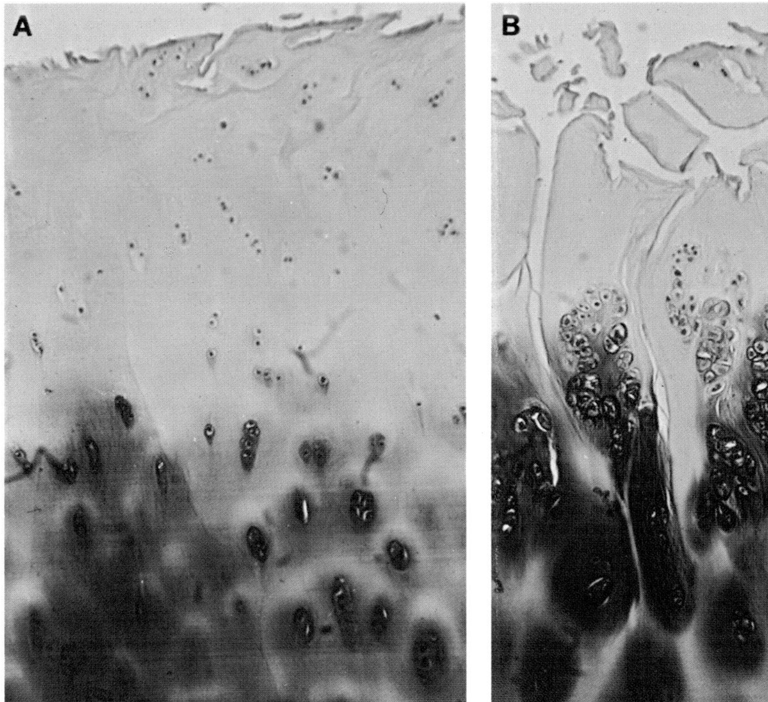

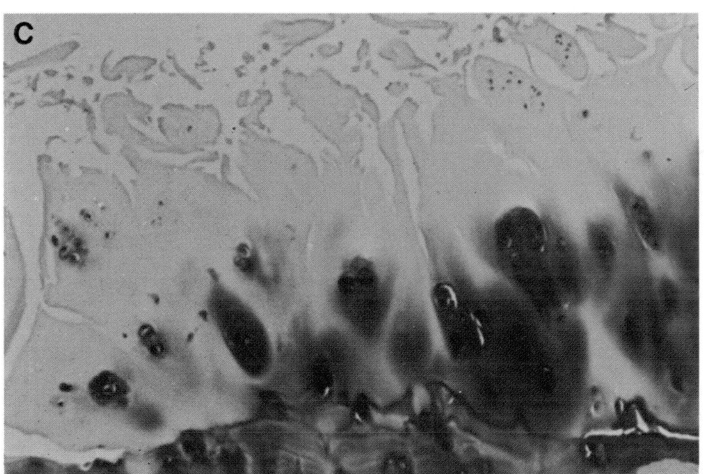

PLATE 13-1. Osteoarthritis, stages of progression of disease in adult human articular cartilage. Stained with safranin-O and counterstained with hematoxylin. (*A*) Early stage. The tangenital zone normally is characterized by lack of safranin-O staining for GAGs. The irregularities and infoldings of the surface are well shown. The lamina splendens is absent. The cells of the superficial zone become rounded and multicellular clones are formed. At the transitional zone, the intercellular matrix is becoming less intensely stained, the main concentrations of mucopolysaccharides occurring in the immediate vicinity of the clones and individual cells. (*B*) Moderately advanced stage. The clefts extend deeply; the surface is markedly disrupted, and the superficial layer is almost acellular. Clone formation is more pronounced in the middle zone, in which the heightened metabolic activity of the chondrocytes is reflected by intense staining in the immediate pericellular matrix whereas in the interterritorial matrix, loss of staining indicates PG depletion. (*C*) Markedly advanced stage. The superficial and transitional zones are acellular and lack staining with safranin-O, and clefts extend to the deep layer, best observed toward the left side of the photomicrograph. Degeneration extends to the deep zone. (Photomicrographs prepared by Dr. Charles Weiss) (See p. 387.)

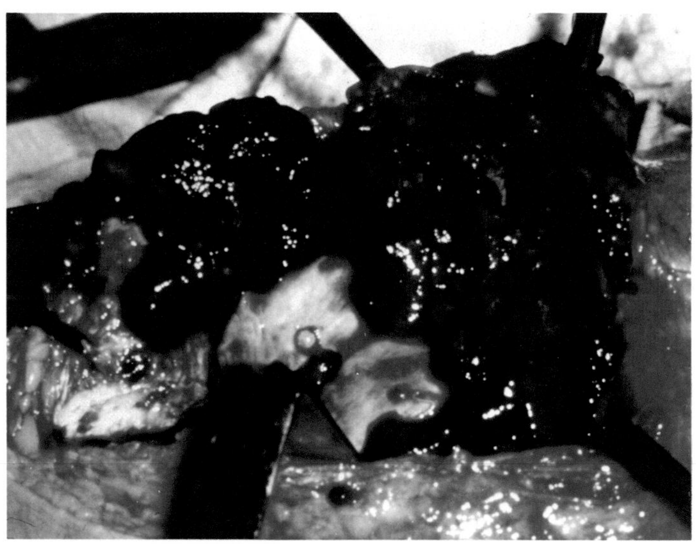

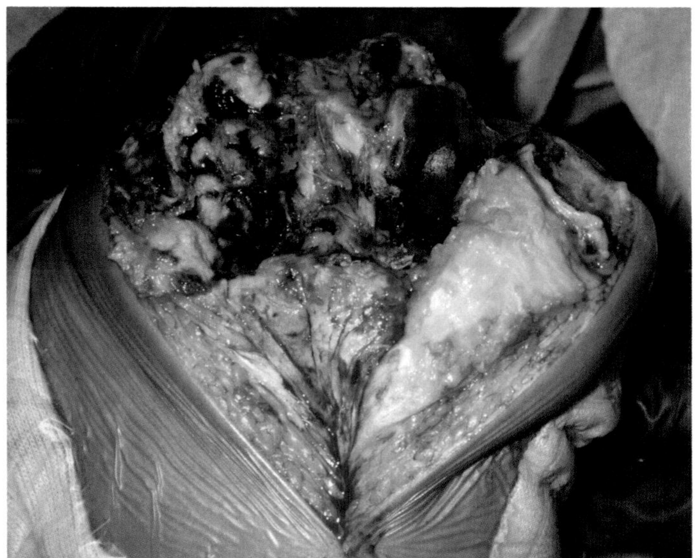

PLATE 13-2. Surgical pathology of hemophilic arthropathy. (*Top*) Stage 3 hemophilic arthropathy of the knee. Note widening of the intercondylar notch (above retractor), preservation of the cartilage, and proliferative synovitis. (*Bottom*) Stage 5 hemophilic arthropathy of the knee. Almost all of the articular cartilage has been destroyed and the eburnated bone on the femoral condyles is stained a deep blue by deposits of hemosiderin. (Arnold WD, Hilgartner MW: Hemophilic arthropathy. J Bone Joint Surg 59A:287, 1977) (See p. 445.)

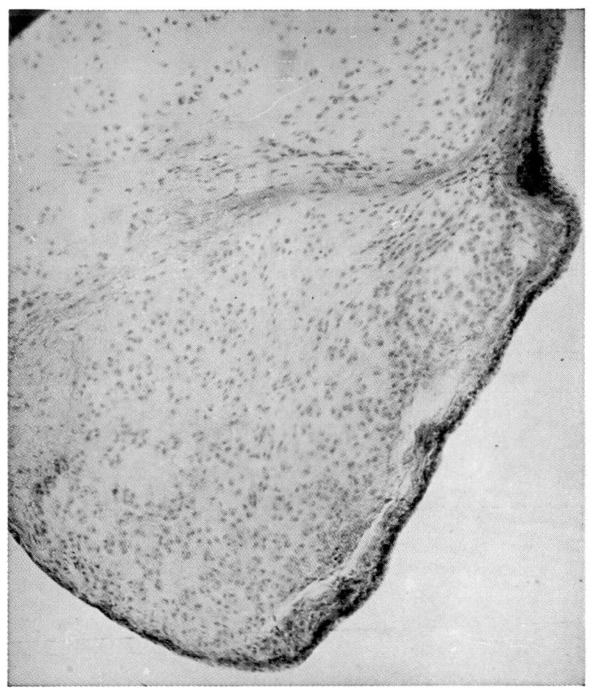

PLATE 13-3. Chondromatosis. Note the synovial lining about the cartilage. (×85) (See p. 455.)

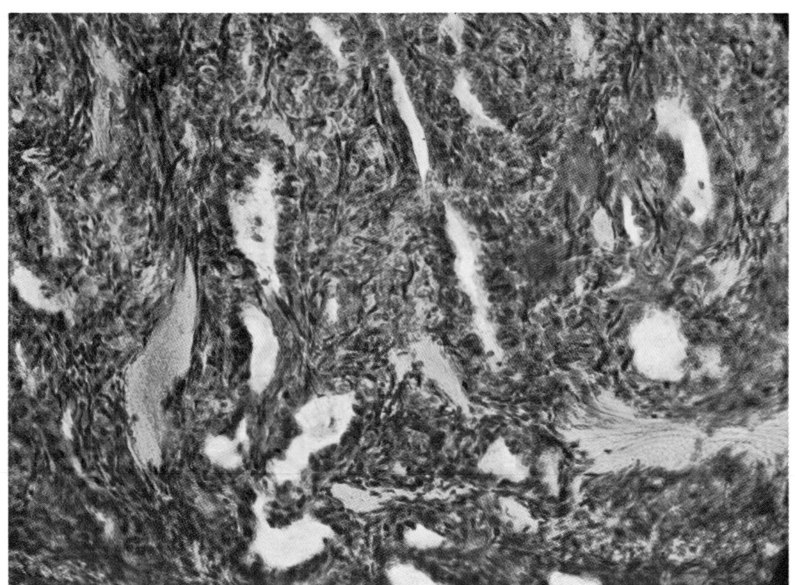

PLATE 13-4. Synovioma. Features include slitlike spaces lined with flattened inconspicuous cells; glandlike spaces lined with larger multilayered cells; homogeneous pink-staining substance in spaces; tendency toward tufting; and sarcomatous appearance of fibroblasts (irregular size, shape, staining, distribution, dense-staining nuclei, and frequent mitoses). (×185) (See p. 457.)

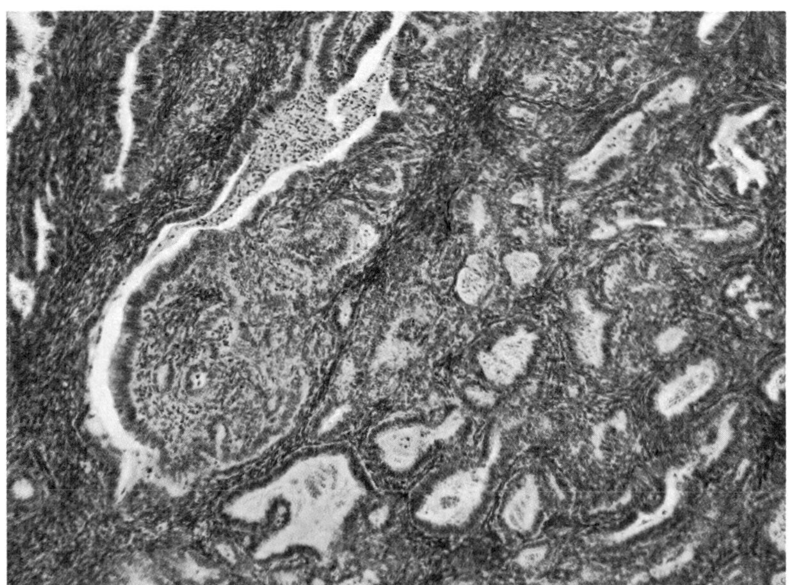

PLATE 13-5. Synovioma. Pseudoadenomatous appearance. The lining cells are cuboidal and columnar. In any tumor, features of glandlike spaces, tufting, and fibrosarcomatous changes should be sought throughout the tumor. One or more features may predominate. (×120) (See p. 457.)

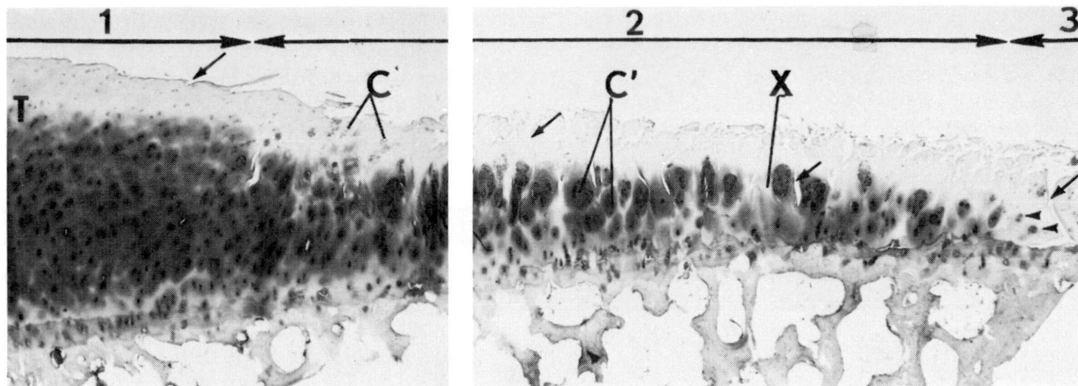

FIG. 13-4. Section from the distal femoral condyle of a 34-year-old man, stained for the presence of mucopolysaccharide with safranin-O (dark stain) and counterstained with fast green (light stain), demonstrating areas of early (*1*), moderately advanced (*2*), and advanced (*3*) osteoarthritic changes in close juxtaposition. Early osteoarthritis has superficial fibrillation (*arrow*), slight hypercellularity, and loss of mucopolysaccharide confined to the upper middle or transitional zone (*T*). Moderately advanced changes have clefts extending deep into the middle zone (*arrows*) and increased numbers of cells in clusters or "clones." Some clones in the superficial and upper middle zones are devoid of a mucopolysaccharide halo (*C*), whereas those in the middle zone show intense safranin-O staining (*C'*). The loss of mucopolysaccharide extends into the middle zone (*X*). Areas of advanced disease contain clefts that extend through the entire thickness of the articular cartilage (*arrow*); the tissue is hypocellular and almost completely devoid of mucopolysaccharide with safranin-O confined to some pericellular areas (*arrowheads*). The subchondral bone lamellae and trabeculae are thickest in the area of advanced osteoarthritis; this reflects more stress in bone and is consistent with the roentgenographic finding of sclerosis. (Weiss C: Ultrastructural characteristics of osteoarthritis. Fed Proc 32:1459, 1973)

the regional veins and is dissipated within 6 minutes. The injection produces little or no discomfort. The measured intraosseous normal pressure (IOP) is 20 mm Hg to 40 mm Hg.[6] In osteoarthritis, injection of the fluid often causes intense pain that is quite similar to the "rest pain" of which the patient complains. The regional veins are poorly visualized or are not visualized at all, the radiopaque medium remaining unabsorbed about the tip of the cannula for more than 20 minutes. The measured intraosseous pressure is high, usually well above 40 mm Hg. When the affected area is decompressed, for example, by osteotomy or fenestration, the intraosseous pressure falls and relief of rest pain is immediate.[4] These facts suggest that intramedullary hypertension secondary to poor venous drainage causes the characteristic rest pain of severe osteoarthritis.

Cysts. The cysts are radiolucent areas restricted to the upper part of the pressure-bearing segment, and they lie within the dense bone deep to the eburnated articular surface.[61] They contain fibrous tissue, which may be loose, myxoid, dense, or fibrocartilaginous. A profusion of large, thin-walled anastomosing venules occupy the bony structure about the cyst, originating from slender arterioles. Within the cyst, few blood vessels are found.

The bony wall of the cyst is formed by thickened trabeculae. When overlying pressure forces are relieved (*e.g.*, by surgery), revascularization of and osteogenic obliteration of the cyst take place.[75]

Stages of Osteoarthritis as Seen Under Light Microscopy. The three microscopic stages are as follows:[82]

Early

Surface irregularities or fibrillations with small clefts not extending beyond the superficial zone; slight hypercellularity; minimum loss of mucopolysaccharides not extending beyond the transitional zone or upper middle zone

Moderately Advanced

More extensive loss of surface; clefts extend into the middle zone and occasionally into the calcified zone; loss of mucopolysaccharides extends into the middle zone; hypercellularity in clusters of cells or chondrocyte clones

Advanced

Thickness of cartilage reduced; clefts may extend down to subchondral bone; mucopolysaccharides markedly diminished throughout entire thickness of articular cartilage; in some areas, complete loss of articular cartilage with exposure of thick, eburnated subchondral bone (see Fig. 13-4)

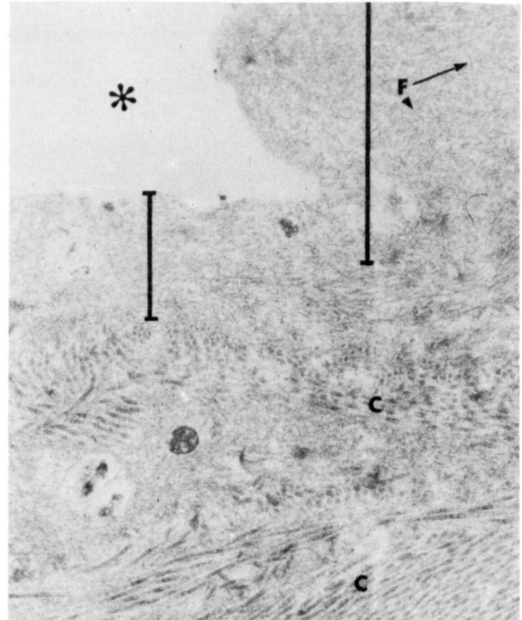

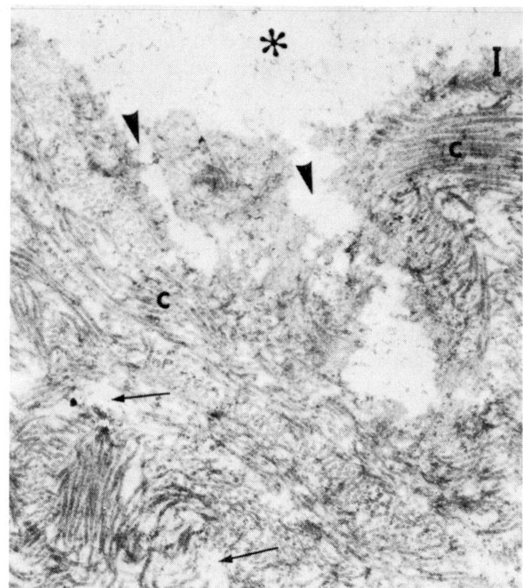

FIG. 13-5. (*Top*) Articular surface of a patient with early osteoarthritis. Note that the minute irregularities of the surface and the fine fibers and filamentous fibrils (*F*), which are 4 nm to 12 nm (40 A–120 A) in diameter, form a layer on the surface up to 3.2μm in depth (*I*) and separating the underlying mature collagen fibers (*C*) from the joint surface (*). Bundles of mature collagen fibers parallel the articular surface. (×20,700) (*Bottom*) Articular surface of a patient 55 years of age with moderately advanced osteoarthritis. Small amounts of amorphous material (*I*) cover the articular surface. Bundles of mature collagen fibers (*C*) with normal periodicity parallel the surface of the clefts (*arrowheads*). Large areas of matrix of low electron density separate individual collagen fibers (*arrows*). (*), joint space (×19,000) (Weiss C, Mirow S: An ultrastructural study of osteoarthritic changes in the articular cartilage of human knees. J Bone Joint Surg 54A:954, 1972)

Histologic Sequence of Progression. Osteoarthritis is a focal disease that shows wide variation in histologic histochemical, biochemical, and metabolic alterations in different selected areas of the same articular cartilage.[70] Therefore, the following descriptions relating to these parameters of the disease reflect the sequence of events as the disease progresses.

The earliest histologic changes of osteoarthritis are loss of surface layers of articular cartilage, a diffuse increase in the number of cells, and a moderate decrease in metachromatic staining, indicative of depletion of PG.[11] An ingrowth of blood vessels takes place from the underlying bone and may extend through the tidemark. The latter phenomenon is highly characteristic of this disorder and may contribute to osteophyte formation.[76]

As the disease progresses, vertical-cleft formation begins at the cartilaginous surface, at first descending through the gliding layer and the closely arranged and tangentially oriented dense collagen bundles, distorting the organization of the latter at this level. As the process advances, the clefts become progressively deeper, extending toward the calcified zone, producing a pattern termed fibrillation and characteristic of chondromalacia. Staining with metachromatic dyes, such as alcian blue, or orthochromatic dyes, such as safranin-O, reveals

FIG. 13-6. Articular cartilage of a 38-year-old with advanced osteoarthritis. The surface is covered by amorphous material (*I*). Mature collagen fibers (*C*) are arranged parallel to the surface of the clefts and are of small diameter (20 nm–30 nm or 200 A–300 A). Membranous (*Mb*) and osmophilic material, probably lipid (*Li*), the remains of degenerated cells, are present just beneath the articular surface. (×6250) (Weiss C, Mirow S: An ultrastructural study of osteoarthritic changes in the articular cartilage of human knees. J Bone Joint Surg 54A:954, 1972)

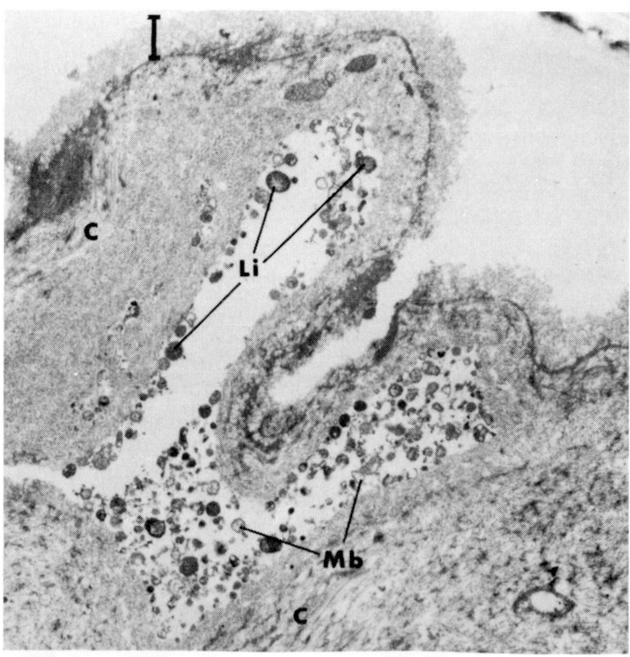

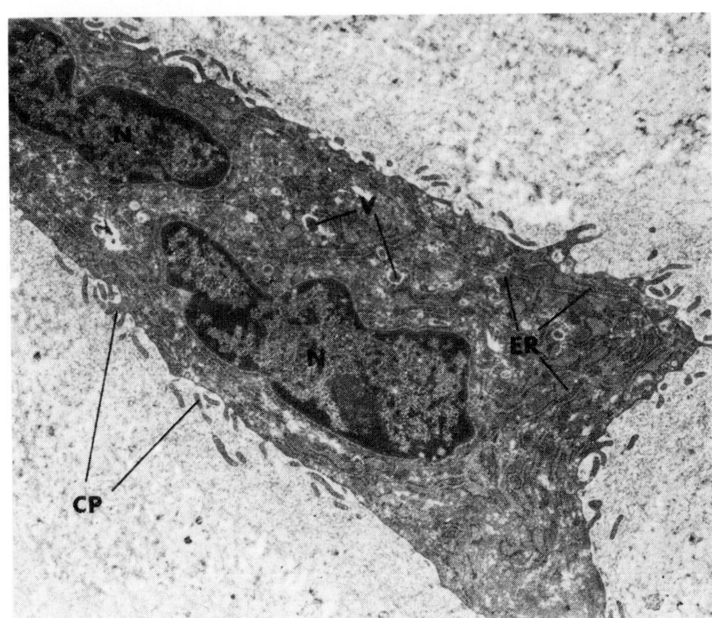

FIG. 13-7. Cell from the superficial zone of the articular cartilage from a 34-year-old with early osteoarthritis. The cell is elongated, with its long axis parallel to the joint surface (*arrow* points toward joint surface), and has long cytoplasmic processes (*CP*). The nucleus (*N*) of this cell is bilobed; the cytoplasm is characterized by dense ground plasm, well-developed rough endoplasmic reticulum (*ER*), and vacuoles (*V*) filled with electron-dense material. (×6275) (Weiss C, Mirow, S: An ultrastructural study of osteoarthritis changes in the articular cartilage of human knees. J Bone Joint Surg 54A:954, 1972)

progressively diminishing intensity of color of the matrix, indicating further depletion of PG. At this stage of the disease, staining is most pronounced immediately about the chondrocytes, which are in a state of hypermetabolic activity. The chondrocytes increase in number and aggregate in clumps or clones, an abnormality highly characteristic of this disease.

In the advanced stage of the disease, the cartilaginous tissue becomes eroded and eventually disappears completely from focal areas of the surface, exposing denuded sclerotic and eburnated bone. Subchondral cysts form, and patches of new cartilage may partially cover eroded areas and extend over marginal osteophytes.

ULTRASTRUCTURAL CHARACTERISTICS

The following description of electron microscopic studies attempts to classify osteoarthritic disease in each zone as early, moderate, and advanced (Figs. 13-5 through 13-11).

Superficial Zone

Matrix

Early. In early osteoarthritis, the articular surface in some areas may still retain an acellular filamentous thin covering, the lamina splendens, which probably represents adsorbed macromolecules of hyaluronic acid or PG. The collagen fibers of the superficial zone with characteristic periodicity and subbanding, and of small diameter, may still be arranged, as in normal articular cartilage, in closely approximated bundles, running at right angles to one another, with little intervening spaces and oriented parallel to the articular surface.

Moderate. The fine filamentous covering of the surface is absent, and numerous infoldings of the articular surface develop. The bundles of mature collagen fibers are arranged parallel to the surface of these folds. The individual collagen fibers and bundles are now separated by large areas of low electron density, reflecting, perhaps, reduced PG content.

Advanced. The surface is covered by amorphous material and is disrupted by clefts which extend deeply. Mature collagen fibers are arranged parallel to the surface of these fibrillations (vertical) and are of small diameter. The interfiber distance is increased and the electron density of the interfiber matrix is reduced.

Cells

Early. The superficial cells are either variable or show evidence of degeneration. Viable cells are large and elongated, with their long axis parallel to the articular surface. Their intracellular organelles are abundant and include an extensive rough endoplasmic reticulum, a prominent Golgi apparatus, vacuoles, and few mitochondria. The nucleus is irregular and often appears bilobed. There are numerous branched cytoplasmic processes. Mature collagen fibers are found adjacent to the plasma membrane. The appearance of the cell is that of a fibroblast, and the increased metabolic activity suggests the synthesis of collagen.

Moderate. Clones of chondrocytes are often found adjacent to the clefts. These clusters lack the homogeneous filamentous or mucopolysaccharide halo seen surrounding the cells and clones of the deeper zones. Instead these are surrounded by collagen fibers of small diameter. The nuclear and cyto-

(Text continues on page 396.)

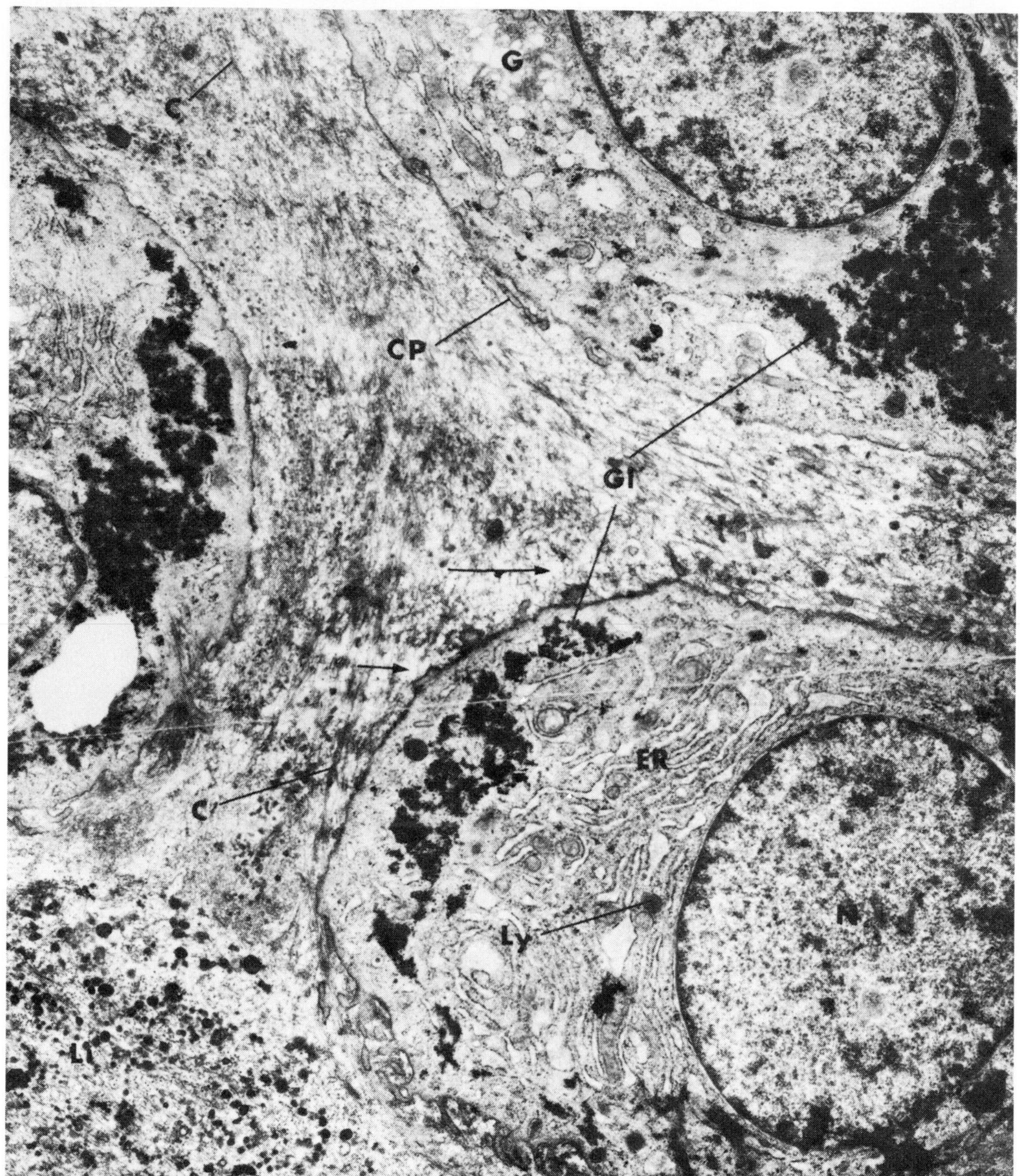

FIG. 13-8. A clone of cells in the superficial zone of the cartilage of a 34-year-old with moderately advanced osteoarthritis. Collagen fibers (*C*) of small diameter (12 nm–20 nm or 120 A–200 A) surround the individual cells as well as the entire clone of cells. Extracellular osmophilic material, probably lipid (*Li*), is present in the vicinity of the cell clump (*lower left*). The interfiber matrix is of low electron density (*arrows*). The cells have short cytoplasmic processes (*CP*). Note the deposits of glycogen (*Gl*), well-developed rough endoplasmic reticulum (*ER*), Golgi apparatus (*G*), the few lysosomallike bodies (*Ly*) in the cytoplasm, and the normal-appearing nucleus (*N*). (×6500). (Weiss C, Mirow, S: An ultrastructural study of osteoarthritis changes in the articular cartilage of human knees. J Bone Joint Surg 54A:954, 1972)

FIG. 13-9. A clone of degenerating chondrocytes in the upper middle zone of the articular cartilage of a 38-year-old with advanced osteoarthritis. Mature collagen fibers (*C*), as well as fibers 12 nm (120 A) in diameter with a beaded appearance (*arrowhead*), are found surrounding the cells. There is a marked decrease in electron density of the interfiber matrix (*arrows*), and extracellular osmophilic material (*Li*) is present. (*Caption continues next page*) ▶

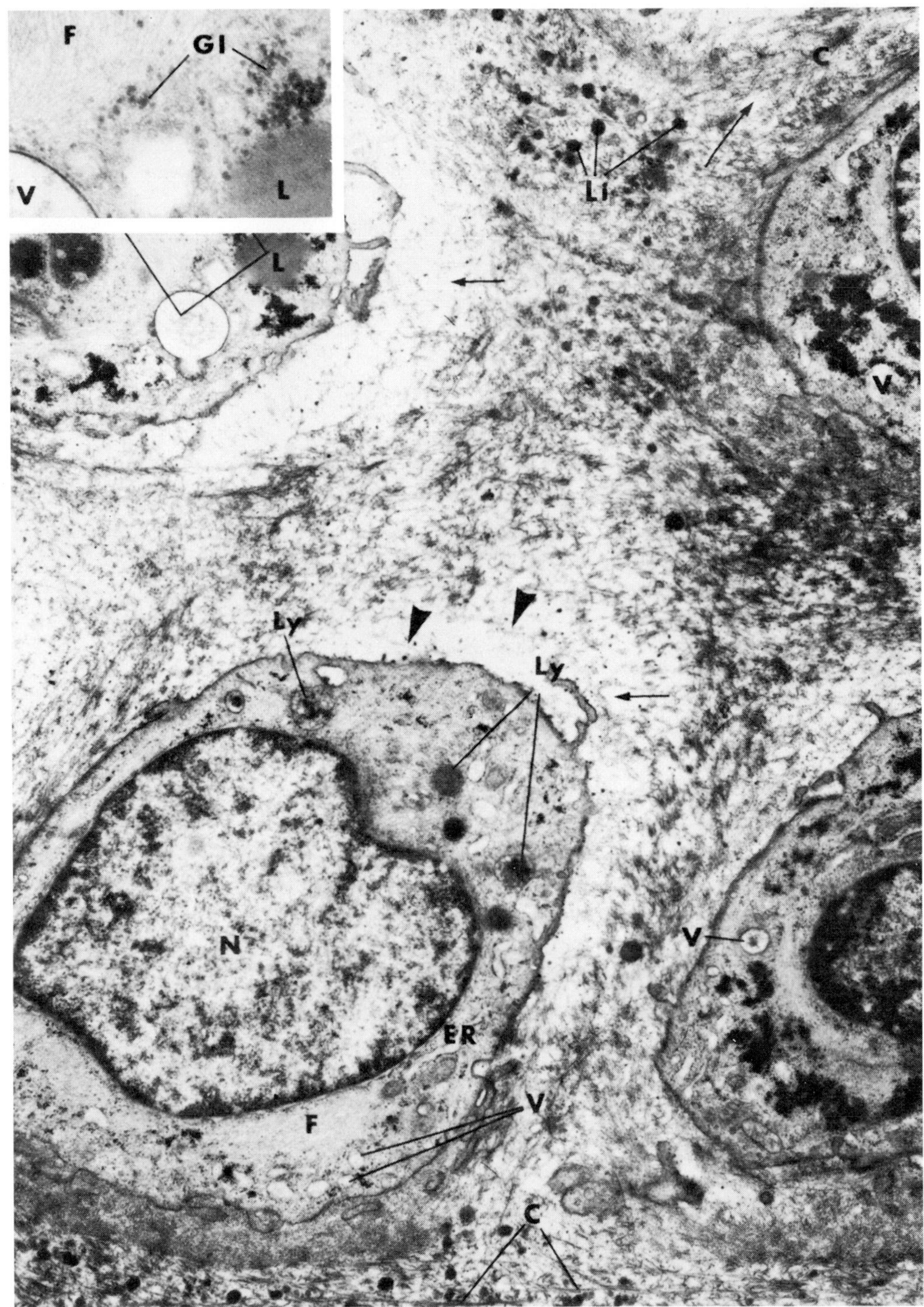

FIG. 13-9 (*Continued*). Nuclei (*N*) have indistinct membranes. Intracytoplasmic organelles are reduced in number (compared with the clump of nondegenerating chondrocytes shown in Figure 13-9) and consist of lysosomallike structures (*Ly*), lipid droplets (*L*), and large vacuoles (*V*). Perinuclear intracytoplasmic filaments (*F*) are very numerous. The rough endoplasmic reticulum (*ER*) is scant. (×8960) (*Inset*) High magnification of the area outlined shows extensive intracytoplasmic filaments 7 nm (70 A) in diameter (*F*), a portion of the lipid droplet, glycogen granules (*G*1), and the vacuole (*V*). (×15,600) (Weiss C, Mirow S: An ultrastructural study of osteoarthritic changes in the articular cartilage of human knees. J Bone Joint Surg 54A:954, 1972)

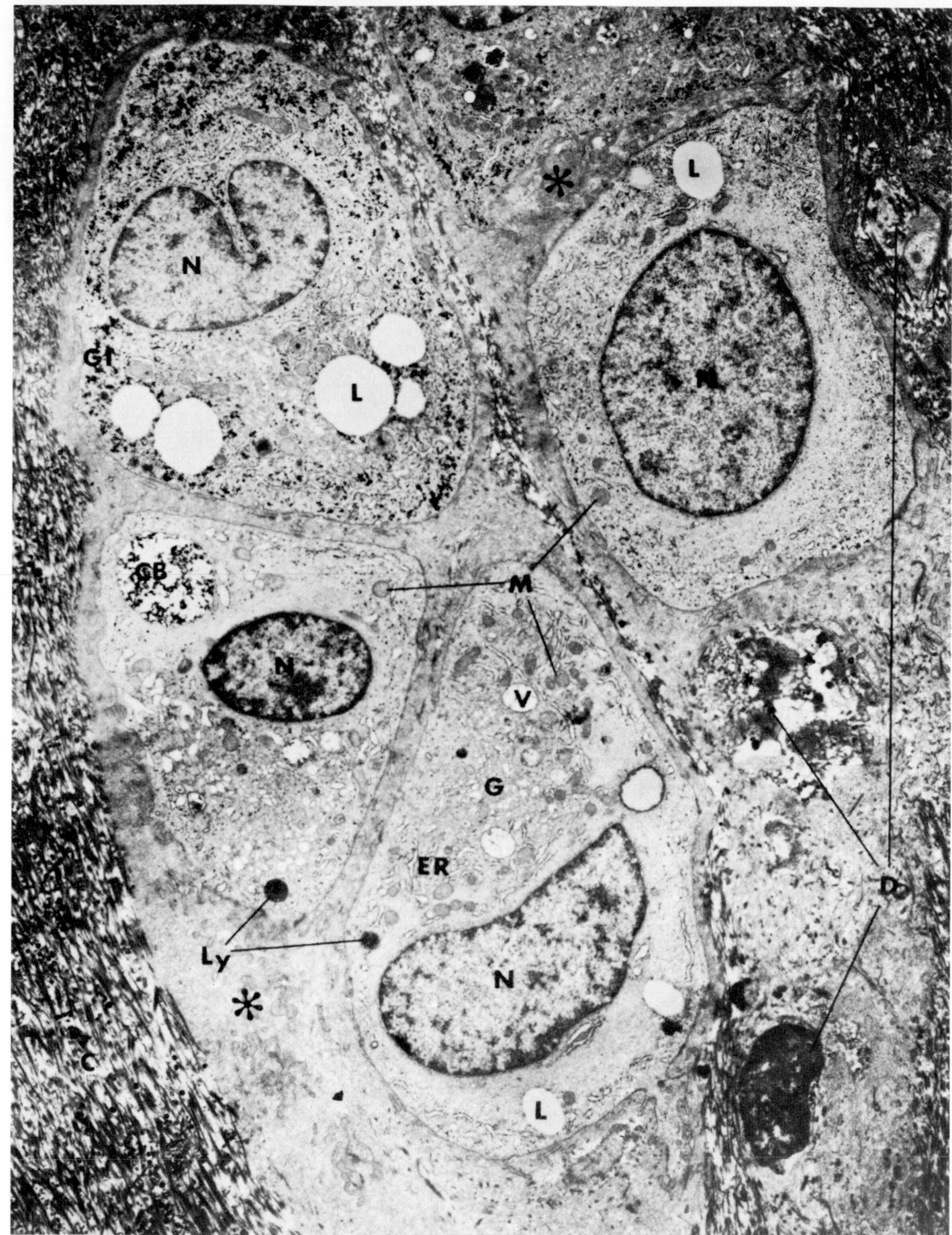

FIG. 13-10. Middle zone chondrocyte clone from a 69-year-old with moderately advanced osteoarthritis. Collagen fibers (*C*) are arranged perpendicular to the joint surface (*large arrow* points in direction of joint surface). The interfiber matrix is of strikingly low electron density when compared with the high electron density of the pericellular halo (*). The presence of remnants of degenerating cells (*D*) in the vicinity of and within the pericellular halo is typical. Chondrocytes have a normal nucleus (*N*), large Golgi apparatus (*G*) with many vacuoles (*V*), well-developed rough endoplasmic reticulum (*ER*), numerous mitochondria (*M*), lipid droplets (*L*), glycogen granules (*Gl*), occasional complex bodies (*CB*), and structures resembling lysosomes (*Ly*). (×4500). (Weiss C, Mirow S: An ultrastructural study of osteoarthritic changes in the articular cartilage of human knees. J Bone Joint Surg 54A:954, 1972)

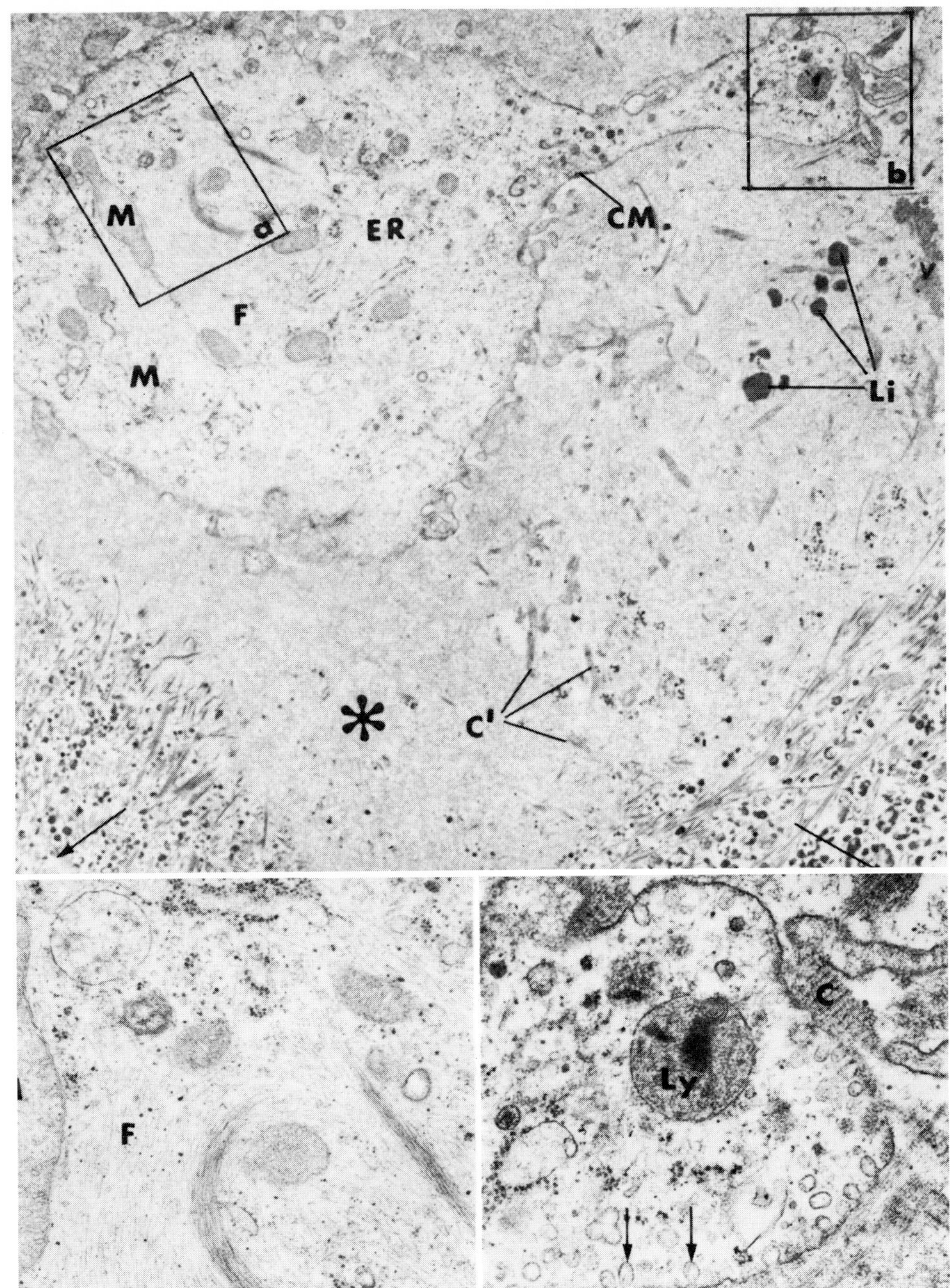

FIG. 13-11. (*Top*) Chondrocytes from the deep zone of articular cartilage of a 55-year-old with moderately advanced osteoarthritis. Collagen fibers (*C*) are arranged perpendicular to the joint surface and are of variable diameter (*large arrow* points toward joint surface). The interfiber matrix is of low electron density (*arrows*), and numerous remnants of degenerating cells (*arrowhead*), especially extracellular lipid (*Li*), are present. Mature collagen fibers of large diameter (*C**) are present within the pericellular halo (*), as are lipid droplets (*Li*). The chondrocyte in this section is in an early stage of degeneration. The cell membrane (*CM*) is intact and mitochondria (*M*) are of unusual shape. There is an abundance of intracellular filaments (*F*), and only the area outlined above (*a*) shows an abundance of intracellular filaments 7 nm (70 A) in diameter and elongated mitochondria. (×18,900) (*Lower right*) At higher magnification the area outlined above (*b*) shows detail of the cytoplasmic process, which contains a lysosomallike structure (*Ly*) and numerous pinocytic vesicles (*arrows*). Mature collagen fibers (*C*) with diameters up to 300 nm (3000 A) are present within the pericellular halo adjacent to the cell membrane. (×22,700) (Weiss C, Mirow S: An ultrastructural study of osteoarthritic changes in the articular cartilage of human knees. J Bone Joint Surg 54A:954, 1972)

plasmic organelles show no degenerative signs: The nuclear and cell membranes are intact, and the rough endoplasmic reticulum, Golgi apparatus, and mitochondria are well developed.

Advanced. Degenerating cells are commonly found in the superficial and deep zones. These are characterized by extensive perinuclear arrangement of intracytoplasmic filaments, numerous lysosomes, and sparse rough endoplasmic reticulum and Golgi apparatus. These degenerating cells are surrounded by large numbers of beaded fibers 12 nm (120 A) in diameter, and mature collagen fibers lie in close proximity to the cell membrane. The number of such degenerating cells increases with the severity of the osteoarthritic lesion and the age of the individual.

Middle Zone

Matrix

Early. The collagen fibers, 20 nm to 160 nm (200 A–1600 A) in diameter, are arranged in random fashion, and there is a wide interfiber distance with spaces of low electron density between the fibers.

Moderate. The collagen fibers are arranged more perpendicular to the articular surface, as contrasted with the normal random arrangement.

Advanced. The perpendicular arrangement of the collagen fibers is even more pronounced.

Cells

Early. The chondrocytes are surrounded by a halo of fine filamentous fibrils. These cells are rounded, have large cytoplasmic volume, and contain many mitochondria, well-developed rough endoplasmic reticulum, and Golgi apparatus, lipid droplets, and an occasional lysosome. Centrioles, which probably indicate cell replication, are present. The largest cells with the most extensive development of organelles are found in the middle zone of cartilage from very elderly people with early to moderately advanced osteoarthritis.

Moderate. The chondrocytes of the middle zone tend to lie in clones composed of from 1 to 20 cells. Individual cells are surrounded by a halo of filamentous fibrils and numerous remnants of degenerating chondrocytes. The cells are often two to three times the size of middle-zone chondrocytes from normal people of a comparable age and show an increased number of organelles.

Advanced. The number of chondrocytes in various stages of degeneration is increased.

Deep Zone

Matrix

Normally in the deep zone the collagen fibers are arranged perpendicular to the articular surface only in cartilage of advanced age, whereas in young cartilage these fibers are randomly arranged. In osteoarthritic cartilage, however, regardless of age, the fibers are arranged perpendicular to the joint surface and are separated by matrix of low electron density, more so than is found in normal young adult human articular cartilage.

Cells

In early osteoarthritis, most chondrocytes exhibit early evidence of degeneration: an increased number of intracellular filaments tending to assume a perinuclear position and a decrease in the amount of organelles. In moderately advanced and advanced disease, almost all cells are in various stages of degeneration and are surrounded by pericellular halos of mature collagen fibers, often of large diameter. The nuclei are often dense, and the cytoplasm contains large whorled filaments, elongated and swollen mitochondria, lysosomelike structures, and sparse amounts of rough endoplasmic reticulum.

In summary, early osteoarthritic changes include minute surface irregularities, loss of the fine fibrillar surface covering (lamina splendens), decreased electron density of the interfiber matrix, cellular changes (notably enlargement of cells in the superficial and middle zones), and increases in the amount of Golgi apparatus and rough endoplasmic reticulum and in the number of centrioles. The number of cells displaying signs of degeneration is increased in the superficial and deep zones. As the osteoarthritic process progresses, the superficial layer infoldings deepen and extend toward the deeper zones. The collagen fibers become arranged parallel to the surface of these clefts in the superficial zone and perpendicular to the joint surface in the middle and deep zones. In these zones, the viable chondrocytes, either singly or in clones, are hypertrophied and have increased numbers of intracellular organelles having to do with synthesis. The number of degenerating chondrocytes increases with the severity of the disease, and these cells often contain large numbers of intracellular filaments and lysosomelike structures. In advanced osteoarthritis, all cells appear degenerated and there are numerous microscars.

BIOLOGIC CHARACTERISTICS OF NORMAL ARTICULAR CARTILAGE

To understand the biologic alterations of osteoarthritic articular cartilage, it is essential first to review the biologic characteristics of normal human articular cartilage. A summary of the points pertinent to this study follows.[42]

Isolation. Articular cartilage is aneural and alymphatic and, except in the developing epiphysis, has no direct contact with the vascular system. Nutrients must pass through two diffusion barriers to reach the chondrocyte. In the mature adult, all nutrients must first pass out of the synovial vascular plexus, traverse the synovial membrane to reach the synovial fluid, and pass through the dense matrix of hyaline cartilage to reach the chondrocyte. In immature animals, the basal layer may receive some nutrients by diffusion from the vascular tree of the underlying bone.[38]

The matrix is freely permeable to nutrients, but diffusion is dictated by the heavy concentrations of its constituent macromolecules, the widely dispersed polyanionic GAG, and a theoretical pore size of 6.8 nm (68 A) has been established.[32,53] In normal articular cartilage, proteins of even low molecular weight diffuse across the matrix very slowly.

Hypocellularity. The cell density of articular cartilage is low. Despite the sparse cellularity and the inert appearance of the chondrocyte, which in fixed sections appears to be small and shrunken with a pyknotic, irregularly shaped nucleus, the chondrocyte is a metabolically active cell that continually synthesizes matrix components as well as participates in the degradation catabolic process. Some matrix components demonstrate a rapid turnover.[47]

Matrix Biochemistry. Normal human articular cartilage is a hyperhydrated tissue whose water content ranges as high as 80%. The remaining constituents are organic macromolecular solids consisting of about equal parts of collagen and PG.[3] The cartilage collagen macromolecule is a triple helix consisting of three $\alpha 1$(II) chains (as contrasted with bone and skin collagen: type I, consisting of two $\alpha 1$ and one $\alpha 2$ chains). Moreover, the $\alpha 1$ $\alpha 2$(II) chains of type II collagen have a different structure than the $\alpha 1$(I) chains of type I in that there is an increased number of hydroxylysine residues and increased glycosylation of hydroxylysine.[57] There are also differences in intramolecular and intermolecular linking.

The PG consist of a series of high-molecular-weight compounds, which are separately synthesized intracellulary, and extracellularly are aggregated through a glycoprotein link about a central hyaluronate core. The smallest PG subunit has a linear protein "backbone" approximately 200 nm (2000 A) long to which are attached, at approximately right angles, 50 or more long side chains of polydimeric sugars (GAGs). At least three distinct species are identified in articular cartilage: chondroitin-6-sulfate, chondroitin-4-sulfate, and keratan sulfate.

Normally, as the animal ages, chondroitin-4-sulfate decreases in concentration to an adult level of less than 5% of the total GAG. Keratan sulfate, present in trace amounts in immature cartilage, is found in increasing concentrations with advancing age, ranging up to 50% in adult human tissue. Chondroitin-6-sulfate is the principal GAG, accounting for 45% to 75% of the sugar component of the tissue.[49] (See Chapter 7.)

Metabolic Activity. Metabolic activity of chondrocytes of normal articular cartilage is quite high.[63] Under the electron microscope, the chondrocytes from the middle zone show extensive networks of rough-surfaced endoplasmic reticulum, dilated cisternae, vacuoles, and Golgi apparatus, suggesting active synthesis of various matrix components.[83] Radioisotopic studies disclose the synthesis and intracellular assembly of components of PGs and collagen, which are then rapidly extruded into the extracellular matrix.[41,67] The process is devoted to a continuous renewal of extracellular matrix. Proteoglycan has a half-life of 8 days and collagen a much slower turnover rate.[47,60] The turnover of PGs is probably mediated through a system of lysosomal and extralysosomal enzymes.[66,84]

DNA Synthesis. Under normal conditions, cell replication can be demonstrated by uptake of tritiated thymidine, but only in immature cartilage. This occurs in two zones: near the surface, where it probably has to do with enlargement of the cartilage mass of the epiphysis during active skeletal growth, and near the basilar layer, where it represents the proliferative zone of a growth plate adjacent to the enlarging bony nucleus of the epiphysis.[39,40] With advancing age, the number of mitotic figures diminishes, at first at the superficial zone, and with maturity DNA synthesis ceases altogether. Mitotic figures are never seen in normal adult articular cartilage. Under certain circumstances (*e.g.*, cartilage laceration or osteoarthritis) the chondrocyte can resume DNA synthesis and cell division.[44,48]

OSTEOARTHRITIC ARTICULAR CARTILAGE

Metabolism. Osteoarthritic human articular cartilage has a considerable increase in synthetic activity.[2,10,46] The increased rate of $^{35}SO_4$ incorporation in osteoarthritic chondrocytes is indicative of an increased rate of synthesis of PG. The rate of synthesis of protein and GAG in osteoarthritic human cartilage is twofold as compared with normal cartilage, the rate of synthesis of PG being directly proportional to the severity of the disease process.[48] As the disease worsens, a point is reached at which the rate of PG synthesis, as measured by the rate of $^{35}SO_4$ incorporation, falls off markedly, indicating that the capacity of the cell to respond has been exceeded, and the reparative function fails.

When DNA synthesis is measured using ^{3}H-thymidine as a substrate to indicate the rate of cellular proliferation, the rate of synthesis parallels the disease severity. During the mild or moderate phases of osteoarthritis, an increased rate of uptake reflects multiple cell divisions as observed histologically as clumps or clones of cells. As the disease becomes well advanced, ^{3}H-thymidine incorporation diminishes rapidly, indicating cessation of cell replication. The reparative process, therefore, fails as the disease reaches the extreme degree.

Biochemical Alterations. The PG content of osteoarthritic cartilage is reduced, and the decrease is proportional to the severity of the disease.[46] This depletion of ground substance is demonstrated by an alteration of the intensity of staining with basic dyes and a decrease in the fixed charge density.[54] Although the total content of GAG is decreased, the individual species of these macromolecules are affected differently: keratan sulfate is relatively decreased and chondroitin-4-sulfate is increased, as compared to the normal state.[49]

The collagen content is unchanged as determined by hydroxyproline measurement.[48] However, changes do occur in the morphology, chemistry, and rate of synthesis. Osteoarthritic chondrocytes synthesize not only type II collagen $[\alpha 1(II)]_3$ chains but also substantial amounts of type I $[\alpha 1(I)_2\alpha 2]$. Therefore, the pattern of collagen synthesis produces fibers more closely resembling those of skin and bone than of normal cartilage. The collagen fibers of osteoarthritis are larger in diameter and their distribution is more variable than in normal tissue, particularly at surface zones.[81]

The water content of normal articular cartilage is approximately 72% to 78%. Osteoarthritic cartilage, on the other hand, has a significant increase in water content. Although the content of hydrophilic PGs is reduced, osteoarthritic cartilage binds freshly administered water more avidly than does normal cartilage. The reason for this phenomenon is not clear. When PG is partially removed from normal cartilage by 4M guanidium hydrochloride, this increased water-binding capacity can be reproduced.[50]

Enzymes Enzyme degradation is a major factor in the production of osteoarthritis. Theoretically, either a hyaluronidase or a protease can act on PG to initiate degradation. An acid cathepsin is present in the lysosomes of chondrocytes and has a powerful hydrolytic action on the protein core of the PPS macromolecule.[66] Since this enzyme is most effective at an acid *p*H, the possibility of another enzyme, a neutral protease, initiating the enzymatic attack at the *p*H of normal tissue would seem more reasonable. Lysosomal activity is markedly increased as reflected by the demonstration of substantial increases of acid phosphatase (a lysosomal marker).

It is apparent that the protein core is cleaved initially. Later, some as yet unidentified enzymes (*i.e.*, polysaccharidases, sulfatases, and hexosaminadases) degrade the GAGs.

Chloroquine is a strong inhibitor of cathepsin D. Cortisone and salicylates are not. Antibodies to cathepsin D can be prepared that are capable of preventing autolysis of cartilage.[85]

Physical Alterations. Biomechanical studies suggest that depletion of the GAG fraction, with subsequent disruption of collagen fibers in the superficial zone, is an early event in the disease process.[16] The creep modulus, a measure of the stiffness of a viscoelastic material, shows a close correlation with the GAG content and a low correlation with the collagen content.[28] Cartilage from visually normal areas showing degenerative changes becomes progressively less stiff (softer) with increasing severity of the disease.[29] Although the osteoarthritic process may appear to be focal in distribution, a generalized decrease in stiffness presages extension of the disease to other areas. The change in the creep modulus precedes the appearance of fibrillation. Since the creep modulus correlates with GAG concentration, it follows that depletion of these constituents precedes, and may cause, the pathologic process.

Fatigue of Cartilage. A mechanical abnormality of a joint can produce secondary osteoarthritis (osteoarthrosis). For example, a meniscectomy will increase contact pressures on the meniscectomized side of the joint, thereby increasing the chances for development of the osteoarthritic process on that side of the joint. Incongruity of the hip joint, either congenital or acquired, increases contact pressures by reducing the contact area, thereby increasing the liability to osteoarthritis.[17]

Unloaded cartilage consists of a hydraulically pressurized PG gel trapped within a collagen meshwork that is prestressed in tension. The pressure is of the order of 3½ atmospheres.[52] Thus, the compressive properties of articular cartilage are proportional to the amount of PG in the matrix, whereas the tensile properties are proportioned to the structure (as well as to the actual amount) of collagen.

The tensile properties of articular cartilage vary from surface to deep layers, and this variation is related to the collagenous composition of cartilage. In the surface layer, the tensile properties are tangential.[26]

A change can be demonstrated in the tensile strength and stiffness of articular cartilage with increasing age.[27] This change takes the form of diminishing strength and stiffness as age advances.

Cartilage in life is loaded cyclically and in compression normal to the surface. Cyclical loading raises the possibility of fatigue failure. Fatigue is the process by which a loaded structure may fail mechanically in the face of a load of the same magnitude applied on numerous occasions, whereas a load of the same magnitude applied on one occasion does not produce failure. Cartilage is prone to fatigue and the fall in fatigue resistance increases with age.[78] A cyclically applied compressive load produces fragmentation of the surface of the loaded cartilage, producing an appearance similar to fibrillation.[79]

These facts suggest that fibrillation and therefore osteoarthritis may be due to fatigue failure in the collagen meshwork of articular cartilage and explains the increased incidence with advancing age.

Although the amount of collagen of cartilage matrix does not diminish with advancing age with the onset of osteoarthritis, the mechanical integrity of the meshwork probably fails. It is entirely possible that the fibers themselves or their cross-links may break. Once the surface becomes fragmented, the meshwork that normally retains the PG is disrupted, and PG depletion may occur by simple leakage.

CLINICAL PICTURE

Despite the generalized changes in the aging process and the frequent occurrence of an advanced degree of the disease, as noted on roentgenograms in many patients, only about 5% of people past 50 years of age have clinical symptoms. The pain is caused by the inflammation in response to joint irritation, whether caused by the mechanical interference by loose bodies, subchondral fractures, cartilaginous debris engulfed by the synovium, or other factors.

SYMPTOMS

The onset is insidious. A continuous, usually mild, aching pain appears. It may be localized to one side of the joint or may be generalized about the joint. It is intensified by lowered barometric pressure, which permits greater synovial swelling. This phenomenon is popularly known as "pain with changes of weather." Stiffness occurs with rest and loosens quickly with activity. This symptom is prominent on arising in the morning. The use of heat and salicylates is almost specific for relief of pain and stiffness.

DIAGNOSIS

Findings. The noninflamed joint displays a dry creaking and grating sensation, both palpable and audible. In the advanced stages with marginal proliferation and capsular thickening, the joint is enlarged. Motion is limited. With extreme destruction, motion is markedly restricted, the joint assuming a fixed deformity corresponding to the destructive process. Complete loss of motion never occurs. When the joint is inflamed, there is an increased amount of synovial fluid, and localized tenderness over the joint interval may be noted. Muscle spasm and atrophy are rarely found. Heberden's node is a characteristic cartilaginous and bony enlargement on the dorsal aspect of the distal interphalangeal joint of a finger. It usually occurs in many fingers. It may occur spontaneously or following trauma, and it commonly develops in women at the menopause. It may be painless, or it may appear rapidly, accompanied by pain, swelling, and tenderness. The swelling may be soft and sometimes cystic, or it may be hard. The enlargement is mainly cartilaginous and therefore not visualized on roentgenograms.

Systemic Manifestations. These are usually absent.

Age. Middle or advanced

Sex. Generalized disease is more common in women and generally makes its appearance soon after the menopause; in men, single weight-bearing joints are most commonly involved.

Joints of Predilection. Terminal interphalangeal joints,lumbar vertebrae, knees, hips, lower cervical vertebrae, sacroiliacs, and elbows

Patient Type. Frequently overweight

LABORATORY FINDINGS

The sedimentation rate is normal, blood counts, blood chemistry and febrile agglutination tests are negative; and the thyroid profile reveals a hypothyroid state in 10% to 30% of patients.

Synovial fluid examination serves to differentiate degenerative joint disease from rheumatoid and infectious arthritis. When a large amount of fluid accumulates within the joint as part of an acute inflammatory response, the fluid has the gross appearance of normal synovial fluid. It is clear, pale yellow, and viscous and does not clot. The cell count rarely exceeds the normal range of 60 to 3000 and consists mainly of mononuclears. The concentration of sugar is identical with that of the blood, and the total protein does not rise above 5.5 g/dl.

In contrast, the synovial fluid from rheumatoid arthritis is thin and turbid and clots on standing. The Ropes test is positive, whereas it is negative in osteoarthritis. The cell count often rises above 3000 and consists mainly of polymorphonuclear leukocytes. Its total protein frequently is above 8 g, and the globulin concentration approaches and often exceeds that of the albumin.

When osteoarthritis is superimposed on rheumatoid arthritis, the synovial fluid accumulation may represent a reaction to either disease. Therefore, a single synovial fluid specimen may define the main offender, although when its characteristics are typical of rheumatoid arthritis, an underlying osteoarthritic process is not ruled out. On the other hand, when the synovial fluid has characteristics of osteoarthritis, the rheumatoid disease may be inactive at the time. When both conditions are suspected, repeated synovial fluid examinations are mandatory.

ROENTGENOGRAPHIC FINDINGS

Early, the x-ray appearance is normal. Then joint narrowing gradually appears, reflecting thinning of the articular cartilage covering opposing subchondral cortices. Finally, with advanced progression of the disease, the joint interval is markedly narrowed, the articular margins are sharp, osseous spurs or osteophytes appear at the margins, the subchondral bone becomes wide and sclerotic, and bone cysts appear in the subchrondral bone at areas of maximum pressure. A negative film does not rule out the disease. On the other hand, a film with typical characteristics of osteoarthritis does not necessarily define this as the primary disease. Degenerative changes are frequently superimposed on other disease, notably gout, infectious arthritis, and rheumatoid arthritis.

TREATMENT

Osteoarthritis is regarded as a benign disease when the involvement is generalized and the joints are minimally affected. In most instances, degenerative joint disease affects many joints, is slowly progressive, and is relatively nondisabling. The patient seeks help either for generalized aching and stiffness or for an acutely painful episode in a single joint. Treatment by nonsurgical measures is aimed at retarding progression, alleviating pain and stiffness, preventing deformity and improving motion and stability.

In exceptional situations in which disease is advanced within an individual joint and function is severely compromised by pain, restricted motion, deformity, and internal derangements of the joint, surgical treatment may become necessary.

CONSERVATIVE

The following discussion on the principles of nonsurgical treatment is applicable to osteoarthritis of single or multiple joints. The operative treatment is described for the individual joint in the appropriate regional section.

1. ***Rest.*** The involved joints are rested to reduce compression and shear stresses and allow the synovial inflammation to subside. Excessive joint use will aggravate symptoms and accelerate degenerative changes. During an acute inflammatory episode of an individual joint, bed rest with the joint placed in such a position so as to relax the capsule and ligamentous structures is advisable, thereby minimizing compression of the articular surfaces.

2. ***Range of Motion.*** The joint is moved through a full range of motion several times daily to prevent capsular contraction. Excessive motion carried to the extreme will impose dangerously high compression of the joint surfaces and must be avoided.

3. ***Weight Bearing.*** Abstinence from weight bearing on involved joints of the lower extremities is accomplished by using crutches or a walker.

4. ***Vertical Load Reduction.*** On weight-bearing joints this is accomplished by weight reduction and use of a cane in the hand opposite to the involved joint. Advanced disease or bilateral joint involvement requires bilateral canes, crutches, or a walker, and the patient should be instructed on proper gait.

5. ***Traction.*** Traction is used during the acute inflammatory phase, particularly of a weight-bearing joint, to separate the joint surfaces and to stretch the contracted capsule until the inflammation subsides.

6. ***Physical Therapy.*** Moist heat is followed by massage and range of motion exercises, both passive and active. Forcible attempts to regain lost motion should be avoided.

   Painful Heberden's nodes are aided by plain hot water soaks or paraffin applications.

   Isometric exercises rather than isotonic are preferred to build muscle power while minimizing joint stress.

7. ***Body Mechanics.*** Good body mechanics is aided by eliminating faulty posture, applying shoe supports, and performing graduated exercises of all joints.

8. ***Orthopaedic Appliances.*** A removable plaster splint secures rest and permits daily physical therapy. For the lower back, a simple plastic or fabric corset may suffice. A brace is a more effective form of immobilization. An ordinary elastic bandage applied around the affected joint restricts the extremes of motion while permitting a little use. For the entire lower extremity, a long ischial-bearing caliper brace reduces the weight-bearing pressures, and the addition of a leather cuff about the knee provides immobilization.

9. ***Iontophoresis.*** Ordinarily, mecholyl or histamine is used. The effect is questionable.

10. ***X-ray Therapy.*** This supposedly acts by reducing inflammation and minimizing scar-tissue formation. Although it has been recommended by some workers, relief of symptoms is inconstant, and it appears to be of little value.[30]

11. ***Corticosteroids.*** A suspension of corticosteroids, sometimes mixed with a soluble form, is injected intra-articularly, reducing pain and swelling within a few hours to a few days and improving motion.[22] No constitutional effects are noted. The steroid acts by its anti-inflammatory action, and the duration of symptomatic relief is variable, lasting from several weeks to many months. A schedule of injections given at regular intervals, guided by the duration of response, keeps the patient comfortable and able to

continue his activity but does not halt progression of the disease.

Intra-articular corticosteroids have been shown to have deleterious effects on articular cartilage, impairing synthetic activity of the chondrocyte and causing a reduction of the proteoglycan content of the matrix.[65] The effect is reversible within 2 weeks, and this suggests the minimal permissible time interval between injections.

Preparations commonly used include hydrocortisone, hydrocortisone tertiary butylacetate, triamcinolone, 6-methylprednisolone, and dexamethasone.

12. ***Warm, Dry Climate***

13. ***Graduated Exercises.*** Muscle imbalance creates abnormally high stresses concentrated on one side of the joint and greatly accelerating the degenerative process. Graded active exercises are designed to improve and balance muscle power acting about the joint.

14. ***Drug Therapy.*** Drugs are used for their analgesic and anti-inflammatory properties, but none has been successful in halting progression of the pathologic process. Salicylates are the preferred drugs. Experimentally, they have been shown to have an inhibitory effect on cartilage degradation, decreasing loss of hexosamine and hydroxyproline, but this has not been confirmed.[19]

Acetylsalicylic acid (aspirin) is both analgesic and anti-inflammatory and represents the drug of choice in osteoarthritis. To be effective, adequate therapeutic levels are required. Doses of 640 mg four times daily may be gradually increased until adequate relief is obtained. Older people are more likely to develop toxic effects and gastrointestinal distress. If tinnitus or impaired hearing occurs, aspirin should be withheld. Gastrointestinal intolerance may be obviated by using enteric-coated aspirin, aspirin-antacid combinations, salicyl-salicylic acid, magnesium salicylate, and choline salicylate.

Acetophenetidin (phenacetin) may be substituted when aspirin is not tolerated. The usual dose is 300 mg given four times a day, but long-term administration is not advisable, since interstitial nephritis may develop.

Acetaminophen is both analgesic and antipyretic and is virtually free of severe toxicity or side-effects. It may potentiate the effects of oral anticoagulants. The dosage for adults is 325 mg to 650 mg. tid; for a child 7 to 12 years of age, 162 mg to 325 mg tid, and from 3 to 6 years of age, 120 mg tid.

Propoxyphene hydrochloride (Darvon), 65 mg, and ethoheptazine citrate (Zactane), 75 mg, are given three times a day or whenever necessary for analgesia.

Pentazocine (Talwin) is given orally for severe pain in doses of 50 mg. Frequent side-effects include nausea, flushing of skin, and light-headedness.

Indomethacin (Indocin) is analgesic and anti-inflammatory.[37] It must be used with caution, especially in patients intolerant of aspirin. A total daily dose of 75 mg to 150 mg is given in divided doses with food or antacids to minimize reactions (gastrointestinal upset or bleeding, occipital headache, light-headedness).[77]

Phenylbutazone (Butazolidin) has a derivative, oxyphenbutazone (Tandearil), that is less toxic. The possible toxic effects include bone marrow depression, upper gastrointestinal tract bleeding, water retention, and dermatitis. If given on a regular basis, repeated blood counts are mandatory.[31]

Liniment application to the affected part presumably causes a "counterirritation" hyperemia and effects relief of pain. Methyl salicylate is commonly used. The effect is likely psychological.

SURGICAL

Surgical measures are aimed at relieving pain, improving and maintaining joint movement, correcting deformity and malalignment, reducing vertical loads and shear stresses, removing inra-articular causes of erosion of articular surfaces, and, in markedly advanced disease, when the proper indications exist, attempting to create a new joint with artificial implants. Arthrodesis is the only certain way of relieving pain and providing stability for function and must be considered when other more conservative forms of surgery are not feasible or have failed. Special surgical considerations are applicable to each joint and are described in the appropriate regional section.

RHEUMATOID ARTHRITIS

Rheumatoid arthritis is a chronic inflammatory systemic disease of young or middle-aged adults, characterized by destructive and proliferative changes in synovial membrane, periarticular structures, skeletal muscle, and perineural sheaths. Eventually, joints are destroyed, ankylosed, and deformed.

ETIOLOGY

The cause is unknown. However, theoretical causes include the following:

Infectious. Hemolytic and nonhemolytic types of streptococci have been isolated from joints and regional lymph nodes.

Endocrine. This is suggested by response to adrenocortical steroids.
Allergic. Rheumatoid arthritics frequently exhibit various allergic manifestations. Eosinophilia is frequent.
Metabolic

THEORY OF PATHOGENESIS

The most widely held theory of pathogenesis is that an immunologic response takes place in the synovial tissues. An unknown, presumably exogenous, antigen encounters the defender cell, the lymphocyte, which is transformed into a larger plasma cell. The plasma cell manufactures antibodies.[22] Antibodies, antigen, and complement combine to form a complex. Scavenger phagocytic cells engulf the complex. These phagocytes contain small enzyme-producing sacs (lysosomes) that destroy the complexes. However, some of the lysosomes escape from the phagocytic cells, and their proteases attack the cartilage and synovium. Destruction of tissue produces debris that calls forth more phagocytic activity to remove the debris. Consequently more phagocytic cells pour out more enzymes which create more destruction and further inflammation, and the arthritic process becomes self-perpetuating.

The inflamed synovium forms a pannus, a granulomatous mass that grows over and destroys cartilage, tendons, and ligaments.

Under the electron microscope, the lining consists of three types of synovial cells: type A cells, which are phagocytic and take up particulate matter and immune complexes from the synovial fluid; type B cells, which resemble fibroblasts and are believed to synthesize protein and hyaluronic acid, which are present in the synovial effusion; and type C, or undifferentiated, cells, which have the properties of both the A and B cells.[113]

In the deeper regions of the synovial membrane, dense nodules of lymphocytes and plasma cells appear to be engaged in the immune response. Large amounts of γ-globulin are synthesized and are deposited with complement and a presumed antigen as antigen-antibody complexes.

In response to human immunoglobulin G (IgG), autoantibodies are synthesized in rheumatoid synovial tissue.[87] These autoantibodies, known as rheumatoid factors, not only react with human IgG, but also cross-react with the IgG of a number of animal species, making it feasible to test for rheumatoid factor with systems such as sheep cells coated with rabbit IgG. Patients with higher titers of rheumatoid factor generally have poorer prognoses.[111]

A procollagenase precursor is liberated in large quantity from viable cells during phagocytosis of aggregated human γ-globulin.[114] The neutrophil is the principal source of the proenzyme, with only small amounts in lymphocytes and lymphoblasts. The proenzyme is activated by trypsin or rheumatoid synovial fluid but not by osteoarthritic fluid. In addition, various other enzymatically active proteases are phagocytically released from human leukocytes, for example, β-glucuronidase, elastase, and neutral proteases, the last-named from lysosomes. The pannus of a rheumatoid joint has the ability to produce an active collagenase and invade and degrade cartilage *in vitro*.[96] These facts imply that collagenase may be a principal factor in the pathology of rheumatoid arthritis. Moreover, it can be shown that iron influences the production of collagenase from leukocytes, thereby explaining the pathogenesis of cartilage destruction in hemochromatoses and hemophilic arthropathy.

Leukocytes have been shown to phagocytose immune complexes present in the rheumatoid joint.[123] The *in vivo* release of procollagenase during phagocytosis and its subsequent activation by the rheumatoid synovial fluid then give rise to active collagenase, which initiates the split in the collagen molecules of joint cartilage.[106] The neutral protease, which is released by the leukocyte during phagocytosis, then completes the degradation of the collagen fibrils of joint cartilage.

PATHOLOGY

The disorder is primarily a synovitis.[97] Early, hyperemia, edema, and swelling occur, lining cells proliferate until they are three or more layers thick, and the underlying tissue is infiltrated with lymphocytes and plasma cells. Villous processes gradually develop and project into the joint cavity. They may become necrotic and extruded into the joint. The typical microscopic lesion is an area of fibrinoid necrosis surrounded by fibroblasts conspicuously arranged radially to the surface of necrosis (Fig. 13-12). Beyond this is an enveloping layer of fibrous tissue. The rheumatoid units and infiltration of round cells are prominent not only in the synovium but also in periarticular structures. The leukocytes frequently are aggregated into round collections that may encircle a blood vessel. An increased amount of clear or slightly turbid fluid accumulates in the joint. The synovium at the periphery forms a pannus of granulation that grows progressively and extends over the articular surface, absorbing and replacing the articular cartilage with fibrous connective tissue. Vascular granulation tissue from the marrow extends toward the articular surface and destroys the cartilage from within the bone. The articular cortex becomes thin and deficient so that fibrous pannus forms the main covering of the bone. The granulation tissue extends toward the opposite articular surface, merging with the pannus there, bridging the joint with granulation tissue. A fibrous ankylosis results. The fibrous tissue may undergo metaplasia into bone. Within the articulating bones, the trabeculae become lessened in number and thinned. The hematopoietic tissue is replaced

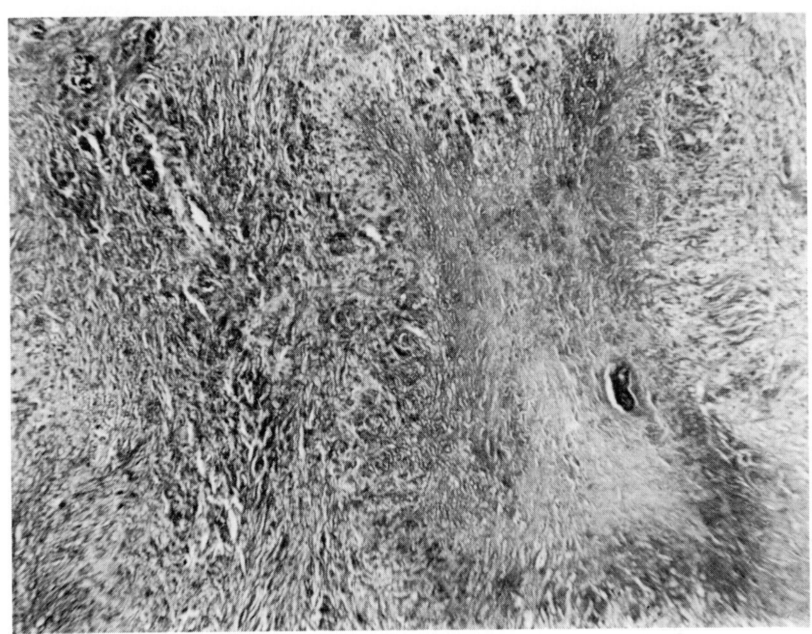

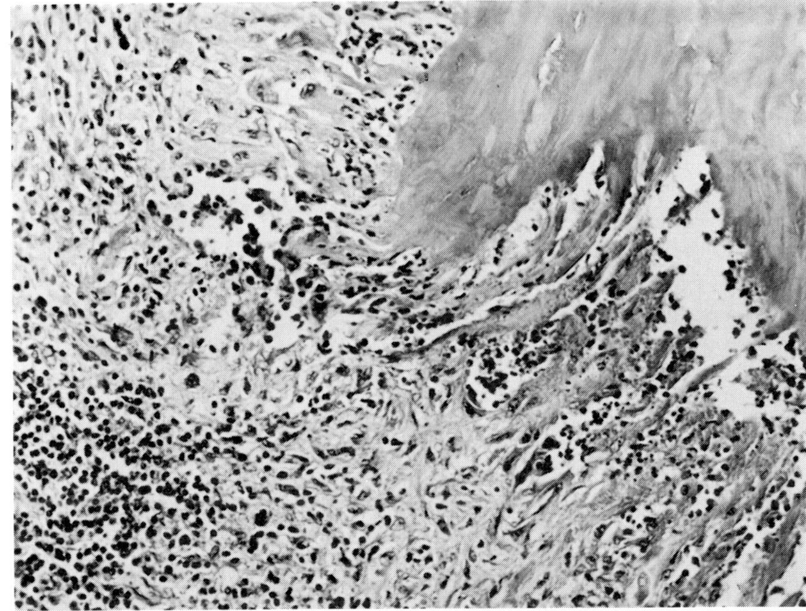

FIG. 13-12. Rheumatoid arthritis. (*Top*) Microscopic appearance showing the area of fibrinoid necrosis surrounded by fibroblasts arranged radially to the surface of necrosis. Round cell aggregations are not prominent in this section. (*Bottom*) High-powered microscopic appearance at the edge of a nodule removed from the olecranon area. Note the radially disposed fibroblasts at the edge of the fibrinoid material and infiltration of round cells.

by a fibrofatty marrow. Fibrous proliferation thickens the capsule.

Muscle Changes. Muscle changes are widely distributed in skeletal muscles; the condition is known as nodular polymyositis. The individual muscle fibers undergo localized or diffuse degenerative changes characterized by increase in size and number of sarcolemmic nuclei, loss of striations, hydropic swelling of fibers, and localized collections of lymphocytes. Similar lesions are formed in the collagen diseases. The degenerated muscle is replaced by fibrous tissue. Loss of muscle elasticity and contractile power is partly responsible for restricted joint motion.

Subcutaneous Nodules. Subcutaneous nodules are composed of the typical basic rheumatoid unit consisting of a central necrotic zone, a surrounding layer of large mononuclear cells radially arranged (palisade formation), and an outer zone of dense connective tissue with marked round-cell infiltration. They are found in 20% of patients, particularly over such pressure points as the elbow or over the subcutaneous surface of long bones, such as over the tibia.

Peripheral Circulation. The arterioles respond poorly to changes of temperature; therefore, the capillaries are empty or blood flow is sluggish. As a result, the distal extremities appear cold and cyanotic.

Lymph Nodes. Lymph nodes exhibit follicular hyperplasia, increased reticuloendothelial activity, proliferation of connective tissue, and lymphocytic invasion of the capsule.

Nerves. In the perineural connective tissue are found areas of focal necrosis, epithelioid reaction, and leukocytic infiltration.

Heart. Rarely, cardiac changes identical with those of rheumatic fever are found.

CLINICAL PICTURE

The onset is insidious, usually before 40 years of age (Table 13-1). Females predominate. Constitutional symptoms consist of weakness, fatigue, and sweating, but no fever. Rarely, the onset may be acute and febrile. Gradually, a number of joints exhibit stiffness and aching; later, there is swelling, pain, warmth, tenderness, and limited motion. Characteristically, the hands, particularly the proximal joints of the fingers, are involved. In the palm of the hand, the lumbrical muscles are palpable as tender swellings that pull the proximal phalanges into flexion. Next in frequency of occurrence are the feet, the knees, and the wrists. Involvement is generally multiple and symmetrical. The swelling of the joint consists not only of increased synovial effusion but also of inflammatory edema of the periarticular structures, so the swelling is maximal about the joint and gradually tapers off at a distance. The overlying skin is stretched, shiny, and thin. A typical fusiform appearance results. The joints assume a semiflexed position, and movement in any direction is painful. The surrounding muscles are in spasm. Direction of deformity of the extremities is favored by posture, but certain typical positions are assumed. The arm is in adduction and internal rotation, the elbow in flexion, the forearm in pronation, the wrist flexed, and the hand deviated ulnarward; fingers are flexed and deviated ulnarward at the metacarpophalangeal joints, and there is extension at the middle interphalangeal

TABLE 13-1 Clinical Differentiation in Rheumatoid Arthritis

	Rheumatoid Arthritis	Osteoarthritis
Geographic distribution	Most common in temperate climates; rare in tropics	Climate not a factor
Family history	Often history of rheumatic fever or rheumatoid arthritis in a member of immediate family	Frequently, history of a similar form of arthritis in one or both parents
Past history	Occasionally, history of rheumatic fever; frequently, history of tonsillitis or sinusitis	Not characteristic; sometimes history of trauma or faulty body mechanics
Age at onset	Any age; over 80% between 20 and 50	Rare before 40 years
Mode of onset	Rarely acute; usually subacute or insidious; often accompanied by migratory pains	Insidious; not accompanied by migratory pains
General condition	Usually undernourished, anemic, and "chronically" ill; frequently slight fever (+99°F) and slight leukocytosis	Well nourished, frequently obese; not anemic; no fever, no leukocytosis
Involvement of joints	Symmetrical and generalized; proximal interphalangeal joints especially involved	Usually weight-bearing joints, spine, hips, knees; distal joints of fingers (Heberden's nodes)
Appearance of joints	Early: periarticular swelling, fusiform fingers Late: ankylosis, extreme deformity, ulnar deflection	Early: slight articular enlargement Late: more pronounced articular enlargement; limitation of motion usually slight; never ankylosis; Heberden's nodes
Muscular atrophy	Often pronounced, particularly in later stages	Not characteristic
Cutaneous changes	Extremities frequently cold and clammy; skin atrophic and glossy; redness of thenar and hypothenar eminences Psoriasis occasionally present	No characteristic features
Subcutaneous nodules	Present in 15% to 20% of patients	Not present

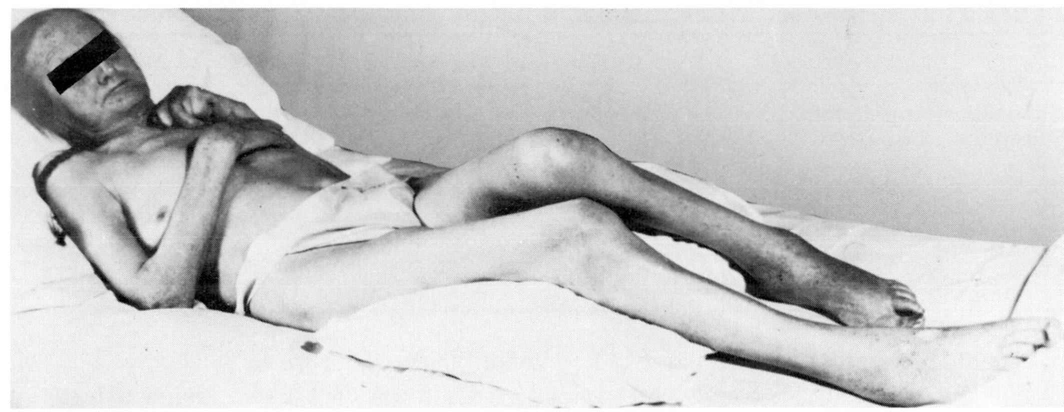

FIG. 13-13. Rheumatoid arthritic derelict, with a severely advanced stage of rheumatoid arthritis.

joints. The hip is flexed and adducted, the knee is flexed, the foot is in equinus, varus, and cavus, and the toes are clawed. With persistence of the disease, these deformities become fixed (Fig. 13-13). Sweating, coldness, and cyanosis of hands and feet are common. Subcutaneous nodules may be found over bony pressure points or may be palpable within muscles (Fig. 13-14). The spleen and the lymph nodes may be palpably enlarged.

The course is one of remissions and exacerbations. Remissions occur, characteristically, during pregnancy and jaundice. With each exacerbation, restriction of joint motion becomes progressively worse, a fixed flexion-adduction deformity develops, and muscles that function about the affected joint become atrophic.

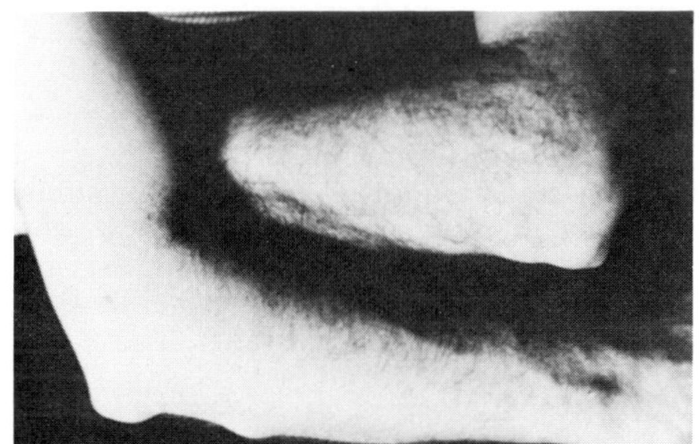

FIG. 13-14. Subcutaneous rheumatoid nodules.

DIAGNOSIS

ROENTGENOGRAPHIC FINDINGS

Early, the joint structures appear to be normal. Then gradually the articulating bones become osteoporotic and, as the disease progresses and articular cartilage is destroyed, the joint interval is narrowed (Table 13-2). The articular cortex becomes thinned and almost indistinct. Finally, bony trabeculations bridge and obliterate the joint space. If the disease stops short of severe destruction, supervening degenerative changes occur, consisting of increased density and irregularity of the articular surfaces and marginal spurring.

LABORATORY FINDINGS

The erythrocyte sedimentation rate (ESR) is elevated, particularly during the active stage. During the periods of remission, the rate continues to increase but to a lesser degree. A hypochromic normocytic anemia is frequently associated. The white cell count is normal.

SEROLOGIC TESTS

Serum from patients with rheumatoid arthritis contains a substance of unknown composition, the rheumatoid factor, which, in the presence of γ globulin, is capable of agglutinating certain strains of streptococci, sensitized sheep cells, and latex particles.[95,118,122] This forms the basis for agglutination tests which are positive in a high percentage of rheumatoid arthritics. The rheumatoid factor may also be present in small amounts in sera of patients with Marie-Strümpell spondylitis and certain collagen diseases and in an occasional normal person.

A convenient laboratory procedure uses a standard suspension of latex particles in a solution of γ-globulin.

1. *Latex fixation test on serum:* unknown serum + γ-globulin-latex suspension

   Agglutination is likely when the unknown serum contains an abundance of the rheumatoid factor. If no agglutination occurs, the unknown serum contains an inadequate concentration of rheumatoid factor, and a second more sensitive test must be performed.
2. *The inhibition test:* rheumatoid serum of known high

TABLE 13-2 Laboratory Differentiation in Rheumatoid Arthritis

	Rheumatoid Arthritis	Osteoarthritis
Agglutination reactions	Positive in over 50% of typical cases	Never definitely positive
Sedimentation rate	Usually greatly increased; tends to return to normal as patient improves	Normal or only slightly increased
Roentgenographic appearances	Early: osteoporosis, periarticular swelling, and joint effusion Late: narrowing of joint space, bone destruction, ankylosis, and deformities	Early: no osteoporosis; slight lipping at joint margins Late: marked lipping, osteophytes, narrowing of joint space, deformation of articular bone ends

agglutinating activity + unknown euglobulin + standard γ-globulin-latex suspension

This test uses the characteristics of euglobulin from the unknown serum. Euglobulin from normal serum neutralizes the rheumatoid factor, thereby inhibiting agglutination. Euglobulin of rheumatoid serum has no effect on the rheumatoid factor and agglutination proceeds unhindered.

The inhibition test is considered to be the most sensitive. It is likely to be positive (agglutination occurs) even when the rheumatoid factor is present in minute amounts. When an unknown serum displays a negative latex fixation test and a positive inhibition test, the arthritis in question may be part of a rheumatoid spondylitis or a lupus erythematosus. The latter disease is of grave import and may be identified by inspecting LE cell preparations.

DETERMINATION OF DISEASE ACTIVITY

Generalized activity may be measured by the sedimentation rate. The rate during exacerbations increases to as high as 100 mm/hour and lessens to as low as 30 mm to 40 mm. It becomes normal only after the disease "burns out." The sedimentation rate as an index is crude, inasmuch as it may be elevated in other conditions, including infection and carcinoma.

Localized activity within a single joint is determined by injection of iodized oil into the joint and by taking arthrograms. In an acutely inflamed joint the oil is absorbed rapidly and passes to the regional lymph nodes in which it is visualized within a few hours to several days. When inflammation is absent and vascularity is reduced, the oil remains unabsorbed for a month or more. It is advisable to perform surgery during periods of minimal activity.[102]

DIFFERENTIAL DIAGNOSIS

The main diseases to be differentiated are the following:

Rheumatic fever. As a rule, large joints are involved. After subsidence of arthritis, the joints return to normal. It is associated with fever, leukocytosis, tonsillitis, and cardiac, pulmonary, and kidney inflammatory lesions. Relatively young people are afflicted. It responds to salicylates. The antistreptolysin-O titer is elevated (after infection with group A hemolytic streptococci).

Osteoarthritis. The older age-group is predisposed. Distal interphalangeal and large weight-bearing joints are chiefly affected, and there are Heberden's nodes—a firm, fibrous nodule about the distal interphalangeal joints. Spurring is seen, but there are no bony ankylosis and no systemic symptoms. The ESR is not elevated.

*Criteria for Diagnosis of Rheumatoid Arthritis**

1. Morning stiffness
2. Pain on motion or tenderness in at least one joint
3. Swelling (soft tissue thickening or fluid; not bony outgrowth alone) in at least one joint continuously for not less than 6 weeks
4. Swelling of at least one other joint
5. Symmetrical joint swelling
6. Subcutaneous nodules
7. X-ray changes typical of rheumatoid arthritis
8. Positive latex fixation test
9. Poor mucin clot
10. Characteristic histologic changes in synovial membrane
11. Characteristic histologic changes in nodules

Classic: Any seven criteria for at least 6 weeks
Definite: Any five criteria for at least 6 weeks
Probable: Any three criteria for at least 4 weeks

* American Rheumatism Foundation.

TREATMENT

Rheumatoid arthritis is an inflammatory disease destructive to joints. Involvement of one joint leads to secondary changes detrimental to other joints in the extremity.

Therefore, the aim of treatment is to keep the inflammatory process at a minimum, thereby preserving joint motion, maintaining health of muscles supplying motor power about the joint, and preventing secondary joint stiffness and deformity. In addition, constitutional defects must be corrected, notably the secondary anemia. The possible deformities must be anticipated and prevented by appropriate splinting. Finally, surgical measures correct the deformities, eliminate pain, and provide stability. A plan of treatment should be outlined and followed through.

CONSERVATIVE

Conservative treatment is outlined below.[104]

Rest. The patient is kept at complete bedrest.

Removal of Foci. Teeth, tonsils, sinuses, and pelvic organs are investigated, and infections are eliminated.

Nutritious Diet. A diet high in calories and high in vitamins is essential.

Transfusions and Hematinics. Transfusions and hematinics are continually necessary during the entire course of the disease.

Hormones. Combinations of estrogen and androgen are administered for their anabolic effect on bone structure.

Dilute Hydrochloric Acid. Dilute hydrochloric acid is necessary to combat the achlorhydria that contributes to the anemia.

Splinting. The inflamed joint is firmly immobilized in a plaster splint. This relieves pain and reduces inflammation quickly.

The position of function is desirable in the event that ankylosis ensues. Several times daily the cast is removed, hot packs are applied, or the patient is placed in a Hubbard tank at 33.7°C to 38.9°C (92.6°F–102°F), and the joints are put through a full range of motion to help maintain joint mobility. While immobilized, muscle-setting exercises combat muscle weakness and atrophy. After removal of the splint, resistance exercises are prescribed to restore joint stability before allowing weight bearing. Recent experience has shown that this treatment reduces the incidence of ankylosis.[93,94]

If weight bearing is permitted on an unstable joint, the instability causes recurrent effusion, muscle wasting, and further instability, a vicious circle.

Positions of Rest for Inflamed Joints. The proper positions are the following:

Shoulder—scapulohumeral angle 45°; forward flexion 45°
Elbow—70° flexion, 15° supination of forearm
Wrist—30° dorsiflexion, support to arches of hand
Fingers—45° flexion
Spine—full extension, good posture
Jaw—open at least 1 inch
Hip—flexion 5°, abduction 5°, neutral rotation
Knee—flexion 5°
Ankle—at right angle, no valgus or varus of foot

Cortisone. In 1935, Kendall, at the Mayo Clinic, isolated compound E (17-hydroxy-11-dehydrocorticosterone) from the adrenal cortex. In 1949, Hench and co-workers discovered the therapeutic effect of compound E, or cortisone. Later, he noted the effect of pituitary adrenocorticotropic hormone (ACTH), which stimulates the adrenal cortex to secrete a cortisonelike substance, probably compound F (17-hydroxycorticosterone). The circumstances leading to the discovery were the observations that there was a remission of rheumatoid arthritis during pregnancy and jaundice and that the adrenal cortex underwent hypertrophy and hyperfunction in pregnancy. Compounds E and F produce a dramatic reduction of inflammation and remission in rheumatoid arthritis. The acute inflammatory swelling of the joints is reduced, and mobility is restored. Unfortunately, cessation of treatment is usually followed by relapse, and continued treatment may cause complications. Cortisone is useful in controlling the disease. It has no curative effect. Its benefit is to reduce inflammation, prevent further destruction, maintain mobility, and avoid muscle atrophy and secondary effects to neighboring joints. One hopes to maintain the integrity of the joints and to prevent deformity until the disease has run its course. The commonly accepted duration is 3 to 5 years.

Effect on Histopathologic Lesions. The synovial membrane tends to revert to normal. The lymphocytes and the plasma cells disappear, vascularity is decreased, and edema subsides. The subcutaneous nodules become smaller and less inflammatory. The central necrotic zone becomes poorly defined, the palisade layer disappears, the outer zone of fibrous tissue becomes more dense, and round cells are sparse. In muscle, the nodules disappear and degenerative changes are less noticeable.[112]

Method of Administration. The use of cortisone is limited by its adverse side-effects. One must weigh carefully the disadvantages against the advantages to be gained by treatment with this compound. Many synthetic steroids have been developed in an effort to reduce the incidence of side-effects, but the compounds vary in their mineralocorticoid and glucocorticoid activity, and the same compound may differ in its potency and side-effects in different patients. Therefore, treatment is preferably initiated in a hospital where the effects can be studied by laboratory procedures and the appropriate drug selected. An adverse effect calls for reduction of dosage of the drug or discontinuance entirely. When a generalized effect is desired, for example, when an acute widespread polyarthritic state exists, the drug is given orally in amounts sufficient to overcome the acute symptoms and then is gradually reduced to the least possible maintenance dose. It is desirable to limit each course of treatment to a period of a few months with rest periods of several weeks between courses. When discontinuing treatment, the drug should be withdrawn gradually to avoid the acute manifestations of the hypoadrenal state. Discontinuance of the hormone frequently is followed by severe exacerbation of the disease. It is during this period of relative adrenocortical insufficiency that the patient is vulnerable to the stress of surgery, trauma, and infection. Therefore, while corticosteroids are being withdrawn in small decrements, ACTH should be administered to overcome atrophy of the adrenal cortex.

When the acute inflammatory process is limited to a few joints, particularly when these are accessible, intrasynovial injection of steroids (esterified prednisolone) will control symptoms without the problem of systemic side-effects.

Systemic Effects. Typical systemic effects are the following:

1. Depresses pituitary ACTH secretion
2. Causes adrenal cortical atrophy (reversible); decreased excretion of 17-ketosteroids
3. Depresses adrenal cortical secretion
4. Inhibits Koch phenomenon
5. Reduces antibody phenomenon
6. Diabetogenic: increases glucogenesis, hyperglycemia, glycosuria, insulin resistance, liver glycogen; increases insulin requirement in diabetics
7. Catabolic: nitrogen-containing tissue destruction shown by negative nitrogen balance; delays development of new bone; bony trabeculae become thinned and general architecture becomes weakened, making bones susceptible to trauma; frequent compression fractures of spine (Fig. 13-15)
8. Results in electrolyte balance effect: serum potassium level falls, cardiac arrhythmias result; sodium retention occurs early, followed later by increased excretion; early edema causes gain in weight, possible hypertension; hypochloremic, hypokalemic alkalosis develops
9. Involutes lymphatic tissue
10. Delays development of granulation tissue
11. Reduces circulating eosinophils
12. Results in Cushing's syndrome features: cutaneous striae, moon facies
13. Produces acute psychosis: euphoria, stimulation, insomnia
14. Increases appetite

Before treatment one must determine the presence of tuberculosis and diabetes, both of which may flare up under the influence of cortisone. Other contraindications are chronic nephritis, acute psychosis, and peptic ulcer. During treatment, a low-sodium diet is prescribed. Increased blood pressure and weight and pitting edema are danger signals indicating sodium retention. Blood sugar, sodium and potassium, and blood counts are checked at intervals. The ESR may be done several times a year to record activity of the disease. After treatment with cortisone, one must exercise caution regarding surgical procedures. The adrenal cortex may be atrophied and unable to respond to the stress of surgery. Sufficient doses should be prescribed, both preoperatively and postoperatively.

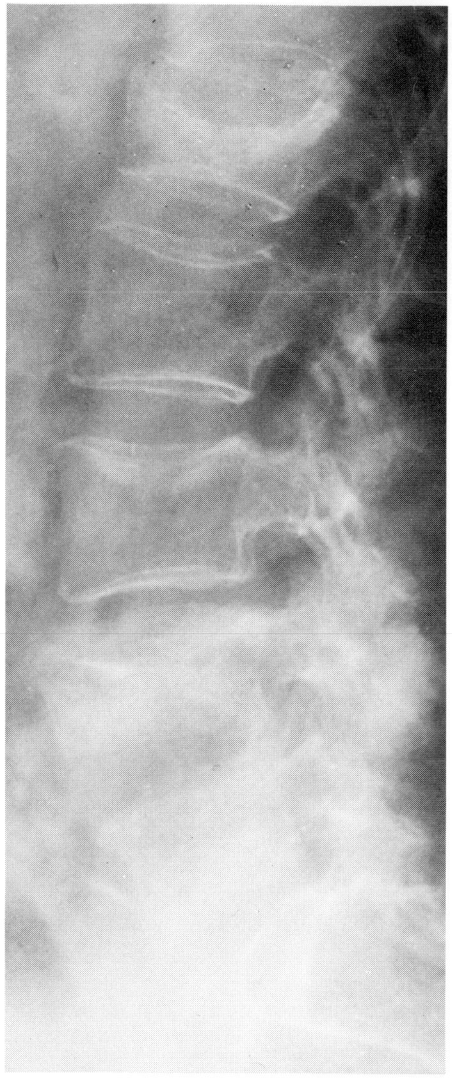

FIG. 13-15. Pathologic fractures of the first and fourth lumbar vertebrae in the course of cortisone therapy. Note that these are not wedge-shaped compressions. The fractures have occurred centrally from expansile force of the disks, a pertinent point establishing this as a pathologic fracture. Until fracture occurs, the vertebral bodies of the rheumatoid spine, in spite of being osteoporotic, tend to retain their size and configuration.

Synthetic Steroids. The main advantage of synthesized compounds is the reduced tendency for salt and water retention, hypertension, and potassium loss, whereas the other hormonal side-effects are similar to, and in some cases greater than, those of the parent steroid cortisone (Fig. 13-15). A number of different compounds should be used before the proper one is selected to suit the individual patient.

Prednisone. Prednisone is derived from cortisone by introduction of a double bond between carbons 1 and 2; it is about four times as potent as cortisone. Although it tends to cause less salt retention, the development of cutaneous ecchymoses and peptic ulceration seems to occur more readily. It is administered orally.

Prednisolone. Prednisolone is derived from hydrocortisone and is about four times more potent. Its salt-retaining property is reduced, and it is administered orally, parenterally, intrasynovially, and topically. The tertiary butyl acetate ester of prednisolone is used for injection into a joint or into soft tissue, because absorption from these sites is insignificant. Therefore, the local anti-inflammatory effect is more pronounced and sustained, whereas the systemic effect is almost nil.

Triamcinolone. The addition of a fluorine atom to prednisolone at the 9a-carbon position multiplies the potency of the parent compound but markedly increases its salt-retaining effect. The latter effect is negated by the addition of a hydroxyl radical at the 16a-carbon position. It has a number of unique side-effects, such as anorexia, weight loss, tissue wasting, muscle weakness, and leg cramps, which may be used to advantage in patients who have excessive appetite and weight gain while on other steroids.

Dexamethasone. The salt-retaining effect of fluorination at the 9a-carbon position is negated by addition of a methyl group at the 16a-carbon position. The potency is more than 25 times greater than that of hydrocortisone. The drug may be administered by any route—orally, parenterally, intrasynovially, topically, or injected directly into soft tissue.

Adrenocorticotropic Hormone (ACTH). The hormone from the pituitary stimulates the adrenal cortex to produce more compound E and F, the effects of the latter being reproduced. The adrenal cortex is hypertrophied, and there is an increase of urinary 17-ketosteroids. The hormone is effective only by parenteral administration. It is prepared in a gelatin menstruum, which retards its absorption from the site of injection and prolongs its action. It is injected in daily doses of 100 mg. The usual precautions are taken.

Salicylates. Salicylates are anti-inflammatory, analgesic, and antipyretic compounds that are the drugs of choice for rheumatoid arthritis. Salicylates have an action comparable to corticotropin or corticosteroids when given in large doses. It has been shown experimentally that salicylates work through the pituitary as the mediator, as proved by the loss of their effect after hypophysectomy. These effects include eosinopenia, inhibition of inflammatory phenomena and tissue sensitivity (immune reaction), depression of γ-globulin and antibody production, retention of sodium chloride and water, loss of potassium and nitrogen, decreased glucose tolerance, increased excretion of uric acid, and increased 17-ketosteroids in the urine; there is also the depletion of adrenal cholesterol and ascorbic acid and even occasional production of Cushing's syndrome.[116]

Acetylsalicylic acid (aspirin, ASA) is the most effective nonsteroidal, anti-inflammatory drug used. It has been shown to decrease the synthesis of prostaglandins and lipoperoxidase, but the relationship of these actions to its anti-inflammatory properties is unclear. After oral administration, acetylsalicylic acid is rapidly absorbed and quickly hydrolyzed to free salicylate by nonspecific esterases.This metabolic process can intensify, and the blood salicylate level may suddenly rise out of proportion to the dose. Consequently, the administration of large doses requires constant monitoring of blood salicylate levels to prevent toxicity. The excretion of unchanged acetylsalicylic acid can be promoted by alkalinization of the urine.

Adverse dose-related effects of acetylsalicylic acid include the early development of tinnitus and decreased hearing, which presage serious toxic effects; such complaints demand immediately discontinuing the drug. Acetylsalicylic acid decreases platelet adhesiveness by preventing release of adenosine diphosphate (ADP). This poses a serious problem in patients with potential bleeding sites (*e.g.*, peptic ulcer, hiatus hernia, or those on anticoagulants). At high doses, acetylsalicylic acid interferes with prothrombin production or function, thus potentiating the effects of anticoagulants. Various gastrointestinal symptoms are generally dose-related direct irritation, although peptic ulceration and serious gastric hemorrhage may occur even at low dosage in susceptible people. To reduce gastric irritation, buffered preparations are often used, although excessive buffer (*e.g.*, $NaHCO_3$) may lead to systemic and urinary alkalosis and increased excretion of the drug. Various allergic reactions and central nervous system symptoms are not uncommon, and excessive diaphoresis is a frequent complaint. The various salicylate salts (*e.g.*, those of choline, sodium, calcium, and magnesium) rarely have these side-effects, but they are not as efficacious.

Aspirin is prescribed in doses that maintain a blood salicylate level of 25 mg to 30 mg/dl. About 10 to 15 300-mg tablets are given daily in four divided doses with meals. The average daily requirement for an adult is three tablets with each of three meals and four or five tablets with a bedtime snack. Sustained-release tablets provide longer relief and may be given at bedtime. Choline magnesium trisalicylate (Trilisate) causes less gastrointestinal irritation, and other nonsteroidal anti-inflammatory drugs cause still less, but these are not as effective as anti-inflammatory agents.

Constant monitoring of blood salicylate levels is mandatory to prevent salicylism. The normal therapeutic blood salicylate level is 20 mg to 30 mg/dl. In children under 10 years of age, levels of 35 mg to 40 mg/dl are permissible. In the adult, toxic levels are reached when blood levels exceed 30 mg/dl, and over the age of 60, these levels should not be permitted to rise above 20 mg/dl. The earliest symptoms of toxicity, tinnitus or reduced hearing, are reversible when the drug is discontinued.

Nonsteroidal Anti-Inflammatory (NSAI) Drugs. Aspirin is the main therapeutic agent, but it often produces undesirable side-effects and can prove ineffective altogether. Various nonsteroidal substitute drugs have been developed that are comparable in effectiveness to aspirin without major side-effects. Many of these compounds are propionic acid derivatives, and some are chemically related to indomethacin. Their actual mode of action is unknown. The pituitary-adrenal axis is unnecessary for their activity. They are known to interfere with the synthesis of prostaglandins, but the effect of this on the disease is unclear. Because prostaglandins are essential to uterine contractility, NSAI drugs are contraindicated in pregnancy.

Propionic acid derivatives have a strong affinity for albumin and may displace other drugs from their albumin-binding sites. Consequently, when NSAI drugs are given to patients receiving hydantoins, sulfonamides, sulfonylureas, or coumarins, these patients should be closely watched for signs of drug overactivity. Many NSAI agents prolong bleeding times by reducing either platelet aggregation or platelet adhesiveness; patients receiving anticoagulants or who are afflicted with a bleeding disorder should be constantly monitored.

Gastrointestinal complaints are common, although milder and less frequent than with aspirin or indomethacin or phenylbutazone. Although gastric ulceration due to nonaspirin NSAI agents is rare, it is known to occur, especially in patients with a history of peptic ulcer and hiatus hernia. Such patients should be monitored for gastrointestinal bleeding.

Cross-sensitivity between NSAI agents is frequent, and the administration of a new agent to a patient who has already demonstrated allergic reactions (*e.g.*, to aspirin) is contraindicated.

Many other less common side-effects can occur with prolonged use of nonsteroidal anti-inflammatory drugs, the most serious of which include fluid retention, impairment of liver function, and adverse effects on renal function. Consequently, the prolonged administration of these agents is best carried out by those proficient in their use.

These aspirin substitutes, because of their high cost, are regarded as a second line of defense against rheumatoid arthritis. Furthermore, they do not alter the course of the disease.

The following drugs are the most common agents currently used.

Sulindac. Sulindac (Clinoril) is an NSAI indene derivative whose mechanism of action is unknown. A dose of 400 mg/day is comparable in action to 3600 mg to 4800 mg/day of aspirin, but with considerably lower incidence of side-effects. It is used mainly for rheumatoid arthritis and may be used in conjunction with gold salts. It may supplant corticosteroids, and the latter may be withdrawn slowly over several months. It may be used for ankylosing spondylitis and has been regarded as effective as indomethacin.

Precautions. Sulindac is an inhibitor of platelet function. It may induce abnormalities of liver function. It is eliminated mainly by the kidneys and should be used cautiously when renal function is impaired. Because it causes fluid retention, it should be administered cautiously when cardiac function is impaired and in hypertension. Concomitant administration of aspirin will decrease plasma levels of its active plasma metabolites.

Dosage. The dose is 150 mg to 200 mg twice a day.

Naproxen. Naproxen (Naprosyn) is an NSAI agent whose properties are similar to those of other NSAI drugs. Its anti-inflammatory, analgesic, and antipyretic effects are not superior to those of aspirin, but its gastrointestinal tolerance is greater and other side-effects are milder. It is principally used in mild or moderate cases of rheumatoid arthritis that are intolerant of, or fail to respond to, a therapeutic serum salicylate level. Because the potential for cross-sensitivity exists, naproxen should not be administered to patients in whom aspirin or other NSAI agents induce allergic reactions. It prevents synthesis of prostaglandin, which is essential for uterine contraction, and therefore cannot be given during pregnancy. Because it displaces other drugs from their albumin-binding sites, caution must be exercised in patients receiving coumarin, warfarin, or a hydantoin, sulfonamide, or sulfonylurea. It decreases platelet aggregation and prolongs bleeding time. The drug is eliminated mainly by glomerular filtration and therefore should be used with proper monitoring when renal insufficiency exists.

Dosage. The long half-life (13 hours) permits administration twice a day. The usual adult dose is 250 mg to 500 mg orally twice a day, in the morning and at bedtime. The benefits do not become apparent before approximately 1 week, and relief is experienced in about 35% of patients. The drug may be used in conjunction with gold or antimalarials and sometimes with low-dose corticosteroids.

Tolmetin. Tolmetin (Tolectin), like indomethacin, is an indoleacetic acid derivative. Unlike indomethacin, its metabolism is not dependent on a hepatic enzyme system, and it has a shorter half-life, is metabolized and excreted rapidly, and is therefore less toxic. In young children in whom the liver enzyme system is not yet fully developed, indomethacin metabolism is faulty and this agent consequently is highly toxic. Therefore, in juvenile rheumatoid arthritis, tolmetin is preferred when indomethacin is considered as an NSAI drug. Symptoms of central nervous system involvement, particularly headache, or gastrointestinal disturbance is far less common with tolmetin than with indomethacin. Tolmetin is comparable to aspirin in efficacy. In the adult, when aspirin cannot be used because of poor response or intolerance to therapeutic serum salicylate levels, and indomethacin provides a good response, tolmetin should be substituted. Tolmetin will prolong bleeding time by decreasing platelet adhesiveness, but it has little effect on platelet aggregation and therefore does not alter prothrombin time when administered with warfarin.

Dosage. The starting adult daily dosage is 1200 mg in divided doses, usually two 200-mg tablets three times a day.

Ibuprofen. Ibuprofen (Motrin), an NSAI agent, is a propionic acid derivative with analgesic and antipyretic properties. It is administered orally, is rapidly absorbed, has a half-life in serum of 2 hours, and is completely eliminated in the urine within 24 hours. Its effect is comparable to aspirin, phenylbutazone, and indomethacin, but it has milder side-effects and a much lower incidence of peptic ulceration and gastrointestinal bleeding. It may be used in conjunction with gold salts or corticosteroids. Because, like other NSAI agents, it is subject to cross-sensitivities, it should not be used in patients who have exhibited allergic reactions to another NSAI drug, including aspirin. In patients with peptic ulcer, hiatus hernia, colitis, and active rheumatoid arthritis, nonulcerogenic drugs (*e.g.*, gold salts) are preferred. Ibuprofen interferes with platelet aggregation and may significantly prolong prothrombin times. It should be used with caution in patients on anticoagulant therapy. Like other NSAI drugs, particularly propionic acid compounds, it has a strong affinity for albumin and may displace other drugs from their albumin-binding sites. Therefore, it should be used with caution in patients receiving hydantoins, sulfonylureas, sulfonamides, or coumarins, and these patients should be closely watched for signs of drug overactivity. Ibuprofen inhibits prostaglandin synthesis and should be avoided during late pregnancy.

Dosage. Food interferes with absorption. The drug, in 300-mg, 400-mg, or 600-mg doses, is given three or four times a day at least half an hour before or 2 to 3 hours after meals. High doses (*e.g.*, up to 3200 mg/day) may be required, and yet the drug may prove to be ineffective. If a clinical response is not apparent within 2 weeks, other NSAI agents should be tried. The agent is effective in only 35% of patients with mild to moderate cases of rheumatoid arthritis.

Piroxicam. Piroxicam (Feldene) is the newest NSAI drug that has a long half-life (mean approximately 5 days) and therefore can be administered once a day. Its main side-effect is gastrointestinal irritation, and it is contraindicated in the presence of peptic ulcer, hiatus hernia, and colitis. Like other NSAI agents, its effect is presumably derived as a result of inhibition of the biosynthesis of prostaglandins; therefore, it should not be administered during the latter stages of pregnancy. It is strongly bound to albumin and may displace other protein-bound drugs, such as coumarins and hydantoin. It should not be given when other NSAI drugs have demonstrated allergenicity.

Dosage. The dose is 20 mg orally daily. The effect may become apparent after approximately 2 weeks.

Indomethacin. Indomethacin (Indocin) is a nonsteroidal indole derivative possessing excellent anti-inflammatory, antipyretic, and analgesic properties; however, its usefulness is limited because of potential serious side-effects. Its mode of action, like that of other anti-inflammatory drugs, is not known. Its therapeutic action is not due to pituitary adrenal stimulation. It is a potent inhibitor of prostaglandin synthesis, but whether this is related to its anti-inflammatory effect is unkown. Indomethacin will reduce the inflammation, swelling, and symptoms of rheumatoid arthritis. After oral administration, it is readily absorbed and quickly attains peak plasma levels. It is eliminated by the kidney and, after liver enzymatic processes, through the biliary tract. Consequently, impaired liver function and renal insufficiency may lead to excessive plasma levels and drug toxicity. In rheumatoid arthritis, the drug is mainly effective for short-term use during acute flare-ups of the chronic disease.

Precautions. Gastrointestinal side-effects are common, and dyspeptic symptoms such as nausea and heartburn should be regarded with alarm because they may be forerunners of such serious problems as ulceration, perforation, and hemorrhage, particularly in the presence of preexisting lesions (*e.g.*, diverticulosis, ulcerative colitis). Both patient and physician must be alerted for adverse symptoms, and the stool should be examined repeatedly for blood. The gastrointestinal effects can be reduced by giving the drug immediately after meals, with food, or with antacids.

Indomethacin is contraindicated in children in whom the hepatic enzyme system is incompletely developed.

Serious visual disturbances due to corneal deposits and retinal disease may develop with prolonged therapy. Because these may occur without symptoms, ophthalmologic examinations at intervals are mandatory.

Common central nervous system symptoms are headache and light-headedness. Platelet aggregation is inhibited, and bleeding times may be prolonged. The drug should be administered with caution to patients with bleeding disorders or those on anticoagulants. Indomethacin is contraindicated in patients who have demonstrated an allergic reaction to aspirin or other NSAI drugs. Because it inhibits prostaglandin synthesis, it is contraindicated during pregnancy.

Dosage. For the acute attack in the moderate to severe type of rheumatoid arthritis, indomethacin is given in 25-mg doses four times a day for several days. For long-term therapy, 25 mg/day can be increased by increments of 25 mg each week to maximal doses of 100 mg to 150 mg/day in divided doses with meals or antacids. Doses above these levels are more likely to produce adverse effects. When the drug is prescribed, appropriate warnings should be given to the patient. The stool is examined repeatedly for blood, blood counts are taken at intervals, and, especially in the long-term therapeutic schedule, repeated ophthalmologic examinations are mandatory.

Because of potential serious side-effects, I do not recommend the use of this drug.

Phenylbutazone. Phenylbutazone (*Butazolidin, Butazolidin Alka*) is a pyrazole compound with excellent anti-inflammatory properties; its usefulness is limited by potentially serious toxic reactions. It can induce gastrointestinal ulceration, perforation, and hemorrhage, and it can suppress the bone marrow, producing aplastic anemia, leukopenia, and thrombocytopenia. Both of these reactions can develop suddenly and without warning symptoms and sometimes can prove fatal. Severe water retention, edema, and serious skin rashes may occur at times. Administration of phenylbutazone requires monitoring by repeated blood counts, examining the stool for blood, and noting the following forewarning symptoms: fever, sore throat, mouth lesions (symptoms of blood dyscrasia), dyspepsia, epigastric pain, progressive anemia, black or tarry stools (symptoms of bleeding gastrointestinal ulceration), skin rashes, weight gain, or edema. The drug is contraindicated in patients with peptic ulcer, hiatus hernia, colitis, unusual bleeding tendency, poor cardiac function, and allergic asthma; in children; during pregnancy or anticoagulant therapy; and in the elderly in whom there is an exceedingly high risk of severe and sometimes fatal reaction.

Phenylbutazone is rarely used in rheumatoid arthritis and is restricted to an acute episode when conventional treatment fails.

Dosage. After a 1-week trial period and no response, the drug should be abandoned. The initial daily dose in an adult is 300 mg to 600 mg/day in divided doses. If the response is adequate, the dose should be reduced to the minimum effective dose, usually less than 400 mg daily. To minimize gastrointestinal irritation, the drug should be taken with milk or meals, or Butazolidin Alka may be used. I do not recommend the use of this drug.

Gold Therapy. Gold salts when used judiciously have a prolonged beneficial effect.[99] In contrast, prolonged benefit from ACTH and cortisone is unusual. The mechanism of action of gold is unknown; its use is empirical. However, experimental use of the radioisotope of gold reveals selective uptake in synovia and other articular tissues, as well as liver, kidney, and spleen.[88] However, in rheumatoid arthritis, the affinity for the synovial tissues is strong. It may also work by altering the immune response because of its affinity for reticuloendothelial tissue.[103] During treatment 75% is retained in the tissues, while 25% is excreted. The amount in the body increases during treatment, and excretion continues for many months after discontinuing treatment. Remission occurs only while gold is in the body and is being excreted. Gold is of value only during the acute stage. The best available preparation at present is gold sodium thiomalate (Myochrysine).

Procedure (with Myochrysine). Injections are given deeply intramuscularly. The first injection is 10 mg; 1 week later, 25 mg; and the third week, 50 mg. The 50-mg dose is repeated weekly over 4 to 5 months until a total of 1 g has been given. A favorable response is indicated by clinical improvement and reduction of the ESR. With each dose, 10 ml of 10% calcium gluconate is given to lessen possibility of reaction. Another course of treatment is given after 6 to 12 months or after a recurrence. If no improvement occurs after 5 months, it is useless to continue. Change of symptoms should be expected between 6 and 15 weeks. Recurrence can occur from 6 months to 5 years.

Toxic Reactions. Eternal vigilance is mandatory to prevent serious toxic reactions. Before each injection the skin is examined for a rash or purpuric spots. Pruritus is a complaint before appearance of the rash. The mouth is examined for stomatitis. The patient is questioned for gastrointestinal symptoms, especially diarrhea. The urine is checked for albumin or microscopic hematuria. A slight amount of albuminuria is permissible. Hematologic reactions include granulocytopenia, thrombocytopenia, and aplastic anemia. These are rare but serious. They are less likely with the small dosage schedule herewith recommended. Every 2 weeks a complete blood count and platelet count is done. The reduction of hemoglobin, leukocytes, and platelets and the tendency to eosinophilia are danger signals, and all treatment must be suspended. If improvement does not occur promptly after discontinuance of treatment, British Anti-Lewisite (BAL) is administered without delay. From 2 mg to 3 mg/kg body weight of 10% BAL (dimercaprol) is injected deeply intramuscularly—six times the first day, four times the second and the third day, then three times daily for 4 days. Parenteral steroids are effective.

Contraindications. Contraindications include hepatic or renal damage and blood dyscrasias.

Combined Cortisone and Gold Therapy. Combined cortisone and gold treatment seemingly would be advantageous, but the percentage of patients improved is only a little greater than when gold is employed alone. The excellent therapeutic response may continue for a long time after the cortisone has been discontinued.[120]

Manipulation. Passive manipulations or wedging casts to overcome contractures are not advisable. It is impossible to estimate the extent of intra-articular adhesions. These adhesions may be torn only to be replaced by more extensive scarring.

The fibrotic inelastic muscles may be damaged. Fracture of the osteoporotic bones is a definite risk. When the articular involvement is considered minimal, gentle prolonged traction or, as in the deformities of the hand, dynamic splinting is permissible. Otherwise, gradual spontaneous correction by active motion is most desirable and the result more lasting. Deformities that are persistent should be treated surgically.

X-ray Treatment. X-ray therapy is used occasionally for relieving pain and low-grade inflammation, particularly when cortisone, ACTH, and gold salts have been ineffective. Its greatest field of usefulness is in rheumatoid arthritis of the spine.

Relief of Muscle Spasm. Hot, wet packs are most beneficial for muscle spasm. Muscle relaxants such as myanesin (Tolserol) and carisoprodol (Soma) are of doubtful value. Small doses of diazepam (Valium) are valuable.

Aspiration. Removal of joint fluid is indicated when effusion is recurrent and causes pain by distention.

Hydrocortisone Injections. When only one or two large joints are involved, compound F injected intra-articularly is effective in rapidly reducing the inflammation and eliminating pain. The local effect is prolonged, and constitutional effects are avoided. A dose of 1 ml of the suspension is injected, and the patient usually experiences some increased discomfort for about a day. Thereafter, improvement is dramatic. The injection is repeated at weekly intervals, then reduced in frequency until the maintenance dose and length of remission are determined.

Intra-Articular Irradiation. Radioactive colloidal gold may be injected into a joint where the β-ray surface irradiation may be used.[109] Since these rays penetrate to a depth of only 1 mm to 2 mm, their radiation effect is mainly against the synovial lining. The procedure has been limited to the knee joint, which is at a distance from vital structures that may be sensitive to radiation. A dose of 10 mc of colloidal gold ^{198}Au is injected into the joint with care to ensure that no radioactive fluid is spilled onto the skin. A reactive increase of effusion develops within the first week and disappears within a few weeks. In most cases the relief of pain and effusion appears to be lasting.

Special Drugs. In patients with progressive rheumatoid arthritis who do not respond to therapy with salicylates or NSAI drugs, stronger and potentially more toxic agents may be considered. The administration of these highly effective but toxic drugs demands an expertise of clinicians and pharmacologists well versed in their use. The following are the most common agents in current use.

Antimalarial Compounds. Chloroquine has been shown to improve rheumatoid arthritis, but, because of potential oculotoxicity, has been supplanted by hydroxychloroquine (Plaquenil) in smaller, safer doses.[89] After treatment is begun, improvement is first seen after an interval of 6 to 12 weeks. The dose of hydroxychloroquine is 2 mg to 4 mg/kg/day, and partial or complete remission can be maintained for years, often on a gradually reduced dosage. Opthalmologic monitoring is necessary to detect corneal deposits or retinopathy. Ocular toxicity is more likely to develop in the elderly but does not necessarily result in impaired vision. After cessation of therapy, arthritis usually recurs within 3 months.

Immunosuppressive Agents. The immunologic abnormalities found in rheumatoid arthritis are that rheumatoid factor is an IgM globulin directed against IgG, IgG–anti-IgG complexes may represent an immune-complex phenomenon, there are cytotoxic lymphocytes, and thymus-derived and bone marrow–derived lymphocytes (T and B cells) are seen in rheumatoid arthritis synovial fluid. These form the rationale for the use of immunosuppressants.[110] The potential susceptibility to infection does not seem to affect rheumatoid arthritis patients.

Azathioprine. Azathioprine (Imuran) is a potent drug used to prevent rejection in renal homotransplantation. It is an imidazolyl derivative of mercaptopurine. It produces decreased antibody response and reduced IgG and IgM synthesis and has an anti-inflammatory action. Its main toxic effect is bone marrow depression. It is effective at doses as low as 1 mg/kg/day. The dose must be reduced when the drug is given concomitantly with allopurinol (Zyloprim) and in the presence of renal insufficiency. It is as effective as gold; it is not as effective as cyclophosphamide, although it is less toxic.

Penicillamine. Penicillamine is a potent, potentially toxic compound whose chemical structure closely resembles the amino acid cysteine and yet is part of the molecular structure of penicillin. It is a lathyritic drug, that is, it interferes with the formation of cross-links between tropocollagen molecules and it cleaves those that are newly formed. Originally used as a chelating agent to remove copper in Wilson's disease and to reduce excess cysteine excretion in cystinuria, it has been found to have a beneficial effect on rheumatoid arthritis comparable to that of gold.

The D-isomer is used because it is less toxic. It can dissociate the rheumatoid factor, an IgM macroglobulin, which might explain its effect on rheumatoid arthritis, but the actual mode of action is unknown.[100,101,108] Its basic toxic effects include marrow suppression (thrombocytopenia, leukopenia), renal toxicity, and foul taste. Fatalities have been reported.

To prevent toxicity, the least effective therapeutic dose is used and renal function and marrow activity are monitored. The drug is administered on an empty stomach, at least 1 hour apart from any other drug, food, or milk. This permits maximum absorption and reduces the likelihood of metal binding. Low oral doses, 250 mg/day, are continued for 30 days. If no adverse effects appear, the dose is gradually increased to 500 mg/day for 30 more days. Usually at this dose after 2 to 3 months of therapy, a therapeutic effect should be noticed. Then the dose is increased and continued at 750 mg/day.[92]

D-Penicillamine therapy is reserved for acute active rheumatoid arthritis unresponsive to conventional forms of treatment and gold therapy. If this drug can be tolerated, it can be used in conjunction with corticosteroids and salicylates and may be continued for years. It should not be undertaken without considering, and taking measures to prevent, the risks.

Cyclophosphamide. Cyclophosphamide (Cytoxan) is a bivalent substituted nitrogen mustard, one of a class of drugs, the alkylating agents, whose mode of action is due to their reaction with cellular DNA. Cyclophosphamide is the most potent alkylating agent known, and it is a powerful immunosuppressive drug, acting on various immune mechanisms, particularly antibody production.[98] The agent is effective at high doses of about 150 mg/day.[91] Severe toxic effects include bone marrow suppression, particularly a leukopenia, which should not be allowed to fall below 3000 to 4000. Other serious problems include chronic cystitis, impairment of ovarian and testicular function, alopecia, and infection. The use of this highly toxic agent should be limited to severe progressive rheumatoid arthritis that is unresponsive to other more conservative means and to second-level drugs (gold, hydroxychloroquine, penicillamine). Azathioprine should be tried first because it is less toxic.

Protozoacides. Because protozoalike structures have been isolated from rheumatoid tissues, protozoacides have been used.[115,121]

Clotrimazole. Clotrimazole can effect dramatic disappearance of active rheumatoid arthritis. It has been shown to induce adrenal hyperplasia. The dose is 10 mg to 12 mg/day, and improvement begins within 24 hours, with reduction of pain, swelling, and stiffness and improvement of joint mobility. Active disease disappears in 3 to 28 days, and after 6 weeks the blood count and ESR become normal. Rheumatoid arthritis factors and autoantibodies disappear from the blood. Occasionally, Herxheimer's reaction occurs: transient increase of joint pain, swelling, heat, and pyrexia, with eosinophilia. This is typical of many parasitic diseases treated with drugs that destroy the causative organisms.

Copper Sulfate. Copper sulfate, 25 mg in 5 ml distilled water three times a day is administered with conjugated bile salts (*e.g.*, dehydrocholin), three to six 250-mg tablets three times a day. The medication should be taken after meals, washed down with milk or orange juice, and continued for 5 to 6 months to prevent recurrences. Loose stools are reduced by administration of Kaopectate or Lomotil. With this combination of drugs, the therapeutic effect takes place more slowly than with clotrimazole, usually after about 3 to 6 weeks.

Other. Less active but also effective protozoacides are chloroquine phosphate, iodoquinol (Diodoquin), and levamisole.

SURGICAL

Treatment by surgery should not be delayed too long.[86,105,119] Smith-Petersen showed that a primarily involved joint, if left deformed and mechanically deficient, will cause secondary changes in other joints, and severe, fixed deformities will ensue. Delay until the disease is "burnt out" increases the difficulty. The muscles become fibrous, ligaments and capsules become masses of scar tissue, and secondary joints undergo degenerative changes. However, one may avoid surgery during a period of activity when constitutional effects are at their height. The period of decline of the ESR is strategic.

Cortisone administered over time induces atrophy and hypofunction of the adrenal cortex. Such a patient is highly susceptible to the shock of surgical trauma. Preoperative preparation demands discontinuing cortisone and giving, instead, daily large doses of ACTH for several weeks until the adrenal cortex has been restored. Transfusions and liver-iron preparations are given to combat anemia. Intraoperatively, corticosteroids are administered intravenously.

Operations in Early Disease. When acute inflammatory disease of a joint is protracted and unresponsive to medical management and conservative orthopaedic measures, surgical synovectomy will temporarily halt the effusions and remove the destructive pannus. The disease process is delayed for an indeterminate period of time. In addition, the following surgical procedures should be considered.

Shoulder. Excision of the anteroinferior portion of the acromion (acromioplasty) and the coracoacromial ligament will free the tendinous cuff from impingement and allows excision of the thick villous subacromial bursa and the intra-articular synovium and its extensions (Neer). At the same time, section of the subscapularis tendon may be added to facilitate overcoming the adduction contracture by postoperative physical therapy.

Elbow. The radial head is excised. Spasm of the biceps, a prominent feature of the early stages, draws the head upward against the capitellum, damages the joint surfaces, and causes pain and further muscle spasm. Synovectomy is done at the same time. The procedure relieves pain quickly and permits free motion.

Knee. Synovectomy is done for recurrent effusion with synovial thickening. If the articular cartilage is eroded extensively, synovectomy alone is useless and may result in an unsound fibrous ankylosis.

Tenotomies and posterior capsulotomy (Wilson) may be performed.

Intermediate and Late Operations.

Elbow. The arthroplasty excision should be thorough to prevent reankylosis. Early considerable instability is counteracted later by periarticular fibrosis. Motion is good but not stable enough for crutch walking.

Arthrodesis may be performed. When fixed in the functional position, a painless strong limb is provided for heavy activity.

Wrist. Radiocarpal fusion in the "grasp position" is accomplished. The wrist is fixed in 10° to 15° of dorsiflexion. If flexion deformities of the fingers due to fibrotic flexors and intrinsics are present, dorsiflexion at the wrist will increase the degree of flexion, making it more difficult to open the hand. Therefore, surgical correction of the hand should logically follow. Wrist fusion should be carried out early, before deformity is extreme and before there is gross destruction at the metacarpophalangeal and the interphalangeal joints.

Resection of the lower end of the ulna corrects limited supination and pronation due to rheumatoid involvement of the distal radioulnar joint.

Hand. Degenerative changes in the joints make fingers easy prey to deforming contractions of muscles acting about the joints.[90] Contracture of these muscles, particularly the intrinsics, results in muscle imbalance between the long extensors, the long flexors, and the intrinsics. (A similar mechanism occurs in ischemic contracture local in the hand, collagen diseases, and various types of arthritis.) Intrinsic contracture flexes the metacarpophalangeal joints and extends at the interphalangeal joints. If the proximal interphalangeal joint is hyperextended, the distal joint is flexed. Contracture of the adductor muscles draws the thumb into the palm toward the third metacarpal. This is the "intrinsic plus" position. The collateral ligaments at the metacarpophalangeal joints are so degenerate that the proximal phalanges are subluxated far anteriorly and fixed there by ligament and muscle contracture. The fingers deviate ulnarward at the metacarpophalangeal joints as the long extensors are displaced into the interknuckle grooves. The thumb is overflexed by the short flexors at the metacarpophalangeal joint, the long extensors hyperextending the distal joint.

Occasionally, the long extensors predominate. The fingers are hyperextended at the metacarpophalangeal joints, flexed at the middle joints, and extended at the distal joints.

In the early stage of muscle irritation and spasm, a reverse knuckle-bender splint and a spring cock-up splint will apply mild elastic traction counteracting deformity.

For a fuller discussion of rheumatoid arthritis of the hand, see Chapter 25.

After the process has become quiescent, surgical intervention may be undertaken. The surgical attack is aimed at removing the diseased tissues (synovectomies), relieving pain, improving function by increasing motion (implant arthroplasty, capsulotomy), providing stability (arthrodesis), restoring muscle balance (tendon transfer), and correcting deformity. A few examples of many possible procedures follow:

- Tenotomy of lateral bands, which allows metacarpophalangeal joints to extend and the distal two joints to flex
- Shortening of metacarpals, which releases tension on all muscles. A segment of bone is removed at the base and fixed temporarily with Kirschner wires. (This procedure is done only when metacarpophalangeal joints can be extended passively.)
- When the metacarpophalangeal joints are destroyed, implant arthroplasties will restore motion, relieve pain, and correct deformity (Swanson). The same procedure may be applicable for severe rheumatoid disease at the proximal interphalangeal joints and at the basal joint of the thumb (trapeziometacarpal joint).
- Shortening of the thumb metacarpal at the base. Fibrotic adductors may be removed and the cleft kept open by pins and subsequent pedicle graft. If adduction is lost, a tendon-T operation is done. Tendon transference may be necessary to restore opposition.
- Radial displacement of extensor tendons to overcome ulnar drift. The luxated tendons are elevated and transferred to the radial side of the knuckle, where they are sutured into a slit in the dorsal aponeurosis.
- Tendon transfer, in which the extensor indicis proprius and extensor digiti quinti proprius are transferred to the lateral band on the radial side of the index and the little fingers, respectively

Hip. The hip is generally involved at a late stage of severe generalized disease. Multiple joint involvement of both lower extremities is the rule, and flexion contractures of hips and knees are common. Some type of arthroplasty or pseudarthrosis is indicated. The objectives are relief of pain, provision of increased motion, and maintenance of stability. It is a basic principle to restore a satisfactory level of function in the distal joints before hip joint reconstruction is attempted.

Total Hip Replacement. Complete prosthetic replacement using both acetabular and femoral components is the ideal procedure. However, certain pathologic features pose considerable surgical obstacles (*e.g.*, severe osteoporosis, thinning of the inner acetabular wall, protrusio acetabuli, and a thin, narrow, fragile femur). The procedure is generally reserved for the adult at middle age and beyond, preferably before the advanced destructive stage of the disease. (See Chapter 27.)

For the young rheumatoid arthritic, mold arthroplasty should be considered, because, in the event of failure, other surgical alternatives are not compromised.

Arthroplasty of Smith-Petersen (1939). A Vitallium (65% cobalt, 30% chromium, 5% molybdenum) mold is interposed, the articular surfaces become lined with smooth glistening fibrocartilage, and the underlying bone becomes more firm. Reankylosis is less likely than when other interposing material, such as fascia lata, is used. Recurrence of stiffness and deformity is greater in rheumatoid arthritis than in degenerative, but some useful motion is gained, permitting ambulation with canes and sitting on a high chair. Rarely, the femoral head and neck within the cup may undergo resorption, subluxation, or dislocation.

The technical principles for arthroplasty are the following:

1. Enlarge the acetabulum, consistent with stability of mold and neck.
2. Excise the entire capsule and diseased synovial tissue.
3. Replace the blood lost, which is considerable.
4. Coagulate raw bone surfaces after reshaping to prevent new bone formation.
5. Adapt modifications to rheumatoid arthritis to gain more mobility in spite of marked fibrosis.
   a. Whitman reconstruction: remove head, reshape neck, displace greater trochanter downward before interposing cup
   b. Colonna: remove head and neck, reshape trochanter, which forms new articulating surface,

detach and reattach trochanteric muscles at lower level

Arthrodesis. Bilateral arthrodesis is not advisable. However, with one freely movable hip joint, the other can be fused, providing stability and freedom from pain.
Pseudarthrosis. The procedures of Girdlestone and Batchelor restore movement and correct deformity. Instability is unlikely or minimal because of surrounding soft tissue fibrosis.
Knee. As a major weight-bearing joint, severe degenerative changes and flexion, valgus, and varus deformities can develop rapidly and become extremely disabling. Early recognition of failure of conservative treatment and aggressive surgical intervention are essential.
Synovectomy. Removal of the synovial membrane before radiologic signs of destruction develop may prevent or delay progression of the disease, and it offers an early opportunity for preserving motion. Most of the membrane can be removed through an anterior approach, and, in the absence of extensive involvement of the posterior compartment, the posterior membrane may be ignored.
Osteotomy. Supracondylar osteotomy is indicated for severe flexion contracture. For varus and valgus deformity, selection of either the upper tibia or the lower femur for a corrective osteotomy will depend on the site of major bone involvement.
Arthroplasty. For advanced destructive disease, particularly when both knees are affected, an attempt should be made to preserve motion in at least one knee by an implant arthroplasty. Prerequisites for this procedure are failure of all treatment short of arthrodesis, bone structure adequate for support of an implant, and intact medial collateral and posterior cruciate ligaments. The patient must be willing to accept an arthrodesis in the event of failure.
Arthrodesis. Fusion of the knee joint will provide a stable, painless joint for good function. When severe rheumatoid destruction is bilateral, at least one knee should be arthrodesed and the other knee should undergo arthroplasty. An essential prerequisite for arthrodesis of the knee is satisfactory function of the ipsilateral hip. The latter situation may be attained by a total hip replacement operation.
Capsulotomies and Tenotomies. These procedures are notably ineffective.
Ankle. Equinus deformity is corrected by lengthening of the Achilles tendon and posterior capsulotomy and, if joint involvement is severe, by arthrodesis.
Foot and Toes. The typical deformity of the foot is a rigid cavus deformity, clawing of the outer four toes, usually subluxated or even dislocated dorsally at the metatarsophalangeal joints and flexed at the proximal interphalangeal joints. In the large toe, destruction of the metatarsophalangeal joint causes severe pain and markedly restricted motion, a pronounced disability for walking. The metatarsal heads are all prominent with overlying painful calluses on the plantar aspect. The rheumatoid disease may also involve the tarsal area and hind foot.

The customary multiple joint involvement requires a number of surgical procedures preferably done at one sitting, and, if necessary, both feet should be corrected by two surgical teams.

If possible, the forward weight-bearing points, the heads of the first and fifth metatarsals, should be preserved, and the head and neck of the second, third, and fourth metatarsals are removed. In extreme deformity, the first and fifth are included. Then the distal flexion contracture of the second to fifth toes is corrected manually. A threaded Kirschner wire is inserted into each toe starting at the base and emerging at the tip while the toe is held straight; then the toe is aligned with the corresponding metatarsal as the wire is passed retrograde into the metatarsal.

For hallux rigidus and valgus deformity, the proximal half of the proximal phalanx is removed (Keller procedure). This effectively relieves pain and corrects the deformity but weakens push-off. A Silastic implant arthroplasty may be performed.

For cavus deformity, distal tarsal resection combined with a triple arthrodesis will effectively correct the deformity while controlling pain due to disease throughout the tarsus.
Spine. Osteotomy corrects the forward stooped deformity at the level of L2 or L3. A V-shaped excision of bone is performed across the line of the articular processes, from interlaminar space to the intervertebral foraminae. Then the deformity is corrected by hyperextension. This is followed by spine fusion and plaster immobilization. (See Marie-Stümpell disease, in Chapter 30).

Miscellaneous procedures include lumbar sympathectomy, which is done in the vasospastic types.[28] It improves peripheral circulation and relieves pain.

JUVENILE RHEUMATOID ARTHRITIS

CLINICAL PICTURE

Rheumatoid arthritis in children (Still's disease, JRA) is a generalized multisystemic disease that can result in severe sequelae, such as crippling joint deformities, heart disease, amyloidosis, and permanent blindness.[128,146] This disease is characterized by certain features that distinguish it from the adult disease: high fever, a characteristic rash, lymphadenopathy, splenomegaly, often involvement of one or a few joints, alterations in the rate of growth of adjacent epiphyseal plates, at times a striking leukocytosis, rarity of rheumatoid nodules, absence of rheumatoid factor in most cases, and chronic iridocyclitis, a major cause of childhood blindness. Any one or more of these characteristics can exist in any combination, producing a variable clinical picture. Further, the arthritis is highly variable as to intensity and extent of involvement. Consequently, the disease varies considerably as to onset, course, manifestations, and prognosis.[140]

The incidence of JRA is about 6 to 8 per 100,000 per year.[15] It is more common in females, in the approximate ratio of 7:3, and can begin at any age from early infancy to puberty, the average being 6 years of age. It starts most commonly between 1 and 4 years of age and as puberty approaches, between 9 and 14 years of age.

DIAGNOSIS

Early diagnosis is essential to preventing serious sequelae. In only 50% of cases, the polyarticular involvement resembling the adult form is unmistakable. In other cases, the arthritic phenomena are misleadingly mild and limited to one or a few joints, while other systemic features are prominent, suggesting other childhood diseases. Therefore, the clinical syndromes should be carefully studied.

PATHOLOGY

The basic pathologic process is similar to that in the adult but is modified by the thick cartilage and by the adjacent epiphyseal growth plates.[127] Because of the thicker cartilage, the subchondral bone is affected late. The disease influences the epiphyseal plate so that longitudinal growth may be accelerated or retarded, or premature epiphyseal closure can occur. The result may be limb-length disparity or shortened stature. Ossification of the epiphysis is delayed.

The arthritis may be mild, moderate, or severe. It may affect one, several, or many joints. When only cartilage degradation has taken place, regeneration and complete recovery are possible. The pannus on both sides of the joint may join to form a fibrous ankylosis, which may later ossify.

In the hand, wrist, and foot, the disease can be compared to the adult disease. Involvement of the hand is more likely when the onset is after 10 years of age.[145] Usually cervical symptoms precede involvement of the hand. Other characteristic sites are the following:

Temporomandibular Joints

This results in inability to open the mouth.

Mandible

Retarded growth of the mandible causes mandibular recession.

Cricoarytenoid Joints

Cervical Spine

This may occur early, prior to involvement of the peripheral joints. The apophyseal joints narrow and become ankylosed, particularly at the upper levels. The ankylosing process is limited to the cervical region, whereas true ankylosing spondylitis involves the entire spine. Atlantoaxial subluxation can occur.

Hip

Ossification of the epiphysis is delayed. A fibrous flexion adduction contracture and ankylosis may develop and, rarely, bony ankylosis. The acetabulum is poorly developed, small and shallow. The femoral head is underdeveloped and small, and the femoral shaft is narrow. With passage of time, protrusio acetabuli results.

Knee

This is the most common site in the monoarticular form of the disease. A flexion contracture and ankylosis and posterior subluxation of the tibia can develop. A tendency to valgus deformity is due to overgrowth of the medial femoral condyle.

Ankle

The subtalar joint is frequently affected. Structures beneath the peroneal retinaculum are often involved by rheumatoid tenosynovitis.

Low Back

The sacroiliac joints are eroded but never develop bony fusion (contrary to Marie-Strümpell disease).

Thoracic and Lumbar Spine

Although the thoracic and lumbar spine are rarely affected, approximately 15% of patients will develop a scoliotic curve of variable degree. The incidence is greater in severe protracted cases toward the end of the growth period and at the terminal stages of the disease.[144]

POLYARTICULAR JRA

Clinical Picture

Polyarticular JRA comprises half of all cases. The disease begins with simultaneous, symmetrical involvement of four or more joints, usually affecting the hands, wrists, feet, ankles, and knees. (Fig. 13-16). The joints are warm and swollen, pain is low-grade, and motion is restricted. Occasionally the joints may be reddened and tender. Swellings of the fingers are typically fusiform. When pain is minimal and the patient is too young to complain, one can observe a protective attitude (*e.g.*, maintaining a flexed position of the joints, limping, or wincing on passive motion).

The condition may be initiated as an acute tenosynovitis that precedes the development of arthritis. Occasionally, arthritis and tenosynovitis develop concurrently.[137,139]

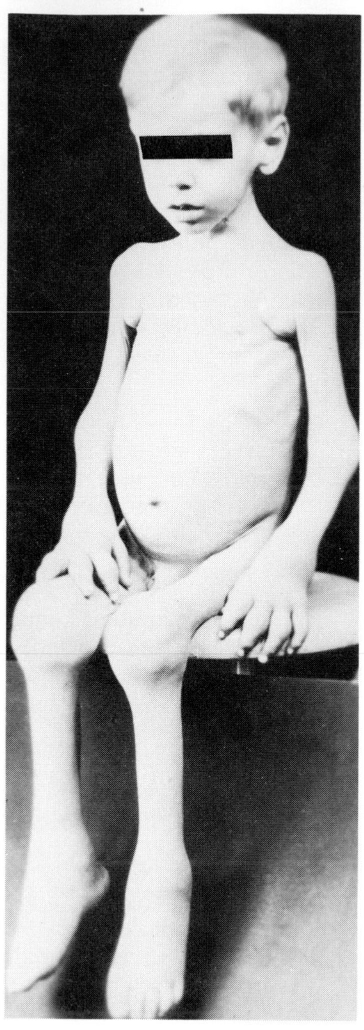

FIG. 13-16. Still's disease, or rheumatoid arthritis, in a child.

Involvement of the cervical apophyseal joints causes limitation of motion of the cervical spine, and typically the head is held projecting stiffly forward. This finding is similar to that seen in ankylosing spondylitis, but the lumbar and dorsal spine are uninvolved, and chest expansion is normal.

When the subtalar joint is involved, the heel is inverted, subtalar motion is limited and painful, peroneal spasm can occur, and a toeing-in gait is observed. A thick, boggy swelling beneath the peroneal retinaculum represents tenosynovial disease.

Retarded vertebral growth results in a shortened trunk. Lack of mandibular development results in a receding chin deformity. Premature epiphyseal closure can produce limb inequality or shortening.

System manifestations include a child who appears ill, is anorectic, and loses weight. Fever is low-grade, usually less than 102° F or 39° C. It is usually the quotidian type of fever with daily peaks, typical of JRA, and occasionally a double quotidian fever with two peaks daily. A maculopapular evanescent rash, generalized lymphadenopathy, and splenomegaly are common. Subcutaneous nodules are rare.

Laboratory Findings

Typical findings include elevated white cell counts (rarely above 20,000; occasionally, count is normal or leukopenic), an elevated ESR, an often positive C-reactive protein test, and rheumatoid factor found in only 10% of children under 12 years of age (higher at later age).

Roentgenographic Findings

At an early stage, there are only nonspecific findings, including articular soft tissue swelling, regional osteoporosis, and perhaps delayed appearance of the ossification centers. In more advanced disease, the relatively characteristic findings are the following:[142]

1. Destruction of joint cartilage revealed as narrowing of the joint interval
2. Destruction of bone revealed as ragged erosion of the adjacent ossification centers or metaphysis. Destruction of both joint cartilage and bone is a late roentgenographic manifestation, particularly in monoarticular arthritis and in the very young child.
3. Bandlike zone of metaphyseal rarefaction, identical to that seen in childhood leukemia, always in proximity to active arthritis. However, contrary to leukemia, these are rarely seen after 2 years of age. In the cervical vertebral bodies, the translucent bands parallel the superior and inferior margins.
4. Periosteal bone apposition, an early finding, particularly common in phalanges, metacarpals, and metatarsals, adjacent to affected joints
5. Flattening of epiphyseal ossification centers, especially of weight-bearing joints and of small joints of hands and feet
6. Typical erosions and "cupping" of ossification centers of proximal phalanges
7. Subluxation of joint, especially of hip and knee
8. Protrusio acetabuli, in long-standing hip disease
9. Bony ankylosis
10. Growth disturbances. Accelerated epiphyseal maturation with overgrowth is common and at the knee results in a ballooned-out appearance of the epiphysis. Retardation of growth can also occur. The abnormal influences acting on the epiphyseal growth plate result in increased or decreased bone length. The small bones of the hands and feet are often foreshortened as a result of premature epiphyseal fusion.
11. Short mandible
12. Temporomandibular joint findings, including shallow fossa, poorly differentiated condyle, limited excursion; best seen in tomograms
13. Cervical apophyseal joints, including erosions, joint

space narrowing, eventual fusion (especially in upper portion of cervical spine), subluxation of atlantoaxial joint

Differential Diagnosis

Polyarthritis is a component of a broad spectrum of diseases. When the composite picture is presented of typical arthritic and systemic manifestations accompanied by confirmatory laboratory findings, the diagnosis is self-evident. The problems of diagnosis arise when the early manifestations are vague and resemble other conditions.[125]

Juvenile Rheumatoid Arthritis. There must be polyarthritis (two or more joints involved) or monoarticular arthritis lasting longer than 3 months. Swelling must be present or two of the following; heat, pain and tenderness, and limitation of motion.

Polyarthritis must be present more than 6 weeks, with one of following:

Rash of JRA

Evanescent, salmon pink, macular pale center; seen on chest, arms, axilla, thighs, and, less commonly, face; most frequently associated with systemic symptoms (high fever, splenomegaly, lymphadenopathy, leukocytosis)

Rheumatoid Factor

Positive in ±15% of patients; seropositivity increases with age; significant only when titer is high, because it can appear in low titer in other diseases

Iridocyclitis

In 20% of JRA patients; insidious onset, detected by slit-lamp examination; may lead to blindness

Cervical Spine Involvement

Two other joints must be involved; limitation of cervical motion may be only finding; may or may not exhibit radiographic evidence of apophyseal disease

Pericarditis

In 10% of JRA cases; usually associated with other systemic manifestations; pericarditis with polyarthritis, in absence of myocarditis or valvular lesions, almost always characteristic of rheumatoid arthritis in children; systemic lupus erythematosus must be excluded

Tenosynovitis

In many patients, involves chiefly the hands, ankles and feet

Intermittent Fever

Various patterns of fever in JRA; a persistent intermittent fever with diurnal variation between 102° F and 106° F with return to normal suggestive of JRA only if other diseases such as sepsis and leukemia excluded

Morning Stiffness

In many children after a period of rest, lasting a few minutes to several hours

Nonspecific features include the following:

Systemic Manifestations

Before arthritis occurs; fever, rash, pericarditis, splenomegaly, lymphadenopathy, weight loss, malaise

Laboratory Findings

Anemia, extreme leukocytosis, and increased acute phase reactants (ESR, C-reactive protein)

Subcutaneous Nodules

Occurs in JRA, rheumatic fever, systemic lupus erythematosus, and sometimes in patients with no discernible disease

Joint Fluid Changes

Fluid clear to turbid with increased opacity may spontaneously clot; total cell count increased moderately, averaging 15,000/cu mm, mainly polymorphonuclear leukocytes

Synovial Biopsy

Nonspecific chronic inflammatory reaction with villous hyperplasia and round-cell infiltration; chief value in monoarticular form of JRA to rule out tuberculosis, infectious disease, neoplasms

Early Roentgenographic Findings

Soft tissue swelling juxta-articular osteoporosis, juxta-articular periosteal new bone formation (late changes: altered epiphyseal growth, erosions, ankylosis)

Rheumatic Fever. Major manifestations are carditis, polyarthritis, chorea, erythema marginatum, and subcutaneous nodules. Minor clinical manifestations are fever, arthralgia, previous rheumatic fever, or rheumatic heart disease. Laboratory findings in the acute phase reaction include ESR, C-reactive protein, and leukocytosis; there is a prolonged P-R interval.

Supporting evidence includes preceding streptococcal infection (increased ASO or other streptococcal antibodies), positive throat culture for group A streptococci and recent scarlet fever.

The presence of two major criteria, or one major plus two minor criteria, indicates a high probability of rheumatic fever if supported by evidence of preceding streptococcal infection. Absence of the latter should make the diagnosis suspect, except when rheumatic fever is first discovered after a long latent period from preceding involvement (*e.g.*, Sydenham's chorea or low-grade carditis).

The patient with polyarthritis and fever with an elevated ESR but no carditis poses a diagnostic problem early in the course of the disease. Strong supporting evidence of a preceding streptococcal infection (increased ASO titer or other streptococcal antibodies, positive throat culture for group A streptococci, or recent scarlet fever) is necessary before making a diagnosis of rheumatic fever. Occasionally, a patient developing early JRA after having a respiratory streptococcal infection may appear to have rheumatic fever. It is only when the arthritis persists beyond the 6-week to 3-month period that the diagnosis is clarified.

The polyarthritis of rheumatic fever is extremely migratory; that of JRA is more stable. The joints of rheumatic fever are more painful. Erosions in rheumatic fever are nonexistent. Polyarthritis lasting more than 5 weeks in rheumatic fever is extremely rare.

Systemic Lupus Erythematosus. Systemic lupus erythematosus is characterized by multisystem involvement: renal involvement, polyserositis, positive LE-cell preparation or positive antinuclear factor, malar flush, hemolytic anemia, thrombocytopenia, Raynaud's phenomenon, and leukopenia. It occurs more frequently in girls and is unusual under the age of 5 years.

A positive LE-cell preparation is significant only when it is markedly positive, because mildly positive LE preparations can occur in about 5% of cases of JRA and in other diseases. The antinuclear factor is a more specific index of antinuclear antibody.

The rheumatoid agglutination tests are positive in 10% to 15% of JRA cases but never in juvenile lupus erythematosus. (In the adult, more than 60% of rheumatoid arthritics have positive rheumatoid factor tests, compared with only about 25% of patients with systemic lupus erythematosus.)

The polyarthritis in systemic lupus erythematosus is milder than in JRA. Destructive or erosive changes in joints are unusual in lupus.

Response to salicylates is rapid in rheumatic fever, slower in JRA and very little or not at all in lupus erythematosus.

Septic Arthritis. Fever is present, and the joint is hot, red, very tender, and extremely painful with movement; prominent effusion is seen. Synovial fluid is turbid, and there is a very high polymorphonuclear cell count, a low glucose content, low viscosity, and poor mucin clot. The source of the organisms is from distant focus, is spread from adjacent osteomyelitis, or is contaminated by direct trauma. Bacteria are revealed by synovial biopsy or by direct smear and culture of synovial fluid.

Leukemia. The predominant presenting symptom is pain of sudden onset, primarily in large weight-bearing joints and frequently also in joints of the fingers, often bilateral, and lasting for several days to several months. The painful, swollen, and tender joints are migratory.

Other clinical manifestations include splenomegaly (in 50%), hepatomegaly (in 37%), lymphadenopathy (in 43%), and purpura (in 20%).

A basic rule in differentiating the arthritic manifestations of leukemia from other forms of arthritis is that the initial peripheral hemogram can be completely normal for several months, while the bone marrow is normal. The articular and bone manifestations can exist for some time before a definitive diagnosis of leukemia can be made.

Roentgenographic changes seen in leukemia are focal destructive lesions, osteosclerosis, subperiosteal new bone formation, and characteristic transverse bands of diminished density at the growing ends of long bones.

Reiter's Syndrome. The symptom complex known as Reiter's syndrome is characterized by polyarthritis, conjunctivitis, and urethritis. It can be found in children, usually between 9 and 16 years of age, generally males. The polyarthritis is indistinguishable from that of rheumatoid arthritis early in the disease, but the disease characteristically lasts only a few weeks to several months, followed by complete clinical recovery. The large weight-bearing joints of the lower extremity are the usual sites of involvement. Considerable synovial effusion occurs, but destruction is unknown. A culture of urethral exudate may reveal typical "L" forms.

Congenital Agammaglobulinemia and Acquired Hypogammaglobulinemia. The γ-globulins, the antibodies that protect against bacterial infections, are diminished or absent. The acquired type in adults occurs as a result of lymphatic or reticuloendothelial disturbances (*e.g.*, lymphoma, chronic leukemia, multiple myeloma, sarcoidosis).

Polyarthritis occurs in both the child and the aduult and is indistinguishable from that in rheumatoid disease. Destructive changes are noted by roentgenogram.[134]

Diagnosis is by protein electrophoresis. Absence of isohemoagglutinins in the serum is characteristic of agammaglobulinemia. Another test is performed by adding the patient's serum to agar containing rabbit or horse antiserum. Normally the human antibody (γ-globulin) combines with the antigen to produce a precipitate. The degree of the precipitate or its absence reflects the amount of γ-globulin present in the serum of the patient. In children the polyarthritis seems to disappear with adequate γ-globulin therapy.

Allergic Reactions. Children with allergic reactions can manifest polyarthritis and systemic symptoms. The joint swellings exhibit periarticular soft tissue swelling and joint effusion. The clinical picture simulates JRA.

The differentiating points are remittent or sustained fever; angioneurotic edema involving an entire foot or hand, periorbital area, or circumoral area; intensely itching urticaria; absence of joint erosions and juxta-articular osteoporosis; joint swelling seldom lasting beyond a few weeks; and relief of all symptoms on removal of the offending antigen.

Viral Diseases. Definite polyarthritis, lasting from a few days to several weeks, can occur preceding, during, or following any number of viral diseases. The arthritis is characteristically transient and not erosive. Among the diseases it may be associated with are rubella, rubeola, mumps, chickenpox, smallpox, infectious mononucleosis, viral influenza, and infectious hepatitis.

Diagnosis is by identifying the offending viral disease, usually by laboratory aids.

Miscellaneous Diseases. Miscellaneous diseases include the following:

Polymyositis and dermatomyositis
Polyarteritis
Scleroderma
Tuberculous arthritis
Gonococcal arthritis
Meningococcal arthritis
Fungal diseases
Hemophilia
Ankylosing spondylitis
Hemoglobinopathies—sickle cell anemia
Sarcoidosis
Plasma cell hepatitis
Juvenile gout

Course. The typical course of polyarticular JRA is intermittent, with exacerbations and remissions continuing over many years. Remissions can be prolonged only to recur after years. The patient should never be regarded as cured.

Occasionally, the disease is unremitting and increasingly severe. Marked deformities of joints develop. The patient is chronically ill. Vasculitis is manifested by peripheral neuropathies and ulcerations of the extremities. As the illness is prolonged, amyloidosis develops and should be suspected when hepatosplenomegaly persists or when proteinuria and hematuria develop and are not related to gold therapy.

MONOARTICULAR JRA

Clinical Picture

In approximately 30% of patients, only a single joint is at first involved, usually the knee, less frequently the hip, elbow, and ankle.

In contrast to the polyarticular type, which causes premature epiphyseal closure, monoarticular JRA often accelerates epiphyseal growth, resulting in increased length of the extremity. The limb-length discrepancy is temporary, however, because the opposite extremity catches up as the arthritis is brought under control.

The onset is usually before 3 years of age and is insidious; symptoms are mild, except for the hip, which may be quite painful.[135] The joint is minimally swollen, stiff, and painful. Objectively, an antalgic limp may be the only finding.

The patient generally looks well. Only rarely will there by lymphadenopathy, splenomegaly, rash, myocarditis, or pericarditis. The clinical picture is deceptively benign, yet monoarticular JRA has the highest incidence of a sight-threatening complication, iridocyclitis.

Chronic iridocyclitis is at first asymptomatic until vision decreases. The earliest manifestation, clumps of cells and protein, can only be detected by slit-lamp examination. The complication may develop many years after the onset of arthritis, even during a remission, and slit-lamp examinations should be carried out at 3-month intervals.

Laboratory Findings

The sedimentation rate, white cell count and hematocrit, and hemoglobin are often normal.

Roentgenographic Findings

Roentgenographic findings are not specific and may show juxtaepiphyseal osteoporosis and, occasionally, periosteal ossification.

Synovial Fluid Examination

When aspirating joint fluid, the syringe should be coated with sterile heparin to prevent clotting prior to analysis. Also the joint fluid should be diluted with normal saline instead of glacial acetic acid for a white cell count. Otherwise, the fluid may coagulate and cause a spuriously low cell count.

The examination should include appearance of the fluid, whether clear, opalescent, or turbid; consistency of the clot (Ropes test); white cell count; types of cells; glucose level compared with blood sugar level; stain for bacteria; and culture (Table 13-3).

Differential Diagnosis

A history of trauma is often obtained in monoarticular JRA. In infectious arthritis, culture and antibiotic sensitivity are indicated. When tuberculous synovitis is suspected, a synovial biopsy will demonstrate granulomas and giant Langhans' cells. Other monoarticular conditions, such as osteochondritis dissecans and meniscal injury, must be ruled out.

Course

In most cases, a few more joints, generally less than four, will eventually become involved. The disease is then termed oligoarticular or pauciarticular arthritis. In about

TABLE 13-3 The Joint Fluid in Monoarticular Arthritis

Cause	Gross Appearance	Mucin Clot	White Cell Count	Percent of Neutrophils	Glucose Difference
Traumatic	Clear or hemorrhagic	Good	5,000	<50	<10 mg/dl
Rheumatoid	Clear to opalescent	Good to poor	15,000 to 25,000	50 to 90	10 mg to 25 mg/dl
Infectious	Cloudy or turbid	Poor	50,000 to 100,000	>90	>50 mg/dl

one fourth of cases, the syndrome becomes the polyarticular type, marked by remissions and exacerbations. Chronic iridocyclitis with resulting blindness always remains a threat.

ACUTE FEBRILE JRA

Acute febrile JRA is characterized by severe systemic manifestations and minimal articular symptoms and findings, generally termed arthralgia. Sometimes the only early indication of joint involvement may be the guarded attitude of the child, sitting or lying in a knee-flexed position.

Clinical Picture

The child appears ill, is irritable, listless, and anorectic, and suffers weight loss. He is feverish and presents lymphadenopathy, splenomegaly, myocarditis, pericarditis, pneumonitis, pleuritis, and rash. Any one or several or all of these findings can occur in any combination.

Fever is typically quotidian or double quotidian, with a daily peak or peaks, usually above 102° F (39° C) and often rising to more than 105° F (40° C). It then falls to normal or subnormal levels. After a month or two, the fever becomes relapsing, periodic, or remittant. The fever may precede joint involvement by days, months, or years.

The rash is more frequent in acute febrile JRA and appears in the late afternoon or evening. It is brought out by rubbing or scratching (Koebner's phenomenon) and can appear long before joint involvement.

Splenomegaly is present in about 50% of patients with acute febrile JRA. Hepatomegaly is often associated.

Lymphadenopathy may be prominent but can be confused with acute leukemia or lymphoma.

Pericarditis is the most frequent form of cardiac involvement. It is benign, detected by electrocardiogram (ECG); the cardiac shadow is enlarged on a roentgenogram, and a friction rub is evident on auscultation. Symptoms include dyspnea, disproportionate tachycardia, and severe stabbing chest pain. The condition generally lasts 1 to 15 weeks. It never causes tamponade.

Myocarditis is the most serious complication. It can cause cardiac dilatation and failure. Treatment is prompt administration of corticosteroids.

Laboratory Findings

Laboratory findings include a striking neutrophilic leukocytosis; an elevated ESR; normocytic hypochromic anemia, usually unresponsive to iron; and, usually, normal serum electrophoresis.[129,143] However, α_2- and γ-globulins may be high.

Differential Diagnosis

The differential diagnosis must exclude other causes of fever, rash, and joint pain.

Systemic lupus erythematosus (SLE) criteria include the following:

- Children younger than 5 years not affected
- Never marked leukocytosis
- Rash not evanescent, not brought out by rubbing
- LE cells, oral lesions, renal abnormalities
- Antinuclear antibodies may be found in both JRA and SLE; in JRA titers are low, in SLE high; absence of antinuclear antibody excludes SLE

The macular rash of polyarteritis, hypersensitivity angiitis, and Schönlein-Henoch purpura is associated with purpura and ecchymosis. Renal manifestations are evident in these vascular disorders but not in JRA.

The symptoms and signs of childhood leukemia are similar to febrile JRA and include severe anemia and purpura. Peripheral blood and marrow study confirm the diagnosis.

Course

About half of patients with the acute febrile onset continue with this disease with remissions and exacerbations each year. As patients approach adulthood, the attacks subside slowly, leaving no deformities.

Half the patients develop the polyarthritic course, which continues into adult life with remissions and exacerbations.

TREATMENT

CONSERVATIVE

A long-range program is designed to control the disease, prevent and correct deformities, preserve joint motion, and avert serious sequelae. This is accomplished by various drugs, rest to acutely inflamed joints, application of casts if necessary, and physical therapy. Treatment is best initiated in a hospital where a team approach includes the pediatrician, orthopaedic surgeon, and physical therapist. The appropriate drug and its dosage is determined and its effect studied. Orthopaedic splinting and supervised non-weight-bearing exercises are carried out. When the disease is brought under control, protective braces are applied and treatment is continued at home. Weight bearing is not permitted until the acute inflammatory phase of the disease has subsided.

Aspirin. Aspirin is the drug of choice. Active disease is suppressed by four to six daily doses that total 90 mg to 130 mg/kg (⅔ to 1 gr/lb). A more frequent and higher dosage is required for patients with more pronounced systemic manifestations. A blood salicylate level of 20 mg to 25 mg/dl is desirable, but a satisfactory clinical response may be obtained with a lower blood salicylate level. One must observe for signs of salicylate toxicity, and the blood salicylate level is monitored. Gastrointestinal irritation is common and can be reduced by enteric-coated capsules or buffered preparations. Gastrointestinal bleeding can occur with prolonged salicylate administration, and periodic blood counts and stool examinations for occult blood are mandatory.

Signs of salicylate toxicity include the following:

1. *Gastrointestinal.* Epigastric pain, peptic ulceration, and chronic blood loss (as much as 6 ml/day can be lost in stool during prolonged administration) are typical signs.

2. *Acid-Base Balance.* Initially, respiratory alkalosis and later metabolic acidosis are seen. It is controlled by discontinuing salicylate administration and then restarting it at a lower dosage.

3. *Other Side-Effects.* Hypersensitivity (allergic rash, anaphylactic shock), excessive perspiration, palpitations, occasionally fluid retention, and rarely lethargy and drowsiness are common signs.

Intra-Articular Corticosteroids. The use of prednisolone as a tertiary butylacetate injected into a joint will give relief for periods lasting from 4 weeks to several months. The chief indication for this treatment is monoarticular disease of a weight-bearing joint, the knee, hip, and ankle.

The synovial fluid is removed and 5 mg to 20 mg of steroid is injected. The injection may be repeated, but preferably at long intervals.

Infrequently, selective injection of a small joint of the hand may be tried.

Systemic Corticosteroids. Steroids are anti-inflammatory agents that do not cure JRA. They are used only when other treatment fails, except in life-threatening situations or in iridocyclitis.

Advantages. Steroids reduce fever, promote a feeling of well-being, improve strength and appetite, reduce swelling and stiffness of joints, suppress inflammation of iridocyclitis, reduce the size of the spleen and the liver, and suppress polyserositis, including pericardial effusion.

Disadvantages. Steroids do not prevent erosion and destruction of joints; they cause severe toxic effects; the dosage must be increased to maintain improvement; and withdrawal symptoms are common.

Contraindications. Steroids are never used when the following apply:

1. A child has JRA with a mild form of articular disease
2. JRA patients respond reasonably well to other agents
3. Severely afflicted JRA patients have not attempted the basic conservative program of therapy and salicylates and other agents
4. Suspected or known sepsis or pyrogenic arthritis is seen
5. Such associated conditions as diabetes, peptic ulcer, central nervous system disease (including neuroses and psychoses), hypertension, and severe chronic renal disease are present.

Indications. Steroids are used when the following apply:

1. Iridocyclitis or uveitis occur, because of threatened blindness
2. High fever and severe peripheral articular disease do not respond to salicylates
3. Severe pericarditis occurs. Relief is secured within 24 hours. The medication must be continued until the heart returns to normal size.
4. The patient is committed to long periods of total immobilization. The patient is unable to perform basic activities and often has fibrous ankylosis and marked weakness and is completely bedridden. The steroid overcomes postural hypotension, increases strength, reduces stiffness and swelling of joints, and makes it possible for physical therapy to be carried out.
5. Severe peripheral articular disease is present. The patient is unable to perform basic activities of daily living. Salicylates and gold have failed.

Dosage. The preferred daily dose at the beginning of therapy is 10 mg prednisone. This should be gradually reduced over the early weeks to the lowest possible maintainance dose. The use of larger doses of corticosteroid every other day will reduce the awesome toxicity potential.[132] As the dosage is reduced, ACTH is given every few days. If steroid dosage is suddenly discontinued completely, serious exacerbation of the disease may follow with serious withdrawal symptoms. With prolonged administration, problems of increased dosage and reduced response are encountered.

Side-Effects. Cushingoid changes (acne, masculinization in females, marked increase of hair on arms and legs), hypertension (can produce encephalopathy and convulsions), edema, osteoporosis with pathologic fractures, masking of infection, delayed healing, peptic ulcer, central nervous system effect (euphoria, convulsions, psychosis), and posterior subcapsular cataracts may be seen.

A rare adverse reaction to corticoids in children is pseudotumor cerebri, a form of intracranial hypertension causing headache, nausea, vomiting, and papilledema. It occurs primarily in children on long-term steroid therapy and is due either to an abrupt decrease in maintenance dose or to a change from one steroid compound to another. Should it occur, one must return to the previous maintenance dose or resume treatment with the original drug.

Gold. A useful drug, gold is capable of inducing a prolonged remission. It is preferred over corticosteroids because its complications are fewer and it is readily controlled. Potentially serious toxic effects such as marrow depression and nephritis can be detected at an early stage by monitoring the blood and urine and can be averted by discontinuing the drug.

Gold therapy is considered only when the arthritis responds poorly to aspirin. The response to gold is not appreciated until at least 3 months have elapsed. Therefore, concurrent treatment with aspirin should be continued until the benefit of gold can be established.

When 25 mg gold sodium thiomalate is injected intramuscularly weekly, an average plasma level of 330μg/dl is maintained. The plasma concentration, after an average level is established, remains constant with continuing weekly dosage. Large amounts of gold are retained in the body during the period of administration, chiefly bound to α_1-globulin as a gold protein complex.[133] The water-soluble compounds are most effective in maintaining constant plasma levels. They tend to deposit more readily in inflamed joints than in normal joints. Excretion of gold is mainly by the kidney.

Method of Administration. Sodium aurothiomalate is an effective preparation. Initially, 10 mg is given intramuscularly, followed by 25 mg weekly for 20 weeks. Then four injections of 25 mg are given at 2-week intervals, then four injections at 3-week intervals, then at monthly intervals thereafter.

A hemogram and urinalysis are performed 1 week after the first dose, then at weekly intervals for a few weeks, then at monthly intervals for 3 or 4 months. If toxicity has not occurred by this time, the hemogram and urinalysis can be done at 3-month intervals or oftener if indicated.

Gold therapy is continued as long as it is beneficial and there are no adverse reactions. Complications are more frequent in children under 6 years of age and in the early months of therapy.

Toxic Effects. In children, significant toxicity is minimal to gold and is less common than with corticosteroids. In Brewer's experience, no children have died as a result of gold therapy.

Dermatitis. The drug rash disappears when the dosage is reduced from 2 mg to 5 mg. Other lesions of the skin and mucous membrane include stomatitis, pharyngitis, vaginitis, and glossitis.

Gastrointestinal Disturbances. Gastritis, colitis, and hepatitis are exceedingly rare.

Central Nervous System Problems. "Nitritoid" reactions characterized by vertigo, giddiness, flushing of the face, and headache were noted with older, probably impure, preparations but not with modern compounds.

Nephritis. Toxic nephritis, manifested by significant hematuria or albuminuria, is extremely rare. Transient albuminuria, consisting of a trace of albumin, occurs at some point during treatment but is of no significance. An occasional patient will have significant hematuria and nephritis. Renal biopsy reveals membranous glomerulonephritis as well as a rare nephroticlike syndrome.

Hematopoietic Toxicity. Bone marrow depression, particularly thrombocytopenia or leukopenia, may occur but disappears when the medication is discontinued.

Exacerbation of Disease. Mild to moderate exacerbation of joint pain and swelling can occur in an occasional patient after each injection of gold. This generally disappears after five or six injections, but a few patients may continue to complain, necessitating discontinuance of the medication.

Treatment of Gold Toxicity. Skin rash, the most common adverse effect requires only reduction of the dose of gold. With severe forms of rash, parenteral steroid is indicated and is effective. No patients require dimercaptopropanol (BAL). Penicillamine may be useful in patients who do not respond to parenteral corticosteroids.

Nephritis responds to discontinuance of the drug, and permanent renal pathology is rare. Thrombocytopenia and leukopenia likewise respond to discontinuance of gold therapy. If necessary, steroids are administered.

Indomethacin. Indomethacin (Indocin) is a NSAI analgesic and antipyretic agent. There is considerable disagreement between rheumatologists as to its efficacy in rheumatoid arthritis, but progressive reduction of joint swelling and tenderness and increased range of motion with improved functional capacity have been reported in more than 50% of patients.[141] Children with rheumatoid arthritis who have serious pyrexia and cannot be controlled with aspirin may often respond dramatically to indomethacin.[126] The drug must be used with great care because of potential serious side-effects. Unexplained fatalities have been recorded in children with rheumatoid arthritis under therapy with indomethacin.[136]

Eye Care. Periodic slit-lamp examinations are carried out at 6-month intervals in all patients with JRA. In monoarticular patients, the most susceptible group, the examinations should be done at 3-month intervals, even while the disease is in remission.

Conservative Orthopaedic Management. The principles that should be observed are as follows:

1. ***Rest.*** Moderate rest facilitates resolution of the inflammation. This can be accomplished by frequent periods of bed rest, but prolonged bed rest must be avoided because it will result in muscle atrophy and flexion contractures. Lightweight bivaled casts are applied to the hand, foot, or knee continuously for about 1 or 2 weeks to allow the acute inflammation to subside. Instead of a cast, a removable heat-malleable plastic splint may be applied.

2. ***Exercise.*** The splint is removed several times daily for active and passive range of motion exercises and for application of heat. The exercises maintain nutrition of the articular cartilage, preserve the range of motion by maintaining adequate length of ligamentous structures and prevent muscle weakness and atrophy.

3. ***Heat.*** Stiffness and painful muscle spasm are relieved by the application of heat.

4. ***Orthosis or plaster cast.*** This is used to rest the acutely inflamed joint and to prevent or correct deformity. Continuous plaster immobilization must be avoided because it encourages muscle atrophy and joint contracture.

The management of rheumatoid arthritis of the knee associated with flexion contracture, a common problem, exemplifies the basic principles of orthopaedic treatment. After the acute inflammation has subsided, the flexion contracture must be overcome using various methods.

Traction can be used. Buck's traction is best avoided because it can encourage posterior subluxation of the tibia. Instead, a modified type of Russell's traction is applied (Fig. 13-17). The upward pull is directed at the proximal portion of the leg through a pin inserted transversely through the tibia. Caution is exercised to avoid the tibial tubercle and growth plate. Longitudinal pull is in line with the tibia.

Serial splinting is useful. Each week the joint is partially positioned toward the corrected position while a new cast is applied.

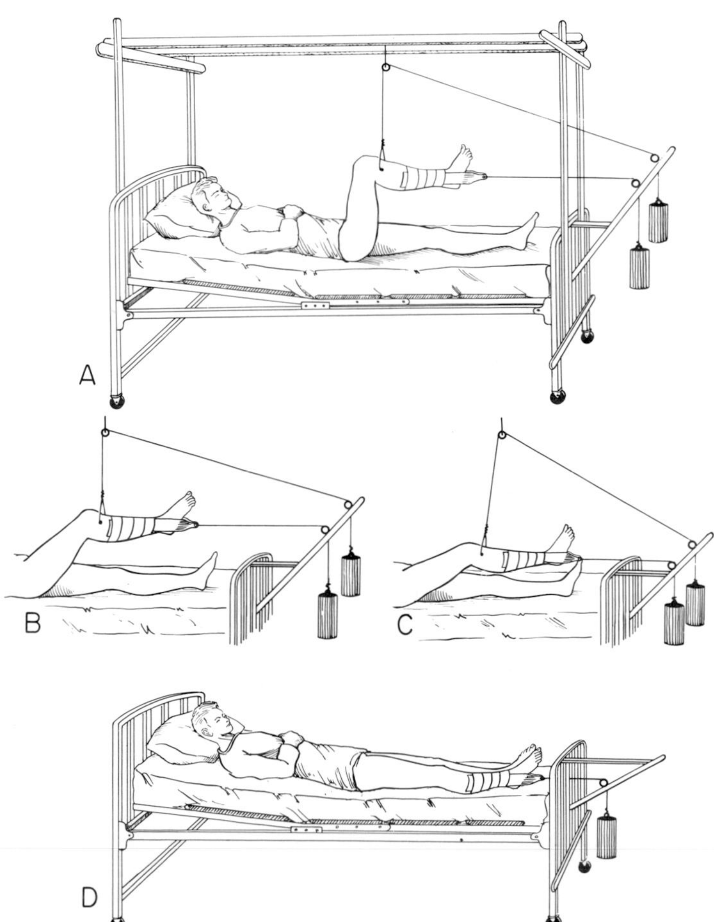

FIG. 13-17. A modified Russell's traction, 90-90, is used. Gradual extension is obtained with upward force on the proximal tibia to correct posterior subluxation as the knee is extended. As the deformity is corrected, the traction must be adjusted accordingly, as illustrated sequentially by *A, B, C, D.*

The three-point pressure principle can be used to correct the deformity. The orthotic appliance developed by Engen is effective (Figs. 13-18 and 13-19).[130] The backward thrust at the apex of the knee should be directed over the lower end of the femur to force the femur posteriorly, thereby stretching the posterior fibers of the collateral and anterior cruciate ligaments. If no pressure is exerted anteriorly over the lower end of the femur, the tibia is merely extended, hinges on the posterior shortened fibers of the collateral and anterior cruciate ligaments, and displaces posteriorly.

This basic orthosis can also be used to correct knock-knee deformity or knock-knee and flexion contracture at the same time.

A wedging cast similarly can be used to correct deformity. However, it is difficult to position the wedge and posterior hinge so as to apply proper points of pressure. An improperly applied wedging cast can force the tibia posteriorly.

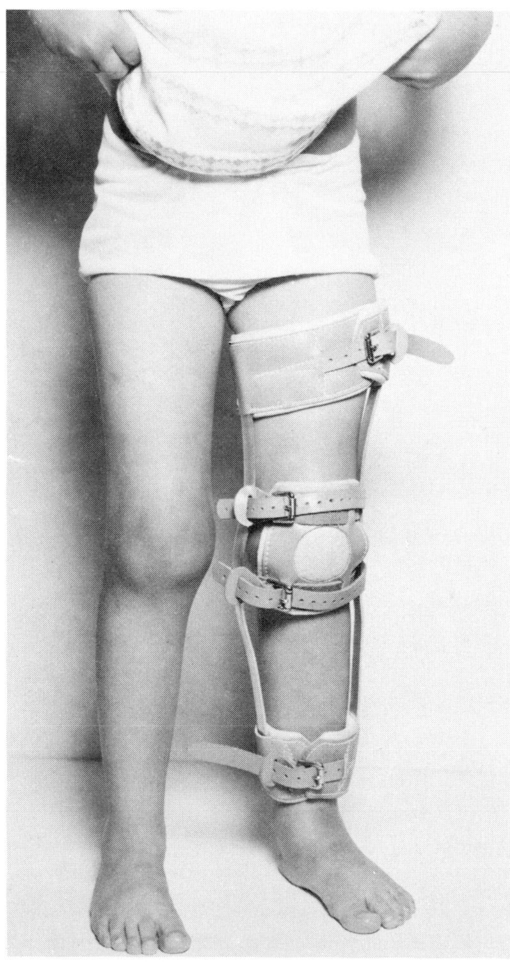

FIG. 13-18. The three-point fixation brace is used to overcome flexion contracture of the knee. (Bianco AJ Jr et al: Juvenile rheumatoid arthritis. Orthop Clin North Am 2:745, 1971)

The same three-point pressure principle can be used to correct other deformities (*e.g.*, flexion of the wrist).

The supple arthritic foot requires adequate support to prevent deformities. During the acute inflammatory stage, the foot is immobilized in a bivalved cast and after pain and swelling have subsided is put through range of motion exercises. Then a well-built shoe with standard inserts (longitudinal and metatarsal pads) is used. Usually a regular last is specified, but for pes cavus a straight last is required. Shoe corrections by wedges, heel lift, or transverse metatarsal bar may be prescribed. Standard leg bracing is useful for severe deformity, joint destruction, or muscle weakness. It may be used while awaiting surgical reconstruction, which preferably is done after full growth is attained.

Weight bearing is not permitted while the disease is acute. After the acute inflammation has subsided, limited weight bearing is permitted, using crutches and gradually increasing the amount of weight borne on the extremity.

Various orthoses will help reduce weight bearing and protect against contracture and deformity. To a high-top lace shoe fitted with a metatarsal bar to prevent cavovarus deformity is attached a patellar tendon–bearing cuff with two uprights. This may be extended upward with an ischial weight-bearing orthosis.

Physical Therapy. The extremity is removed from the bivalved cast twice daily for heat and exercises.

Heat Application. Moist heat is most efficacious for relieving the severe stiffness that develops after rest and for reducing pain and swelling. The modalities used are warm tub baths, hot packs (hot towels or Hydrocollator pack) to single joint, a paraffin bath for small joints of the hands and feet, and an electric blanket.

The Therabath* is a commercially available paraffin bath that can be used at home. A mixture of paraffin and oil is kept at a properly controlled temperature at all times. The hand or foot is dipped into the mixture and withdrawn immediately. It is cooled until there is no dripping, and then it is immersed again. This is repeated until a thick coating of paraffin is formed, usually about 10 to 12 times. The treated area is then wrapped in plastic and covered with a turkish towel for about 10 minutes. At the end of this time, the paraffin is peeled off and replaced in the Therabath, and the involved joints are exercised.

Exercises. Range of motion and strength of musculature are maintained by exercise. The range of motion is lost rapidly in involved joints that are not exercised to a complete range daily. Active and active assistive exercises are done slowly and smoothly. In addition, the shortened muscles are stretched. During acute exacerbations, exercises are gentle and non–weight bearing, with increased intervals of rest.

* W. R. Medical Electronics Co., St. Paul, Minnesota.

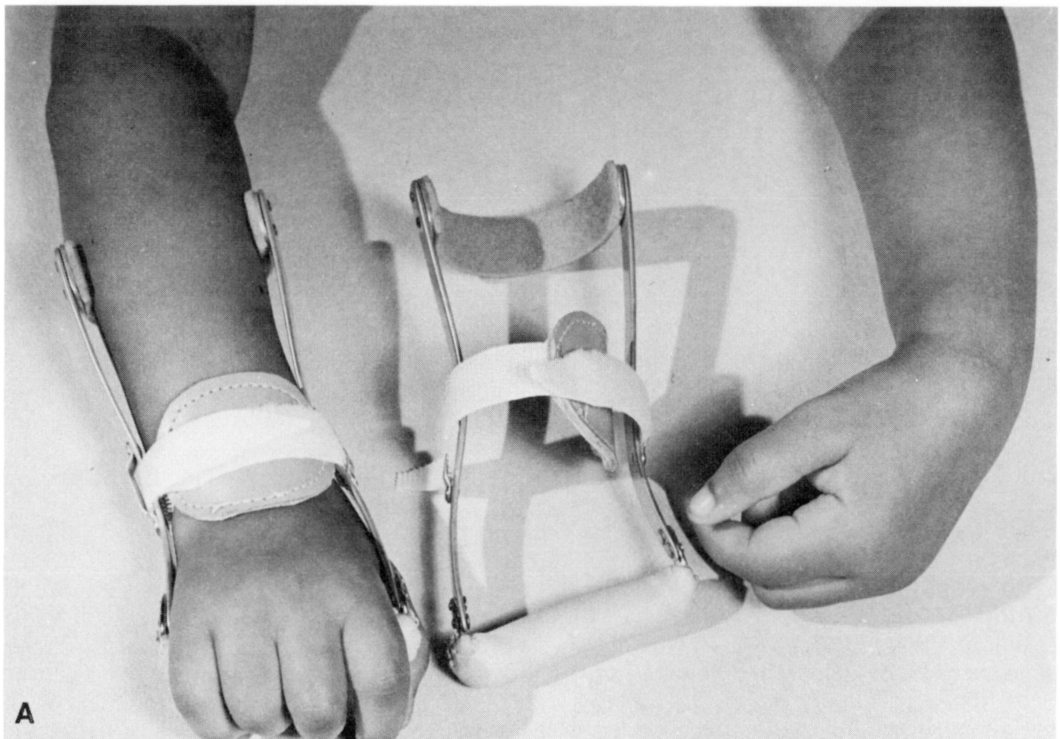

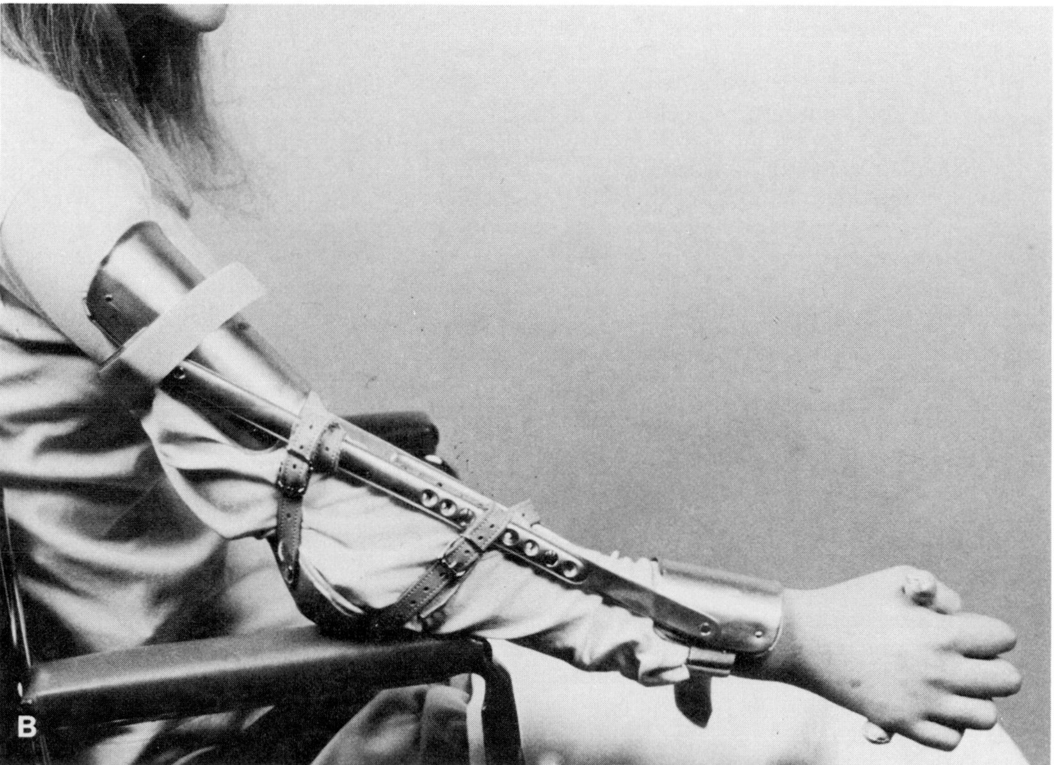

FIG. 13-19. The Engen extension orthosis is based on the three-point pressure corrective principles. (*A*) Correcting flexion deformity of the wrist. (*B*) Correcting flexion deformity of the elbow.

The patient is instructed on proper gait and maintaining correct posture. Positions of stress and strain are avoided. Swimming is the best form of exercise for children.

SURGICAL

The indications for surgical intervention in JRA are gradually being enlarged. Synovectomy will retard or halt progressive articular destruction and often will improve the general well-being of the patient. After contractures have developed, various soft tissue procedures can be done to correct deformity (*e.g.*, capsulotomy, tenotomies). After destruction of the joint has taken place, arthroplasty or arthrodesis is done. The following procedures are the most commonly indicated.

Early Synovectomy. Early synovectomy removes the diseased tissue and prevents destruction of cartilage. Synovectomy may or may not improve the range of motion but can be expected to relieve pain and retard or halt progress of the disease. In children, the possibility of an excellent or good joint following early synovectomy is greater when surgery is performed after 7 years of age. The most successful results are obtained in the monoarticular or pauciarticular class.[138]

The indications for synovectomy are as follows:[131]

Persistence of active synovitis for more than 18 months without roentgenographic evidence of destruction and without significant loss of motion, in the face of adequate nonsurgical therapy.

Presence of active synovitis with roentgenographic evidence of destruction, regardless of duration of disease.

Presence of active synovitis with significant loss of motion in the face of prolonged nonsurgical treatment.

Late Synovectomy. The main benefit is halting active disease. Improvement of motion and relief of pain are less likely when destructive changes are already visible on roentgenograms.

Total Hip Replacement. When disease onset is below the age of 5 years, the acetabulum is underdeveloped, the femoral head is small, and the femoral shaft is narrow. In those cases in which onset is over the age of 10 years, erosions and protrusio acetabuli tend to develop quickly. A few hips progress to bony fusion. Hip involvement is common in patients whose onset is between 16 and 21 years of age.

Surgery is best performed after full growth is attained. Surgical problems are posed by long-term corticosteroid therapy: osteoporosis, general poor development of the acetabulum and femur due to growth failure, poor skin healing, and increased risk of wound infection. The acetabulum is small and shallow in many cases. If the hip is fused, it may be difficult to find the plane of the old acetabulum. A narrow femoral shaft will require a modified stem of the femoral component.[124]

Anesthetic technical problems are presented because of ankylosing spondylitis of the neck, inability to open the mouth because of temporomandibular disease, and inability to pass an endotracheal tube, because the arthritis may affect the cricoarytenoid joints. One should be prepared for a tracheotomy.

The smallest prosthesis is used. The short femoral neck prothesis is often required; otherwise, the trochanter cannot be reattached owing to contractures of the glutei. Flexion and adduction contracture requires tenotomies.

The results are good to excellent in 85% of patients.

Osteotomy. Sometimes osteotomy is required in older children to correct a severely fixed flexion or valgus deformity of the knee or a flexion-adduction deformity at the hip. This can also be done when the joint is ankylosed to place it in a more functional position.

Arthrodesis. Arthrodesis is reserved for the joint that is severely damaged and when no other surgical procedure, such as arthroplasty, is likely to be successful. Rheumatoid arthritis of the cervical spine is often complicated by an acute case of chronic atlantoaxial subluxation. Immediate atlantoaxial arthrodesis is indicated to prevent catastrophic cord compression (see Chronic Atlantoaxial Subluxation) (Fig. 13-20).

Correction of Flexion Contracture of the Knee. Before advanced destruction of the joint has taken place, correction of flexion contracture can be accomplished by posterior soft tissue release. The approach is through a lazy-S incision over the lateral aspect of the knee. A step-cut tenotomy of the biceps tendon is done. Then the posterior capsular fat and areolar tissue are separated from the lateral side of the knee toward the medial side, and the posterior capsule is incised in a longitudinal manner. The peroneal nerve is isolated and protected and is closely observed while the knee is gradually extended. The interior of the joint can be approached through the same lateral incision, and a synovectomy is done.

If the medial hamstrings are contracted, they may be sectioned or lengthened through a small medial incision. The tibia must be pushed anteriorly, and this may require section of the posteromedial capsule.

THE RHEUMATOID VARIANTS

Certain diseases that are similar to, but distinct from, rheumatoid arthritis can be designated seronegative spondyloarthropathies and have clinical features in common, including a negative test for serum rheumatoid factor; absence of rheumatoid nodules; inflammatory

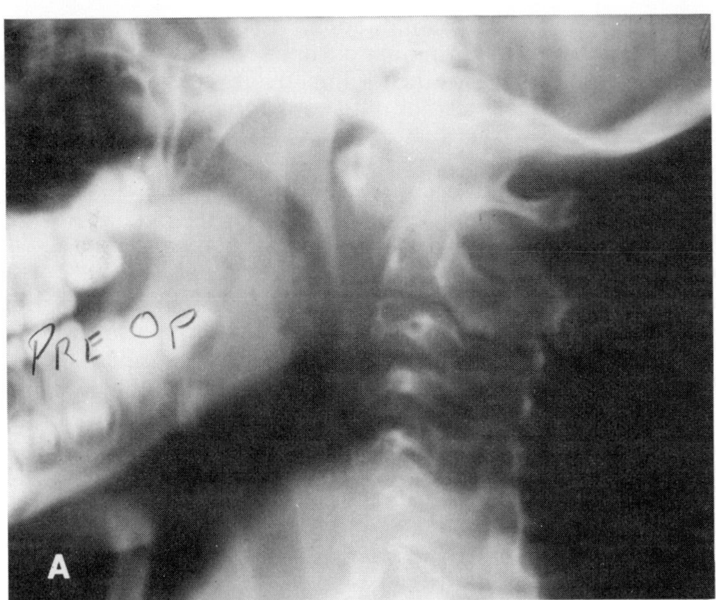

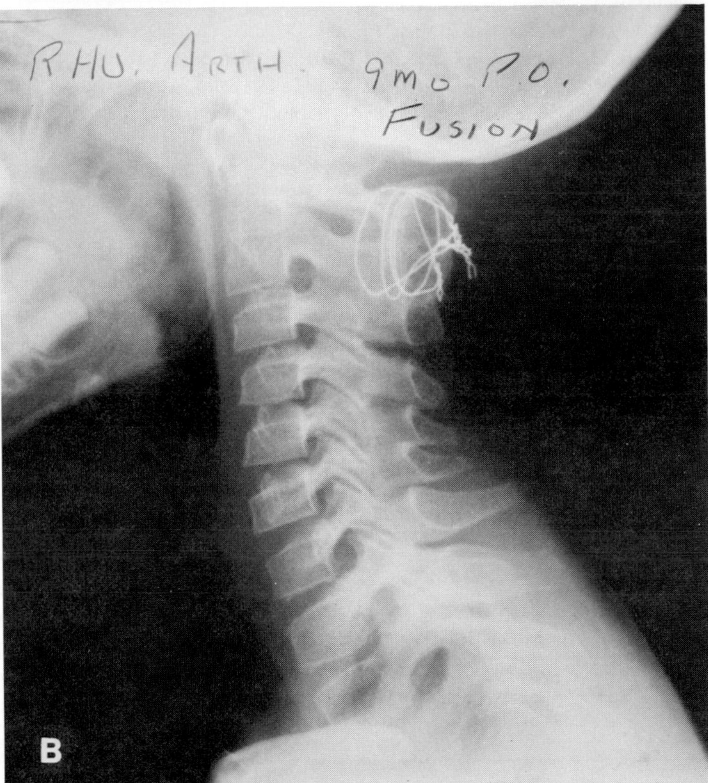

FIG. 13-20. (*A*) A roentgenogram of the cervical spine in a child with rheumatoid arthritis demonstrates anterior subluxation of the atlas on the axis. Note the increased distance between the anterior ring of the atlas and the odontoid process. (*B*) Lateral view of the cervical spine 9 months following posterior fusion using iliac bone grafts. The subluxation has been reduced and immobilized in the corrected position. (Bianco AJ Jr et al: Juvenile rheumatoid arthritis. Orthop Clin North Am 2:745, 1971)

peripheral arthritis, often asymmetrical; roentgenographic evidence of sacroiliitis, with or without spondylitis; associated gastrointestinal, ocular, genital, or cutaneous abnormalities; a tendency to occur frequently within the same family; and a frequent association of HLA-B27, a specific histocompatibility antigen, particularly when the axial skeleton is involved.[152,162,187] These diseases include ankylosing spondylitis, Reiter's syndrome, the arthropathy associated with inflammatory bowel disease, psoriatic arthritis, and certain patterns of juvenile rheumatoid arthritis.

During the early stages of development of these

diseases, their clinical manifestations are highly variable and easily mistaken for rheumatoid or infectious arthritis. The identification of the histocompatibility antigens is, therefore, a valuable test for differentiating this category of disease, because rheumatoid arthritis lacks the specific antigen.

HLA antigens are specific protein determinants on the membrane surfaces of many mammalian cells, including platelets, fibroblasts, and leukocytes. In humans these protein determinants are under the control of two closely associated gene loci on the sixth autosomal chromosome. Because autosomal chromosomes are paired, each person has a total of four genes, or two allelic pairs, one pair inherited from the father and the other pair inherited from the mother. One allelic pair codes for two membrane antigens, so that each person has a specific set of up to four HLA antigens on his leukocytes, just as he has a specific set of blood-group antigens on the membrane surfaces of his red blood cells. If a person is exposed to HLA antigens different from his own, he forms antibodies to these. Therefore, the HLA type can be determined on the basis of specific protein determinants on each persons's leukocytes. His specific HLA pattern can be identified in the tissue-typing laboratory by means of the microdroplet lymphocytotoxicity test. Thus far, about 30 different antigens have been recognized. One pair of loci may be coded for the first segregant series of 12 antigens, and the second pair of loci may be coded for the second segregant series of 18 antigens.

In studies of the genetics of immunity, it has been shown that certain diseases may be associated with specific HLA types. When an experimental animal is challenged by a well-defined protein antigen (*e.g.*, bovine insulin), the intensity of the antibody response is under genetic control. Therefore, some animals when challenged produce a high titer of antibody and others only a small one. It was noted that a particular immune response was often associated with a given HLA pattern. Hence, the gene loci governing the intensity of the immune response, called immune response genes, are closely linked to specific HLA genes.

TABLE 13-4 Frequency of HLA-B27 Among Seronegative Spondyloarthropathies

Disease	HLA-B27 Positive (%)
Ankylosing spondylitis	90
Reiter's syndrome	95
Inflammatory bowel disease with spondylitis	70
Juvenile chronic polyarthritis (overall)	35
Juvenile chronic polyarthritis with spondylitis	95
Psoriasis and peripheral arthritis	25
Psoriasis and spondylitis	35

(Goldin RH, Bluestone R: HLA-W27 antigens and sacroiliitis. Comp Ther 2:23, 1976)

Significant associations of certain HLA types occur among populations of patients having diseases in which immunologic aberrations are a feature. Rheumatic diseases in particular appear to bear a relationship between a given disease and a specific HLA type. For example, HLA-B27 antigen is found only in 6% to 7% of a normal white population and in 4% of a normal Afro-American population. The antigen is virtually absent among black Africans. However, more than 90% of patients with ankylosing spondylitis are positive for HLA-B27.[52] Moreover, this antigen is often associated with other disorders of the seronegative spondyloarthropathy group. Consequently, the presence or absence of the HLA-B27 antigen when testing a patient's lymphocytes is of diagnostic importance. It should be noted that the HLA-B27 antigen is absent in rheumatoid arthritis and acute rheumatic fever.

Whenever a clinical picture is suggestive but not diagnostic of a seronegative spondyloarthropathy, the presence of HLA-B27, detected by lymphocyte typing, would increase the probability of the patient's having one of these entities. However, absence of the antigen does not rule out such a diagnosis (Table 13-4).

Tissue typing can predict the probability of a family member of a patient with ankylosing spondylitis developing a related disease or of a patient with inflammatory bowel disease developing ankylosing spondylitis.

PSORIATIC ARTHRITIS

Psoriatic arthritis is an inflammatory erosive arthritis remarkably similar to rheumatoid arthritis; it possesses a broad spectrum of involvement, varying from oligoarticular to polyarticular disease, but predominantly affects in asymmetrical fashion the small joints of the hands and feet. This condition was first described in detail in 1888.[166] Psoriatic arthritis is included among the group of rheumatoid variants, which also includes Reiter's disease, idiopathic ankylosing spondylitis, and the arthritis associated with inflammatory bowel disease, because all have certain characteristics in common, such as a hereditary influence, a negative test for rheumatoid factor, spondylitis, and sacroiliitis. When the rheumatoid factor is rarely detected in psoriatic arthritis, it represents that normally found in low titer in approximately 5% of the general population.[191]

Psoriatic arthritis develops in 5% to 10% of cases of psoriasis of the skin.[196] The arthritis manifestations usually appear about 10 to 12 years after the skin changes first appear and are more likely to develop when skin involvement is extensive. Rarely, psoriatic arthritis may appear to precede psoriasis of the skin, but careful examination usually reveals "hidden" lesions. Almost invariably, pitting disease of the nails is associated.[196] Psoriasis with or without arthritis is probably determined genetically in a multifactorial manner.[178,197] Environmental factors such as trauma may trigger the arthritis in the genetically predisposed.[179] similar to other seronegative spondyloarthropathies, an increased frequency of the histocompatibility antigen HLA-B27 has been found. When the antigen is detected, particularly in a male patient, the development of sacroiliitis or spondylitis is highly probable, occurring in approximately half of all cases of psoriatic arthritis.[153,177] In pure cutaneous psoriasis (without arthritis), HLA-B27 is absent. Psoriatic arthritis is capable of evolving in Reiter's syndrome and vice versa.[177]

PATHOLOGY

The fundamental process consists of a chronic inflammation with edema and round cells followed by intense fibrous replacement.[189] The inflammatory tissue erodes the cortex and the articular cartilage at the periphery of the articular end of the bone. The destruction extends centrally and exposes the cancellous bone. Dense fibrous tissue eventually occupies the entire joint. The inflammatory tissue extends along the surface of the shaft, which is eroded from without, causing the characteristic scalloped appearance. In contrast to rheumatoid arthritis, pannus formation, dense accumulations of round cells, and osteoporosis are never observed. Rarely, complete bony ankylosis may result, but fibrous ankylosis with dislocation and subluxation, especially at the metatarsophalangeal joints, is more common.

CLINICAL PICTURE

Skin changes usually precede arthritic manifestations by months to years, but rarely skin and joints appear to be involved simultaneously. When arthritis appears to develop independently, a careful search often discloses hidden areas of psoriasis, such as in the scalp, natal cleft, axilla, and navel. Disease of the nails is associated in a high proportion of cases.

The initial symptoms usually appear in a single joint; often, the interphalangeal joint of a finger or toe is the earliest site.[179] The onset may be insidious and the arthritis mild, or the initial episode may develop acutely, the finger or toe swelling up within a few hours, becoming tense, livid, and shiny, closely resembling an acute attack of gout, especially when the large toe is involved.[189] The syndrome evolves in exacerbations and remissions. Recurring effusions are common, particularly when the knee is involved.[169] During an attack, severe, transient, migratory aches and pains develop in several joints, especially about the sacroiliac joints and lower spine. In the early stages, the involvement is typically oligoarticular, sometimes affecting but a single joint, the inflammation is mild, and remissions are complete. Later, residual damage becomes apparent as deformity and limitation of motion develop.

In the hand, the distal interphalangeal joints and later the proximal interphalangeal joints and, rarely, the metacarpophalangeal joints are affected. The deformities that are typical of rheumatoid arthritis, such as ulnar deviation at the metacarpophalangeal joints and boutonnière and swan-neck deformities at the proximal interphalangeal joints, are relatively uncommon.[169] Occasionally, the distal radioulnar joint is involved, causing dorsal subluxation of the ulna and often associated with a neighboring tenosynovitis. The intensity of involvement of the fingers is highly variable. Tenosynovial effusion may cause generalized swelling of the finger, producing a typical sausagelike digit (Fig. 13-21). The distal interphalangeal joint may become generally swollen, red, and tender, resembling the acute phase of osteoarthritis with Heberden's nodes. Severe destructive and deforming changes and acro-osteolysis of the tufts of the distal

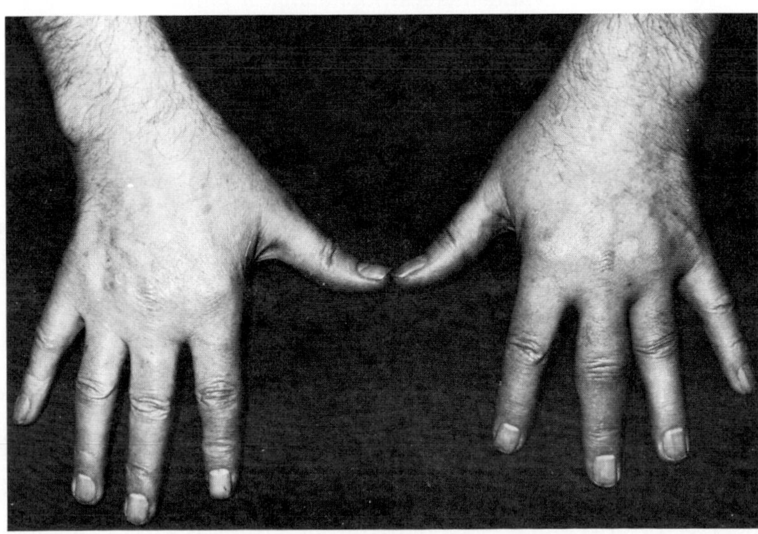

FIG. 13-21. Psoriatic arthritis, oligoarticular pattern. Note the sausage-shaped swelling of the left middle finger and asymmetrical involvement of only a few joints. (Wright V, Moll JMH: Seronegative Polyarthritis. Amsterdam, Elsevier/North-Holland, 1976)

phalanges produce an extreme unstable deformity of many digits, the so-called arthritis mutilans.[156]

In the foot, the distal and then the proximal interphalangeal joints and finally the metatarsophalangeal joints are affected. The toes are frequently subluxated and dislocated dorsally at the metacarpophalangeal joints. The tarsus and ankle joints are spared. When the large toe is involved, severe destruction of the interphalangeal joint is typical and may be mistaken for gouty arthritis, especially when associated with hyperuricemia.

Characteristically, the disease affects more and more joints with each exacerbation, but true migratory involvement does not occur. The large joints of the extremity are rarely affected.

In approximately half the cases of psoriatic arthritis, sacroiliitis or spondylitis develops, causing pain and stiffness of the lower back and tenderness over the sacroiliac joints. The symptoms are generally mild and often overlooked.

Five clinical groups can be identified:

Classic Psoriatic Arthropathy (5%)

Predominantly affects the distal interphalangeal joints

Arthritis Mutilans (5%)

Severe osteolysis affects the distal interphalangeal joints, proximal interphalangeal joints, and metacarpophalangeal joints of the hand. The severe osteolysis produces marked digital telescoping or the *doigt en lorgnette* deformity.

Symmetrical Polyarthritis (15%)

Similar to rheumatoid arthritis but lacks rheumatoid nodules and serology is negative

Asymmetrical Oligoarticular or Monoarticular Arthritis (70%)

Affects scattered distal interphalangeal, proximal interphalangeal, and metacarpophalangeal joints. A digit may be sausage shaped because of associated effusion of a flexor tendon sheath.

Ankylosing Spondylitis or Sacroiliitis (5%)

Similar to idiopathic ankylosing spondylitis but back pain is remarkably minimal or lacking[166,178]

COURSE

The arthritis is extremely variable in its behavior. In some patients there is a complete and permanent remission after the initial attack. Other patients continue to suffer remissions and exacerbations, each episode becoming increasingly worse. Fortunately, only a few pursue an unrelenting course with progressive destruction, but it is rare for complete crippling to ensue. When the histocompatibility antigen is present, especially in a male, the risk of developing sacroiliitis or spondylitis is enhanced.[177]

All types share common clinical characteristics, such as their occurrence in family members and the development of complications such as iridocyclitis. Psoriatic arthritis is highly vulnerable to trauma, the resulting inflammation tending to persist for lengthy periods.

ROENTGENOGRAPHIC FINDINGS

A wide spectrum of features include erosive changes and narrowing of small finger and toe joints; dissolution of terminal phalangeal tufts (acro-osteolysis); whittling of phalanges, metacarpals, and metatarsals; cupping of the proximal ends of phalanges, metacarpals, and metatarsals (when the end of a whittled bone articulates with the cup-shaped erosion of the distal bone, the typical deformity is called "pencil-in-cup" deformity); ankylosis of various small joints of the hands and feet; lack of symmetry; severe destruction of an isolated joint causing marked widening of the joint interval; predilection for distal interphalangeal and proximal interphalangeal joints, with relative sparing of metacarpophalangeal joints; sacroiliitis with gradual osseous obliteration of the joints; and ankylosing spondylitis (Figs. 13-22 and 13-23).[148,179,182]

Most of these features are relatively uncommon, except asymmetry and destruction of small isolated joints and an oligoarticular involvement. In the early phase of the disease, the only roentgenographic abnormality may be juxta-articular soft tissue swelling and minimal joint erosion. The changes of sacroiliitis are identical with those observed in idiopathic ankylosing spondylitis. In the spine, the syndesmophytes are asymmetrical. The classic "bamboo spine" of idiopathic ankylosing spondylitis is uncommon.

LABORATORY FINDINGS

The incidence of HLA-B27 is high when psoriasis is associated with arthritis, even more so in the presence of sacroiliitis. The ESR is normal in pure cutaneous psoriasis and is elevated when psoriatic arthritis develops. Anemia is very common and parallels the severity of the arthritis.[169] Hyperuricemia is also very common; it does not necessarily imply the presence of gouty arthritis. Antinuclear antibodies are occasionally positive, more often in association with very extensive psoriasis with destructive joint disease.

DIFFERENTIAL DIAGNOSIS

Psoriatic arthritis must be differentiated from rheumatoid arthritis; psoriatic arthritis lacks the rheumatoid factor. However, rarely the rheumatoid factor is present in low titer, but this represents that usually detected in approximately 5% of the general population.[191] Rheumatoid nodules are never found. Hand deformities typical of rheumatoid arthritis, such as ulnar deviation of the

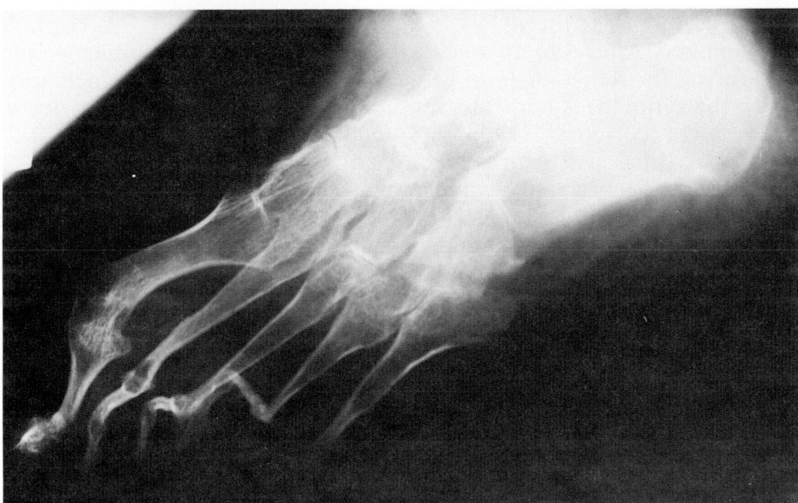

FIG. 13-22. Psoriatic arthritis. Note the "whittling" of all metatarsals, metatarsophalangeal (MTP) ankylosis of the hallux and second MTP joint, and "cupping" of the proximal end of the base of the fifth proximal phalanx. (Wright V, Moll JMH: Seronegative Polyarthritis. Amsterdam, Elsevier/North-Holland, 1976)

fingers, swan-neck deformity, and boutonnière deformity, rarely ever develop.[169] When the HLA-B27 antigen is present (in 30% of patients with psoriatic arthritis), rheumatoid arthritis can be ruled out because the antigen is invariably absent in this disease. Antinuclear antibodies are found in some psoriatic arthritics and therefore have no diagnostic significance.

Hyperuricemia occurs in 10% to 20% of all patients with psoriasis, presumably reflecting increased purine metabolism in the skin.[159] However, true gouty arthritis is unusual and can be confirmed only by finding urate crystals in joint aspirates and by noting the response to colchicine.

Following an injury, when a "traumatic" arthritis fails to recover within a reasonable period, underlying psoriatic disease should be suspected and hidden lesions sought in such areas as the scalp, natal cleft, and umbilicus.

TREATMENT

Early arthritis requires only simple analgesics such as aspirin or the nonsteroidal anti-inflammatory drugs. Phenylbutazone and indomethacin may produce serious side-effects and are best avoided. A small dose of a corticosteroid (*e.g.*, 2.5 mg or 5 mg prednisolone) may be given at night. A good clinical remission can be achieved by relatively large doses of prednisolone (40 mg–60 mg daily) or ACTH (40 units–50 units daily).

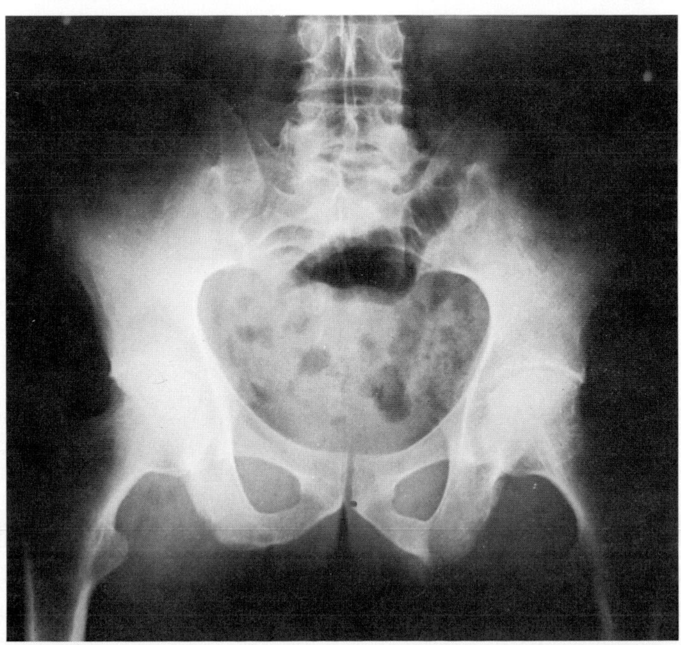

FIG. 13-23. Psoriatic spondylitis showing end stage of sacroiliitis with disappearance of bilateral sclerosis and complete ankylosis of both sacroiliac joints. (Wright V, Moll JMH: Seronegative Polyarthritis. Amsterdam, Elsevier/North-Holland, 1976)

Then the dose is reduced to the amount necessary for maintenance. After 6 to 10 weeks, the drug is gradually withdrawn, the remission lasting for 6 weeks to 6 months. When the synovitis is refractory, an intra-articular injection of a corticosteroid is helpful. Sometimes, treatment of the skin disease with ultraviolet light and preparations of coal tar (Goeckerman treatment) will simultaneously control skin and joint symptoms.[185]

Progressive cases require energetic measures to prevent advanced crippling disease. The various drugs used for rheumatoid arthritis cannot be used for psoriatic arthritis. Neither gold nor penicillamine is of value. Antimalarial preparations are contraindicated because they may produce exfoliative dermatitis.

For long-term control, antimetabolites may be used with appropriate safeguards. These include methotrexate, 6-mercaptopurine, azathioprine, and azaribine.[150,160,167,170] Present regimens for treating psoriasis, such as photochemotherapy (ultraviolet light plus methoxsalen), may also benefit the arthritis.[183]

The surgical treatment is similar to that used for rheumatoid arthritis. Psoriatic placques may form about an operative wound but do not affect healing, nor do they predispose to infection.

REITER'S DISEASE

Reiter's disease is an idiopathic syndrome characterized pathologically by an asymmetrical arthritis similar to that of rheumatoid arthritis and characterized clinically by the highly characteristic tetrad of abacterial urethritis, conjunctivitis, arthritis, and mucocutaneous lesions.[164,184,194] The association of arthritis with two other members of the tetrad is sufficient to make a diagnosis. Reiter's disease is one of the group of diseases classified as seronegative spondyloarthropathies, otherwise known as rheumatoid variants, with such common clinical characteristics as absence of the rheumatoid factor, a family history, the frequent association of the histocompatibility antigen HLA-B27, ankylosing inflammation of the sacroiliac joints and spine, and similar cardiac and ophthalmologic complications.

ETIOLOGY

The exciting cause is unknown. The predisposing causes are the following:

Sex. Men are predisposed in a ratio of 50:1.

Enteric Infection. The syndrome often follows outbreaks of dysentery, most commonly due to *Shigella, Yersinia,* and *Salmonella.*[175,181,186,190] Organisms are never cultured from joints.

Heredity. There is a high incidence of HLA-W27 histocompatibility antigen.

Mycoplasma. This is a filterable, pleomorphic, ultramicroscopic, pleuropneumonialike organism, the L-forms, which can be cultured from the urethral discharge.[172] They are mycoplasmalike structures lacking cell membranes and therefore are not affected by penicillin. They grow on culture plates adjacent to the colonies of nonpathogenic bacteria, and they are presumed to be latent forms of the latter organisms. These formless structures are known to be inhabitants of the genitourinary tract of both male and female, and therefore transmission by sexual contact is suggested. The onset of the initial episode often follows, after an interval of days, sexual intercourse. This cause is regarded as controversial.

Age. The disease occurs most commonly between 20 and 40 years of age.

CLINICAL PICTURE

Typically, the condition occurs in men between 20 and 40 years of age. An attack averages about 3 months, ranging from 2 weeks to 1 year; there is recurrence in approximately half of the patients, the recurrence rate diminishing with time. The remainder undergo a complete remission following the initial attack.

The initial episode varies in severity and duration. The onset may be spontaneous, may follow (several days to a few weeks) sexual intercourse, or may be associated with an epidemic of dysentery. The first symptoms are those of urethritis and cystitis (*i.e.,* dysuria, frequency, and mucoid or mucopurulent discharge). Acute prostatitis is frequently associated, and the prostatic secretions contain large numbers of neutrophils.

Within a few days, a mild catarrhal conjunctivitis makes its appearance and causes lacrimation, photophobia, and discharge. This condition may be so mild and evanescent that it may pass unnoticed, subsiding without sequelae.

Within 2 weeks after the onset of urethritis, an acute polyarthritis develops accompanied by a slight elevation in temperature daily. The weight-bearing joints, particularly the knees and ankles and the small joints of the feet, are most commonly involved. The joints are hot, swollen, and tender. The periarticular edema characteristic of gonorrheal arthritis does not occur. Synovial fluid is abundant and clear or slightly turbid. Mucous membrane ulcerations form within the oral cavity and about the glans penis. Those within the mouth are relatively asymptomatic, are evanescent, and, unless looked for, escape notice. Keratotic skin lesions form, especially over soles and palms.

The initial attack is self-limited, generally lasting about 4 to 6 weeks and subsiding slowly within about 6 months. The acute episode may appear to undergo a remission but instead smolders indefinitely as a chronic process. In approximately 50% of patients, recurrences are usual and represent acute exacerbations of a chronic process.

Prolonged courses are likely to be complicated by ankylosing disease of the sacroiliac joints and spine, not unlike that of idiopathic ankylosing spondylitis. Morning low back pain and aching referable to the sacroiliac joints, morning stiffness, anterior chest pain, and restricted chest expansion, so characteristic of ankylosing spondylitis, are apt to develop during an acute episode; rarely, pain and stiffness may affect other areas of the spine. Deforming dorsolumbar kyphosis, another characteristic of idiopathic ankylosing spondylitis, does not develop in Reiter's disease. Often the spondylitis and sacroiliitis may be asymptomatic and discovered on roentgenograms.

The late inactive stage is represented by a variable combination of deformities, usually involving the lower extremities and lower back. A typical clinical pattern is one that includes a stiff lumbar spine, deforming arthritis of various small joints of the feet, and often a painful heel spur. The spondylitis is generally mild, nondeforming, asymmetrical, and ultimately progressing to ankylosis of the involved segments.[163]

Urinary Tract Involvement. Acute nonspecific urethritis. Abacterial mucopurulent discharge; the specimen is best obtained in the morning. Occasionally, prostatitis, seminal vesiculitis, trigonitis, or cystitis. Epididymitis never occurs.

Ocular Involvement. Mild conjunctivitis develops during the initial attack and clears within a few days. Acute iritis usually develops as a late event, even years afterward, in about 10%; rarely, it occurs during the first attack. Of all rheumatoid variants, Reiter's disease has the greatest incidence of this serious complication.

Mucocutaneous Lesions. Superficial ulcerations of the mouth are asymptomatic, evanescent, and often overlooked. Ulcers of the glans penis have circinate raised margins and become confluent. Hyperkeratotic papules develop prominently over plantar surfaces but also may be found over the palms, over the trunk extremities, and, in the circumcised patient, over the glans penis. Subungual brownish yellow hyperkeratotic lesions elevate and may separate the nails.

Joint Involvement. The lower extremities are mainly involved, clinically resembling rheumatoid arthritis. Typically, involvement is asymmetrical and polyarticular; rarely, it is symmetrical. It may be monoarticular. One knee joint is almost always affected. Involvement is not migratory as in rheumatic fever but is sustained in affected joints for the duration of the attack. An attack is rarely severe and may resemble gouty arthritis, especially when the large toe is involved. Reiter's disease does not respond to aspirin, corticosteroids, and gold as does rheumatoid arthritis.

Various forms of soft tissue involvement are often associated, most commonly Achilles tendinitis, plantar fasciitis, tenosynovitis of the fingers, periostitis, and spur formation of the heel.

Pain referable to the lower back and sacroiliac joints is usually present sometime during the acute attack.

After the acute attack subsides, subtle, intermittent symptoms develop about the lower back, representing sacroiliac and spondylitic inflammation, or involvement at these sites may progress silently, and it is only when roentgenograms are taken that extension of the disease becomes apparent.

COURSE

A single acute attack may undergo a complete and permanent remission without residual. In about half of the patients, recurrences are frequent, the rate of recurrence approximating 15% a year.[157] A complete remission of the individual attack may not take place, and the disease may persist and fluctuate in severity. Ongoing low-grade rheumatic activity in these chronically inflamed, destroyed, and deformed joints is represented by persistent synovial swelling, an elevated sedimentation rate, and progressive roentgenographic changes. A highly characteristic site of involvement is the plantar aspect of the calcaneus, where a painful periostitis produces a bony overgrowth.[149]

After repeated severe attacks, a striking and typical deformity of the foot develops, the so-called Launois deformity, consisting of dorsal subluxation and lateral deviation of the toes associated with a pes cavus.[158]

COMPLICATIONS

Aortic insufficiency and atrioventricular block are the most common late sequelae of Reiter's disease. The lesions resemble those usually associated with idiopathic ankylosing spondylitis. They are manifested late, generally in middle-aged men with atheromatous disease.[164]

During the acute phase of the disease, neurologic complications may develop, such as meningoencephalitis, acute psychosis, and cranial nerve lesions. The chronic phase of the disease may be accompanied by various neuropsychiatric disorders, most commonly seizures, personality changes (especially paranoia), and peripheral radiculopathies.

ROENTGENOGRAPHIC FINDINGS

Early, in mild arthritis, slight soft tissue thickening and minimal subchondral osteoporosis may be detected and are reversible. Later, the subchondral osteoporosis becomes pronounced and persistent, erosions develop, and the joint space narrows. Finally, destructive changes may ultimately lead to ankylosis. The roentgenographic features are indistinguishable from rheumatoid arthritis.

Peripheral Joints. There are destructive changes, usually about the interphalangeal and metacarpophalangeal joints of the toes and the knee and ankle, subluxation and lateral deviation of the toes, and cavus deformity (Fig. 13–24). The joints of the fingers and wrist are less commonly involved. Occasionally, there is ankylosis of small joints. Periosteal new bone formation is seen over the plantar aspect of the calcaneus (Fig. 13-25).

Sacroiliac Joints. Loss of definition and erosions of joint margins are seen. Early, there is periarticular sclerosis. Ultimately, bony ankylosis results and the adjacent bony sclerosis disappears (Fig. 13–26).

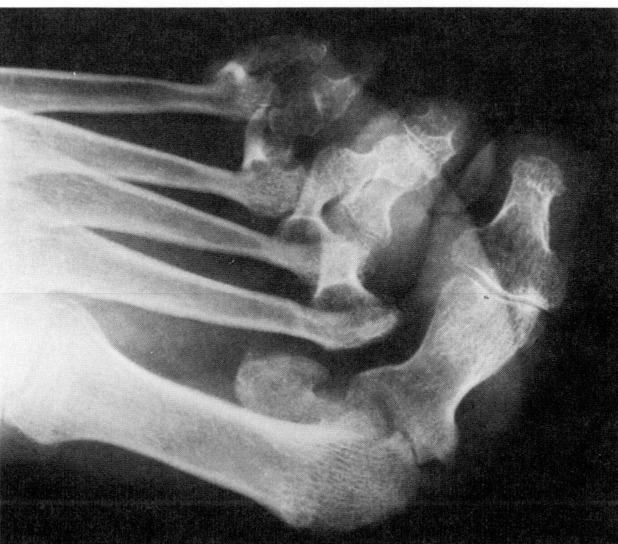

FIG. 13-24. Roentgenogram of a deformed foot in a patient with Reiter's disease. (Good AE: Reiter's disease: A review with special attention to cardiovascular and neurologic sequelae. Semin Arthritis Rheum 3:253, 1974)

Lumbar Spine. Focal asymmetrical changes about the apophyseal joints lead to bony ankylosis, mainly about the lower lumbar spine. Numerous syndesmophytes form as nonmarginal bony bridges that bypass the margins of the vertebral bodies as they vault to join each other (see Fig. 13-26). Teardrop-shaped paravertebral ossifications are characteristic.

LABORATORY FINDINGS

The laboratory findings are as follows:

- Negative tests for rheumatoid factor
- Normal synovial fluid complement levels
- Positive HLA-B27 histocompatibility antigen
- Biopsy of mouth, penile, and cutaneous lesions[168]
- Positive stool cultures for *Shigella, Yersinia,* or *Salmonella* organisms, especially following dysentery epidemic

DIFFERENTIAL DIAGNOSIS

In contrast to rheumatoid arthritis, Reiter's disease lacks the rheumatoid factor and antinuclear antibody, no rheumatoid subcutaneous nodules are found, and a high incidence of the histocompatibility antigen HLA-B27 is found. It should be emphasized that a small percentage of cases exhibiting the rheumatoid factor in low titer represents that normally found in the general population. Synovial biopsy is not helpful.[168]

Gonorrheal arthritis is excluded by absence of organ-

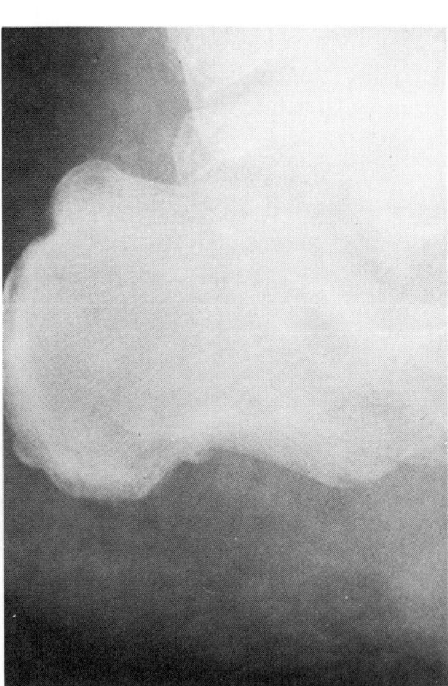

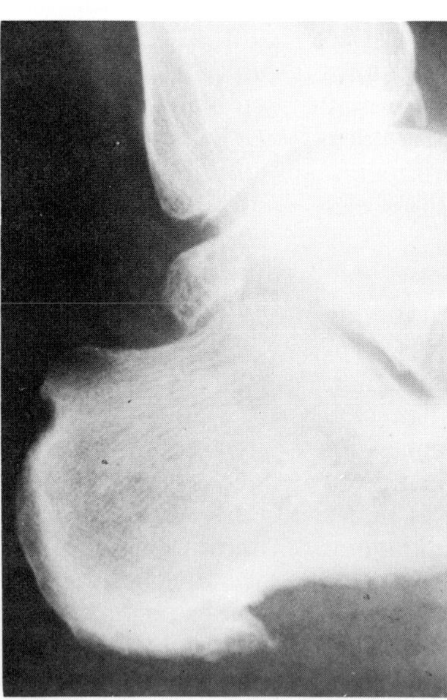

FIG. 13-25. Reiter's disease. Typical heel spur forming over a period of 5 years. (Courtesy of Dr. Armin E. Good)

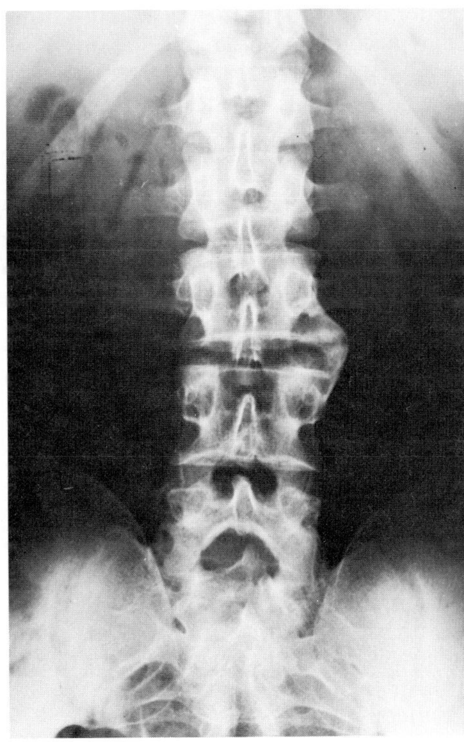
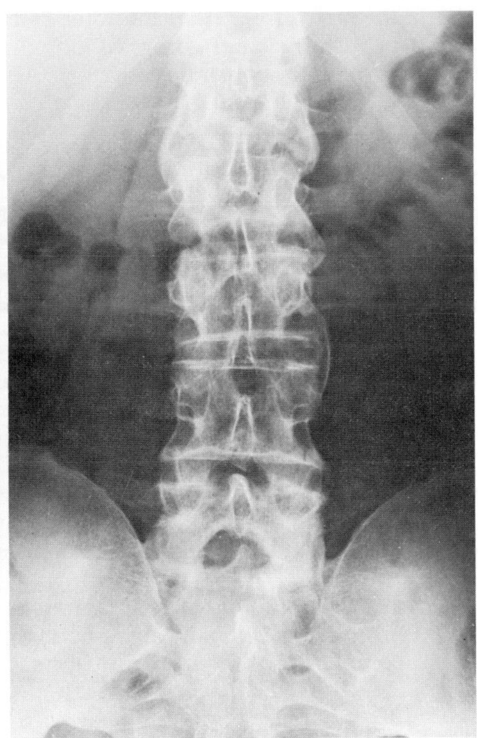

FIG. 13-26. Roentgenographic features of the lumbosacral spine in Reiter's disease. (*Left*) Five years after the onset of disease, a single beaked bony bridge is seen at the left margin of the third lumbar interspace. (*Right*) Nineteen years after Reiter's disease, the bridge has been remolded into a typical syndesmophyte, similar in appearance to intervertebral calcifications, which have appeared at T12–L1, L1–2, and L2–3. Note that the syndesmophytes typically bypass the margins of the vertebral bodies as they vault toward each other. The progression of sacroiliac changes from indefinable joint margins and juxta-articular sclerosis to complete ankylosis is well illustrated. (Good AE: Reiter's disease and ankylosing spondylitis. Acta Rheum Scand 11:305, 1965)

isms in synovial fluid. When an abacterial arthritis represents a reactive synovitis of true gonorrheal urethritis, the HLA-B27 antigen is usually absent and the disease readily responds to antibiotics. The histocompatibility antigen is normally present in approximately 7% of the general population.

TREATMENT

There is no specific treatment for Reiter's disease. Each acute attack is self-limited, and treatment is directed toward relieving pain and minimizing potential deformity. Although corticosteroids and ACTH may temporarily alleviate symptoms, the disease progresses, and their use in a self-limited condition is unwarranted. Occasionally, a single intra-articular injection of a long-acting corticosteroid preparation is permissible. Contrary to rheumatoid disease, Reiter's arthritis does not respond to gold injections. Administration of antibiotics is of no benefit.

The main objectives of orthopaedic treatment during an acute phase are prevention of deformity and preservation of mobility. The patient is placed at bed rest, and weight bearing is forbidden. Nonsteroidal anti-inflammatory drugs are prescribed, and a splint is applied and is removed at intervals for exercises and application of hot packs. During the chronic phase, residual deformity is managed in a manner identical to that for rheumatoid disease.

Medical management involves visceral, neurologic, and ophthalmologic complications. Monitoring of the eye during the acute stage and for years thereafter is prudent. During an acute attack, unless a secondary infection supervenes, prostatic massage is contraindicated, because it tends to provoke an acute exacerbation of symptoms.

In the vast number of instances, without treatment, the disease is self-limited, all symptoms ultimately subsiding with little or no residual.

ARTHRITIS OF INFLAMMATORY BOWEL DISEASE

Arthritis is a frequent manifestation of various inflammatory conditions of the intestine and is considered a seronegative spondyloarthropathy or rheumatoid variant similar to other diseases with certain characteristics, notably absence of rheumatoid factor, prevalence in males, a familial history, and a high incidence of the HLA-B27 histocompatibility antigen, particularly when the development of ankylosing inflammation of the spine is imminent.

CHRONIC INFLAMMATORY BOWEL DISEASE

In ulcerative colitis and regional enteritis (Crohn's disease), one of the major extraintestinal manifestations is a seronegative peripheral arthritis (10%–20% of cases).[165]

Erythema nodosum, oral ulcerations, and anterior uveitis (iridocyclitis) are other complications that may accompany flare-ups of bowel disease.[173,198] Ankylosing spondylitis or sacroiliitis also may develop (5%–15% of cases), but these are unrelated to the activity of the bowel disease.[165,199]

A mild oligoarticular arthritis usually follows the onset of the inflammatory bowel disease; rarely, the joint involvement may precede bowel symptoms. The knee, ankle, and wrist are the joints most often affected, and usually the inflammation is mild, although infrequently severe degrees of involvement may occur. About two or three such episodes occur during the course of the disease, each attack lasting a few months and subsiding completely or with minimal residual limitation of motion. Occasionally, an active arthritis may persist for years with partial remissions and exacerbations, but the prognosis for joint function is good even with recurrent attacks.[173] The radiographic changes are minor, consisting of soft tissue swelling, juxta-articular osteoporosis, and small erosions.

An ankylosing spondylitis or sacroiliitis indistinguishable from idiopathic ankylosing spondylitis is occasionally a complication of chronic inflammatory bowel disease. The HLA-B27 antigen, usually absent in patients with inflammatory bowel disease with peripheral arthritis, is present in most patients who ultimately develop ankylosing spinal disease or anterior uveitis. Consequently, the detection of this genetic marker in a patient with chronic inflammatory bowel disease indicates that the patient is at high risk for the ultimate development of these serious complications.[180]

Treatment. The peripheral arthritis generally responds to successful treatment of the bowel disease, including bowel resection.[198] Symptomatic treatment includes rest, application of hot packs, and administration of nonsteroidal anti-inflammatory drugs if well tolerated. A blood salicylate level of about 20 mg to 30 mg/dl is desirable if not contraindicated by the bowel problem. A single intra-articular injection of a long-acting corticosteroid preparation is effective.

The spondylitis and sacroiliitis are managed similar to idiopathic spondylitis. A single spinal dose of irradiation (600 rads–700 rads) may alleviate disabling pain and stiffness but should be reserved only for the rare patient unable to tolerate medication.

DYSENTERIC ARTHROPATHY

Sterile seronegative arthritis may infrequently be a complication of intestinal infection with *Shigella* or *Salmonella* and as many as 30% of cases of *Yeresinia.*[147,154,193] The joint symptoms follow a definite diarrheal illness, is usually mild and often prolonged, and may be accompanied by fever. Sometimes the arthritis is the only manifestation of the intestinal infection, and the latter can be detected only by stool cultures and agglutination tests. The typical course is one of a polyarthritis or arthralgia, usually asymmetrical, following within weeks the manifestations of abdominal pain and diarrhea, and subsiding over a period of weeks or months. The knee, ankle, and wrist are most commonly involved; ultimately, the sacroiliac joints and spine may develop an ankylosing inflammation. The arthritis fluctuates in activity and may be migratory, subsiding in some joints and appearing in others, not unlike rheumatic fever.

Carditis not infrequently accompanies the arthritis of *Yersinia enterocolitica.*[147] However, this is benign, is never accompanied by murmurs, and is detected only by transient electrocardiographic changes.

Diagnosis of dysenteric arthritis is made by stool cultures and agglutination tests.[147,193] Significantly, approximately 90% of patients with dysenteric arthropathy have the HLA-B27 histocompatibility antigen, generally reflecting the impending development of ankylosing spondylitis. A typical syndrome comparable to Reiter's disease seldom develops, and then usually with *Shigella* infection.

Treatment. Treatment with antibiotics is ineffective. Low-dose steroids and the nonsteroidal anti-inflammatory drugs provide symptomatic relief. The steroids should be used with caution for fear of precipitating a septicemia.

MISCELLANEOUS INTESTINAL DISORDERS

Arthritis and arthralgia are component manifestations of many syndromes in which pathology of the bowel is a prominent part of the disorder. A seronegative arthropathy may resemble and need to be differentiated from rheumatoid arthritis. The following are examples.

Whipple's disease is rare; it occurs most commonly in middle-aged men and is characterized by gastrointestinal cramping pain, diarrhea, and occult blood loss (89%); arthralgias (65%–90%); weight loss (60%); hypotension (63%); lymphadenopathy (52%); and various atypical symptoms, including spondylitis. Up to 30% of patients with Whipple's disease develop their joint pains 5 to 10 years before the onset of abdominal symptoms.[171,174] The diagnosis is made by finding densely packed periodic acid–Schiff (PAS)-positive macrophages in a small-bowel biopsy. Formerly regarded as a fatal disease, the disease can be cured by antibiotics.[171]

Behçet's syndrome is a rare multisystem disorder characterized by painful oral and genital ulcerations and iritis and frequently associated with arthritis of large joints and gastrointestinal manifestations. The colon displays discrete ulcerations reminiscent of ulcerative colitis, but the latter disease is not complicated by oral and genital ulcers or involvement of the central nervous system.

Episodes of oligoarticular, asymmetrical arthritis frequently involve the knee, ankle, wrist, and elbow, and each attack is often associated with malaise, low-grade fever, exacerbation of oral and genital ulcerations, and erythema nodosum. Multiple exacerbations and remissions of arthritis take place over the years, although the synovitis may persist unabated for many months. Despite the prolonged smoldering synovitis, the outlook for preservation of joint function with little or no deformity or roentgenographic change is good. Sacroiliac and axial spinal involvement are rare. In marked contrast, ankylosing inflammation of these joints is common in ulcerative colitis.[155,176]

Arthritis is a well-recognized complication of jejunocolic or jejunoileal bypass procedures (25% of cases) done for morbid obesity with hyperlipidemia. Articular involvement, most often affects the knees, wrists, ankles, and fingers. In most cases, the joint symptoms remit spontaneously or respond, within a few weeks, to low-dose steroids or nonsteroidal anti-inflammatory drugs. Weeks or months later, however, the symptoms may recur. The symptoms subside completely after 2 or 3 years. When surgical restoration of bowel continuity is done, the arthropathy is relieved. The arthritis is rarely minimally erosive or deforming.[161,192]

PALINDROMIC RHEUMATISM

Palindromic rheumatism is a rare, benign condition characterized by multiple recurring attacks of painful inflammation affecting joints and adjacent tissues.[200,201] The cause is unknown. Each attack lasts but a few hours to 1 or 2 days and is followed by a complete remission. All joints are liable to involvement, but the finger joints are predisposed. The typical attack begins very suddenly, usually late in the afternoon. Within a few minutes a joint may become painfully swollen, reaching its intensity within a few hours. The periarticular soft tissues are reddened and swollen, the overlying skin stretched and shiny. Disability is mild. No constitutional effects are associated (as contrasted with weight loss, anemia, fever in rheumatoid arthritis). Involvement of the soft tissues overlying muscles consists of a painful swelling, an inch or more in diameter, which is brawny, firm, and tender but does not itch or burn (in contrast with the swelling of angioneurotic edema). Favored sites of swellings are the bottoms of heels, finger pads, distal phalanges, flexor surfaces of forearms, thumb pads, and Achilles tendons. Occasionally, a subcutaneous nodule may be palpable in the hand. Laboratory and roentgenographic findings are negative. Pathology consists of low-grade inflammation that completely subsides without residual damage. No treatment is known, although gold compounds have been used successfully.[202] The condition is chronic but may be cured spontaneously or reduced in severity in a majority of cases over the years.

NEUROARTHROPATHY

A neuropathic joint (Charcot's joint) is one associated with central or peripheral nerve lesions and characterized pathologically by extreme destruction, pronounced new bone formation, and elongation of the supportive structures and clinically by painlessness and abnormal mobility.

ETIOLOGY

Ninety percent of cases occur in conjunction with tabes dorsalis and occur mainly in the lower extremity. Most of the remainder are associated with syringomyelia and are seen mainly in the upper extremity. Rare cases apparently are related to peripheral nerve lesions (including leprosy) and various spinal cord and cerebral lesions, notably arteriosclerotic degenerative disease.

The actual mechanism of production is unknown. Eloesser showed experimentally that trauma to an anesthetic joint will result in changes comparable with a Charcot joint.[203] Unexplained, however, is involvement of a single joint in an extremity, whereas the other equally anesthetic joints remain undisturbed.

Males are predisposed. The areas of predilection in decreasing order of frequency are knee, foot, ankle, hip, spine, elbow, shoulder, and wrist.

PATHOLOGY

The picture is typified by destruction, reactive sclerosis, large exostoses, multiple loose intra-articular bodies, deformity, subluxation and dislocation, and marked parosteal ossification. When destruction and osteoporosis predominate, the atrophic or degenerative type is present. The hypertrophic or proliferative type is characterized by excess bone formation in the form of extremely dense sclerosis, large osteophytes, and parosteal ossification. Usually, both types are present in the same joint.[204,207]

GROSS APPEARANCE

The capsule is thickened and hyperplastic. It is stretched by repeated effusions of large amounts of synovial fluid until it becomes redundant. Its attachments about the joint margins become progressively displaced distally as the articulating bone ends are destroyed. The articular aspect of the capsule is lined by a ragged synovial membrane from which villi grow inward, particularly at the joint line. The membrane contains cartilaginous and bony plaques some of which are partially extruded, remaining attached by a pedicle, while others are completely separated and lie free within the joint cavity. The ligaments are stretched, permitting unusual mobility of one bone upon the other. The articular cartilage is degenerate and worn away. The exposed subchondral bone is necrotic, fractured, and compressed or eroded. The underlying cancellous bone may be porous and filled with debris. More commonly, reactive sclerosis forms dense bone that replaces the cancellous bone. A pannus of granulation tissue may extend over and absorb the articular cartilage. Marginal exostoses form by reactivated endochondral ossification and are usually massive. The joint cavity is filled with debris of pieces of necrotic bone and cartilage. In the neighboring muscles and fascia, heterotopic bone formation takes place.

MICROSCOPIC APPEARANCE

The capsule exhibits fibroblastic proliferation, organizing hemorrhage due to tears, and bone formation by metaplasia or preceded by cartilage formation. The articular cartilage displays typical degeneration (*i.e.*, loss of matrix, fibrillations, and fissuring). Where it is not worn away by bony contact, it is eroded by a pannus. Within the bone, multiple small fractures and areas of necrotic bone are seen. In some areas osteoclastic resorption of dead bone takes place. In the immediate vicinity, active bone formation replaces the cancellous trabeculae with dense laminated compact bone. When bone replacement is deficient, the marrow spaces become filled with amorphous debris and subject to erosion.

CLINICAL PICTURE

Trauma with or without fracture frequently initiates the condition. A large amount of synovial fluid greatly distends the joint, and the overlying tissues appear edematous. The fluid when aspirated is abundant, yellow, and viscous and clots rapidly. The cell count is 500 to 2000/cu mm, mainly lymphocytes. Gradually, the swelling subsides, leaving a relaxed capsule and an abnormally mobile joint. For example, the knee will display lateral mobility or can be hyperextended. Over the ensuing weeks or months the joint becomes enlarged and deformed and even more unstable. Repeated joint effusions occur. Pain is notably absent. Examination of the joint reveals marked irregularities identified as bony projections from the articulating bones and bone formations in the surrounding soft tissues. Palpation of the redundant, soft, thickened capsule reveals many intra-articular bodies similar to a "bag of bones." The joint can be passively and painlessly moved in all directions.

In tabes dorsalis, the lower extremities and the spine are prone to involvement. Associated signs of tabes includes ataxia, Argyll Robertson pupils, absent knee reflexes, and absent deep position, vibration, and pain sense. Symptoms complained of are lancinating pains, girdle pains, paresthesias, gastric crises, and loss of bladder control.

In syringomyelia, glial proliferation and cavitation occur about the central canal of the cord in the lower cervical and upper dorsal region. Therefore, the arthropathy is confined mainly to the upper extremities. Clinically, one finds sensory dissociation—loss of pain and temperature, and preservation of touch. Deep sensation is undisturbed. Progressive muscle atrophy in the arms and fibrillations and trophic changes in the fingers are added findings. Most commonly, the elbow is involved. It is swollen with excess fluid, is destroyed, and displays abnormal lateral mobility, and bony masses in the soft tissues are greater than in tabes. The cervical spine when involved causes a kyphosis or scoliosis, but the cord is not involved.

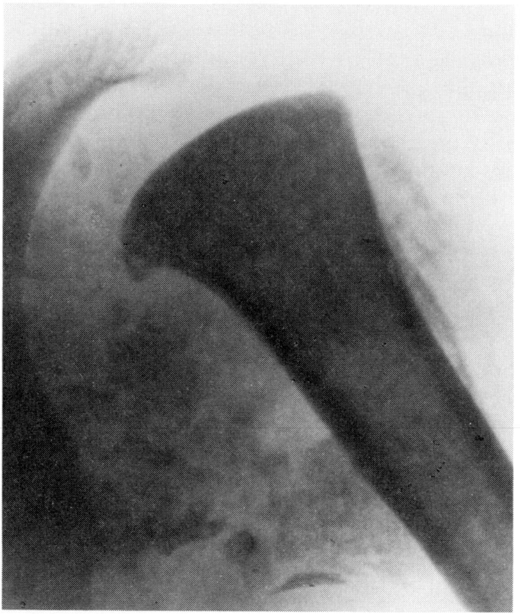

FIG. 13-27. Neurotrophic joint.

FIG. 13-28. Charcot knee.

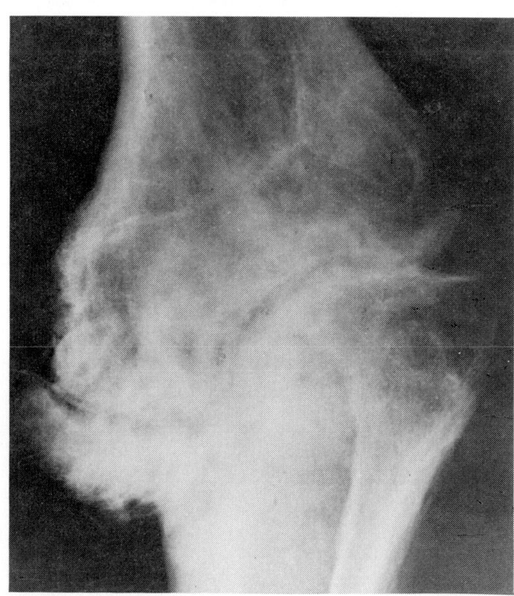

ROENTGENOGRAPHIC FINDINGS

At the time of the initial swelling, the roentgenograms are unrevealing. Gradually, over the ensuing weeks the joint surfaces become denser and yielding at points of bony contact and pressure. The surfaces disintegrate. Bone shadows appear in the periarticular soft tissues. The bone architecture beneath the articulating cortex becomes sclerosed. Free ossific bodies appear within the joint cavity. Large marginal exostoses develop. Pathologic fractures heal with considerable callus. In the knee, the medial femoral condyle is often the site of earliest changes. In the foot, the midtarsal joints are affected most frequently. Disintegration of the ankle may follow a Pott's fracture. Subluxation, dislocation, and deformity are late findings (Figs. 13-27 through 13-29).

TREATMENT

In the acute stage, the joint should be shielded from trauma of ordinary motion and weight bearing. The fluid should be aspirated and the limb immobilized in a cast. The limb is elevated until swelling is reduced. After the acute stage, the articulating bones are hardened and can be used with the proper support.[205]

Useful measures are as follows:

Knee. A straight caliper with an ischial fitting ring may be used. A leather corset about the knee may be added. In severe cases, arthrodesis is best but is difficult to obtain. A preliminary operation to improve circulation consists in drilling holes through the areas of sclerosis.[208] Several weeks later arthrodesis is done. The irregular sclerotic surfaces are resected, and two flat ends are apposed. Two cross grafts are inserted from femur to tibia after the method of Brittain. The compression apparatus of Charnley is applied, and the limb is suspended on a Thomas splint. Compression is gradually increased over the ensuing weeks until early fusion can be demonstrated. This is followed by prolonged immobilization in a cast, which is discontinued only when good bony bridging has occurred.

Ankle. A brace or ankle corset is used for mild cases, and crutches may be worn. Arthrodesis is best. The principles of drilling, grafts, fixation, compression, and prolonged immobilization should be followed.

Foot. Destruction is in the distal tarsal area where fusion is almost impossible. Special shoes with steel arch supports plus a cane will permit ambulation. The danger of trophic ulcers with secondary infection is great. Weight

FIG. 13-29. Charcot ankle and foot.

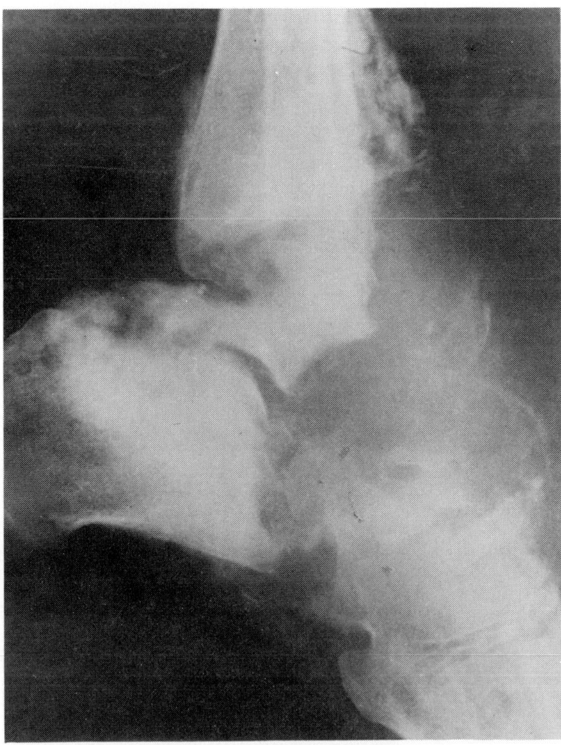

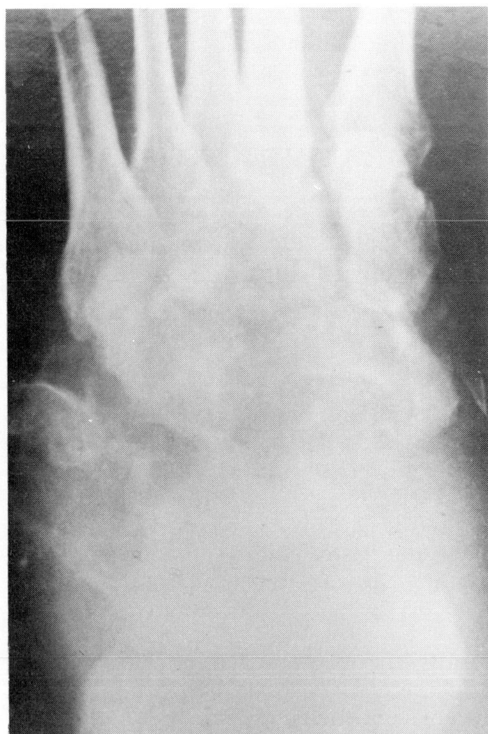

bearing should be limited or avoided and a metatarsal bar worn on the shoe. Extreme destruction warrants amputation.

Hip. Extreme destruction followed by subluxation with loss of stability is usual. A subtrochanteric Shanz osteotomy with 30° of abduction provides stability.

Spine. A corset or jacket may be worn. However, progression of deformity is usual. A spine fusion is indicated.

Elbow. Disability is minimal. A leather-hinged corset that permits only flexion and extension movement improves function.

NEUROGENIC ARTHROPATHY ASSOCIATED WITH DIABETES MELLITUS

In diabetic patients of advanced age, with severe arteriosclerosis and poorly regulated diabetes of long standing, a Charcot type of arthropathy may occur.[206] The foot is prone to involvement, a painless swelling without inflammatory signs appearing in the tarsal area. Roentgenograms reveal destruction and fragmentation. Trauma frequently initiates the condition. Additional symptoms of night pain and paresthesias and findings of loss of reflexes and vibratory sense imply peripheral nerve changes. The spinal fluid protein and cell count are increased. Inadequate circulation makes conservative treatment mandatory.

SUPPURATIVE ARTHRITIS

An acute arthritis (pyrogenic arthritis) due to specific bacteria and productive of purulent exudate is designated a suppurative arthritis.

ETIOLOGY

Predisposing Factors. Children are most commonly affected. An infective focus frequently precedes. Trauma to the joint often initiates the onset.

Exciting Factors. *Staphylococcus aureus* or *Staphylococcus albus* and hemolytic streptococci are the most common exciting causes. Less common are pneumococcus, meningococcus, gonococcus, and typhoid.

Mode of Infection. The mode is often hematogenous from an infective focus. Less commonly, it is spread from an adjacent focus, especially osteomyelitis, or by direct introduction through a wound.

Areas of Predilection. The most common sites are the knee, hip (especially in infants), and shoulder.

PATHOLOGY

Basically, the condition is an acute synovitis that varies in degree, depending on the virulence of the organism and the resistance of the tissues. In a mild case the synovium is congested, edematous, and infiltrated with polymorphonuclear leukocytes. Serum exudes into the joint cavity where it admixes with an increased amount of synovial fluid and deposits flakes of fibrin over the inner lining of the joint. The serous fluid is clear or slightly opaque and contains a slight amount of polymorphonuclear leukocytes. The synovial sac is greatly distended by the large amount of fluid. The condition is designated as serous arthritis or, when precipitation of fibrin is excessive, as serofibrinous arthritis. When inflammation is more intense, congestion, edema, and leukocytic infiltration are greater in degree. Areas of vascular thrombosis and focal necrosis occur. The joint exudate contains a large number of polymorphonuclear leukocytes, as high as several hundred thousand per cubic millimeter, and therefore is very opaque, thick, and gray or yellowish gray. Proteolytic enzymes originating from the polymorphonuclear leukocytes dissolve the articular cartilage and may even erode the bone. The intense intra-articular pressure causes necrosis and destruction of intra-articular soft tissues and capsule, the exudate erupting into the surrounding soft tissues and even through the skin. This is the typical purulent arthritis characteristic of staphylococcal infections. When a hemolytic streptococcus is the causative organism, the infection is fulminating and quickly destructive. The synovial inflammatory signs are intense, vascular thrombosis and necrosis are extreme, and hemorrhagic extravasations are seen. The defenses are not as adequate as in the case of staphylococci, so polymorphonuclear leukocytes are not as numerous. The exudation into the joint consists of a bloody serous fluid typical of serosanguineous arthritis. The danger of a fatal septicemia is greatest in this type.

Healing in the mild serous form takes place by resolution. The serous exudate is resorbed, and inflammation of the synovium subsides, the joint returning to normal. The more serious destructive arthritis requires not only the resorption of purulent exudate but also repair by granulation tissue (resolution and organization), which bridges the joint and eventuates in fibrous ankylosis. The capsule becomes fibrotic, thickened, and inelastic. Loss of articular cartilage exposes the bone to mechanical trauma, resulting in degenerative arthritis.

Acute suppurative arthritis of the hip, which occurs most often in infants, presents an unusual situation. The femoral head is composed almost entirely of cartilage that lies completely within the articular cavity. The distention of the capsule by the exudate shuts off the circulation to the head, and the enzymatic action dissolves the cartilage. In consequence, the femoral head disintegrates, and subluxation and dislocation result. Because the ossification center does not normally appear until the sixth or seventh month and may be delayed by the infection, a pathologic dislocation of the hip may not be recognized until the walking age.

CLINICAL PICTURE

A history of antecedent trauma and infection may be obtained.

Symptoms. Pain gradually increases in intensity over several hours, eventually becoming excruciating. It is accentuated by joint movement and, in the case of the lower extremity, by weight bearing. Constitutional symptoms of an acute infection include chills, fever, sweats, malaise, anorexia, and, in infants, nausea and vomiting.

Findings. The patient limps if the lower extremity is involved. Usually, only one joint is affected. The joint is swollen, red, warm, and tender throughout, and the position is one of partial flexion. The swelling consists of increased joint fluid, which may obliterate the markings. In the case of the knee, the patella is floating. In a gonorrheal arthritis, a peculiar soft tissue edema surrounds the joint. The muscles are in protective spasm. The temperature is elevated, spiking daily as high as 104° F.

In the hip the thigh is held in flexion, abduction, and external rotation, because this is the position of greatest relaxation of the capsule. Pain is referred along the inner side of the thigh to the medial aspect of the knee.

LABORATORY FINDINGS

Aspirated joint fluid is serous, serosanguineous, or frankly purulent. Microscopically, the offending organism may be identified. The fluid is cultured, and the bacteria are tested for susceptibility to antibiotics.

There is a high leukocytosis, with polymorphonuclear leukocytes predominating, an increased sedimentation rate, and a positive C-reactive protein.

ROENTGENOGRAPHIC FINDINGS

Films are generally negative at the outset. However, ballooning of the synovial sac may be interpreted from the rounded soft tissue outlines and density peculiar to purulent exudate. If the infection persists, osteoporosis of all bones adjacent to the joint takes place. With destruction of cartilage, narrowing of the joint interval occurs. Degenerative arthritis supervenes as a late sequela. A neighboring osteomyelitis may be revealed.

The obturator sign is diagnostic of hip involvement. A soft tissue shadow is normally seen over the lateral wall of the pelvis and medial to the acetabulum. When the joint is distended by fluid, the shadow bulges inwardly, becoming very prominent by comparison with the opposite side. The obturator internus is presumably the structure involved. The sign affords a valuable diagnostic aid in infants.

TREATMENT

Drainage. In suppurative joint disease, immediate and free, dependent drainage is mandatory. The proteolytic action and pressure of the exudate are very destructive. Fatal septicemia, bone infection, and, if infection is overcome, a disabling ankylosis are complications that can be avoided by early diagnosis and instituting drainage. Aspirations are mentioned only to be condemned. The exudate rapidly reaccumulates, and destruction continues. Repeated insertion of a needle may introduce additional infection. One should not judge an infection as "mild" and depend on aspirations and antibiotics. Although many cases can be handled by such conservative treatment, an occasional case will progress and threaten local structures and even life itself. Energetic surgical measures should not be executed as an afterthought. As with any other surgical infection, given the opportunity the body defenses will eliminate the infection. The joint is opened on two sides to provide through-and-through gravity drainage. Gutta-percha drains may be inserted to prevent premature closure and are removed in 24 to 48 hours. The synovium is not sutured. It will close spontaneously and rapidly when infection is controlled. The only exception to surgical drainage is gonococcal infection, which responds promptly to penicillin.

Antibiotics. Antibiotics are given in adequate amounts. Penicillin or a cephalosporin, which combats most gram-positive organisms, may be combined with an aminoglycoside, which is effective against gram-negative organisms. Administration of aminoglycosides (*e.g.*, tobramycin) requires monitoring for ototoxicity and nephrotoxicity. In adults, 3 to 5 mg/kg/day of tobramycin sulfate is administered intravenously or intramuscularly in three or four equal doses. In children 6 to 7.5 mg/kg/day is given in equally divided doses every 8 hours. High doses of penicillin or cephalosporin are likewise administered. The so-called broad-spectrum antibiotics, such as chlortetracycline and oxytetracycline, may be substituted. Because antibiotics do not readily pass through inflamed synovium, the antibiotics may be introduced directly into the joint by constant drip. Meanwhile, culture and sensitivity studies will identify the offending organism and the appropriate antibiotic.

Immobilization. The limb is immobilized in a removable splint such as a folded blanket and is elevated. The position of function must be maintained in the event that ankylosis ensues. Movement during the acute stage is forbidden.However, in the subacute subsiding stage the joint should be moved gently and passively each day as a precaution against formation of ankylosing adhesions. When the hip or the knee is involved, traction is advisable. It immobilizes the joint, distracts the articular surfaces, thereby reducing damage due to pressure, and affords convenience for changes of dressings.

Supportive Therapy. Supportive treatment includes fluids, transfusions, a highly nourishing diet, and sedation.

The temperature usually falls to normal, drainage subsides, and the wounds close spontaneously. In rare instances, if the infection progresses unabated and constitutes a serious menace to life, amputation is indicated.

A nonfunctional ankylosis resulting from suppurative arthritis should be treated with respect. Results of arthroplasty, except in cases in which the joint has been preserved, are disappointing. Arthrodesis in the position of function is best.

Pathologic dislocation of the hip can be handled by subtrochanteric osteotomy or arthrodesis.

GONOCOCCAL ARTHRITIS

Gonorrhea and its complicating arthritis has become an uncommon disease since the introduction of antibiotics. However, one must be on guard to recognize and treat immediately the occasional case of gonorrheal infection because of its destructiveness to the joint. It is possible for gonorrhea to lie dormant for many years and suddenly make its appearance as a genitourinary infection, arthritis or conjunctivitis. Pelvic surgical procedures and urethral instrumentation have been known to provoke the infection. The appearance of an arthritis following these procedures should arouse suspicion.

PATHOLOGY

The process is similar to other forms of suppurative arthritis. The synovium is congested, edematous, and infiltrated with polymorphonuclear leukocytes. The articular cartilage is digested by the tryptic substances in the pus. A large amount of synovial fluid contains a preponderance of polymorphonuclear leukocytes. Sugar content of the fluid is decreased. Healing takes place by fibrosis of the synovium, and fibrous adhesions bridge the joint, resulting in ankylosis. Bony ankylosis is uncommon.

CLINICAL AND LABORATORY FINDINGS

Usually within 3 weeks after an acute gonorrheal urethritis, a polyarticular arthritis develops, most commonly in the knees, the wrists, and the ankles. The joints become hot, swollen, reddened, tender, and distended with a large amount of fluid. The periarticular tissues present a peculiar diffuse edematous boggy swelling. Pain becomes severe. Tenosynovitis, particularly about the ankles and the wrists, is a frequent accompaniment. The temperature rises as high 104° F. A high polymorphonuclear leukocytosis and an increased sedimentation rate are laboratory findings. The complement fixation test is not of value unless a negative test becomes positive during the course of the disease. After a few days, the arthritic symptoms and findings subside but may persist in one joint as a resistant monoarthritis. If untreated, the destruction of articular tissues eventuates in ankylosis. Typical gonorrheal arthritis is self-limited and runs its course in about 3 months.

DIAGNOSIS

The organism is identified on a direct smear of aspirated fluid or by culture.

TREATMENT

The gonococcus is highly susceptible to penicillin. It is unnecessary to inject the antibiotic intra-articularly. The affected joints are put at rest by splinting. The splints are removed daily for passive motion to break up soft newly formed adhesions. The position of function is sought in the event that ankylosis takes place. After the acute stage, physical therapy is instituted to restore full motion to the joint and strength to the atrophied muscles.

Ankylosed joints, particularly when destruction is not too far advanced, are suitable candidates for arthroplasty. When loss of joint surfaces has resulted in a painful degenerative arthritis or a deformity, arthrodesis in the functional position is best.

HEMOPHILIC ARTHRITIS

Hemophilia is a hereditary coagulatory disorder characterized by the occurrence of hemorrhages that appear spontaneously or as a result of insignificant trauma; these are most common in a joint and result from prolonged coagulation time of the blood.[213,220,226]

ETIOLOGY

The condition is genetically determined, is due to a deficiency of factors VIII, IX, or XI, and most often has a sex-linked mendelian recessive transmission from the affected male through the unaffected female offspring to another male. This is a rare condition, and the incidence is approximately 3 to 4 per 100,000.

Hemophilia may be classified according to the specific factor deficiency.

HEMOPHILIA A

Also known as classic hemophilia, hemophilia A constitutes 80% of cases. It is due to a congenital deficiency of factor VIII, the antihemophilic factor or antihemophilic globulin. This is a large protein molecule that must be administered intravenously because it undergoes degradation when given by oral or intramuscular routes.

Classic hemophilia occurs in the male, and the gene is carried on the X chromosome and is transmitted by the unaffected female. Theoretically, the female offspring of a hemophiliac father and a carrier mother can be affected, but this must be an extreme rarity.

HEMOPHILIA B

Also known as Christmas disease, hemophilia B is caused by a deficiency of factor IX, the plasma thromboplastin component or Christmas factor. It too is transmitted by a gene linked to the X chromosome and is clinically identical to hemophilia A. It comprises 15% of cases.

HEMOPHILIA C

Hemophilia C is a mild form of the disease that occurs in both males and females. It is due to a deficiency of factor XI, the precursor of thromboplastin termed plasma thromboplastin antecedent. It has an autosomal dominant inheritance.

VON WILLEBRAND'S DISEASE

von Willebrand's disease is the syndrome that develops when both factor VIII and platelets are deficient.

PATHOLOGY

Blood mixed with synovial fluid acts as an irritant to the synovial membrane. Removal of blood from the joint is achieved by the synovium, where hemosiderin can be seen intracellularly within the superficial cellular layer, and by macrophages and leukocytes in the subsynovial stratum, where erythrocytes can be seen disintegrating. This is the normal resorptive mechanism, which eventually becomes exhausted, and hemosiderin accumulates in large amounts both in the synovium and in the articular cartilage. The synovial membrane, reflecting its increased function, undergoes hyperplasia and villous formation at the surface, becomes hypervascular, and develops reactive granulation tissue and fibrosis. Perivascular cuffing with both polymorphonuclear leukocytes and mononuclears is reminiscent of similar findings in rheumatoid arthritis. The reactive granulation tissue forms a pannus that absorbs the articular cartilage at its peripheral margins, but not to the degree seen in rheumatoid arthritis.

Because of deposition of iron within the cartilage, there is interference with chondrocytic metabolism. Moreover, diffusion of nutrient substances and lubrication of the articular cartilage become ineffective. It has been demonstrated that neutrophilic leukocytes in particular, and lymphocytes and mononuclears to a lesser degree, on engulfing the foreign products, release a procollagenase, which in turn is converted to a collagenase.[114] In addition, various other enzymatically active proteases are phagocytically released from human leukocytes (*e.g.*, β-glucuronidase, elastase, and neutral protease). The pannus of a rheumatoid joint, and perhaps that of a hemophiliac joint, has the ability to activate the collagenase precursor and to invade and degrade the articular cartilage.[222] As a consequence, the cartilage loses its matrix components; becomes soft, yellowish, and mechanically unable to withstand stresses, particularly vertical loads; microscopically develops vertical clefting and chondron formation similar to that seen in osteoarthritis; and breaks down. Loss of surface cartilage as it is eroded occurs in an irregular manner so as to produce a highly characteristic maplike appearance (Color Plate 13-2). The subchondral cortex, instead of developing reactive sclerosis typical of primary osteoarthritis, becomes thinned and worn through. Subchondral hemorrhages in the porotic bone are presumed to produce cysts by engulfing the fine trabeculae, which, deprived of their circulation, necrose and absorb. The process of bone resorption has not been clearly defined.

During the growth period, perhaps because of the hyperemia, the epiphyses about the affected joint become enlarged, often asymmetrically producing gross deformity (*e.g.*, varus or valgus). The rate of longitudinal growth may be increased or retarded, but early closure of the epiphyseal plate is usual.

Irregularities of the opposing articular surfaces lead to secondary osteoarthritic changes. At the hip joint, breakdown of the acetabular roof invites subluxation. The femoral head, when affected during the early growth period, develops changes mimicking Legg-Calvé-Perthes disease. At the knee joint, progressive capsular contracture causes marked restriction of motion and posterior subluxation of the tibia. At all joints the chronic deformity is generally a flexion contracture.

Hemorrhages may occur as large, progressive accumulations of blood within muscles or between muscles and their sheaths or in the vascular subperiosteal area where they remain as slowly enlarging "pseudotumors" or "hemophilic cysts," becoming encircled by a fibrous capsule and often developing ossifications, especially when the pseudotumor extends beneath and strips up the periosteum.[219] These are potentially life-threatening situations because they may suddenly expand, erode the surface of the bone so as to invite a pathologic fracture, or extend outward, bursting through the skin and resulting in a fatal hemorrhage or becoming secondarily infected. Moreover, the pseudotumor may compress vital nerve or vascular structures. Ill-advised attempts to aspirate the swelling or attempt a biopsy through a small incision often cause uncontrollable secondary infection, septicemia, and death. Immediate removal may be indicated.

Hemorrhage within the iliacus muscle is common in hemophiliacs, causing distention within its sheath and forming an enlarging mass in the iliac fossa. This is a closed compartment that contains the femoral nerve and the iliacus muscle, so therefore the femoral nerve is often involved and occasionally the iliac bone is eroded. Should the bleeding continue, the hematoma extends into the psoas sheath with which the iliacus sheath communicates, and a second fusiform tumorlike mass forms. At surgery, the femoral nerve is observed to traverse the cavity and is completely surrounded by the blood clot. The iliac vessels lie in front of the iliacus sheath and are displaced forward by the hematoma but are not completely occluded.

A hemorrhage may develop within a firmly closed fascial space, such as the volar compartment of the forearm and the posterior compartment of the leg, and unless immediately recognized and decompressed will lead to Volkmann's contracture or at least partial muscle fibrosis and contracture. Since the iliacus sheath is easily distensible, ischemic necrosis of the muscle does not take place, and following resorption of the hematoma, complete muscle recovery can be anticipated.

CLINICAL PICTURE

A history of bleeding occurring spontaneously or as a result of trivial trauma is typical. The patient is a man who describes many incidents of uncontrollable hemorrhage following tooth extraction or minor cuts and bruises and most commonly into and about joints. Acute hemarthrosis occurs in one joint as a rapid effusion, with marked swelling developing within a few minutes to several hours. The knee is involved most often; less often involved are the ankle, the elbow, and the hip. The swelling follows the outline of the synovial cavity. The pain is severe; the joint feels warm, and its position is one of maximal relaxation of the capsule (*e.g.*, partial flexion at the knee and elbow; partial flexion and slight abduction and external rotation at the hip). The acute phase lasts for a few days to several weeks. After the blood is absorbed, the chronic synovitis persists for many weeks and months as a tender, sore, painful, and swollen joint, and the swollen, boggy synovial tissue may be palpable most prominently at the suprapatellar area of the knee. With each attack, joint motion becomes progressively more limited and the joint becomes more thickened and deformed, generally in a fixed flexion position. Additionally, at the hip and shoulder, rotation is likewise restricted. Degenerative arthritic changes supervene at an early age, and the symptoms and findings correspond to the joint involved and its deformity. A fibrous ankylosis may ensue. The musculature about the joint becomes atrophied; this is most pronounced in the quadriceps femoris. The final picture of deformity may resemble the end stage of rheumatoid arthritis.

Large bulbous tumorlike hematomas may develop along the shafts of long bones or within the large muscles that envelop these bones, producing the characteristic hemophilic pseudotumors or hemophilic cysts mentioned earlier. The large accumulation of blood may destroy the overlying muscles and skin, with terminal external hemorrhage; it may form a chronically oozing sinus that becomes secondarily infected, leading to a fatal septicemia; it may erode the bony cortex and partially destroy the shaft, producing deformity and susceptibility to fracture; or, when hemorrhage appears to be subperiosteal in origin, it may be delimited for a long time by the thick periosteal covering, causing reactive periosteal ossification, and may be palpable as a slowly growing and deceptively benign tumor. It may suddenly rupture out of its retaining envelope and as a massive hemorrhage cause necrosis of overlying soft tissues and extension through the skin. The mass may compress vital nerve and vascular structures.[219,224]

The pseudotumors most often occur within, or are related to, powerful muscle groups, such as the iliopsoas, quadriceps femoris, triceps surae, gluteus maximus, and forearm muscles.

Hemorrhage within the iliacus muscle is common and easily distends the overlying iliacus sheath, forming an enlarging mass in the iliac fossa. Clinically, the initial complaint is severe and constant pain at the groin, spreading upward to the lumbar area or distally along the thigh. Spasm of the iliacus muscle causes the hip to be held in a curled-up position for comfort (*i.e.*, flexion and external rotation), and any attempt to extend the hip intensifies the pain. Under anesthesia, the hip can be fully extended, thus differentiating the deformity from a hemarthrosis within the hip joint. Femoral nerve palsy is a frequent, although not invariable, accompaniment because the femoral nerve traverses the iliacus compartment. The quadriceps femoris is paralyzed, the patellar reflex is absent, and loss of cutaneous sensation is limited to the area of distribution of the femoral nerve (anterior aspect of the distal two thirds of the thigh and anteromedial aspect of the proximal two thirds of the leg). When sensory loss is minimal because of nerve overlap, the skin over the patella is always anesthetic. Rarely, the lateral femoral cutaneous nerve is involved. A mass in the iliac fossa becomes palpable after a few days and obliterates the normal concavity to the inner aspect of the ilium. Occasionally, a second mass develops within the psoas sheath and is palpable medial to the first mass. Under appropriate factor-replacement therapy, the iliacus pseudotumor recedes, the flexion deformity at the hip subsides, and the femoral nerve deficit clears up gradually over a number of months.

Hemorrhage within firm fascial compartments, such

as the volar compartment of the forearm and the posterior compartment of the leg, causes severe local pain due to ischemic necrosis of muscle, and as it recedes it leaves a weak, fibrotic, and contracted muscle, Myostatic contracture of forearm muscles results in Volkmann's contracture and that of calf muscles results in an equinus deformity that yields only to lengthening of the Achilles tendon.

When hemarthrosis occurs in the hip before puberty, changes occur in the epiphysis similar to those in Legg-Calvé-Perthes disease, resulting in a stiff hip limp and limitation of abduction and internal rotation. Bleeding into the hip during the adult period results in changes described as secondary osteoarthritis.

ROENTGENOGRAPHIC FINDINGS

Roentgenographically visible joint changes first become apparent at about 6 years of age, after several bleeding episodes.[226] When medical treatment is inadequate, the changes develop rapidly. However, in the severe form of hemophilia, when the plasma level of circulating factor is below 5%, the arthropathy may continue to progress despite adequate treatment.[214] The process may be categorized roentgenographically according to early changes that are reversible and late changes of destruction (Fig. 13-30).

Early Stage. The initial acute hemarthrosis is characterized by a rounded, bulged-out soft tissue density produced by the hemorrhage-distended capsule. No para-articular skeletal abnormalities are seen.

Chronic Intermediate Stage. Persistent, hyperplastic, congested, boggy, swollen synovium and reactive para-articular skeletal changes produce the following roentgenographic features: osteoporosis, particularly of the epiphyses; overgrowth, sometimes asymmetrical, of the epiphyses; occasional early closure of the epiphyseal plate; and preservation of the joint interval (cartilage thickness unchanged). Later, subchondral cavities (cysts) form and may communicate with the joint space. There is squaring of the patella, and the intercondylar notch of the femur and the trochlear notch of the ulna are widened. This is the final stage at which the arthropathy is reversible by treatment.

End Stage of Destruction. At first, gradual narrowing of the joint interval reflects progressive loss of articular cartilage. Then the subchondral cortex becomes irregular, interrupted, and indistinct. Subchondral bone cysts become pronounced. The ends of the bones become markedly disorganized. When surgery is performed at this stage, one finds little or no recognizable synovium, and the articular cartilage is absent over a widespread area, exposing irregular demineralized bone. At the late stage of fibrous ankylosis, degenerative changes supervene (*e.g.*, sclerosis, osteophyte formation).

At the site of a pseudotumor, a bulbous opacity lies in close approximation to the cortex of the adjacent bone, and a bony defect varies from a slight saucer-shaped defect to a deep erosion; however, the circumscribed soft tissue density may appear to lie within the soft tissues remote from the bone. It may evolve slowly or rapidly, or an apparent indolent mass may suddenly enlarge. The most common locations for a hemophilic pseudotumor are the anterior thigh, calf, inner aspect of the ilium, and volar aspect of the forearm. When an iliacus tumor is suspected, an angiogram may reveal that the iliac vessels are displaced forward but are not occluded.

TREATMENT

With the discovery of factor deficiencies and the availability of lyophilized concentrates, the outlook for control of bleeding episodes and their destructive phenomena has dramatically improved. It is now possible to intervene surgically, not only for acute situations (*e.g.*, fractures) that pose massive life- and limb-threatening hemorrhages, but also on an elective basis (*e.g.*, total joint replacement). A multidisciplinary approach to treatment is led by the hematologist and orthopaedic surgeon. The orthopaedic management of any problem requires a hematologist who is skilled in the treatment of coagulation disorders and has access to a laboratory capable of performing accurate factor assays.

MEDICAL MANAGEMENT

Hemostasis is best achieved by replacement of the missing factor using concentrates of the needed clotting factor obtained from fresh frozen plasma.[211,231] A lyophilized cryoprecipitate containing either factor VIII or factor IX permits administration in small volume, decreasing the risk of circulatory overload. Although the lyophilized preparations are obtained from large donor lots, significant titers of A and B isoagglutinins may be present and may cause a hemolytic anemia in patients with red cell type A, B, or AB. Moreover, despite screening of donors, hepatitis is still a problem, especially when factor IX concentrates are given.

Before administering the deficient factor, it is necessary to determine the presence of inhibitors (antibodies) in the recipient. Inhibitors are said to occur in 6% to 20% of hemophiliacs. The efficacy of factor replacement may be reduced or rendered entirely ineffective by circulating antibodies, and their presence is a distinct contraindication to open surgical procedures. The inhibitor titer must be determined 7 to 14 days after a test dose of concentrate is administered.

REPLACEMENT THERAPY

The dosage needed to correct a factor deficiency is calculated on the basis of the patient's weight and

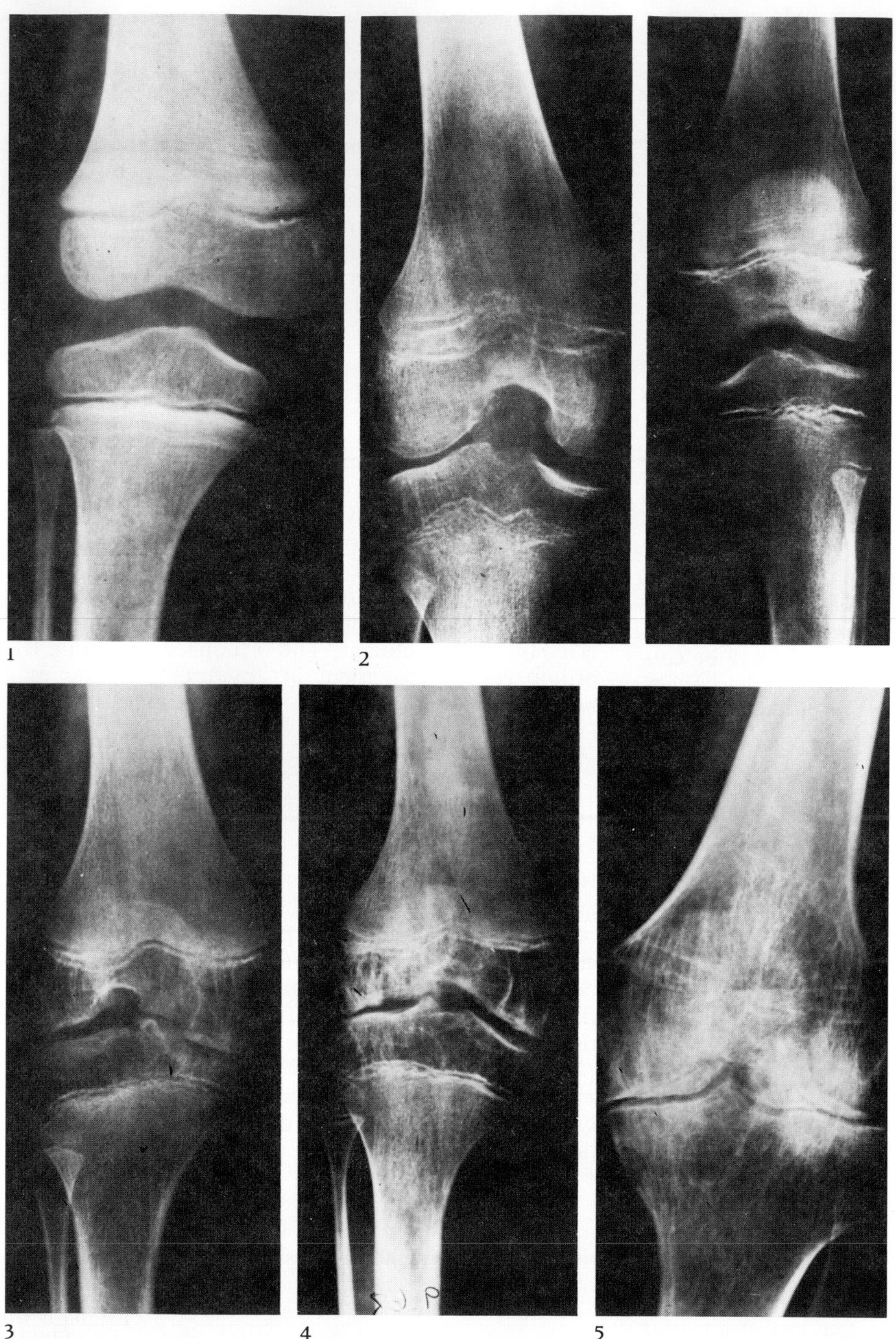

FIG. 13-30. Roentgenographic stages of hemophilic arthropathy. Stage 1: Soft tissue swelling (synovial thickening, blood in joint). Stage 2: Epiphyseal overgrowth, osteoporosis (integrity of joint space maintained). Stage 3: Marked epiphyseal overgrowth and osteoporosis, early incongruity (beginning cartilaginous destruction). Stage 4: Narrowing, cyst formation (advancing cartilaginous destruction); the femoral intercondylar notch is widened. Stage 5: Severe loss of joint space associated with a fixed fibrous contracture. Stages 1, 2, and 3 are largely reversible and can be maintained with medical treatment. Stages 4 and 5 are irreversible. (Hilgartner M: Hemophilic arthropathy. Adv Pediatr 21:139, 1975)

assumed plasma volume. As a general rule, 1 unit of factor VIII per kilogram of body weight will raise the patient's plasma level of factor VIII activity by 2%, while one unit of factor IX per kilogram of body weight will raise the patient's plasma level of factor IX activity by 1.5%. It is necessary to make serial determinations of factor levels to establish the rate of fall after administration. In the patient who is not bleeding, the biologic half-life of factor VIII is 6 to 12 hours, while that of factor IX is 8 to 18 hours. Therefore, for maintenance therapy doses of factor VIII must be repeated every 8 hours and doses of factor IX, every 12 hours, to maintain the desired plasma level.

For the control of an acute hemarthrosis, a single

infusion to raise the plasma level to 40% to 50% of normal will achieve hemostasis and, allowing for further decay, will provide further protection for about 24 hours.[209] A single dose combined with non–weight bearing, ice bags, and immobilization is usually adequate to relieve pain and restore motion within 24 hours.

Hematomas and muscle hemorrhages require raising the plasma level of factor VIII or IX to 20% to 30%. This is adequate when combined with ice bags and a compression bandage. Bleeding into the triceps surae, because scarring and contracture rapidly lead to resistant equinus deformity, need higher levels, approximatley 40% to 50%.

Serious hemorrhages, such as bleeding into the nasopharynx, retroperitoneal area with nerve involvement, or central nervous system, require prompt treatment with sufficient concentrate to achieve levels of 80% to 100% of normal.

The medical management of a hemophiliac requiring surgery requires precise assays of factor levels at frequent intervals. Elective surgery should not be undertaken until the patient has been thoroughly investigated for factor VIII and IX inhibitors. Many patients may have a low-titer inhibitor, the production of which is not stimulated by the routine transfusions but which may appear after the long-term high-dose therapy required for lengthy postoperative care.

One aims to achieve 100% plasma levels at the time of the surgical procedure and to maintain a level of more than 60% of normal for the first 4 days after operation and of more than 40% for at least 4 more days. A level of 100% is also necessary for manipulation of a fracture or joint under anesthesia or for removal of pins or a similar procedure. Levels of 20% are maintained for postoperative physiotherapy for as long as 4 to 6 weeks after major surgery.

ORTHOPAEDIC NONSURGICAL MANAGEMENT

Hemophilic Arthropathy. For acute hemarthrosis occurring at the earliest stage (acute hemarthropathy), a single infusion of the appropriate factor is given to achieve a plasma level of 40% to 50%. The extremity is elevated and the joint immobilized for 24 hours in a posterior plaster splint, bivalved cast, or pillow splint, in such a manner to permit constant monitoring of the skin and neurovascular function. Ice bags are applied. Within a short time after the factor has been administered, pain is controlled, and by 24 hours motion is restored.

Aspiration should be avoided for fear of reducing the intra-articular counterpressure and introducing infection. Occasionally, aspiration may be necessary when swelling is substantial and the skin is under extreme tension.[225] Proponents of aspiration suggest that removal of the blood lessens the degree of arthropathy. Before aspiration is attempted, the plasma level must first be elevated to 30% to 40%.

When appropriate replacement therapy fails to control the acute hemarthrosis, or when repeated hemarthroses develop within a short period, and the joint continues to display persistent warmth; thick, boggy synovial swelling; and restriction of motion, the stage of subacute arthropathy can be said to exist. Factor replacement and immobilization must be continued. Small doses of corticosteroids may be given for a few days. At this stage the probability is great that chronic progressive arthropathy will develop.

Chronic repeated and persistent hemarthroses ultimately lead to severely restricted joint motion, deformity, flexion contracture, and substantial muscle atrophy. The resulting instability of the joint further encourages bleeding, which in turn hastens serious joint destruction. For this reason prolonged immobilization in a brace is indicated; muscle atrophy should be prevented, joint motion encouraged, and repeated hemarthrosis controlled.[229] Replacement therapy (level 20% to 30%) is combined with physical therapy for 6 weeks. Isometric exercises are initiated and followed by graduated range of motion exercises. When the lower extremity is involved, crutch non-weight-bearing walking is mandatory, and no weight bearing is permitted until all inflammatory signs have abated and good muscle power is restored. This may require months to a year. Manipulation and massage are avoided. Intra-articular injections of corticosteroids are contraindicated. If the chronic synovitis and chronic hemarthrosis are brought under control, the program can be stepped up to include light daily activities such as swimming and hiking. The brace support must not be discontinued until all evidence of inflammation has subsided.

Knee Flexion Contracture. Knee flexion contracture may develop even prior to the development of chronic hemophilic arthropathy. The deformity may be overcome by gentle traction and by a turnbuckle-type cast composed of leg and thigh sections connected by an adjustable semicircular fixed hinge that can be straightened gradually.[228] It is essential that the axis of this hinge be located level with the midpoints of the femoral condyles, corresponding to the instant centers of rotation. Roentgenograms are taken every few days to ensure that posterior subluxation of the tibia is not taking place.

Alternatively, split Russell's traction may be used. Longitudinal traction is applied to the leg while overhead pull is exerted through a sling beneath the proximal portion of the leg.

Manipulation may occasionally be indicated. Adequate levels of the deficient factor must first be attained, and a gentle manipulation is carried out under general anesthesia.

ORTHOPAEDIC SURGICAL MANAGEMENT

Principles. Surgery is to be avoided when other options are available.[231] Replacement of deficient factor now permits surgical intervention in handling both acute life-

and limb-threatening hemorrhages (*e.g.*, pseudotumors, fractures) and elective procedures such as osteotomy, arthrodesis, and total joint replacement. Preoperatively, the presence of inhibitors (antibodies) must be determined; if present, surgery is contraindicated. The inhibitor titer must be checked 7 to 14 days after a test dose of factor is administered. If no inhibitors are present, the deficient factor must be brought to a level of 80% to 100% on the day of surgery. Provision is made for whole blood or washed packed red cell replacement. Postoperatively, the plasma must be assayed at frequent intervals during factor-replacement therapy, particularly with cryoprecipitate, because this preparation varies greatly in potency. A level of at least 60% must be maintained for 4 days after surgery and of above 40% for at least 4 more days. If bleeding persists, the problem is usually the presence of circulating antibodies or thrombocytopenia induced by multiple blood transfusions. If inhibitors are absent and the platelet count is normal, the cause for bleeding must be sought elsewhere.

Because multiple operative sessions increase the risk of developing inhibitors, one should attempt as many procedures at one session as the patient will tolerate. A pneumatic tourniquet is used. Vessels are ligated rather than electrocoagulated, and tube suction is necessary for 24 hours. Drugs that affect the clotting mechanism should be avoided (*e.g.*, aspirin, antihistamines, guaiacolate).

Hemophilic Pseudotumor. Also known as hemophilic cyst, hemophilic pseudotumor consists of a massive hemorrhage; the hemorrhage may be beneath the periosteum of a long bone and extend secondarily into the surrounding musculature, or it may initially develop within the muscle itself or between the muscle and its sheath.[219,221] As the hemorrhagic mass slowly enlarges, a fibrous wall forms about it, creating a cystlike structure containing recent blood clots, residues or disintegrating blood cells, and serum. The expanding mass may compress vital structures. Because the femoral nerve is enclosed by the iliacus sheath and the median nerve by the carpal tunnel, these are the nerves most often affected. The iliacus muscle is the most common site for the formation of a pseudotumor. Wherever the hemorrhagic tumor mass forms in a limb, extension poses the threat of ultimately penetrating the overlying skin, resulting in either a fatal hemorrhage or a draining sinus, which inevitably becomes infected. When the pseudotumor develops within a closed fascial compartment (*e.g.*, volar aspect of forearm), ischemic necrosis of muscle and fibrosis produce a myostatic contracture.

Attempts to aspirate the mass are unsuccessful and may result in a secondarily infected sinus tract, spread of infection, and increased susceptibility to recurrent hemorrhage. For these reasons, aspiration is unwarranted. If the mass appears to be static, a period of watchful waiting is permissible to determine whether the mass will recede and be replaced by fibrosis. However, procrastination is dangerous. Preliminary replacement therapy and adequate provision for blood transfusions should immediately be followed by excision. At surgery the use of human antihemophilic globulin locally as a paste and an antibiotic, plus booster doses of the deficient factor, will control bleeding. Prior to closure, the tourniquet is deflated and the bleeding vessels are ligated. Electrocoagulation should be held to a minimum. Postoperatively, replacement therapy is continued for at least 3 weeks.

Under cover of replacement therapy, most pseudotumors can be successfully removed. However, when replacement therapy fails and circulation is marginal, amputation may be necessary.[233]

Radiation therapy is suitable for small inaccessible pseudotumors, the rationale being to destroy the vessels feeding the mass.[223] Care must be exercised to shield the epiphyseal plate. A dosage of 750 rads is given at 125 rads daily, and healing usually occurs within a few weeks. Higher dosage may be given for lesions of the femur and tibia.[212]

An iliacus pseudotumor usually responds to conservative treatment. Traction is applied to the leg, and high levels of the deficient factor are maintained. The frequently associated femoral nerve deficit subsides gradually over a number of months.

Synovectomy. The indications for synovectomy are repeated uncontrollable hemarthroses and chronic synovitis. Chronic hypertrophied synovial tissue may liberate enzymes (*e.g.*, collagenase) that cause destruction of articular cartilage. Early synovectomy significantly reduces bleeding episodes and eliminates the thick, boggy synovium, but unless performed before there are extensive joint changes, the arthropathy will progress.[217,231]

Fractures. Hemophiliacs are unusually susceptible to fractures because of osteoporosis and the limited joint motion that accompanies the arthropathy.[218,227] Treatment of the fracture should not be delayed because procrastination invites rapid formation of antibodies to the offending deficient factor.[210] The principles of treatment include immediate vigorous replacement of the deficient factor, maintenance of hemostasis, particularly during the first 7 to 10 days, and absolute immobilization. Aggressive replacement therapy aims at achieving at least 40% to 60% of normal plasma levels during the early days and 20% to 30% for several weeks thereafter. A stable fracture in an adult, or almost any fracture in a child, may be treated by immobilization in a plaster cast. Unstable fractures may produce uncontrollable bleeding if treated by nonsurgical methods and threaten nerve and vascular compromise. Moreover, nonunion is a possibility. Therefore, the unstable fracture in the adult should be treated early by internal fixation once adequate levels of the deficient factor are achieved and before untenable antibody titers arise. Union generally takes place at a normal rate or sooner, usually with a minimum of periosteal callus.

A neighboring pseudotumor may erode the bone and produce a pathologic fracture. Intramedullary or other internal fixation plus bone grafts are necessary.[232]

Supracondylar Osteotomy. Supracondylar osteotomy is done to correct a severe flexion contracture of the knee that does not respond to conservative treatment.[211] The deformity is often associated with some degree of valgus and external rotation. A useful range of motion is a prerequisite.

Arthrodesis. Arthrodesis may be indicated for severely destroyed joints.[230] Percutaneous pins for compression devices should be avoided as they cause continuous bleeding about the pin tracts and invite infection.

Total Joint Replacement. The indications for total replacement of a joint are pain and an advanced state of arthropathy.[215,216,231] One must first eliminate the possibility that pain may be due to persistent bleeding. A program of replacement therapy, a short course of steroids, and physiotherapy are carried out. If this fails, pain is considered the result of mechanical changes in the joint, and a total joint replacement is indicated.

Achilles Tendon Lengthening. Bleeding into the calf often results in contracture of the triceps surae and equinus deformity of the foot. Surgery at this site requires rigid adherence to hematologic principles to avoid major complications. Surgical correction is generally good and lasting.

Neurapraxia. By definition, neurapraxia is a physiological rather than an anatomical interruption of the nerve.[211] The nerves involved in decreasing order of frequency are the femoral, peroneal, sciatic, median, and ulnar. Femoral nerve involvement is usually due to bleeding about the iliacus.

Treatment is usually nonsurgical, consisting of factor-replacement therapy to achieve plasma levels of 80% to 100% of normal for several days and tapering the dose to maintain levels of 40% while recovery is taking place. The extremity is splinted, followed later by physical therapy using electrical stimulation. Where hyperplastic synovium is suspected of causing compression of the nerve (*e.g.*, at the ulnar groove or carpal tunnel), a synovectomy may be necessary.

When the nerve lesion is localized to a closed fascial compartment, such as the volar compartment of the forearm, immediate decompression is mandatory. If nerve conduction loss is partial, a waiting period is permissible while adequate replacement therapy is carried out.

TRAUMATIC ARTHRITIS

Direct trauma to a joint causes the soft tissues, particularly the synovial membrane, to become congested, edematous, and hemorrhagic (contused). At the same time an increased outpouring of synovial fluid occurs. The latter may contain serum and fibrin, which impart a deep amber color to the fluid. If tissues are torn, extravasation into the joint cavity varies from a minute amount, detected microscopically or chemically, to frank hemorrhage. Synovial fluid interferes with the clotting mechanism of blood so that the mixture to a large extent remains liquid. Healing takes place by resolution of synovial inflammation and absorption of joint fluid, the joint returning to normal over a period of several days to weeks.

Various factors militate against restoration of normal joint physiology and anatomy. If fibrin or blood clots are deposited in the depths of synovial folds, they become organized into adhesions. The fibroblastic process heals tears and hemorrhage within the synovium, producing a permanently thickened, inelastic, and inextensible lining membrane, its inner fold obliterated. This is labeled chronic synovitis. The capsular covering too may be severely contused and torn and healed by scarring, becoming adherent to overlying and subjacent structures. Particularly when this capsule is composed in part of movable musculotendinous structures, as in the shoulder and the knee, the motion of the joint is restricted. The muscles about the joint atrophy rapidly. This condition is called periarthritis.

During the acute inflammatory stage, the articular cartilage, in consequence of lack of nourishment from synovial fluid, becomes soft, unelastic, and fragile, losing its resistance to mechanical pressures. Microscopically, degenerative changes take place. Over succeeding months, surface cartilage is worn away, and the exposed subchondral bone undergoes reactive sclerosis. Irregular joint surfaces lead to abnormally high surface loads and frictional forces. Degenerative arthritis almost always follows severe direct trauma to a joint. The degree of these changes depends on the following:

1. The severity of impact
2. Tearing of soft tissue structures (ligaments, menisci), with resultant instability
3. Associated bone injury, producing irregular joint surfaces
4. A preexistent degenerative arthritis
5. Obesity, in the case of the lower extremities. The condition may be designated late secondary osteoarthritis.

Prolonged distention of the joint by fluid has been said to cause healing of ligaments in the elongated position, resulting in an unstable joint. This is the rationale for aspiration. On the other hand, it is questionable whether the pressure is sufficient in degree or duration to have such an effect. Removal of fluid is generally followed by rapid reappearance of fluid in the joint.

CLINICAL PICTURE

There is a history of direct trauma. A gradual onset, over hours, of swelling, pain, and limitation of motion implies increased effusion with a minimum of blood. An acute onset, over minutes to an hour, indicates intra-articular hemorrhage.

Swelling is mainly intra-acticular, due to fluid accumulation. In the knee, the patella is ballotable. Edema and tenderness are localized over the site of trauma. The position is one of semiflexion. Motion is limited in all directions, owing to obstruction of fluid. Abnormal mobility in a lateral direction indicates torn collateral ligaments. Evidence of other soft tissue injury should be sought. These findings are described in Chapters 21 through 30.

LABORATORY FINDINGS

Joint fluid aspirate varies from a clear amber to bloody. Its removal, in the absence of complicating soft tissue injuries, should restore complete motion to the joint.

ROENTGENOGRAPHIC FINDINGS

Early Roentgenograms are negative. By definition, traumatic arthritis implies that soft tissue injury is not apparent on stress views and by arthrography. Routine roentgenograms and tomograms rule out bone injury. The changes due to developing osteoarthritis gradually appear over many months and to a greater degree than a similar process that may affect other joints.

ARTHROSCOPY

Invasive diagnostic arthroscopy is not indicated unless symptoms are intractable. If an internal derangement is defined by arthroscopic examination, the term "traumatic arthritis" is no longer tenable.

TREATMENT

The joint is placed at rest by a metal or plaster splint. A compression dressing and an icebag retard hemorrhage. Muscle-setting exercises are practiced while the splint is worn, to reduce the muscle atrophy and to prevent periarticular adhesions. Removal of fluid by aspiration to relieve pain or the introduction of compound F is not justified. Infection is a definite danger. Bloody joint fluid is an excellent medium for the growth of organisms introduced by the aspirating needle. As the swelling is subsiding, gentle passive exercises and later active non-weight-bearing exercises are practiced. Mobility of the joint and integrity of the musculature are maintained. A severely injured joint should not be subjected to weight bearing until all signs of inflammation have subsided. This precaution against damage to articular surfaces may require several weeks. When recurrent effusions occur with repeated attempts at weight bearing, an intra-articular mechanical impediment should be suspected. Arthrography may demonstrate a cartilaginous joint mouse. Occasionally, exploratory arthrotomy may be necessary to identify the cause. One should not wait until degenerative changes have set in before resorting to such measures. When a periarthritis has resulted after an acute traumatic arthritis, physical therapeutic measures are required. Forceful stretching should be avoided, since tearing of soft tissue and formation of more adhesions further restrict motion.

When ambulation with full weight bearing is resumed, muscle weakness causes joint instability, which may lead to strains and reactive synovitis. An elastic compression bandage should be worn.

ALTERATIONS IN COMPOSITION AND FUNCTION OF SYNOVIAL TISSUES RELATED TO TUMOR FORMATION

The intimal layer of the articular capsule is made up of specialized mesenchymal cells that have the capacity of regulating the passage of substances between the articular and the vascular fluids and of secreting mucin. Similar tissues line the tendon sheaths and the bursal spaces. Under certain mechanical influences (*e.g.*, irritation over a bony prominence), a synovia-lined bursal space will form. The synovial lining of a joint varies from dense connective tissue lined by inconspicuous flattened cells to a membrane comprised of many layers of round, oval, or cubical cells that are supported by a loosely textured and highly vascular connective tissue. These latter areas may contain recesses or crypts, as well as permanently formed papillary projections called villi. With flexion and extension of the joint, temporary folds are also produced in the synovia-lining layer of cells and its supporting subsynovial tissues. Another function is the transportation of colloidal and particulate matter across the synovial membrane. Continuous or intermittent bleeding into the articular cavities leads to extensive storage of hemosiderin in the phagocytes of the subsynovial tissues or in the synovial-lining cells. Lipoids and other phagocytosed substances may also accumulate in these tissues under certain abnormal circumstances.

Under the influence of injury and persistent irritation, neoplasmlike overgrowths of the synovial tissues will result. Some lesions are heavily pigmented with hemosiderin, others may contain large amounts of lipoid alone or in combination with hemosiderin. The structural peculiarities of synovium are reproduced in the new growth. Therefore, fibrous connective tissue elements are the main component in one tumor, whereas another would display prominent tufting or villous overgrowths. In still another, the lining cells are prominent and multiply so that several layers of cells are seen. These new growths can occur also in regions far removed from joints, since the mesenchymal tissue always has a synovia-forming capacity.[234]

PIGMENTED VILLONODULAR SYNOVITIS

Pigmented villonodular synovitis (synovial xanthoma, villous synovitis) is the name applied by Jaffe and associates to an idiopathic villous overgrowth and pigmentation of the synovial membrance of a single joint. Many names have been applied to these xanthomatous lesions, which are characterized by their yellow or yellowish brown color due to deposits of cholesterol and hemosiderin. Since bursae and tendon sheaths are related to synovium in their origin, they too are the site of xanthomatous growths.[235]

PATHOLOGY

The joint may be distended by a chocolate-colored mass with small or large, soft or hard, nodular masses on a base of fibrous connective tissue having the consistency of rubber. The cut surface resembles fine sponge rubber and displays a mixture of gray and pale yellow. Microscopically, fibrous connective tissue contains many cells, the nuclei of which are vesicular but vary in size and shape. Some are oval, some spindle-shaped, and others polyhedral (Fig. 13-31). Scattered yellow pigment may be contained in large oval or polyhedral cells, resembling large monocytes or histiocytes. Cells containing lipoid material, the foam cells, occur in varying amounts. Occasional giant cells of the epulis type occur about areas of destruction and debris. The synovium is thrown into folds, the stroma is edematous and markedly vascular, perivascular cuffs of lymphocytes may be seen, and, in the later stages when fibrous tissue proliferation occurs, the cells are squeezed out, becoming sparse, and the vascularity is lessened.

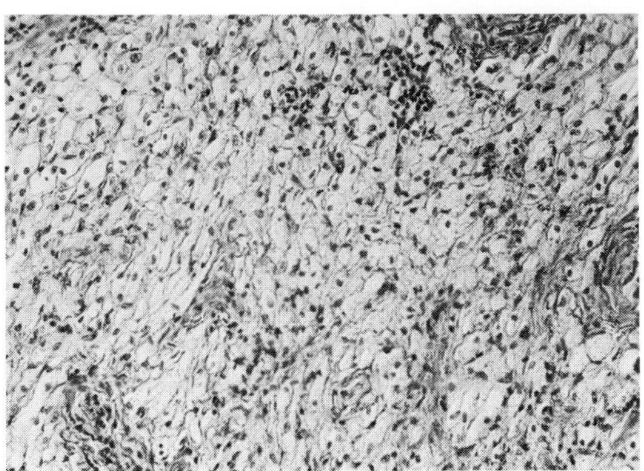

FIG. 13-31. Xanthoma cells or foam cells. They are large and polyhedral and contain a small, central, usually pyknotic nucleus and transparent, foamy cytoplasm. Lipoid bodies are dissolved out in hematoxylin-eosin stains and are demonstrable by fat stains. Foam cells exist in varying proportion with fibroblasts and collagenous fibrils. When fibrous tissue is abundant, xanthoma cells are enveloped and difficult to demonstrate, the lesion being termed a fibroxanthoma. The characteristics of a fibroxanthoma are foam cells; fibrocellular stroma with short, blunt, spindle-shaped cells containing a pale, slightly elongated nucleus; multinucleated giant cells of the epulis type, containing five to 40 nuclei; blood pigment, coarse yellow or brown pigment of hemosiderin scattered throughout the groundwork, situated principally intracellularly in macrophages or foam cells; blood vessels, mainly small abundant capillaries; and, when xanthomatous tumors develop within the synovium of joints (nodular synovitis), synovial villous formation. (DeSanto DA, Wilson PD: Xanthomatous tumors of joints. J Bone Joint Surg 21:531, 1939)

THEORIES OF PATHOGENESIS

Jaffe and co-workers favor the theory that xanthoma represents an inflammatory response, the causative agent being unknown; the xanthoma or foam cells are derived from the macrophages of the reticuloendothelial system and are modified to contain cholesterol. These workers do not believe in bacterial, lipoid metabolic, and hemorrhagic causes, because the condition cannot be reproduced experimentally.[235] They reject the theory of Geschickter and Copeland, who state that the lesion develops through proliferation of osteoclasts in associated sesamoid bones.[236] However, Young and Hudacek experimentally produced the growth in dogs.[237]

CLINICAL PICTURE

Age. The condition is usually seen in the young adult from 20 to 40 years of age. The diffuse villous form occurs in the second and third decades; the circumscribed nodular growth occurs in the third to fifth decades.

Sex. Men most commonly

Area of Predilection. Knee joint, a few in the ankle; rare elsewhere

Trauma. History occasionally obtained, relationship doubtful

Duration of Symptoms. From 1 day to many years

Course. Usually the symptoms are gradual onset of pain, mild to moderate, intermittent, and associated with a limp. Mechanical interference causes stiffness, locking, limitation of motion usually in extension, and a snapping sensation at times. In the more localized form, the symptoms are mild and develop very gradually; therefore, as a rule, patients do not seek advice early.

Findings. A soft tissue swelling enlarges the entire joint. The effusion may be pronounced, the patella floating, and moderate generalized tenderness may be present. In the localized form, a palpable small tumor may suggest a joint mouse. Usually, in this type the tumor is not palpable, and only after arthrography or on arthroscopy is the true nature of the disease defined. The swelling is slight and intermittent. Effusion is minimal.

Aspiration. A thick orange brown fluid containing cholesterol in large amounts is pathognomonic. In the localized form, however, the effusion is not abundant, is straw colored, and is sterile.

LABORATORY FINDINGS

Laboratory findings are not diagnostic. The blood cholesterol is at the upper limits of normal. No alteration of the cholesterol-cholesterol ester ratio exists.

ROENTGENOGRAPHIC FINDINGS

Direct films of the joint are usually negative or may display general soft tissue enlargement. Occasionally, moderate decalcification from tumor pressure is noted. An air or double-contrast arthrogram reveals, in the diffuse type, a bubbly flocculent effect within the synovial cavity. In the localized type, a soft tissue shadow encroaches upon the synovial pouches, most commonly in the posterior part of the suprapatellar area (Fig. 13-32).

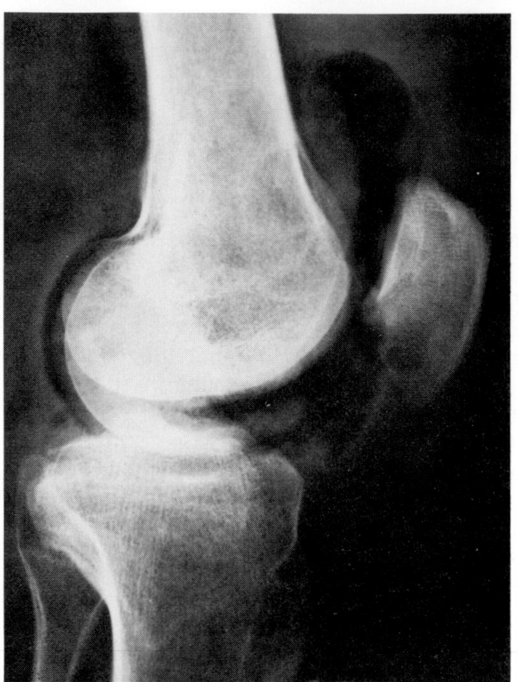

FIG. 13-32. Pigmented villonodular synovitis. Note the nodular density in the suprapatellar pouch demonstrated by air arthrography.

ARTHROSCOPY

Direct arthroscopic visualization of the interior of the joint will demonstrate the highly characteristic gross pathologic picture of villonodular synovitis.

TREATMENT

Surgical excision is indicated. Recurrences are common but are adequately handled by x-ray irradiation. No malignant degeneration has ever been reported.

HEMANGIOMA OF A JOINT

Hemangioma of the synovial membrane is a rare vascular tumor occurring in young people, located predominantly in the knee, and characterized clinically by a long history of recurrent episodes of pain in the knee.[238–240]

PATHOLOGY

The tumor appears as a dark blue grapelike mass that bulges beneath a shiny synovial covering (Fig. 13-33). The cut section of the tumor is typically spongy, but thrombosis and organization may cause it to be indurated. When localized and pedunculated, the mass may produce obstruction to joint motion manifested clinically as locking. A more diffuse and sessile type of tumor occasions only periodic pain and swelling. Microscopically, a profusion of vascular spaces is seen. These are usually thin walled and small (capillary) or distended (cavernous). Rarely, the spaces resemble small veins.

CLINICAL PICTURE

The patient usually is an adolescent or a young adult, and the knee is most often involved. A long history of joint disability dates from early childhood and consists of spontaneously recurring episodes of painful locking or diffuse, poorly localized pain accompanied by swelling.

Physical findings include tenderness, which is either diffuse throughout the joint or well localized over a palpable soft mass, pain on motion, and visible quadriceps atrophy. Often the symptoms are vague, no mass can be made out, and the tenderness is poorly defined.

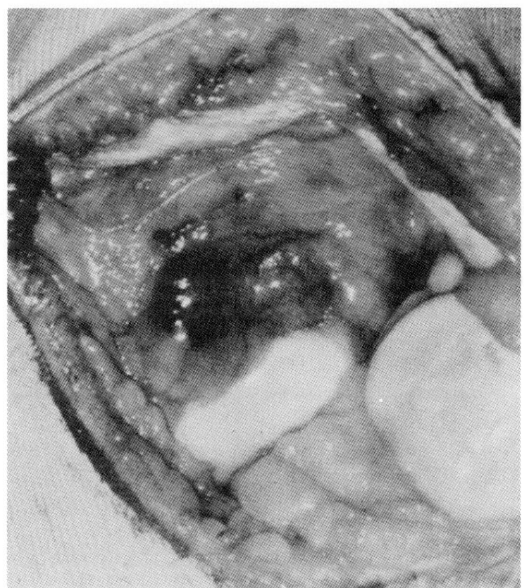

FIG. 13-33. Hemangioma of the synovial membrane, gross appearance. The tumor lies in the subsynovial tissue. (Lewis RC, Coventry MB, Soule EH: Hemangioma of the synovial membrane. J Bone Joint Surg 41A:264, 1959)

ROENTGENOGRAPHIC FINDINGS

A double-contrast arthrogram will usually outline the tumor, provided that it is sufficiently prominent.

ARTHROSCOPY

Arthroscopy defines the nature of the growth preoperatively.

TREATMENT

Surgical excision is the treatment of choice.

OSTEOCHONDROMATOSIS

In this disease, cartilaginous or osteocartilaginous bodies develop in the synovial membrane of joints or their communicating bursae.

ETIOLOGY

The condition is considered to arise from embryonic rests. Both synovial membrane and articular cartilage develop from the same mesenchymal tissue.

PATHOLOGY

Hyaline cartilage forms in the stratum synoviale of the synovial membrane, particularly at the points of reflection of the membrane (Color Plate 13-3). Multiple isolated areas of synovium are affected so that a tremendous number, even hundreds, of spheroid cartilaginous nodules protrude into the joint cavity (Fig. 13-34). Each cartilaginous body may remain unchanged or may become calcified; the calcified cartilage may be transformed to bone, particularly at its center, by metaplasia or by the process of endochondral ossification. The body gradually is extruded into the joint cavity, where it is attached, at first, by a synovial pedicle. Nutrition carried through the pedicle enables both cartilage and bone to hypertrophy. The body may be torn free from its attachment, its bony center undergoing aseptic necrosis. However, it continues to grow by hypertrophy of its cartilaginous covering, which derives its nutrition from synovial fluid. The repeated trauma to the articular surfaces by these loose bodies causes multiple erosions and eventually degenerative arthritic changes.

CLINICAL PICTURE

Sex. Males predominate

Age. 30 to 50 years

Location. in order of frequency: knee, elbow, ankle, hip and shoulder

Symptoms. Dull ache, stiffness, transient locking episodes, grating sensations and in the case of the knee, a giving way

Findings. Generalized joint tenderness, thickening of the soft tissues through which the nodules may be palpable, and marked audible and palpable crepitus.

ROENTGENOGRAPHIC FINDINGS

Only when the bodies are calcified or ossified are they visible on a direct film (Fig. 13-35). Even so, because many are composed only of cartilage, the number is always much greater than one would suspect from the film. When all bodies are chondromatous, air or double-contrast arthrography is necessary for visualization.

TREATMENT

Loose joint mice must be removed immediately to halt further damage to articular surfaces. The patient should be forewarned that a certain amount of degenerative

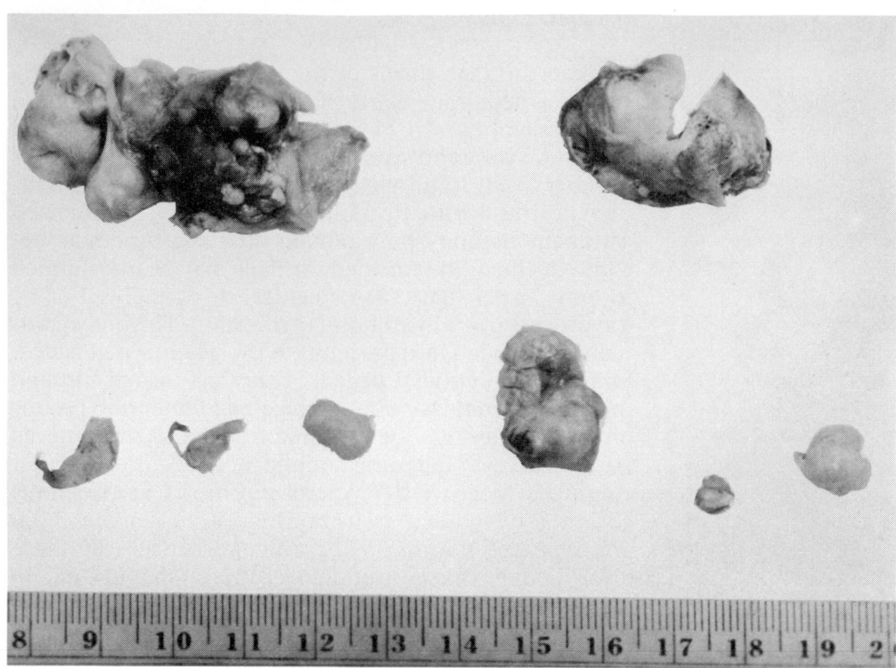

FIG. 13-34. Osteochondromatosis. These loose bodies were recovered from a knee joint.

FIG. 13-35. (*A*) Osteochondromatosis of the shoulder joint. (*B*) Osteochondromatosis of the ankle.

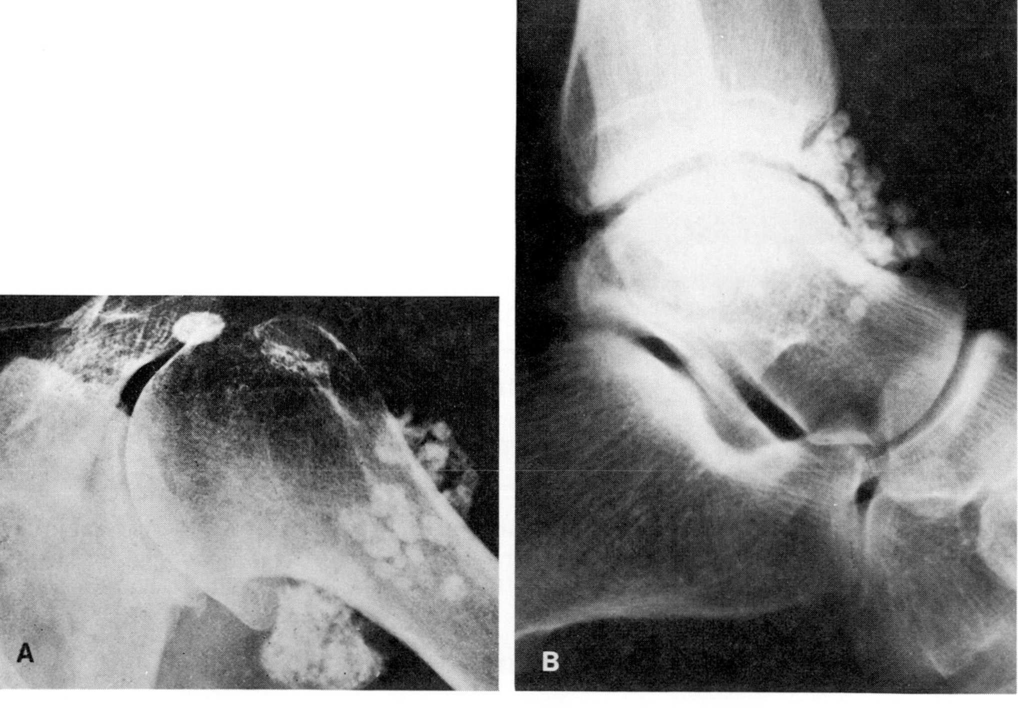

arthritis is already present and may cause residual symptoms. In addition to removal of loose bodies, a complete synovectomy is performed. All communicating bursae, as demonstrated by air arthrography, are also excised. As a general rule, the menisci are damaged, requiring removal. The outlook for permanent cure is excellent.

SYNOVIOMA

The normal synovial membrane consists of an intima, which varies from a multilayered membrane of round, oval, or cuboid cells to an incomplete lining of flattened cells, and a subintima, a supporting layer of connective tissue that varies from loose vascular tissue to dense fibrous connective tissue. When a multilayered type of membrane rests on a loose supporting stroma, tufts or villi tend to form. A malignant tumor may arise from any one or all of these elements. The supporting layer may be the origin of a tumor indistinguishable from fibrosarcoma. A tumor arising from the intima displays flattened synovial or adenomatouslike elements mixed with fibrosarcomatous features. In any one tumor, either the adenomatous or the fibrosarcomatous element may predominate, but as a rule the tumor is composed of a mixture of both. The synovioma (synovial sarcoma, synovial sarcomesothelioma, cancerous synovial tumor) is a slowly growing malignant tumor occurring in juxtaposition to and often attached to synovial tissue, but almost invariably lies outside the joint.[241–244]

PATHOLOGY

GROSS APPEARANCE

Grossly, the tumor can rarely be identified as a synovioma, since a synovial attachment is difficult to find. The tumor is sharply circumscribed, rounded, and lobulated (Fig. 13-36). As it grows expansively, it compresses the surrounding tissue, which becomes attenuated to form a pseudocapsule. Often the tumor is densely adherent to adjacent structures. Occasionally, it may be possible to trace a connection with a tendon sheath or joint. The tumor seldom forms within a joint cavity. Instead, it lies in close proximity to tendons and tendon sheaths, bursae, and joint capsules. The cut section of tumor is firm and grayish pink and often contains dark blood-stained or yellowish brown areas of necrosis.

MICROSCOPIC APPEARANCE

Three basic patterns indicating a synovial origin are seen (Color Plates 13-4 and 13-5):

1. Formation of tissue spaces. These vary from slitlike clefts lined with flattened cells to well-formed glandular spaces lined with cuboid or columnar cells, often multilayered. A homogeneous mucinouslike fluid often occupies the slitlike clefts.
2. Formation of cell tufts. Compact groups of oval or

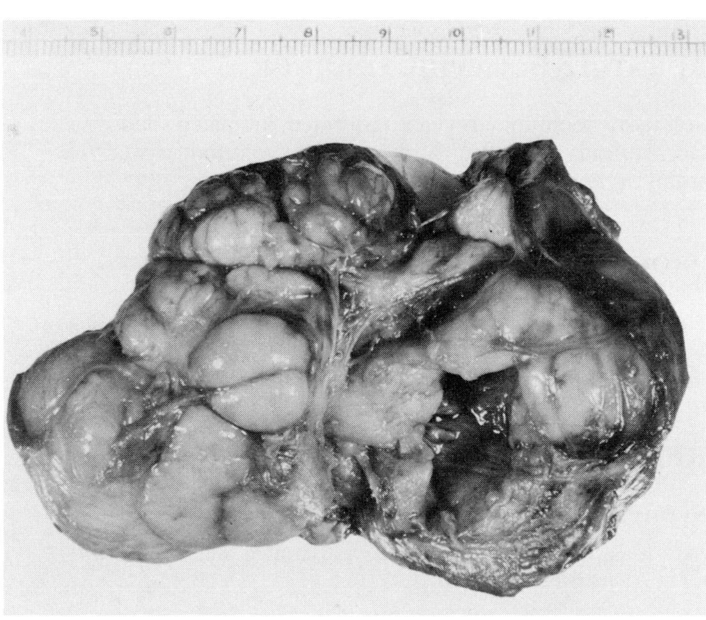

FIG. 13-36. Synovial sarcoma removed from the popliteal space. The tumor was indurated and, although well localized, was densely adherent to the surrounding structures.

polygonal cells are arranged in tuft-like formations, occurring either in the solid portions of the tumor or as papillary projections extending into the glandlike spaces.
3. Epitheliallike cells on a supporting stroma of compact tissue. The cells are elongated and contain small dark nuclei.

Evidence of malignancy is observed in the fibrosarcomatous stroma. Occasionally, the tumor consists almost exclusively of fibrosarcoma, and only after an exhaustive search for synovial elements is the true origin of the tumor revealed. Basically, the tumor is identified by clefting, tufting, villous formations, and glandlike spaces with secretion.

CLINICAL PICTURE

Age. Young adults, rare after 40 years

Area of Predilection. Lower extremity, especially about the knee

Position. In soft tissue outside of joint

Symptoms and Findings. Painful swelling begins in a periarticular or peritendinous site; it increases slowly over years before the swelling is large and pain severe; swelling is firm or soft, moderately tender

Course. Very slow, metastasizes eventually to the lungs

ROENTGENOGRAPHIC FINDINGS

Soft tissue technique reveals a rounded, lobulated shadow. Occasionally, stippling is observed if the tumor contains small areas of calcification.

PROGNOSIS AND TREATMENT

The tumor is very slow growing and metastasizes late. Local excision is inadequate. Radical amputation is indicated.

REFERENCES

Synovial Fluid

1. Ropes MW: Examination of synovial fluid. Bull Rheum Dis 7(Suppl):S21, 1959

Degenerative Joint Disease

2. Anderson CE et al: Composition of the organic component of human articular cartilage. J Bone Joint Surg 46A:1176, 1964
3. Anderson CE, Ludowieg J, Harper H et al: The composition of the organic component of human articular cartilage: Relationship to age and degenerative joint disease. J Bone Joint Surg 46A:1176, 1964
4. Arnoldi CC, Linderholm H: Intracalcaneal pressure in patients with different forms of dysfunction of the venous pump of the calf. Acta Chir Scand 137:21, 1971
5. Arnoldi CC, Linderholm H, Müssbichler H: Venous engorgement and intraosseous hypertension in osteoarthritis of the hip. J Bone Joint Surg 54B:409, 1972
6. Azuma H: Intraosseous pressure as a measure of hemodynamic changes in bone marrow. Angiology 15:396, 1964
7. Barnett CH, Cochrane W, Palfrey AJ: Age changes in articular cartilage of rabbits. Ann Rheum Dis 22:389, 1963
8. Bennett GA, Waine H, Bauer W: Changes in the knee joint at various ages. New York, The Commonwealth Fund, 1942
9. Bluestone R, Bywaters EGL, Hartog M et al: Acromegalic arthropathy. Ann Rheum Dis 30:243, 1971
10. Bollet AJ: Connective tissue polysaccharide metabolism and the pathogenesis of osteoarthritis. Adv Intern Med 13:33, 1967
11. Collins DH: The Pathology of Articular and Spinal Diseases. London, Arnold, 1949
12. Collins DH, McElligott TF: Sulfate ($^{35}SO_4$) uptake by chondrocytes in relation to histological changes in osteoarthritic human articular cartilage. Ann Rheum Dis 19:318, 1960
13. Dymock JW: Arthropathy of hemochromatosis: Clinical and radiological analysis of 63 patients with iron overload. Ann Rheum Dis 29:469, 1970
14. Ekholm R: Articular cartilage. Acta Anat 11:1, 1951
15. Frankel VH, Burstein AH: Orthopaedic Biomechanics: An Introduction to the Engineering Fundamentals of Orthopaedic Surgery. Philadelphia, Lea & Febiger, 1967
16. Freeman MAR: The pathogenesis of primary osteoarthrosis. In Apley AG (ed): Modern Trends in Orthpaedics. London, Butterworth & Co, 1972
17. Freeman MAR: The fatigue of cartilage in the pathogenesis of osteoarthrosis. Acta Orthop Scand 46:323, 1975
18. Freeman MAR, Meachim G: Aging, degeneration and remodelling of articular cartilage. In Freeman MAR (ed): Adult Articular Cartilage. New York, Grune & Stratton, 1972
19. Ginsberg JM: Protective effects of salicylates on cartilage degeneration. J Bone Joint Surg 52A:831, 1970
20. Hamilton E et al: The arthropathy of idiopathic hemochromatosis. Q J Med 37:171, 1968
21. Harrison MHM, Schajowicz F, Trueta J: Osteoarthritis of the hip: A study of the nature and evolution of the disease. J Bone Joint Surg 35B:598, 1953
22. Hollander JL: Intra-articular hydrocortisone in arthritis and allied conditions. J Bone Joint Surg 35A:983, 1953
23. Honner R, Thompson RC: The nutritional pathways of articular cartilage. J Bone Joint Surg 53A:742, 1971
24. Jaffe HL: Metabolic, Degenerative and Inflammatory Diseases of Bones and Joints. Philadelphia, Lea & Febiger, 1972
25. Kellgran JH: Osteoarthrosis in patients and population. Br Med J, p 1, July 1961
26. Kempson GE: Mechanical properties of articular cartilage. In Freeman MAR (ed): Adult Articular Cartilage, p 171. New York, Grune & Stratton, 1972
27. Kempson GE: The mechanical properties of articular cartilage and their relationship to matrix degeneration and age. Ann Rheum Dis 34(Suppl 2):111, 1975
28. Kempson GE et al: Correlations between stiffness and chemical constituents of cartilage in the human femoral head. Biochem Biophys Acta 215:70, 1970

29. Kempson GE et al: Patterns of cartilage stiffness on normal and degenerative human femoral heads. J Biomech 4:597, 1971
30. Kuhns JG, Morrison SL: Twelve years experience in roentgenotherapy for chronic arthritis. N Engl J Med 235:399, 1946
31. Kuzell WC et al: Phenylbutazone (Butazolidin) in rheumatoid arthritis and gout. JAMA 149:729, 1952
32. Kyriazis AP, Tsaltas TT: Studies in permeability of articular cartilage in New Zealand albino rabbits: The effect of ageing, papain, and certain steroid hormones. Am J Pathol 62:25, 1971
33. Lasker FH, Sargison KD: Ochronotic arthropathy. J Bone Joint Surg 52B:781, 1970
34. Lawrence JS et al: Osteoarthrosis: Prevalence in the population and relationship between symptoms and x-ray changes. Ann Rheum Dis 25:1, 1966
35. Levene C: The patterns of cartilage canals. J Anat 98:515, 1964
36. Little K, Pimm LH, Trueta J: Osteoarthritis of the hip: An electron microscopic study. J Bone Joint Surg 40B:123, 1958
37. Lutfi AM: Mode of growth, fate and function of cartilage canals. J Anat 106:135, 1970
38. McKibben B, Holdsworth FW: The nutrition of immature joint cartilage in the lamb. J Bone Joint Surg 48B:793, 1966
39. Mankin HJ: Localization of tritiated thymidine in articular cartilage of rabbits: I. Growth in immature cartilage. J Bone Joint Surg 44A:682, 1962
40. Mankin HJ: The calcified zone (basal layers) of articular cartilage of rabbits. Anat Rec 145:73, 1963
41. Mankin HJ: The Articular Cartilages: A review. Am Acad Orthop Surg Instr Course Lect, Vol 19, pp 204–224. St. Louis, CV Mosby, 1970
42. Mankin HJ: The reaction of articular cartilage to injury and osteoarthritis. N Engl J Med 291:1285, 1335, 1974
43. Mankin HJ, Baron PA: The effect of aging on protein synthesis in articular cartilage of rabbits. Lab Invest 14:658, 1965
44. Mankin HJ, Boyle CJ: The acute effects of lacerative injury on DNA and protein synthesis in articular cartilage. In Bassett CAL (ed): Cartilage Degradation and Repair. Washington, D.C., Natl Acad Sci, Natl Research Council 1967
45. Mankin HJ, Conger KA: The acute effects of intra-articular hydrocortisone on articular cartilage in rabbits. J Bone Joint Surg 48A:1383, 1966
46. Mankin HJ, Dorfman H, Lippiello L et al: Biochemical and metabolic abnormalities in articular cartilage from osteoarthritic human hips: II. Correlation of morphology with biochemical and metabolic data. J Bone Joint Surg 53A:523, 1971
47. Mankin HJ, Lippiello L: The turnover of adult rabbit articular cartilage. J Bone Joint Surg 51A:1591, 1969
48. Mankin HJ, Lippiello L: Biochemical and metabolic abnormalities in articular cartilage from osteoarthritic hips. J Bone Joint Surg 52A:424, 1970
49. Mankin HJ, Lippiello L: The glycosaminoglycans of normal and arthritic cartilage. J Clin Invest 50:1712, 1971
50. Mankin HJ, Zarins A: Water binding in normal and osteoarthritic cartilage. Annual Meeting of Orthopaedic Research Society, Dallas, Texas, 1974
51. Mankin HJ, Zarins A, Jaffe WL: The effect of systemic corticosteroids on rabbit articular cartilage. Arthritis Rheum 15:593, 1972
52. Maroudas A: Fluid transport in articular cartilage. Ann Rheum Dis 34(Suppl 2):55, 1975
53. Maroudas A, Bullough P: Permeability of articular cartilage. Nature 219:1260, 1968
54. Maroudas A, Evans H, Almeida L: Cartilage of the hip joint: Topographical variation of glycosaminoglycan content in normal and fibrillated tissue. Ann Rheum Dis 32:1, 1973
55. Meachim G: Age changes in articular cartilage. Clin Orthop 64:39, 1969
56. Meachim G, Collins DH: Cell counts of normal and osteoarthritic articular cartilage in relation to the uptake of sulfate ($^{35}SO_4$) in vitro. Ann Rheum Dis 21:45, 1962
57. Miller EJ: Isolation and characterization of a collagen from chick cartilage containing three identical alpha chains. Biochemistry 10:1652, 1971
58. Mills K: Pathology of the knee in rheumatoid arthritis. J Bone Joint Surg 52B:746, 1970
59. Moskowitz RW, Davis W, Sammarco J et al: Experimentally induced corticosteroid arthropathy. Arthritis Rheum 13:236, 1970
60. Repo RU, Mitchell H: Collagen synthesis in mature articular cartilage of the rabbit. J Bone Joint Surg 53B:541, 1971
61. Rhaney K, Lamb D: The cysts of osteoarthritis of the hip. J Bone Joint Surg 37B:663, 1955
62. Rodnan GP et al: Postmortem examination on an elderly severe hemophiliac, with observations on the pathologic findings in hemophiliac joint disease. Arthritis Rheum 2:152, 1959
63. Rosenthal O, Bowie MA, Wagoner G: Studies in the metabolism of articular cartilage. I. Respiration and glycolysis of cartilage in relation to its age. J Cell Comp Physiol 17:221, 1941
64. Salter RB, Field P: The effects of continuous compression on living articular cartilage. J Bone Joint Surg 42A:31, 1960
65. Salter RB, Gross A, Hall JH: Hydrocortisone arthropathy: An experimental investigation. Can Med Assoc 197:374, 1967
66. Sapolsky L, Altman RD, Woessner JF et al: The action of cathepsin D in human articular cartilage on proteoglycans. J Clin Invest 52:624, 1973
67. Schubert M, Hamerman D: A Primer on Connective Tissue. Philadelphia, Lea & Febiger, 1968
68. Silberberg M, Silberberg R, Hasler M: Ultrastructure of articular cartilage of mice treated with somatotrophin. J Bone Joint Surg 46A:766, 1964
69. Sokoloff L: Elasticity of ageing cartilage. Fed Proc 25:1089, 1966
70. Sokoloff L: The Biology of Degenerative Joint Disease. Chicago, University of Chicago Press, 1969
71. Sokoloff L et al: The genetics of degenerative joint disease in mice. Arthritis Rheum 5:531, 1962
72. Stecher RM: Heredity of osteoarthritis. Arch Phys Med 46:178, 1965
73. Steinberg ME, Cohen RW, Cogen FC: Effects of intra-articular anti-metabolites. Arthritis Rheum 10:316, 1967
74. Stockwell RA: The cell density of human articular and costal cartilage. J Anat 101:753, 1967
75. Trias A: Effect of persistent pressure on the articular cartilage. J Bone Joint Surg 43B:376, 1961
76. Trueta J: Studies of the Development and Decay of the Human Frame. Philadelphia, WB Saunders, 1968
77. Wanka J, Dixon AS: Treatment of osteoarthritis of the hip with indomethacin. A controlled clinical trial. Ann Rheum Dis 23:288, 1964
78. Weightman B: Tensile fatigue of human articular cartilage. J Biomech 9(4):193, 1976
79. Weightman B, Freeman MAR, Swanson SAV: Fatigue of articular cartilage. Nature 244:303, 1973

80. Weiss C: Ultrastructural study of ageing human articular cartilage (abstr). J Bone Joint Surg 53A:803, 1971
81. Weiss C: Ultrastructural characteristics of osteoarthritis. Fed Proc 32:1459, 1973
82. Weiss C, Mirow S: An ultrastructural study of osteoarthritic changes in the articular cartilage of human knees. J Bone Joint Surg 54A:954, 1972
83. Weiss C, Rosenberg L, Helfet AJ: An ultrastructural study of normal young adult human articular cartilage. J Bone Joint Surg 50A:663, 1968
84. Weissman G, Spilberg IL: Breakdown of cartilage protein-polysaccharide by lysosomes. Arthritis Rheum 11:162, 1968
85. Weston PR et al: Specific inhibition of cartilage breakdown. Nature 222:285, 1969

Rheumatoid Arthritis

86. Badgley CE: The orthopedic treatment of arthritis. Am Acad Orthop Surg Lect 5:314, 1948
87. Bartfeld H, Epstein WV: Conference on rheumatoid factors and their biological significance. Ann NY Acad Sci 168:1, 1969
88. Bertand JJ, Waine H, Tobias CA: Distribution of gold in the animal body in relation to arthritis. J Lab Clin Med 33:133, 1948
89. Bunch TW, O'Duffy JD: Disease modifying drugs for progressive rheumatoid arthritis. Mayo Clin Proc 55:161, 1980
90. Bunnell S: Surgery of the rheumatic hand. J Bone Joint Surg 37A:759, 1955
91. Cooperating Committee of the American Rheumatism Association: A controlled trial of cyclophosphamide in rheumatoid arthritis. N Engl J Med 283:883, 1970
92. Dixon ASJ et al: Synthetic D(−)penicillamine in rheumatoid arthritis: Double-blind controlled study of a high and low dosage regimen. Ann Rheum Dis 34:416, 1975
93. Duthrie JR: Discussion during symposium on management of rheumatoid arthritis. Br Orthop Assoc Ann Meeting 1951
94. Duthrie JR: Medical treatment of rheumatic diseases. J Bone Joint Surg 34B:211, 1952
95. Hall AP, Mednis AD, Bayles TB: The latex agglutination and inhibition reactions. N Engl J Med 258:731, 1958
96. Harris ED Jr et al: Collagenase and rheumatoid arthritis. Arthritis Rheum 13:83, 1970
97. Herbut PA: General Pathology. Philadelphia, Lea & Febiger, 1955
98. Hersh EM: Immunosuppressive agents. In Sartorelli AC, Johns DG (eds): Handbook of Experimental Pharmacology, vol 38, part 1, pp 577–617. New York, Springer-Verlag, 1974
99. Hersperger WG: Gold therapy for R. A. Ann Intern Med 36:571, 1952
100. Idem: Comparison of the effect of plasmaphoresis and penicillamine on the level of circulating rheumatoid factor. Ann Rheum Dis 22:71, 1963
101. Jaffe IA: Intra-articular dissociation of the rheumatoid factor. J Lab Clin Med 60:409, 1962
102. Kelikian H: Surgery in the treatment of chronic arthritis. Surg Clin North Am 29:87, 1949
103. Kersley GD: The present status of gold therapy in R. A. Practitioner 161:158, 1948
104. Kuhns JG: Non-surgical treatment of arthritis. Am Acad Orthop Surg Inst Course Lect 6:292, 1949
105. Law WA: Surgical treatment of the rheumatic diseases. J Bone Joint Surg 34B:215, 1952
106. Lazarus GS et al: Role of granulocyte collegenase in collagen degradation. Am J Pathol 68:565, 1972
107. McGregor DD, Mackaness GB: Life and function of lymphocytes. In Zweifach BW, Grant L, McCluskey RT (eds): The Inflammatory Process, 2nd ed, vol 3. New York, Academic Press, 1974
108. Mahammed I et al: Effect of penicillamine therapy on circulating immune complexes in rheumatoid arthritis. Ann Rheum Dis 35:458, 1976
109. Makin M, Robin GC: Chronic synovial effusions treated with intra-articular radioactive gold. JAMA 188:725, 1964
110. Mason M et al: Azathioprine in rheumatoid arthritis. Br Med J 1:420, 1969
111. Mellors RC et al: Rheumatoid factor and the pathogenesis of rheumatoid arthritis. J Exp Med 113:475, 1961
112. Norcross BM, Lockie LM, Constantine AG et al: The effect of cortisone and ACTH on the histopathologic lesions of rheumatoid arthritis. Ann Intern Med 36:751, 1952
113. Norton W, Ziff M: Electron microscopic observations on the rheumatoid synovial membrane. Arthritis Rheum 9:589, 1966
114. Oronsky AL et al: Phagocytic release and activation of human leukocyte procollagenase. Nature 246:417, 1973
115. Otterness IG, Niblack JF: Clotrimazole and rheumatoid arthritis. Lancet 1:148, 1976
116. Pfizer Spectrum: In JAMA 151:(No. 9 Adv.), 1953
117. Shutkin NM: Note on the use of nitrogen mustard in rheumatoid arthritis. J Bone Joint Surg 33A:265, 1951
118. Singer JM, Plotz CM: Latex fixation test. Am J Med 21:888, 1956
119. Speed JS: Campbell's Operative Orthopedics. St. Louis, CV Mosby, 1949
120. Thompson HE: Cortisone and gold therapy in chronic rheumatoid arthritis. Ann Intern Med 36:992, 1952
121. Wyburn-Mason R: Clotrimazole and rheumatoid arthritis. Lancet 1:489, 1976
122. Ziff M, Brown P, Baden J et al: Hemiagglutination test for rheumatoid arthritis with enhanced sensitivity using euglobulin fraction. Bull Rheum Dis 5:75, 1954
123. Zucker-Franklin D: The phagosomes in rheumatoid synovial fluid leukocytes: A light, fluorescence, and electron microscope study. Arthritis Rheum 9:24, 1966

Juvenile Rheumatoid Arthritis

124. Arden GP et al: Total hip replacement in juvenile chronic arthritis and ankylosing spondylitis. Clin Orthop 84:130, 1972
125. Brewer EJ Jr: Juvenile Rheumatoid Arthritis. Philadelphia, WB Saunders, 1970
126. Colgan MT, Mintz AA: The comparative antipyretic effect of N-acetyl-p-aminophenol and acetylsalicylic acid. J Pediatr 50:552, 1957
127. Collins DH: The Pathology of Articular and Spinal Diseases, p 202. London, Edward Arnold & Co, 1947
128. Cornil V: Memoire sur des coincidences pathologiques du rhumatisme articulaire chronique. CR Mem Soc Biol (Paris), 3:3, 1864
129. Ebaugh FG et al: The anemia of rheumatoid arthritis. Med Clin North Am 39:489, 1955
130. Engen TJ: Adjustable knee or elbow extension orthosis: A new orthotic development. Orthop Prosthet Appl J 15:45, 1961
131. Eyring EJ et al: Synovectomy in juvenile rheumatoid arthritis. J Bone Joint Surg 53A:638, 1971
132. Fisher DA et al: Intermittent corticosteroid therapy of juvenile rheumatoid arthritis. Arthritis Rheum 7:413, 1964
133. Freyberg RH: Gold therapy for rheumatoid arthritis. In Hol-

lander JL: Arthritis and Allied Conditions, ed. 7th Philadelphia, Lea & Febiger, 1966
134. Good RA et al: The simultaneous occurrence of rheumatoid arthritis and agammaglobulinemia. J Lab Clin Med 49:343, 1957
135. Griffin PP, Tachdjian MO, Green WT: Pauciarticular arthritis in children. JAMA 184:145, 1963
136. Jacobs JC: Sudden death in arthritic children receiving large doses of indomethacin. JAMA 199:932, 1967
137. Jacobs JH et al: Rheumatoid arthritis presenting as tenosynovitis. J Bone Joint Surg 39B:288, 1957
138. Kampner SL, Ferguson AB Jr: Efficacy of synovectomy in juvenile rheumatoid arthritis. Clin Orthop 88:94, 1972
139. Kellgren JH, Ball J: Tendon lesions in rheumatoid arthritis. Ann Rheum Dis 9:48, 1950
140. Laaksonen AL: A prognostic study of juvenile rheumatoid arthritis. Acta Paediatr Scand (Suppl)55:166, 1966
141. Lockie LM, Norcross BM: Salicylates, phenylbutazone, chloroquines, and indomethacin in treatment of rheumatoid arthritis. In Hollander JL: Arthritis and Allied Conditions. Philadelphia, Lea & Febiger, 1966
142. Martel W et al: Roentgenologic manifestations of juvenile rheumatoid arthritis. Am J Roentgenol Radium Ther 88:400, 1962
143. Roberts FD et al: Evolution of anemia of rheumatoid arthritis. Blood 21:470, 1963
144. Rombouts JJ, Rombouts-Lindemans C: Scoliosis in juvenile rheumatoid arthritis. J Bone Joint Surg 56B:478, 1974
145. Sairanen E: On rheumatoid arthritis in children: Clinicoroentgenologic study. Acta Rheum Scand 2:1, 1958
146. Still GF: On a form of chronic joint disease in children. Med Chir Trans 80:47, 1897

The Rheumatoid Variants

147. Ahvenen P: Human yersiniosis in Finland: II. Clinical features. Ann Clin Res 4:39, 1972
148. Baker H: The Relationship Between Psoriasis, Psoriatic Arthritis, and Rheumatoid Arthritis: An Epidemiological, Clinical and Serological Study. M.D. thesis, University of Leeds, 1965
149. Baron JM: Reiter's disease. Br J Clin Pract 14:679, 1960
150. Baum J: Treatment of psoriatic arthritis with 6-mercaptopurine. Arthritis Rheum 16:139, 1973
151. Bourdillon C: Psoriasis and Arthropathies. Paris, Thése, 1888
152. Brewerton DA et al: Ankylosing spondylitis and HLA-W27. Lancet 1:904, 1973
153. Brewerton DA et al: HLA-W27 and arthropathies associated with ulcerative colitis and psoriasis. Lancet 1:956, 1974
154. Cahn A, Fries JF: An "experimental" epidemic of Reiter's syndrome revisited: Follow-up evidence on genetic and environmental factors. Ann Intern Med 84:564, 1976
155. Chajek T, Fainarr M: Behçet's disease: Report of 41 cases and a review of the literature. Medicine 54:179, 1975
156. Clarke O: Arthritis mutilans associated with psoriasis. Lancet 1:249, 1950
157. Csonka GW: Recurrent attacks in Rieter's syndrome. Arthritis Rheum 3:164, 1960
158. Csonka GW: Reiter's syndrome. Ergeb Inn Med Kinderheilkd 23:125, 1965
159. Eisen AZ, Seegmiller JE: Uric acid metabolism. J Clin Invest 40:1486, 1961
160. Feldges DH, Barnes CG: Treatment of psoriatic arthropathy with either azathioprine or methotrexate. Rheumatol Rehabil 13:120, 1974
161. Ginsburg JH, Quismorio FP, Mongan ES et al: Articular complications after jejunoileal shunt: Clinical and immunological studies. Arthritis Rheum 19:797, 1976
162. Goldin RH, Bluestone R: HL-A W27 antigens and sacroiliitis. Compr Ther 2:23, 1976
163. Good AE: Involvement of the back in Reiter's syndrome. Ann Intern Med 57:44, 1962
164. Good AE: Reiter's disease: A review with special attention to cardiovascular and neurologic sequelae. Semin Arthritis Rheum 3:253, 1973–1974
165. Haslock I, Wright V: The musculo-skeletal complications of Crohn's disease. Medicine 52:217, 1973
166. HILL AGS: Sacro-iliac joint in adult rheumatoid arthritis and psoriatic arthropathy. Ann Rheum Dis 20:247, 1961
167. Kersley GD: Amethopterin (methotrexate) in connective tissue disease—psoriasis and polyarthritis. Ann Rheum Dis 27:64, 1968
168. Kulka JP: The lesions of Reiter's syndrome. Arthritis Rheum 5:195, 1962
169. Leonard DG, O'Duffy JD, Rogers RS III: Prospective analysis of psoriatic arthritis in patients hospitalized for psoriasis. Mayo Clin Proc 53:511, 1978
170. Levine E, Paulus HE: Treatment of psoriasis with azaribine. Arthritis Rheum 19:21, 1976
171. LeVine ME, Dobbins WO III: Joint changes in Whipple's disease. Semin Arthritis Rheum 3:79, 1973
172. McCormack WM, Braun P, Lee YH et al: The genital mycoplasmas. N Engl J Med 288:78, 1973
173. McEwen C, Lingg C, Kirsner J: Arthritis accompanying ulcerative colitis. Am J Med 33:923, 1962
174. Maizel H, Ruffin JM, Dobbins WO III: Whipple's disease: A review of 19 patients from one hospital and a review of the literature since 1950. Medicine 49:175, 1970
175. Masbernard A: Le syndrome de Fiessinger-Leroy-Reiter: Enseigments par l'étude de 80 cas observés en Tunisie. Rev Rhum 26:21, 1959
176. Mason RM, Barnes CG: Behçet's syndrome with arthritis. Ann Rheum Dis 28:95, 1969
177. Metzger AL et al: HL-A W27 in psoriatic arthritis. Arthritis Rheum 18:111, 1975
178. Moll JMH: A Family Study of Psoriatic Arthritis. D.M. thesis, University of Oxford, 1971
179. Moll JMH, Wright V: Psoriatic arthritis. Semin Arthritis Rheum 3:55, 1973
180. Morris RT, Metzger AL, Bluestone R et al: HL-A W27—a useful discriminator in the arthropathies of inflammatory bowel disease. N Engl J Med 290:1117, 1974
181. Noer HR: An "experimental" epidemic of Reiter's syndrome. JAMA 198:693, 1966
182. O'Duffy JD: Psoriatic arthritis. Postgrad Med 61:165, 1977
183. Parrish JA et al: Photochemotherapy of psoriasis with oral methoxsalen and longwave ultraviolet light. N Engl J Med 291:1207, 1974
184. Reiter H: die Reiterische Krankheit. Dtsch Med Wochenschr 82:1337, 1957
185. Rosenthal M et al: Letter: Psoriatic arthritis. N Engl J Med 195:1204, 1976
186. Schittenhelm A, Schlecht H: Uber Polyarthritis enterica. Dtsch Arch Klin Med 126:329, 1918
187. Schlosstein L et al: High association of an HL-A antigen, W27, with ankylosing spondylitis. N Engl J Med 208:704, 1973
188. Serre H, Simon L, Sany J: Le rhumatisme psoriasique. J Med Montpellier 4:3, 1969
189. Sherman M: Psoriatic arthritis: Observations on the clinical,

roentgenographic and pathological changes. J Bone Joint Surg 34A:831, 1952
190. Solem JH, Lassen J: Reiter's disease following *Yersinia enterocolitica* infection. Scand J Infect Dis 3:83, 1971
191. Waller M, Toone EC: Normal individuals with positive tests for rheumatoid factor. Arthritis Rheum 11:50, 1968
192. Wands JR, LaMont JT, Mann E et al: Arthritis associated with intestinal-bypass procedure for morbid obesity. N Engl J Med 294:121, 1975
193. Warren CP: Arthritis associated with *Salmonella* infections. Ann Rheum Dis 29:483, 1970
194. Weinberger HJ, Ropes MW, Kulka JP et al: Reiter's syndrome, clinical and pathological observations: A long term study of 16 cases. Medicine 41:35, 1962
195. Wilke G: Polyneuritiden nach chronischer Enterocolitis, insbesondere nach Ruhr Dtsch Med Wochenschr 69:443, 1943
196. Wright V: Psoriasis and arthritis. Ann Rheum Dis 15:48, 1956
197. Wright V, Moll JMH: Psoriatic arthritis. Bull Rheum Dis 21:627, 1971
198. Wright V, Watkinson G: The arthritis of ulcerative colitis. Br Med J 2:670, 1965
199. Zvaitler NJ, Martel W: Spondylitis in chronic ulcerative colitis. Arthritis Rheum 3:76, 1960

Palindromic Rheumatism

200. Boland EW, Headley NE: Treatment of so-called palindromic rheumatism with gold compounds. Ann Rheum Dis 7:246, 1948
201. Hench PS, Rosenberg EF: Palindromic rheumatism. Arch Intern Med 73:293, 1944
202. Hench PS et al: (Rheumatism Review). Ann Intern Med 28:66, 309, 1947

Neuroarthropathy

203. Eloesser L: On the nature of neuropathic affections of joints. Ann Surg 66:201, 1917
204. Ghormley RK (ed): Orthopedic Surgery, p 375. New York, Nelson, 1938
205. Key JA: Treatment of Charcot's joint. Urol Cutan Rev 49:161, 1945
206. Lippman EM, Grow JL: Neurogenic arthropathy associated with diabetes mellitus. J Bone Joint Surg 37A:971, 1955
207. Luck JV: Bone and Joint Diseases, p 243. Springfield, Charles C Thomas, 1950
208. Soto-Hall R: Fusion in Charcot joint of the knee. Ann Surg 108:124, 1938

Hemophilic Arthritis

209. Abildgaard CF: Current concepts in the management of hemophilia. Semin Hematol 12:223, 1975
210. Ahlborg A, Nilsson IM: Fractures in haemophiliacs with special reference to complications and treatment. Acta Chir Scand 133:293, 1967
211. Arnold WD, Hilgartner MW: Hemophilic arthropathy. J Bone Joint Surg 59A:287, 1977
212. Brant EE, Jordan HH: Radiologic aspects of hemophilic pseudotumors of bone. Am J Roentgenol 115:525, 1972
213. Brinkhous K (ed): Handbook of Hemophilia. Amsterdam, Excerpta Medica, 1975
214. Creveld S van, Heedmaeker PJ, Kingma MJ et al: Degeneration of joints in haemophiliacs under treatment by modern methods. J Bone Joint Surg 53B:296, 1971
215. D'Ambrosia RD et al: Total hip replacement in patients with hemophilia and hemorrhagic diathesis. Surg Gynecol Obstet 139:381, 1974
216. Duthie RB et al: The Management of the Musculoskeletal Problems in the Hemophilias, p 48. Oxford, Blackwell Scientific Publications, 1972
217. Dyszy-Laube B et al: Synovectomy in the treatment of hemophilic arthropathy. J Pediatr Surg 9:123, 1974
218. Feil E, Bentley G, Rizza CR: Fracture management in patients with haemophilia. J Bone Joint Surg 56B:643, 1974
219. Fernandez de Valderrama JA, Matthews JM: The haemophilic pseudotumor or haemophilic subperiosteal hematoma. J Bone Joint Surg 47B:256, 1965
220. Ghormley RK, Clegg RS: Bone and joint changes in hemophilia. J Bone Joint Surg 30A:589, 1948
221. Goodfellow J, Fearn CB, Matthews JM: Iliacus haematoma: A common complication of haemophilia. J Bone Joint Surg 49B:748, 1967
222. Harris CO Jr et al: Collagenase and rheumatoid arthritis. Arthritis Rheum 13:83, 1970
223. Hilgartner MW, Arnold WD: Hemophilic pseudotumor treated with replacement therapy and radiation. J Bone Joint Surg 57A:1145, 1975
224. Hussey HH: Editorial: Hemophilic pseudotumor of bone. JAMA 232:1040, 1975
225. Ingram GIC, Mathews JA, Bennett AE: Controlled trial of joint aspiration in acute haemophilic hemarthrosis (abstr). Ann Rheum Dis 31:423, 1972
226. Jordan HH: Hemophilic Arthropathies. Springfield, IL, Charles C Thomas, 1958
227. Kemp HS, Matthews JM: The management of fractures in haemophilia and Christmas disease. J Bone Joint Surg 50B:357, 1968
228. McDaniel WJ: A modified subluxation hinge for use in hemophilic knee flexion contractures. Clin Orthop 103:50, 1974
229. McKay SR: Early management of joint and soft tissue bleeding. In Committee on Prosthetic Research and Development (ed): Comprehensive Management of Musculoskeletal Disorders in Hemophilia, p 72. National Academy of Science, 1973
230. Patel MR, Pearlman HS, Lavine LS: Arthrodesis in hemophilia. Clin Orthop 86:168, 1972
231. Post M, Telfer MC: Surgery in hemophilic patients. J Bone Joint Surg 57A:1136, 1975
232. Rosenthal RL, Graham JJ, Selirio E: Excision of pseudotumor with repair by bone graft of pathological fracture of femur in hemophilia. J Bone Joint Surg 55A:827, 1973
233. Staas WE et al: Lower extremity amputation in hemophilia: Case report and review of surgical principles. J Bone Joint Surg 54A:1514, 1972

Alterations in Composition and Function of Synovial Tissues Related to Tumor Formation

234. Bennett GA: Malignant neoplasms originating in synovial tissues. J Bone Joint Surg 29:259, 1947

Pigmented Villonodular Synovitis

235. Jaffe HL, Lichtenstein L, Sutro CJ: Pigmented villonodular synovitis. Arch Pathol 31:731, 1941

236. Minear WL: Xanthomatous joint tumors. J Bone Joint Surg 33A:451, 1951
237. Young JM, Hudacek AG: Experimental production of pigmented villonodular synovitis in dogs. Am J Pathol 30:799, 1954

Hemangioma of a Joint

238. Bennett GE, Cobey MC: hemangioma of joints. Arch Surg 38:487, 1939
239. Cobey MC: Hemangioma of joints. Arch Surg 46:465, 1943
240. Lewis RC Jr, Coventry MBV, Soule EH: Hemangioma of the synovial membrane. J Bone Joint Surg 41A:264, 1959

Synovioma

241. Bennett GA: Malignant neoplasms originating in synovial tissues. J Bone Joint Surg 29:259, 1947
242. Berger L: Synovial sarcoma in serous bursae and tendon sheaths. Am J Cancer 34:501, 1938
243. Haagaensen CD, Stout AP: Synovial sarcoma. Ann Surg 120:826, 1944
244. Tillotson JF, McDonald JR, Janes JM: Synovial sarcomata. J Bone Joint Surg 33A:459, 1951

14

Orthopaedic Neurology

Section I
Neurodiagnosis

For accurate diagnosis of the level and type of nerve involvement in an orthopaedic disability, there is no substitute for familiarity with the anatomy of the spine and cord, with the various deep and superficial reflexes and the nerve centers through which they pass, and with the dermal sensory pattern. With the systematic investigation of these parameters and the interpretation of electrodiagnostic findings, the localization of neurologic dysfunction should be a reasonably routine procedure for the examiner and the treatment and prognosis should be clarified.

ANATOMY OF THE SPINAL CORD

The spinal cord, a direct downward continuation of the medulla oblongata, starts at the upper border of the atlas and ends at the lower border of the first lumbar vertebra as the conus medullaris.[1] Although cylindrical, it is slightly flattened in its anteroposterior diameter. Corresponding to the large nerves supplying the upper and the lower limbs is a cervical enlargement from C3 to T2 and a lumbar enlargement from T9 to T12. From the lowest end of the spinal cord (the conus medullaris) extends a delicate median prolongation, the filum terminale interna, which ends with the dural sac at the second sacral vertebra. Its extradural prolongation, the filum terminale externa, ends at the coccyx (Fig. 14-1).

The spinal cord is enveloped by the dura, the arachnoid, and the pia mater. External to the dura is the epidural space, which is filled by a thin layer of fat, areolar tissue, and veins. The arachnoid and the subarachnoid spaces are filled with fluid, which cushions the spinal cord. The pia mater intimately surrounding the spinal cord also has lateral extensions to the inner dural surface. These are equally spaced between nerve roots and are known as dentate ligaments.

In fetal life, the spinal cord fills the entire length of the vertebral canal and the spinal nerves run in a horizontal direction. As the vertebral column elongates with growth, the spinal cord is drawn upward, and therefore the roots assume an increasingly oblique and downward direction toward their foramina of exit, forming at its lowest portion the cauda equina.

The spinal nerves emerge from the spinal cord in pairs: 8 in the cervical region, 12 in the thoracic region, 5 in the lumbar region, 5 in the sacral region, and 1 pair of coccygeal nerves, making a total of 31 pairs of spinal nerves. These also correspond to varying segments of neuromeres of the spinal cord.

Each spinal nerve has an anterior and a posterior root, the latter showing an oval enlargement called the ganglion. These nerve roots joint to form plexuses:

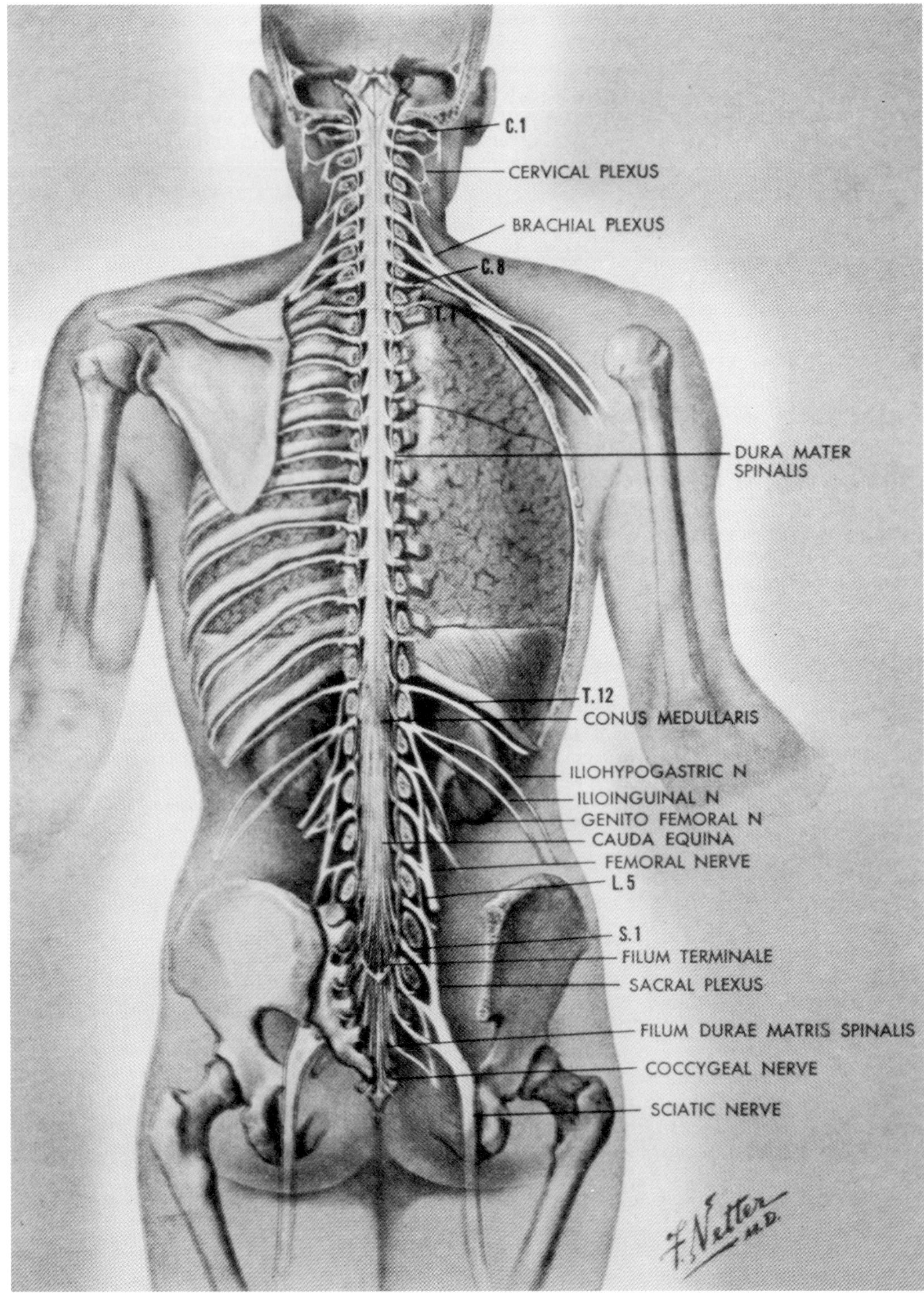

FIG. 14-1. The spinal cord *in situ.* (Drawing by F. Netter *in* The central nervous system. Clinical Symposia 1:186, No. 6, 1949)

The cervical plexus, formed by the anterior divisions of the upper four cervical nerves
The brachial plexus, formed by the anterior divisions of nerves C5 to C8 and by the first thoracic nerve
The lumbar plexus, formed by the anterior divisions of nerves L1, L2, and L3 and the greater part of L4
The sacral plexus, formed by the roots of L4 and L5 and of S1, S2 and part of S3
The coccygeal plexus, formed by nerves S3 to S5

In addition to the 12 pairs of intercostal nerves, some of the most significant nerves are the iliohypogastric nerve arising from the first lumbar root; the ilioinguinal nerve arising also from the first and the second lumbar roots; the sciatic nerve, which is the main nerve of the sacral plexus, and the coccygeal nerve, which also receives filaments from the fourth and fifth sacral nerves.

EXIT OF SPINAL NERVES

As the anterior root of the spinal cord emerges from the anterior and lateral gray columns, it traverses the surrounding membranes of pia, arachnoid, and dura. The posterior root, which is attached to the posterolateral portion of the spinal cord, originates from two bundles of fibers in the spinal ganglion. Both anterior and posterior roots pierce the dura separately as they make their exit through their respective intervertebral foramina. As a rule, the posterior root is thicker and larger than the anterior root. They are enclosed in a common dural sheath just beyond the spinal ganglion, where they become the spinal nerve and are surrounded by epineurium. (Color Plate 14-1).

The spinal ganglia, which lie at the outer portion of the intervertebral foramina, are oval and vary in size corresponding to their nerve roots.

The spinal nerves lie horizontally in the cervical region, but below these segments they assume an increasingly oblique and downward direction as they approach the lumbar region where they are almost vertical, forming the cauda equina. At the lower thoracic level there is a difference of two vertebral segments between the origin of the spinal nerve and the level of exit.

From each sympathetic trunk ganglion, which lies on the posterolateral surface of the vertebral body, a branch (gray ramus communicans) joins the adjacent spinal nerve.

Efferent, preganglionic sympathetic fibers (white ramus communicans), which originate in the lateral columns, pass along with the anterior root to the corresponding sympathetic ganglion or along its trunk to the sympathetic plexus.

Shortly after emerging from the intervertebral foramen, each spinal nerve turns back through the same foramen to supply the spinal cord membranes, blood vessels, intervertebral ligaments, and joint surfaces.

The spinal nerve then divides into two branches, each with fibers from both roots.

The anterior division supplies anterior and lateral portions of the trunk and the limbs. In the thoracic region it spans the space between the pleura and the intercostal membranes, runs below the lower rib margin, and supplies the intercostal muscles and adjacent skin. In the cervical and lumbar regions the anterior divisions form plexuses.

The posterior division is directed backward shortly beyond the formation of the spinal nerve. Its medial branch supplies the multifidi, the longissmus, the semispinalis, and the trapezius muscles and then proceeds along the spinous process and supplies the skin. Its lateral branch traverses the longissimus muscle and supplies the intercostal muscle and adjacent skin. In the lumbar region the medial branches of the posterior division hug the articular processes of the vertebrae and end in the multifidi, the lateral branches supply the group of sacrospinalis muscles, adjacent fascia, and skin.

SECTIONS THROUGH THE SPINAL CORD

Cross sections of the spinal cord at various levels show considerable variation in size and shape. The proportion of gray to white matter also varies and is much greater in the cervical and the lumbar regions and greatest in the conus medullaris. The anterior and the posterior gray columns in the thoracic region are equally thin, but in the cervical region the anterior gray columns are larger; in the lumbar region and below, both gray columns are about equally wide and in much greater proportion to the white matter (Color Plate 14-2).

Through the entire length of the spinal cord runs the central canal, which is lined with ciliated ependymal cells. Superiorly, it opens into the fourth ventricle and inferiorly extends into the filum terminale. The horizontal gray matter that joins the gray columns surrounds the central canal and is divided by it into anterior and posterior gray commissures.

TRACTS

Through the spinal cord run fibers carrying impulses to and from various portions of the brain. These fibers group themselves into tracts. Only those of known clinical importance will be described.

Funiculus Gracilis (Goll) and Funiculus Cuneatus (Burdach). These fibers carry muscle and joint sensations and lie between the posterior median and the posterolateral sulcus. In the cervical and the thoracic regions these tracts are separated by a septum at the lower portion of which is found the comma tract of Schultze.

Lateral Spinothalamic Tract. This tract mediates pain and temperature sensation. It arises in the posterior column, crosses to the opposite side in the anterior commissure, and ascends in the lateral funiculus to the thalamus.

Ventral Spinothalamic Tract. This tract transmits impulses of touch. It also arises in the posterior column, crosses in the anterior commissure to the opposite side, and ascends in the anterior funiculus to the thalamus.

Dorsal Spinocerebellar Tract. This tract transmits impulses from leg muscles and trunk between the C6 and the L2 segments. It is located on the lateral surface ventral to the posterolateral sulcus and ascends to the cerebellum by way of the restiform body.

Ventral Spinocerebellar Tract (Gower's). This tract carries impulses to the cerebellum by way of the medulla, the pons, and the anterior medullary velum. It lies at the periphery on the ventrolateral aspect of the cord.

Spinotectal Tract. This tract arises from cells in the posterior gray column, crosses over and ascends in the lateral funiculus, and ends in the corpora quadrigemina.

Rubrospinal Tract. This tract carries impulses for cerebellar reflexes. It arises in the red nucleus and crosses over and descends near the center of the lateral funiculus.

Lateral Pyramidal Tract. This tract carries impulses to the primary motor neuron. It arises from large cells in the precentral gyrus and, after decussation in the medulla, enters the lateral funiculus, lying between the dorsal spinocerebellar tract and the lateral funiculus.

Direct Pyramidal Tract. This tract is small; it arises from cells in the central motor area, passes down the same side close to the anterior median fissure, then crosses in the anterior commissure to the opposite side and at various levels ends by synapses with the anterior horn cells.

Tectospinal Tract. This tract mediates optic and auditory reflexes. It arises in the superior colliculi and crosses and then descends in the anterior funiculus to end in the motor cells of the anterior column.

SPINAL MEMBRANES AND NERVE ROOTS

The spinal cord is enveloped by membranes that are a direct continuation of those surrounding the brain (Color Plate 14-3).

Dura Mater. This membrane extends direct from the cranial dura, beginning at the foramen magnum and continuing as far down as the second sacral vertebra. It adheres anteriorly to the posterior longitudinal ligament and corresponds in shape to the enlargements of the spinal cord. The dura also invests the spinal nerves as they leave the lateral margins of the spinal cord to their points of exit.

Subdural Space. This is a potential space containing a minute quantity of fluid and is found between the arachnoid and the dura.

Arachnoid and Subarachnoid. These structures consist of a delicate meshwork of mesothelial cells with spaces filled with cerebrospinal fluid. These membranes also envelop the spinal nerves to their intervertebral foramina.

Pia Mater. This delicate fibrous layer intimately invests the spinal cord. At its lateral margins the pia forms denser pointed prolongations to the inner dural surface. These are spaced equally between the nerve roots and also separate the anterior from the posterior spinal roots.

Although there are no visible demarcations, the spinal cord is said to be made up of segments of varying lengths. These segments correspond approximately to the attachments of a pair of spinal nerves. The widest segments are in the midthoracic region.

On cross section of the spinal cord one can see the white matter on the periphery, which is made up of medullated nerve fibers held together by neuroglia. In the central portion of the spinal cord is the gray matter, which has the form of the letter *H*. This consists of numerous nerve cells and nonmedullated nerve fibers held together by neuroglia.

Spinal Nerves. These nerves consist of an anterior and a posterior spinal root with its ganglion. They are attached to the corresponding gray matter of the spinal cord.

Anterior Root. The anterior root arises from nerve cells in the anterior and lateral columns of the gray matter. As they pass through the white matter they become medullated. They leave the spinal cord in two or three irregular rows (fila) to efferent pathways.

Posterior Root. The posterior root arises from the medial afferent fibers of the spinal ganglion and reaches the posterolateral sulcus in the form of six or eight fasciculi (fila).

Spinal Ganglia. These ganglia are enveloped by the continuation of the dural sheath and contain irregularly spherical cells. The cells give off a unipolar coiled axon that divides into a medial and a lateral portion. The former is directed toward the spinal cord and becomes the posterior root, whereas the latter is directed peripherally to sensory end organs of muscles, joints, skin, and viscera.

Anterior Median Fissure. This fissure is lined by an overlapping fold of pia and dips into the greater part of the anterior portion of the spinal cord.

Anterior Lateral Sulcus. This fine depression lies about midway between the anterior median fissure and the lateral margin of the spinal canal and marks the exit of the fila of the anterior roots.

ARTERIES OF THE SPINAL CORD

The spinal cord derives its blood supply from the vertebral artery and a series of spinal rami that enter the intervertebral foramina at successive levels (Color Plate 14-4).

Posterior Spinal Artery. This branch of the vertebral artery begins near the lateral margin of the medulla oblongata and descends on the dorsolateral surface of the spinal cord posterior to the spinal roots. In its downward course to the cauda equina, the posterior spinal artery receives a succession of small arterial branches that enter the spinal canal through the intervertebral foramina. These vessels and their branches anastomose freely around the posterior roots and with the corresponding vessels on the opposite side, dipping also into the substance of the spinal cord; in the midline they form the posterior central artery.

Anterior Spinal Artery. This artery is formed by the union of two branches from the terminal portion of the vertebral artery at the level of the foramen magnum. The artery descends as a single trunk on the anterior aspect of the spinal cord to the conus medullaris. It continues along the cauda equina and ends as a fine arteriole accompanying the filum terminale. At successive levels, it, too, is reinforced by spinal branches entering through the intervertebral foramina. Along its course small twigs from this artery enter the substance of the spinal cord, and in the anterior median fissure these form the anterior central artery.

Spinal Branches. These branches arise at various levels from the sacral, iliolumbar, intercostal, inferior thyroid, and vertebral arteries, which enter the spinal canal through the intervertebral foramina. Each spinal branch divides into two rami: (1) a peripheral ramus, which, after entering the spinal canal, divides into an ascending and a descending branch and then anastomoses with the one above and below to form two lateral chains on the posterior surfaces of the vertebral bodies near the junction of the pedicles and (2) a central ramus, which supplies the spinal cord and it membranes by dividing into anterior and posterior arteries that anastomose with the anterior and the posterior arteries of the spinal cord.

VENOUS DRAINAGE OF SPINAL CORD AND VERTEBRAL COLUMN

Outside and inside the vertebral canal, running along the entire length, are series of venous plexuses that freely anastomose with each other and end in intervertebral veins.

Two groups of venous plexuses are found outside the vertebral canal: (1) the anterior group, which lies in front of the vertebral bodies and receives some venous tributaries from vertebral bodies and communicates with the basivertebral and the intervertebral veins, and (2) the posterior group, which forms a network of venous plexuses spreading over the spinous processes, laminae, facets, and adjacent deep musculature. In the cervical region these veins communicate with the deep cervical occipital and cerebral veins.

The venous plexuses inside the vertebral canal lie between the dura and the inner vertebral surfaces. These veins receive tributaries from the adjacent bony structures and the spinal cord. Although they form a close network, running vertically within the spinal canal, they may be subdivided into a pair of anterior internal venous plexuses of veins, which lie on either side of the posterior longitudinal ligament and into which basivertebral veins empty, and into a single posterior internal venous plexus of veins, which lies anterior to, and on either side of, the vertebral arches and the ligamentum flavum, which anastomoses with the posterior external veins.

These plexuses form almost a series of venous rings at the level of each vertebra, found most strikingly at the foramen magnum.

Tunneling the bony structure of each vertebral body is the basivertebral vein, which has a small valvelike opening as it joins the anterior internal venous plexus.

The intervertebral veins leave the spinal cord through the intervertebral foramina in company with the intercostal, the lumbar, and the sacral veins.

The veins of the spinal cord are minute and delicate. They emerge from the anterior median fissure as the anterior central vein and from the posterior sulcus as the posterior central vein. There are also two lateral longitudinal veins, on either side of the spinal cord, and they all empty into the intervertebral veins. However, those near the foramen magnum empty into the inferior petrosal sinus of cerebellar veins.

DERMAL SEGMENTATION

Sensation from the outside world reaches consciousness through sensory impulses. Most of these are carried by afferent nerve fibers to the spinal cord and up to the brain.

The nerve fibers that carry sensation of pain, temperature, touch, vibration, position sense, and other discriminatory sensibilities have their cells of origin in the

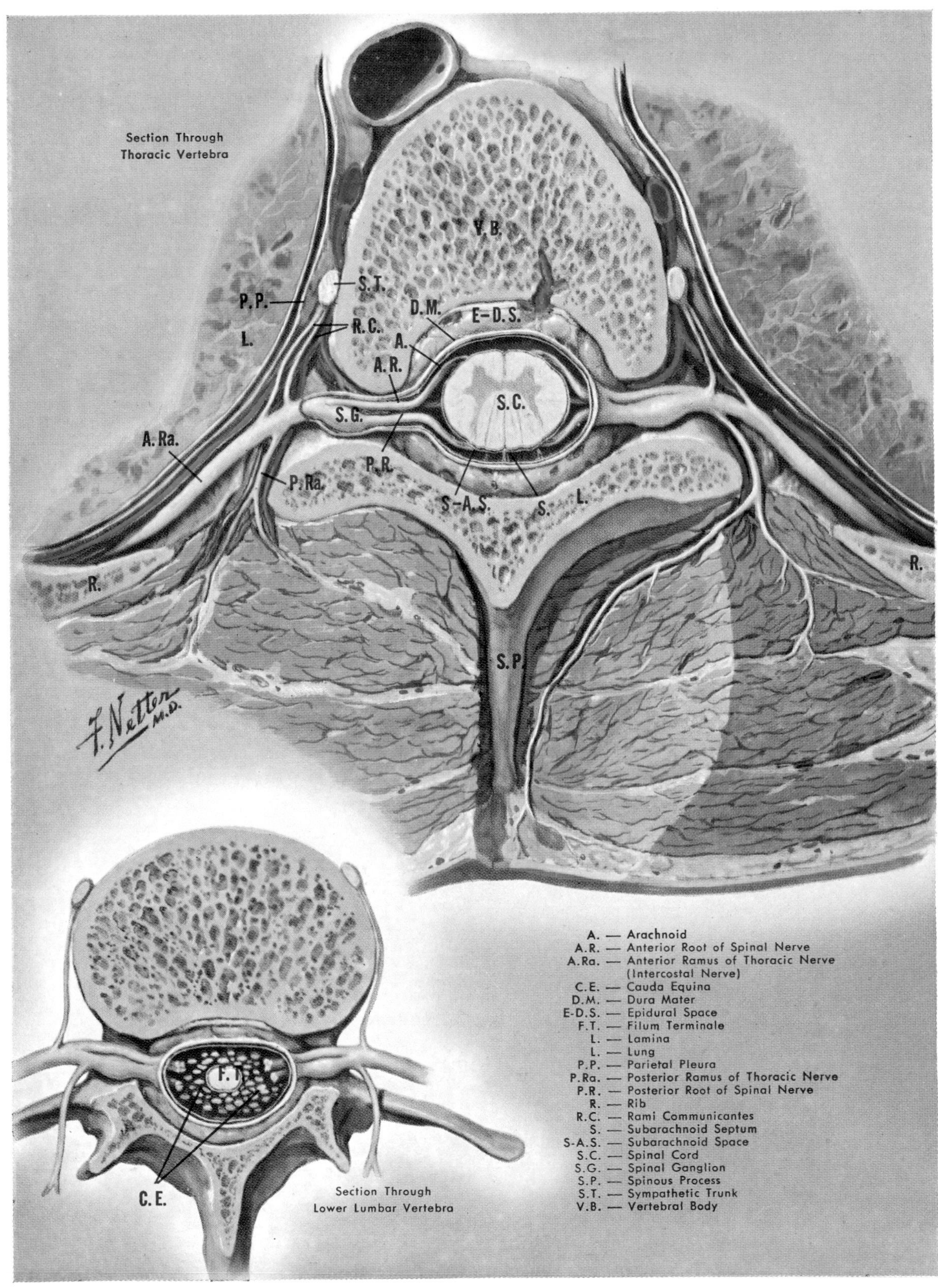

PLATE 14-1. Exit of spinal nerves. (Drawing by F. Netter *in* The central nervous system. Ciba Clinical Symposia 1:187, No. 6, 1949) (See p. 466.)

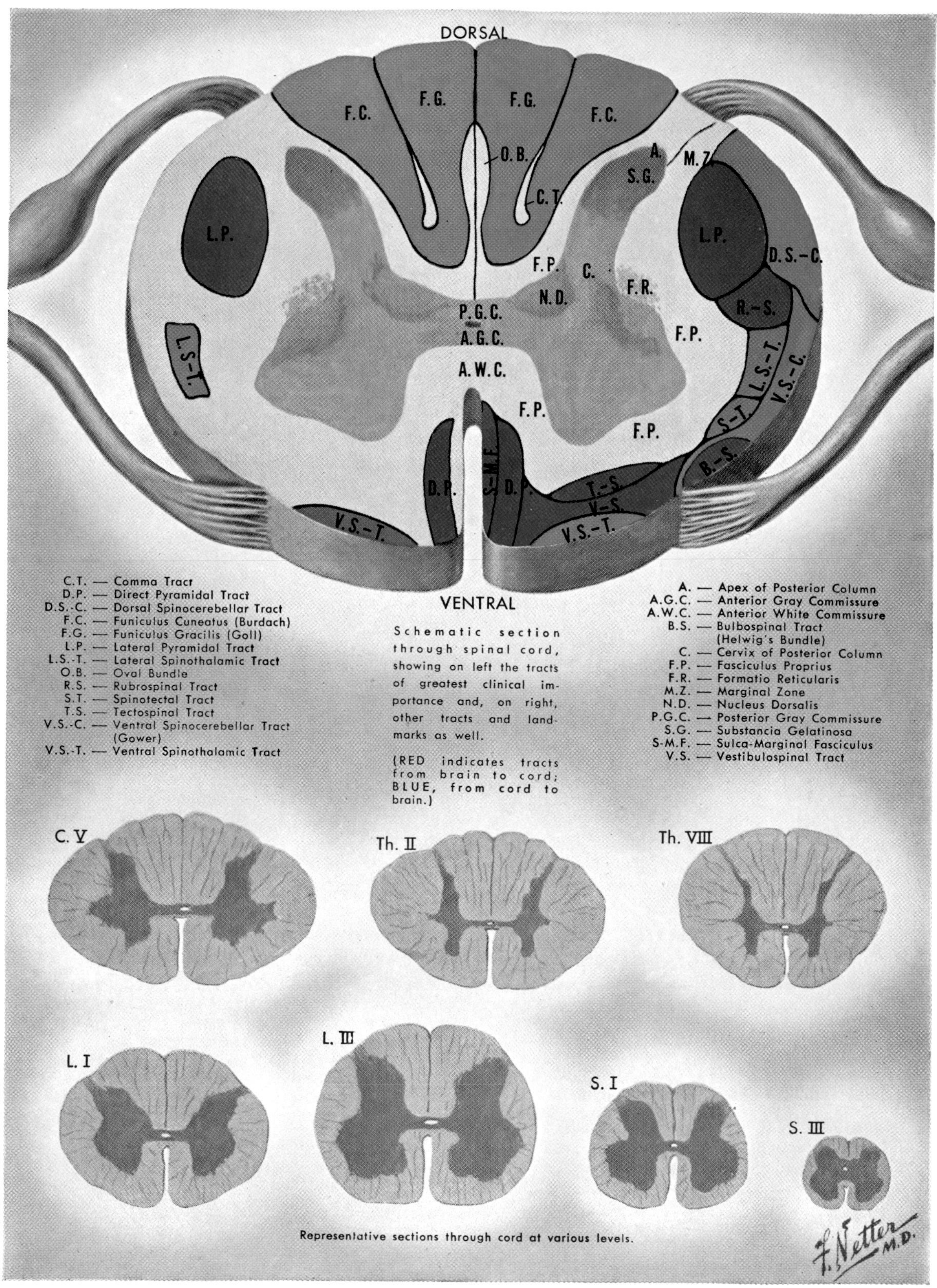

PLATE 14-2. Sections through the spinal cord. (Drawing by F. Netter *in* The central nervous system. Ciba Clinical Symposia 1:188, No. 6, 1949) (See p. 466.)

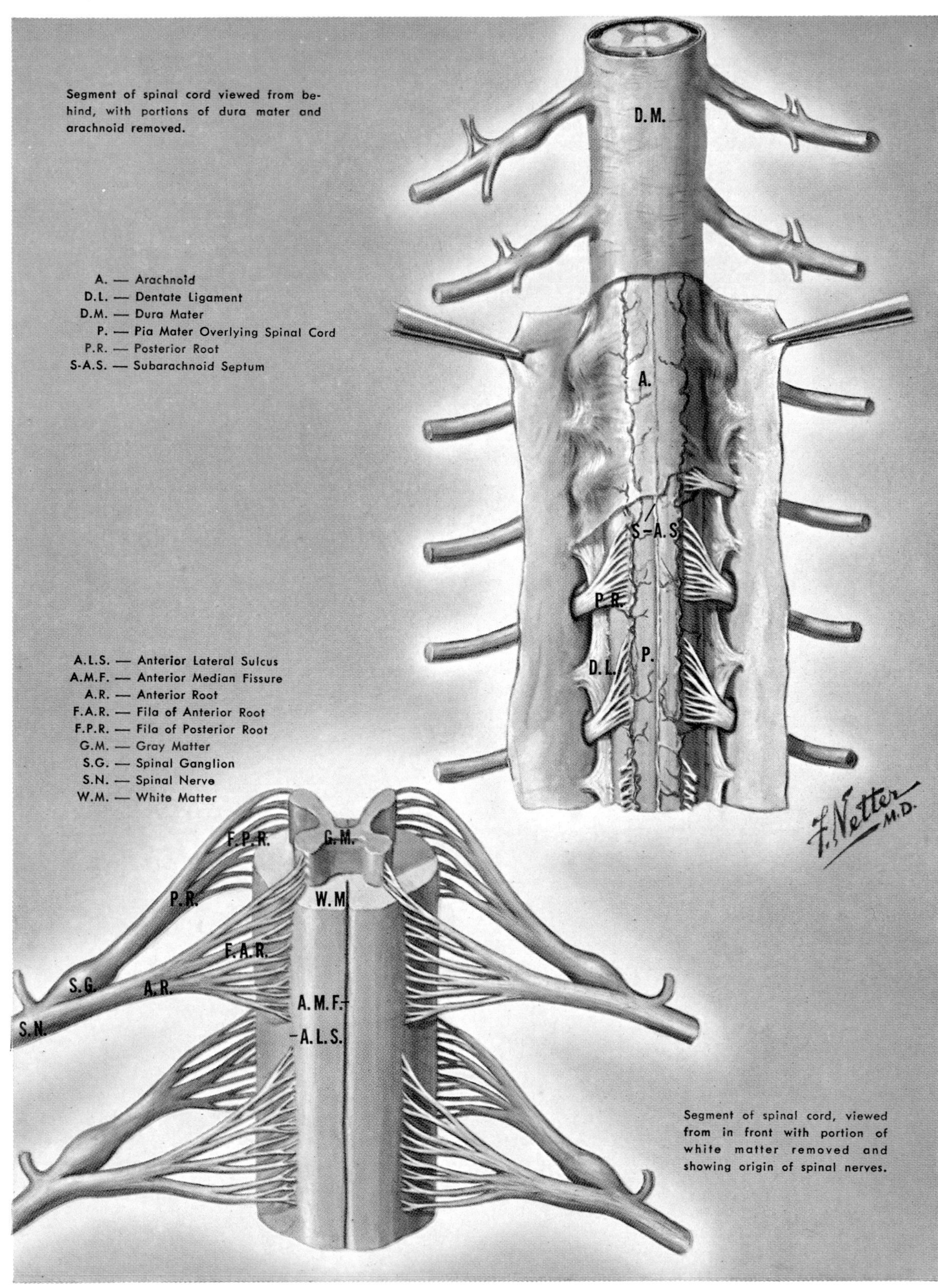

PLATE 14-3. Spinal membranes and nerve roots. (Drawing by F. Netter *in* The central nervous system. Ciba Clinical Symposia 1:189, No. 6, 1949) (See p. 467.)

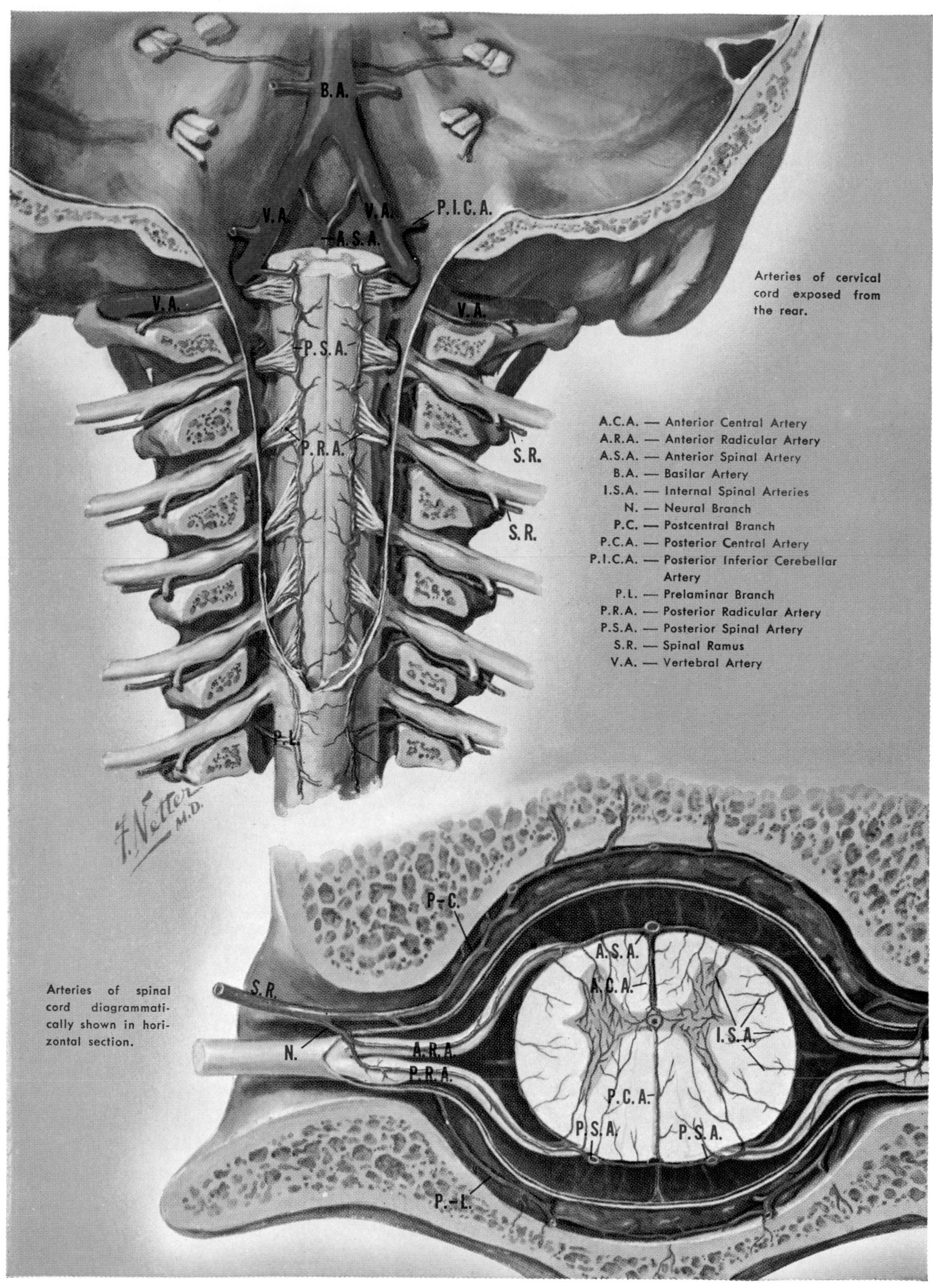

PLATE 14-4. Arteries of the spinal cord. (Drawing by F. Netter *in* The central nervous system. Ciba Clinical Symposia 1:190, No. 6, 1949) (See p. 468.)

spinal ganglia, from which fibers also arise to make up the dorsal root.

The fibers that carry the impulses of sensation from the skin, the muscles, and the joints are arranged in segments, which in simplest form are found in the thoracic region as broad bands. In the upper and the lower limbs the sensory arrangement is more complicated but follows a vertical pattern in each limb.

It has been found that if a dorsal root is sectioned, complete anesthesia of the involved dermal segment does not follow because of an overlapping of sensation by the nerves above and below the affected dermal segment. It has been further established that each sensory nerve carries impulses not only from its own dermal segment but also from the ones above and below. This overlapping of cutaneous sensation is known as metamerism.

If one is familiar with the cutaneous distribution of various nerve roots, it is possible to localize with great accuracy the site and the level of any pathologic disturbance.

A chart outlining the exact sensory dermal segments is a good reference (Fig. 14-2), but it is valuable to remember some surface landmarks that will serve as a general guide to localization:

The clavicle is supplied by C3 sensory root.
The deltoid is supplied by C5 sensory root.
The nipple area is supplied by T4 sensory root.
The intercostal margin is supplied by T7 sensory root.
The umbilicus is supplied by T10 sensory root.
The groin region is supplied by T12 sensory root.
The lateral aspect of the forearm and hand is supplied by C6 and C7 sensory roots.
The inner aspect of the forearm and hand is supplied by C8 and T1 sensory roots.
The anterior surface of the thigh and inner surface of the leg is supplied from above down by L1, L2, L3, and L4.
The outer and posterior surfaces of the legs are supplied by L5 and S1 and S2 sensory roots.
The perineum is supplied by S3, S4, and S5 sensory roots.

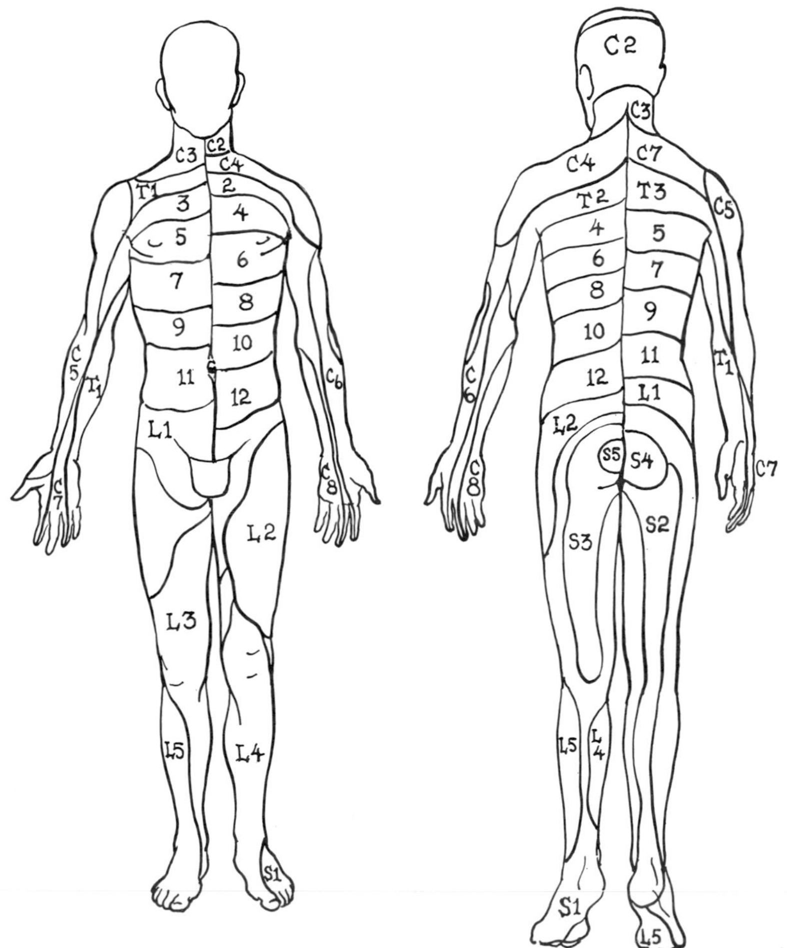

FIG. 14-2. Distribution of spinal dermatomes. Considerable overlap occurs; consequently, involvement of a single spinal segment may not be evident.

NEUROLOGIC DIAGNOSIS

Diagnosis of orthopaedic conditions requires a basic understanding of neurology.[2] A simple neurologic examination ordinarily suffices to differentiate the majority of neurologic disorders.

MOTOR FUNCTION

Disturbance of muscle power varies from paresis (weakness) and paralysis (complete loss) to hyperkinesia (increased muscular movements). The patient may be able to move a muscle; yet paresis may be demonstrated by inability to perform a movement against resistance. Monoplegia defines paralysis of a single extremity; hemiplegia is paralysis of a unilateral half of the body; diplegia or brachial paraplegia is paralysis of both upper extremities; and paraplegia is paralysis of both lower extremities. The paralysis is due to either an upper or a lower motor neuron lesion.

The upper motor pyramidal cells of the cerebral precentral cortex send fibers through the corticobulbar and the corticospinal tracts to the motor cells of the cranial nerves and of the anterior horns of the spinal cord on the opposite side. These tracts undergo partial decussation at the caudal end of the medulla before continuing distally into the spinal cord. The major portion of the fibers cross to the opposite side, forming the lateral corticospinal tract; the smaller uncrossed portion continues downward as the ventral corticospinal tract. The lower motor neurons are also under the influence of various other motor centers in the brain, located chiefly in the basal ganglia and the cerebellum.

LESIONS

Upper motor neuron lesions produce a spastic paralysis characterized by increased muscle tone, increased deep reflexes, diminished or absent superficial reflexes, and demonstrable pathologic reflexes such as the Babinski, the Oppenheim, the Gordon, and the Chaddock. These findings are explained by the removal of the inhibitory impulses of the cerebral centers.

A *lower motor neuron lesion* is characterized by a flaccid paralysis (loss of muscle tone), absent deep reflexes, muscle atrophy, and the reaction of degeneration. This type of paralysis may be produced by disease or injury to the anterior horn cells, the anterior roots, the peripheral nerves, the nerve plexuses, or the cauda equina.

Hyperkinesia is a condition of excessive, involuntary, purposeless movements.

Tremors are rhythmic, oscillating movements affecting all or groups of muscles. *Intention tremors* are characteristic of multiple sclerosis.

Tonic spasms are prolonged, intense, muscular contractions. *Clonic spasms* are rapid, repeated contractions of muscles.

A *cramp* is a tonic spasm localized to one muscle. Persisting spasm of a muscle eventually leads to its contracture. Continued spasm of a group of muscles overcoming their antagonists may cause joint contracture.

Choreiform movements are quick, uncoordinated, irregular, and arrhythmic; they are characteristic of chorea, which commonly follows rheumatic fever.

Athetosis, which is due to basal ganglia damage and often associated with hemiplegia, is characterized by a recurring series of slow, vermicular, ''pill-rolling'' movements of the hands.

Myotonia is a condition of increased muscle tonus that is brought on by emotion and attempts at movement.

Lesions of the corpus striatum are commonly associated with cerebral palsy. They are characterized by athetochoreic movements, rigidity, tremor, loss of associate movements, and masked facies.

Synergic movements are governed by the cerebellum. *Adiodokokinesis* is the inability to accomplish synergic movements (*e.g.*, the patient is unable to perform rapidly and alternatingly supination and pronation with both hands at the same time).

Hypotonia is a decrease of muscle tonus associated with muscle atrophy. Hypotonia also arises when lesions interrupt transmission of deep sensation (*e.g.*, in tabes dorsalis).

Complicated coordinated movements are examined by observing the manner of walking to check for *gait disorders.* Paresis will produce a slow, guarded, short-stepped, shuffling gait. Paralysis of the anterior tibial muscles, especially by an anterior horn or peripheral nerve lesion, causes a dropfoot and produces a steppage gait. To avoid tripping over the plantar flexed foot, the extremity is advanced with knee and hip hyperflexed. With spasticity, the legs are advanced slowly with shortened steps and the toes scraping the ground. Adductor tightness produces a scissors gait, by which the legs are alternately crossed. In the ataxic or tabetic gait, because of absence of deep position sense, the patient must constantly observe the placing of his feet; The hip is hyperflexed and externally rotated, and the forefoot is strongly dorsiflexed before being thrown down with the heel striking the ground first. The patient is unable to stand with eyes closed. In contrast, the cerebellar ataxic is not aided by visual assitance. The gait is stumbling, drunken, swaying from side to side, and there is a tendency to fall toward the side of the lesion.

Muscle coordination in the lower extremity may be tested by having the patient, while his eyes are closed, place the heel of one foot upon various points on the opposite leg. The upper extremities are tested by asking the patient to touch the tip of his nose with the end of the index finger.

REFLEXES

The simplest spinal reflex consists of a primary sensory and motor neuron and a synapse in the anterior gray matter of the spinal cord. It is composed of a receptor, or peripheral sensory nerve ending; an afferent conductor; a synaptic center; an efferent conductor; and the effector mechanism or muscle fibers. One or more intermediate neurons are interposed between the primary neurons. The latter may remain localized to one side of the cord (association neurons), pass to the opposite side of the cord (commissural neurons), or extend proximally or distally to complete an intersegmental reflex arc. Each reflex is contained within a definite segment of the cord (Fig. 14-3).

Deep Reflexes. Reflexes requiring stimulation of the tendons (*e.g.*, patellar, Achilles, biceps and triceps) are termed *deep reflexes.*

Superficial Reflexes. Others requiring cutaneous stimulation (*e.g.*, abdominal and cremasteric) comprise the superficial reflexes. Destruction of either limb of the reflex arc or the spinal cord segment abolishes the reflex response. If the lesion extends across the entire spinal cord segment, elimination of inhibitory impulses from cerebral centers causes an exaggeration of deep reflexes below the level of the lesion. Superficial reflex arcs involve the cerebral cortex, thereby explaining their absence in upper motor neuron lesions.

Pathologic Reflexes. Destruction of the upper motor neurons or pyramidal tracts is indicated by pathologic reflexes. The Babinski phenomenon is elicited by stroking the plantar surface of the foot. Normally, all the toes flex plantarward. A pathologic response is a dorsiflexion of the large toe. An exaggerated deep reflex is only of significance if associated with absent superficial reflexes, pathologic reflexes, and sustained clonus. Sphincter disturbances are often present, manifest by difficulty in starting the urinary stream, urinary retention, or incontinence.

Argyll Robertson Pupil. The pupil of the eye contracts when exposed to light and when accommodating for a near object. When the pupil reflexly contracts to accommodation but not to light, it is the Argyll Robertson pupil, which is characteristic of central nervous system lues.

Reflex Centers. The centers of various reflexes of importance to the orthopaedic surgeon are:

Deep reflexes	
Biceps	C5
Triceps	C6
Radial	C7
Ulnar	T1
Patellar	L2-L3
Achilles	L5-S1
Superficial reflexes	
Upper abdominal	T8-T10
Lower abdominal	T10-T12
Cremaster	L2
Sphincteric reflexes	
Bladder	S3-S4
Anus	S3-S4

Mass Reflexes. In normal humans, the motor response to an afferent impulse is localized and specific. In lower vertebrates the response, usually a flexor spasm, is more widespread and constitutes a protective reflex. When, in

FIG. 14-3. Elements of the spinal reflex arc. (After Ranson)

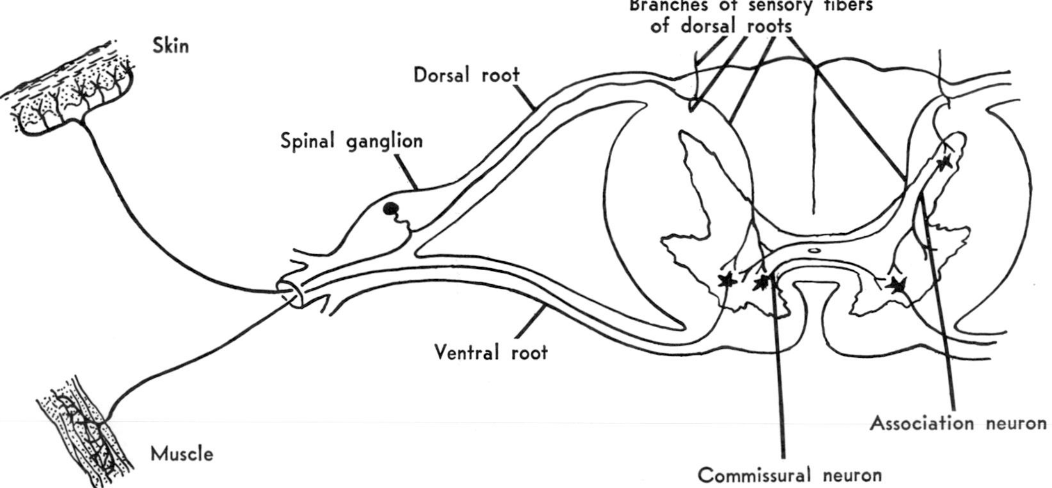

the human the spinal cord is completely transected, the distal portion temporarily loses and then regains its reflex excitability. The reflex response is now primitive. Specificity of response is lost, and stimulation occasions a widespread motor reaction. For example, stroking the plantar surface of the foot produces flexion at the hip and the knee, dorsiflexion of the foot, and emptying of the bladder. This is the "mass reflex" characteristic of complete interruption in continuity of the spinal cord. The center for this reflex is located low down in the spinal cord and is independent of cerebral control.

SENSATION

Objective evidence of sensory loss defines the site of the lesion and should be compared with normal areas. Changes of sensation form an accurate indication of improvement or progression. Light touch is determined by stroking the skin with a wisp of cotton. The hair on the skin produces sensation other than light touch and should first be removed. Pressure touch is tested by use of a blunt instrument. Pricking the skin with a needle elicits superficial pain. Temperature sensation is determined by applying a test tube filled with hot water and another with cold water. Vibration sense is tested with a tuning fork.

Epicritic or discrimination sensibility is the ability to discriminate between two points. When this sensation is reduced, the points of a compass may have to be widely separated before the stimulus can be recognized as dual. Position is tested by placing a part of an extremity such as the large toe in a certain attitude and asking the blindfolded patient to describe the position. Stereognosis, the sensation of size, shape, and form, the center for which exists in the parietal lobe, is determined by placing familiar objects in the patient's hand. Disease of the posterior columns of the cord produces loss of muscle and joint sensibility in the hands and, therefore, a loss of stereognosis.

Sensations conducted through peripheral nerves consist in deep sensation, the ability to discern pressure, position, and vibration; protopathic sensation, the recognition of painful stimuli and the distinction between extremes of hot and cold; and epicritic sensation, the ability to discriminate between two points and to distinguish between finer grades of temperature.

Severance of a cutaneous nerve produces a loss of all forms of superficial sensation, touch, pinprick, two-point discrimination, and distinction between hot and cold. The sense of deep position, pressure, and vibration is preserved. Epicritic sensory loss is well defined. Protopathic sensory loss after division of a peripheral nerve is smaller because of enormous overlapping in innervation from several nerves. Therefore, in determining peripheral sensory loss, testing superficial touch with a wisp of cotton is more accurate than testing pain perception with a pin. Destruction of nerves closer to the spinal cord increases the extent of loss to painful stimuli.

Afferent sensory fibers pass through the dorsal root to enter the spinal cord. Each fiber passes to the posterior gray column, where it divides into a long ascending and a short descending branch. Thus synapses are made not only with neurons at the same level but also at other levels as high as the medulla. Through relays, afferent impulses reach the cerebral cortex and the cerebullum.

The impulses of movement, position, and vibration pass upward within the cord on the same side as their point of entry. Impulses of touch, pain, and temperature cross to the opposite side of the cord before ascending.

A transverse division of the spinal cord causes loss of sensation below the level of the lesion. At the upper level of sensory loss there exists a band of hyperesthesia due to sensory root irritation at the level of the lesion.

Sensory supply to the body is made up of a regularly spaced series of dermatomes, which correspond to spinal cord segments. If one imagines the body in the quadruped position and then intersects the body at regular intervals, beginning at the neck and ending at the coccyx, the segmental nerve distribution will be apparent. In this position the thumbs and the large toes are in a more advanced position than the small finger and toe. Therefore, the radial side of the upper extremity is represented by a higher segmental level of the spinal cord than the ulnar side, the medial side of the thigh and the leg are of a higher segmental level than the external side of the lower extremity. By finding the sensory loss in a specific dermatome, the level of the spinal cord lesion is localized.

The viscera are generally lacking in sensory fibers. Disease in a viscus supplied by a certain spinal cord segment will produce referred pain in the cutaneous distribution of that segment. Thus, gallbladder disease causes interscapular pain; subdiaphragmatic disease causes pain in the shoulder.

The type of pain should be noted. Tabes dorsalis causes lightning pains; neuritis causes a burning pain; arthritis, an aching pain and sense of stiffness; and spinal disease, a girdle pain.

THE AUTONOMIC NERVOUS SYSTEM

From various centers in the central nervous system, fibers pass through the spinal nerves by way of rami communicantes to ganglia; the latter in turn innervate viscera, glands, heart, blood vessels, and smooth muscles. The sympathetic trunk, on each side of the body, extends along the lateral aspect of the spinal column from C2 to the coccyx. It is composed of 21 to 22 ganglia: 3 cervical (superior, middle, inferior), 10 or 11 thoracic, 4 lumbar, and 4 sacral. Gray and white rami communicantes connect the sympathetic trunk with the spinal nerves. The gray rami are composed of unmyelinated fibers, originating in the sympathetic ganglia and distributed through peripheral nerves to blood vessels (vasomotor), sweat glands (secretory), and smooth muscles of hair follicles (pilomotor). The white rami consist of myelinated fibers, which originate from cells in the intermediolateral column of the spinal cord and form preganglionic fibers, which synapse with ganglionic cells. The abdominal portion of the sympathetic trunk supplying the lower extremity and the inferior, or stellate, ganglion of the cervical trunk supplying the upper extremity are of importance to the orthopaedic surgeon. A great portion of sympathetic fibers innervating blood vessels pass distally in the vessel walls and are independent of peripheral nerves.

Preganglionic fibers, which originate in the brain and the sacral region, run directly to ganglia and their plexuses, which lie distally near the innervated organ. These react similarly to pilocarpine and are termed *parasympathetic.* Preganglionic fibers originating in the thoracolumbar region of the cord pass to ganglia in the sympathetic chain, which lies next to the spine and at a distance from the innervated part. These react to epinephrine and are termed *sympathetic.*

Most structures are innervated from both sympathetic and parasympathetic divisions, the action of such supply counteracting each other. Thus, a blood vessel will undergo spasm from action of adrenergic drugs but relaxes on administration of cholinergic drugs.

TROPHIC INNERVATION

A trophic center in the anterior horn is concerned with nutrition of all parts of the body. A lesion affecting this center or its peripheral nerve results in trophic changes. An acute irritative lesion produces herpes zoster. A chronic irritative lesion produces a thickened, rough, scaly skin. A destructive lesion causes a poorly nourished skin, which appears thin, glossy, and dry and ulcerates easily. The nails become ridged and brittle. The muscles become atrophic, and bones undergo osteoporosis. Severe, painless destruction of joints associated with tabes dorsalis and syringomyelia is thought to be trophic in origin.

ELECTRODIAGNOSIS

The electrical examination, an essential adjunct to neurologic diagnosis, provides an objective evaluation. It helps to determine the site of disease or injury of a peripheral nerve, whether impairment of function is due to contusion or division, the loss of nerve conductive capacity, and whether degeneration or regeneration is occurring. It aids in differentiating organic from hysterical paralysis, upper from lower motor neuron disease, and peripheral nerve involvement from muscular disease.[4,6]

Normal nerves and muscles respond to electrical stimuli in a prescise and uniform manner. These responses are altered by disease processes in a manner that is often characteristic of disease. Contraction of the muscle may be induced by percutaneous stimulation of its motor nerve or by direct stimulation of the muscle. When a nerve is divided, the distal end loses its power of conduction completely within 2 to 4 weeks, following which stimulation of the nerve no longer causes a muscular contraction. However, the muscle remains capable of contracting in response to direct stimulation by certain types of current (*e.g.*, galvanic).

The two procedures mainly used are electromyography (EMG) and electrical stimulation of a muscle and its motor nerve. In certain situations, electrical stimulation of a sensory cutaneous nerve provides diagnostic information. These procedures are concerned primarily with disease or trauma that affects the lower motor neuron, its axon, the neuromuscular junction, and the skeletal muscle fibers that it supplies. These components together comprise the *motor unit.*

The electromyogram records the variations of the electric potential or voltage detected by the needle electrode inserted into the skeletal muscle. The electrical activity is displayed on a cathode-ray oscilloscope and played over a loud speaker for simultaneous visual and auditory analysis. In normal muscle at rest, no electrical activity develops, but during voluntary contraction, the action potentials of motor units appear. In the presence of disease of the motor unit, electrical activity of various types may appear in resting muscle, and, with voluntary contraction, the forms and patterns of the action potentials become abnormal.

The electrical activity visualized on the electromyogram is produced by muscle fibers and may be designated *muscle action potentials.* The action potential of a normal muscle fiber originates at the motor end-plate and is triggered by the arrival of the nerve impulse at the neuromuscular junction. The action potential sweeps along the muscle in both directions from the motor end-plate at a velocity of approximately 4 meters/sec, exciting the contractile mechanism, the contraction beginning after an interval of about 0.001 sec. The contraction itself produces no electrical activity. During voluntary contraction, all muscle fibers innervated by a single lower motor neuron act together, their tiny action potentials summating to produce the larger action potential of the complete motor unit.

In muscle at rest, motor units are inactive and no electrical activity is detected. During a weak voluntary contraction, only a single motor unit may be active in the vicinity of the needle electrode. Its action potential recurs in a rhythmic fashion at the rate of 5 to 10/sec. As voluntary contraction increases, the rate at which the motor unit fires increases. Other units join in, acting rhythmically and independently, to increase the strength of contraction, so that during a strong contraction many motor units are active. Their rhythmically recurring action potentials are so numerous that they are superimposed on one another on the recording and cannot be distinguished from each other. The resulting record is designated as an *interference pattern.*

To properly analyze the abnormal electrical response of a muscle, it must be correlated with measurements of nerve conduction velocity, tests of neuromuscular transmission, and results of the clinical examination.

ELECTROMYOGRAPHY

When muscle fibers contract, they generate an electric current, which can be seen and heard on the cathode-ray oscilloscope and its amplified loud speaker (Fig. 14-4). The needle electrode is inserted into the muscle, and the minute voltages are amplified, converted into visible patterns by means of the cathode-ray oscilloscope, and transformed into sound energy, causing sounds that are characteristic of the type of action potentials produced. The screen images of the action potentials and their patterns are photographed, and a permanent record is made. Moreover, a television tape recorder can record both graphic images and sound for a permanent playback record.[6]

Between 14 days to 28 days after denervation of a muscle, the individual muscle fibers will begin to twitch in a rhythmical manner. These involuntary rhythmical contractions are collectively termed *denervation fibrillation.* True denervation fibrillation cannot be observed clinically through the intact skin, inasmuch as it represents contraction of the individual muscle fibers. Therefore, to detect its presence electromyography is employed. The voltages generated by fibrillating denervated muscle fibers have a short magnitude, ranging from 5μv to 100μv, and are termed *denervation fibrillation voltages* (Fig. 14-5). Their form is diphasic and their frequency varies from 2 to 30/sec. Each wave has an extremely short duration of 1 to 2 msec, which is responsible for the characteristic clicking sound.

Because fibrillation potentials are not visible for at least 2 weeks, and possibly as long as 4 weeks, it is not evident immediately following a severe nerve injury that causes complete interruption of motor nerve function. The electromyogram at this stage has limited usefulness in determining whether the nerve is intact (neurapraxia) or is completely divided and requires surgical repair. It may detect minimal residual innervation, which suggests continuity of the nerve and is justification for conservative treatment.

The earliest sign of reinnervation is the appearance during voluntary effort of low-amplitude motor unit potentials, many of which are polyphasic and of slow duration. They appear many weeks before clinical evidence of recovery. When regeneration of the motor nerve takes place, the reactivated muscle generates motor unit voltages, which produce highly complex polyphasic waves.These polyphasic waves are also characteristic of demyelinating diseases of the anterior horns, namely, poliomyelitis, amyotrophic lateral sclerosis, and progressive muscular atrophy. Therefore, these complex polyphasic waves represent early nerve degeneration or early nerve regeneration. The complexity of the highly polyphasic wave is probably caused by muscle fibers that are either denervated or reinnervated at different times so that contractions cannot occur synchronously. The complex motor unit voltages range in magnitude from about 1000μv to 1500μv and vary in frequency from 2 to 30/sec; the duration of each wave is from 5 to 15 msec. Irregularity of these motor unit voltages gives rise to a very rough-sounding noise.

Because denervation fibrillation takes place only after wallerian degeneration of its nerve has occurred, it is a valuable objective sign of lower motor neuron disease. Its presence differentiates between upper and lower motor neuron disease, myopathy, and atrophy secondary to peripheral nerve involvement and between functional and organic paralysis.

Denervation fibrillation is also useful for localization of the site of a lower motor neuron lesion. For example,

FIG. 14-4. Electromyogram of normal biceps brachii muscle. The records are photographs of the trace on the cathode-ray oscilloscope. An upward deflection is caused by a change of voltage in the negative direction at the needle electrode. (Clinical Examinations in Neurology, 4th ed. Philadelphia, WB Saunders, 1976)

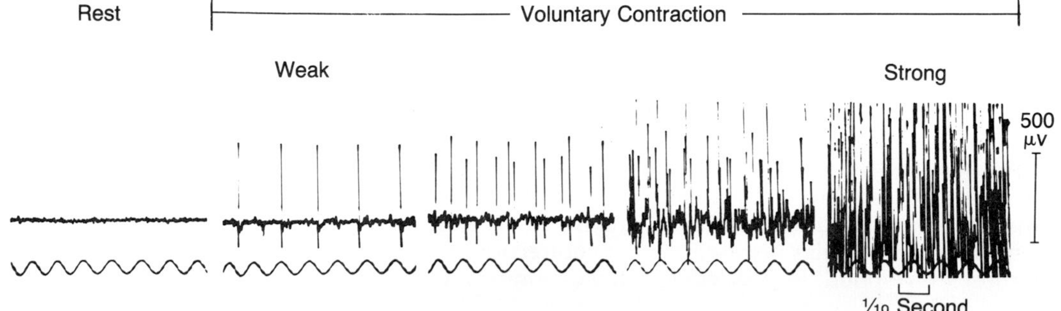

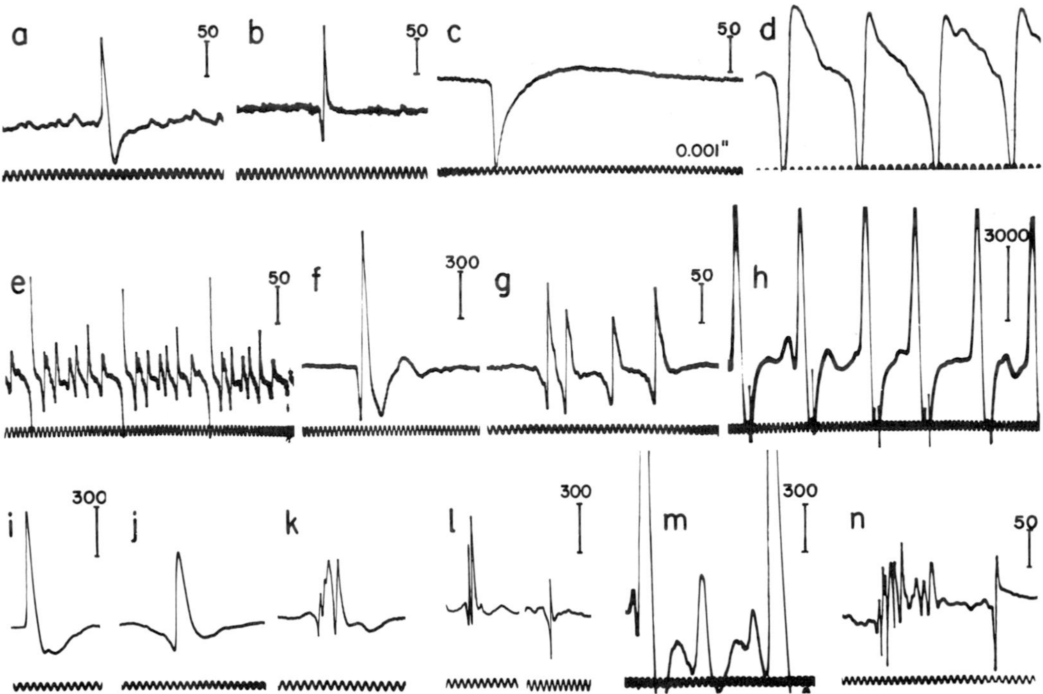

FIG. 14-5. Action potentials in electromyography: End-plate (*a*) noise (small negative deflections) and an associated muscle fiber spike from normal muscle; fibrillation potential (*b*) and positive wave from denervated muscle (*c*); high-frequency discharge in myotonia (*d*); bizarre repetitive discharge (*e*); fasciculation potential, single discharge (*f*); fasciculation potential (*g*), repetitive or grouped discharge; synchronized repetitive discharge in muscle cramp (*h*); diphasic (*i*), triphasic (*j*), and polyphasic motor unit action potentials from normal muscle (*k*); short-duration motor unit action potentials in progressive muscular dystrophy (*l*); large motor unit action potentials in progressive muscular atrophy (*m*); highly polyphasic motor unit action potential (*n*) and short-duration motor unit action potential during reinnervation. Calibration scales are in microvolts. All time scales are 1000 cycles/sec. An upward deflection indicates a change of potential in the negative direction at the needle electrode. (Clinical Examinations in Neurology, 4th ed. Philadelphia, WB Saunders, 1976)

compression of a nerve root can be identified by fibrillation in a group of muscles constituting the innervated myotome. Both posterior and anterior primary divisions of the nerve root and their muscles of supply are involved. When the C5 nerve root is involved (*e.g.*, by a herniated disk), fibrillation is present in the paraspinal muscles between the fourth and fifth cervical vertebrae (posterior primary division), rhomboids, supraspinatus, infraspinatus, deltoid, biceps, and brachioradialis (anterior primary division). In disk protrusion at the lumbosacral level, compression of the S1 nerve root will cause fibrillation and abnormal action potentials in the gastrocnemius, the hamstrings, the gluteus maximus (anterior primary division), and the paraspinal muscles between the first and second sacral vertebrae (posterior primary division). Electromyographic changes are most pronounced when root injury is severe and prolonged. In diagnosing a root compression syndrome, electromyography must be used in conjunction with myelography and a neurologic examination.

When a peripheral nerve, such as the median, is involved, denervation fibrillation will be observed only in those muscles supplied by that nerve and must be confirmed by nerve conduction studies. When involvement of peripheral nerves occurs at a proximal level (*e.g.*, about the plexus), absence of abnormal fibrillation or motor action potentials in the paraspinal muscles places the lesion beyond the nerve root.

Fasciculations are twitches of portions of muscle. They represent spontaneous contraction of a motor unit and are accompanied by action potentials comparable in size to those of a motor unit. They occur in two forms:

1. Single action potentials are the most common, are brief, occur sporadically at rates of 1 to 30 per minute, and are common in normal people. They also occur in irritative lesions of the lower motor neuron and are limited to muscles innervated by that nerve. They are invariably associated with degenerative diseases of the anterior horn (*e.g.*, amyotrophic lateral sclerosis

and progressive muscular atrophy). They are polyphasic spikes of relatively short duration.

2. Fasciculation action potentials, which are briefly repetitive, are caused by a brief tetanic contraction of a motor unit that is more prolonged than a single twitch. Such momentary discharges are characteristic of irritative or compressive lesions, such as nerve root compression by a disk and in carpal tunnel syndrome. When they are numerous and prolonged, they produce undulation of the surface of the muscle, a condition called myokymia.

In muscular dystrophy, instead of the normal simple motor unit potentials on voluntary effort, the waves are of lesser magnitude (up to 150μv) and shorter (1 to 2 msec). When the patient is relaxed completely, no fibrillation is noted (Fig. 14-6).

In myotonia, on voluntary effort a burst of impulses may continue for 30 to 50 seconds, but there is no fibrillation.

In myasthenia gravis, there is first a burst of impulses that rapidly diminish in amplitude, duration, and frequency. Characteristically, the administration of neostigmine or edrophonium (Tensilon) causes restoration of normal motor unit potentials.[8]

It should be recognized that fibrillation potentials indistinguishable from those of denervated muscle are commonly found in patients with polymyositis and dermatomyositis and occasionally in those with progressive muscular dystrophy. Differentiation will require other tests and a clinical examination.

Although denervation fibrillation indicates that some of the muscle fibers are without innervation, it also indicates that these fibers are still capable of contractility. Therefore, the nutrition of these muscles theoretically may be preserved by interrupted galvanic stimulation, massage, and heat; irreversible fibrotic changes are thereby prevented until, as in the case of a peripheral nerve lesion, regeneration takes place.

ELECTRICAL STIMULATION OF NERVE TRUNKS

Stimulating electrodes are placed over a selected point of the nerve, and a single pulse of electricity, somewhat greater than that required to produce a maximal response of the muscle, is administered once to produce a muscle twitch or repetitively to produce a tetanic contraction. The muscle response is recorded for measurement through electrodes placed over the muscle, whose action potential is amplified and displayed on a cathode-ray oscilloscope. A stimulus artifact appears on the graph at the moment of stimulation of the nerve and is followed, after several milliseconds, by the action potential. The delay between the stimulus artifact and the action potential is the conduction time of the impulse along the length of nerve between the point of stimulus and the muscle fibers. The action potential of the muscle response as displayed on the graph represents the summation of the potentials of all responding muscle fibers. Its magnitude is determined by the number of fibers that respond and should be compared with the corresponding muscle on the opposite side of the body. Serial records taken at regular intervals

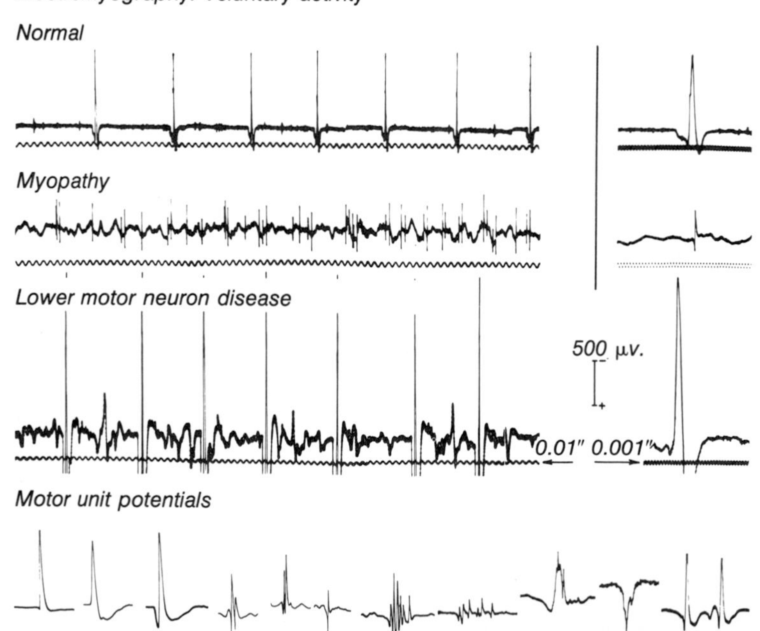

FIG. 14-6. Differentiating myopathy from lower motor neuron disease. (*Top*) Motor unit action potentials during weak voluntary contraction (m. biceps brachii) in a normal person. (*Middle*) In progressive muscular dystrophy (myopathy). (*Bottom*) In amyotrophic lateral sclerosis (lower motor neuron disease). Action potentials on the left are recorded with a slow time base (time signal is 100 cycles/sec.). Action potentials on the right are recorded with a more rapid time base (time signal is 1000 cycles/sec.). (Clinical Examinations in Neurology, 4th ed. Philadelphia, WB Saunders, 1976)

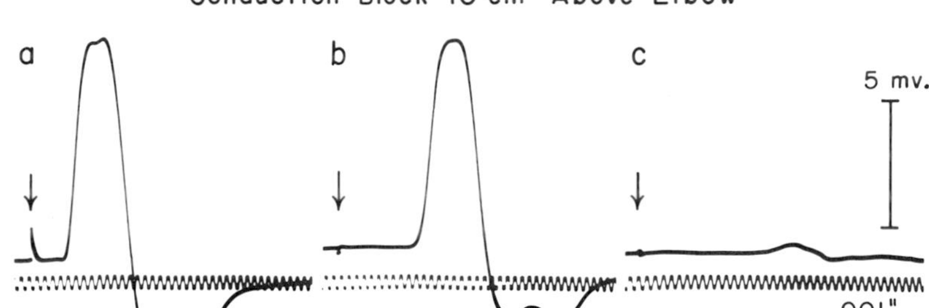

FIG. 14-7. Location of the site of block of nerve conduction. The action potential of the hypothenar muscles was recorded as an indication of the response to maximal stimulation of the ulnar nerve. A normal response occurred when the nerve was stimulated at the wrist (*a*) or at the elbow (*b*). A greatly diminished response was obtained when the nerve was stimulated 11 cm or more above the elbow (*c*). Surgical exploration revealed compression of the nerve at a point 10 cm above the elbow as the cause of paralysis of voluntary contraction. The stimulus artifact (*arrow*) designated the exact time of initiating the stimulus. Time scale is 1000 cycles/sec. (Clinical Examinations in Neurology, 4th ed. Philadelphia, WB Saunders, 1976)

may disclose changes that indicate either progress in reinnervation or advancing denervation.

The procedure also aids in localization of the point of nerve injury or disease. A normal muscle response indicates that the nerve lesion is proximal to the point of stimulation, either in the proximal portion of the nerve trunk, plexus, or root, or at a higher level in the central nervous system. If the point of nerve stimulation is placed at successively proximal points along the nerve, and a reduction of conduction time suddenly appears at a certain point of application, the lesion is situated just beyond this level (Fig. 14-7).

The portion of a nerve trunk beyond the level of a severe nerve injury, regardless of whether complete interruption of the nerve is physiologic or anatomical, remains normally excitable to nerve stimulation for 2 to 3 days after the injury; then it becomes progressively less excitable until it is completely inexcitable just prior to the appearance of fibrillation potentials in the muscle. Therefore, the electrical response within the first 10 days is no indication of the degree of nerve injury.

Motor Nerve Fibers. Conduction velocity of motor nerve fibers is reduced in peripheral neuropathies caused by either trauma or disease and is reflected on the electromyogram as an increase in the conduction time from the point of stimulation to the muscle, as an increase in the duration of the action potential of the muscle (because reduction of conduction velocity does not uniformly affect all nerve axons within the trunk), or as both of the above.

In conditions that affect the anterior horn cells, such as amyotrophic lateral sclerosis and progressive muscular atrophy, conduction velocities are usually within the normal range or only slightly below the average normal conduction velocity for the nerve tested. Marked slowing of conduction velocity to within 5% to 60% of the normal average is found only in conditions affecting the peripheral nerve. These include chronic nerve compression (*e.g.*, carpal tunnel syndrome), severe nerve injury or neuritis which is undergoing recovery, and chronic neuropathies, particularly those primarily demyelinating disorders such as Guillain-Barré syndrome and Charcot-Marie-Tooth atrophy of the neuropathic type. The low conduction velocity during reinnervation of a muscle after a severe nerve injury or neuritis is related to the small diameter of regenerating nerve fibers.

The conduction velocities at birth are about one-half of adult values, increase to adult values by 3 to 5 years of age, and then slow progressively after 20 to 30 years of age, becoming about 5 to 10 meters/sec slower by 80 years. Conduction velocities are decreased by low temperatures and insufficient circulation in the extremity.

For example, to determine the conduction velocity of the ulnar nerve in the forearm, a stimulating electrode is placed over the nerve at the wrist and the other electrode is placed over the hypothenar muscles. The distance between electrodes is determined in millimeters. The time between the stimulus artifact and the action potential on the graph is determined in milliseconds (Fig. 14-8). Next, the stimulating electrode is placed over the nerve at the elbow and the procedure is repeated. These values of distance and time for the elbow to the hand are recorded, and the values of the wrist to the hand are subtracted, yielding values from elbow to wrist. Millimeters and milliseconds are transposed to meters and seconds, yielding the conduction velocity as meters per second for the ulnar nerve from the elbow to the wrist (Table 14-1).

Afferent Nerve Fibers. Conduction in afferent nerve fibers[5] is a more sensitive indication of involvement of large myelinated fibers than are tests of conduction in motor fibers. This is determined by recording the action potential evoked in a cutaneous nerve by a maximal electrical stimulus. A small triphasic action potential, usually less than $50\mu v$ in amplitude, represents the action potential of large myelinated fibers. The nerve action potential is recorded by electrodes at standard positions along the course of the nerve. For example, in compression of the median nerve at the wrist, the stimulating electrodes are placed about the index finger (digital

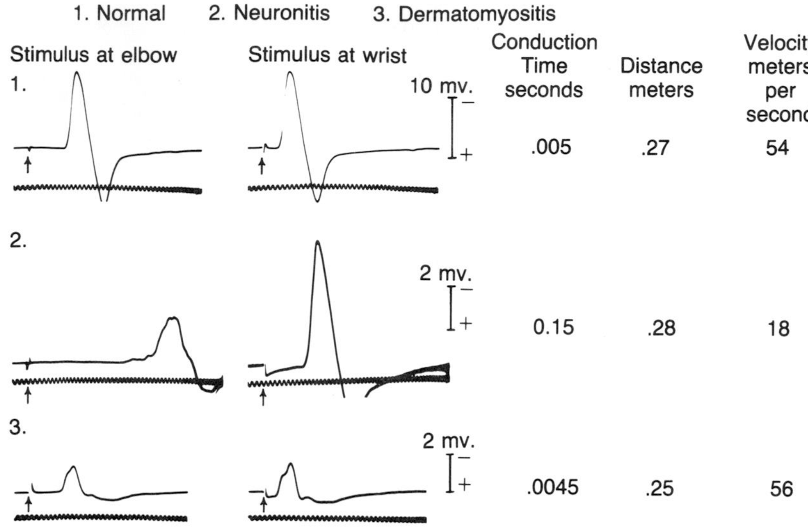

FIG. 14-8. Measurement of conduction velocity of the ulnar nerve in a normal person (*1*), in chronic polyneuropathy (*2*), and in dermatomyositis (*3*). The action potential of the hypothenar muscles was recorded as an indication of the response to stimulation of the ulnar nerve at the elbow and at the wrist. The arrows indicate the stimulus artifact. The time scales are 1000 cycles/sec. The conduction time, conduction distance, and conduction velocity of the nerve impulse between elbow and wrist are indicated in columns at the right. The conduction time between elbow and wrist is the difference conduction time from elbow to hand and wrist to hand. (Clinical Examinations in Neurology, 3rd ed. Philadelphia, WB Saunders, 1971)

nerve) and the recording electrodes over the median nerve at the wrist (Fig. 14-9). The cutaneous nerve action potential may be small, absent, or delayed in neuropathy even though the results of the neurologic examination reveal little or no sensory deficit, and the accompanying motor unit response may appear normal.

The cutaneous nerve action potential is normal in myopathies and diseases of the anterior horn cells. It is also preserved in lesions proximal to the dorsal root ganglion; thus it is preserved despite loss of sensation after avulsion of a nerve root. It is therefore a valuable aid in detecting severe brachial plexus traction injuries in which nerve roots are avulsed.

The nerve action potential can be consistently recorded in cutaneous nerves such as the digital, radial, and sural nerves. Reduction in amplitude, slow conduction, and the absence of nerve action potential are indicative of an abnormality. It can also be applied to a mixed nerve, such as the ulnar and median, when recorded motor unit potentials appear normal or equivocal.

TABLE 14-1 Summary of Means and Standard Deviations of Conduction Velocities of Various Nerves in Normal Persons

Nerve	Conduction Velocity (Meters per Second)
Peroneal	50.1 ± 7.2
Median	53.0 ± 6.4
Ulnar	55.1 ± 6.4
Posterior tibial	50.2 ± 9.3

(Johnson EW, Olsen KJ: Clinical value of motor nerve conduction velocity determination. JAMA 172:2030, 1960)

Fatigability of Muscle. Repetitive stimulation of a peripheral nerve with supramaximal stimuli may disclose unusual fatigability of a muscle. Since the action potential is a measure of muscle response, a progressive decline in amplitude after the first few responses indicates that fewer muscle fibers respond even though the stimuli are continued at rates that normal muscle can endure for long periods. This test is used chiefly in the diagnosis of myasthenia gravis. The abnormal action potentials can be temporarily corrected by administering neostigmine or edrophonium.

STRENGTH DURATION CURVES

Strength duration curves[9] are used to determine the excitability of muscle to progressively shorter times of the application of electrical current. The procedure can provide early evidence of degeneration after a nerve injury and in chronic lower motor neuron disease in the anterior horns in which spontaneous fibrillation is often absent or difficult to detect.

The muscle is stimulated by a constant voltage type of electrical stimulator with a maximal output of 200 volts, the longest duration of application being 300 msec and the shortest being 0.01 msec. It provides a square wave stimulus.

The amount of current needed to cause a barely perceptible muscle contraction is measured at the longest pulse duration of the stimulator, 300 msec. This is the rheobase, which, by definition, is the least amount of current flowing for an infinite time required to cause a barely perceptible contraction. Since a time longer than 300 msec will never lower the current needed to produce

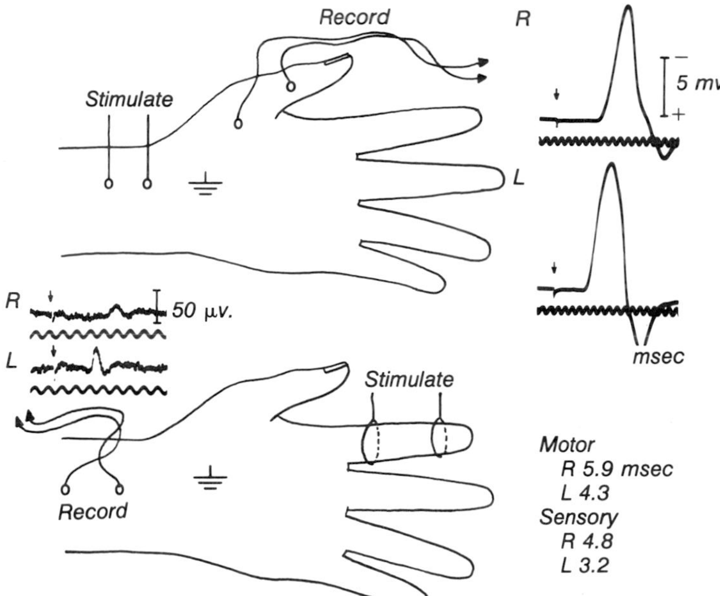

FIG. 14-9. The carpal tunnel syndrome, latency of muscle and nerve action potentials. Nerve action potentials evoked by stimulation of digital nerves in index finger are detected by surface electrodes over median nerve at the wrist. The action potentials of thenar muscles evoked by stimulation of the median nerve at the wrist are recorded by surface electrodes over belly and tendon of abductor pollicis brevis. Latency of both responses (to start of muscle action potential and to peak of nerve action potential) is prolonged on the right side. (Clinical Examinations in Neurology, 3rd ed. Philadelphia, WB Saunders, 1971)

the smallest contraction, this is the longest time utilized. The rheobase is therefore a measure of the electrical threshold of the tissue. Below this threshold, regardless of the length of time the current is applied, the muscle will not contract.

After the voltage for a minimal contraction at 300 msec is determined, the voltage values are then determined as successively shorter pulse durations: 100, 30, 10, 3, 1, 0.3, 0.1, 0.03 and 0.01 msec. The strength of stimulus required to produce minimal contraction is determined at each duration, and the values are plotted on a graph to obtain a curve, termed the *strength duration* (or *intensity duration*) *curve* (Fig. 14-10). This relates strength and duration of the pulse required to produce minimal contractions.

In normally innervated muscle, the same amount of current will produce the same minimal response at each successively shorter duration. The same voltage will produce the same barely perceptible contraction at 1 msec as it does at 300 msec. At extremely short durations, only a slight increase of voltage is required. The resulting plotted line is essentially straight except for a minimal curve at extremely short durations.

In contrast, denervated muscle requires progressively increased intensity of current with successively shorter duration periods, starting almost immediately at times shorter than 300 msec. The resulting curve rises steeply. Denervated muscle contracts sluggishly, and it may fail to respond at all before the shortest duration times have been reached.

The strength duration studies (SD curve) provide objective evidence of progression of denervation or reinnervation at an earlier date than is clinically apparent. It therefore becomes a valuable diagnostic and prognostic tool for the orthopaedic surgeon.

Within 2 to 3 days after a clinically complete nerve injury, the SD curve begins to rise, indicating denervation, and the curve of complete denervation becomes fully developed at 14 days. *If the SD curve remains normal 7 days after injury, a neurapraxia exists and a good outlook is probable.*

The earliest sign of reinnervation in the SD curve is the appearance of a discontinuity or kink in the curve, and as regeneration is proceeding, with more muscle fibers becoming reinnervated, the kink becomes wider, the curve shifts to the left, and the slope becomes shallow. If the curve of a nerve lesion shows no change over a period of 6 weeks, it may be concluded that reinnervation has ceased, and surgical exploration may be indicated.

It should be reemphasized that the early signs of denervation on the SD curve may precede clinical evidence of weakness and sensory loss by many weeks. Moreover, it provides a method for following the progress of recovery by serial examinations. It should be correlated with the electromyographic studies and the neurologic examination.

Although denervation fibrillation indicates that some of the muscle fibers are without innervation, it also indicates that these fibers are still capable of contractility. Therefore, the nutrition of these muscles may be preserved theoretically by interrupted galvanic stimulation, massage, and heat; irreversible fibrotic changes are thereby prevented until, as in the case of a peripheral nerve lesion, regeneration takes place.

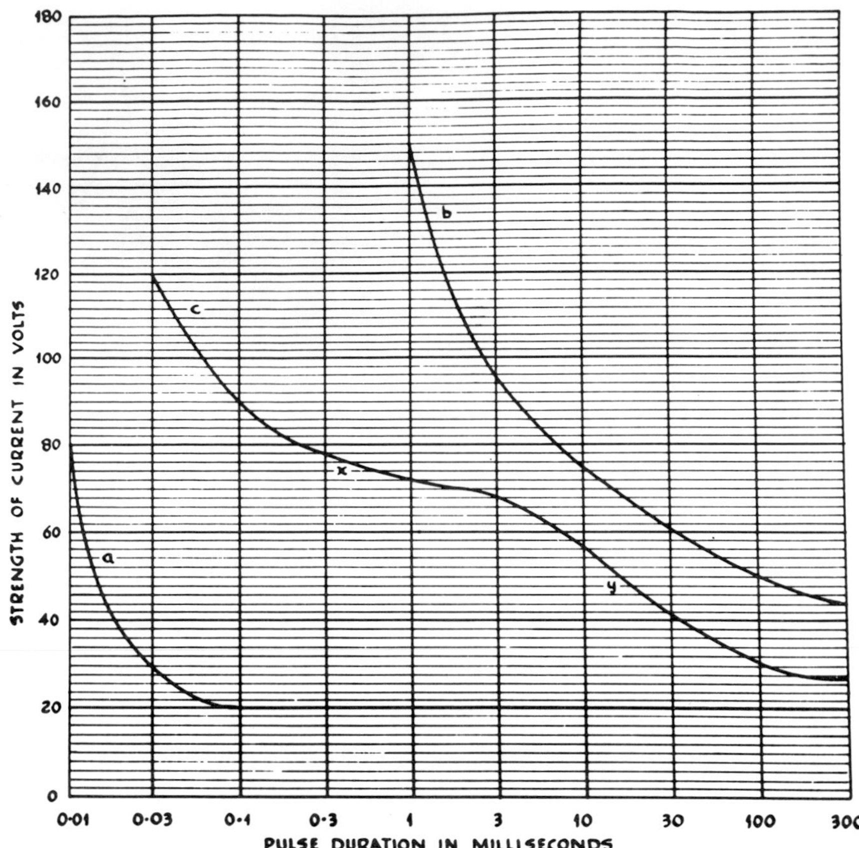

FIG. 14-10. Strength duration curves on normal (*a*), denervated (*b*), and partially innervated muscle (*c*). That part of the curve (*c*) marked *x* represents the innervated component (response of nerve) and that part marked *y* represents the denervated component (response of muscle). (Wynn Parry CB: Electrodiognosis. J Bone Joint Surg 43B:222, 1961)

LOCALIZATION OF SPINAL CORD LESION

BASIC ANATOMY

The pyramidal, or motor, tracts that have already crossed above the spinal cord descend in the lateral columns of white matter. Anterior and lateral to these fibers are the lateral spinothalamic tracts, which carry impulses of pain and temperature upward from the opposite side of the body. The posterior white columns transmit upward both deep (joint, muscle, bone) and superficial tactile sensations uncrossed.

TYPES OF LESIONS

The various types of lesions include the following.

Lower Motor Neuron Lesion. In this lesion limbs are flaccid, deep reflexes are absent, and muscles are atrophied. This lesion may be in the anterior horn, the anterior spinal root, or in a peripheral nerve. If sensory changes are absent, the peripheral nerve is excluded. Anterior poliomyelitis is the most common cause.

One must remember that a sudden traumatic lesion of the spinal cord produces at first a flaccid paralysis below the level of the lesion, but eventually spastic paralysis develops.

Upper Motor Neuron Lesion. This condition is characterized by increased muscle tone and spasticity, hyperreflexia, clonus, absent superficial reflexes, and positive pathologic reflexes. Bilateral spastic paralysis is due most commonly to cerebral palsy.

Combined Upper and Lower Motor Neuron Lesion. Spastic paralysis in the lower extremities and flaccid paralysis in the upper extremities, with a reaction of degeneration and no sensory loss, indicate a combined lesion of the anterior horns and the corticospinal tracts. The disease is amyotrophic lateral sclerosis. When this combination is associated with loss of pain and temperature sense, while tactile sense is preserved, the cause is syringomyelia or an intramedullary tumor. The central lesion destroys the centrally crossing fibers of pain and temperature, while tactile fibers ascend in the posterior columns unharmed.

Lesion of Posterior Spinal Root. This lesion involves

absence of deep reflexes, loss of all sensation, and spontaneous lightning pains. Loss of joint and muscle sense results in ataxia. The disease is due to tabes dorsalis (locomotor ataxia). The posterior columns undergo secondary degeneration.

Combined Lesion of Posterior Columns and Pyramidal Tracts. In addition to loss of joint and muscle sense and an ataxia, a spastic weakness with hyperreflexia is present. Subacute combined degeneration is due to pernicious anemia. Increased mean corpuscular volume (MCV) and mean corpuscular hemoglobin (MCH), macrocytosis, and achlorhydria are confirmatory.

Transverse Lesion of the Spinal Cord. At the corresponding segmental level, the deep reflex is absent; flaccid paralysis, muscle atrophy, and electrical evidence of denervation are present. Below this level, one finds spastic paralysis, hyperreflexia, absent superficial reflexes, pathologic reflexes, complete sensory loss, or sphincteric constriction with urinary retention. The cause of the pathology includes myelitis, tumor, fracture-dislocation of the spine, thrombosis, hemorrhage, abscess, and vertebral disease. When the onset is sudden, vascular or traumatic lesions are probable. Tumors and infections cause slowly progressive symptoms.

Section II
Miscellaneous Affections of the Nervous System

SPINAL CORD TUMORS

To the orthopaedic surgeon the identification of a spinal cord tumor is important as a source of pain about the spine or of pain referred to other regions. Symptoms about the chest and the abdomen may cause confusion with visceral disease. Especially important is the differentiation from other causes of pain in the upper or lower extremity, particularly intervertebral disk protrusion.

PATHOLOGY

Spinal cord tumors are intramedullary, originating from and involving the substance of the cord itself, and extramedullary, occurring in the meninges and the surrounding tissues.[12] The intramedullary tumors are most frequently ependymomas and less often multiform glioblastomas and medulloblastomas. The extramedullary tumors include meningiomas, angiomas, lipomas, glands of Hodgkin's disease, tuberculomas, syphilomas, cysts of the spinal cord, and metastatic tumors. An ependymoma of the filum terminale forms a giant-sized mass, which compresses the roots of the cauda equina. Multiple neurofibroma of von Recklinghausen's disease may form in the cauda equina. The extramedullary tumor is more frequent, and the vast majority are benign and accessible to surgery. Intramedullary tumors occur most often in the cervical and the lumbar enlargements. A glioma of the cervical enlargement may become cystic and produce a syringomyelic cavity.

CLINICAL PICTURE

Symptoms are caused by direct pressure on the cord and the nerve roots, by pressure against the opposite side of the cord that is pushed against the bony wall, and by changes in blood vessels with altered blood and spinal fluid flow.

Pain

Pain is the most frequent symptom and usually is felt in the region supplied by the involved posterior root.[13] Thus a neuralgic pain may extend down a limb or be situated about the chest or the abdomen as a girdle pain. The usual pain of an intraspinal lesion may precede any other symptom by months or years and may be constant or intermittent. It characteristically is most pronounced at rest and is reduced in intensity by exercise. It usually persists in a well-localized area because of definite nerve root involvement. Commonly, it is lancinating and aggravated by coughing, sneezing, lifting, and straining during bowel movement. It invariably awakens the patient 4 to 6 hours after he has retired and often becomes so severe as to compel the patient to walk the floor or to sleep in a sitting position.

Pain may be confined to the back, where it is generally situated about the site of the lesion. However, involvement of the cauda equina anywhere in its course from the upper lumbar canal often causes low back pain. Referred pain from the cervical area involves the upper extremity. Within the thoracic spinal canal, a lesion at a definite vertebral level will involve the dermatome several segments below. Thus, a neurofibroma at the T5 level often causes pain in the subcostal area of the abdomen, where it may be mistaken for gallbladder disease. Cauda equina tumors cause sciatica as well as low back pain, with a ruptured disk often being diagnosed.

Involvement of a motor nerve may cause painful spasms of the muscle that it innervates.

Motor Signs

Eventually, motor signs appear in the form of muscle weakness at the level supplied by the involved segment of the cord and usually on the same side. Involvement of the pyramidal tracts causes a spastic paralysis with hyperactive deep reflexes, absent superficial reflexes, and presence of pathologic tendon reflexes below the level of the lesion. As spinal cord compression continues, the opposite side is implicated likewise.

When the cauda equina is involved, the paralysis is flaccid and both knee and ankle reflexes are lost.

Sensory Changes

Sensory changes are varied. Compression of the posterior columns causes a loss of deep sensation, position, and vibration sense. When the lateral columns are compressed, the spinothalamic tracts are affected and pain and temperature sensation is lost on the opposite side below the level of the lesion.

Brown-Séquard Syndrome

When pressure of the tumor compromises the function of one half of the spinal cord, a syndrome results that corresponds to hemisection of the cord. Pain and temperature sense is lost on the opposite half of the body, and position, vibration, deep pain, and light touch, as well as motor function, are lost on the ipsolateral side.

Hyperesthesia and Hyperalgesia

Because of irritation of the posterior roots, hyperesthesia and hyperalgesia are often found at the level of the lesion.

Additional Signs

Sphincter weakness with incontinence of urine and feces often develops with severe compression. Impotence is commonly associated. Trophic ulcers and bedsores may occur. Perspiration is generally reduced or lacking below the level of the lesion. Special localizing signs include the following:

Cervical lesions: occipital pain, neck rigidity, pain in the upper extremities, paralysis of the diaphragm when C3 to C6 are involved

First dorsal lesions: Horner's syndrome: enophthalmos, anhidrosis, and ptosis of the upper lid (opposite effect is secured when lesion is irritative)

Dorsal lesions: paraplegia, most often in flexion, with pain radiating to chest and abdomen anteriorly

Lumbar lesions: shooting pains down legs, low back pain, loss of knee or ankle reflex; tumor high within lumbar enlargement may cause spastic paralysis below level of lesion; tumor low within lumbar enlargement may also compress nerve roots, causing flaccid paralysis of muscles corresponding to this level.

Cauda equina lesions: sciatic pain, low back pain, loss of both ankle and knee reflexes, flaccid paralysis

Conus lesions: severe sphincteric weakness and impotence, saddle anesthesia due to involvement of lowest sacral and coccygeal nerves

DIAGNOSIS

Spinal Fluid Examination

Changes in intraspinal pressure and chemical composition of the fluid are essential to diagnosis.

Manometric Test. The patient is placed in the lateral recumbent position, a lumbar puncture is performed, and a manometer is attached to the needle. The following observations are made:

Initial pressure. It is normally 80 to 150 mm.

Oscillation. These are of two types: a slow rise and fall of the fluid level corresponds to respirations; a more rapid, smaller rise and fall occurs coincident with the pulse.

Jugular compression. An assistant compresses both jugular veins momentarily. Normally, this causes an immediate rise of the column of spinal fluid which varies from 220 mm to 400 mm, followed by an immediate fall to the initial level. A space-consuming intraspinal lesion interferes with the free flow of spinal fluid as well as the free flow of blood through the veins of the spinal cord and roots. Increase of intracranial tension by jugular compression will not cause the normal rise in spinal fluid pressure when a mass is interposed between the cranium and the lumbar sac. Jugular compression will not effect the normal height of rise and, on release of compression, the fluid level falls slowly.

Abdominal straining. The patient strains momentarily as though at stool. This causes an immediate high rise and fall, regardless of the presence of a tumor.

Removal of fluid for examination

Spinal Fluid Changes. There is a marked increase of albumin content just below the level of the lesion and sometimes just above the level. The total protein is much greater than that found with disk rupture. The diagnostic Froin's syndrome (xanthochromia, spontaneous coagulation, and no cells) may appear below the level of the lesion.

Roentgenographic Findings

Localized erosion and demineralization of adjacent bony structures may be found. Attention is directed especially to the pedicles, which may be flattened in contour, the width of the spinal canal being correspondingly wider at this level. Large expanding lesions, such as an ependymoma of the cauda equina, are likely to effect bone changes. Destruction of an adjacent vertebra may indicate a malignant metastasis. Metrizamide injection helps to localize the lesion. Characteristic shadows produced by certain tumors have been described but are not reliable.

Myelography is essential for determining the presence of a space-occupying mass and localization for surgical removal. It may aid in detecting a congenital malformation such as a tight filum terminale and diastematomyelia.

Computed tomography combined with myelography will disclose an extraordinary enlargement of the spinal cord or cauda equina, an extramedullary compressive mass, and secondary erosive bone changes. A bone scan may localize a vertebral neoplastic lesion.

Importance of a General Examination

Carcinomas of thyroid, breast, prostate, and adrenal gland are prone to metastasize to the spinal column. These sites should be investigated thoroughly before exploration of the spine is attempted.

TREATMENT

Surgery aims at relief of compression of the spinal cord. The mortality rate is less than 4%. Most tumors are extramedullary and after their removal symptoms subside to a remarkable degree. Intramedullary tumors are surgically inaccessible. Even when the lesion cannot be removed, laminectomy reduces pain and prolongs life by relief of pressure. It often prevents bladder paralysis and ascending urinary infection.

CAUDA EQUINA TUMORS

Tumors of the cauda equina are especially important to orthopaedic study because they produce a subtle clinical picture that often is erroneously treated as being due to musculoskeletal disease. Failure to recognize this possibility at an early stage results in irremediable paralysis. The early symptoms are often mistakenly attributed to a lumbar disk protrusion. The following points aid in recognition and should be carefully studied and correlated with a complete neurologic examination including diagnostic procedures (*e.g.*, electrodiagnosis, myelography).

Early pain is a cardinal symptom. It develops early and continues long before neurologic signs appear. Its radiation varies: back of thighs, front of thighs, perineum, sciatic distribution, or limited to the low back.

Later symptoms are muscle weakness; flaccid paralysis; and impaired sensation of all forms, including pain and temperature sense. In the male there is impaired erection and ejaculation. Deep tendon reflexes are absent. Sphincter loss and saddle anesthesia, when it occurs early and is severe, points to a high lesion about the conus; when it develops late, the lesion is low in the cauda equina. A lesion of the epiconus typically causes early paralysis of the feet.

Symptoms suggesting tumor rather than a disk protrusion include insidious onset, spontaneous, no prior trauma; unremitting, progressive course; sphincter involvement; and constant pain, unrelieved by recumbency and severe at night.

Common presenting symptoms in order of frequency are low back pain, unilateral sciatica and numbness of legs.

Common physical findings in order of frequency are diminution of ankle jerks and sensory changes.

The myelogram reveals a space-occupying mass. There is markedly high spinal fluid total protein in 70% of tumor cases. In 30% of cases, the total protein is not elevated.

Malignant tumors include leiomyosarcoma, lymphoma, myxofibrosarcoma, metastatic carcinoma, and neurogenic fibrosarcoma. Benign lesions include neurilemmoma, ependymoma, neurofibroma, meningioma, fibrous cyst, ependymal cysts, chordoma, lipoma, and fibrosis.

FILUM TERMINALE SYNDROME

Progressive spastic paralysis (filum terminale or cord traction syndrome) can occur in Arnold-Chiari syndrome, scoliosis, and other spinal malformations. The mechanism appears to be abnormally short filum terminale, which pulls the cord distally as the vertebral column grows in length. In Arnold-Chiari syndrome, the hindbrain is pulled into the narrow foramen magnum. In scoliosis, the cord is pulled over the angulation. Typically, symptoms appear during periods of rapid growth, from 13 to 19 years of age. A shortened cauda equina is often a component of spina bifida and is responsible for restricting ascent on the conus medullaris during growth. Treatment is by sectioning the filum, which gradually improves the patient. In Arnold-Chiari syndrome, decompression of the foramen magnum produces the same result.[14,15] This latter condition consists of herniation of the hindbrain and the cerebellum through a narrowed foramen magnum. It occurs during the growth period when the spinal cord is prevented from ascending by a tight filum terminale. The constriction of the hindbrain interferes with the exit of spinal fluid from the ventricles, and hydrocephalus results in infants, with signs of increased intracranial pressure and spastic paralysis in older children. In addition, the discrepancy in growth between the spinal cord and the spinal column results in reversal in the course of the cervical spinal nerve roots, which become angulated over their point of exit at the intervertebral foramina.

When progressively increasing weakness in the lower extremities, deformities of the feet, sphincter weakness, root pains in the upper extremities, and headaches develop in an actively growing child, a tight filum terminale and the Arnold-Chiari deformity should be suspected. The fibrous tissue formation about a spina bifida occulta is often the aggravating factor (see Spina Bifida, Chapter 30).

SPINAL MUSCULAR ATROPHIES OF UNKNOWN ETIOLOGY

Recognition of spinal muscular atrophies of unknown etilogy is important to the orthopaedic surgeon, who must differentiate them from peripheral neuropathies and central nervous system diseases of known etiology, which have a more favorable outlook. In certain of these rare diseases, such as peroneal atrophy and Friedreich's ataxia, the severe disability caused by skeletal deformities and muscle imbalance can be improved by surgical procedures.

PROGRESSIVE SPINAL MUSCULAR ATROPHY

Progressive spinal muscular atrophy is characterized by progressively increasing weakness and atrophy that usually begin in the small hand muscles and extend to the arms and the lower extremities. The cause is unknown.

PATHOLOGY

The cervical spinal cord is affected most severely, but eventually all portions become involved. The anterior horn cells degenerate, disappear, and are replaced by glial tissue. Occasionally, the medulla may be involved.

CLINICAL PICTURE

Symptoms develop insidiously in a middle-aged person, usually a man. Weakness and awkwardness in use of the hands is often the first complaint. Pain is absent. The small muscles of the hand atrophy, producing a characteristic clawhand. Gradually, the weakness and atrophy increase in degree and spread to the arms and the shoulders and after a long period of time involve the legs. The process may involve one hand at first, but eventually becomes symmetrical. It rarely starts in the lower extremities but invariably spreads to the upper extremities.

Examination reveals atrophy, muscle fasciculations, absent deep reflexes, and a reaction of degeneration. Sensation is intact. The nerve conduction velocities are normal or only slightly decreased. Electromyography shows large motor unit action potentials of long duration, characteristic of disease of the anterior horn cells. These are frequently ten times the amplitude of normal muscles. Fibrillation is minimal or absent.

PROGNOSIS

The course is slow and protracted, often as long as 25 years. Rarely is death caused by bulbar symptoms.

FAMILIAL PROGRESSIVE SPINAL MUSCULAR ATROPHY

Familial progressive spinal muscular atrophy (also called Werdnig-Hoffman disease) is a rare form of progressive degeneration of the anterior horn cells. It is characterized by a familial incidence, onset of flaccid paralysis in early infancy, and progression to a fatal termination in about 5 years. Symptoms typically start in the trunk and spread peripherally along the extremities.

AMYOTONIA CONGENITA

In amyotonia congenita (also called Oppenheim's disease) the anterior horn cells, particularly those in the lower half of the spinal cord, fail to develop. As a result the lower extremities of the newborn display a flaccid weakness or paralysis with absent deep reflexes. The condition tends to improve a little with time.

AMYOTROPHIC LATERAL SCLEROSIS

Amyotrophic lateral sclerosis is characterized by rapid progression of degeneration of the anterior horn cells and pyramidal tracts involving both the spinal cord and the brain stem. It appears most often in middle-aged men. Symptoms include weakness, atrophy and flaccid paralysis in the upper extremities, spastic paralysis in the lower extremities, and bulbar paralysis, which at first is manifested as difficulty in swallowing and talking. Atrophy involves all muscles. The gait is typically spastic. Sensory disturbances are absent. The disease is rapidly progressive, with death occurring in 2 to 5 years in most instances.

PERONEAL MUSCULAR ATROPHY

Peroneal muscular atrophy (also known as Charcot-Marie-Tooth disease or hereditary muscular atrophy) is characterized by slowly progressive symmetrical muscular atrophy and weakness of the legs and the feet, with eventual involvement of the forearms and the hands. Involvement of the peroneal muscles is typical.

ETIOLOGY

The cause is unknown. Males are affected more often than females. The disease is transmitted as a dominant, recessive or sex-linked characteristic.

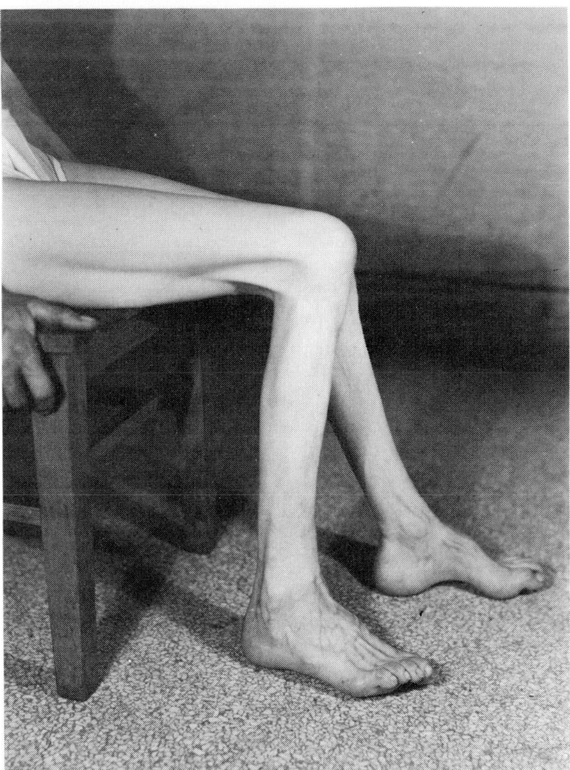
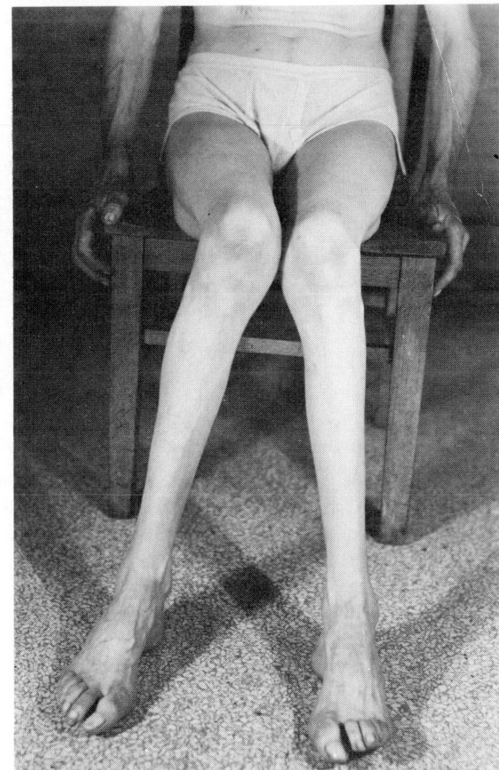

FIG. 14-11. Charcot-Marie-Tooth peroneal muscular atrophy. Note the "stork legs" and pes cavus. (Courtesy of Dr. Alexander T. Ross)

PATHOLOGY

A degenerative process without an inflammatory reaction affects the anterior horn cells and the peripheral nerves and, to some extent, the posterior columns.

CLINICAL PICTURE

The onset of symptoms tends to appear at about the same age in childhood in the afflicted members of the family. Initially, the gait is clumsy and peroneal weakness is demonstrable in frequent ankle inversion strains. Pains and paresthesias are common in the legs. Very slowly over many years there develops the typical picture of atrophy of the leg muscles and the intrinsic muscles of the feet (Fig. 14-11). At first a dropfoot and inversion of the ankle develop into a fixed equinocavovarus deformity with clawed toes. The gait is steppage. The peroneals usually show the greatest amount of weakness. A comparable muscle atrophy and deformity later develop in the upper extremity, causing thinning of the forearms and clawed hands. The deep reflexes are lost. Loss of tactile, temperature and proprioceptive sensations is variable in degree. The face, the trunk, and the pelvic and shoulder girdles are not affected.

ELECTRODIAGNOSIS

The conduction velocities of the peroneal nerves are markedly slowed. Electromyography shows a steadily decreasing number of normal motor unit action potentials. Serial strength duration studies (SD curves) disclose progressive reduction of muscle response to electrical stimulation. This study will establish when advance of disease has been halted.

PROGNOSIS

The course is slow and protracted but may become stationary at any time. The patient may live out the normal life expectancy.

TREATMENT

Neostigmine (Prostigmin), 15 mg three times daily, is often helpful in lessening weakness and ataxia. A spring dropfoot brace and dynamic splinting of the hand prevent contracture. When deformity is extreme, surgical procedures are necessary. Surgery should be delayed until progression of the disease has been halted and there has been no evidence of muscle involvement for at least 2 years.

Before the gastrocnemius is involved, a fixed equinocavovarus deformity develops. The equinus consists in weakness of anterior tibial muscles and dropped forefoot and contracture of plantar fascia, causing cavus deformity. A Lambrinudi foot stabilization procedure corrects the equinus. Achilles tendon lengthening is contraindicated because the calf muscles are needed for adequate push off. Muscle imbalance must be corrected and dorsiflexion provided or reinforced. The posterior tibial tendon is rerouted through the interosseous membrane and inserted into the third cuneiform. The procedure may be done as early as 7 years of age, although it is preferable to wait until bone maturity is attained. The operation should always be preceded by plantar stripping.[16,18]

When the calf muscles are inadequate, a panastragalar arthrodesis plus tarsal wedge resection is necessary.

Surgical procedures are also available for overcoming intrinsic muscle paralysis and contracture in the hand (see Chapter 25).

FRIEDREICH'S ATAXIA

Friedreich's ataxia (hereditary spinal ataxia) is a hereditary and familial disease and is characterized by progressive degeneration of the corticospinal, the spinocerebellar, and the posterior columns of the spinal cord.

ETIOLOGY

The cause is unknown. Transmission occurs through affected and unaffected people and usually by an autosomal recessive gene.

PATHOLOGY

A demyelinizing process occurs in the pyramidal tracts, in the spinocerebellar tracts and especially in the posterior columns. When destruction is severe and extensive, the anterior horn cells may be involved.

CLINICAL PICTURE

The average age at onset is 10 years. Initially, the complaints include awkwardness of gait, stumbling, frequent falling, frequent twisting of the ankles, foot fatigue, and difficulty in obtaining comfortable shoes. The shoes wear out rapidly and become misshapen as foot deformity gradually develops. Typically, a symmetrical clawfoot forms, with marked elevation of the longitudinal arch, prominent metatarsal heads, widening of the forefoot, and hyperextension and clawing of the lesser toes. An equinus is apparent and is due to dropping of the forefoot at the midtarsal area. Muscle weakness becomes apparent in the peroneals and the anterior tibials. This clinical picture is quite common and may not progress beyond this point, thereby constituting an abortive form of the disease.

In typical Friedreich's ataxia, symptoms and findings slowly progress over the years. The gait becomes ataxic, and Romberg's sign is positive. Cerebellar signs include failure to perform the finger-to-nose test and adiodokokinesis. Deep pain, position, and vibration sense are impaired, attesting to a posterior column lesion. The deep tendon reflexes are lost early. Later, as the pyramidal tracts are involved, the reflexes may become hyperactive and the Babinski sign is positive. Speech becomes halting and explosive. Muscle weakness and atrophy affect particularly the intrinsic muscles of the feet and the legs, especially the peroneals and the anterior tibials. An extreme equinocavovarus deformity may develop and in itself, regardless of the ataxia, is very disabling. Eventually, usually at about 30 years of age, the patient becomes bedridden. A kyphoscoliosis is an additional deformity in 80% to 90% of cases, usually in the thoracic region, and is progressive

Cardiac abnormalities occur in approximately 30% of cases. A toxic, chronic, progressive myocarditis produces a diffuse interstitial fibrosis and round cell infiltration, cardiomegaly, and occasionally coronary artery atherosclerosis. The cardiac disease may precede neurologic symptoms and may be mistaken for rheumatic heart disease until central nervous system signs develop. Congestive heart failure is rare but may develop at a late stage of Friedreich's ataxia in the adult, responds poorly to the usual treatment, and may prove to be the terminal event.[20,21]

TREATMENT

Surgical intervention is indicated both for the mild abortive form and the severe type of the disease.[19] In the latter, provision of a stable, corrected foot will greatly aid ambulation and may add many useful years to the lifespan of these persons.

The basic procedure consists of a triple arthrodesis with adequate wedging resection to overcome deformity. Because the equinus is limited to the forefoot, Achilles tendon lengthening is contraindicated. Instead, the midtarsal resection and subcutaneous fasciotomy, if necessary, will suffice. When anterior tibial function is inadequate, the extensor hallucis longus is transferred to the neck of the first metatarsal, and the interphalangeal joint of the large toe is fused. Bone surgery should be postponed until bone maturity is adequate.

SYRINGOMYELIA

Syringomyelia is a slowly progressive disease of the spinal cord and the medulla oblongata that is caused by cavitation and gliosis and is characterized clinically by dissociated sensory loss and muscular atrophy.

ETIOLOGY

The cause of true syringomyelia is unknown. Pseudosyringomyelia is cavitation that is localized and secondary to vascular lesions, intramedullary tumors, or trauma to the cord.

PATHOLOGY

The essential lesion is the slowly progressive destruction of the central portion of the cervical enlargement of the spinal cord, from where it extends downward to involve the thoracic and the lumbar segments and upward into the medulla oblongata.[17] The central lesion is a cavitation that extends into the posterior and the anterior gray columns and then compresses and sometimes destroys the posterior and the lateral white columns. Microscopically, abnormal masses of ependymal cells lie in close relationship to thin-walled blood vessels, suggesting a choroid plexus that secretes cerebrospinal fluid. It is the accumulated fluid that forms the cavity and extends along lines of least resistance. When the choroid plexus–like structure is destroyed, fluid no longer forms and progress of the degenerative process is arrested. Similarly, surgical drainage of the syrinx with provision of a permanent external communication, or spontaneous perforation into the central canal, stops progress of the disease.

CLINICAL PICTURE

The onset is insidious. Weakness and atrophy of the intrinsic muscles of the hands are often the initial symptoms and findings. Pain (sharp, shooting, or burning) throughout the upper extremities is common. The loss of painful sensation is first disclosed by unnoticed burns and injuries. Examination reveals loss of pain and temperature sense, usually extending in a shawllike distribution over the arms and the shoulders. Tactile sensation is undisturbed. Reduced sensation to touch, when present, is associated with loss of proprioception and signifies extension of the lesion into the posterior white columns. When spasticity, hyperactive reflexes and pathologic reflexes are present in the lower extremities, the lesion has compressed the pyramidal tract laterally. Progression of the lesion may halt at any time. Involvement of the medulla oblongata (syringobulbia) is indicated by aphonia and dysphagia. Charcot's joint develops in approximately 20% of cases in the upper extremity. Scoliosis is a frequent deformity.

PROGNOSIS

Although slowly progressive, the disease may become stationary at any time. Bulbar involvement is of serious import.

TREATMENT

Drainage of the cavity is indicated. A platybasia with an Arnold-Chiari deformity is a not uncommon cause of pseudosyringomyelia. This should be investigated and decompressed if necessary. A Charcot joint at the shoulder or the elbow may require stabilization.

DIFFERENTIAL DIAGNOSIS OF THE MUSCLE ATROPHIES

Progressive Spinal Muscular Atrophy. The upper extremity, especially the hand, is chiefly affected. The disorder is painless, sensation is intact, and onset occurs in middle age, with very slow progression.

Peroneal Atrophy. The condition is familial, with several members of the family afflicted. Lower extremities are earliest and chiefly involved. Shoulder and pelvic girdles escape involvement. Pain is often associated, and peroneal paralysis is characteristic. Onset is in childhood, and the disorder is rarely fatal.

Familial Progressive Spinal Muscular Atrophy. The condition is familial but has its onset in early infancy, starting in the trunk and progressing rapidly to involve the extremities; death results in a few years.

Amyotonia Congenita. Flaccid paralysis of lower extremities already present at birth is seen; there is a tendency toward some improvement.

Amyotrophic Lateral Sclerosis. The onset is in middle age when flaccid paralysis in the upper and spastic paralysis in lower extremities occurs. The disorder is rapidly progressive, involving the medulla; it is fatal in a few years.

Syringomyelia. Atrophy is associated with loss of pain and temperature sense and preservation of tactile sense in the upper extremities.

Poliomyelitis. Preceded by a febrile disturbance, paralysis is often transient in some areas; atrophy is assymetrical, spotty, and nonprogressive.

Cervical Cord Tumor. Root pain and atrophy may be unilateral and become progressively worse. Sensory impairment affects all forms. Headache is common. Spinal fluid studies may show subarachnoid block and an increase of total protein.

Friedreich's Ataxia. Muscle atrophy affects the leg and foot, causing typical severe equinocavovarus deformity. Onset is in childhood. Ataxia, loss of proprioception, pyramidal tract signs, and nystagmus occur. The disorder is hereditary and familial.

PERIPHERAL NERVES

FUNCTION OF A PERIPHERAL NERVE

Peripheral nerve fibers conduct sensory, motor, and trophic impulses. Sensation includes coarse and light touch, pain, temperature, stereognosis, and deep tissue sense (pain, position, vibration). Motor fibers innervate muscles. Trophic fibers are supplied to all tissues, including skin, tendons, joints, and muscles.

BASIC NERVE UNIT

The motor fibers originate from neurons in the anterior horn of the spinal cord. Sympathetic neurons in the lateral columns of the gray matter give rise to vasomotor and trophic fibers. All fibers combine and emerge as myelinated fibers from the anterolateral aspect of the cord as a common white ramus. A ganglion located outside the dorsolateral aspect of the cord is connected with the latter by a dorsal gray nerve root. It contains the neurons for sensory perception.

PATHOLOGY FOLLOWING SEVERANCE OF A PERIPHERAL NERVE

All functions distal to the point of severance are interrupted. At the end of the proximal nerve segment the axons multiply and attempt to grow distally. However, a connective tissue bulblike growth envelops the end of the nerve and obstructs the path of these fibrils, which become arranged in disorderly fashion. The connective tissue and fibril growth is called a neuroma. The distal nerve segment swells to twice its original size and undergoes wallerian degeneration. This process is complete in about 1 month. Its proximal end displays only a small enlargement, consisting only of fibrous tissue. Occasionally, the connective tissue growths at the end of each segment may unite, and some of the fibrils may successfully penetrate the mass and grow distally. Partial function may thereby be restored.

SYMPTOMS AND FINDINGS FOLLOWING COMPLETE NERVE INJURY

Stereognosis, the most specialized perception of shape and texture is lost. The specialized touch corpuscles (Meissner's, Pacini's, Ruffini's) located in the hand, most particularly in the median nerve distribution, are linked with the stereognostic center on the opposite side of the brain.

Superficial sensation to touch, pain, and temperature is lost. This includes epicritic sensation (light sensation), by which two points of a compass are distinguished, and coarse sensation, such as pain.

Deep sensation to muscle and joint movements, position, deep pressure, and vibration travels mainly in motor nerves and if these nerves are injured, sensation is lost. Bunnell describes an excellent method of mapping anesthetic areas by an electric skin resistance machine consisting of a battery, a galvanometer, and two electrodes placed near one another. Anesthetic skin is electroresistant because the sweat glands are dry. Placed on normal skin, this apparatus is a detector of malingerers, since the galvanometer will show normal conductivity. A person who claims to have pain will show excellent conductivity, because pain stimulates the sweat glands. No reaction is obtained on anesthetic skin.

Loss of motor supply to a muscle results in progressive atrophy and fibrous degeneration of that muscle. A muscle is partially paralyzed when nerve severance is incomplete and is revealed by a limited amplitude of motion and decreased force against resistance.

Deep reflexes are diminished and lost.

Electric stimulation of the nerve no longer causes the muscle to contract. However, the muscle may be well stimulated directly by faradic current. This response gradually diminishes until after 2 weeks no response to faradism is obtainable. Nevertheless, the muscle continues to respond to galvanic current by a slow vermicular contraction, greater in amplitude and followed by slow relaxation. This chain of events, namely, early loss of response to faradism and increased continued response to galvanism, is known as the reaction of degeneration and is characteristic of peripheral nerve interruption. After the muscle has undergone complete fibrous degeneration, no further electric reaction is obtainable. Each muscle responds best electrically at the point at which the nerve enters the muscle. Normally, it contracts strongly to faradic current and gives a quick twitch to galvanic. (See Electrodiagnosis.)

Trophic influence is lost. All tissues in the supplied area undergo atrophy. The skin is thin and glossy, red, or cyanotic. Hair and nails are brittle. Bone is osteoporotic. Joint cartilage is thinned, and ligaments are contracted and inflexible, resulting in decrease of motion due to contracture of the joint. Healing of wounds is slow. This picture should be differentiated from the condition of reflex sympathetic dystrophy, which is characterized by a generally painful, swollen, cold, cyanotic part and typical mottled osteoporosis.

DETERMINING THE SITE OF NERVE INJURY

The particular nerve involved is revealed by the muscles paralyzed and the area of anesthesia. The point of interruption is located by the history of accident, by the location of the nerve, and by Tinel's sign. The last is performed by percussing or tapping over the severed nerve end, causing tingling in the area of distribution of the nerve. In the course of regeneration the sign can be elicited further distally, indicating the level to which the new axons have grown.

REGENERATION OF NERVES

Severed nerves will bridge a gap of 1 cm or a little more. At operation a nerve stripped of its surrounding tissues loses its blood supply and function temporarily. Scar tissue will strangulate a nerve and obstruct peripheral growth. Repair of a peripheral nerve demands accurate approximation in exact rotation; otherwise, sensory fibers may grow down motor pathways, and vice versa, and so are wasted. Regeneration occurs at a rate of 1 mm or 2 mm/day. Motor recovery can occur after 2 or 3 years, and sensory return occurs from 3 to 5 years after nerve severance. In the arm, the radial nerve regenerates better than the median and the median, better than the ulnar. Sensation recovers before motor function. Protopathic precedes the epicritic sense. Deep sensibility returns with the epicritic sense and, finally, stereognosis occurs. The proximal portions of the anesthetic area disappear first. Tinel's sign can be elicited by tapping anywhere over the newly formed nonmyelinated axons. The sign disappears in 1 or 2 years as the axons become myelinated. The quality of sensation early after return is not normal. Paresthesia is felt in response to stimuli. Reactivation of muscles occurs later, the most proximal ones returning first. The early flicker of motion increases until a large portion of the muscle contracts, although it moves the part through a limited amplitude and is easily fatigued. Strength and coordination in movement are acquired eventually. Trophic changes progress even after nerve severance; these start to regress when sensation begins to appear. Serial electromyographic and strength duration studies will often demonstrate beginning recovery of muscle excitability to electric stimulation long before clinical signs of reinnervation become apparent. These electrodiagnostic tests can be used to follow the rate of nerve regeneration.

THE DEGREE OF NERVE INJURY

Neurapraxia is a physiological injury to a nerve. No anatomical damage is present. The paralysis is transient, sensory loss is slight, no reaction of denegeration is obtainable, and recovery is complete within a few hours to days.

Neurotmesis is complete physiological and anatomical interruption of the nerve fibers and their sheaths. Recovery generally is obtainable by surgical approximation.

Axonotmesis is interruption of nerve fibers within their sheath. The Schwann tubes remain in continuity so that spontaneous cure eventuates. It is necessary to distinguish between neurotmesis and axonotmesis to determine whether to intervene surgically.

Traction nerve injuries are often severe and are essentially a neurotmesis. Although anatomical continuity may appear to be preserved, extensive intraneural scar formation occurs. Direct compression injuries at a fracture site usually have a good prognosis for spontaneous cure. This is especially so in the case of the radial nerve. Involvement of the axillary nerve has an unfavorable prognosis. It is necessary to preserve muscle and joint function by galvanic stimulation, passive motion, and daily massage until the nerve regenerates. Inasmuch as axons grow down 1 mm/day, one can estimate the time required to reach the most proximally involved muscle (*e.g.*, the brachioradialis in case of the radial nerve). If reinnervation does not occur at the expected time, surgical exploration of the nerve should be undertaken. Electromyographic evidence of motor unit action potentials is found in the most proximal muscle some weeks before a flicker of voluntary power is ascertained clinically.

POLYNEURITIS

Polyneuritis (multiple neuritis) is applied to a painful, degenerative, often inflammatory process in a neuron and its fiber.[12] When any portion of a neuron, whether axon or cell body, is involved, the remainder of the cell invariably undergoes changes. Therefore, the painful degenerative process, regardless of its initial situation, causes functional loss of the entire unit.

Neuritis is very common and is caused by many conditions. The principal causes are listed in Table 14-2 under those causing mononeuritis and others causing polyneuritis. Neuritis of a single nerve most often stems from local causes, which are described under their respective sections. The following discussion applies mainly to multiple neuritis.

PATHOLOGY

In most forms of polyneuritis, a noninflammatory degeneration of the peripheral nerves takes place. The

TABLE 14-2 Principal Causes of Neuritis

Generalized Polyneuritis

VIRUS	BACTERIOTOXIC	DEFICIENCY OR METABOLISM	CHEMICAL
Measles	Focal infections	Pellagra	Mercury
Smallpox	Rheumatism	Pernicious anemia	Lead
Chickenpox	Erysipelas	Sprue	Silver
Parotitis	Scarlet fever	Beriberi	Arsenic
Herpes	Rheumatic fever	Alcoholic neuritis	Phosphorus
Acute febrile	Chorea	Korsakow's psychosis	Methyl alcohol
Acute infective	Septicemia	Pernicious vomiting	Ethyl alcohol
Landry's	Puerperal fever	Hunger edema	Ethyl iodide
Poliomyelitis	Gonorrhea	Pregnancy	Trichlorethylene
Encephalomyelitis	Meningitis	Chronic colitis	Carbon tetrachloride
Epidemic (lethargic) encephalitis	Diphtheria	Cancer with cachexia	Trinitrotoluene
Erythroedema	Typhoid fever	Tuberculosis with cachexia	Dinitrobenzene
Acute rabic myelitis	Paratyphoid fever	Senility with cachexia	Triorthocresyl phosphate
	Typhus fever	Diabetes	Aniline
	Influenza	Myxedema	Sulfonethylmethane, barbital, etc.
	Pneumonia	Hematoporphyrinuria	Chloral, chlorbutanol
	Malaria	Recurrent polyneuritis	Carbon monoxide
	Relapsing fever	Chronic progressive polyneuritis	Carbon bisulphide
	Serum sickness	Chronic bacillary dysentery	
	Acute enteric fever		

Localized Neuritis

MECHANICAL	INFECTIOUS
Pressure	Diphtheria
Tumor	Tetanus
Edema	Streptococci
Arthritis	Leprosy
Fibrosis	
Trauma	
Saturday night paralysis	
Volmann contracture	
Meralgia paresthetica	

myelin sheath swells, breaks up into fatty globules, and disappears, while the axis cylinder remains intact. If the process is halted at this stage, regeneration is rapid. If the process of degeneration advances, the axis cylinder shows an increase in Schwann cells, then disintegrates. Lacking its coverings, the axon undergoes degeneration (wallerian degeneration). Regeneration occurs after removal of the debris, regrowth of the cylinder, regrowth of the unmyelinized axon at the rate of 1 mm to 2 mm/day, and finally restoration of the myelin sheath.

The rate of regeneration is inversely proportional to the extent of degeneration of the enveloping sheaths. When the nerve cylinder and myelin sheath appear intact, regeneration is rapid.

CLINICAL PICTURE

Symptoms pertain to both motor and sensory divisions of the peripheral nerve.

Sensory Findings. Pain is common and often severe. It varies in intensity and character and may be sharp, burning, or boring. It always follows the course or distribution of the nerve and disappears when the nerve is severed at its proximal portion. Paresthesias often precede and follow the pain. The nerve is tender along its entire course. All forms of sensation, including pain, touch, temperature, position, and vibration, are reduced or entirely lost.

Motor Loss. Impairment varies from paresis to paralysis. Muscles are flaccid and lack the resiliency of muscles with tone. Atrophy develops. The deep reflexes are reduced or absent.

Electric Reactions. Nerve conduction velocity is reduced or absent.

Cramps and Muscle Spasm. Occasionally these symptoms occur at the onset because of an irritative lesion.

Autonomic Changes. The efferent autonomic fibers run through the motor nerves. The vasomotor, pilomotor, sudomotor, and trophic nerve fibers are involved. The skin becomes thin, glossy, cyanotic, and cold. Hyperhidrosis or hypohidrosis, hypertrichosis, and nail changes may occur.

Muscular and Joint Contractures. Contractures may develop as a result of unbalanced muscle pull.

INFECTIOUS POLYNEURITIS

Infectious polyneuritis (also known as Landry's ascending paralysis, Guillain-Barré syndrome, encephalomyeloradiculitis, infectious neuronitis, polyneuritis with facial diplegia) is a clinical syndrome characterized by an acute onset of widespread, progressive, symmetrical, frequently ascending paralysis of peripheral and cranial nerves. It is often associated with facial diplegia, shows relative absence of sensory findings, and is often accompanied by a high spinal fluid protein level. It is frequently preceded by a respiratory infection and sometimes by gastroenteritis. Almost complete recovery occurs in patients who survive. The mortality rate is variously reported at from 20% to 35% and results from respiratory failure.[41,45,47,58,84]

Etiology

The exciting cause is unknown, but the frequent history of an antecedent respiratory or gastrointestinal infection, and the common association with diseases of known viral etiology (*e.g.*, influenza, infectious hepatitis, infectious mononucleosis) suggests that a filterable virus is at fault. However, attempts to isolate a virus have been unsuccessful, and the pathologic changes are not typical of those viral diseases affecting the nervous system. Studies indicate that it is probably an autoimmune disease.[36]

The disease affects individuals at any age, and the sexes are equally affected. Infectious polyneuritis is second only to alcoholic polyneuritis in frequency of the polyneuritides.

Pathology

The pathology consists of degenerative changes affecting the spinal and cranial nerves, with retrograde changes in the motor cells of the spinal nerve and cranial nerve nuclei. Perivascular accumulations of mononuclear cells are observed in the endoneurium and epineurium. Wallerian degeneration of axons and proliferation of Schwann cells are seen.

In patients who die within a few days of the onset, pathologic changes are almost impossible to detect.

Clinical Picture

In about two thirds of cases, a mild upper respiratory infection, less commonly a gastroenteritis, precedes the onset of neuritis. After an interval of 5 to 12 days, pains appear in the back and the legs are the initial symptoms of developing neuritis. The first objective neurologic finding is usually symmetrical weakness of the lower extremities, most often first affecting the distal portions and ascending to involve the remainder of the lower and then the upper extremities and the facial muscles within 24 to 72 hours. Paresthesias usually precede the weakness. The weakness increases in intensity within a few days but may develop over a period of 2 to 3 weeks. Paralysis of the cranial nerves is frequent, including facial diplegia (80%), dysphagia, and dysarthria (50%).

Motor weakness of the trunk and extremities is usually severe, and a flaccid quadriplegia is not uncommon. Extreme weakness of the muscles of respiration occurs in about one fourth of cases, necessitating a tracheotomy and respirator.

Sensory changes are not a prominent feature and consist mainly of hypoesthesia. Severe loss of cutaneous sensation is rare.

The muscles and nerves are moderately tender. The deep tendon reflexes are diminished or absent. Plantar and abdominal reflexes are generally preserved or show no response.

Laboratory Findings

The cerbrospinal fluid pressure is elevated in severe cases. Characteristically, the spinal fluid protein is markedly elevated, although not invariably so, sometime reaching 1000 mg/dl. A slight pleocytosis is found in 20% of cases.

Course and Prognosis

Symptoms reach their maximum as a rule within a week of onset but may sometimes progress over several weeks. Recovery generally occurs over 3 to 4 weeks; it may be delayed for a number of months and is either complete or results in minimal residual weakness. Formerly regarded as a benign disease with a good prognosis, it is now known that a fatal termination from respiratory failure occurs in 20% to 35% of cases.

Treatment

Bulbar involvement requires urgent measures. Early tracheotomy and the use of a respirator can be lifesaving. Positive pressure ventilation may be necessary. The corticosteroids and adrenocorticotropic hormone may be tried, but their effect is questionable.[27,77] During the acute stage, warm wet packs are applied to the extremities, followed by passive range of motion exercises. During the convalescent stage, recovery of muscle strength is aided by a planned program of exercises.[72] When resolution of muscle weakness is delayed, the use of orthotic devices prevents deformities of muscle imbalance, and a walker assists ambulation. Corrective surgery for residual deformity and to restore muscle balance is rarely necessary and should observe the principles described in the section on poliomyelitis and flaccid paralysis.

BACTERIOTOXIC POLYNEURITIS

Many bacterial diseases are often associated with a transient peripheral neuritis. The mechanism of causation may be bacterial, toxic, and vitamin deficiency. The following are especially important:

Septicemic polyneuritis. Symptoms are similar to those caused by alcohol. In addition to pain, tenderness, and hyperesthesia of the skin, paresthesias are frequent and trophic changes of the fingers occur. The cranial nerves may be involved.

Diphtheritic polyneuritis. Cranial nerve involvement occurs within a few weeks after the sore throat. Bulbar symptoms include aphonia, nasal regurgitation of liquids, dysphagia, and abductor paralysis of the vocal cords. Facial and ocular paralysis; limb paralysis, particularly of the extensor muscles; and respiratory and cardiac paralysis may develop. The paralysis usually develops first in the vicinity of the diphtheritic membrane, hence the frequency of cranial nerve involvement. Spread of infection is apparently by way of perineural lymphatics. The palatal, pharyngeal, and laryngeal paralyses clear up in a few weeks; ocular palsies last longer; while those of the extremities last a long time.

Enteric and paratyphoid polyneuritis. Neuritis is asymmetrical and often starts with severe pains about the shoulders, followed by atrophy of the trapezius or the serratus magnus. Dietary vitamin deficiency is the probable cause.

Serum disease neuritis. Whether the serum or the treated disease is the cause is debatable.

Puerperal polyneuritis. This occurs several weeks before term. The causative factor is prolonged avitaminosis associated with hyperemesis gravidarum.

Rheumatic polyneuritis. This designation is given to a mild type of polyneuritis associated with rheumatoid arthritis. It generally disappears with improvement of the arthritis, leaving atrophic stiff muscles. Intrinsic muscle contracture of the hand, a frequent residual of rheumatoid arthritis, may be partly a residual of neuritis.

DEFICIENCY OR METABOLISM POLYNEURITIS

Some unknown factor causes inflammatory changes in the peripheral nerves and degenerative changes in the spinal cord. The mechanisms at work include lack of digestive juices in the stomach, lack of vitamin B, failure of absorption from the gastrointestinal tract, and inadequate diet.

Beriberi

Beriberi, formerly seen in India and Japan, is due to thiamine deficiency. The onset is acute with cardiac dilatation and tachycardia but no fever. Edema is prominent about the body but chiefly affects the lower extremities. Nausea, vomiting, and depression are followed by polyneuritic pains, areflexia, sensory disturbances, and muscle atrophies. The course lasts from a few weeks to several months, and death occurs from cardiac failure or intercurrent disease. Edema may be absent.

Subclinical vitamin B_1 deficiency develops with dietary inadequacy, anorexia, failure of assimilation, or increased requirement in thyrotoxicosis, pregnancy, and lactation.

Diabetic Polyneuritis

This syndrome affects diabetics over 40 years of age and consists of signs and symptoms of involvement of the peripheral nerves: pains, paresthesias, motor weakness, and loss of deep tendon reflexes in the lower extremities. Although ascribed to arteriosclerosis of nerves, vitamin B deficiency, or interference with carbohydrate metabolism, the actual cause and pathogenesis are unknown.

The pathology consists of degenerative changes in the peripheral nerves, posterior roots, and posterior columns of the spinal cord. Retrograde degenerative changes may be found in the anterior horn cells.

Sensory symptoms predominate and are characteristic of diabetic neuritis: paresthesias, severe nocturnal burning sensations (*e.g.*, about the heels), spasmodic lightninglike pains, and hyperesthesia of the lower extremities.

The deep tendon reflexes are lost, and when proprioception is lost and ataxia is associated, the symptom complex resembles tabes dorsalis (pseudotabes). A perforating ulcer may form in the foot.

The polyneuritic syndrome may cause slight temporary weakness, rarely paralysis, of the lower extremities. This is in contrast to single nerve involvement (mononeuritis) in diabetes, which is probably due to sudden arterial occlusion within the nerve and which causes permanent paralysis. The femoral and anterior tibial nerves are most frequently affected by mononeuritis.

The outlook for polyneuritis in the diabetic is good, with improvement taking place over several weeks to a few months. Occasionally, burning pain about the heels may persist as a very distressing symptom and keeps the patient awake at night.

The symptoms of occlusive arterial disease (intermittent claudication, numbness, rest pain) should not be confused with those of diabetic polyneuritis.

Treatment consists of control of severe painful spasms by use of narcotics, bed rest, and warm moist packs. The administration of various components of vitamin B in large amounts seems to shorten the course and lessen the intensity of the pain. The diabetes should be well controlled.

CHEMICAL POLYNEURITIS

Lead Neuritis

Lead poisoning differs from other forms of polyneuritis in causing involvement of the central nervous system, especially the anterior horn cells. Painters, plumbers, plasterers, and typesetters are predisposed. Cosmetics, hair dyes, and many other substances contain lead.

The degenerative neuritis is limited to motor nerves, especially those to the extensors of the hand and the forearm. However, the forearm flexors and the deltoid finally are involved. Usually, the brachioradialis and sometimes the extensor and the abductor of the thumb are spared. When the lower extremity is involved, the peroneals are more likely to be affected than the anterior tibial. The course is chronic, and the outlook is good when the offending agent is removed.

Arsenical Polyneuritis

The source of arsenic includes medications, wines, and insecticides. Symptoms resemble those of alcoholic polyneuritis. Pain in the limbs and numbness of the hands and the feet are followed by wristdrop and footdrop. The muscles atrophy rapidly. Cutaneous anesthesia, pains, and hyperesthesias are more severe than in alcoholic polyneuritis, and mental symptoms are rare.

Associated features of arsenical poisoning include abdominal pain, vomiting and diarrhea, skin pigmentation, keratoses, and herpes zoster.

The diagnosis is established by recovering arsenic from the urine and the hair.

Recovery requires 2 to 3 years.

Mercurial Polyneuritis

Polyneuritis due to mercury poisoning resembles other forms of polyneuritis, but renal damage and gingivitis are additional findings.

Alcoholic Polyneuritis

This type of polyneuritis occurs in patients who are chronically addicted to alcoholic intake for many years. Because their dietary intake is also inadequate, the cause appears to be a combination of the toxic effect of alcohol and a nutritional deficiency. Moreover, most patients suffer from achlorhydria, with loss of intrinsic factor and malabsorption, which may explain the frequently associated anemia and posterior column involvement in the spinal cord. The condition is best described as an alcohol–vitamin deficiency polyneuritis, but the actual pathogenesis is unclear. It is the most common form of polyneuritis and occurs about five times more frequently in men than in women.

Symptoms develop slowly over weeks to months, but they may develop rapidly over a few days. The first symptoms are pain in the legs and paresthesias in the hands and feet. These are soon followed by weakness of the legs, dropfoot, and ataxia. Unless the condition is recognized and the process halted by treatment, the legs gradually become paralyzed and muscle weakness spreads to involve the trunk and upper extremities. In extreme cases, optic neuritis, extraocular paralysis, and weakness of facial muscles and those of other cranial nerves develop. Muscle weakness is greatest in the distal portions of the extremities, and the extensors are more severely affected than the flexors. Anesthesia and hypoesthesia are most pronounced over the distal parts of the extremities, whereas cutaneous sensibility is preserved elsewhere. Proprioception is impaired. The nerve trunks and muscles are tender. The deep tendon reflexes disappear, especially in the legs. Plantar and abdominal skin reflexes are unresponsive. Drying, scaling, and pigmentation of the skin on the back of the hands and wrists, and swelling of the ankles, suggests a pellagralike component.

Korsakoff's syndrome is a combination of polyneuritis and a mental state characterized by confusion, disorientation, loss of memory, and a tendency to confabulate. Most often it is associated with alcoholic polyneuritis, but it may occur with other forms of polyneuritis and, in alcoholics, can occur in the absence of polyneuritis. Signs of liver damage and convulsive seizures are not infrequent. The mortality rate in untreated cases is about 50%, with death occurring within the first few weeks after the symptoms become severe. Recovery is slow and incomplete.

The course of alcoholic polyneuritis is prolonged, especially if paralysis has already developed before treatment is instituted. In uncomplicated cases, the mortality is low but is increased proportionate to the degree of cerebral involvement.

The pathology, as in the majority of other forms of polyneuritis, is mainly a noninflammatory degeneration of the peripheral nerves. In the initial stages there are swelling and fragmentation of the myelin. As the destructive process advances, the axis cylinders also become involved, and the axons undergo disintegration. Retrograde changes are found in cells of the anterior horns (axonal reaction). In chronic cases, the posterior funiculi show degeneration of the ascending fibers.

Treatment. Thiamine and vitamin B complex given intravenously in large doses greatly reduce the mortality. The medical regimen aims at gradual withdrawal of alcohol and increasing the diet, which is supplemented by vitamins. Correction of the anemia and malabsorptive defect is essential.

Orthopaedic treatment consists of splinting of the extremities during the acutely painful stage to prevent stretching of the paralyzed muscles. Physical therapy includes warm moist packs and passive range of motion exercises. Later, when voluntary movements begin to return, increasing active exercises, electrical stimulation, and muscle training help to restore strength and coordination. Orthoses and walking aids may be necessary for months. Recovery may take as long as 2 years.

INDIVIDUAL PERIPHERAL NERVES

MERALGIA PARESTHETICA

The lateral femoral cutaneous nerve arises from the posterior divisions of the second and third lumbar nerves. It makes its appearance at the lateral border of the psoas and passes obliquely across the iliacus to the anterior-superior iliac spine, where it proceeds beneath the inguinal ligament to enter the anterolateral aspect of the thigh.

Any syndrome manifesting numbness, paresthesias, and pain over the lateral and anterolateral aspect of the thigh suggests an inflammatory, degenerative lesion of the lateral femoral cutaneous nerve and is designated meralgia paresthetica (lateral femoral cutaneous neuropathy). The sensations experienced are described variously as burning, tingling, hyperesthesia, numbness, or severe pain. Often pain occurs after activity or direct pressure against the thigh and is relieved by rest. Reduction of tactile sensation is demonstrable over the lateral aspect of the thigh.

In most instances, the condition is idiopathic. Some cases are due to kinking and constriction of the nerve at its point of emergence from the pelvis. Normally, the nerve courses beneath the inguinal ligament and in front of the sartorius muscle. Instead, the lateral femoral cutaneous nerve may penetrate between two fasciculi of the inguinal ligament. Consequently, when the hip is fully extended, the nerve is compressed by the posterior fibers of the ligament (Fig. 14-12).

Treatment. Symptoms may persist for many months but almost invariably subside. If pain is persistent and intolerable and is relieved by injection of a local anesthetic about the nerve at its point of emergence from the pelvis, surgical relief may be accomplished by division of the portion of the inguinal ligament lying posterior to the nerve or by removal of the nerve.

Otherwise, the lesion presumably must be located proximal to this point. It is essential to seek pathology lying along the route of the nerve, whether intraspinal, retroperitoneal, abdominal, or pelvic.

AXILLARY NERVE

Anatomy

The axillary nerve springs from the posterior cord of the brachial plexus and runs alongside the radial nerve behind the axillary artery, separating the latter from the subscapularis muscle on the floor. At the lower border of the muscle, it leaves the radial nerve and turns posteriorly, in company with the posterior humeral circumflex artery, through the quadrangular space to the

FIG. 14-12. Lateral femoral cutaneous nerve (LFCN) of the thigh. (*Top*) Normal course of LFCN passing under the inguinal ligament medial to the anterior superior iliac spine (ASIS). (*Bottom left*) LFCN passing through a split in the inguinal ligament. (*Bottom right*) LFCN astride the iliac crest lateral to the ASIS. (*FN*, femoral nerve; *IL*, inguinal ligament) (Edelson JG, Nathan H: Meralgia paresthetica. Clin Orthop 122:255, 1977)

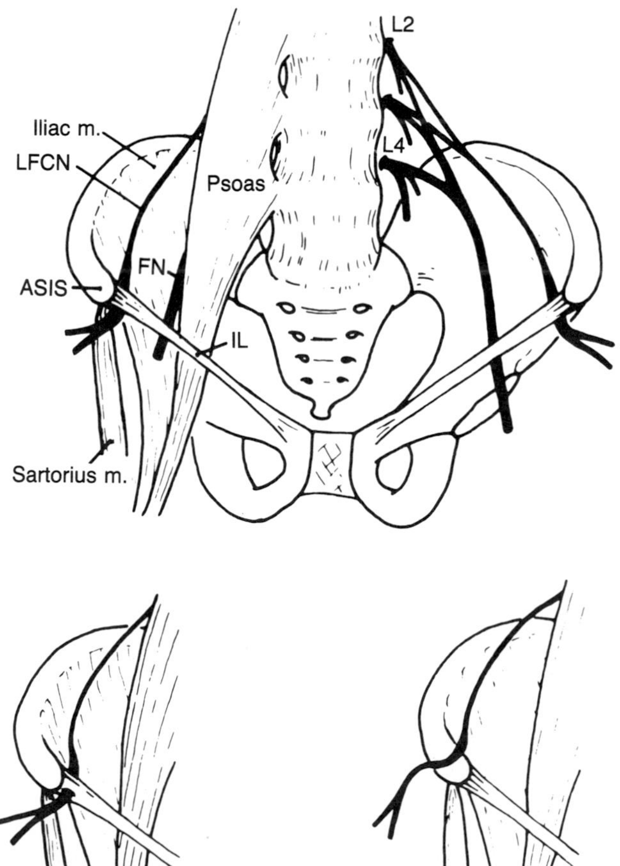

posterior aspect of the humerus, where it divides into anterior and posterior branches. The posterior branch gives off the nerves of supply to the teres minor and the posterior part of the deltoid before it curves around the posterior border of the deltoid to supply the skin over the lower half of the deltoid (upper lateral cutaneous nerve of the arm). The anterior branch proceeds laterally and anteriorly beneath the deltoid and in contact with the surgical neck of the humerus about 2 inches below the upper attachment of the deltoid, giving off numerous twigs to the muscle throughout its course. The nerve of supply to the shoulder joint originates from the main nerve in the quadrangular space (Fig. 14-13).

Clinical Picture

Injury to the axillary nerve occurs by a direct contusion or actual severance of nerve fibers in the course of surgical reflection of the deltoid from its attachment to the acromion, the clavicle and the scapular spine. Involvement of the main nerve in the axilla or at the surgical neck of the humerus produces complete paralysis of the deltoid with loss of abduction at the shoulder plus anesthesia of a small patch of skin over the lower half of the deltoid. The first 20° to 30° abduction is initiated by the musculotendinous cuff, chiefly the supraspinatus component. The amount of this range of motion varies with the condition of the rotator cuff muscles. Occasionally, even with complete reaction of degeneration and atrophy of the deltoid, the supraspinatus may hypertrophy in compensation and restore abduction. When the anterior branch is interrupted, the muscle anterior to the point is paralyzed. Partial muscle paralysis is frequently compensated for by hypertrophy of the supraspinatus and the activity of the pectoralis major, especially with the arm above the horizontal plane.

Treatment

Prophylactic treatment consists chiefly of avoiding unnecessary extension of operative incisions and rough handling of the deltoid muscle. When the nerve has been contused, spontaneous regeneration may take place in 4 to 6 months, during which time the deltoid must be relaxed on an abduction frame and light massage and electric stimulation administered. Daily active exercises are done in an attempt to strengthen the cuff muscles. Operative repair of this nerve is exceedingly difficult and frequently impossible. Conservative treatment is advised unless severance of the main large nerve is evident.

Operative exposures of the shoulder should avoid muscle-splitting incisions. If unavoidable, the incision should be confined to the anterior third of the deltoid and not beyond 1½ inches distal to the acromioclavicular joint.[22]

Arthrodesis. Complete deltoid paralysis, when not compensated by other muscle action, requires arthrodesis of the shoulder. The trapezius and the serratus anterior will raise the arm effectively.

Harmon Operation. When the anterior portion of the deltoid is paralyzed, the muscle may be seriously weakened, particularly in forward flexion, and the humeral head may even dislocate or subluxate anteriorly.[45] This condition is remedied by transposing the posterior origin of the functioning muscle to a new anterior position.

FIG. 14-13. Nerve supply to muscles of the upper extremity.

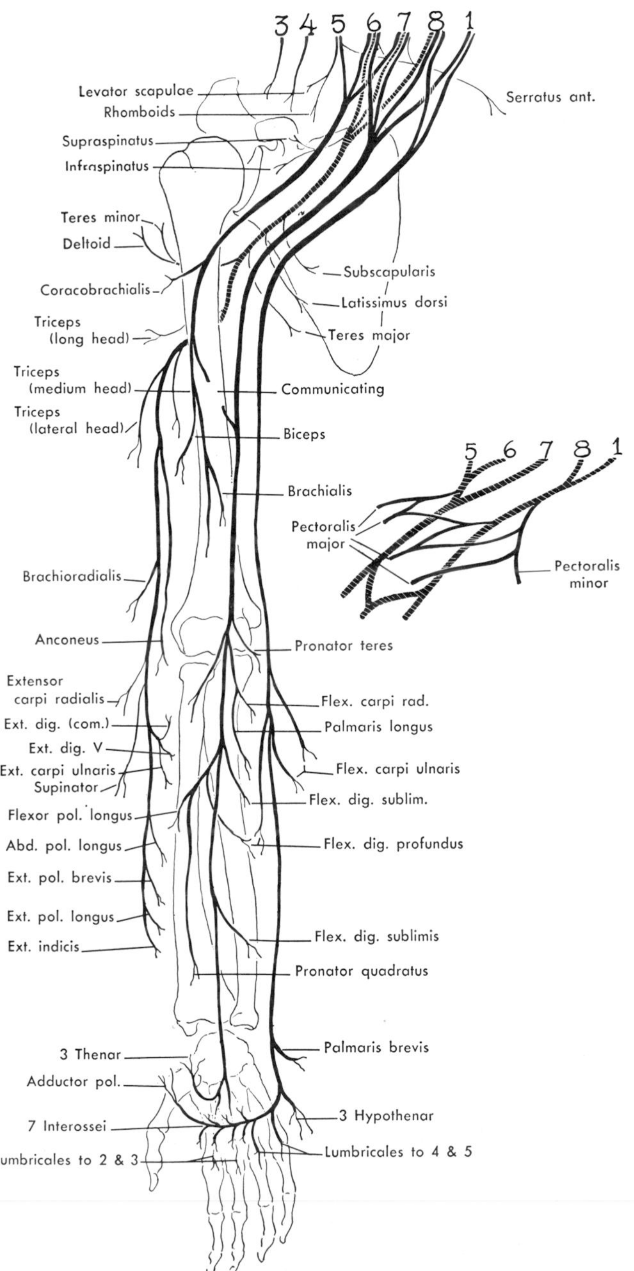

Trapezius Tendon Transplant. The trapezius muscle insertion is transferred by fascia lata strip extensions to the deltoid tubercle.[59] The prerequisite is good power in all scapular muscles, including trapezius, serratus anterior, pectoralis major, rhomboidei, and levator scapulae muscles. The main contraindication is subluxation of the shoulder joint.

Biceps and Triceps Transference. The tendons of the short head of the biceps and the long head of the triceps are fixed to the anterior and the posterior rims of the acromion.

MEDIAN NERVE

Anatomy

The median nerve extends from the junction of the lateral head (from the anterior divisions of the fifth, the sixth, and the seventh cervical nerves) and the medial head (from the eighth cervical and the first thoracic nerves). It enters the axilla lateral to the axillary artery and lies between the musculocutaneous nerve laterally and the ulnar nerve medially. The nerve descends in the arm with the brachial artery and other nerves in a groove just medial to and slightly behind the biceps muscle and gradually crosses over in front of the artery (rarely, it crosses behind) until it lies medial to the artery before it reaches the elbow. The pulsations of the artery can be felt throughout its course in the arm and provide an excellent anatomical landmark for approaches to the nerve.

No branches are given off in the arm, except occasionally when the nerve to the flexors of the forearm has a high origin. At the elbow it lies deep to the bicipital aponeurosis (lacertus fibrosus) and the median cubital vein. It enters the forearm by passing between the larger humeral and the smaller ulnar head of the pronator teres, descending in the medial part of the forearm between the sublimis and the profundus muscles. Above the wrist it is radial to the sublimis and directly beneath the palmaris longus tendon. Then it passes beneath the transverse carpal ligament and after giving off the motor branch to the thenar muscles (opponens, abductor brevis, superficial head of the flexor brevis) it inclines volarward to supply by six terminal branches the thumb, the index, the middle, and the ring fingers. In the hand it lies in a plane superficial to the tendons and deep to the superficial vessels, although its branches to the fingers are volar to the vessels.

The first branches arising from the nerve just above the elbow are those to the humeral head of the pronator teres. Then, below the elbow, branches supply the rest of the pronator teres, the flexor carpi radialis, the palmaris longus, and the flexor digitorum sublimis. At the upper border of the pronator teres a large interosseous branch arises, also penetrates between the pronator heads, supplies the radial portion of the flexor profundus and the flexor pollicis longus, and then descends on the interosseous membrane along with the anterior interosseous artery to end in the pronator quadratus.

In the hand, the median nerve gives off five palmar digital nerves. The first three supply both sides of the thumb and the radial half of the index finger. Each of the other two divide at the clefts distally to supply the opposing halves of the index and the middle fingers and the middle and the ring fingers. Motor branches to the lumbricals of the index and the middle fingers are given off from these digital nerves. (The ulnar nerve supplies the other two lumbricals, all the interossei, the adductor pollicis, and the deep head of the flexor pollicis brevis.) The motor and the sensory distributions of the median and ulnar nerves frequently overlap. Occasionally, even the opponens may be supplied by the ulnar. Normally, the median nerve supplies the palmar surface of the thumb, the index, the middle and the radial half of the ring fingers, and the dorsal surface of the distal thirds of these fingers. The distal ends of the index and middle fingers, volar and dorsal, invariably have no overlap of sensory supply from radial or ulnar nerves, and absence of sensation in this area in median nerve severance is usually complete.

Findings After Median Nerve Injury

Severance above the elbow results in loss of flexion of the thumb, the index finger, and the middle finger; wrist flexion is weak and deviates ulnarward from unopposed action of the flexor carpi ulnaris; pronation is weak or absent; the thumb is in a position at the side of the hand and cannot be brought forward into a position of opposition; the upper forearm and the thenar area lose their normal convexity because of atrophy; loss of sensation is experienced in the volar aspect of thumb, index and middle fingers, and radial half of ring finger. Occasionally, the opponens function may be intact because of anomalous ulnar nerve supply, but this function is generally inadequate in that the thumb cannot be rotated so that its nail is parallel with the palm. The appearance of the hand is similar to the flat hand of the monkey and therefore is called simian hand. Trophic disturbances occur chiefly at the distal end of the index finger, which becomes thin and conical. Injuries of the median nerve above the elbow, in addition to severance by missiles or sharp instruments, may result from the jagged edges of a supracondylar fracture.

Lesions at the wrist occur frequently from accidental cuts by knives or broken dishes or suicide attempts. The nerve may be compressed against the nonyielding transverse carpal ligament by a dislocated semilunar bone or by strongly grasping an object, particularly with the wrist in flexion, whereby the flexor tendons are strongly displaced volarward. Inflammatory synovial swelling, most commonly caused by rheumatoid arthritis or neoplasm, encroaches on the carpal tunnel and constricts the nerve. A lesion at the wrist level is beyond the level of supply to the long flexors of the thumb, the index finger, and the middle finger; the radial carpal flexor; and the pronators. The paralysis affects the short abductor (inability to bring the thumb far forward opposite the index finger), the opponens, the superficial part of the short flexor, and the lumbricals to index and middle fingers. The loss of sensation is the same as in higher lesions.

Partial nerve injury or irritation of the median nerve is the most common cause of *causalgia.* This disorder is characterized by severe burning pain in the extremity, especially the hand, that is aggravated by physical or emotional stimuli. The hand initially may be swollen, red, warm, perspiring, and hyperesthetic. Gradually, the skin becomes thinned, glossy, cold, cyanotic, and dry. The hand is held fixed with the fingers extended and the thumb adducted, and the joints may ankylose in this position. Pain becomes extremely distressing. Keeping the part moist seems to reduce the symptoms temporarily.

Surgical Treatment

Decision should be made as to whether conservative or surgical treatment is to be done. In nerve suture, better results obtain from early intervention. Late suture generally leads to partial restoration, particularly of sensation, and paresthesias. The nerve should be explored and the ends obtained and sutured in exact rotary apposition. Gaps between nerve ends can be overcome in the palm by flexing the metacarpophalangeal joint. Above the wrist the nerve is freed and the wrist is flexed. If the elbow is also flexed and the nerve is gently pulled distally, a 3½-inch gap can be overcome. For larger gaps, it is necessary to dissect the nerve in the upper arm and reroute it superficial to the elbow structures by detaching the humeral head of the pronator teres. A plaster cast maintains flexion of the joints, and very gradual extension is obtained over a period of 1 month. If a graft is needed, the sural nerve may be used. This extensive surgery is justified by the serious disability caused in workers by loss of the important tactile sense in the median nerve area. If opposition is inadequate after nerve suture, the movement may be restored by a pulley operation around the insertion of the flexor carpi ulnaris.

At exploratory operation in causalgic states,[25] the nerve displays a lesion in continuity (*i.e.,* intraneural scarring). Complete division of a nerve rarely causes causalgia. In wartime series, high velocity missiles or bomb splinters were the main causes, with the injury practically always being above the elbow in the case of the median nerve (above the knee in the lower extremities). Treatment consists of sympathectomy, which is preceded by procaine block of the second thoracic ganglion. Complete anhidrosis and increase in warmth of the hand appearing 10 minutes after the block demonstrates effectiveness of the block. Pain is relieved for 1 to 3 hours. A preganglionic sympathectomy is most effective. The white rami communicates to the second and the third thoracic ganglia and the sympathetic trunk below the third are divided.

RADIAL NERVE

Anatomy

The radial nerve is the continuation of the posterior cord that is formed by the posterior divisions of the brachial plexus. In the axilla it lies directly behind the axillary artery and with the other neurovascular structures runs on a floor formed by the subscapularis muscle proximally and the latissimus dorsi and the teres major distally. The axillary (circumflex) nerve, which originates from the posterior cord, descends alongside the radial nerve, then leaves it at the lower border of the subscapularis, where it passes backward through the quadrangular space.

Beyond the teres major, the radial nerve proceeds posterior to the humerus by entering an interval between the long and medial heads of the triceps and reaching the spiral groove between the medial and lateral heads of the muscle. It passes around the back of the humerus to the lateral side, where it pierces the lateral intermuscular septum to reach the anterior aspect of the arm. Here it lies in an interval between the brachialis medially and the brachioradialis and the extensor carpi radialis longus laterally. At this level it gives off branches of supply to the lateral half of the brachialis, to all of the brachioradialis and the extensor carpi radialis longus, and to the posterior interosseous nerve.

It then continues distally in the foream under cover of the brachioradialis until a level about 2 inches above the wrist is reached. Here it pierces the deep fascia and turns laterally and dorsally, crossing superficial to the tendons of the long abductor and the short extensor of the thumb and gaining the dorsum of the hand, where it supplies digital branches of sensation to the dorsum of the thumb, the index finger, the middle finger, and the radial half of the ring finger as far as the middle phalanges. In the spiral groove the radial nerve gives off the posterior cutaneous and the lower lateral cutaneous nerves of the arm, the posterior cutaneous nerve of the forearm, and muscular branches to the triceps and the anconeus.

The posterior interosseous nerve springs from the radial nerve at the level of the lateral epicondyle. It descends under cover of the brachioradialis and gives branches to the extensor carpi radialis brevis and the supinator. Then it penetrates the supinator and passes obliquely around the lateral aspect of the shaft of the radius to reach the back of the forearm and travels distally on the surface of the abductor pollicis longus and under cover of the extensor digitorum. Then it lies on the interosseous membrane under cover of the extensor pollicis longus and proceeds distally to supply the wrist joint. In the back of the forearm it supplies the remainder of the extensor muscles and the abductor pollicis longus. Therefore, it supplies all muscles on the lateral and the dorsal aspects of the forearm except the brachioradialis and the extensor carpi radialis longus, which are supplied directly by the radial nerve.

Clinical Picture

The extent of motor and sensory findings depends on the level of the injury and the degree of trauma. When the radial nerve is interrupted at the axilla where it is usually involved by direct compression, such as by the arm resting over the back of a chair (Saturday night palsy) or by pressure of a crutch (crutch palsy), the extensors of the elbow, the extensors and the supinators of the forearm, the extensors of the wrist, the extensors of the metacarpophalangeal joints of the fingers, and the extensors and the long abductor of the thumb are paralyzed. A strip of the posterior and the posterolateral surface of the arm, the posterior third of the forearm, and an autonomous zone on the dorsum of the hand over the first interosseous space are anesthetic.

The typical picture is one in which the patient holds the extremity at the side, the elbow is slightly flexed, the forearm is pronated, the hand is dropped at the wrist, and the fingers are dropped at the metacarpophalangeal joints. The thumb is turned forward into the palm and interferes with flexion of the fingers. The patient cannot make a fist because the wristdrop tenses the extensors of the fingers and thereby opposes their flexion.

Involvement of the nerve in the spiral groove may be immediate and caused by the sharp jagged edge of a fracture fragment; or it may be delayed by formation of callus about and incarceration of the nerve. An injury to the nerve beyond the spiral groove permits the function of the triceps and the anconeus and preserves sensation at the back of the arm and the forearm. The autonomous area at the back of the hand supplied by the superficial radial nerve is anesthetic.

Injury to the radial nerve in the interval between the brachioradialis and the brachialis involves the brachioradialis and the extensor carpi radialis longus. The brachialis, which has a dual nerve supply, continues to function. The autonomous sensory area of the hand is affected. Gunshot and stab wounds are main offenders at this level. These muscles escape, and hand sensation is preserved when the injury is at the level of the radius, where the posterior interosseous nerve encircles the bone 1 fingerbreadth below the head of the radius. Surgical trauma is the frequent etiologic agent. Beyond this level, the supinator brevis is permitted to function, whereas a wristdrop, a fingerdrop at the metacarpophalangeal joints, and the thumb rolled forward into the palm are the deformities. The thumb extensors and the long abductor gain their branches of supply a little more distally than the extensor digitorum communis and the wrist extensors, so that it is possible to have the thumb alone involved by a properly placed point of trauma.

Missiles and stab wounds produce most nerve injuries in the forearm. When the superficial radial nerve alone is severed, the loss is restricted to sensation in the autonomous zone. This area is the main site of pain when a causalgic state results from incomplete lesions of the superficial radial. Partial paralysis of one or several muscles and hypoesthesia or hyperesthesia rather than anesthesia indicate that the nerve lesion is incomplete and continuity of the nerve is preserved.

Automatic movements at the wrist should not be interpreted as preservation of the wrist extensors. When the fingers are flexed, the extensor tendons are tightened and the hand is drawn backward at the wrist.

Examination of extension of the fingers should be limited to the metacarpophalangeal joints. The lumbrical muscles supplied by the median and the ulnar nerves extend the distal two phalanges at the interphalangeal joints.

By force of gravity, the elbow is extended in spite of triceps paralysis. Examination is performed by keeping the arm horizontal and the forearm dependent and by attempting to extend the elbow actively; or the entire extremity may be supported on a flat surface with the elbow flexed, and active extension is attempted.

Treatment

Regardless of the level or the cause of nerve injury, the affected muscles should be kept in a state of relaxation by supportive splints and their tone maintained by galvanic stimulation and light massage until the nerve regenerates. An anterior molded splint counteracts the wristdrop and should extend beyond the metacarpophalangeal joints to support the proximal phalanges. An additional extension from the splint holds the thumb in complete extension and dorsal abduction.

If paralysis is immediate and complete, the nerve should be explored and sutured promptly. Good results are proportionate to early repair. Nothing is lost by venturing an early exploratory operation and finding the nerve intact.

Gaps between nerve ends may be overcome by flexing the elbow, by externally rotating and adducting the arm and by freeing various branches. If the distance is extensive, occasionally the nerve may be transposed anteriorly. Shortening of the humerus is sometimes justified to aid approximation.

Compression injuries, no matter how extensively the muscle is involved, are generally temporary, and almost complete restoration of function is the rule. Various texts also include in this category radial nerve injuries due to fractures at the middle third of the humerus. However, the possibility of complete nerve tears and their serious implications certainly warrant operative exposure of the fracture site, whereupon both nerve and bone injuries can be dealt with at the same time.

Electrodiagnostic studies of nerve conduction and muscle response correlated with the results of the neurologic examination should clearly define whether surgical or conservative measures should be undertaken. Following complete severance of a nerve, the nerve conduction velocity begins to slow after 2 or 3 days and is maximal at 2 weeks. Therefore, within 48 to 72 hours, eliciting this finding justifies surgical exploration. On the other hand, if no conduction impairment develops by 1 week, nerve interruption is physiological (apraxia) rather than anatomical, and a nonsurgical regimen is pursued. During the ensuing weeks, physical therapy measures include electrical stimulation, heat and massage to maintain muscle tone, splinting to relax affected muscles, and range of motion exercises while awaiting spontaneous recovery. At the same time, serial strength-duration studies afford excellent objective evidence of recovery long before actual clinical response is noted. If muscle response to electrical stimulation does not improve after 6 weeks, exploration of the nerve is indicated.

When a causalgic state arises in the distribution of the radial nerve, an incomplete nerve lesion should be suspected, the nerve explored, and the pathologic process dealt with. A neuroma should be resected, if necessary, by removal of a portion of the nerve, followed by reapproximation, or adhesions may be freed and the nerve surrounded by fatty tissue or paratenon or imbedded in adjacent muscle. The Tinel sign may reveal the exact site of initiation of pain impulses.

Prognosis

The prognosis in radial nerve repair is usually very good. However, failure of some portion to regenerate necessitates tendon transplantation. Triceps paralysis needs no compensation other than that provided by gravity. Extension at the elbow is rarely ever required. Such an instance is the need for use of crutches, whereupon the brachioradialis or latissimus dorsi transferred to the triceps tendon and olecranon will provide satisfactory elbow extensor power.

Supination of the forearm may be restored by osteotomy of the radius and by rotating the distal fragment. The Tubby operation transplants the insertion of the pronator teres from the volar to the dorsal aspects of the radius. Extension of the thumb, and particularly abduction (which stabilizes the digit at the carpometacarpal joint), is necessary for proper apposition of the thumb to the fingers in the functions of pinch and grasp. The flexor carpi radialis may be transplanted to the long abductor and both extensors. The flexor carpi ulnaris is transferred to the finger extensors.

If no tendons are available for transference, dorsiflexion of the wrist is provided either by arthrodesis of the wrist or by severing the tendons of the extensor cummunis and tenodesing the proximal ends of the distal segments to the dorsum of the radius. Active flexion at the metacarpophalangeal joints thereby tightens these tenodesed tendons and automatically dorsiflexes the wrist. The carpometacarpal joint of the thumb may also be stabilized by arthrodesis.

ULNAR NERVE

Anatomy

The ulnar nerve is the largest branch of the medial cord of the brachial plexus, arising under cover of the pectoralis minor and descending along the medial side of the axillary artery and the proximal half of the brachial artery. At the level of insertion of the coracobrachialis at the middle of the humerus, it leaves the brachial artery and, in company with the ulnar collateral artery, it passes backward through the medial intermuscular septum to the posterior aspect of the arm. Then it descends along the medial head of the triceps to the back of the medial epicondyle and passes between the heads of the flexor carpi ulnaris to enter the forearm. There, under cover of the flexor carpi ulnaris (which it supplies), it lies on the flexor digitorum profundus (supplies its medial half) and is immediately lateral to the ulnar artery.[35]

Near the pisiform bone it emerges through the deep fascia lateral to the flexor carpi ulnaris and descends anterior to the flexor retinaculum, where it divides into superficial and deep branches. The deep branch passes medial to the hook of the hamate and, with the deep branch of the ulnar artery, enters the interval between the abductor and the flexor of the little finger to gain the deep area of the palm. It gives off branches of supply to the hypothenar muscles, then turns laterally across the palm deep to the flexor tendons, giving off three branches, each of which runs distally in front of the interosseous space, supplying the interosseous muscles. The medial two branches also supply the medial two lumbrical muscles. At the lateral side of the palm, the main deep branch of the ulnar nerve ends by breaking up into nerves of supply to the adductor pollicis and the first dorsal interosseous muscle. The superficial branch of the ulnar nerve runs under the palmaris brevis, which it supplies, and then divides into two digital branches, which provide sensation to the palmar aspect of the little finger and the ulnar half of the ring finger.

The dorsal branch of the ulnar nerve arises from the latter at the middle of the forearm and descends with the parent nerve to the carpus, where it becomes superficial and inclines backward to gain the dorsum of the hand. Here it divides into two dorsal digital nerves, which supply the skin of the medial third of the back of the hand and the little finger and the ulnar half of the ring finger as far as the second phalanx.

Clinical Picture

When the flexor carpi ulnaris is paralyzed (on attempting flexion at the wrist, the hand deviates radialward), interruption of the ulnar nerve has occurred above the elbow. Preservation of this muscle's function places the lesion distal to the elbow. Otherwise, ulnar nerve paralysis is typified by the following: the ring and little fingers are extended at the metacarpophalangeal joints and flexed at the proximal interphalangeal joints, because of loss of lumbrical action. When the lesion is sufficiently low in the forearm, the flexor profundus is spared and, unopposed by the intrinsics, exerts strong flexion on the distal phalanges; clawing of the ring and little fingers is pronounced.

When the flexor carpi ulnaris and the ulnar portion of the flexor profundus are paralyzed by a high lesion, the ensuing atrophy over the ulnar aspect of the forearm is very apparent. In this instance, flexor power to the distal phalanges of the ring and little fingers is lost. This is demonstrated best by placing the hand palm down when the inability of the little finger to scratch the surface of the table is evident. The hypothenar eminence is thinned, and the hollowing of the interosseous spaces attests to atrophy of the paralyzed interossei, the thumb adductors, the inner head of the flexor pollicis brevis, the hypothenars, and the two lumbricals on the ulnar side. Abduction and adduction of the fingers is lost to a great extent. The index and the middle fingers may still abduct because their lumbrical innervation through the median nerve is still intact.

Pinch between the thumb and the index finger normally depends on the ability to stabilize the metacarpophalangeal joint in flexion (adductors and flexor brevis) so that such action is strong and the apposed fingers form the letter O. In ulnar paralysis, the proximal phalanx becomes hyperextended, the interphalangeal joint of the thumb hyperflexes, and the pinch is weak. Failure of stabilization at the carpometacarpal joint by the abductor pollicis longus will likewise interfere with pinch. Loss of thumb adductors is demonstrated by inability of the thumb to scrape across the distal palm. Instead, it comes forward into the opposed position. Another test is failure to resist attempts to extract a sheet of paper held between the apposed sides of the thumb and index finger. On the volar aspect, sensation is lost over the ulnar portion of the hand and all of the little finger and the ulnar half of the ring finger. On the dorsum, the entire little finger, the ring finger, the ulnar half of the long finger, and the ulnar third of the hand are involved. However, because of overlap from adjacent nerves, loss of sensation is variable; the distal two thirds of the little finger are independent and invariably involved.

Trophic changes in the ring and little fingers reflect the loss of sensory innervation. Very frequently innervation from the median nerve preserves function of the intrinsics and the thumb adductors. Fibers innervating these muscles may proceed distally in the median nerve to the distal third of the forearm and by a connecting branch enter the ulnar nerve before the latter reaches the hand. In such an instance, a high ulnar lesion fails to eliminate intrinsic action.

Treatment

Repair of the ulnar nerve should be done with care. The nerve contains both motor and sensory fibers, and accurate coaptation will prevent sensory fibers from growing down motor pathways, and vice versa. Gaps are overcome by flexing the wrist and the elbow. The nerve at the elbow may be transposed anteriorly, and branches are freed, thereby permitting mobilization distally. Recovery of function requires more than a year and occurs in the following order: forearm muscles, sensation, hypothenar muscles, interossei, and thumb adductors. During this long recovery period, the hand is splinted with the metacarpophalangeal joints in flexion and the interphalangeal joints in extension to keep the paralyzed muscles in a relaxed state and prevent joint contractures. A stretched muscle will become fibrotic and void the result of nerve suture.

When ulnar nerve paralysis is permanent, tendon transplantation is the treatment of choice. Necessary prerequisites are mobile joints and good muscles for transfer.

Surgical Repair of Clawed Fingers. A clawhand deformity is due to intrinsic muscle paralysis while the long extensors and the long flexors are still functioning.[69] The loss of flexor power on the proximal phalanges allows the extensors to pull the proximal phalanges into hyperextension; tension on the long flexors pulls the distal phalanges into flexion, unopposed by the lost extension of the intrinsics.

Extension of the distal two phalanges takes place synergistically by the long extensors and the intrinsics (Fowler). The action of the long extensors is lost when the proximal phalanx is hyperextended. Any procedure that prevents hyperextension of the proximal phalanx preserves extension of the distal two phalanges and eliminates the claw deformity. The following procedures are the most commonly used:

Bunnell technique. This operation transplants multiple slips of sublimis tendons through the lumbrical canals into the aponeurotic expansion. This procedure is not effective in clawhand of long standing in which the patient has developed the habit of flexing the wrist to extend the distal phalanges automatically, thereby rendering the sublimis impotent.

Fowler technique. This procedure splits the extensor indicis proprius and the extensor digiti quinti into two strands each; next, each individual slip is passed through the interosseous space anterior to the transverse metacarpal ligament and inserted into the aponeurosis.

Riordan technique. This is a tenodesis procedure. Half of the extensor carpi radialis longus and the extensor carpi ulnaris is separated from the parent tendon and left attached to the insertion into the base of the second and the fifth metacarpals, respectively. Each half is split longitudinally into two slips, and then each slip is passed and attached as in the Fowler operation. The tendon should be under tension at the conclusion of the operation so as to obtain restriction of extension.

Postoperatively, the hand is immobilized in a pressure dressing, maintaining the wrist in dorsiflexion, the metacarpophalangeal joints in flexion, and the distal two joints in extension. Tendon transplantation is unsuitable in deformity with skin and joint contractures. These require joint arthrodeses.

Restoration of Thumb Adduction and Carpal and Metacarpal Arches. When grasping small round objects, the hand cups into an arch and enables the fingers to converge during flexion; thus strength of grasp is obtained. These arches are produced mainly by the thenar and hypothenar muscles. They are reduced considerably in ulnar paralysis and are completely flattened in combined median and ulnar paralysis. It is essential to restore the functions of pinch and grasp.

Tendon Loop Operation. The tendon of the extensor communis to the index finger is removed just before its insertion and is prolonged by a tendon graft around the ulnar border of the hand, placed volar to the hypothenars and beneath the finger flexors and inserted into the ulnar side of the base of the proximal phalanx of the thumb. The distal remaining stump of the tendon is attached to the extensor indicis to avoid adduction and rotation deformity of the index finger. This procedure restores only adduction and is suitable only in pure ulnar paralysis.

Tendon T Operation. This procedure provides strong adduction to both thumb and index fingers and re-forms the carpal and the metacarpal arches. A tendon graft is placed transversely across the palm beneath the flexor tendons and is attached to the neck of the fifth metacarpal and the ulnar side of the base of the proximal phalanx of the thumb. To its center is attached a motor tendon, usually one of the sublimis tendons. Contraction of the motor tendon pulls on the cross member and apposes the thumb and the index finger. This procedure is done when median nerve paralysis is associated with ulnar involvement and it is necessary to correct thumb opposition also. (See also Chapter 25.)

Compression of the Ulnar Nerve at the Elbow

Also known as traumatic ulnar neuritis, tardy ulnar nerve palsy, and ulnar neuropathy at the elbow, injury to the ulnar nerve at the elbow may occur by diverse means:

Chronic repetitive blunt trauma. The ulnar nerve courses superficially within the postcondylar groove between the olecranon and the medial epicondyle of the humerus. Here it is vulnerable to a single, severe direct blow or to repeated external pressures, such as sustained under occupational conditions.

Post fracture. The nerve is held firmly within the groove against the subjacent bone by firm dense fascia. Roughening of the bone resulting from a fracture imposes frictional forces against the gliding nerve.

Cubitus valgus deformity (Fig. 14-14). The nerve is supposedly stretched over the medial prominence at the elbow. The deformity may be congenital and associated with anterior dislocation of the radial head, retarded growth of the lateral portion of the lower humeral physis following trauma or infection, or malunion of fracture.

Arthritis of elbow joint. Osteoarthritis may produce irregularities of the postcondylar groove or may compress the nerve by a prominent osteophyte or protruding ganglion. Rheumatoid synovium may penetrate the medial capsule and compress the nerve.[67]

Recurrent subluxation or dislocation of nerve. When the fascial covering of the ulnar groove is thin and lax, the ulnar nerve moves out of its groove onto the tip of the medial epicondyle when the elbow is completely flexed, returning to its normal location

FIG. 14-14. Cubitus valgus, the result of malunion of fracture at the lower end of the humerus. Degenerative arthritis has supervened. Stretching of the ulnar nerve over the medial prominence is a common sequel.

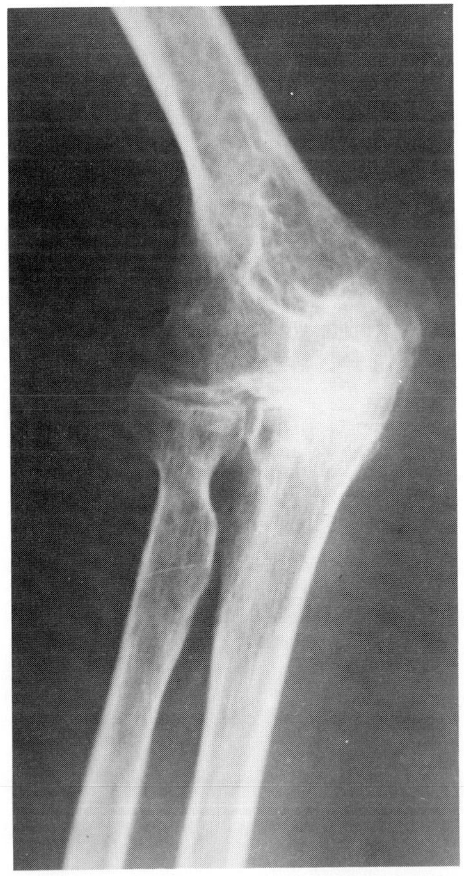

when the elbow is extended.[34] Repetitive subluxations of this nerve normally occur in approximately 16% of the population, are generally asymptomatic, but may be the underlying factor that produces symptoms when trauma is superadded.

Acute trauma, infection. Severe direct trauma of neighboring infection may produce scarring, which can incarcerate the ulnar nerve.

Muscle compression. Compression by an accessory muscle, the anconeus epitrochlearis, which bridges the groove, is said to cause compression of the nerve.[56]

Idiopathic. It is not unusual to fail to detect the cause of the neuropathy on surgical exploration.

Pathophysiology. About 2 cm distal to the medial epicondyle, an aponeurotic arch (arcade) passes between the two heads of origin of the flexor carpi ulnaris, one firmly attached to the medial epicondyle and the other loosely attached to the olecranon, with the aponeurotic arch forming the roof of the "cubital tunnel" (Fig. 14-15).[64,65] The floor of the tunnel is formed by the medial capsule of the elbow. During flexion of the elbow, the space of the tunnel through which the ulnar nerve courses is diminished by tightening of the aponeurotic arch and by outward bulging of the capsule. Narrowing the caliber of the cubital tunnel, especially while the ulnar nerve is placed under tension, compresses and damages the nerve. The intraneural pressure is increased threefold when the elbow is flexed while the wrist is extended; by abducting and externally rotating the arm (*e.g.*, as when placing the hand behind the head), intraneural pressure increases to six times that of the relaxed nerve.[66] Such pressures are well above the normal nerve's interstitial perfusion pressure and are capable of damaging the nerve. Additional sites of nerve compression have been described, such as a band distal to the edge of the aponeurotic arch[39] and another proximal to it.[48]

FIG. 14-15. The cubital-tunnel syndrome, demonstrating the mechanism of compression of the ulnar nerve by the arcuate ligament. (*Left*) The arcuate ligament extending between the two heads of origin of the flexor carpi ulnaris and forming the roof of the tunnel is slack when the elbow is fully extended. (*Right*) When the elbow is flexed, the aponeurotic covering becomes taut, the medial capsule bulges outward, and the ulnar nerve is compressed. (Wadsworth TG: The Elbow. Edinburgh, Churchill Livingstone, 1982)

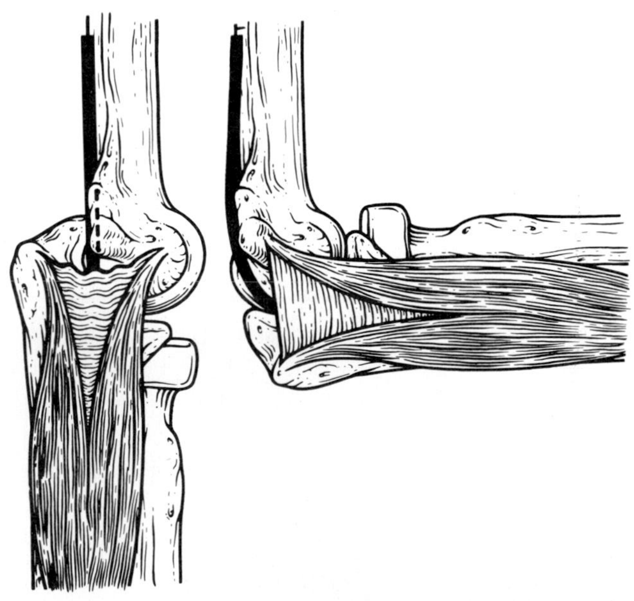

The aponeurotic arch, also known as the arcuate ligament, is slack in extension and tightened up on flexion,[80] when it compresses the underlying nerve. When the aponeurotic band is divided, the underlying nerve is often found to be flattened, and proximally it presents a fusiform enlargement.[80,82]

Normally, the ulnar nerve elongates by approximately 5 mm at the postcondylar groove during flexion, and it glides freely in the groove. Encroachment on the groove or the cubital tunnel (*e.g.*, by an osteophyte or synovial protrusion) will produce friction, pressure, and tension, which compromises intraneural vascularity and results in edema and ultimate scarring.[85] Once intraneural fibrosis is established, the neurophysiology is permanently altered. Consequently, long-delayed surgical correction is less likely to relieve symptoms.

The symptoms resulting from external neural compression are highly variable, ranging from subjective dysesthesias to a combination of a sensory and motor deficit in the area of distribution of the ulnar nerve. The flexor carpi ulnaris and the ulnar half of the flexor digitorum profundus muscle are usually spared.[82] This may be explained by the fact that the nerve fibers to these muscles are deeply situated within the ulnar nerve at the elbow and are generally unaffected by external compression.[80]

Clinical Picture. The history often discloses a predisposing factor, such as a cubitus valgus deformity, severe direct trauma to the superficially located nerve, or repetitive trauma to the ulnar groove.

Symptoms are related to the severity of involvement. Minimal nerve irritation causes subjective dysesthesias in the ulnar distribution and perhaps a sensation of clumsiness of the hand.

Moderate involvement produces pronounced subjective pain and paresthesias and definite objective findings such as interosseous weakness and atrophy. The flexor carpi ulnaris and the flexor profundus to the distal phalanges of the little and ring fingers are rarely affected. The nerve may be tender and palpably enlarged at the postcondylar groove.

Severe nerve lesions are rare. The interossei are very weak and atrophied, and the flexor carpi ulnaris and ulnar half of the flexor profundus are partially weakened. Sensory loss varies from marked hypoesthesia to anesthesia in the ulnar distribution of the hand, both over the volar and dorsal aspects. Sweating in this area is reduced, although hyperhydrosis is not infrequent.

The cubital tunnel syndrome, which is produced by compression of the ulnar nerve by the arcuate ligament, is characterized by symptoms provoked by prolonged flexion attitudes of the elbow, such as during sleep, and improved by extension positioning of the elbow. Sometimes the symptoms can be elicited by acutely flexing the elbow for about 5 minutes (elbow flexion test).[82]

Recurrent ulnar nerve subluxations at the elbow may be a cause of ulnar neuritis.[34] Such repetitive displacements occur frequently in the general population and are usually asymptomatic unless trauma is superimposed. The fascial roof over the postcondylar groove is lax, permitting the nerve to slip out and forward over the epicondyle when the elbow is flexed and to return when the elbow is extended. Complete anterior displacement is exceptional. The condition is nearly always bilateral. The enlarged tender nerve can be felt to slip beneath the examining finger during flexion and extension of the elbow. A symptomatic nerve is usually tender, and the chief complaints are referable to the hand.

Diagnosis. Traumatic ulnar neuritis at the elbow must be differentiated chiefly from ulnar nerve compression at the wrist. The exact distribution of sensory changes is of great diagnostic significance. The dorsal cutaneous branch of the ulnar nerve leaves the parent nerve beyond the elbow. Consequently, sensory impairment in the dorsal ulnar aspect of the hand localizes the lesion proximally. Contrariwise, absence of this finding does not necessarily implicate the ulnar nerve at the wrist, because the nerve may be only partially involved at the elbow.

Electrodiagnostic studies will reveal slowing of conduction of the ulnar nerve at the elbow.[43] Similar studies will establish whether the nerve is involved proximally (*e.g.*, at the thoracic outlet) or distally at the wrist.

Preoperatively, it is important to determine the presence of a compressive bone lesion about the ulnar groove. In addition to routine roentgenograms of the elbow, a special view is taken to outline the groove (Fig. 14-16). The externally rotated arm is placed against the cassette while the elbow is acutely flexed, and the central x-ray beam is directed vertically.[82]

Prognosis. The prognosis depends largely on the degree of nerve involvement and on the time interval between the onset of symptoms and the surgical intervention.[57,60,74] If the nerve is minimally affected with no detectable muscle weakness, transposition of the nerve,

FIG. 14-16. The cubital-tunnel syndrome. (*Left*) Roentgenogram taken with the humerus flat on the plate, the elbow fully flexed, and the humerus externally rotated; the tube was centered 1 inch distal to the point of the elbow and overlying the olecranon. (*Right*) Operative findings. (*a*, ulnar nerve; *b*, arcuate ligament; *c*, medial epicondyle; *d*, olecranon) (Wadsworth TG: The Elbow. Edinburgh, Churchill Livingstone, 1982)

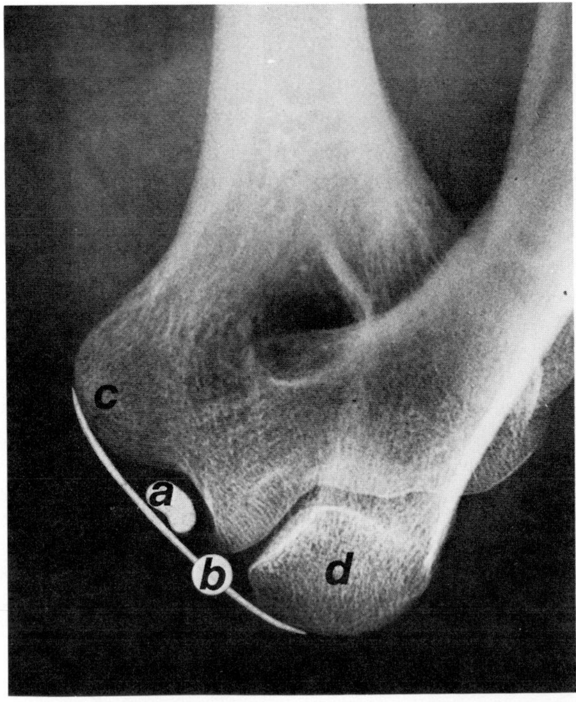

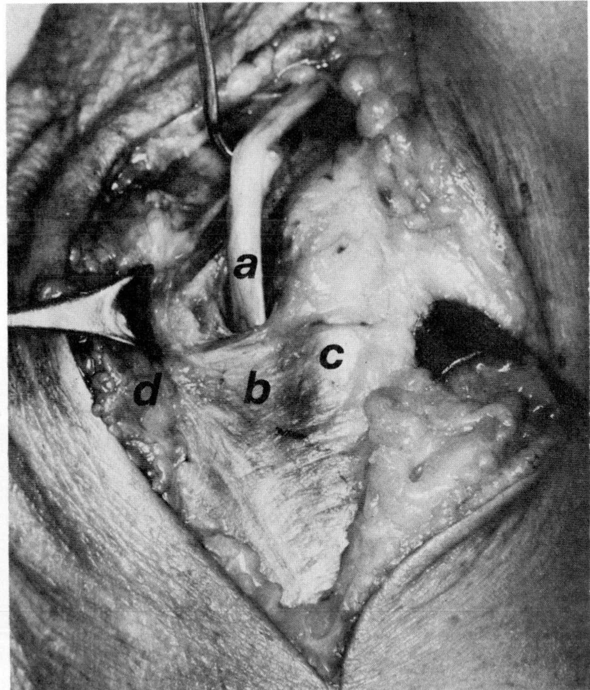

if properly performed, leads to almost immediate relief of local discomfort and peripheral paresthesias. With moderate sensory and motor impairment, following surgery the hand becomes stronger, but variable weakness and sensory impairment persist in some. When there is advanced paralysis of ulnar innervated muscles, anterior transposition will result in partial recovery of motor power in some, but sensory recovery is better; normal function is never regained.

Long duration of symptoms prior to surgery carries an adverse prognosis. Within a few months, recovery is fairly good, regardless of whether anterior transposition or an aponeurotic release is done. After 1 year, only about one fourth of patients will achieve a satisfactory recovery after anterior transposition and improvement after simple aponeurotic release is poor.[46]

Muscle power may continue to improve over 6 months to a year, the long flexor muscles recovering more completely than the intrinsic muscles. A variable sensory deficit often persists. Complete recovery is rarely attained if the course exceeds 3 months, and the chance for any recovery is poor when symptoms have existed for 1 year. Nevertheless, persistence of symptoms after operation is a definite indication for reexploration of the nerve.

Treatment. While it is possible for minimal involvement of the ulnar nerve to spontaneously recover, the hazards of prolonged watchful expectancy dictate that immediate surgical decompression must be done as soon as the diagnosis is established. The nerve must be transposed anteriorly, where its course is shorter. Sites of potential kinking should receive appropriate attention. The medial intermuscular septum extending proximally from the epicondyle must be adequately resected. The aponeurotic band extending between the heads of origin of the flexor carpi ulnaris is released. Care is required to ensure that the nerve is not kinked where it dips down between the flexor carpi ulnaris and the flexor digitorum superficialis. The nerve should not be laid into a groove cut in the muscle, because the scarring and intermuscular septa become adherent to the nerve. The origin of the common flexor-pronator tendon should be elevated, the nerve placed beneath the muscle mass, and the tendon origin restored.

Occasionally, it may be possible to remove a locally compressing lesion such as a ganglion or osteophyte without the need for anterior transposition.

Technique. The nerve is lifted out of its groove by incising the fascial roof, and it is dissected distally to partially free its branches entering the muscle. By freeing each branch proximally from the parent trunk, the nerve is more easily mobilized. Then a large segment of the medial intermuscular septum extending proximally from the medial epicondyle is removed. The epicondylar attachment of the common flexor-pronator tendon is removed and reflected distally, and the aponeurosis extending between the two heads of the flexor carpi ulnaris is incised. The ulnar nerve is then brought anteriorly and placed alongside the median nerve; it is then rerouted deep to the flexor-pronator muscle mass whose tendon is then resutured to the epicondyle. Postoperatively, the elbow is immobilized in 90° of flexion, with the forearm fully pronated and the wrist slightly flexed. The cast is removed at 3 weeks.[32,55,57,74]

An alternative procedure consists of releasing the aponeurotic arch of the flexor carpi ulnaris with local neurolysis. The aponeurosis may be resutured deep to the nerve.[64] This operation is suitable only when the findings at operation point to definite nerve compression at this site, especially when the floor of the cubital tunnel is compromised by an osteophyte, cyst, or synovial rheumatoid extension, for example. This is a limited procedure that is applicable only when symptoms are of recent origin.

Ulnar Nerve Compression at the Wrist

At the level of the wrist, the ulnar nerve courses through a tunnel anterior to the flexor retinaculum just lateral to the pisiform bone, then divides into a superficial (mainly sensory) branch and a deep branch as it proceeds distally beneath a fascial roof that bridges the interval between the pisiform and the hook of the hamate. The floor of the narrow canal is formed by the ligaments between pisiform, triquetrum, and hamate. Because of the limited diameter of this tunnel, the ulnar nerve is vulnerable to lesions that encroach on the canal (*e.g.*, osteoarthritic osteophyte, ganglion, rheumatoid pannus). When the nerve is compressed at a site proximal to the point of bifurcation, both sensory and intrinsic muscle deficits result. Since the dorsal branch of the ulnar nerve leaves the ulnar nerve proximal to the wrist, sensation to the medial third of the back of the hand and the entire dorsal surface of the little finger and ulnar half of the ring finger as far as the second phalanges is preserved. When nerve compression takes place within the tunnel distal to the point of branching, only the deep branch is affected; the hypothenar muscles are often spared, and the ulnar intrinsic muscles are denervated. Of diagnostic importance, the function of the flexor profundus to the little and ring fingers and of the flexor carpi ulnaris is unaffected. The patient is still capable of scratching the surface of the table with the little and ring fingers.

Anatomy. The ulnar artery and nerve enter the hand by passing through a triangular space (Guyon's canal), which is bordered medially and proximally by the flexor carpi ulnaris tendon and pisiform bone, anteriorly by the thin volar carpal ligament blended with the tendinous insertion of the flexor carpi ulnaris, and posteriorly by the transverse carpal ligament overlying the pisotriquetral articulation (Figs. 14-17)[75,80] Distal to Guyon's canal, under cover of the palmaris brevis muscle, the nerve divides into superficial and deep branches. The superficial branch supplies the overlying muscle and passes through

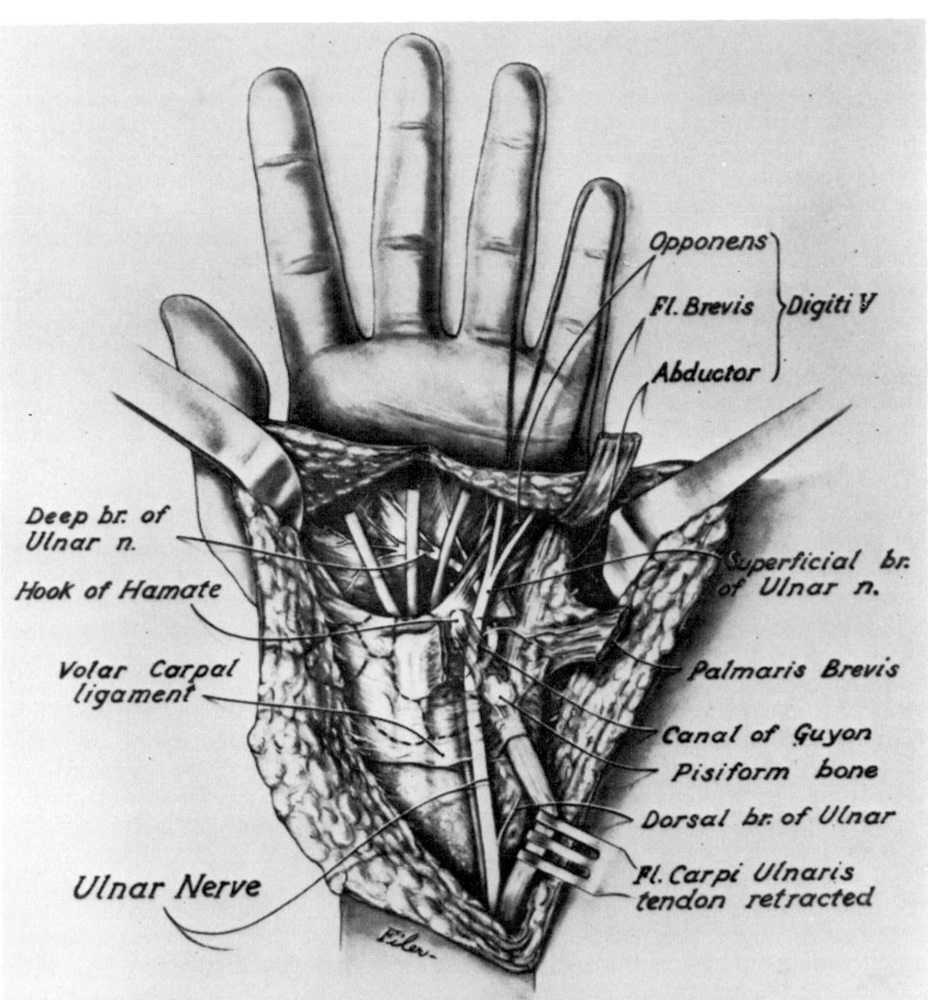

FIG. 14-17. Anatomical relationships of the ulnar nerve at the wrist and hand. Note that the nerve branches beneath the thin fascial covering that bridges the interval between the pisiform and hamate bones. (Shea JD: Ulnar nerve compression syndromes at and below the wrist. J Bone Joint Surg 51A:1095, 1969)

a fat pad; it then courses distally and subcutaneously to provide sensory innervation to the ulnar side of the palm and the volar aspect of the little and ulnar half of the ring fingers, extending onto the dorsum of these fingers over the distal phalanges.

The deep palmar branch passes lateral to the pisiform, then medial to the hook of the hamate, where it makes an abrupt turn as it dips deeply between the origins of the abductor and flexor of the little finger; it is accompanied by a deep branch of the ulnar artery. It enters a narrow fibro-osseous tunnel that is bounded proximally by the pisohamate ligament. Before it passes into this extremely narrow tunnel, the deep palmar branch supplies the motor nerve to the hypothenar muscles; then it passes through the opponens and turns laterally under cover of the deep flexor tendons along the line of the deep palmar arch and supplies branches to the following muscles: interossei, third and fourth lumbricals, adductor pollicis, and deep part of the flexor pollicis brevis (32% of the time[81])[71]. Although there are numerous variations of the motor supply between median and ulnar nerves, the adductor pollicis is almost invariably supplied by the ulnar nerve. As the deep branch passes across the palm, it lies in close relationship to the proximal end of the metacarpals, providing a hard surface against which the nerve may be compressed.[71]

Within Guyon's canal, the ulnar nerve lies on the medial side, the ulnar artery is on the lateral side, and the remainder of the space is occupied by fat globules.[44] Here the nerve is subject to compression within a confined space, but compression is more likely as the nerve passes through the distal narrow, relatively rigid fibro-osseous canal between the origins of the small muscles to the little finger and the pisohamate ligament. Beyond this point, as the nerve courses deep in the palm, the nerve is most often damaged by a penetrating injury.

The intraneural arrangement of the nerve bundles within the ulnar nerve at the proximal level of the wrist is such that the motor fibers to the intrinsic muscles are located posteriorly and the sensory fibers are found anteriorly. Theoretically, if compression against the posterior aspect of the nerve occurs, motor weakness should prevail over sensory loss. However, this is not borne out clinically, because both motor and sensory deficits develop concomitantly when the ulnar nerve is injured proximal to the point of bifurcation. Because the dorsal cutaneous branch leaves the main nerve 6 cm to 8 cm proximal to the wrist, an injury beyond this level spares the dorsal ulnar distribution.

Pathology. Ganglia produce the largest number of compressive lesions at the wrist.[30,68,73] These lesions may arise proximally near the radioulnar or pisotriquetral joint or distally from the triquetrohamate or pisohamate joint deeply within the palm. Osteoarthritis is frequently the underlying condition,[53] which gives rise to the ganglion, an extruded osteophyte, or a loose ossicle.[80] Often a history is obtained of blunt trauma to the base of the hypothenar eminence, perhaps sustained by a single severe blow from using the hand as a hammer or by a fall on the outstretched hand, or of repetitive trauma, such as occurs in an occupation requiring the use of a vibrating tool or a pneumatic hammer.[24,50] The pisiform appear to sustain the brunt of the injury, and frequently osteoarthritic changes develop at the pisotriquetral joint.

Scarring may develop weeks to months after an injury about the hypothenar eminence, with the cicatrix enveloping and incarcerating both the ulnar nerve and ulnar artery within Guyon's canal.[37,40,49] At operation, edematous fibrous tissue and thrombosed vessels are found. They appear to constrict the nerve, and, provided that the collateral circulation is adequate, resection of scar tissue and the affected segment of ulnar artery and freeing the nerve will relieve neurologic symptoms.[80]

The ulnar artery, because of its superficial location in close relationship to the pisiform and hamate, is vulnerable to injury. A single or repetitive blunt trauma may damage the intima, resulting in thrombosis; the trauma may be severe enough to disrupt the elastic fibers and smooth muscle of the media, resulting in a progressively enlarging fusiform aneurysmal dilatation, the true aneurysm; or a penetrating injury may partially section the artery, producing a localized hemorrhagic mass whose interior becomes recanalized, developing a cystic, bulbous false aneurysm whose cavity communicates with the lumen of the artery (Fig. 14-18).

Regardless of whether the ulnar artery is thrombosed, forms an aneurysmal dilatation, or is affected by disease, (*i.e.*, arteritis, thromboangiitis), ulnar neuritis invariably is associated, whether by direct compression or by irritation. The majority of cases produce paresthesias, sometimes objective sensory loss, but rarely involvement of the deep branch of the ulnar nerve. The neurapraxia responds to resection of the involved segment of artery.[33,37,52,54,78] Rarely, an aneurysm of the hand may form as a result of atheromatous occlusion of a main artery and represents a poststenotic dilatation.[79]

A neuroma may form immediately proximal to the site where the deep branch of the ulnar nerve dives deeply into the palm through the tight tunnel beneath the hook of the hamate.

Many rare causes of involvement of the ulnar nerve at the wrist and hand have been described.[75] It should be emphasized that severe trauma to the base of the hand may cause fracture of a carpal bone, such as the hamate,[49] pisiform, or triquetrum, lying in the path of the nerve, and may be easily overlooked unless diligently sought for.

Clinical Picture. The symptoms and findings are dependent on the site and degree of injury.[28,31] The lesions fall into two anatomically related patterns: (1) a lesion situated proximal to the pisohamate ligament that causes both sensory and motor involvement and (2) a lesion arising deeply in the palm distal to the pisohamate ligament that affects the interossei and ulnar lumbricals

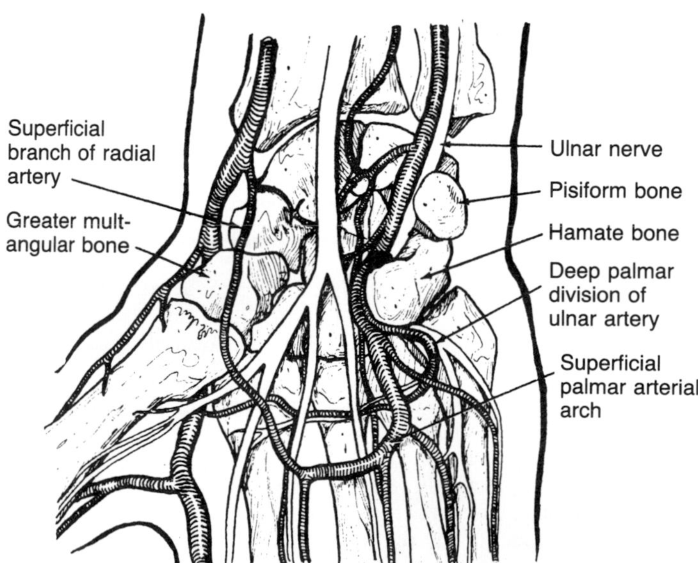

FIG. 14-18. The superficial arterial arch of the hand demonstrating the two sites most vulnerable to injury. One site is the hypothenar eminence adjacent to the hamate bone, and the other site is on the thenar eminence where the greater multangular lies beneath the superficial branch of the radial artery. Neither site has the protection of the palmar aponeurosis. These are the most common locations for the development of traumatic palmar aneurysms. Note that the ulnar component is relatively fixed beneath the hook of the hamate by its deep arterial branch. The superficial radial artery is held to a definite course over the greater multangular by its passage between the abductor brevis and opponens muscles. The artery is damaged by compression between the overlying force and the underlying bony anvil. (Smith JW: True aneurysms of traumatic origin in the palm. Am J Surg 104:7, 1962)

but spares the hypothenar muscles and volar ulnar sensation.

Compression at the level of Guyon's canal presents the following features:

The compressive tissue is sometimes palpable (*e.g.*, ganglion, rheumatoid pannus, bone fragment).
Sensory loss occurs over volar ulnar distribution but spares the dorsal area except over the distal phalanges.
Motor involvement affects the hypothenar, ulnar two lumbricals, and interossei.
Clawing of the little and ring fingers is seen.

A compressive lesion that exerts pressure only on the deep branch as it passes through the narrow tunnel between the origins of the flexor and abductor digiti minimi enroute to the deeper layers of the palm produces a purely motor weakness of the interossei but spares the hypothenar muscles. An abducted attitude of the little finger results from the unopposed action of the abductor to the finger. The sensory nerve is spared. Clawing of the little and ring fingers sometimes occurs. The compressive lesion, often a ganglion, is seldom palpable and usually is first encountered at operation. In general the development of the compressive lesion and its effects take place silently (*i.e.*, without pain).

A frequent predisposing condition is osteoarthritis of the wrist. Precipitating injuries are encountered in certain occupations (*e.g.*, repetitive pressures of a pneumatic tool, or frictional forces over the base of the hand, such as in motorcycling). A tender callus at the base of the palm about the pisiform suggests an external traumatic cause.[24]

A penetrating injury within the palm is self-incriminating.[28] Only motor structures beyond the point of nerve interruption are affected. The adductor pollicis and the first dorsal interosseous are muscles supplied by the terminal branches of the deep branch of the ulnar nerve.

When osteoarthritis of the pisotriquetral joint is the source of compression, the clinical features are usually provoked by direct trauma such as a fall on the outstretched hand. They include pain and tenderness over the pisiform, and crepitus and pain elicited by passively moving the pisiform from side to side. Active ulnar deviation and flexion of the wrist against resistance reproduce the pain. Roentgenographic confirmation is required.

Rarely, the superficial branch may sustain a direct injury over its superficial course or may be compressed by a loose bone fragment (*e.g.*, from a fracture of the hook of the hamate).[75] Clinically, this is characterized by pain over the ulnar side of the palm and little and ring fingers, where sensory loss may be detected, by no sensory loss over the proximal portion of the dorsal aspect of these fingers, by positive Tinel's sign, and by roentgenographic evidence of bone fragment. The intrinsic muscles are not affected.

It should be emphasized that arteritis or thromboangiitis of the ulnar artery at the wrist will produce, in the majority of instances, the clinical features of involvement of the superficial branch alone; less often, both sensory and motor components are involved. Persistent aching pain at the base of the hypothenar eminence and ischemic symptoms of a finger are sometimes associated.[52]

Diagnosis. Muscle weakness and wasting in the ulnar-innervated intrinsic muscles is common to a whole host of neurologic and myopathic conditions. Before a peripheral neuropathy can be suspected, it is necessary to rule out not only the myopathies but also various neurologic entities that are situated at the level of the spinal cord, nerve roots, and brachial plexus. Then localization of the site of ulnar nerve involvement becomes all important.

When symptoms suggest distal ulnar nerve involvement, the differential diagnosis must follow a logical sequence. Inquiry is made into possible occupational factors. An injury such as a laceration, despite a time lapse, is recorded. Generalized disorders such as collagen disease are sought for. Disorders of the cervical spine thoracic outlet, shoulder, and elbow must be excluded. A detailed sensory examination may serve to distinguish between nerve compression at the elbow from injury to the distal portion of the ulnar nerve. When sensation is lost over the volar ulnar sensory distribution, but sensation is intact over the dorsal ulnar area, the injury is localized distal to the point of origin of the dorsal sensory branch (*i.e.*, 6 cm to 8 cm above the wrist).

Muscle examination must be detailed because, except for loss of manual dexterity, intrinsic muscle weakness and wasting may not be apparent. Electromyographic studies of the first dorsal interosseous muscle may show fibrillation potentials indicative of denervation at least of the deep branch. However, this is generally a late finding when overt clinical findings are so obvious. It is possible to obtain very early evidence of a neurapraxia long before fibrillation potentials become apparent by plotting strength-duration curves of the first dorsal interosseous or adductor pollicis muscle.

Nerve conduction delay between the wrist and the first dorsal interosseous or adductor pollicis, when nerve conduction velocity proximal to this site is normal, is highly diagnostic and must be clearly demonstrated prior to surgical intervention. When fibrillation potentials are already present on electromyographic studies, denervation is far advanced. Reinnervation and muscle recovery after surgical decompression or nerve repair is indicated by the appearance on the electromyogram of numerous polyphasic motor units, improved nerve conduction velocity, and return to normal strength-duration patterns.

Following trauma, whether a single severe blunt injury or repetitive trauma, particularly to the base of the hypothenar eminence, persistence of pain and exquisite tenderness at the site of injury should lead one to suspect involvement not only of the ulnar or median nerve (depending on the location) but also of the neighboring ulnar or superficial branch of the radial artery, respectively. Thrombotic occlusion or aneurysmal dilatation of the artery (especially the ulnar artery) may be detected by Allen's test and angiography. It is important to determine the state of the collateral circulation before embarking on surgery.

Roentgenograms of the wrist and hand, including special carpal tunnel and pisiform views, are necessary to determine the presence of osteoarthritis, fracture, and neoplasm (Fig. 14-19).

Treatment. Immediate decompression of the ulnar nerve is mandatory. At operation, the nerve is isolated adjacent to the tendon of the flexor carpi ulnaris distally in the forearm and then freed progressively by severing the volar carpal ligament and then the fascial roof overlying the interval between the pisiform and the hook of the hamate, beneath which the nerve divides into superficial and deep branches before the latter enters the narrow tendinous interval between the origins of the abductor and flexor digiti minimi. The compressive lesion is identified and removed. This may include, for example, a ganglion, osteophyte, loose ossicle, or rheumatoid pannus. When osteoarthritis of the pisiform-triquetral joint is present, or the pisiform is dislocated, the bone may be removed without impairing the power of wrist flexion. In most instances, the compressive neuropathy constitutes a neurapraxia, which gradually recovers over several months to as long as 2 years.

When the possibility of severance of the deep palmar branch by a penetrating injury exists, the nerve should be explored beneath the flexor tendons in the palm and repair carried out.[28]

The presence of an ulnar artery lesion and the state of the collateral circulation should be clearly defined before operation. Thrombotic occlusion of the ulnar artery at the wrist requires segmental arterial resection. Aneurysm of the artery requires excision of the aneu-

FIG. 14-19. Position of the wrist for roentgenography of the pisiform-triquetral joint. Osteoarthritis of this joint is often responsible for the synovial protrusion that compresses the deep branch of the ulnar nerve. The ulnar side of the forearm lies in contact with the cassette. The wrist is dorsiflexed and abducted, and the hand is supinated as far as possible without losing contact with the cassette. The dorsal surface of the forearm lies at an angle of approximately 60° with the cassette. (Jenkins SA: Osteoarthritis of the pisiform-triquetral joint. J Bone Joint Surg 33B:532, 1951)

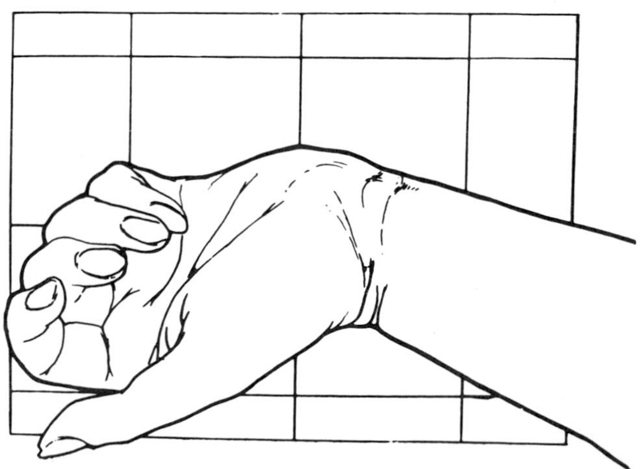

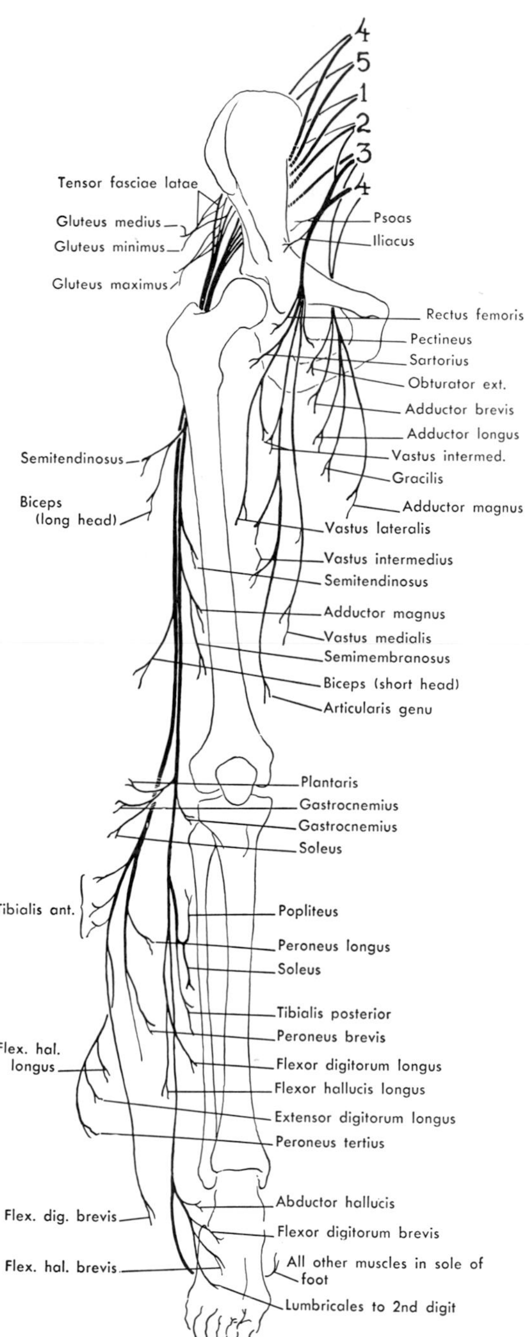

FIG. 14-20. Nerve supply to muscles of the lower extremity.

rysmal sac. Before the aneurysm is removed, its arterial tributaries are temporarily clamped and adequacy of distal blood flow is established. If the collateral circulation is insufficient, restoration of arterial continuity by end-to-end anastomosis or a vein graft is necessary. Formerly, temporizing was advocated to permit the development of additional collaterals before resecting an arteriovenous aneurysm or a false aneurysm.[29,38] Current opinion holds that delay will increase the incidence of complications: trophic changes in the fingers, rupture of the aneurysm, pressure on an adjacent nerve, and propogation of the thrombus with distal digital embolization.[76] (See Aneurysms of the Hand.)

SCIATIC NERVE AND SCIATICA

Anatomy

Sciatica is the term applied to the condition of pain in the area of distribution of the sciatic nerve. It is due to a large variety of intraspinal, intrapelvic, and extrapelvic causes. Therefore, knowledge of the anatomy is a necessary prerequisite to making a differential diagnosis (Figs. 14-20 and 14-21).

The sciatic nerve arises from the L4 and L5 and S1 through S3 nerve roots. These nerve roots, after emergence from the spine, form the sacral plexus within the pelvis. The fourth and fifth lumbar nerves form the large

FIG. 14-21. Lumbosacral plexus. Note the position of individual nerves as they emerge from under cover of the psoas major muscle. Involvement of these nerves by visceral disease in the lumbar region is reflected in sensory disturbances in the lower abdominal, the inguinal, and the lateral femoral areas. Involvement by pelvic disease refers dysesthesias to the anterior femoral area (femoral nerve) and the posterior aspect of the entire lower extremity (lumbosacral trunk).

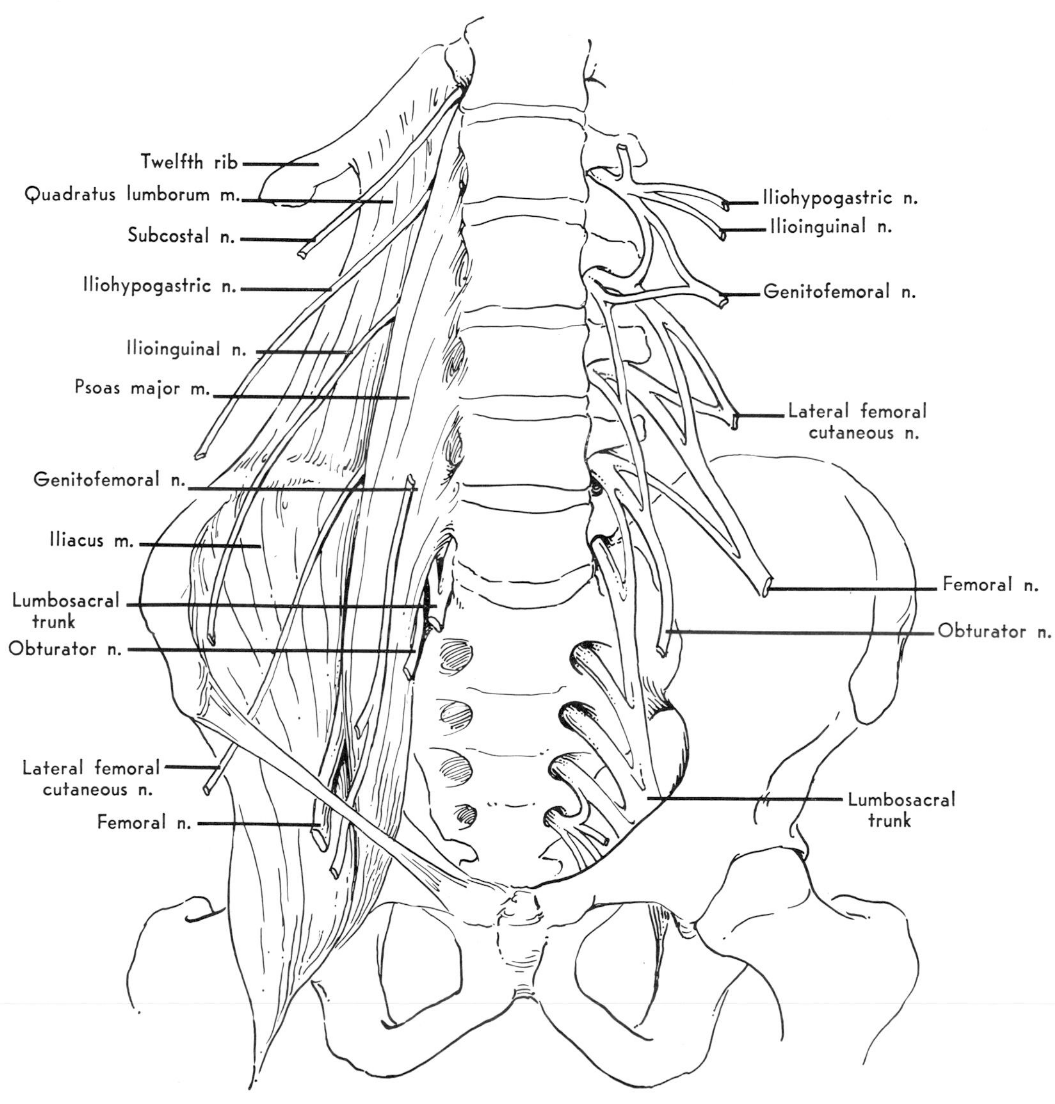

lumbosacral trunk, which appears at the medial margin of the psoas major and descends downward over the pelvis brim to join the first sacral nerve.

The plexus lies on the posterior wall of the pelvis between the piriformis behind and the hypogastric vessels, the ureter, and the sigmoid colon in front. The plexus gives rise to nerves to the gluteal muscles and the external rotator muscles of the hip, then converges distally toward the greater sciatic foramen as a large flattened band, the sciatic nerve.

The nerve emerges from the foramen at the lower border of the piriformis and comes to lie between the other external rotators anteriorly and the gluteus maximus posteriorly. The rotators and the nerve are situated in a groove between the ischial tuberosity medially and the greater trochanter laterally. At this point it is exposed to pressure from the posteriorly displacing femoral head in dislocations.

The sciatic nerve descends beneath the obliquely placed biceps femoris long head and lies on the adductor magnus, very close to the back of the femur. In this position it is easily compressed between the bone and a hard chair seat and gives rise to the sensation of the foot falling asleep; or it may be involved in tumor or callus formation. Sharp jagged edges of fragments may sever the nerve. Branches springing from the sciatic nerve supply the hamstrings and the posterior part of the adductor magnus. Nerves of supply to the biceps and the semitendinosus arise quite high so that these muscles are generally spared in lesions of the sciatic nerve and knee flexion is preserved. A lower branch to the semitendinosus and a common branch for the adductor and the semimembranosus complete the distribution in the thigh. In the lower third of the thigh, the sciatic divides into the tibial (medial popliteal) and the common peroneal (lateral popliteal) nerves.

The tibial nerve in the popliteal space lies to the lateral side of the large vessels, then crosses over them and comes to lie medially. In the lower fossa, branches are given off to both heads of the gastrocnemius and to the soleus, the popliteus, and the plantaris. A cutaneous nerve, the sural, is given off here and descends superficially in the calf to the lateral side of the foot and the little toe. At the lower end of the popliteal fossa, it exits through the tendinous arch in the soleus and descends in the leg under cover of the muscle, lying on a floor that is formed by the posterior tibial and the flexor digitorum longus muscles.

At the lower third of the leg it lies in intimate contact with the posteromedial surface of the tibia, where it may be easily affected by bony lesions. Then it passes under the flexor retinaculum behind the medial malleolus and enters the sole of the foot, where it divides into medial and lateral plantar nerves. These supply the small muscles to the toes and the skin of the sole, except the extreme medial and lateral borders.

The tibial nerve, throughout its course in the leg, lies just behind and lateral to the tibial vessels and together with the latter are held in intimate contact with the deep calf muscles by an enveloping layer of fascia. At the level of the medial malleolus, the neurovascular bundle lies 1 fingerbreadth posterior to the malleolus.

The common peroneal nerve originates at the upper end of the popliteal fossa and passes distally and laterally toward the head of the fibula in close relationship to the posterior border of the biceps tendon. At the level of the fibular head it lies in a groove between the head, to which the biceps inserts, and the gastrocnemius. Here it gives off the lateral sural cutaneous nerve, which supplies the skin on the posterior and the lateral surfaces of the leg. Then it passes around the neck of the fibula where, under cover of the origin of the peroneus longus, it divides into the superficial and the deep peroneal nerves. These branches are in close contact with the bone and are easily damaged. Surgery in this area demands mobilization of the nerves by first securing the common peroneal above and behind the biceps, then loosening it distalward. Finally, by severing the posterior attachment of the peroneus longus, the main nerve and the branches may be displaced forward with the muscle out of harm's way.

The deep peroneal nerve passes obliquely forward beneath the extensor digitorum longus to the front of the interosseous membrane and comes into intimate relationship with the anterior tibial artery, with which it descends distally to the front of the ankle joint. Here it divides into medial and lateral terminal branches; the former supplies the dorsal surfaces of the apposing aspects of the large and the second toes; the latter innervates the extensor digitorum brevis. In the leg, the deep peroneal supplies the anterior tibial, the extensor hallucis, and the extensor digitorum longus muscles at a high level, so that a lesion in the distal portion of the leg affects the foot extensor power very little. Above the ankle, the neurovascular bundle is found in the interval between the tibialis anticus and the extensor digitorum longus.

The superficial peroneal nerve originates about the neck of the fibula and innervates the long and the short peroneal muscles as it descends distally in close contact with the bone. Then it runs superficial to the brevis and passes obliquely forward between the peronei and the extensor digitorum longus and divides into a medial and an intermediate dorsal cutaneous nerve. The former supplies the skin on the medial side of the great toe and the adjacent sides of the second and the third toes; the latter supplies the adjacent sides of the third and the fourth toes and the fourth and fifth toes. The lateral side of the fifth toe is supplied by the sural nerve.

Clinical Picture

Sciatica, defined, is pain in the area of distribution of the sciatic nerve (*i.e.*, over the buttock, the posterior thigh, the posterior or posterolateral leg, and the foot, dorsal or plantar). The most important causes of sciatic nerve pain are the following:

Primary nerve disease
- Inflammatory: alcoholic, avitaminosis, infection (spread from pelvis, hip)
- Degenerative: heavy metals
- Metabolic: diabetes

Secondary nerve involvement
- Intraspinal:
  - Intervertebral disk compression of nerve root
  - Hypertrophic arthritis
    - Osteophyte compression
    - Edema at foramina
  - Posttraumatic arachnoiditis, fracture
  - Vertebral disease
    - Tumor
    - Infection
  - Intraspinal tumor
  - Congenital deformities (spondylolisthesis)
- Extraspinal
  - Intrapelvic
    - Tumors (*e.g.*, prostate)
    - Infection (*e.g.*, postabortive)
  - Extrapelvic
    - Trauma (*e.g.*, gunshot, dislocated hip)
    - Tumors (*e.g.*, pressure of osteochondroma)
    - Infection

Reflex nerve pain
- Tumors (*e.g.*, episacral lipoma, osteoid ossteoma)
- Trauma, particularly low back strains

These are by no means all the causes of sciatica, but the outline is designed to aid in the differential diagnosis.

The sciatic nerve carries not only the described motor and sensory fibers but also sympathetic fibers. Each motor supply is to a definite muscle or group of muscles. The sensory fibers supply a definite area also, and in spite of overlap from adjacent peripheral nerves there is an autonomous zone of sensory loss that defines the particular nerve involvement. When the peripheral nerve is irritated, a constant burning pain in the area of distribution results. Also, the stimulation of sympathetics causes vasoconstriction (pallor) and increased sweating in the autonomous area. When the nerve is injured further so that function is lost, in addition to paralysis there results anesthesia in the autonomous zone, increased warmth (vasodilation), and dryness. Trophic lesions are common. Next to the median nerve, the sciatic nerve is a frequent source of causalgia.

Lesions proximal to the lumbar plexus (*i.e*,. at the level of the nerve roots) cause an incomplete sensory loss corresponding to a dermatome or segment. Muscle weakness or paralysis involves a group of muscle fibers, not necessarily anatomically distinct muscles, corresponding to a myotome. No vasomotor or sudomotor functions are lost. This picture contrasts sharply to that of peripheral nerve lesions. Thus, the clinical picture of a disk compressing a nerve root at the lumbosacral interval may display hypoesthesia over the lateral lower leg, slight weakness of dorsiflexion at the ankle when attempted against resistance, and no change in color, warmth, or moisture in the skin.

When the sciatic nerve is inflamed, pressure over the nerve by the palpating finger will accentuate the pain. The nerve is most accessible to examination at the groove between the greater trochanter and the ischial tuberosity; at the popliteal space; at the posterior edge of the biceps tendon; and at the neck of the fibula. Any stretching of the nerve, as when performing the Lasègue maneuver, will increase the pain when the nerve is inflamed, so that the test does not necessarily point to a low back lesion. When the test is positive in the absence of nerve tenderness, it suggests that the nerve is displaced over a prominence (*e.g.*, a disk or a bone tumor).

Differential Diagnosis

The differential diagnosis of sciatica should begin at the proximal areas and proceed distally. The back is inspected for deformities and abnormal posture. Inequalities in length of the lower extremities are determined. Evidence of hip dislocation and instability should be sought. The soft tissues about the lower back, particularly at the posterior-superior iliac spine, are examined for tender lipomatous masses. Local anesthesia of a suspected mass will temporarily relieve reflex sciatic pain if this is the cause. A roentgenogram of the spine demonstrates bony lesions and narrowing of disk spaces. One should remember that narrowing of the disk space and concomitant degenerative arthritic changes about the facets at the same level are late results of a disk long since gone by rupture or degeneration. Consequently, nerve root compression by a herniated disk at this level is less likely. Oblique views of the lumbar spine will show interruption in continuity of the pars interarticularis that is characteristic of spondylolysis and spondylolisthesis; encroachment on the foramina by osteophytes can be seen. Pantopaque myelography may display defects characteristic of various space-occupying lesions. Spinal fluid studies give further information, such as the increased protein content of tumors and disks, manometric evidence of a spinal block, and tests for syphilis.

Computed tomography of the lumbosacral spine may detect an intradural or extradural compressive lesion. Sonography of the pelvis and retroperitoneal space may reveal a mass that compresses the sacral plexus.

The abdomen is examined for evidence of lesions that by their involvement of the lumbosacral plexus could produce sciatic pain. The male genitourinary system may reveal a prostatic tumor that by spread backward could encompass the nerve trunks. Similarly, the tumors peculiar to the female reproductive system, such as endometriosis, are causative. Bony lesions in the pelvis may compromise the nerve before or after it emerges from the greater sciatic foramen. At the level of the hip, the most common causes are traumatic posterior dislocation and the large osteochondral growths peculiar to this region. Beyond this site, fractures of the femoral shaft may injure the nerve. Direct compression of the nerve against the unyielding underlying bone may entirely destroy nerve function, or irritative lesions will result in the causalgic state. At the neck of the fibula, the peroneal nerve is affected by compression, as by a cast, or by improper surgical approaches. The investigation always should include thorough roentgenography of the entire extremity. An unsuspected bony tumor, such as an osteoid osteoma, which exerts its influence reflexly, may thereby be revealed.

When the sciatic nerve is interrupted in the thigh, usually the ability to flex the knee is not lost, because the biceps femoris and the semitendinosus are innervated very high. A flaccid, dangling, and anesthetic foot results, and the anesthesia extends to the posterior and the lateral aspects of the leg. When the common peroneal nerve is involved, the ability to dorsiflex the foot and the toes and to evert the foot is lost. Sensory loss is found over the dorsum of the foot and the toes except on the lateral side of the little toe. The superficial peroneal nerve injury results in loss of eversion of the foot and reduced sensation over the medial aspect of the big toe and the apposing surfaces of the second and the third toes, the third and the fourth toes, and the fourth and the fifth toes. The deep peroneal (anterior tibial) nerve must be injured high in the leg in order that innervation to the foot and toe extensors be interrupted. Otherwise, the only effect is loss of sensation between the large and the second toes.

In contrast to the peroneal nerve, which is the most exposed of the sciatic components, the tibial nerve is rarely injured. Its loss results in paralysis of the calf and the plantar muscles and their obvious atrophy. Peculiarly enough, the gait is little disturbed, and the functional defect becomes apparent only when fast walking or running is attempted; then loss of takeoff is demonstrable. Clawfoot deformity results from the unopposed pull of the extensors at the metacarpophalangeal joints, because of paralysis of the interossei and the lumbricals. The loss of extension at the interphalangeal joints by these muscles causes flexion deformity of the toes. The deformity is comparable with that seen in the hand. The sensory loss includes the sole of the foot and the plantar aspect of the toes. If the sural nerve is also involved, the posterolateral leg and the lateral border of the foot and little toe are also anesthetic.

The autonomous zones should be sought and outlined by the starch-iodine test or by determining the skin resistance by an instrument such as the dermometer. In the case of the sciatic nerve, the autonomous zone includes the entire dorsum and plantar surfaces of the foot, except a small medial area, and the lower lateral aspect of the leg. The autonomous zone of the peroneal nerve is extremely variable over the dorsum of the ankle and the foot. The zone for the tibial nerve exists over the sole of the foot and the toes and the lateral surface of the heel.

Treatment

Because of the great length of the sciatic nerve, regeneration is prolonged, and repair should be undertaken at the earliest possible date. The site of injury can be localized by Tinel's sign and by segmental nerve conduction velocity studies.

The incision begins at the posterior-superior iliac spine and is carried obliquely downward and outward to a point medial to the great trochanter. Then it is curved medially at the gluteal fold to the midline of the thigh and continued distally to a point just above the popliteal fossa. At the upper end of the incision, the gluteus maximus is split in line with its fibers, and laterally it is severed from its insertion into the iliotibial band. The muscle is reflected medially, exposing the nerve as it emerges at the lower border of the pyriformis. By severing the outer end of that muscle, the latter is elevated to afford further access to the nerve as it emerges from the sciatic notch. In exposing the nerve in the thigh, the deep fascia is cut with care, since the posterior cutaneous nerve lies just below its deep surface. The biceps is displaced medially; the nerve is identified where it lies deeply and is traced distally beneath the biceps. After the nerve branches, the incision is curved downward and laterally toward the fibular head if the exposure of the peroneal nerve is desired, or it is curved medially and distally along the medial side of the leg if the tibial nerve is sought. Mobilization of the nerve is obtained by flexion of the knee and hyperextension of the hip. The position is maintained by a cast for several weeks until the nerve has firmly united; the cast is discarded; and the nerve is gradually stretched by straightening out the knee.

The peroneal nerve is picked up at the medial border of the biceps tendon and traced distally. The posterior attachment of the peroneus longus is severed and lifted forward, thereby exposing the branches about the fibular neck. The superficial nerve continues distally in contact with the bone in the interval between the peroneus longus and the extensor digitorum longus. Then it runs superficial to the peroneus brevis and goes obliquely forward to the anterior aspect of the ankle and the dorsum of the foot. The deep peroneal nerve proceeds distally beneath the extensor digitorum longus, then behind the tibialis anticus where it is found with and lateral to the vessels. Mobilization of the peroneal nerve is obtained by flexing the knee. If necessary, the neck of the fibula may be resected to aid in approximation.

In approaching the posterior tibial nerve, the two heads of the gastrocnemius are split apart in the midline, exposing the tendinous arch of the soleus beneath which the nerve and the vessels pass. The arch is then cut in the midline, and the soleus is spread, revealing the neurovascular bundle where it lies snugly against a floor of the posterior tibial muscle. Distally, it comes to lie 1 fingerbreadth behind the medial malleolus, and then passes beneath the medial retinaculum to enter the sole of the foot. The nerve always lies lateral to the artery. The numerous small vessels with which it is intimately associated make mobilization of the nerve difficult. First, the nerve must be isolated in the thigh and the muscular branches stripped upward, and then the knee is flexed.

PERONEAL NERVE

The common peroneal nerve and its divisions, the superficial and deep peroneal nerves, may be injured by stretching, compression, and severance.

The nerve may be stretched by a force that adducts the leg at the knee,[83] by an internal torsional injury of the lower leg, which generally produces a spiral fracture of the tibia,[63] and by forcible inversion of the foot at the ankle, which produces a sprain[51] or fracture of the ankle. Excessive traction exerted on the common peroneal nerve disrupts the neural structures to a variable degree. Most often the axons are torn apart within their intact sheath, so that on gross inspection the nerve appears normal. The interruption in continuity, usually at the level of, or just proximal to, the head of the fibula, is not demonstrable until the sheath is incised. Rarely, disruption of the nerve sheath itself is apparent and localizes the site of injury. Clinically, the nerve deficit is immediate. A variable degree of motor loss (dorsiflexion and/or eversion of the foot) and sensory loss (dorsum of foot) can be detected and should be sought for, because surgical exploration and repair of the nerve is most urgent.

At operation the damaged portion of the nerve is excised and the nerve is sutured. By flexing the knee, approximation of the nerve ends is facilitated. If, after incising the sheath at the level of the fibular head, the nerve appears normal, the dissection should be extended proximally as high as the point of bifurcation of the sciatic nerve. At this level an artery entering the epineurium may be torn within the sheath, producing hemorrhage within the closed compartments, which compresses the nerve. This latter condition should be suspected when, after an above-described injury, gradually increasing severe pain and peroneal weakness develop in the lower leg and foot. After ligation of the vessel and evacuation of the clot, relief of symptoms is rapid and often dramatic.

The common peroneal nerve in its superficial location where it winds about the neck of the fibula is susceptible to compression or accidental surgical division. The nerve may be compressed by an external force such as a tightly fitted cast. Encroachment on the nerve from within the leg by a disease process produces gradually increasing symptoms of peroneal weakness. A cyst may arise from the posterior aspect of the upper tibiofibular joint and press on and even actually invade the nerve. In any case of spontaneous peroneal nerve involvement, surgical exploration should include visualization of the entire posterior tibiofibular juncture. Removal of an extraneural cyst effects rapid abatement of symptoms. In the case of intraneural invasion by the cyst, merely incising the sheath and freeing the nerve will often effect considerable improvement. (See Chapter 28.)

Peroneal paralysis that develops quickly after a period of unusually excessive walking activity suggests ischemic compression within the anterior tibial or peroneal compartment. Decompression of the compartment by incision of the fascial covering is urgent, but, if it is delayed, the typical grayish white appearance of muscle necrosis is immediately apparent.

In traction or surgical injuries in which actual interruption in continuity can be demonstrated, the outlook for recovery is poor.[26] At the other extreme, good recovery may be anticipated when a compressive lesion is removed. If, after a traction injury, surgical exploration is delayed for several months, adhesions and pigmentation found within the sheath may represent the residual of a hematoma. In such a situation, careful neurolysis may effect a variable degree of slow recovery.

OBTURATOR NERVE

Anatomy

The obturator nerve arises from the second, third, and fourth lumbar ventral divisions of the lumbar plexus, which is situated retroperitoneally and behind the psoas major muscle. It descends within the fibers of that muscle and emerges from its medial border near the brim of the pelvis. Then it passes behind the common iliac vessels and lateral to the hypogastric vessels and the ureter; when proceeding toward its point of exit from the pelvis, it runs along the lateral pelvis wall above the obturator vessels to the upper part of the obturator foramen. While within the foramen, it divides into anterior and posterior branches.

The anterior division enters the thigh above the upper border of the obturator externus and then runs distally on the anterior aspect of the adductor brevis, where it divides into branches of supply to the adductor brevis, the adductor longus, and the gracilis. One branch proceeds beyond as a cutaneous branch to the medial side of the thigh. Near the obturator foramen, the anterior division gives off a twig to the hip joint (Fig. 14-22).

The posterior division pierces the upper part of the obturator externus and descends behind the adductor brevis and in intimate contact with the adductor magnus which is supplies. It gives off an articular branch, which pierces the lower part of the magnus and supplies the back of the knee joint.

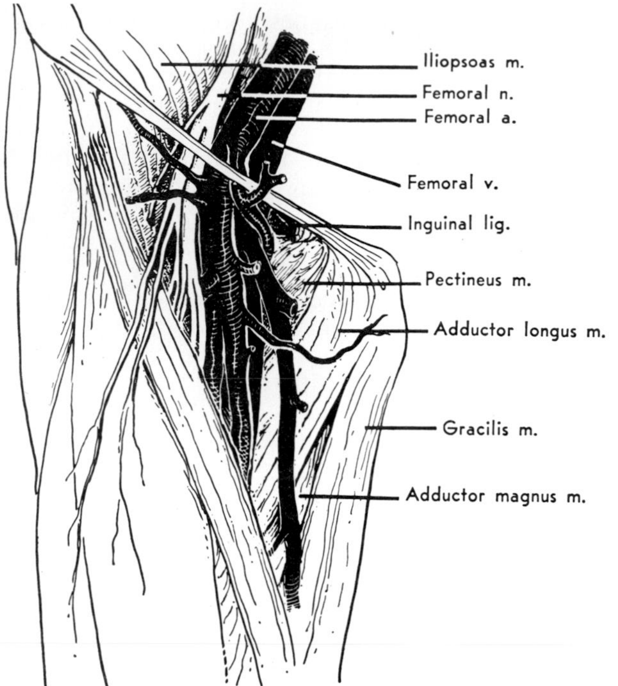

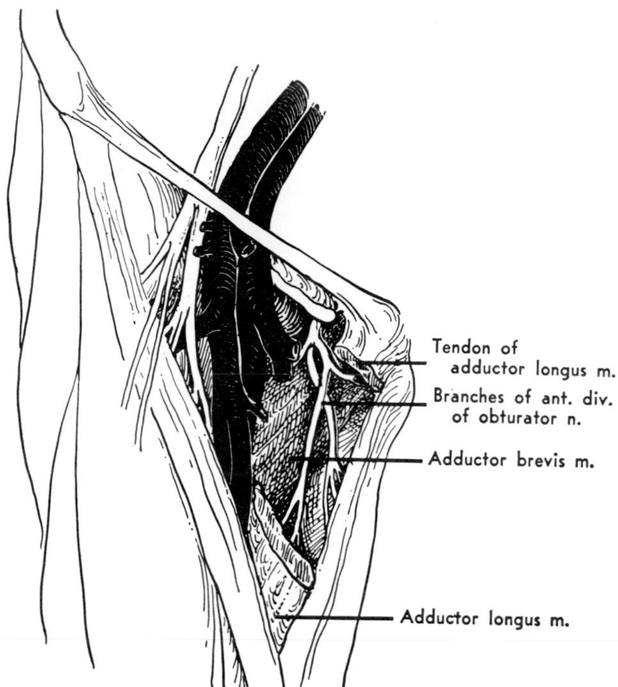

FIG. 14-22. Approach to the extrapelvic portion of the obturator nerve. (*Left*) Superficial anatomy. The incision is made over the adductor longus tendon, which is palpable as a tight prominent cord beneath the skin. The superficial veins are ligated, and the large vessels laterally are avoided. (*Right*) Intermediate level. The tendon of the adductor longus is severed and elevated, bringing into view the adductor brevis to which the branches of the anterior division of the obturator nerve intimately cling. These are resected, and the brevis is severed and elevated. The branches of the posterior division lie on the surface of the adductor magnus, which lies at the deepest level.

Clinical Picture

Interruption in continuity of the obturator nerve or its divisions is very rare, but when it occurs it would cause paralysis of all the adductors except the magnus, which has a dual nerve supply (obturator and sciatic). Disability is nil, since the pectineus as well as the magnus preserves some adductor function. Sensation is reduced or absent over the inner aspect of the lower thigh. Overlap from the saphenous nerve would preserve sensation. Although the obturator nerve runs during part of its course through the psoas muscle, destruction of the nerve by infection in a tuberculous abscess is unlikely. However, irritation of the nerve may cause spasm of the adductors and pain along the inner aspect of the lower thigh, signs pointing to psoas muscle involvement. This combination of spasm and pain may also occur reflexly in disease of the hip. Vague complaints of discomfort over the inner aspect of the knee should draw one's attention to the hip joint, particularly in the absence of clinical findings in the knee.

The most common involvement in the obturator nerve distribution occurs as a result of an upper motor neuron lesion, particularly in cerebral palsy. In this typical scissors gait the limbs cross over each other in marked adduction as forward progression is attempted. Passive attempts to abduct the limbs at the hips are strongly resisted, and the taut adductor longus tendon stands out prominently.

Treatment

Repair of a severed obturator nerve within the lesser pelvis is difficult and is generally unnecessary, inasmuch as some adductor function is spared and disability is not great. When hyperactivity of the adductors interferes with gait, one or both divisions of the nerve and the adductor longus and brevis may be severed at their tendinous attachments. (see Fig. 14-59). Pain due to degenerative arthritis of the hip referred to the obturator nerve distribution theoretically may be relieved by section of the articular branch. However, this has not worked out well in actual practice.

NERVE TUMORS

The ordinary benign nerve tumor is called a *neurinoma.* The constituent of the nerve from which it originates is debatable. If it arises from the connective tissue perineurium, it is designated a *perineurial fibroma or fibroblastoma.* If it arises from the Schwann cells of the sarcolemma sheath, the proper designation is *schwannoma.* Disregarding the site of origin, the conventional term to use is *neurofibroma.*

Common Features. Microscopically, these tumors display long, slender, wirelike fibers with elongated nuclei that have a tendency to be arranged in parallel rows or palisades. Palisading always suggests a nerve sheath origin. The nuclei are grouped in streams, flowing columns, or whorls. These features are lost in the more malignant tumors.

Types. Nerve tumors are divided into neurofibroma, neurofibromatosis (von Recklinghausen's disease), and neurogenic sarcoma.

Neurofibroma. Neurofibroma is a round or fusiform, firm, white mass attached to the sheath of a nerve and not containing nerve fibers.

Neurofibromatosis. Neurofibromatosis consists in large numbers of tumors, especially in the fine cutaneous nerves, skin pigmentations, hypertrophy of part or all of a limb, and various bone deformities such as scoliosis. Microscopically, palisading and whorls are seen with the addition of nerve fibrils penetrating the mass.

Neurogenic sarcoma. Neurogenic sarcoma arises from a nerve, probably from a preexistent neurofibroma. Ewing believes that most fibrosarcomas are really neurogenic in origin. They are single slow-growing tumors in the intermuscular tissue. Microscopically, in addition to the palisading and whorls, curling, rippling, or waviness of the nuclei are characteristic. The malignity is demonstrated by the swelling and the pleomorphism of the cells, mitotic figures, and less tendency to palisading. (See Chapter 15).

Section III
Poliomyelitis and Related Affections

Although the incidence of poliomyelitis has been markedly reduced so that only sporadic cases are encountered, this condition best portrays the principles that apply to any disease with residuals of flaccid paralysis. As an example, muscle imbalance resulting from a partial brachial plexus injury may require surgical measures to restore muscle balance, overcome deformity, and provide stability to improve prehensile function of the upper extremity. Moreover, a considerable number of patients continue to require orthopaedic treatment for sequelae of poliomyelitis acquired prior to the advent of immunization. This study should therefore be interpreted as a model for innumerable similar problems of orthopaedic interpretation and management.

Poliomyelitis (infantile paralysis) is an acute infectious disease caused by a virus that inflicts typical temporary or permanent destructive changes in the central nervous system and results in paralysis and deformities.

ETIOLOGY

The cause of poliomyelitis is a filterable virus with the following characteristics:[150]

- Isolated often from brain and spinal cord
- Found in nasal secretions and rectal washings of both active cases and healthy contacts and also in flies
- Destroyed by weak disinfectants; resistant to glycerol; preserved in frozen dried state; persists in water despite chlorination
- Several strains: type I (Brunhilde), type II (Lansing), and type III (Leon)
- Reproduced in the rhesus monkey
- Culture in human embryonic tissues, producing visible changes in growing cells that are inhibited by immune serum.

EPIDEMIOLOGY

Since the widespread use of oral vaccine, paralytic poliomyelitis is no longer epidemic. Only five cases of paralytic poliomyelitis were reported in 1974. It is extremely sporadic, and when it occurs, it is mainly during the warm months. The method of transmission and portal of entry are unknown, but the disease is probably spread by infected fecal matter or food. The virus presumably enters through the gastrointestinal and respiratory tracts, reaching the central nervous system through the hematogenous route.

A viremia is probably present during the incubation period before the onset of paralysis. This is suggested by the fact that the virus is regularly found in the blood of orally infected primates, with the onset of paralysis occurring 3 to 7 days later. Usually, only one case occurs per family. Infants, adolescents, and adults as well as all races and classes are affected. The bulbar type commonly has a history of a recent tonsillectomy. A history of swimming and bathing is often elicited.

RELATIONSHIP OF COXSACKIEVIRUSES

The virus is a member of an enterovirus group that includes coxsackieviruses and the echoviruses. Other members of this group can produce a paralytic syndrome mimicking poliomyelitis. These individual viruses may be isolated and identified on tissue culture and serologic studies.

Coxsackieviruses are frequently found in association with the poliomyelitis virus. Both are found in the human pharynx and the stools, and both are similarly distributed in nature. However, each is immunologically distinct. The coxsackievirus is isolated from paralytic and nonparalytic poliomyelitis, from sewage and flies in areas in which poliomyelitis is prevalent, and in a variety of clinical syndromes, including aseptic meningitis, encephalitis, epidemic pleurodynia, and influenza. In poliomyelitis, the neutralizing antibody titers to poliomyelitis and coxsackieviruses rise together during convalescence. Their relationship is unexplained. Coxsackieviruses are characterized by causing paralysis in newborn mice and hamsters.

PATHOLOGY

The portal of entry and the method of dissemination are unknown. Presumably the virus enters through the gastrointestinal and respiratory tracts and is disseminated by the hematogenous route to the central nervous system.[94,144]

The extraneural pathology is limited to the reticuloendothelial system, with hyperplasia and congestion of the spleen and lymph nodes.

The intraneural pathology chiefly involves the motor nerve cells. Insterstitial changes consist of congestion, edema, and small punctate hemorrhages. The neurons may be directly damaged by a cytotoxic substance elaborated by the virus or indirectly damaged by the increased capillary permeability, which causes local edema and hemorrhages.

Anterior horn neuron changes early show swelling of the cell, enlargement of the nucleus, and disappearance of the Nissl bodies. Next, the nucleus undergoes chromatolytic degeneration, and basophilic granules fill the cytoplasm. These changes may recede at this stage, with reversibility and restoration of the cells, or the destruction of the cell may progress to completion. The interstitial tissues display marked hemorrhage, edema, perivascular mononuclear infiltration (cuffing), and glial invasion followed by fibrosis. The meninges also are congested and diffusely infiltrated with cells. The degenerating neurons are surrounded and absorbed by the mononuclear cells and replaced by glial cells.

Cellular infiltration and congestion are also seen in the posterior ganglia and posterior nerve roots and may be responsible for peripheral neuritic pains. Efferent nerve fibers from destroyed neurons degenerate, and their innervated muscles atrophy and become fibrotic. The anterior horns of the cervical and lumbar enlargements of the spinal cord are most severely affected. Involvement is spotty and asymmetrical. Each muscle is innervated by a column of cells, which extend longitudinally up and down the cord. Destruction of a portion of the column leaves sufficient cells to maintain at least innervation of a portion of that muscle. Muscles that characteristically are supplied by shorter columns (*e.g.*, the tibialis anterior) are more subject to permanent paralysis because of insufficient residual functioning neurons.

The intermediate or internuncial cell group is regularly involved.[119] These are situated just dorsal to the anterior horn and are concerned with synaptic relays. Through these cells impulses, including those coming from higher centers, are relayed to motor neurons of the anterior horn. Control from the higher regulatory or inhibitory centers may explain the most frequent symptom of spasm, which occurs in all but totally paralyzed muscles.

Changes in the higher centers (medulla, pons, basal ganglia, tegmentum) display perivascular cuffing, lymphoid infiltration and thrombosis.[133] These changes are usually reversible and transitory. Thus, basal ganglia lesions may explain the phenomenon of incoordination and asynergic contraction of muscles. Reversible cerebral lesions partially explain the transitory paralysis as a loss of voluntary cerebral control.

The bones become slender and rarefied. Longitudinal growth is reduced in affected extremities. Fasciae become thickened and contracted. Subluxations and dislocations occur in weight-bearing joints. Scoliosis is common.

CLINICAL PICTURE

Following an unknown period of incubation, generalized constitutional involvement lasting a few days, known as the systemic phase, is manifest by fever, irritability, sweating, and respiratory and/or gastrointestinal inflammation. Next, the virus invades the central nervous system with evidence of meningeal irritation (*e.g.*, stiff neck and back, headache, vomiting, muscle tenderness, and severe neuritic pains). Spinal fluid changes are now evident, and convalescent serum therapy is indicated. As the disease involves the anterior horn cells, paresis or flaccid paralysis is evident—the so-called paralytic stage. This acute stage lasts a few days to a week, the temperature subsides, and a variable amount of muscle recovery begins. This latter convalescent stage lasts as long as 2 years. Generally, the maximum improvement takes place within the first 6 months.

SYSTEMIC STAGE

The systemic stage is characterized by prodromal upper respiratory infection and/or gastrointestinal inflammation, fever, malaise, apprehension and cervical lymphadenopathy. There are no spinal fluid changes. The patient may recover completely or may worsen.

STAGE OF MENINGEAL IRRITATION (PREPARALYTIC STAGE)

The second stage is marked by involvement of the central nervous system, sudden onset, high fever, prostration, headache, and pain in the back and neck. The patient is irritable and sensitive to touch. The child objects to being held. Very painful spasms of various muscles occur;

almost invariably the quadriceps is involved. Then coarse tremors, sweating, and neck rigidity follow. The head-drop sign consists of backward dropping of the head as the recumbent child is lifted from the table. The back becomes rigid. Kernig and Brudzinski signs are positive. The earliest reflexes to disappear are the superficial. Next, the deep reflexes disappear in a variable and spotty manner.

The spinal fluid exhibits a ground-glass appearance and has a cell count of about 250/cu mm, chiefly polymorphonuclear leukocytes at first, but later lymphocytes and mononuclear cells predominate. The count may vary from 10 to 1000 cu mm. Albumin and globulin levels are moderately increased; the sugar content is normal or increased; and the fluid is sterile. It is important to note that poliomyelitis may be present without characteristic spinal fluid changes.

Recovery from this stage may occur without the advent of paralysis.

PARALYTIC STAGE

Spinal Type. The constitutional and meningeal signs continue. To these are added flaccid muscle weakness and paralysis with corresponding reduced deep reflexes. The involvement is spotty and asymmetrical. Opposing muscles are often in spasm, and their unopposed action, if left untreated, encourages deforming contractures. The extremities, the back, the abdomen, and the muscles of respiration are affected.

Bulbar Type. The bulbar type is often associated with encephalitis and runs a more fulminating course. Constitutional and meningeal symptoms are extreme. Somnolence, stupor, and emesis are common. Other symptoms of bulbar involvement include nasal speech, regurgitation of food through the nose, inability to swallow, and accumulation of mucus in the throat, which may be aspirated. The gag reflex is absent. The medullary respiratory center may be involved.

RESPIRATORY PARALYSIS

Spinal Type. In this type of respiratory paralysis, the intercostal muscles supplied by T1 to T12, and the diaphragm, supplied by C3 to C5, are paralyzed. Respiratory excursion movements are shallow, the alae nasae dilate, and the accessory muscles of respiration are used. When the diaphragm is paralyzed, paradoxical respiration is noted (*i.e.*, the abdomen sinks inward on inspiration). When the intercostals are paralyzed, inspiration causes a sinking inward of the chest. Fluoroscopic examination reveals the extent of diaphragm involvement.

Encephalobulbar Type. The encephalobulbar type causes arrhythmic respirations, although the intercostals and the diaphragm are intact. Respiration may suddenly fail without warning.

SHORTENING OF MUSCLES

A number of muscles are increasingly irritable and in spasm, as can be demonstrated by abnormal action potentials.[135] If spasm is allowed to persist, permanent shortening and contracture ensue. If such a muscle is the antagonist to a paralyzed muscle, the latter is stretched and weakened. Typical sites of involvement of "tight" painful muscles are the back, the hamstrings, and the calf.

THE ABORTIVE CASE

Usually recognized only during an epidemic, the abortive case appears as a nonspecific illness with symptoms of a mild infectious disease, mild fever, headache, vomiting, and drowsiness. The diagnosis is proved by spinal fluid findings during the convalescent stage.

DIFFERENTIAL DIAGNOSIS

The following diseases must be considered in the differential diagnosis:

- Conditions causing systemic symptoms (*e.g.*, upper respiratory infection)
- Conditions causing meningeal irritation
  - Suppurative meningitis
  - Virus encephalitis
  - Toxic encephalitis (*e.g.*, complication of pneumonia)
  - Lymphocytic choriomeningitis
  - Tuberculous meningitis
  - Injury
  - Acute rheumatic fever, causing painful extremities
  - Trichinosis, causing muscular pain
- Conditions simulating paralytic poliomyelitis
  - Acute rheumatic fever ("pseudoparalysis")
  - Bone and joint inflammation
  - Scurvy
  - Infectious polyneuritis of Guillain-Barré
  - Peripheral neuritis
  - Acute encephalomyelitis: viral; vaccinal
  - Botulism; confused with bulbar poliomyelitis; however, meningeal signs are absent and spinal fluid proved negative.

PROGNOSIS

Severe widespread paralysis is often associated with high spinal fluid cell counts. Low cell counts accompany encephalobulbar disease. The mortality is high in bulbar poliomyelitis, with death being due to respiratory failure. However, rapid and complete recovery is often seen in this type. Paralysis of the muscles of deglutition rarely lasts more than 1 or 2 months. Some recovery of muscle power occurs up to 3 years after the acute phase, but the maximum degree of muscle power returns within the first 6 months. Complete loss of all motor neurons supplying a muscle can be strongly suspected if muscles supplied by the same and adjoining spinal cord segments are paralyzed. Thus, the outlook for recovery of a completely paralyzed anterior tibial muscle is poor if the quadriceps and the posterior tibial are likewise involved.

COMPLICATIONS

Bronchopneumonia is most common in the bulbar type and often is the result of aspiration. Atelectasis occurs in respiratory muscle paralysis. Contractures and deformities develop gradually about joints subjected to severe muscle imbalance. Prolonged inactivity causes mobilization of calcium, resulting in hypercalcemia, hypercalciuria, renal calculus, and impairment of kidney function.

TREATMENT

PREVENTIVE TREATMENT

Live, oral poliovirus vaccine (OPV) contains attenuated poliovirus grown in monkey kidney tissue culture or in human cell culture; it is available both in trivalent or monovalent preparations containing types I, II, and III.[87] It produces an immune response resembling that induced by natural poliovirus infection (*i.e.*, it multiplies in the lower intestinal tract and stimulates intestinal immunity as well as increasing circulating antibodies). The immunity is longer lasting than that following administration of killed poliovirus vaccine. The type-specific serum neutralizing antibody titer begins about 1 week after ingestion of monovalent vaccine, and reaches a peak about 3 weeks later. A primary series of three adequately spaced doses of trivalent oral poliovirus vaccine produces an immune response to the three virus types in over 90% of recipients. Of the 22 cases of paralytic polio reported in 1972, 4 were "recipient vaccine-associated" and 6 were "contact vaccine-associated." Paralysis has occurred in those receiving oral poliovirus vaccine, or in close contact, within 2 months following administration. The vaccine should not be given during any illness, nor should it be given to members of a household in which poliomyelitis has just occurred for fear of provoking paralytic complications in individuals who may already be incubating the virus.

Immunization by oral vaccine is now widespread and has virtually eliminated epidemics of the disease. When rarely the disease is acquired in the immunized individual, the degree of paralysis is markedly reduced.

TREATMENT OF THE ACUTE STAGE

During the acute stage, treatment is primarily the responsibility of the pediatrician or internist. In severe degrees of the disease associated with paralysis and respiratory and cardiac complications, especially when the vital centers of the medulla oblongata are involved, the expertise of pulmonary function and cardiologic disciplines is enlisted. At the earliest sign of central nervous system involvement, the orthopaedic surgeon assumes an active role, which includes serial muscle evaluations, physiotherapeutic measures for the relief of muscle pain and spasm, and positioning to prevent deformities of contracture and muscle imbalance. When the acute febrile phase has passed and paralytic residuals are apparent, the orthopaedist must assume the dominant role in the management of the musculoskeletal system until maximum rehabilitation has been attained.

MEDICAL TREATMENT

The patient is placed at absolute bed rest in isolation, and adequate fluid intake is provided. Sedatives are contraindicated because of their depressant effect on the central nervous system. The benefit of convalescent serum is questionable, but when available may be administered in adequate dosage (60 ml plus 1 ml/kg). This dose is repeated every 12 hours.

Paralysis of the shoulder girdle is a warning of probable respiratory muscle failure due to involvement of the cervical spinal cord segments which innervate the diaphragm (C3, C4, C5). Intercostal muscle paralysis stems from involvement of the thoracic spinal cord. A tracheotomy is performed immediately, and the patient is placed on a respirator. The Trendelenburg position aids drainage of bronchial mucus. Respiratory negative pressure of 12 cm to 18 cm water maintains adequate ventilation. Removal from the respirator should be gradual, and the patient should be trained on movements of normal respiration. The rocking or oscillating bed, which alternates the Fowler and Trendelenburg positions, favors the return of normal breathing rhythm; the abdominal contents alternately push and pull on the diaphragm, producing a tidal movement of air. Accumulation of mucus in the pharynx endangers the patient, since aspiration pneumonia and atelectasis may develop. Frequent aspirations are necessary. At the first sign of dyspnea, cyanosis, rapid pulse, and rise in temperature, atelectasis is suspected and confirmed by roentgenograms. Tracheotomy, endotracheal aspiration, administration of oxygen, and use of the respirator constitute emergency measures. Ethyl alcohol may be incorporated into the oxygen circuit as an aerosol. Mucolytic agents aid liquefaction and expulsion of the mucus plug. Antibiotics are given.

Patients with bulbar involvement do very poorly on the respirator.[153] The irregular inefficient respirations cannot be overcome. More competent measures include tracheotomy, repeated aspirations, postural drainage, and administration of parenteral fluids and oxygen. The electrophrenic respirator is a device by which an intermittent stimulus to the exposed phrenic nerve causes rhythmic contractions of the diaphragm and inhibits the abnormal respiratory movements.

ORTHOPAEDIC TREATMENT

During the acute phase, treatment is directed toward relief of muscle pain and spasm and prevention of deformity. An inventory of muscles is initiated after the febrile period has passed and is repeated at 2- to 3-day intervals. This information is necessary to determine at the earliest moment the development of respiratory paralysis, whether spinal in origin or due to brain stem involvement, and the areas of muscle imbalance and developing contractures. Usually paralysis develops 2 to 3 days after the onset of fever and increases in degree over several days, ceasing only after the patient has become afebrile.

Positioning in a functional position is designed not only to prevent deformity but also to secure a functionally advantageous position should contractures occur. Muscle imbalance requires relaxing of paralyzed muscles and stretching of spastic ones. the bed should be firm with boards placed beneath the mattress. A padded footboard maintains a neutral position and prevents a footdrop deformity. The standing reflex is stimulated and the frequently involved anterior tibial muscles are relaxed. The thighs are placed in abduction, neutral rotation, and slight knee flexion with the feet at right angles to the legs. The arms are placed outward to relax the deltoid muscles and are in neutral rotation. Paralyzed muscles must be kept in a state of relaxation, and the resting position may be varied to meet this requirement.

In the supine position, the knees are kept flexed with rolls behind the upper part of the tibia to prevent genu recurvatum and posterior subluxation of the tibia. Excessive and prolonged flexion will lead to contracture and should be avoided.

Tender, painful muscles tend to develop myostatic contractural shortening, causing deformity of joints on which they act. True spasm does not occur, and therefore the stretch reflex is unobtainable. The cause of muscle pain and sensitivity is unknown but is presumably due to inflammation of the posterior ganglia, or of the internuncial neurons and fibers, which are situated dorsal to the anterior horns.

Warm salt baths relieve muscle and nerve pain. The buoyancy of salt water reduces the effect of gravity and permits the few recovering muscle fibers to inaugurate contraction of the muscle.

Hot, wet packs relax and extend the muscles and relieve the pain. Following a 20-minute heat application, the joint should be put through a full range of motion. After the febrile period has passed, the patient is placed in the Hubbard tank.

Splints and braces, theoretically, maintain the muscles in a relaxed state. A stretched muscle become relatively ischemic and fibrotic so that it will not respond to regenerated nerve impulses. Conversely, a splint prevents the physiological stretch necessary to reflex contraction, which maintains normal muscle tone. The present tendency is to avoid splints except when paralysis is regarded as permanent and function must be aided.

Massage is necessary to encourage circulation and is preceded by application of heat by baking or infrared or moist packs. The massage strokes are directed centrally.

Exercises improve muscle strength. At first they are assistive, then active without gravity, then against gravity, and finally against resistance. A chart of individual muscles is kept, and improvement is noted. The suggested method to define muscle strength is:

0 = no contraction
1 = trace of contraction
2 = movement without gravity
3 = movement against gravity
4 = movement against gravity and with slight resistance
5 = movement against strong resistance
6 = normal movement and strength

Absolute immobilization should be avoided if possible. The buoyancy of water aids movement of weak muscles. The Hubbard tank is useful for this (Fig. 14-23). Exercises are passive at first; later they are active (Fig. 14-24). Hot moist packs reduce muscle spasm and pain. Painful tight muscles should be stretched repeatedly, with the aid of curare if necessary. A paretic muscle, because it fails to develop effective tension, tends to atrophy.[151] Inactivity retards muscle regeneration, whereas early muscle use promotes it. Therefore, early and frequent galvanic electric stimulation encourages development of muscle size and strength. Respiratory muscles are strengthened by exercises. Coughing aids the diaphragm. Positive inflation of the lungs several times daily counteracts development of a "frozen" thorax and prevents atelectasis. Tracheotomy and aspiration are continued as long as necessary. Intratracheal instillation of mucolytic agents reduces the viscosity of mucus. Atelectasis is an ever-present danger as long as respiratory muscle weakness exists.

REHABILITATIVE TREATMENT

Deformity may be caused by an intact, spastic or contracted muscle, which is the antagonist of a paralyzed muscle. For example, tight hamstrings in the presence of a paralyzed quadriceps result in a flexion deformity of the knee. The ligamentous structures tighten and the active muscles shorten so that an actual contracture of the joint is the inevitable result. Contracture of the fascial structures likewise causes deformity. The iliotibial band causes pelvic obliquity, flexion at the knee, and external rotation of the leg. Improper posture in the presence of

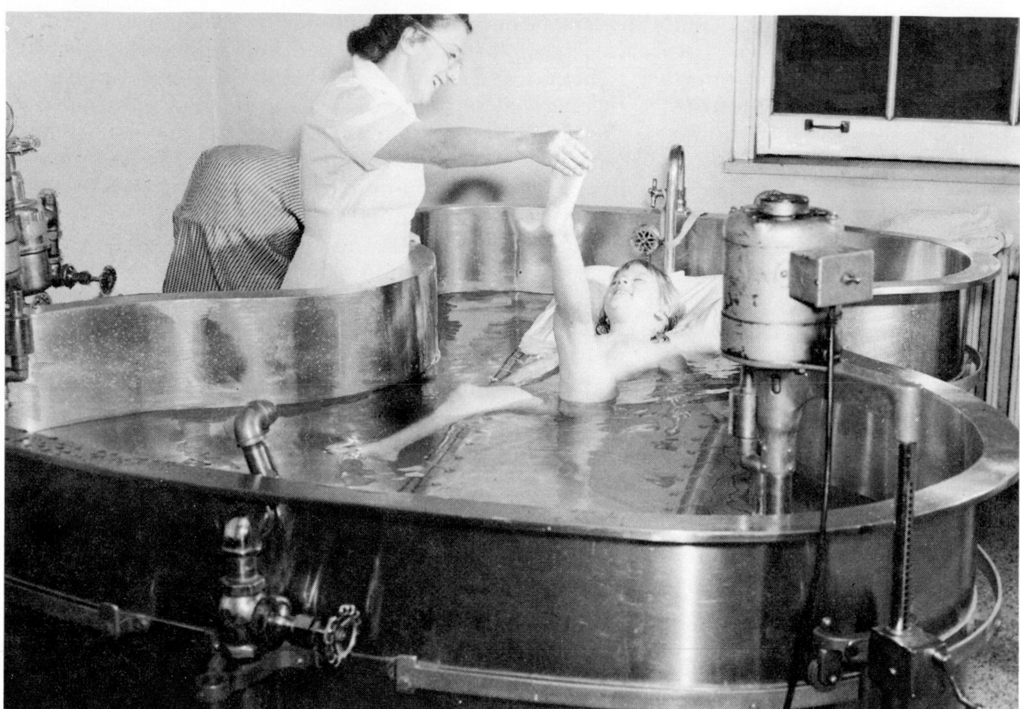

FIG. 14-23. The Hubbard tank.

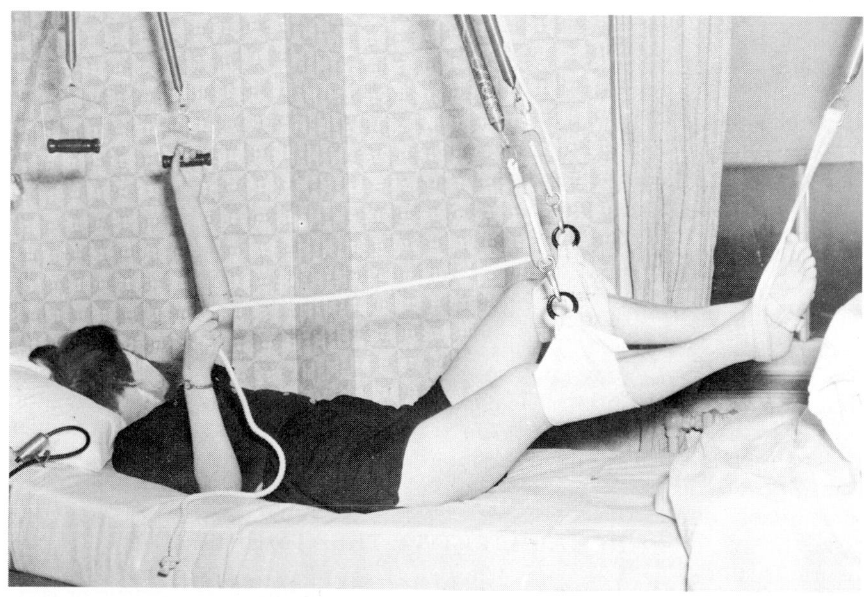

FIG. 14-24. Demonstrating assistive and resistive exercises, using springs. These exercise springs may be obtained at a sporting goods store.

paralyzed muscles favors contractural deformity. When the foot dorsiflexors are paralyzed, a neglected footdrop leads to shortening of the calf muscles and a contracted posterior capsule of the ankle joint. The most common deformities are scoliosis, knee flexion, adduction and internal rotation of the shoulder, flexion of the hips, talipes equinocavovarus, and hyperextension of the metacarpophalangeal joints. When it becomes apparent that muscle imbalance exists, prevention of deformity is imperative and is accomplished by splinting, proper positioning and stretching of the antagonists. If paralysis persists, operative measures are indicated to restore muscle power, correct deformity, and provide stability. Surgery can be done 6 months after the acute phase, because maximum recovery will have taken place by that time. Before the age of 10 years, only soft tissue surgery is permissible, because ossification is not complete enough for bone reconstruction. A poliomyelitic extremity generally has a reduced rate of longitudinal growth and is atrophied. Inequality of the lower extremities requires temporary or permanent epiphyseal arrest of the longer extremity. The fragile bones are susceptible to fracture, but callus formation and union are normal.

Tendon transference is done to substitute for a paralyzed muscle and to restore muscle balance. The transferred muscle must have sufficient power, and its tendon should be attached to the bone as near to the insertion of the paralyzed muscle as possible. The tendon should be retained within its own sheath, or in that of the paralyzed muscle, or should pass through the subcutaneous fat to afford a proper gliding substance. The nerve and blood supply should be protected. All contracted tissues should be released, and the joints over which the transferred muscle acts should be mobilized before transfer. Normal physiological tension in the transferred muscle should be retained.

Peabody stated that a deformity may be dynamic (*i.e.*, caused by muscle imbalance) or static.[132] Therefore, arthrodesis to correct a dynamic deformity during the growth period will most likely be ineffective, because the imbalanced muscle forces continue to act, and the deformity will recur. Tendon transference must be added to provide muscle balance. This can be done before 10 years of age and later supplemented with a bone procedure, if necessary, when skeletal maturity has advanced sufficiently. If the deformity is static, tendon transfers are insufficient and a bone reconstruction procedure is necessary.

RECONSTRUCTIVE SURGERY

THE SHOULDER

Knowledge of the mechanism of abduction and flexion is essential to intelligent treatment. During the first 30° of abduction and 60° of flexion, the scapula finds a position of stability in relation to the humerus. The scapula shifts slightly outward to attain this position. Beyond this point the scapula moves with the humerus in a ratio of 1:2. Therefore, the loss of scapular motion decreases abduction by one third. About 20° of rotation occurs at the acromioclavicular joint. Therefore, its restricted motion diminishes a corresponding amount of abduction. Resection of the outer end of the clavicle is valuable for increasing the range of abduction.

Abduction is performed by the deltoid, whereas the supraspinatus holds the head firmly against the glenoid and establishes the necessary fulcrum. The infraspinous muscles pull the head downward. The scapula rotates by virtue of the force exerted by the trapezius and the serratus anterior. The clavicular portion of the pectoralis major acts with the deltoid and the supraspinatus in forward flexing the humerus. At the same time, the serratus anterior moves the scapula forward.

The humeral head must be depressed during abduction and flexion. This is accomplished by the infraspinous muscles (subscapularis, infraspinatus, teres minor) and the long head of the biceps as its tendon passes over the humeral head.

Stability of the scapula is secured by the rhomboids and the middle portion of the trapezius.

A head depressor mechanism is essential to abduction. Transplantation of the latissimus dorsi and the teres major to the posteroinferior aspect of the greater tuberosity restores this component. Otherwise a Nicola procedure is necessary. Only the clavicular portion of the pectoralis major, which normally functions as a flexor, can be used as an abductor. The levator scapulae, the rhomboids, and the trapezius are necessary to scapular rotation and can be replaced by a fascial transplant from a lower cervical spinous process to the base of the scapular spine.

Restoration of motion requires adequate muscles available for transfers. Otherwise, arthrodesis is done, provided that strong scapular rotation is possible. Extensive paralysis of the forearm and hand is a contraindication to these procedures.

SERRATUS ANTERIOR PARALYSIS

Serratus anterior paralysis results in displacement of the scapula medially during abduction, materially weakening that movement. Winging of the scapula is characteristic. Surgical treatment consists of transferring the pectoralis minor tendon to the inferior angle of the scapula. The thoracodorsal nerve to the latissimus dorsi must be visualized and protected during the procedure.[136] If this muscle is not available, a fascial strip is attached at one end to the inferior angle of the scapula and at the other to the inferior border of the pectoralis major.

RHOMBOID AND TRAPEZIUS PARALYSIS

The scapula lacks fixation and moves forward by the unopposed action of the serratus. A fascial strip attached to the inferior scapular angle is attached to the thoracic spine or the spinal muscles medially. The insertion of the levator scapulae at the superior angle is transferred to a more forward position to elevate the acromion, thereby restoring the lost function of the upper trapezius.

DELTOID PARALYSIS

With the arm elevated, fascial strips connect the trapezius with the deltoid insertion. First, the humeral head must be stabilized by attaching the tendons of the latissimus dorsi and the teres major to the posteroinferior aspect of the greater tuberosity. An alternative is to perform the Nicola procedure. If the posterior portion of the deltoid remains active, it may be detached and transferred to a more favorable position at the outer end of the acromion (Fig. 14-25).

MULTIPLE TENDON TRANSPLANTATIONS

The usual presenting situation is a varying degree of involvement of many muscles about the shoulder. Therefore, transferring only one muscle to restore deltoid function is doomed to failure. It becomes necessary to use all available muscles. A prerequisite is effective scapular control by a functioning trapezius and serratus anterior, or an effective muscle or fascial substitute. Often the posterior portion of the deltoid is preserved and is transferred to a more forward position. In addition, the clavicular portion of the pectoralis major, the short head of the biceps, and the long head of the triceps are transferred to the acromion. At the second stage, the insertion of the clavicular head of the pectoralis major is transferred to the deltoid tubercle to function more

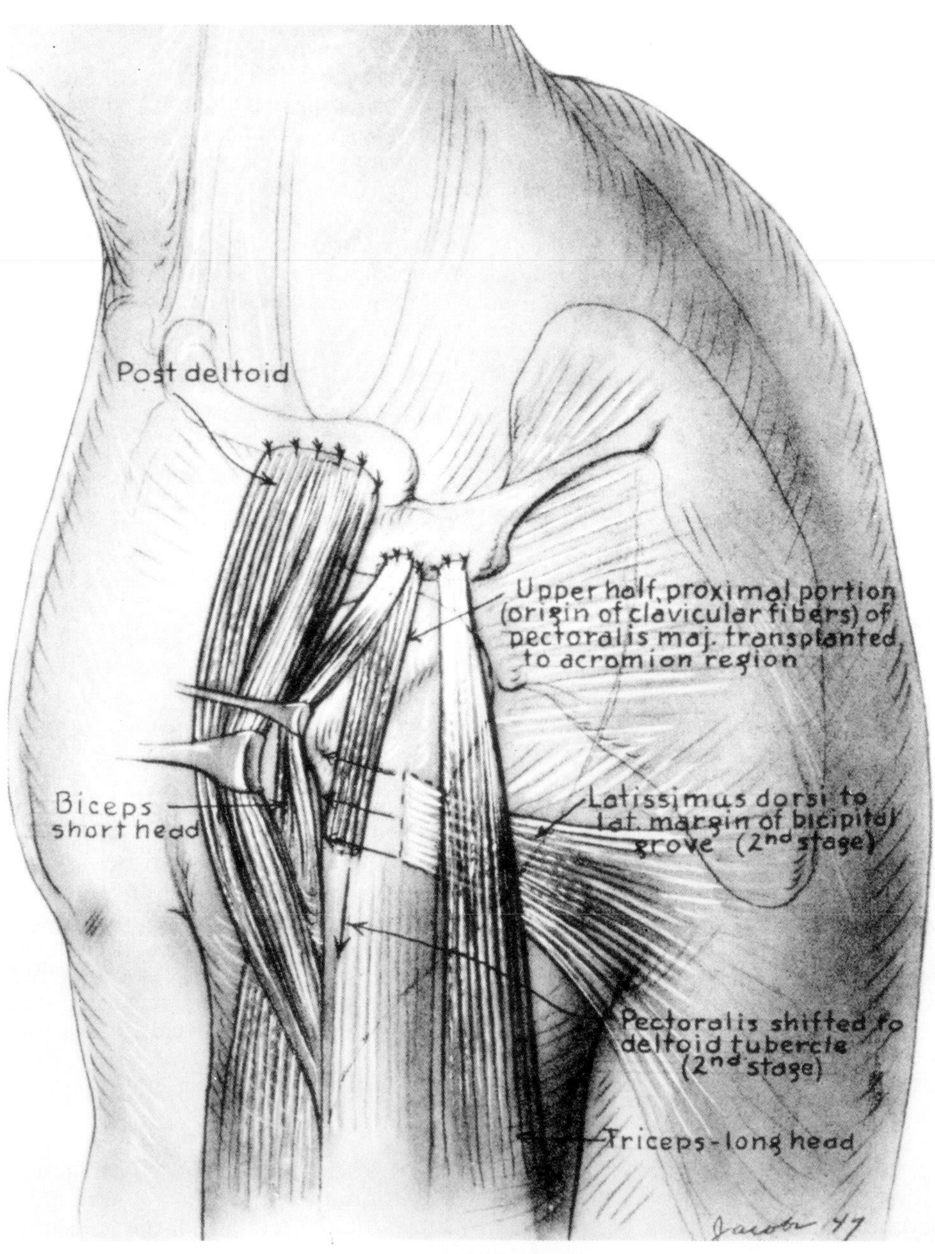

FIG. 14-25. Multiple muscle transplantations for deltoid paralysis. Partial paralysis of all muscles is usual; therefore, several muscles are utilized to provide strong abduction. The posterior portion of the deltoid is often spared and is transferred to a more functional position anteriorly. The operation is carried out in two stages: First stage: (1) Origin of clavicular fibers of pectoralis major (upper half of muscle) transplanted to the acromion. (2) Origin of posterior deltoid shifted to acromion tip. (3) Origins of long head of triceps and short head of biceps transferred to tip of acromion. Second stage: about 3 weeks later. (1) Insertion of clavicular fibers of pectoralis major transferred to region of deltoid tubercle. (2) Insertions of latissimus dorsi and teres major transplanted over lateral surface of the humerus to the lateral margin of the bicipital groove. (Harmon PH: Surgical reconstruction of the paralyzed shoulder by multiple muscle transplantations. J Bone Joint Surg 32A:583, 1950)

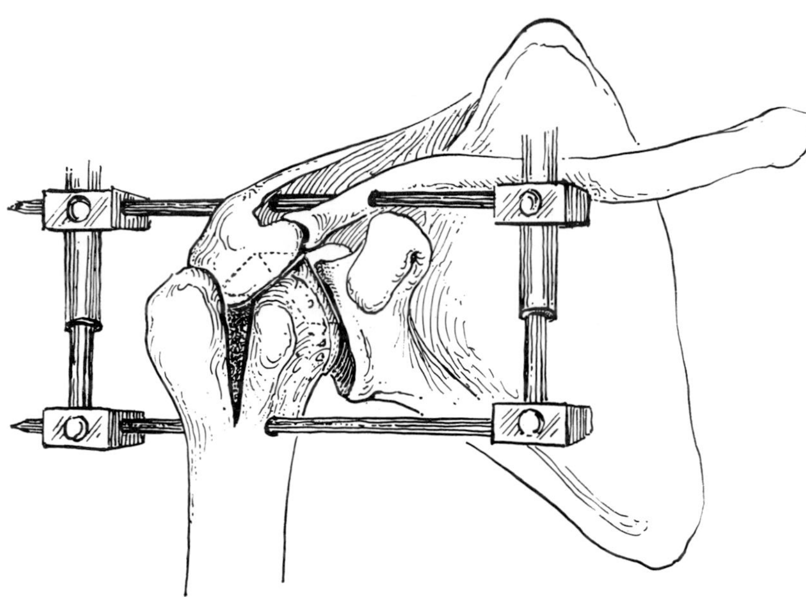

FIG. 14-26. Charnley compression arthrodesis of the shoulder.

efficiently as an abductor. At the same time the latissimus dorsi insertion into the medial side of the bicipital groove is removed and the tendon is rerouted about the humerus and attached to the lateral margin of the groove. This furnishes the external rotator.[109,129]

ARTHRODESIS OF THE SCAPULOHUMERAL JOINT

An absolute requirement is adequate power in the trapezius and serratus anterior muscles. Internal fixation is usually necessary. The optimum position for shoulder arthrodesis is 50° abduction, 20° flexion, and 25° internal rotation. This position is functional; it will provide the ability to reach the face and top of the head while the elbow is flexed and will allow reaching into the trouser pocket. Fusion will increase the power of flexion and extension at the elbow, providing adduction power, which will enable the patient to grasp an object between the arm and the body. This latter movement is facilitated by resecting the outer end of the clavicle at a later date.

If a lesser degree of abduction is preferred (*e.g.*, to avoid winging deformity of the scapula), this can be compensated for by fusion with the arm in further internal rotation. A greater degree of fusion in abduction is permissible in the child in whom epiphyseal growth does not appear to be endangered (Figs. 14-26 and 14-27).

THE ELBOW

Active flexion at the elbow is necessary to satisfactory prehension and function of the entire upper extremity. When the brachialis anticus, the biceps and the brachioradialis muscles are weakened or paralyzed, good active

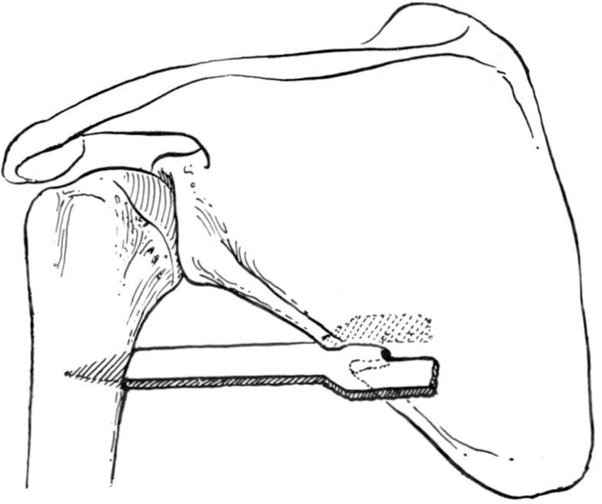

FIG. 14-27. Brittain compression arthrodesis of the shoulder.

flexion must be restored by reinforcement of the weakened muscles or substitution for the paralyzed ones. The function of the hand depends highly on satisfactory elbow flexion, and, unless hand function is acceptable or can be restored by reconstructive procedures, attempts to regain useful elbow flexion are not indicated.

Before deciding on a given transfer, the power of the remaining muscles must be accurately determined. The selected muscle should possess sufficient power to flex the elbow against gravity, either independently or when reinforcing a weak muscle, usually the biceps. The effectiveness of such a transfer is increased if a flexion deformity of the elbow already exists, either as a result of a flexion contracture or by a surgically constructed posterior bone block, which limits extension by 30° to 60°.

Many types of transfer can be used. The procedures most commonly used are described below.

PROXIMAL TRANSPLANTATION OF FLEXOR OR EXTENSOR ORIGINS OF FOREARM MUSCLES OR BOTH

The Steindler flexorplasty, the operation of choice, often uses the common tendon of origin of the flexor pronator group (includes flexor carpi ulnaris, palmaris longus, flexor carpi radialis, flexor digitorum sublimis and superficial head of the pronator teres).[143] The common tendon of origin is detached and transferred to a more proximal point on the humerus. The method is rendered more effective by creating a posterior bone block on the lower end of the humerus, thereby limiting extension of the elbow to 90°. The chief disadvantage of this procedure is that a pronation deformity of the forearm frequently develops. The best results are obtained when the elbow flexors are only partially paralyzed and the finger and wrist flexors are normal (Fig. 14-28).

TRANSFER OF PECTORALIS MAJOR TO THE BICEPS

Transfer of Pectoralis Major Muscle Tendon of Insertion

The Brooks-Seddon procedure[95] is most useful when the clavicular portion of the pectoralis major remains strong whereas the distal or sternal portion is paralyzed (the

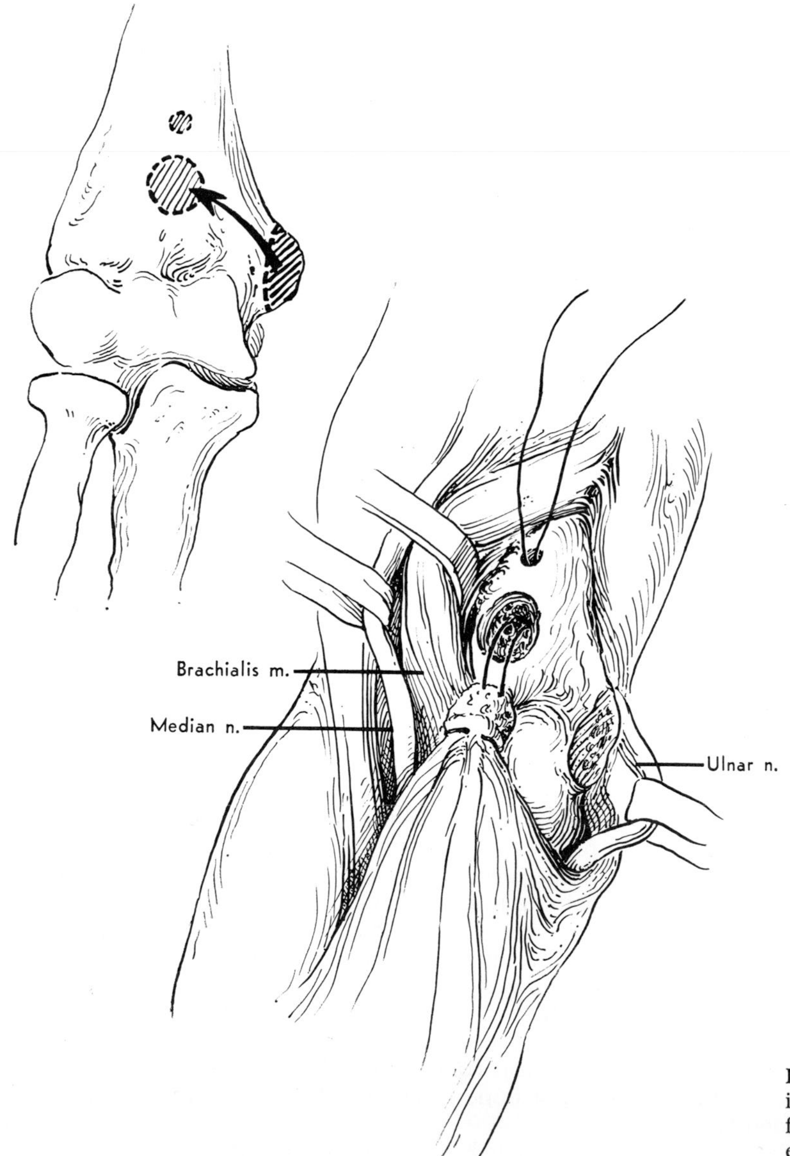

FIG. 14-28. The Steindler operation restores flexion to the elbow. The common tendon origin of the flexor-pronator group is removed with the medial epicondyle and transferred to a higher level.

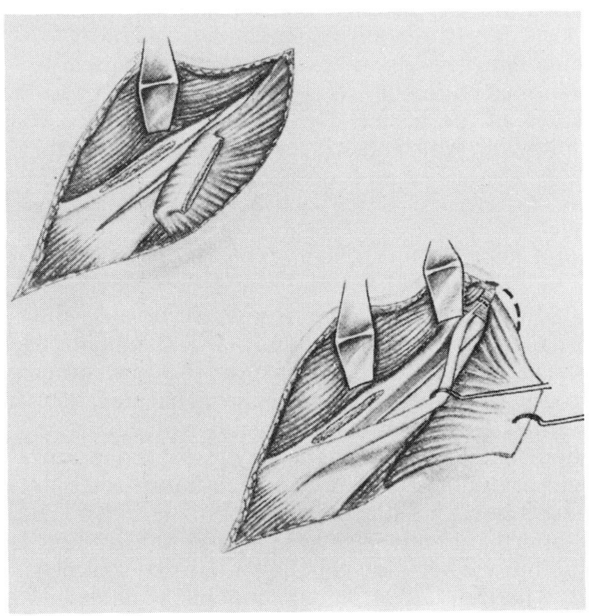

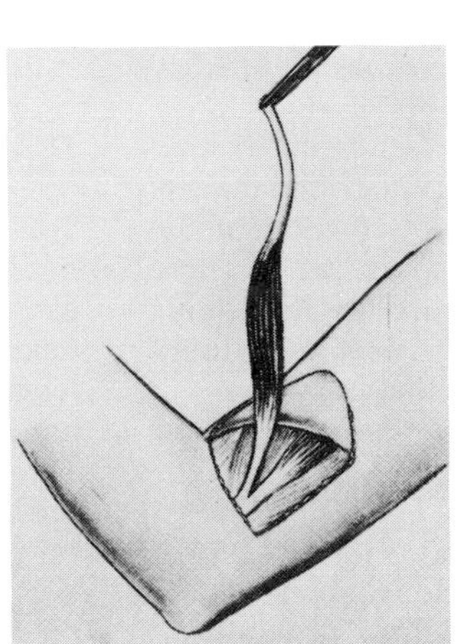

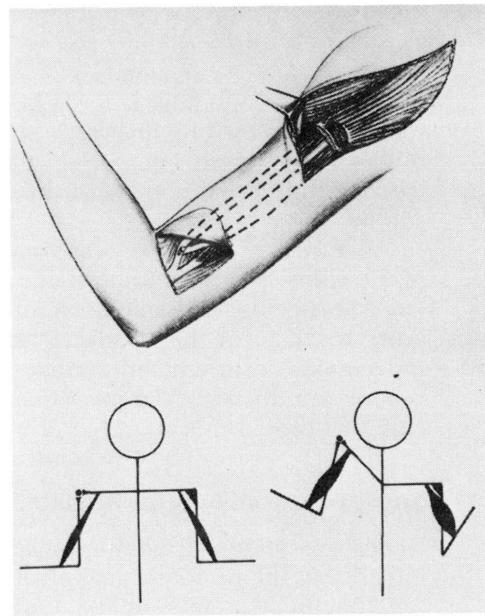

FIG. 14-29. Brooks-Seddon transfer of pectoralis major tendon for paralysis of elbow flexors. (*Top, left*) Insertion of pectoralis major is detached as close to bone as possible. (*Bottom, left*) Tendon of long head of biceps is exposed and divided at proximal end of bicipital groove. (*Center*) Tendor and muscle of long head of biceps are completely mobilized distally to tuberosity of radius by dividing all vessels and nerves that enter muscle proximal to elbow. (*Top, right*) Long head of biceps is passed through two slits in pectoralis major, is looped on itself so that its proximal tendon is brought into distal incision, and is sutured through slit in its distal tendon (*Bottom, right*) To avoid undesirable movements of shoulder during elbow flexion after this transfer, muscular control of shoulder and scapula must be good or shoulder must be fused. Left shoulder shown is flail; right has been fused. When transfer on left contracts, some of its force is wasted because of lack of control of shoulder, but on right, transfer moves only elbow. (Brooks DM, Seddon HJ: Pectoral transplantation for paralysis of the flexors of the elbow. J Bone Joint Surg 41-B:36, 1959)

clavicular and sternal portions have separate innervations). Its insertion is attached to the long head of the biceps. The latter muscle is converted into a long fibrous cord resembling tendon by severing most of its neurovascular connections (Fig. 14-29).

Technique. Two incisions are made: one extends from the lower end of the deltopectoral groove down to the junction of the upper and middle thirds of the arm, the second is L shaped and situated over the anteromedial aspect of the elbow.

Through the first incision the insertion of the pectoralis major is detached as close to the bone as possible. The muscle is mobilized from the chest wall by blunt dissection toward the clavicle. The deltoid is then retracted laterally and upward to allow exposure of the tendon of the long head of the biceps. The tendon is severed at the upper end of the bicipital groove and withdrawn into the wound. The belly of the long head of the biceps is freed from the short head by blunt and sharp dissection, and all vessels entering the muscle belly are ligated and divided. By retraction it is possible to mobilize the muscle to the lowest third of the arm. The remaining neurovascular connections are divided so that the tendon and muscle are completely free down to the tuberosity of the radius. The whole of the long head is then withdrawn through the lower incision. It will be found that in longstanding paralysis the muscle belly is adherent to the overlying fascia and that sharp dissection is required to free it. Until this has been done it may not be possible to flex the elbow by traction on the proximal tendon of the long head. The long head of the biceps is then replaced and its tendon, now visible through the upper incision, is passed through two slits in the pectoralis major and looped on itself so that the proximal tendon can be brought down again into the distal incision. The proximal tendon is then buttonholed into the distal tendon with the elbow acutely flexed. Silk stitches are inserted at the level of the tendon of the pectoralis major and at the distal junction of the tendons.

A plaster cast is retained for 3 weeks. Then reeducation is started, but care is taken to extend the elbow gradually so that active flexion above the right angle is maintained. It may be 2 or 3 months before full extension of the elbow is possible.

Transplantation of Part of Pectoralis Major Muscle

The Clark method consists of detaching the lowermost or sternal portion of origin of the pectoralis major from the chest wall and mobilizing the muscle toward the axilla as far as the nerve and blood supply will allow.[98] The muscle mass is then passed down the arm and attached to the biceps tendon.

This part of the muscle has a nerve and blood supply separate from the proximal part, and in certain instances other than poliomyelitis (*e.g.*, upper brachial plexus lesions) the sternal portion of the pectoralis major may still be active.

After transfer of the pectoralis major, attempted flexion of the elbow produces undesirable shoulder movements (*e.g.*, shrugging, adduction, or internal rotation of the arm) so that the hand strikes the chest wall. These movements occur when muscular control of the scapula is poor, and the shoulder joint should therefore be fused either before or after this type of transfer.

Total Pectoralis Major Muscle Transplant

Under exceptional conditions when the full functional integrity of the pectoralis major muscle is preserved and the functional ability of the entire limb depends on restoration and control of strong elbow flexion, the entire pectoralis major muscle can be mobilized and positioned in a manner so as to provide a very efficient muscle substitute.[121] The entire mass of muscle with its overlying fascial envelope is dissected free of clavicular and chest attachments down to the two neurovascular bundles of supply. The muscle is then rotated 90° about these pedicles, and its proximal portion attached to the acromion. The tendon of insertion is brought subcutaneously down the arm and anchored under maximum tension to the distal biceps tendon and/or biceps tuberosity of the radius, with the elbow flexed 135°. The muscle is now positioned so that it acts co-linear with the normal vector force of the biceps. The position is held for 6 weeks, following which muscle reeducation exercises are begun.

TRANSFER OF LATISSIMUS DORSI MUSCLE

Transfer of the latissimus dorsi is possible because the neurovascular bundle is long and can be mobilized easily.[113] The muscle is ideally suited to providing strong flexion to the elbow because its cross-sectional area, fiber length, and excursion compare favorably with either the biceps brachii for flexion or the triceps for extension. The origin of the latissimus dorsi, when transplanted to the biceps tendon (or radial tubercle), or to the olecranon process, directs the muscle so as to act in a straight line. When the muscle belly is too bulky, it must be trimmed medially. The free lateral border must not be violated, since a large branch of the thoracodorsal nerve runs adjacent to this edge. Dissection to free the muscle must proceed from below upward by carefully sweeping the finger beneath the muscle in such a manner as to avoid hooking the finger between the muscle and the thoracodorsal nerve and vessels (Fig. 14-30).

Technique. The patient is laid on the unaffected side. The incision starts in the loin, then extends onto the lateral margin of the latissimus dorsi and reaches the

FIG. 14-30. Hovnanian transfer of latissimus dorsi muscle for paralysis of biceps and brachialis muscles. (*Left*) Normal anatomy of axilla; note that thoracodorsal nerve and artery are long and can be easily mobilized. (*Top, right*) Skin incision. (*Bottom, right*) Origin and belly of latissimus dorsi have been transferred to arm, and origin has been sutured to biceps tendon and to other structures distal to elbow joint. (From Hovnanian AP: Latissimus dorsi transplantation for loss of flexion or extension at the elbow. Ann Surg 143:493, 1956)

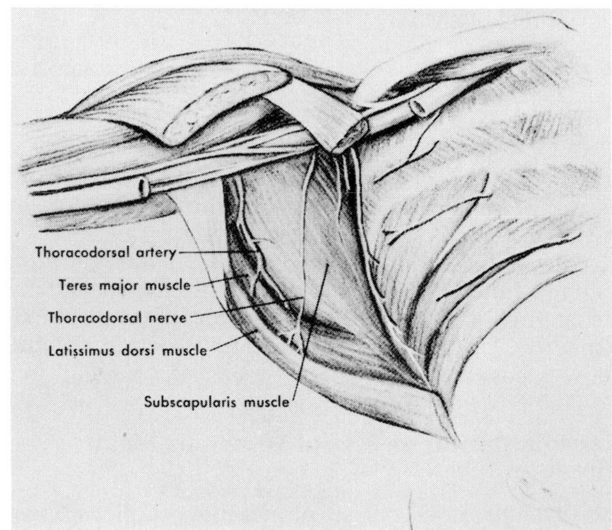

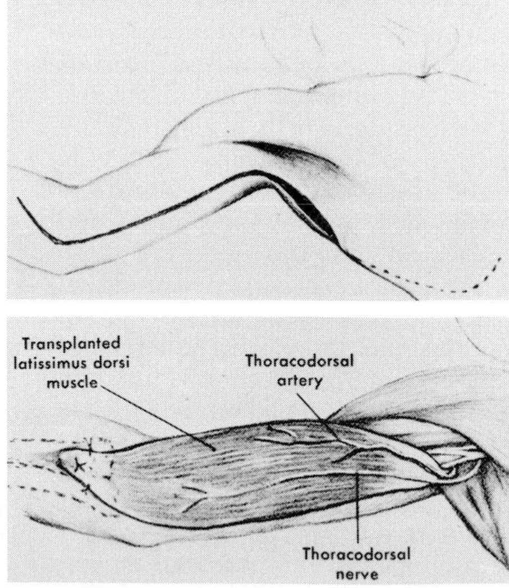

posterior axillary fold. From here the incision is prolonged across the neurovascular bundle of the arm and extended into the antecubital fossa.

The dorsal and lateral aspects of the latissimus dorsi are carefully dissected, leaving its fascial investment intact. The muscle is cut at the aponeurotic junction and detached from underlying abdominal muscles, severing several slips arising from the lower four ribs and the lower angle of the scapula. The upper margin is freed. In the upper third, where the neurovascular bundle enters the muscle belly, extreme caution is exerted to protect these vital structures—the thoracodorsal nerve and vessels running parallel between the serratus anterior and the latissimus dorsi supplying this muscle and the teres major. The anastomosing branches with the lateral thoracic vessels are ligated adjacent to the chest wall. The thoracodorsal nerve to the latissimus dorsi arises from the posterior cord of the brachial plexus, derives its fibers from the sixth, seventh, and eighth cervical roots, and is easily identified and freed. Its trunk is about 15 cm long and runs from the apex of the axilla toward the undersurface of the latissimus dorsi belly.

The muscle is freed from its origin and swung carefully to its bed in the arm. The vessels and nerve are protected from kinking. The intercostobrachial nerve and the lateral cutaneous branches of the third and fourth intercostals are divided. The rim of fibrous aponeurotic fascia of the muscle origin is now sutured to the biceps brachii tendon and the periosteal tissues of the radial tubercle. Firm fixation is ensured by several sutures in the lacertus fibrosus.

Postoperatively, the forearm is kept in flexion and pronation, and the arm is bandaged to the thorax, maintaining adduction. Passive and active exercises are started at the third or fourth week.

Certain principles of technique must be strictly observed to improve the mechanical efficiency of the transplanted muscle and provide strong elbow flexion. The caudal end (origin) of the latissimus dorsi must be removed with a segment of fascia to provide strong tissue, which must first be sutured to the biceps tendon of insertion at the elbow. Then the tendon of insertion of the latissimus dorsi is routed beneath the intact tendon of insertion of the pectoralis major and brought proximally and is fixed at the junction of the coracobrachialis with the coracoid process. The length of the transplant must be adjusted so that the elbow in its resting attitude maintains the elbow at 100° of flexion and the forearm in complete supination after both ends have been sutured. If the transplanted muscle is bulky, the biceps and brachialis muscles may be resected, creating an adequate defect within which the latissimus dorsi may be laid. This method of transplantation provides an effective bipolar transplant that acts in a direct line. Care should be exercised to avoid kinking or twisting of the neurovascular pedicle. (The reader should review the anatomical studies and surgical technique described by Zancolli and Mitre.[155])

Active strong extension of the elbow is required only under exceptional circumstances, such as for crutch walking, push-up support of the hands, as when rising from a bed or chair, or thrusting and pushing motions. When reaching overhead, extensor power only needs to be sufficiently strong to act against gravity. Otherwise weakness or paralysis of the triceps is of no significance, since gravity extends the elbow.

When good strength of elbow extension is necessary, only the latissimus dorsi appears to possess the required characteristics. Following such a transfer, the patient is often capable of performing push-ups.[102,113,138] When this muscle is unavailable, or strong power of extension is not essential, the brachioradialis alone or reinforced with the extensor carpi radialis can furnish the motor.

Technique of Latissimus Dorsi Transfer to Restore Elbow Extension. The procedure for freeing the latissimus dorsi and mobilizing its neurovascular pedicle is the same as that described for transfer to restore elbow flexion (Fig. 14-31).[113] The incision on the arm, however, is carried from the posterior axillary fold onto the posteromedial aspect of the arm without crossing over the brachial neurovascular bundle. After reaching the medial epicondyle, it is curved laterally over the posterior aspect of the shaft of the ulna.

After preparation of the arm bed for receiving the latissimus dorsi muscle belly, its aponeurotic fascia at the free end, representing the original origin of the muscle, is sutured to the triceps tendon, the periosteum of the olecranon, and the fascial covering over the extensor surface of the forearm.

The arm is immobilized in extension and bandaged to the side of the body. Exercises are started at the fourth week.

THE FOREARM

Fixed pronation is the main disabling deformity of the forearm. Supinator function may be restored by tendon transference to the dorsal and radial aspects of the radius. The pronator teres and the flexor carpi radialis are commonly used as motors. Their tendons are sutured together and routed subcutaneously about the ulnar side of the forearm and then dorsally across to the opposite side, and finally they are fixed to the radius on its radial and volar aspects.[149]

WRIST AND HAND

Following poliomyelitis, as a rule, both flexors and extensors are involved and rarely is the paralysis so isolated that a sufficiently strong muscle is available for transference. Arthrodesis of the wrist will overcome a flexion deformity and provide a mechanical advantage for weakly functioning finger flexors. Any functioning wrist flexors or extensors can then be used for transfers.

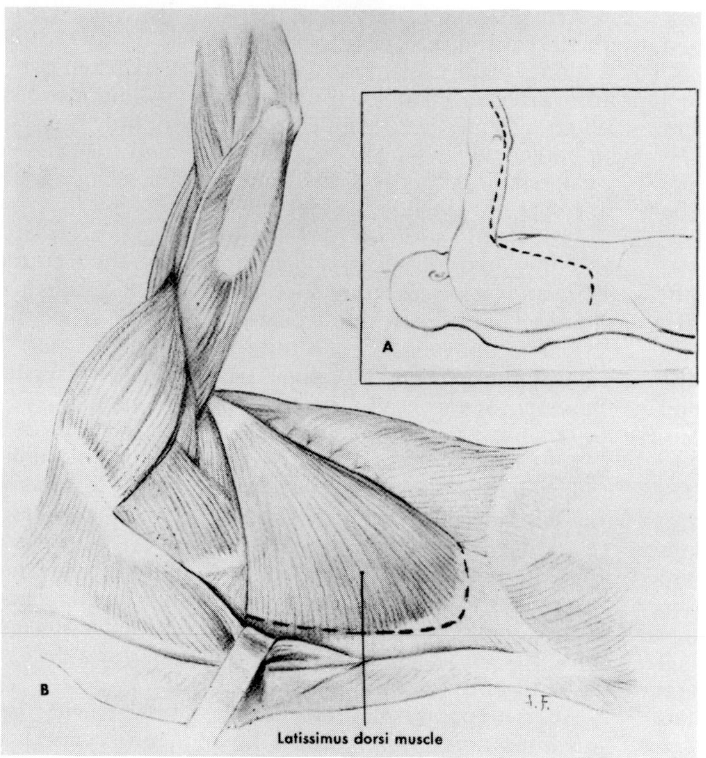

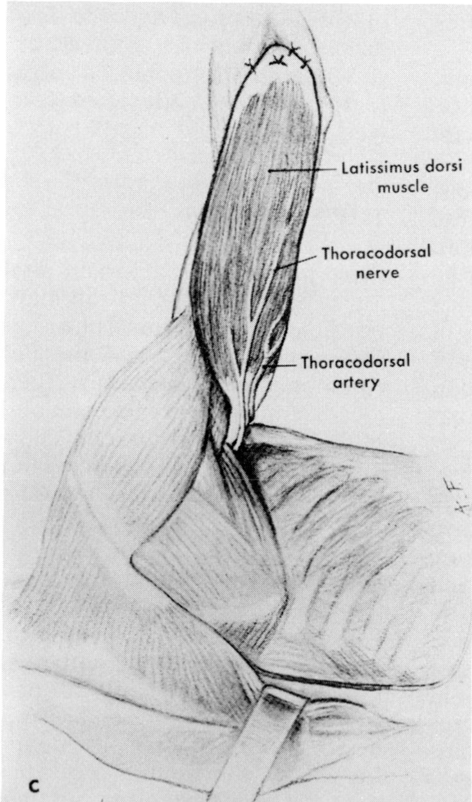

FIG. 14-31. Hovnanian transfer of latissimus dorsi muscle for paralysis of triceps. (*A, Broken line*) Skin incision, (*B, Broken line*) incision to free origin of latissimus dorsi. (*C*) Origin and belly of latissimus dorsi have been transferred to arm, and origin has been sutured to triceps tendon, periosteum of olecranon, and connective tissue septa on extensor surface of forearm. (Hovnanian AP: Latissimus dorsi transplantation for loss of flexion or extension at the elbow. Ann Surg 143:493, 1956)

Restoration of opposition to the thumb is essential for pinch and grasp. (See Chapter 25.)

THE LOWER EXTREMITY

A wide variety of deformities develop in poliomyelitis as a result of muscle imbalance and widespread soft tissue contractures (Fig. 14-32). During the acute and convalescent stages of poliomyelitis, the patient lies supine in the so-called frogleg position with the hips flexed, abducted, and externally rotated; the knees flexed; and the feet in an equinovarus position. This position may be assumed because of muscle spasm involving the hamstrings, hip flexors, tensor fasciae latae, and hip abductors. Initially, contracture of the intermuscular septae and the fasciae enveloping the muscles takes place. Within their covering fascia, the muscles may not be involved at all in causing the contracture, since at surgery after the fascia is incised and retracts, the muscle is found to be in a state of relaxation. Later, a partially paralyzed muscle becomes shortened because the paralyzed fibers are replaced by fibrous tissue. Adaptive shortening of muscles develops even later. Longstanding deformities caused by muscle imbalance and soft tissue contractures, and which develop mainly during the growth period of infancy and childhood, gradually develop structural bone changes that resist correction by soft tissue procedures alone.[90]

The most common deformities of the lower extremity in the postpoliomyelitic child include the following:

Hip flexion-abduction deformity
Pelvic tilt or obliquity, as a result of hip abduction contracture; the opposite side of the pelvis rides high, and the hip is adducted and may subluxate.
Exaggerated lumbar lordosis and anterior inclination of the pelvis secondary to hip flexion contracture. Clinically, this is demonstrated by placing the child recumbent with the lower extremities fully extended and the lordotic spine arching forward from the surface of the examining table. When the affected hip is fully flexed, the lordosis is reduced and the back lies flat against the tabletop. Another method of demonstrating lumbar lordosis is to place the child in the prone position with the lower extremities hanging dependent over the end of the table. This eliminates the lordosis, but when the affected hip is extended and placed in line with the trunk, the lordotic curve becomes manifest. When the deformity is of long standing, structural bone changes develop about the lumbosacral area and these maneuvers fail to change the deformity.
Lumbar scoliosis, convex toward the affected side.
External torsion of the leg on the femur
Genuvalgum and flexion
Equinovarus of the foot

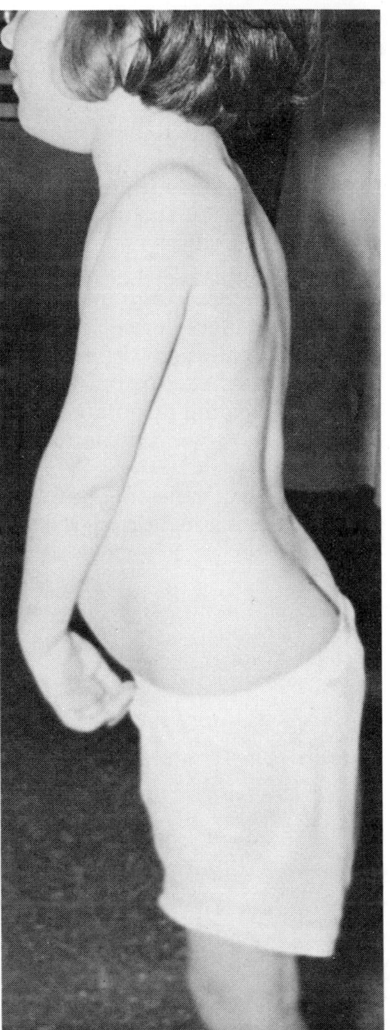

FIG. 14-32. Postpoliomyelitis. Scoliosis, weak abdominals and intercostals, pelvic tilt, and iliotibial band contracture are evident.

Prevention of deformities during the acute and convalescent stages can be accomplished by skilled nursing care and physical therapy. Bivalved casts maintain the joints in the neutral position. A horizontal bar between the casts controls rotation at the hips and legs. The knees should be in slight flexion to prevent recurvatum deformity. Minimal contractures can be overcome by passive stretching daily. Once the deformity has developed, surgical procedures are the only means of correction.

Surgical Principles. These deformities are due to muscle imbalance; to contractures of fascial structures, especially of the iliotibial band, and, to a lesser degree, of muscles, and, with the passing of time, particularly during the growth period; and to structural changes in the bones and joints. Changes in bone architecture develop concomitantly with increasing severity of the contractures, so that it is essential to recognize and treat the deformity at an early date by soft tissue procedures. At a late date, coxa valga and anteversion develop at the hip; in the opposite hip, the femoral head may repeatedly erode the acetabular rim and may subluxate and dislocate. The pelvis and lumbar spine become distorted and therefore prevent full correction of scoliosis and forward pelvic inclination by release of soft tissue contractures. At the knee, abnormal anterior inclination of the upper tibial surface is associated with genu recurvatum and posterior subluxation. Within the foot, contractures of the calf muscles and of the plantar aponeurosis are frequently associated, and structural bone changes develop in long-standing muscle imbalance (*e.g.*, calcaneus deformity in paralysis of the triceps surae). After structural bone changes have created a rigid unyielding deformity, bone resections are required in addition to soft tissue procedures.

A deformity can reduce the effectiveness of a muscle that is only partially paralyzed. For example, a hip flexion contracture in the presence of a weak gluteus maximus will interfere with the action of residual functioning muscle fibers. Once the hip flexion deformity is overcome, gluteus maximus power can be redeveloped.

The multiplicity of deforming factors throughout the lower extremities makes it mandatory that the potential for correcting each be properly evaluated and a schedule of procedures in the proper sequence be prepared. The objective is to improve good balance, stability, and gait.

Correction of hip deformity and reestablishing muscle balance appears to have priority before the feasibility of other surgical procedures about the knee, foot, and lower back can be considered. Overcoming a hip flexion deformity and providing good abductor and extensor power about the hip is absolutely essential to restoring good body balance and should precede the correction of the scoliosis and lordosis. Spine fusion can be undertaken only after deformities of the hip and knee are corrected. If the spine fusion is done initially, the scoliotic and

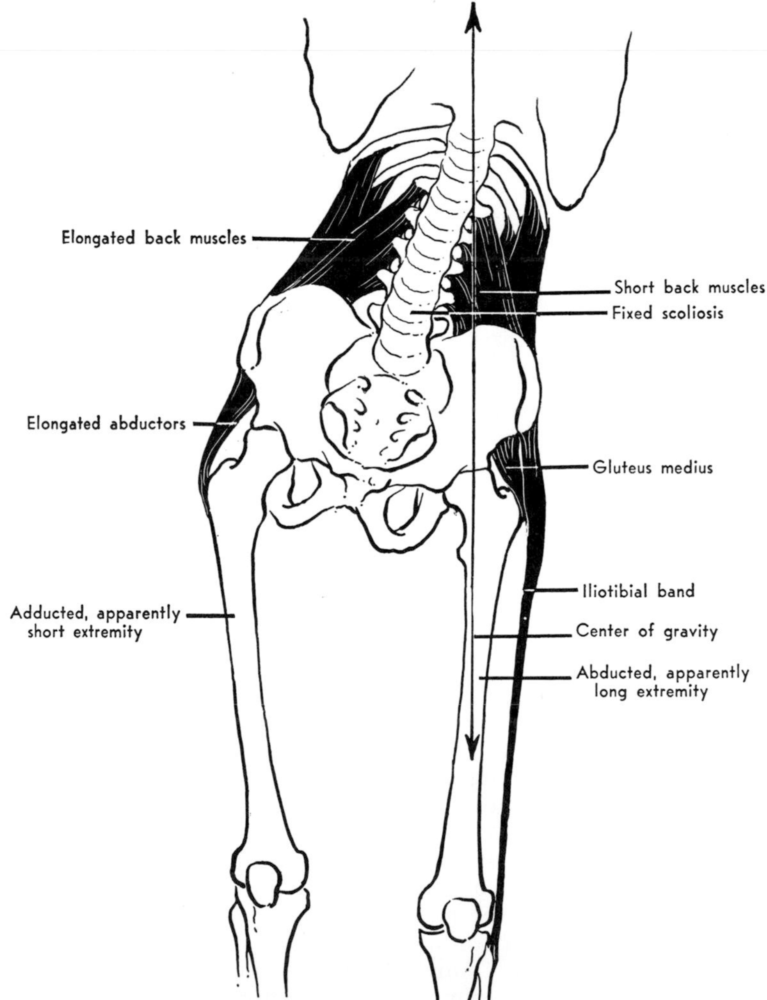

FIG. 14-33. Iliotibial band contracture, showing pelvic obliquity, lumbar scoliosis, displacement of the center of gravity, and stretched, elongated contralateral muscles.

lordotic deformity will recur in the presence of these other deformities. Following anterior soft tissue release at the hip and reinforcement of extensor-abductor power by tendon (or fascial extension) transfer (*e.g.*, iliopsoas, erector spinae, external oblique, tensor fasciae latae) a spine fusion may not be necessary.

Resection of contracted fascial structures are insufficient in correcting more than minimal deformities. Shortened muscles must be released or lengthened, and muscle balance restored. Resection of the iliotibial band will reduce hip flexion-abduction and knee flexion–external tibial rotation deformity only about 50%. Soft tissue release over the front of the hip and tendon transfers is necessary. After bone structural changes have taken place, bone resections must be supplemented by tendon transfers and removal of active deforming muscle forces; otherwise, the deformity will recur.

THE HIP

Flexion and abduction contracture with a variable degree of external rotation is the most frequent deformity about the hip and is due mainly to:

Contracture of the iliotibial band (Fig. 14-33). The band runs anterior and lateral to the hip joint so that its shortening causes flexion of the hip joint. Early in mild contracture, correction can be secured by partial resection of the iliotibial band. At the distal end of the thigh, several centimeters of the band and its attached lateral intermuscular septum are resected.[154] For moderate contracture, extensive removal of the iliotibial band and the lateral intermuscular septum is required.

Contracture of anterior soft tissues at the hip. These include the fascia enveloping the muscles, contracture of the rectus femoris, tensor fascia femoris, sartorius, and iliopsoas and the capsule.

Weakness or paralysis of the gluteus maximus and medius. Paralysis of each muscle alone is rare. Paralysis of the gluteus medius results in loss of abductor power so that when the weight is borne on the affected extremity, the trunk lists over the affected hip for balance, while the opposite side of the pelvis sags (positive Trendelenburg). A side-lurching gait is typical. Paralysis of the gluteus maximus causes the pelvis to incline forward, exaggerating the lumbar lordosis since the trunk must bend backward for balance. Since the innervation of both gluteus maximum and medius is similar, their involvement is coexistent as a rule.

Flexion-Abduction Contracture of the Hip

Prevention. During the acute and convalescent subacute stages, the patient lies supine on a firm mattress, with the hips in neutral rotation, slight abduction, and extension. A posterior plaster shell is applied to the trunk and both lower extremities or just to the lower extremities where the shells are connected by a bar to control rotation. The knees are slightly flexed to prevent recurvatum. All joints are placed through a full range of passive motion. If contracture of the iliotibial band can be detected early, the deformity can no longer be corrected by conservative means.[115] Simple local resection of the iliotibial band and its corresponding attached portion of the lateral intermuscular septum[154] is effective for minor contractures, but recurrences are frequent. Therefore, anterior hip soft tissue release (Soutter) should be combined with removal of the entire iliotibial band and followed with corrective casts. Since complete correction in severe contracture deformity cannot be attained by these procedures alone, tendon transfer to reinforce the gluteus medius and maximum should be added.

The iliopsoas muscle is the most effective muscle for transfer, because its innervation is quite different from that of the glutei, is often preserved in poliomyelitis, possesses good power, and when transferred acts in a direct line to the greater trochanter. When the gluteus medius is chiefly involved and abductor power is the chief requirement, the Mustard procedure of iliopsoas transfer is appropriate. When both glutei are involved, and both abduction and extension must be provided, the Sharrard method of transfer is best. The muscle is transposed through a large hole in the ilium to a new position from the point at which the tendon is drawn through the greater trochanter from posterior to anterior.

When the iliopsoas is not suitable for transfer, the alternatives are the following:

For abduction—external oblique of the abdomen and transposing the tensor fasciae latae to a new origin over the posterior portion of the iliac crest

For extension—the erector spinae muscle extended by a fascial transplant brought upward from iliotibial band and fixed to a subperiosteal tunnel or bone groove just distal to base of greater trochanter

It should be stressed that release of contracted soft tissue structures over the anterior aspect of the hip must always precede or be done at the same time as resection of the iliotibial band and tendon transfers.

Release of Soft Tissue Contractures at the Hip Joint. Through an iliofemoral incision, all fascial limiting structures are incised transversely, and, if necessary, contracted muscles are released at their origins, or their tendons of attachment are severed.[141] Following this procedure, the flexion deformity should be considerably corrected.

At the iliac crest, the origins of the tensor fascia lata and gluteus medius and minimus are exposed. The fascial investments of these muscles may be sectioned transversely, or the muscle origins may be severed, and the muscle reflected from the ilium, and allowed to displace distally. The fascia overlying the sartorius is often very tight and is incised transversely. Similarly, the rectus femoris covering fascia may require incision; or the anterior superior spine with its attached sartorius may be resected along with the origin of the sartorius, and the direct and reflected heads of the rectus femoris may be sectioned.

If the hip cannot be extended at this point without increasing the lumbar lordosis, the capsule must be divided obliquely from proximally to distally. Usually the iliopsoas insertion need not be disturbed unless the muscle is to be used as a motor to restore abduction and extension.

If the ilium has been completely denuded about the crest, the bare bone is resected before the abdominal muscles are sutured to the edge of the gluteal muscles and the tensor fasciae latae over the remaining rim of the ilium.[96] To preserve the iliac apophysis in the skeletally immature child, the bone is resected as a wedge from beneath the anterior portion of the apophysis.

Treatment of the Iliotibial Band. Irwin has stated:

> The iliotibial band with its allied structures is probably the greatest deforming factor in the lower trunk and lower extremity involvement following an attack of poliomyelitis. This is true only in those cases which had no care or in which treatment was inadequate during the acute and early convalescent stage.[115]

Pathologic Anatomy. The iliotibial band is a thickened portion of the fascia lata along its lateral aspect. The fascia lata arises from the coccyx, the sacrum, the iliac crest, Poupart's ligament, and the pubic ramus. Between two layers it encloses the gluteus maximus and the tensor fascia femoris, giving attachment to the latter muscle and most of the former. The fibers of the fascia converge to form the iliotibial band along the lateral side of the thigh. It is continuous medially with the lateral intermuscular septum, which attaches to the linea aspera. Distally, it gives origin to the short head of the biceps. At the level of the knee joint, it spreads out and attaches to the lateral tibial condyle and the head of the fibula. The iliotibial band lies in a plane anterior to the hip joint and posterior to the knee.

Involvement of the attached muscles is responsible for the increased tension under which it is placed during the acute and convalescent states. The taut band is perceived by deep palpation while adducting and extending the thigh. Spasm in the gluteus maximus is demonstrated by resistance to passively flexing the hip while the knee is fully extended. Spasm in the short head of the biceps is demonstrated by flexing the hip (which relaxes the iliopsoas band) and finding resistance to extension at the knee. The patient assumes the most comfortable position in which the thigh is flexed, abducted, and externally rotated at the hip while the knee is flexed. This relaxes the tension on the band. If tension is not overcome by stretching during the acute stage, band contracture becomes progressive and permanent deformity ensues, including the following:

Flexion and abduction contracture of the hip, because the band lies in a plane anterior and lateral to the hip

External rotation of the thigh. The external rotators of the hip become contracted in the position which the patient assumes for comfort.

Genu valgum and flexion contracture of the knee. The compression forces acting on the outer half of the epiphyseal plates probably retard longitudinal growth laterally while growth on the medial side continues unimpeded. The band lying in a plane posterior to the knee and spasm of the short head of the biceps exerts a flexing force.

External rotation of the tibia. The direction of the lowest fibers obliquely downward and forward to insert on the anterolateral aspect of the tibia produces a torsional force. The tibia may subluxate posteriorly.

Short leg. This may be due to compression forces acting on the lower femoral and the upper tibial epiphyseal plates.

Varus deformity of the foot. Because the axes of the knee and the ankle do not lie in the same horizontal plane, any above-knee orthosis in which the lateral uprights are straight fitted to such an extremity will force the foot into varus. Varus deformity is also associated with loss of evertor power in the foot.

Pelvic obliquity, increased lumbar lordosis, scoliosis. When the extremity is positioned in the weight-bearing position, the contracted flexed hip will incline the pelvis forward and carry the lumbosacral junction forward, increasing the lumbar lordosis. The opposite end of the pelvis displaces upward and the lumbar spine deviates toward the affected hip.

Treatment. Prevention demands energetic stretching of the iliotibial band during the acute and convalescent stages. Treatment is continued until the hip and knee joints can be carried through their full range of motion. The full length and extensibility of the iliotibial band is thereby preserved.

Surgical treatment is necessary when increased tension and progressive contracture become evident. A section of the iliotibial band and its attached lateral intermuscular septum must be resected and the deformities corrected by traction and casts. This procedure should be preceded or accompanied by release of soft tissue contractures over the anterior aspect of the hip joint. If the deformities are severe, and gluteal weakness or paralysis is demonstrable, tendon transfers are indicated.

To resect the iliotibial band and correct the deformity two short leg casts from the tibial tubercle to the toes are applied the day before operation. At surgery a 7-cm portion of the band is removed just proximal to the knee and a portion of fascia lata covering the vastus lateralis is either divided or excised. The corresponding portion of the lateral intermuscular septum is excised to its attachment to the femur. Contracture of the septum also contributes to flexion deformity of the knee. If necessary, the lateral patellar retinaculum is also divided.

When external rotatory subluxation at the knee is present, the biceps femoris should be lengthened, and often Z-lengthening of the fibular collateral ligament may also be necessary. At this point an attempt at reduction is made by forcibly extending and internally rotating the knee.

A Kirschner wire is passed transversely through the supracondylar area of each femur, and the short leg casts are reapplied and extended to the upper thighs, incorporating the wires in the casts. The affected thigh is held in abduction and flexion, and traction is applied through a Kirschner bow to the unaffected leg to bring the pelvis to the horizontal level. The body portion of a spica cast is applied and attached to the well-leg cast. The trunk, the pelvis, and the well leg are now held securely. Next, the contracted leg is adducted, extended, and internally rotated until considerable resistance is felt and the double spica is completed. Further wedging of the cast on the affected side at intervals of 3 to 5 days secures complete correction.

Reduction of deformity requires less force and is more effective if release of soft tissue contractures at the front and lateral aspects of the hip is done as a preliminary step, or is done at the same time. Moreover, in severe deformity with gluteal weakness, tendon transfer, particularly of the iliopsoas, adds a dynamic corrective force, which greatly increases the degree of correction while providing stability for the hip.

Iliopsoas Transfer. Only the iliopsoas possesses sufficient strength to replace a paralyzed gluteus muscle, although it never can imitate the powerful action of the replaced muscle.[127,128] At the most, although the gluteal limp is lessened, normal balance is never restored. The operation has its greatest usefulness only when the glutei are partially paralyzed, so that reinforcement markedly improves stability and gait. The strength and range of abduction is materially improved. The ideal situation for lateral iliopsoas transfer is a patient with weak hip abductors but good gluteus maximus, sartorius, iliopsoas, quadriceps, and abdominal muscles.

Mustard Procedure. The Mustard procedure is indicated when the power of abduction must be improved. (Fig. 14-34). The hip is approached by a Smith-Petersen incision. The origins of the sartorius and the rectus femoris are removed. The femoral nerve and vessels are retracted medially. The insertion of the iliopsoas at the lesser trochanter is severed, removing a flake of bone with the tendon. Tendon and muscle are reflected upward. A notch is cut in the ilium between the superior and inferior iliac spines that is large enough to accommodate the muscle belly, which is drawn through and attached to the greater trochanter. Postoperatively, the hip is maintained in abduction for several weeks until the new attachment is secure.

Sharrard Procedure. The iliopsoas muscle is transferred posterior and lateral to the hip joint to provide extension as well as abduction, thus balancing the remaining flexors (sartorius, rectus femoris, pectineus) and adductors (Fig. 14-35).[140] The operation is especially indicated when hip flexors and adductors are strong, but the abductors and extensors are weak or paralyzed. The procedure is also indicated for the more common abduction-flexion deformity of the hip of the poliomyelitic patient, particularly when some abductor power is present and the gluteus maximus is paralyzed.

In the presence of strong flexors and adductors at the hip, a normal iliopsoas muscle, particularly in the presence of a valgus deformity of the femoral neck, produces a strong external rotatory force which is capable of inducing the femoral head to subluxate or dislocate anteriorly out of the acetabulum.[142] Posterior transfer of the iliopsoas eliminates this deforming force and provides a corrective force, which prevents this complication.

For an adduction deformity, the operation is preceded by an adductor tenotomy. A varus osteotomy may be added. Flexion deformity may require anterior soft tissue release.

The incision passes along the anterior two thirds of the iliac crest and follows the medial border of the sartorius. Incision of the gluteal fascia along the middle and posterior thirds of the iliac crest reveals the underlying atrophic gluteus medius. The fascia covering the tensor fascia femoris may be left untouched, unless it needs release for a fixed-flexion contracture. The gluteus medius and minimus are elevated subperiosteally from the outer surface of the ilium, exposing the posterior surface of the bone through which the iliopsoas will later be transplanted.

In the thigh, incising the deep fascia exposes the sartorius. The lateral cutaneous nerve of the thigh is identified and preserved. A small vessel that crosses the origin of the sartorius is divided. For severe fixed-flexion deformity, the origin of the sartorius is divided from the anterior-superior iliac spine and the tendon of the rectus femoris may be divided, especially when extension deformity of the knee is present.

The lower border of the inguinal ligament is defined and the layer of deep fascia extending distal to it is cleared away to expose the femoral nerve as it emerges from the pelvis. The femoral nerve is mobilized toward the lateral side. All its branches except one pass downward and laterally. The sensory branch passing medially may be divided if necessary.

The inner aspect of the false pelvis is exposed by detaching the abdominal muscles from the anterior two thirds of the iliac crest. In the young child it is convenient to detach the cartilaginous apophysis of the iliac crest to provide a firm base for suturing at the conclusion of the operation. The whole of the abdominal wall and its

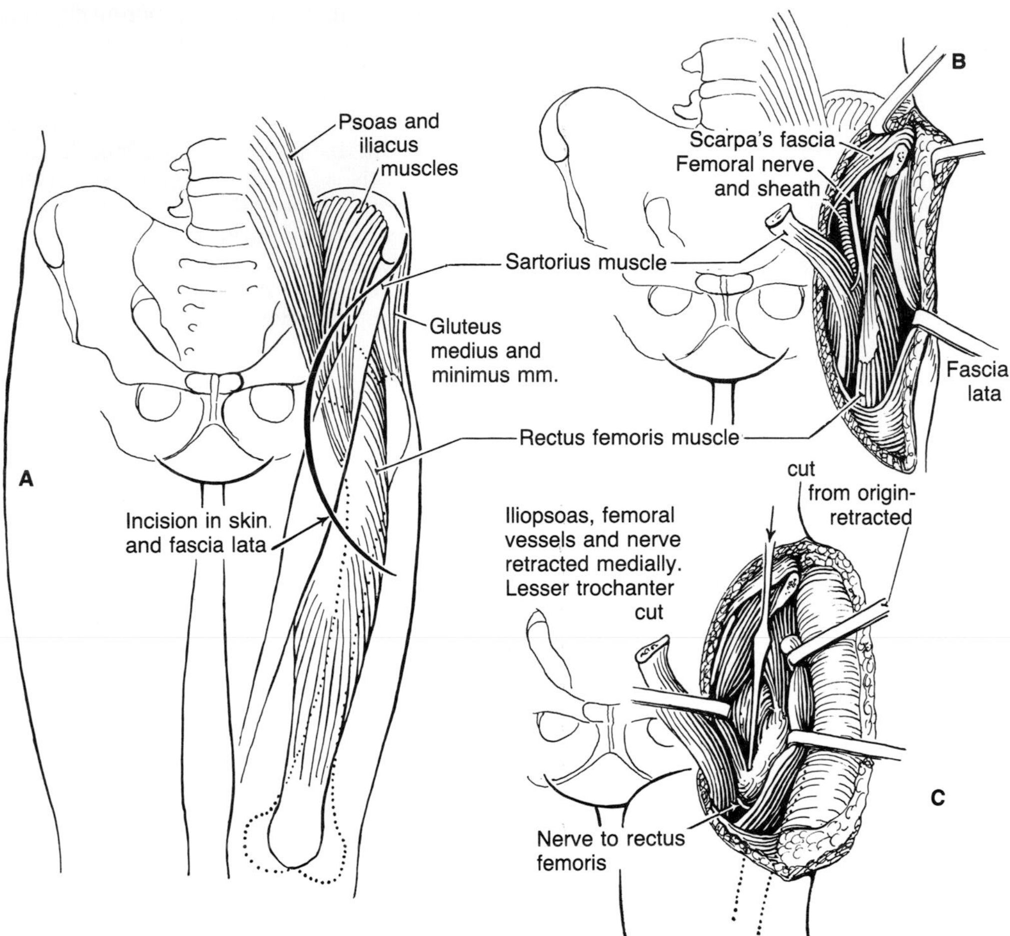

FIG. 14-34. Iliopsoas transfer. (Mustard WT: Iliopsoas transfer for weakness of hip abductors: Preliminary report. J. Bone Joint Surg 34A:647, 1952) (*Continued on facing page*)

contents, including the inguinal canal, can then be displaced upward, with the dissection following the plane between the extraperitoneal fat and fascia and the iliacus. Only one small vessel passes between the two surfaces and requires division. Retraction allows the whole of the iliacus and the pelvic course of the femoral nerve and psoas muscle to be exposed.

The psoas muscle is followed distally and its tendon is defined as it passes over the hip joint. Distal to this the tendon dives back steeply toward the lesser trochanter between the femoral nerve and vessels. The hip is flexed and laterally rotated to bring the lesser trochanter forward. By careful retraction medially of the femoral vessels and laterally of the femoral nerve, it is possible in some limbs to reach and define the lesser trochanter without ligation of the lateral femoral circumflex vessels. In others these vessels should be very carefully dissected out, ligated, and divided. The whole of the iliopsoas tendon can now be seen. Only half of the tendon is attached to the lesser trochanter itself; the remainder separates off into a deeper layer after it has passed across the hip joint to be attached to the shaft of the femur. The lesser trochanter with its attached portion of psoas tendon is detached with an osteotome. The deeper separate portion of the psoas tendon is then divided and the whole psoas tendon mobilized upward into the pelvis, the bursa deep to it indicating the plane of separation. The fibers of the iliacus that are inserted into the iliopsoas tendon are preserved, but that part of the iliacus whose fibers proceed independently toward the femoral shaft is cut at the level of the inguinal ligament.

Dissection proceeds up into the false pelvis. The femoral nerve is mobilized from the iliacus and psoas, with care being taken to preserve the nerve supply to the iliacus, which usually arises by two branches; one is given off soon after the femoral nerve enters the pelvis and the other about halfway through its pelvic course. The distal branch may have to be dissected up to some

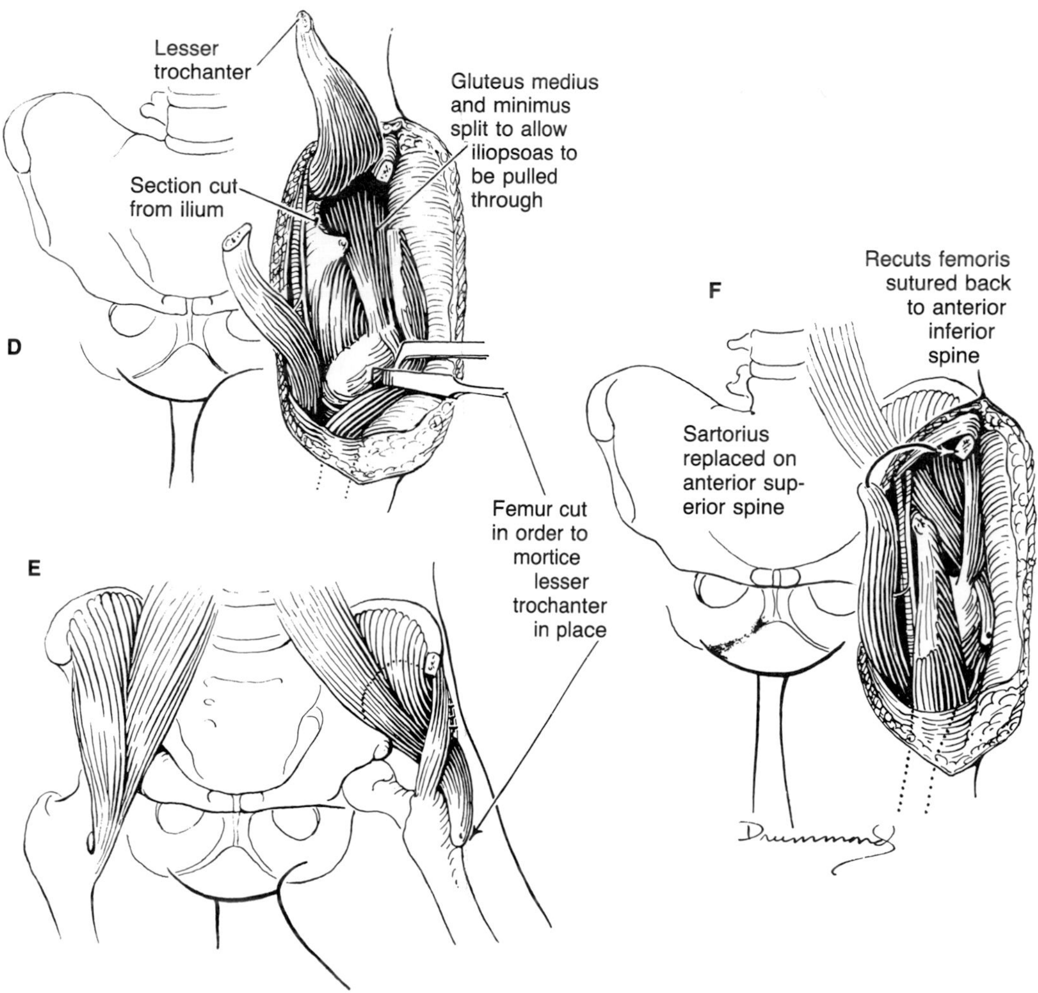

FIG. 14-34. *(Continued)*

extent from the main nerve. The hip is flexed to relax the femoral nerve so that the iliopsoas tendon and the attached trochanter can be passed beneath it to its lateral side. The origin of the iliacus is detached extraperiosteally from the inner aspect of the false pelvis by blunt and sharp dissection. It detaches easily, its origin being from the periphery of the pelvis, but it is important that it be separated from the ilium posteriorly so that the whole of its origin is free. When this has been achieved, the whole false pelvis, the anterior aspect of the sacroiliac joint, the brim of the true pelvis and the extraperitoneal fat lateral to the fifth lumbar vertebra can be seen. The iliacus has now been detached at both ends, although it still retains all its nerve supply and a sufficient blood supply, particularly on its deep surface, from branches of the iliolumbar vessels. In older children, one branch from vessels supplying the deep surface of the iliacus passes into the nutrient foramen on the inner surface of the iliac wing, and this vessel needs to be divided and coagulated. Most of the anterior two thirds of the iliac bone is now exposed on both sides.

With an angled osteotome, a hole is made in the ilium immediately lateral to the sacroiliac joint. The width of the hole should be slightly more than one third of that of the iliac wing. It should be oval, its length being about half as much again as its width and its long axis lying in the longitudinal plane. The iliopsoas tendon and the whole of the iliacus muscle are then passed through the hole. To ensure ease of passage, the origin of the iliacus is passed through the hole first; the iliopsoas tendon and psoas muscle easily follow. The whole of the iliacus muscle now lies outside the pelvis, but it is still attached to its nerve and vessels, which also pass through the bone opening.

The new insertion of the iliopsoas tendon is the posterolateral aspect of the greater trochanter. By passing a finger from the gluteal region distally into a bursa deep to the gluteus maximus tendon, the posterolateral aspect

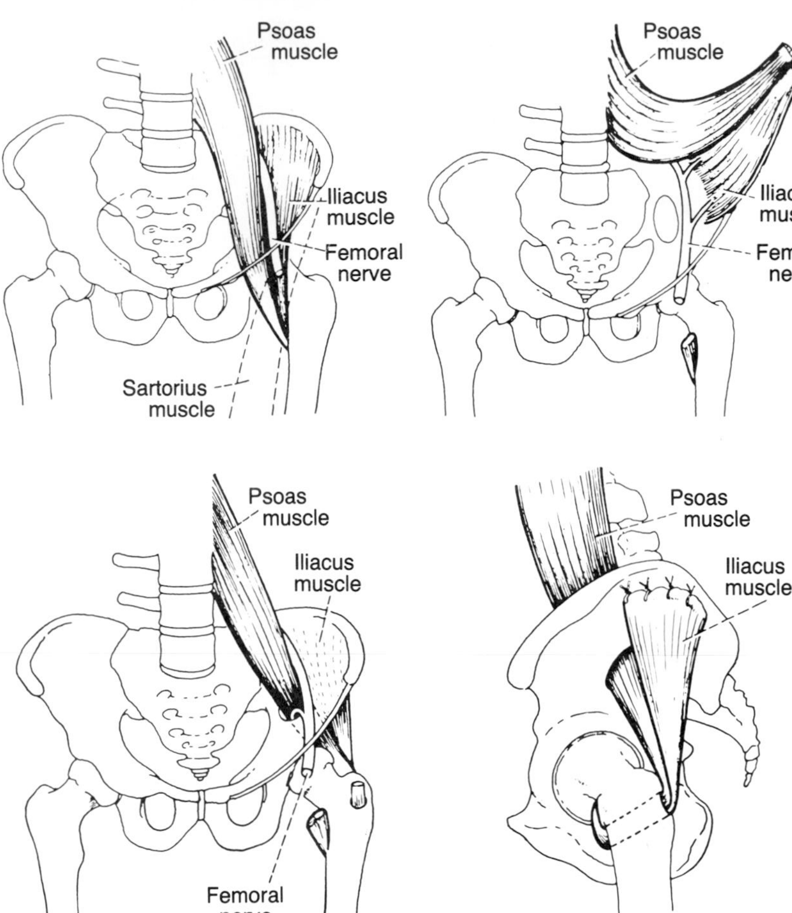

FIG. 14-35. Iliopsoas transfer, Sharrard procedure. (*Top, left*) Normal anatomy. (*Top, right*) Psoas and iliacus muscles freed and foramen constructed in ilium anterior to sacroiliac joint. Branches of femoral nerve protected. (*Bottom, left*) Entire iliacus brought outside of ilium keeping its nerve of innervation free; psoas muscle and iliopsoas tendon brought through; both muscles passed beneath the femoral nerve. (*Bottom, right*) Final result. The origin of the iliacus is attached proximally near crest of ilium. The iliopsoas tendon is attached through a hole in the femur and brought from posterior to anterior. (Sharrard WJW: Posterior iliopsoas transplantation in the treatment of paralytic dislocation of the hip. J Bone Joint Surg 46B:426, 1964)

of the greater trochanter is identified by touch. The corresponding anterior aspect of the trochanter is exposed by dissecting through the fascia lata. A hole is drilled or bored through the greater trochanter from anterior to posterior. A strong silk suture is attached by a clove hitch to the fragment of lesser trochanter and to the iliopsoas tendon, which is then passed through the greater trochanter from behind forward. A wire-passer cannula is inserted in the bone tunnel until its point protrudes in the gluteal region. A wire is then inserted in the cannula, is attached to the silk suture, and pulls the tendon through the cannula. The tendon is brought to the front of the greater trochanter. While the hip is extended and abducted in neutral rotation, the tendon is made taut and is fixed to the anterior surface of the trochanter by several strong sutures. It is important to ensure that the line of tendon pull is straight from within the abdomen through the hole in the ilium to the greater trochanter.

When the iliopsoas tendon has been firmly fixed to the femur, the origin of the iliacus is sutured to the ilium just below the iliac crest in a position corresponding to the origin of the gluteus medius. After tendon fixation, the hip should be gently moved in abduction and adduction and in flexion and extension to demonstrate that the psoas muscle is moving correspondingly inside the pelvis.

Closure is achieved by suturing the abdominal muscles and gluteal fascia back to the iliac crest. The space between the inguinal ligament and the pubic bone is closed by suturing the inguinal ligament to the iliopectineal line. Deep fascia, fat, and skin are sutured. A plaster spica extending to the toes of the affected side is applied with the hip joint in full abduction and extension and in neutral or medial rotation, depending on the degree of femoral neck anteversion. All fixation is discarded after 4 or 5 weeks.

Gluteus Maximus Paralysis. The major extensor force to the hip joint is provided by the gluteus maximus (the hamstrings by their attachment to the ischial tuberosity also extend to the hip). The loss of extensor power while the flexors are active causes the pelvis to incline forward, and flexion contracture of the hip ensues. The exaggeration of the lumbar lordosis caused by pelvic inclination is further increased by contracture of the erector spinae and its investing fascia. In gait, the body lurches backward to attain body balance.

Gluteus maximus weakness can be demonstrated by

placing the patient in the prone position with the lower extremities hanging downward from the edge of the examining table and the knees flexed to nullify hamstring action. The patient is then asked to extend at the hip against gravity and resistance. When extension of the hip against gravity is impossible, lesser degrees of muscle power can be brought out by placing the patient in the side-lying position to eliminate the effect of gravity.

With paralyzed hip extensors and residual power in the flexors, hip flexion deformity recurs following release of the anterior structures of the hip or fasciotomy of the iliotibial band, or both procedures, despite careful post-operative treatment. Restoration of extensor power to the hip can be achieved by erector spinae transfer to the greater trochanter. The fascia of the iliotibial band is used to extend the tendon of insertion to the trochanter. When the tensor fascia femoris with its attached iliotibial band is also attached to the trochanter, it acts with the erector spinae transfer to stabilize the hip as a "digastric muscle." Even when no significant extensor power from the erector spinae can be detected, the transferred fascial band behaves as a dynamic fasciodesis to maintain correction of the deformity.

To accomplish erector spinae and tensor fascia femoris transfer (Fig. 14-36) two separate thigh incisions are made.[90,92,112,141] One starts anterior to the head of the fibula and is carried proximally to above the supracondylar level. The second is made along the lateral aspect of the hip joint. The distal end of the iliotibial band is sectioned transversely at the supracondylar level. A wide flap is created by two longitudinal parallel incisions, is mobilized, and is passed proximally beneath the skin to the proximal incision where the flap is extended proximally to include the distal half of the tensor fascia femoris, preserving its neurovascular bundle. Medial to this flap, the lateral intermuscular septum is divided from its attachment to the femur and is removed.

Release of the contracted structures over the anterior aspect of the hip is then carried out. Fascial and muscular structures are divided as necessary while the hip and knee are held in as much extension as possible. The sartorius and rectus femoris may be tenotomized if they are severely contracted and paralyzed. As a rule it is not necessary to divide the iliopsoas insertion, but if this should become necessary it should be transplanted to the anterior aspect of the hip at the intertrochanteric region. If the capsule is contracted it, too, may be divided.

Next, a subcortical groove is made beneath the proximal attachment of the vastus lateralis, and the proximally mobilized iliotibial band is placed in the groove and sutured to the soft tissues, including the vastus lateralis, while the hip is held in extension.

The longitudinal lumbar incision is made 5 cm to 8 cm lateral to the spinous processes of the fourth and fifth lumbar and first sacral vertebrae and medial to the posterior superior iliac spine. The incision is deepened through the lumbodorsal fascia, exposing the erector spinae muscle. The muscle is split longitudinally between its medial third and lateral two thirds, and by blunt dissection, the lateral two thirds of the muscle is mobilized and is freed from its iliac and sacral attachments by sharp dissection. Since the nerve and blood supply to this muscle is segmental, one or two of the most distal neurovascular bundles may need to be severed in order to mobilize an adequate length of muscle.

The free end of the iliotibial band is passed proximally beneath the gluteal fascia to enter the lumbar incision just medial to the posterior-superior iliac spine. The gliding deep surface of the fascia should face ventrally. With the hip placed in extension, the fascia is attached, under moderate tension, to the free end of the mobilized muscle. The ventral surface of the muscle is placed on the subcutaneous surface of the fascial band, passing the suture in the end of the fascia through the muscle as far proximally as possible. Then the fascia is folded about the end of the muscle and held by several sutures passed into the muscle. Thus the distal end of the muscle is enveloped in fascia the deep surface of which is the gliding surface of the fascia. The incisions are closed. The hip is immobilized in plaster in extension.

After 2 weeks, the remaining contractures are gradually stretched out by repeated manipulations and casts, followed by assistive reeducation exercises. A bivalved long spica cast is applied in the corrected position and is worn at night for several months. Walking with crutches is permitted when the transplant functions satisfactorily, usually about 6 weeks postoperatively.

Poliomyelitic Dislocation of the Hip

The primary cause of dislocation of the hip is muscle imbalance resulting from weak abductors and extensors and normal flexors and adductors.[117] As a result of loss of abductor power, the greater trochanter apophysis contributes little to growth, whereas growth from the capital femoral epiphysis continues unabated. As a consequence, the femoral neck gradually assumes a more vertical position (valgus), at times becoming so extreme as to appear in line with the femoral shaft (valgus = 180°). A small degree of anteversion deformity also develops but never attains the severity seen in congenital dislocation of the hip. Thus, the deformity of the femoral neck contributes the second factor influencing subluxation and dislocation as weight bearing causes the head to stretch the capsule and ride out of the acetabulum superiorly. The acetabulum retains its normal depth and contour for several years, but eventually, because it lacks the pressures of weight bearing from a concentrically apposed femoral head, it becomes shallow, and the acetabular roof becomes increasingly oblique.

In pelvic obliquity caused by a flexion-abduction contracture, the opposite higher side of the pelvis contains a femoral head that by its position is functionally in valgus as related to the acetabulum and may eventually erode the superior rim of the acetabulum, resulting in subluxation and dislocation.

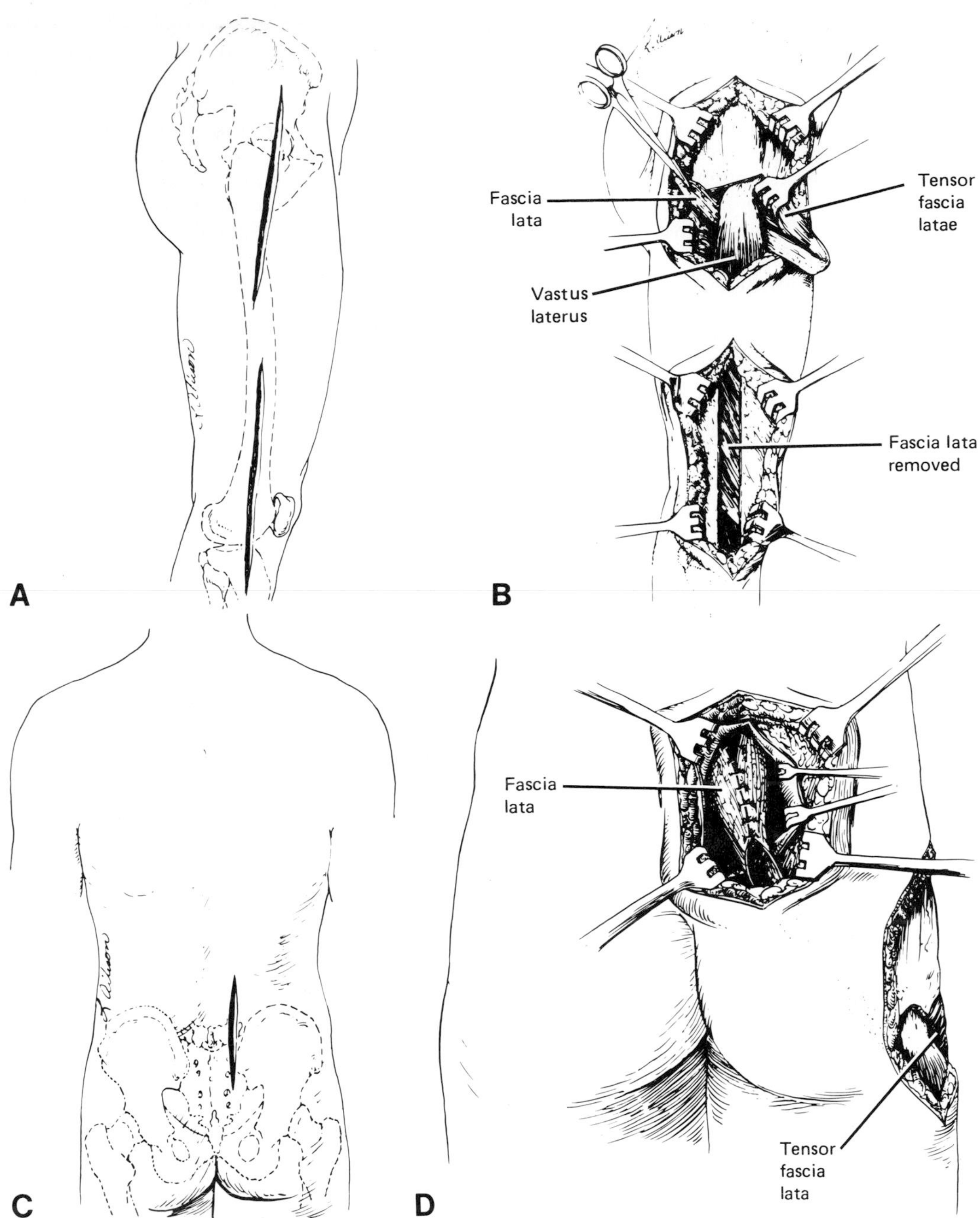

FIG. 14-36. Erector spinae muscle transfer to greater trochanter. (*A*) Lateral thigh incisions. (*B*) Iliotibial band and tensor fascia femoris brought beneath the origin of the vastus lateralis and extended proximally and medially beneath the gluteal fascia. (*C*) Posterior incision. (*D*) Operation completed. The freed distal end of the erector spinae has been enveloped in fascia lata, which glides within the gluteal compartment and extends the tendon of insertion toward the greater trochanter. (Barr JS: Poliomyelitic hip deformity and the erector spinal transplant. JAMA 144:813, 1950)

Dislocation of the completely paralyzed hip is rare and does not occur once weight bearing has been established.[123]

Treatment. Dynamic muscle balance must be restored. When this can be accomplished within the first few years of age, a valgus deformity will correct itself with further growth. Some principles of treatment are listed below.

1. Reduction of dislocation
   a. Early: is easily reduced by abduction.
   b. Later: after contracture of flexors and adductors has taken place, traction and abduction are required.
   c. Late: contracture is severe and requires tenotomy and skeletal traction. If irreducible, skeletal traction is continued until the femoral head is opposite the acetabulum and 30° of abduction is possible. Then open reduction should be done.
2. Correct muscle imbalance: to restore abduction and extension, preferably by iliopsoas transfer (Mustard, Sharrard).
3. Varus femoral osteotomy: to correct valgus deformity. The deformity recurs with further growth unless muscle imbalance is corrected.
4. Acetabuloplasty: to provide adequate roof and depth for stability (Salter, Pemberton, Chiari).
5. Pelvic support osteotomy: is rarely ever done.
6. Arthrodesis: for painful, degenerated hip of adult; when bone reconstructive procedures or tendon transfers have failed. It will relieve pain, achieve stability, decrease limp, and reduce the need for orthoses.
   a. Prerequisites: adequate abdominals and quadratus lumborum, sound knee ligaments (good quadriceps not necessary if no flexion contracture exists), stable foot and ankle, preferably in equinus (may require pantalar arthrodesis), and a functioning opposite lower extremity.
   b. Contraindications: progressive lumbar scoliosis, trunk instability (abdominal muscle weakness), and marked shortening of lower extremity

The Flail Hip

The flail hip is one completely lacking muscle power. Such total paralysis is often associated with extensive involvement of the lower extremity and requires multiple orthotic devices and supports through the upper extremities to make ambulation possible. In spite of such apparatus; the gait is lurching; the extremity remains unstable; endurance is poor; and, lacking support from the opposite extremity and weak upper extremities, ambulation may be impossible. Although a flail hip rarely dislocates, except in infancy, a flexion-abduction contracture of the opposite hip will elevate the flail hip, placing its femoral head in a relative valgus position, encouraging subluxation. This may eventuate, with passing of time, in a painful degenerated hip joint.

Treatment. Arthrodesis of the hip will improve gait, provide stability, and increase endurance and may eliminate the need for an external support.

Principles. If the hip is stabilized to prevent hip flexion, the knee will be extended during weight bearing, provided that the center of gravity of the body is in front of the knee joint and dorsiflexion of the ankle is prevented by either functionally active plantar flexors of the foot or by arthrodesis in slight equinus (Fig. 14-37).[139]

Hip fusion alone or combined with ankle fusion in slight equinus provides good stability for the flail or extensively involved lower extremity. The procedure can be done in children, but the optimum for fusion is 10 to 14 years of age. After the early years of life, the proximal femoral epiphysis contributes only a small amount to the growth in length of the lower extremity. A significant degree of shortening does not occur after a hip fusion. However, it should be noted that if postoperative immobilization is unnecessarily prolonged, the lower femoral epiphysis may prematurely close. A requirement for fusion is good abdominal muscle power or a strong opposite gluteus medius, providing hip-elevating power. Good knee ligaments and absence of flexion contracture of the knee are necessary.

A satisfactory method of fusion involves combined intra-articular and extra-articular fusion, supplemented by internal fixation. A lengthy Smith-Petersen nail is driven through the femoral neck into the ilium. A

FIG. 14-37. Diagram of completely flail lower extremity. (*Left*) The principal of dynamic knee stabilization with the hip and ankle fixed, compared with (*right*) the collapsible knee and flail hip and ankle. (Sharp N, Guhl JF, Sorenson RI, Voshell AF: Hip fusion in poliomyelitis in children. J Bone Joint Surg 46A:121, 1964)

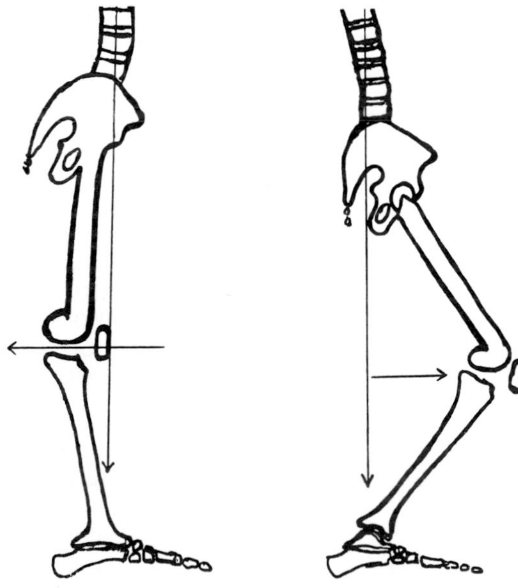

subtrochanteric osteotomy allows postoperative adjustment of the position under roentgenographic control and facilitates early fusion.[147] The best position for fusion is neutral rotation, no adduction or abduction, and 30° of flexion. For biologic function in females, and for short extremities, abduction of 15° is preferred.

Ankle fusion should be delayed until late childhood to avoid injury to the lower tibial epiphyseal plate, which contributes a significant rate of growth.

A walking spica and a standing table are used to prevent supracondylar fractures during the early weeks.

Fixed Pelvic Obliquity

When iliotibial band contracture and its associated tilted pelvis and ipsolateral scoliosis persist over a long period of time, adaptive bony changes, particularly of the spine, render the deformity permanent and not amenable to release of the contracted soft tissues. The affected limb is abducted and apparently long. The opposite hip is adducted and apparently short; its hip abductor is stretched and weakened. The lumbar spine deviates toward the contracted side so that the trunk, and therefore the center of gravity, comes to lie over the affected hip. The contralateral trunk muscles become elongated, and their contractility is impaired. The patient must widely abduct the affected extremity in order to take a step. Obviously, the adducted extremity, its weakened abductors, and stretched abdominal muscles on this side make it difficult to attain balance and to raise the opposite hip when bringing the "long" extremity forward in walking. (This is similar to the disability caused by severe gluteus medius paralysis.) To overcome this situation, it becomes necessary to lengthen the "short" extremity; abducting it at the hip will obtain apparent length and bring the weight-bearing line nearer the center of the body. This is accomplished by a subtrochanteric osteotomy of the "short" extremity and abduction of the distal segment.

Scoliosis per se is also a cause of pelvic obliquity, as is weakness of the lateral abdominal muscles.

Treatment. Roentgenographic studies of the lumbar spine determine whether the pelvic obliquity and scoliosis are fixed. The subtrochanteric region of the femur is exposed. A heavy Steinmann pin is inserted just below the greater trochanter. Below this a wedge-shaped section of bone with its base directed laterally is removed; the medial femoral cortex is left intact to avoid displacement. The removed section of bone is broken up into small fragments and replaced into the defect. A double spica cast is applied, incorporating the pin. After 4 weeks a wedge is removed from the cast below the level of the pin, and the distal limb is abducted as the medial cortex is fractured. The soft callus about the osteotomy site prevents displacement. The cast is repaired with plaster, and immobilization is continued for 8 more weeks.

When pelvic tilt is extreme and the trunk is markedly shifted over the contracted hip, this hip must be osteotomized in the subtrochanteric area and the femoral shaft adducted to shorten its effective length.

Abdominal Muscle Paralysis

Insufficiency of the anterior abdominal muscles results in abdominal bulging, increased lumbar lordosis, and inadequate bowel and bladder expulsion. Stability of the pelvis in front, essential to flexion of the hips, is weakened. When the rectus abdominis is paralyzed, the pelvis tilts anteriorly, resulting in exaggerated lumbar lordosis. Rectus weakness is demonstrated by Beevor's sign; when the head is raised against resistance, the umbilicus shifts toward the actively contracting muscles. If both recti are inactive, the umbilicus remains immobile. Weakness of the transversus and the obliques is diagnosed by inability to initiate the movement of turning over. Paralysis of the quadratus lumborum results in inability to stabilize and raise the lateral aspect of the pelvis while abducting the hip. The pelvis tilts downward and pelvic obliquity is

FIG. 14-38. Fascial transplants for paralyzed abdominal muscles. One transplant from the lower costal margin to the opposite anterior-superior iliac spine, another from the lower costal margin to the symphysis, and the third from the lowermost rib laterally to the middle of the iliac crest represent the different types used. Various combinations are employed, depending on the site of abdominal muscle deficiency. The lateral abdominal fascial transplant is useful for overcoming quadratus lumborum paralysis associated with paralytic scoliosis and pelvic obliquity.

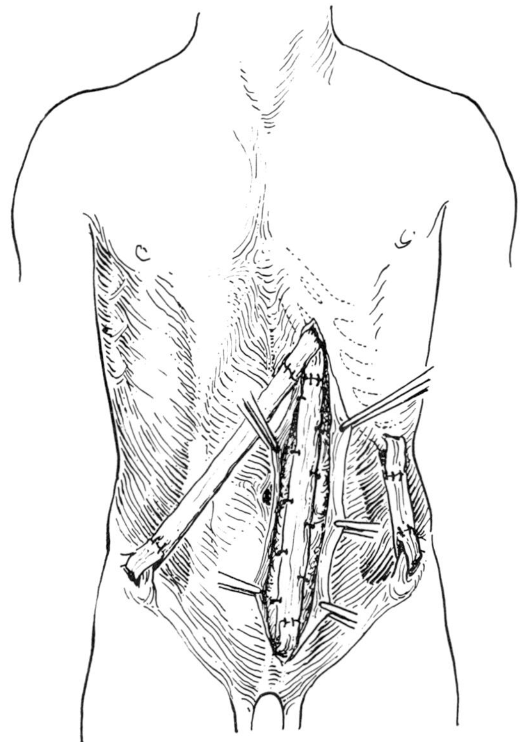

the result. The lumbar spine deviates toward the ipsolateral side. Quadratus lumborum weakness is identified by inability to pull the pelvis proximally against the resistance offered by the examining physician pulling the extremity distally.

Fascial Transplantation. Strengthening the abdominal wall and stabilizing the spine and the pelvis against the deforming influence of unopposed functioning muscles is possible only by transplanting strips of fascia (Fig. 14-38).[124,126] Fascia lata reinforces or entirely replaces the insufficient muscle and not only hypertrophies but also grows in length. After several years it is visible as a prominent subcutaneous band. The procedures employed most commonly are:

Rectus and Oblique Weakness. Two strips of fascia, each measuring 1 × 9 inches, are placed subcutaneously in crisscross fashion across the abdomen. Each is fastened at its proximal end to the periosteum and the soft tissues about the lower costal margin. The distal end is fastened to an osteoperiosteal tunnel in the opposite iliac crest near the anterior-superior iliac spine. When only the lower portion of the rectus is paralyzed, a fascial strip is extended from the functioning muscle above to the pubic symphysis below. If the upper rectus is deficient, the strip extends from the functioning muscle below to the xiphoid above. Paralysis of the obliques is demonstrated by localized abdominal bulging. The fascial strip is fixed to the rectus aponeurosis near the umbilicus. The other end is attached to the costal margin above or the iliac crest below.

Lateral Abdominal Wall Paralysis and Pelvic Obliquity. A wide band of fascia lata is attached to the ninth rib above and to the anterior iliac crest and Poupart's ligament below; or the tensor fascia lata, with iliotibial band attached may be transposed upward and attached to the ninth rib, providing a dynamic corrective force (Fig. 14-39).[99]

Quadratus Lumborum Paralysis. The fascial strip is attached above to the erector spinae at the level of the dorsolumbar junction and below to the posterior half of the iliac crest.

FIG. 14-39. (*Left*) Isolation and mobilization of musculotendinous transplant. (*Right*) Transposition of musculotendinous transplant. (Clark JMP, Axer A: Muscle-tendon transposition for paralysis of abdominal muscles. J Bone Joint Surg 38B:475, 1956)

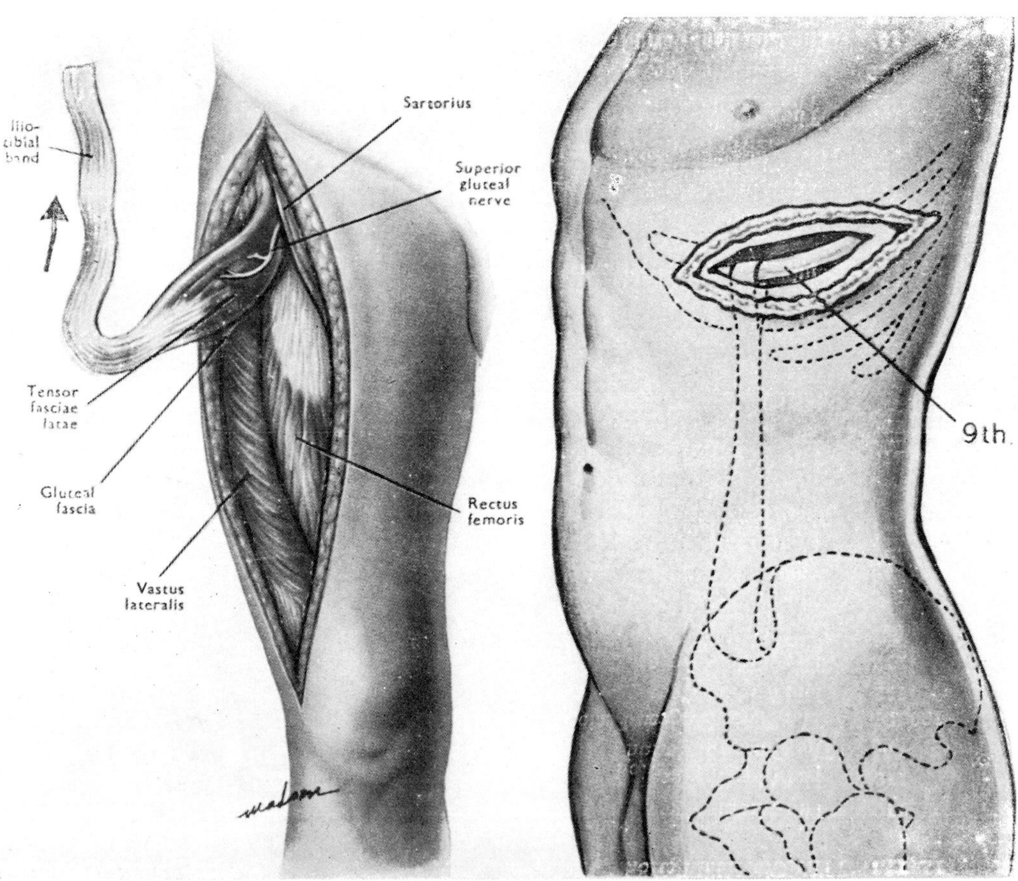

THE SPINE

Postpoliomyelitic scoliosis is due to asymmetrical paralysis of paraspinal muscles (Fig. 14-40).[120] The muscle imbalance is a continually operating mechanism, thereby explaining the development of scoliosis in spite of continuous recumbency. However, the upright position aggravates the curve by adding the factor of gravity. When paralysis is extreme and symmetrical, scoliosis may not develop. Spinal curvatures may be divided into two types:

1. Convexity of curve toward stronger muscle groups (*e.g.*, the iliopsoas, the gluteus medius, the gluteus maximus, the latissimus dorsi, the rhomboids, and the deltoid)
2. Concavity of curve toward stronger muscle groups (*e.g.*, the abdominals, the sacrospinalis, and the quadratus lumborum)

Contracture of the pelvitrochanteric muscles and the iliotibial band with resultant fixed pelvic obliquity deviates the spine toward that side.

A theoretical added factor is a neurogenic element that results in structural changes in the spine. Five percent of poliomyelitis patients develop scoliosis.

The curvature, contrary to the idiopathic type, may develop and progress even after growth is completed. It may make its appearance at any time within 10 years after the acute phase and tends to become severe. Therefore, the postpoliomyelitic patient should be checked every 6 months for several years. Three major types of curve are seen: (1) high cervicodorsal kyphoscoliosis, (2) long dorsolumbar scoliosis, and (3) lumbar curve.

Treatment. Preventive treatment consists in prolonged recumbency, as long as 6 months, in patients with paralysis of trunk and abdominal muscles. The spine should be examined roentgenographically in the standing position every 3 months. Recumbency is maintained until stability of the curve is attained or until progression indicates the need for correction. Lying on a concave frame favors weak abdominals. On resuming ambulation, if asymmetrical involvement of the abdominals and hip muscles exists, the use of crutches with a tripod gait is mandatory. An alternating gait is permissible only if one is certain that the asymmetrically involved trunk muscles will not increase the scoliosis. A postpoliomyelitic scoliosis brace is shown in Figure 14-41.

Surgical treatment consists in correction of the curve and fusion and is particularly indicated in young patients with gross asymmetric involvement and a rapidly progressing curve. Early fusion should be avoided, since a lordosis may develop. Many paralytic curves become

FIG. 14-40. Paralytic scoliosis, demonstrating the effect of unequal muscle pull. (*A*) Rhomboid muscle paralysis. (*B*) Trapezius muscle paralysis. (*C*) Sacrospinalis and deltoid paralysis. (*D*) Sacrospinalis and quadratus lumborum paralysis. (Redrawn from Kleinberg S: Scoliosis. Baltimore, Williams & Wilkins, 1951)

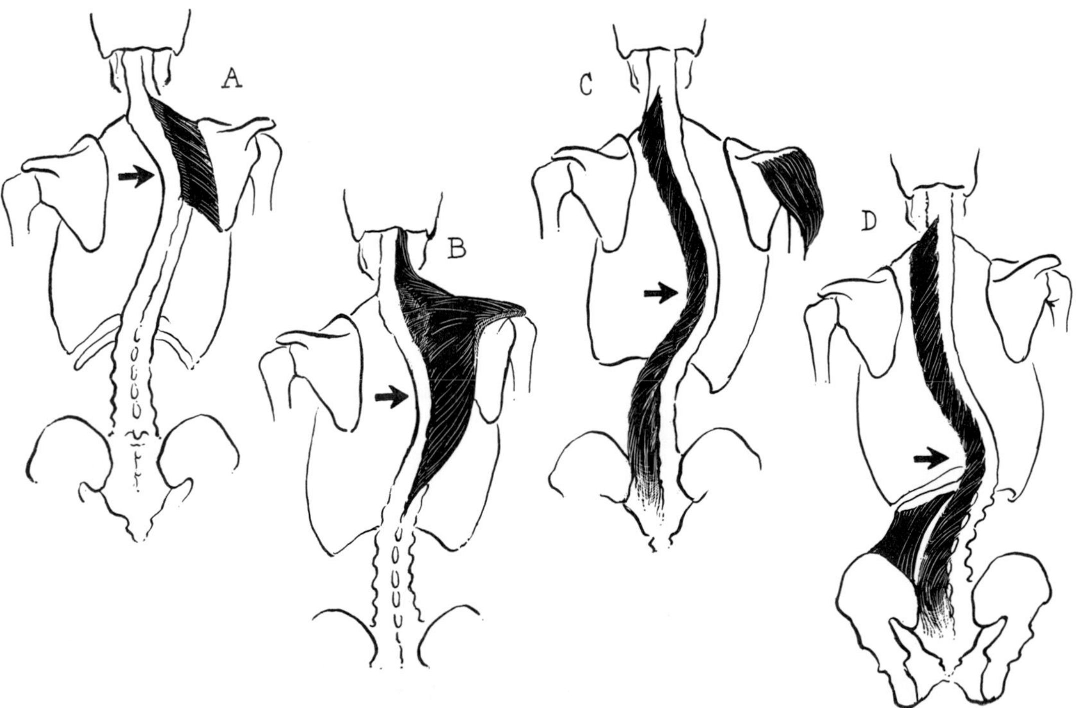

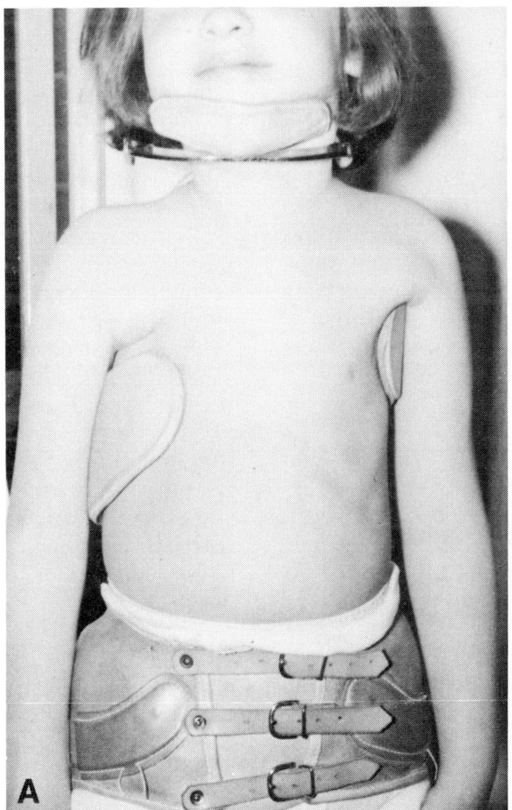

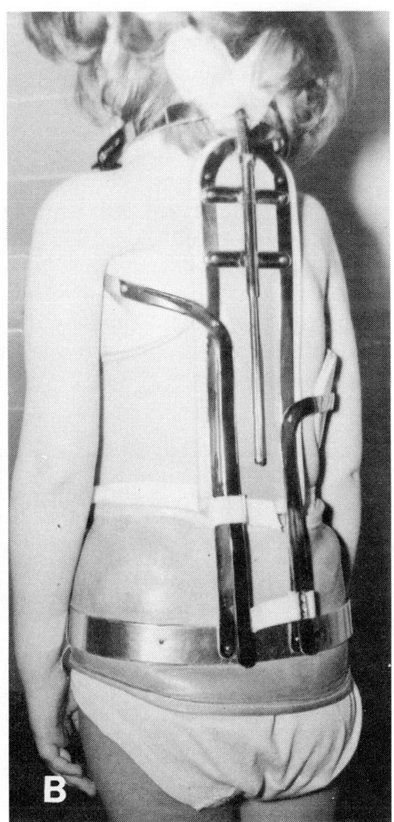

FIG. 14-41. (*A*) Postpoliomyelitic scoliosis brace, anterior view. Open front permits unrestricted chest expansion and abdominal breathing. (*B*) Brace for postpoliomyelitic scoliosis. Note lateral compression pads. Head support is extensible, providing distraction. The Milwaukee brace (see text) is probably better suited for patients with impaired cardiopulmonary function. It allows for chest expansion and corrective exercises and is adjustable to allow for growth.

static and stable and require no fusion. When the curve is of recent vintage, and isolated muscle involvement can be detected, special methods are available to halt further progression of the curve.

1. Pelvic obliquity is treated by iliotibial band resection
2. Abdominal and quadratus lumborum muscles are treated by fascial transplants
3. Scapular elevator muscles. For high cervicothoracic curves, two strips of fascia are attached to the scapular spine, one to the cervical muscles at the apex of the curve on the concave side; the other to the spinous process of the first thoracic vertebra.
4. Rhomboids and levator scapulae normally pull the scapula upward and inward and exert tension on the upper four dorsal and cervical vertebrae. When these are paralyzed, the spine is pulled to the opposite side. Fascial transplants are attached to the vertebral border of the scapula and into the spinal muscles and the latissimus dorsi.

THE KNEE

When the knee is fully extended, it is stable even in the absence of quadriceps function. The position is favored by an equinus position of the foot, either fixed or as a result of an actively controlled plantar-flexor force of strong triceps surae muscles, while standing. With weight bearing, the equinus and the backward pull of the soleus forces the leg and knee posteriorly, thereby extending the knee.

The loss of active extension at the knee in the presence of strong hamstrings favors the development of a flexion contracture of the knee. The opposite situation, a strong extensor and weak flexors, encourages the development of a recurvatum deformity—in reality, hyperextension. A strong biceps (which inserts on the fibular head), plus other weakened hamstrings, and insufficiency of the quadriceps result in a flexion, abduction (valgus), and external rotation deformity of the knee. The same deformity is produced by a contracted iliotibial band, which attaches to the head of the fibula and the lateral tuberosity of the tibia. Persistence of deformity during the growth period results in adaptive bony structural changes, which render the deformity permanent.

Quadriceps paralysis is the only indication for tendon transference about the knee. Before tendon transfers can be done, all deformity about the knee must be corrected. Slight flexion contracture can be overcome by stretching and wedging casts. Severe flexion deformity is treated by supracondylar osteotomy. Subcondylar osteotomy of the tibia will correct genu valgum and tibial torsion. Flexion contracture of the hip and Achilles tendon contracture must first be overcome. The latter procedure should not weaken the calf muscles, and minimal residual equinus is desirable to stabilize the knee in extension. The biceps, the strongest hamstring, is used most frequently for transfer to the patella. In order that this transfer does not displace the patella laterally, a semitendinosus transfer to the medial aspect of the patella is added to balance the pull and lessen the incidence of patellar dislocation (Fig. 14-42). The other hamstrings are too weak to be effective. It is necessary that some flexion power be preserved by at least one functioning hamstring and gastrocnemius; the hip flexors must be adequate for lifting the extremity against gravity; otherwise a severe disability will result.

Flexion Contracture of the Knee

Flexion contracture is caused by the following:

- Iliotibial band contracture, which also causes valgus of knee and external rotation deformity of tibia on femur. Treatment is by resecting the iliotibial band and lateral intermuscular septum proximal to the knee.
- Paralysis of quadriceps, and normal hamstrings. When the biceps is stronger than the medial hamstrings, genu valgum and external rotation of the tibia develop. The tibia may subluxate posteriorly.

Before tendon transfer is attempted, a full range of passive extension must be established. For mild to moderate flexion contracture, wedging casts or an Engen extension orthosis (see below) will stretch the posterior soft tissue structures. For severe flexion contracture, especially when associated with posterior subluxation of the tibia, split Russell traction will overcome the deformity. The vertical portion of the traction is exerted behind the upper end of the leg, and the horizontal component is in the direct longitudinal line of the leg.

Severe flexion contracture sometimes requires surgical correction (*e.g.*, posterior capsulotomy, fractional hamstring tenotomies or lengthening, and supracondylar osteotomy).

FIG. 14-42. Transference of biceps femoris for paralysis of the quadriceps. The semitendinosus must also be transferred from the medial side to reinforce extensor power.

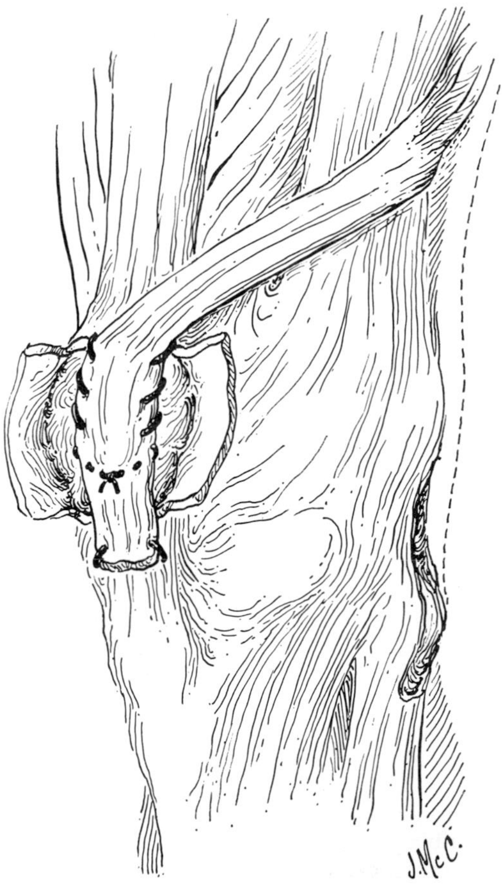

Quadriceps Paralysis. Quadriceps paralysis with slight recurvatum deformity may cause little disability while the triceps and hip flexors are active. The soleus fixes the foot in equinus while forcing the knee backward, and the gastrocnemius prevents extreme hyperextension. The hip flexors raise the extremity off the floor during the swing phase.

Paralysis of the quadriceps in the presence of fixed-flexion contracture of the knee results in lack of stability of the knee, a severe disability which during the stance phase causes the knee to buckle forward. Tendon transfers are necessary to reinforce a weak or paralyzed quadriceps muscle. Before tendon transfers are done, all deformities must be corrected, including flexion contracture of the knee and hip, genu valgum, and equinus deformity of the foot. The available muscles for transfer include the biceps femoris, semitendinosus, sartorius, and tensor fasciae latae.

Before a hamstring is transferred, it is desirable to have another functioning flexor such as the hip flexors and the triceps surae, so that the thigh may be raised while the knee is flexed by gravity and the gastrocnemius. To ensure a satisfactory result of hamstring transfer, especially if the biceps femoris is reinforced by the semitendinosus, it is mandatory to have good hip flexors to raise the extremity from the floor and a good triceps surae and gluteus maximus. When the biceps alone is transferred, lateral dislocation of the patella is a frequent complication. This is less likely when the pull is balanced by a semitendinosus transfer to the medial side.

Recurvatum can develop after hamstring transfer. This complication may be averted by a strong triceps surae; avoiding postoperative immobilization in hyperextension; correcting talipes equinus prior to weight bearing; and strengthening flexor power by physical therapy.

Transfers for Quadriceps Paralysis. Transfer of the biceps femoris to the lateral side of the patella and of the semitendinosus to the medial side is the procedure of choice. Through a lateral longitudinal incision the biceps muscle and tendon are exposed at its insertion on the head of the fibula. The common peroneal nerve, which skirts the medial border of the biceps tendon, is isolated and retracted. The tendinous insertion is severed, with caution not to disturb the additional insertion of the fibular collateral ligament. The biceps tendon and muscles are freed up to the point of entrance of nerves and vessels into the muscle belly. The tendon is routed subcutaneously obliquely forward. The iliotibial band and the intermuscular septum are resected to provide free access of the muscle to the anterior thigh. Through a medial longitudinal incision, the tendon of the semitendinosus is likewise severed at its insertion, freed upward, and routed subcutaneously forward. Both tendons are embedded within a tunnel gouged from the anterior aspect of the patella and sutured to the soft tissues. Postoperatively, a spica cast is applied with the hip fully extended to relax the hamstrings. At 3 weeks, exercises may begin. A brace is worn to maintain extension until the transferred muscles demonstrate their conversion from the swing phase to the stance phase, typical of the quadriceps phase action, and have acquired adequate power.

Genu Recurvatum

Genu recurvatum can be severely disabling when it is more than mild in degree. When this deformity arises as a result of poliomyelitis, it is generally the result of two mechanisms described below.

Quadriceps Paralysis. In order to lock the knee in hyperextension during the stance phase of walking, the triceps surae, by soleus contraction, purposely limits dorsiflexion at the ankle, and the gastrocnemius relaxes permitting vertical weight-bearing forces from above to extend the knee. Over a period of time, with repetitive hyperextension forces, the posterior capsule stretches, the hamstrings and gastrocnemius become inadequate to resist these forces, and the knee progressively hyperextends. The vertical loads are brought to bear chiefly on the anterior aspect of the tibial surfaces, causing the tibial condyles to become depressed anteriorly and enlarged posteriorly. The articular surfaces therefore slope downward and forward, and the proximal portion of the tibial shaft may bow posteriorly. Partial posterior subluxation of the tibia may ensue. This deformity develops very slowly.

Treatment of this type generally brings satisfactory results. The skeletal deformity is initially corrected, and then one or more hamstrings are transferred to the patella.

Weakness of Triceps Surae and Hamstrings. The knee becomes hyperextended because the posterior soft tissues become stretched. Calcaneus or calcaneovalgus deformity is usually associated, and the gait is characterized by the lack of push-off. This deformity develops rather rapidly. Treatment by methods other than arthrodesis is generally unrewarding. No tendon transfers are available, and soft tissue shortening procedures (*e.g.* tenodesis) provide temporary benefit. In spite of protective orthoses, the tissues become stretched out.

Bone reconstructive procedures that preserve joint motion are limited to the first type, quadriceps paralysis with good hamstrings and triceps surae. Essentially this consists in a high tibial osteotomy. When performed during the growth period, the level of osteotomy should be beyond the tibial tubercle to avoid compromising the growth plate. Either an anterior open-wedge osteotomy or a posterior closed-wedge is done. The proximal fragment is kept in hyperextension while the distal fragment is angulated backward and aligned with the femur. Fixation is achieved by various methods (*e.g.*, pins, cortical grafts) until union occurs (Fig. 14-43).

If possible, surgery is best postponed until after skeletal maturity. The osteotomy can then be done proximal to the tibial tubercle through cancellous bone where union is rapid.[100,146]

Various soft tissue procedures have been devised.[110,111] Generally, these consist of using tendon or fascial grafts which are anchored in slots or drill holes in the posterior portions of the femoral condyles and tibial condyles proximal and distal to the epiphyseal plates, respectively. These constitute artificial ligaments, which are held taut while the knee is held in flexion and immobilized in a cast for 6 weeks. The operation is indicated only when the quadriceps is strong enough to lock the knee in extension and when walking without a brace is possible.

THE FOOT AND ANKLE

Paralysis of the muscles acting about the foot and ankle results in various types of functional loss and corresponding deformities, depending on the muscle imbalance between the involved muscles and the remaining musculature. The loss of motor power acting about the joints results in loss of stability of these joints, which worsens as ligamentous and capsular support is lost. Eventually adaptive bony structural changes occur, rendering the deformity permanent. Moreover, the plantar aponeurosis is prone to develop contracture in poliomyelitis, producing, in combination with intrinsic and extrinsic muscle-loss, a cavus deformity.

The plantar flexors of the foot are the triceps surae, flexor hallucis longus, and posterior tibial. The dorsiflexors are the anterior tibial, extensor hallucis longus, extensor communis of the digits, and peroneus tertius. The invertors include the posterior tibial, flexor hallucis longus, and anterior tibial. The evertors are all of the peronei. The plantar flexors provide the force for forward propulsion, push-off, or toe-off. The dorsiflexor muscles

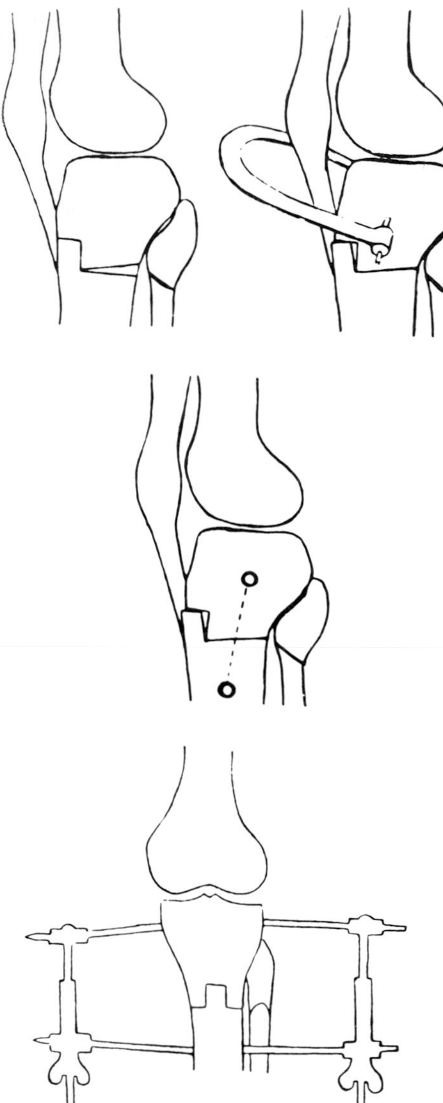

FIG. 14-43. Genu recurvatum, showing methods of surgical correction. (*Top*) Irwin's procedure. (*Center*) Støren's modification of Irwin's method. (*Bottom*) Application of compression by Charnley device. (Støren G: Genu recurvatum: Treatment by wedge osteotomy of the tibia with use of compression. Acta Chir Scand 114:40, 1957)

clear the foot during the swing phase of gait to approach heel-strike.

Tendon Transfer About the Foot

Tendon transfer is required to correct muscle imbalance and prevent deformity resulting from loss of power of the evertors (peronei), invertors (posterior tibial), dorsiflexors (anterior tibial, extensor hallucis longus), and plantar flexors (gastrocnemius, soleus).

Before 10 years of age, bone resections and joint stabilizations are contraindicated because of skeletal immaturity; only tendon transfers are permissible. However, the results of tendon transfers are better in patients above 10 years of age. At a younger age, the child should be examined regularly, and at the earliest indication of developing deformity, in spite of conservative treatment, surgical corrective measures are necessary. Tendon transfers are initially carried out, but surgical resections and stabilization must be added once skeletal maturity is reached.

After 10 years of age, tendon transfers about the foot and ankle must be preceded by stabilizing procedures, with bone resections if necessary to correct structural deformity, to provide stability resulting from loss of power in the evertor and invertor muscles. These dynamic deformities will recur despite stabilization, especially during the growth period, unless accompanied or followed by muscle-balancing transfers.

After tendon transfers and foot stabilization, other deformities of the extremity (*e.g.*, genu valgum must be corrected; otherwise the foot deformity may recur.

The principles of tendon transfer must be strictly observed:

- The transferred muscles or muscle must be equal in power to the paralyzed muscle.
- The tendon must pass in a direct line from its muscle to the point of insertion.
- To preserve gliding, the tendon must pass through subcutaneous fat, through its own sheath, or through the sheath of the paralyzed muscle.
- Pulleys are fully utilized for maximal mechanical efficiency, (*e.g.*, the transverse crural ligament).
- The muscle must be under normal physiological tension.
- Nerve and blood supply must be preserved and protected.
- The transfer must be attached to the tendon or actual point of insertion of the paralyzed muscle, or to the point which will restore balance and overcome deformity.
- Contracted structures must be overcome and joints mobilized.
- Bone operations must precede tendon transfers, if possible.
- The range of excursion of transferred muscle tendon should be similar to that of the muscle being reinforced or replaced.
- Since agonists are preferable to antagonists, they should, if possible, normally act during the same phase of the gait cycle. However, phase conversion is possible.

Combinations of Paralysis

Extensor-Invertor Insufficiency. Extensor-invertor insufficiency is due mainly to paralysis of the anterior tibial muscle resulting in an equinus and planovalgus deformity. The extensor hallucis longus and extensor digitorum longus attempt to compensate for loss of anterior tibial function in dorsiflexing the ankle. Although the toes become clawed and hyperextended the metatarsal heads are depressed. The triceps surae become contracted so that passive dorsiflexion of the ankle becomes limited. Occasionally, the peroneus longus may unopposedly depress the distal end of the first metatarsal, producing a cavus deformity.

Early treatment requires stretching of calf muscles to retain a good range of dorsiflexion at the ankle. A dorsiflexion assist orthosis is worn during the day and a splint may be worn at night. If equinus at the ankle resists stretching, wedging casts may be tried. Surgery initially is limited to posterior capsulotomy, but heel cord lengthening is avoided to retain maximum calf muscle strength. The peroneus longus is transferred to the base of the second metatarsal, and the peroneus brevis must be sutured to the stump of the peroneus longus. The long toe extensors may be transferred to the necks of the metatarsals.

In longstanding deformity and paralysis, after structural changes have supervened, and when insufficient peroneal power requires reinforcement by additional transfer of the posterior tibial, a triple arthrodesis is done after 10 years of age. This provides stabilization while making the peroneals and posterior tibial available for transfer. The posterior tibial, transferred through a window in the interosseous membrane, provides a more direct and effective dorsiflexor for the foot. It may be reinforced by adding the flexor hallucis longus.

Evertor Insufficiency. Evertor insufficiency is due to paralysis of the peroneus longus and brevis. The medial aspect of the foot is pulled into inversion by the posterior tibial, which inserts beneath the scaphoid, and by prolongations to the bases of the inner metatarsals. As the forefoot is adducted, the calcaneus is drawn into inversion. A varus deformity of the foot is produced.

Normally, the anterior tibial elevates the distal end of the first metatarsal, and the peroneus longus depresses it. When the peroneus longus is paralyzed, the distal end of the first metatarsal is drawn dorsally by the unopposed action of the anterior tibial. The dorsally prominent head of the first metatarsal forms a "dorsal bunion" and articulates with the plantar flexed large toe.

Treatment consists of lateral transfer of the anterior tibial to the base of the second metatarsal. In longstanding severe deformity of the first ray, osteotomy of the base of the first metatarsal may be required. After structural changes of the bone have taken place, wedge resections and triple arthrodesis become necessary but are postponed until after 10 years of age and should always be accompanied by lateral transfer of the anterior tibial; otherwise with further growth the deformity will recur.

Loss of Both Invertors and Evertors. By definition, the anterior tibial as well as the posterior tibial, constituting the invertors, and the peronei, constituting the evertors, are paralyzed. Therefore, dorsiflexion power is markedly weakened, as is active mediolateral movement. The foot is severely unstable. Stabilization by the Lambrinudi procedure or a posterior bone block at the ankle limits plantar flexion at the ankle. Dorsiflexion power can thereafter be restored by tendon transfer. As a rule, the proximal attachment of the extensor hallucis longus to the neck of the first metatarsal (Jones procedure) does not provide adequate power, and no other medial or lateral tendon is available. If the flexor hallucis longus tendon is functioning, it can be routed through a window in the interosseous membrane and transferred to reinforce the extensor hallucis longus.

Calf Muscle Insufficiency (Paralysis of Triceps Surae). The triceps surae is the strongest muscle of the body and provides the main force for plantar flexion of

FIG. 14-44. Calcaneus foot. (*Top*) Dorsiflexion apparently exaggerated. (*Bottom*) Abnormally high longitudinal arch.

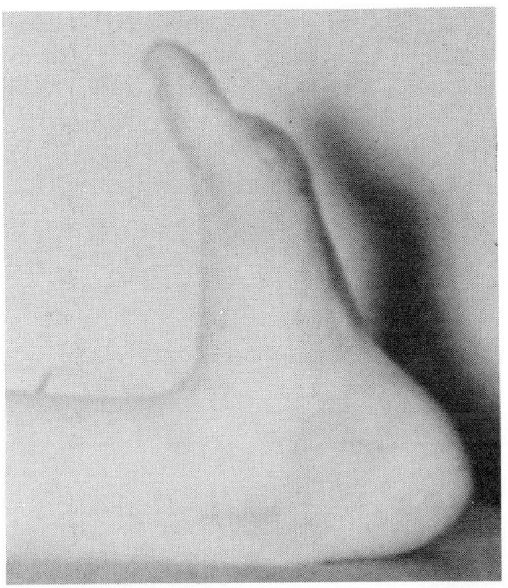

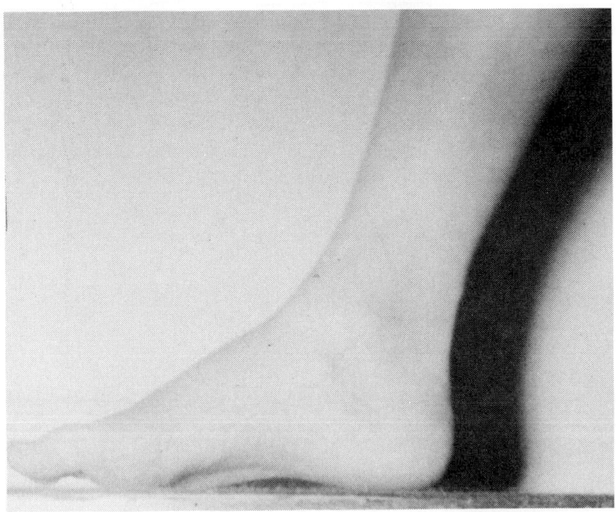

the foot. When the triceps surae is severely weakened or paralyzed, the calcaneus cannot be actively plantar flexed, so that the body weight cannot be borne on the metatarsal heads and push-off in walking is lost. When active dorsiflexion at the ankle remains unopposed, the triceps surae, its tendo Achillis, and the posterior capsule of the ankle are stretched and become lax.

If the long and short toe flexors and the intrinsics remain intact, as walking is attempted their pull on the posterior end of the calcaneus is unopposed; the heel rotates so that the apophysis is directed plantarward, the forefoot is pulled plantarward, and a cavus deformity develops. The plantar aponeurosis becomes contracted and, in the skeletally immature foot, structural changes of the bones and joints occur as further growth proceeds. A rapidly progressive talipes calcaneus deformity develops. The final deformity, usually a calcaneocavus deformity, and the lack of push-off form a combination that is extremely disabling (Fig. 14-44).

Treatment is very difficult because of lack of suitable tendon transfers and the need for correction of the extreme deformity. If the state of muscle imbalance and increasing deformity in the skeletally immature foot can be recognized at an early stage, various measures can immediately be instituted that will ultimately reduce the degree of disability.

When deformity is mild, and residual calf muscle function is present, conservative measures are preferable. Exercises are designed to restore some degree of useful muscle power to the triceps surae and to those muscles concerned with mediolateral stability of the foot, while at the same time maintaining flexibility of the foot. An orthosis is worn that assists plantar flexion at the ankle while limiting dorsiflexion.

When rapid progression of deformity is defined, tendon transfers should be done early. Unfortunately, rarely are the transferred muscles strong enough to restore normal push-off, and, in spite of multiple tendon transfers, some type of support is required to enable the patient to actively rise on the ball of the foot.

The objectives of surgery in the skeletally immature foot are to halt progression of the deformity and to restore the power of push-off. Later, after skeletal maturity has been reached, foot stabilization is necessary.

The plantar fascia should be stripped, and the tendons of the posterior tibial and peroneus longus and brevis are transferred to the apophysis of the calcaneus. If these muscles are inadequate, the anterior tibial can be transferred by routing it through the interosseous membrane. Then the long toe extensors can be transferred to the necks of the metatarsals for better dorsiflexor power and to prevent equinus.[132]

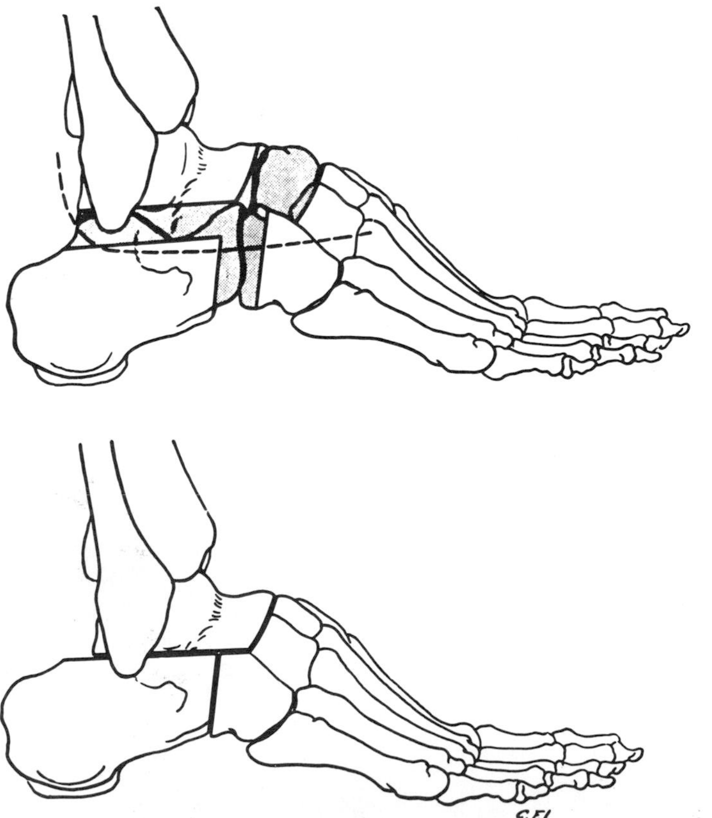

FIG. 14-45. Dunn arthrodesis. Shaded area represents the amount of bone to be resected. Following removal of the navicular, the foot can be displaced posteriorly, providing a longer lever arm for the triceps surae. (Crenshaw AH (ed): Campbell's Operative Orthopaedics. St. Louis, CV Mosby, 1971)

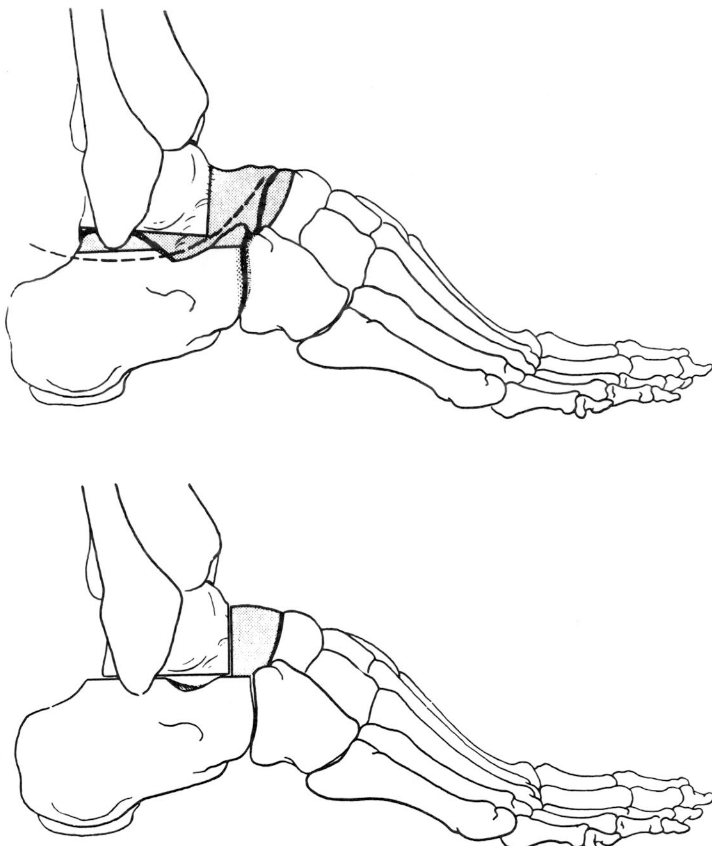

FIG. 14-46. Hoke arthrodesis. The talar head and neck are removed, reduced in size by resection of bone, and replaced. This permits backward displacement of the foot but jeopardizes the blood supply to the talus. The Dunn operation is preferred for stabilization when posterior displacement of the foot is desirable prior to tendon transfers to the triceps surae. (Crenshaw, AH (ed): Campbell's Operative Orthopaedics. St. Louis, CV Mosby, 1971)

In the skeletally mature foot, plantar fasciotomy and stabilization procedures are indicated. Wedge resections of bone correct both the calcaneus and cavovarus deformities. The foot should be displaced as far posterior as possible to provide a longer posterior lever arm, thereby lessening the muscle power required to raise the heel. The long toe extensors, particularly the extensor hallucis longus, are transferred proximally to the metatarsal necks.

Approximately 6 weeks following the stabilization procedure, multiple tendon transfers are done.

When instability is severe, and muscles for transfer are not available, a pantalar arthrodesis is indicated. The operation is done in two stages to preclude development of avascular necrosis.[130]

When the foot must be displaced as far as possible posteriorly to provide a lengthened lever arm and a mechanical advantage for the weak triceps surae, either the Hoke or the Dunn procedure is used (Figs. 14-45 and 14-46). The latter permits slightly more displacement.[114] Wide resection of the head and neck of the talus and their replacement, as is done in the Hoke operation, is not desirable, since this may contribute to avascular necrosis of the talus.[125]

Stabilization of the Foot

Obliteration of the subastragalar, the astragaloscaphoid, and the calcaneocuboid joints, popularly known as "triple arthrodesis" (Fig. 14-47), is necessary to correct instability of the foot due to muscle imbalance. Better stability is afforded if the foot is displaced posteriorly to provide a better lever arm for a weakly functioning calf muscle. Where possible, tendon transfers should be added to reestablish muscle balance. The operation is done only in patients over 10 years of age; before that time the structures are mainly cartilaginous. Deformity of the foot, with or without instability, is an indication for a triple arthrodesis. Resection of bone should be wedge shaped, the base of the wedge being directed toward the convexity of the deformed foot, the apex toward the concavity. For example, in equinovarus deformity, the base of the resected bone is superior and lateral, its width corresponding to the degree of the deformity. Bony overgrowth generally occurs in the tarsals in the direction of the convexity and must be resected. The final position requires that the heel be in slight valgus. If the deformity be planovalgus, the astragalus is plantarflexed, the astragalar head forms a medial and plantar bony prominence,

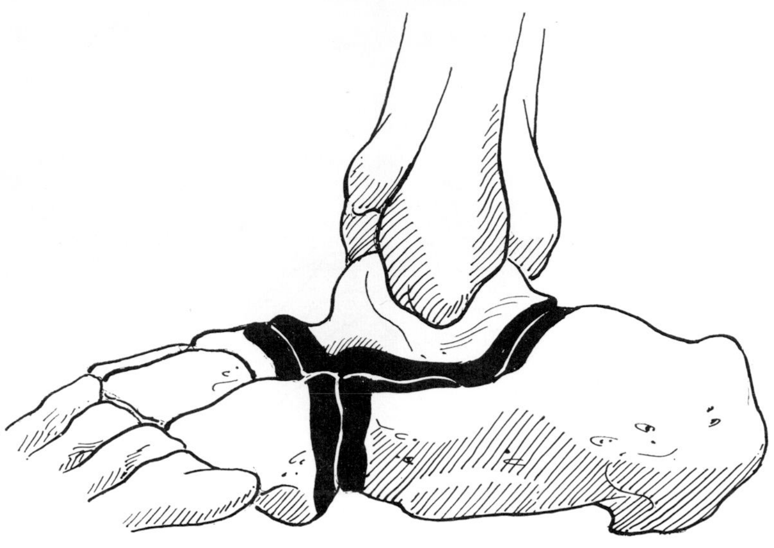

FIG. 14-47. Triple arthrodesis. The talocalcaneal, the talonavicular, and the calcaneocuboid joints are fused.

and the longitudinal arch is flattened. After arthrodesis, positioning the calcaneus more medially beneath the astragalus supports the latter and restores the arch. Calcaneocavus can be corrected by adequate midtarsal resection, displacing the foot posteriorly, and transferring the tendons of the functioning muscles to the Achilles tendon or the calcaneus (Fig. 14-48).

Extra-Articular Arthrodesis of the Subastragalar Joint. Paralysis of the tibials, particularly the posterior tibial, produces a planovalgus deformity, which at first seems to be mild but rapidly becomes severe despite bracing and supports. At first it is possible to correct passively the calcaneal eversion and the talar plantar flexion. Later, the deformity becomes resistant as the contours of the tarsals develop in adaptation to the malposition. It may seem desirable not to defer surgery until an age when a triple arthrodesis may be performed. The Grice[106,107] procedure makes possible correction of deformity and maintaining the correction at an earlier age. It aims at replacing the calcaneus beneath the talar head, positioning the calcaneus in slight eversion, overcoming equinus of the talus, and providing support to the talonavicular junction. Because the arthrodesis is extra-articular, subsequent bone growth is not interfered with. Therefore, correction of deformity is feasible at an

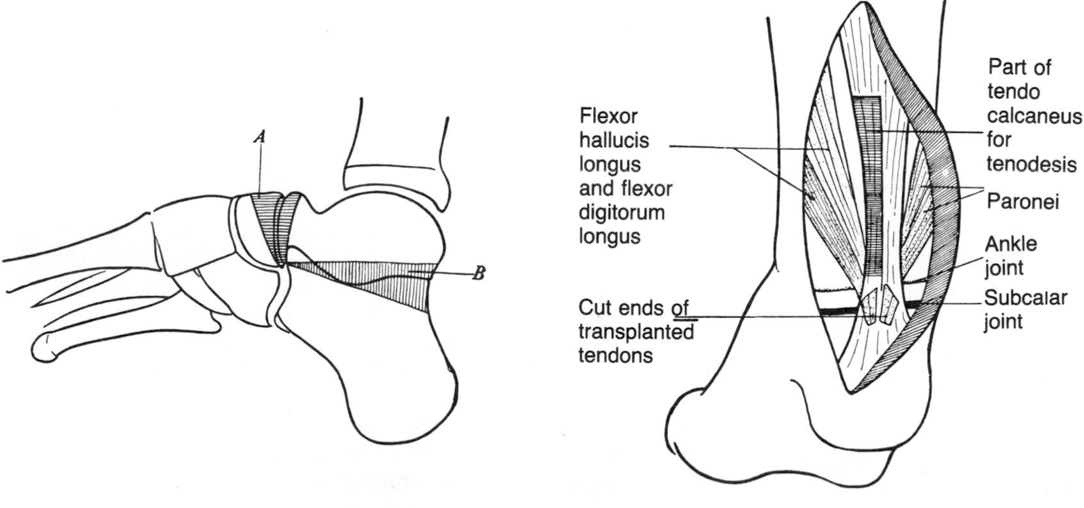

FIG. 14-48. Elmslie's operation. (*Left*) Wedges of bone removed; at first stage (*A*); at second stage (*B*). (*Right*) Transplanted tendons. (Cholmeley JA: Elmsie's operation for calcaneous foot. J Bone Joint Surg 35B:46, 1953)

early age. Muscle imbalance must be corrected, in addition, to prevent recurrence of deformity.

Technique. An oblique incision over the lateral aspect of the foot is used to approach the subastragalar joint (Fig. 14-49). The sinus tarsi is cleared of adipose tissue, and the lateral talocalcaneal ligaments are removed. When the foot is placed in equinus, the calcaneus can usually be replaced beneath the astragalus by inverting the foot. When the deformity has been present a long time, it may be necessary to cut the posterior capsule of the subastragalar joint or remove a slight amount of bone from the lateral articular surface before the calcaneus can be positioned properly. A bed for the grafts is prepared by removing a thin layer of cortical bone from the undersurface of the astragalus and the superior surface of the calcaneus. These slots should be deepened to the level of the cancellous bone.

Two small trapezoid-shaped pieces of corticocancellous bone are removed from the upper tibial metaphysis. The corners at the broad base of each graft are cut away so that the bone segments can be countersunk to prevent displacement. While the calcaneus is held in a slightly overcorrected position, the grafts are placed in their beds in the sinus tarsi. The grafts are positioned in a slightly oblique direction, their anchorage in the calcaneus being somewhat anterior to that in the talus. This alignment corresponds to a right angle to the axis of motion through the subastragalar joint. Compression is maximal, and the grafts are securely locked in place as the foot is everted. Postoperatively, a cast is applied from the toes to the groin with the knee flexed and the foot in maximal dorsiflexion.

Fusion generally requires 6 weeks, after which residual equinus must be overcome by wedging casts or Achilles tendon lengthening. Later, either peroneus brevis or longus is routed about the neck of the talus and beneath the talonavicular ligament and inserted into the navicular bone.

Panastragalar Arthrodesis. When leg muscles are too weak to control the foot at the ankle, and foot instability exists, ankle arthrodesis is performed in addition to a triple arthrodesis. The two procedures may be combined at one operation. The astragalus may be completely removed, thoroughly denuded of cartilage and cortex and replaced. However, circulation to the bone is compromised by the latter procedure, aseptic necrosis often supervenes, and many months of abstinence from weight bearing are necessary before complete replacement occurs. Therefore, ankle fusion and triple arthrodesis should be done as separate operations. Postoperatively, the astragalus should be positioned in equinus, the degree depending on the height of the heel to be worn. When quadriceps paralysis is present, an added degree of equinus favors hyperextension and stability of the knee.

Astragalectomy. Complete excision of the astragalus is useful for severe calcaneal deformity and flail feet in children before the age at which foot arthrodesis can be performed. The deformity is corrected, and the distal end of the tibia articulates directly with the calcaneus and the scaphoid. The range of dorsiflexion and plantar flexion is small, and lateral motion is nil, so that good stability is afforded. However, the foot is weakened, the extremity shortened and a painful pseudarthrosis may ensue. If the triceps surae or the tibials are functioning, the procedure is contraindicated, since equinus or varus deformity, respectively, will result. If adequate functioning muscle is available, tendon transference is more desirable as a temporary measure until stabilization can be done at a later date.

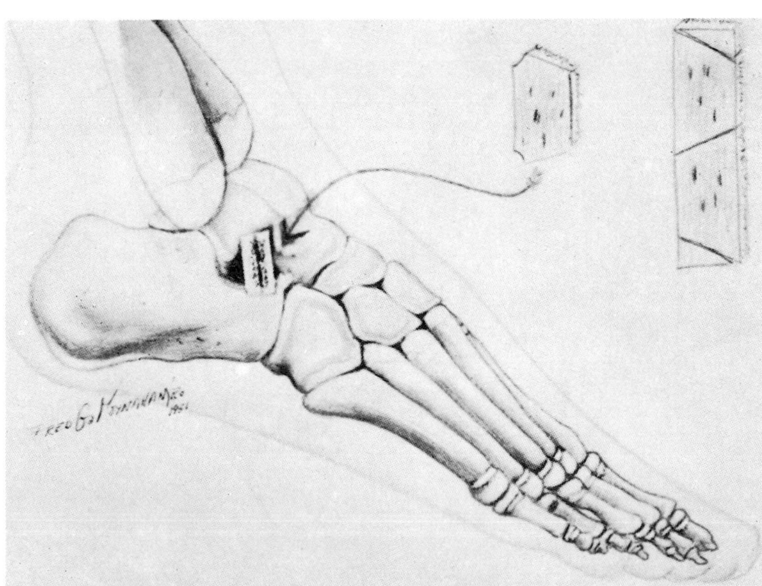

FIG. 14-49. The Grice operation. The bone struts are placed lateral to the talocalcaneal joint and maintain the calcaneus in inversion. Because this procedure does not interfere with subsequent growth, it can be done at an early age.

Loss of Dorsiflexor Power at the Ankle. Paralysis of the anterior group of leg muscles results in inability to dorsiflex the foot actively (dropfoot, paralytic equinus). The Achilles tendon secondarily becomes contracted. The equinus must be overcome for proper ambulation. When calf muscles as well as the anterior group are paralyzed, a flail ankle results, and panastragalar arthrodesis is indicated. If calf muscles are sufficiently strong to aid propulsion, the equinus can be prevented by a posterior bone block operation or by a triple arthrodesis procedure of the Lambrinudi type. Complete correction of the equinus is not desirable when quadriceps paralysis is present. Achilles tendon lengthening should be avoided so as not to weaken the power of push-off.

Posterior Bone Block of Campbell. A longitudinal incision along the medial border of the Achilles tendon extends upward from the os calcis for several inches.[97] The tendon is lengthened, if necessary, by a Z-plasty. By blunt dissection the posterior surface of the lower tibia is exposed without opening the periosteum. The flexor hallucis tendon is retracted medially. On passively dorsiflexing the foot, the posterior capsule of the ankle and the subastragalar joints are rendered taut. These are cut transversely. The posterior edge of the astragalus is visible and is resected. Below this a wedge-shaped cavity is gouged from the os calcis into which a strong cortical graft is inserted so that it extends upward and abuts on the posterior surface of the tibia. This is reinforced by surrounding it with multiple small pieces of cancellous bone. the soft tissues are closed snugly about the grafts, and a cast is applied, the ankle being positioned at a right angle (Fig. 14-50).

Tarsal Plastic of Lambrinudi. Normally, the posterior tuberosity of the astragalus abuts on the posterior rim of the tibia and acts as a block to complete plantar flexion. By resecting a sufficient wedge from the anterior end of the astragalus, the tarsus may be displaced dorsally, so that when the astragalus lies in extreme equinus the tarsus will lie at a right angle to the tibia.[122] Therefore, a strong triceps surae is a necessary prerequisite.

An oblique incision extends from the front of the lateral malleolus distally to the base of the third metatarsal. The sinus tarsi is cleaned out, and the extensor digitorum brevis is elevated from the os calcis. Capsular structures are excised from the astragaloscaphoid and the calcaneocuboid joints, and cartilage and cortex are removed from the apposing articular surfaces. Next, the subastragalar joint is exposed. Cartilage and cortex are removed from the superior aspect of the os calcis. A large wedge-shaped section is removed from the head, the neck and the body of the astragalus, including cartilage, cortex and cancellous bone. The base of the wedge is directed distally, the osteotome or saw blade emerging at the superior rim of the astraglar head. The width of the wedge depends on the amount of equinus to be overcome. Multiple slivers of cancellous bone are gouged up from all apposing surfaces to afford maximal area contact. Next, the tarsals and the foot are displaced upward so that the scaphoid comes to lie almost completely dorsal to the distal end of the astragalus. A notch cut in the inferior aspect of the scaphoid helps to maintain the displacement. This position is held while the soft tissues are closed and a cast is applied (Fig. 14-51).

The Elevated First Metatarsal. Normally, the anterior tibial muscle, which attaches to the first cuneiform and the base of the first metatarsal, acts to elevate the metatarsal. The antagonist is the peroneus longus. When the latter is weak, the first metatarsal displaces upward (dorsal bunion). To obtain the push-off in walking, the

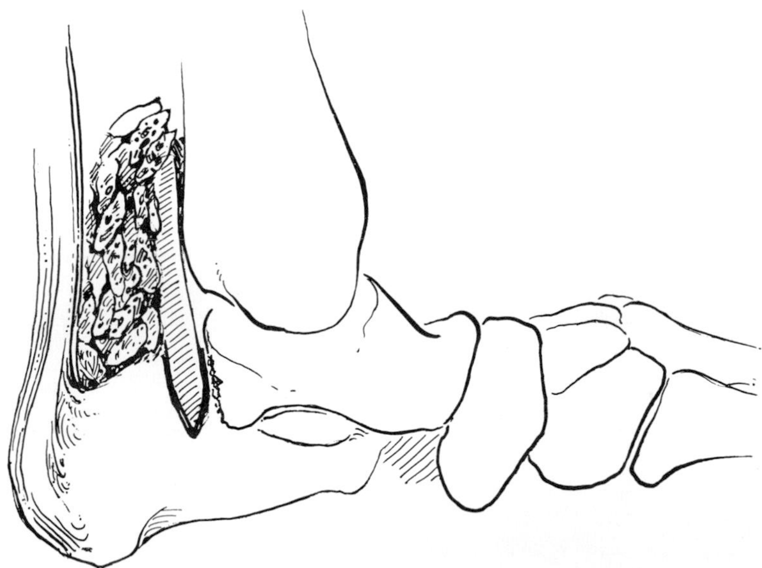

FIG. 14-50. Campbell's posterior bone block operation for equinus deformity due to paralysis of the anterior leg muscles.

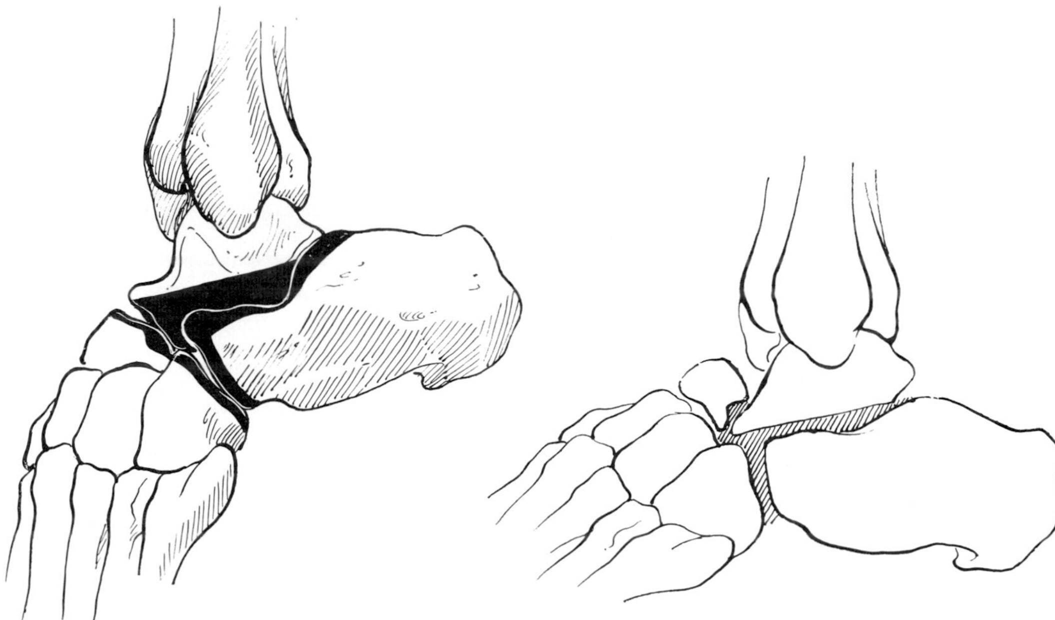

FIG. 14-51. Lambrinudi arthrodesis. A wedge with the base anteriorly is removed from the talus and a notch is cut from the scaphoid, which is displaced dorsally.

large toe is flexed actively downward. Therefore, the deformity is most apparent at first only with weight bearing, but eventually the deformity becomes fixed. The plantar capsule of the metatarsophalangeal joint and the flexor hallucis brevis become contracted. The head of the metatarsal is prominent dorsally where a bony excrescence, the bunion, develops. Removal of the peroneus longus for transfer in the presence of a good anterior tibial is a common cause of the deformity. The anterior tibial should be removed and transferred more laterally about the third cuneiform.

When the dorsiflexors of the great toe are paralyzed and the flexors are intact, the toe is strongly flexed downward to attain stability and push-off. Secondarily the metatarsal displaces upward.

Wedges of bone are removed from the metatarsocuneiform and the scaphocuneiform joints with the bases directed plantarward, and fusion is obtained in the corrected position. The plantar capsule of the metatarsophalangeal joint is released, and the dorsal capsule is severed and imbricated. The flexor hallucis longus tendon may be severed at its insertion and fixed to the neck of the metatarsal to act as an active corrective force. Muscle imbalance should be evaluated. An overacting tibialis anticus is attached to the midline of the foot. Occasionally, arthrodesis of the metatarsophalangeal joint is desirable.

Cavus Foot and Claw Toes

Clawing of the toes is a frequent and characteristic poliomyelitic deformity. It consists of hyperextension at the metatarsophalangeal joint and flexion at the interphalangeal joint. It is due to overaction of the toe extensors, the antagonists of the intrinsics. Excessive tension of the extensors is brought about by the following:

Weakness of the foot extensors allows the forefoot to drop, the toes being drawn up more so by the patient's attempt to dorsiflex the foot by the toe extensors (Fig. 14-52). By passively displacing the forefoot dorsally, the extensor tendons are relaxed and the toes fall downward to their normal position.

Contracture of the plantar aponeurosis pulls the fore-

FIG. 14-52. Typical poliomyletic deformity of foot. Weak anterior tibial and tight heel cord. Dorsiflexion is ineffectively accomplished by extensor hallucis longus. Cavus deformity is developing.

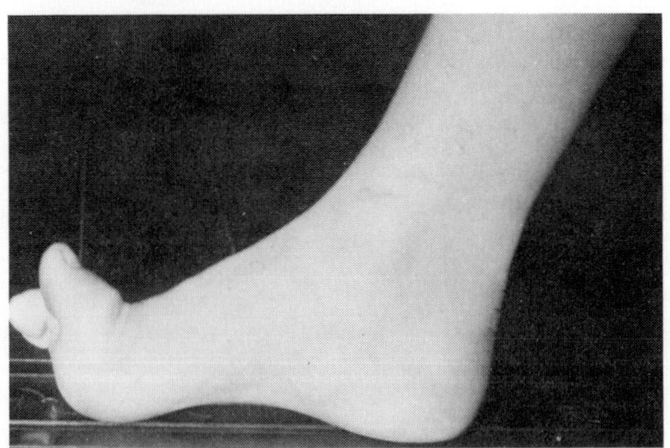

foot plantarward, the extensor tendons being rendered taut. A high longitudinal arch (cavus) is created. The former mechanism is immediately evident, whereas the latter develops insidiously. If the deformity persists, it is rendered permanent by joint contractures. The depressed metatarsal heads on the plantar surface, the dorsal angulation at the proximal interphalangeal joints, and the tips of the toes pointing downward create points of pressure over which painful calluses form.

Paralysis of the intrinsics likewise produces this deformity. As a rule, all five toes are contracted. A cavus and claw toe deformity less commonly develops secondary to spina bifida and other diseases of the central nervous system.

Treatment. The deformity can often be prevented by recognizing and treating the causative factor. A dropfoot should be supported by a brace. Constant manipulation can overcome the effect of contracture of the plantar aponeurosis. When the deformity is fixed, surgical measures are necessary.

Clawing of the Large Toe. The long extensor tendon is severed at its insertion and fixed to the neck of the first metatarsal to supply an active force, elevating the head of the bone. The interphalangeal joint is straightened by a wedge-shaped resection and arthrodesed (Jones operation).[118]

Clawing of Lesser Toes. The base of each proximal phalanx is removed; the interphalangeal joints are resected, straightened, and fixed with intramedullary pins. This results in some loss of flexor power, which does not interfere with walking.

Cavus. The mild early deformity (clawfoot) is little more than an exaggerated longitudinal arch and slight flexion of the toes that is obliterated on weight bearing. Painful calluses over the plantar aspect of the metatarsal heads disappear when pressure is relieved by a metatarsal pad or a metatarsal bar on the sole of the shoe. Arch strain is overcome by an arch support. Severe deformity requires surgical correction.

Surgical Treatment. When clawed toes are the major deformities, removal of the base of each proximal phalanx allows the toes to drop down. The interphalangeal joints must be straightened and fused. The long extensors may then be transferred to the necks of the metatarsals. An alternative is the removal of the outer four metatarsal heads. More commonly, the plantar fascia is thick and contracted, and bony deformity at the tarsus is extreme and fixed. Therefore, it is necessary to resect a bony wedge from the tarsus with its base directed dorsally (Fig. 14-53). At the same time, stripping of the plantar aponeurosis from the plantar surface of the calcaneus is done. Finally, the tarsal area is arthrodesed. Overcorrection must be avoided, since flatfoot or rocker-bottom foot results.

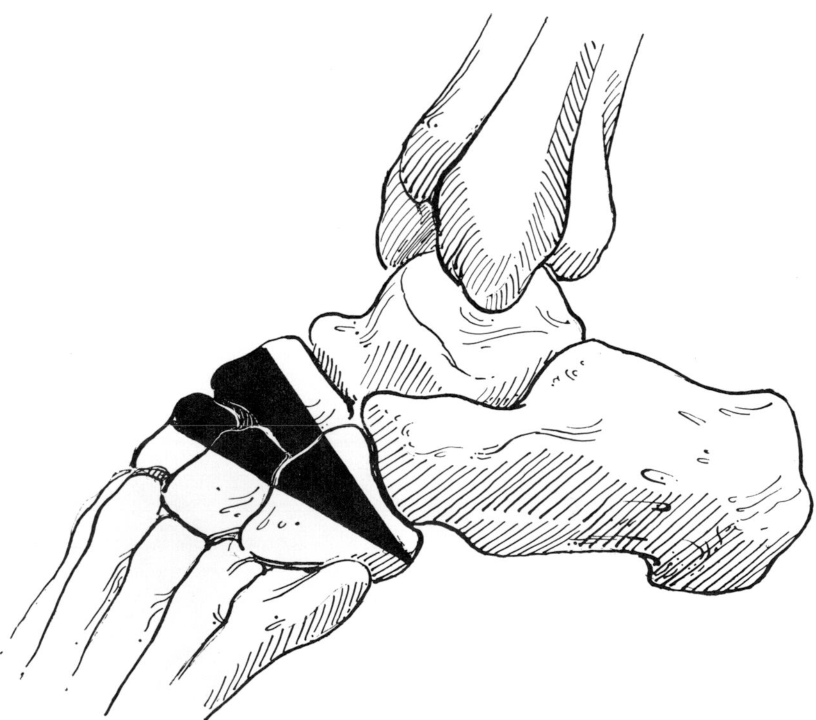

FIG. 14-53. Wedge osteotomy of the tarsus for cavus deformity.

When muscle imbalance is present, and correction is attempted during the growth period, some recurrence of deformity may be anticipated, even though arthrodesis is done. This may be prevented by transferring the toe extensors to the necks of the metatarsals, thereby creating an active dorsiflexing force.

Avoidance of Achilles Tendon Lengthening

Dropping of the forefoot, in contrast to the calcaneus, which remains in its normal horizontal position, produces an apparent limitation of dorsiflexion at the ankle. By elongating the Achilles tendon, the anterior end of the calcaneus will displace upward and reproduce the cavus deformity. Unless the calf muscles are actually contracted, lengthening of the Achilles tendon is contraindicated.

The Short Lower Extremity

Many factors can slow the rate of growth in a long bone of the growing child, such as paralysis, a fracture that traverses the epiphyseal growth plate, infection adjacent to the growth plate, or genetic factors. In both adult and child, a short extremity may result from extensive bone loss due to trauma, infection, and the deformity of disease. Prior to the advent of prophylactic immunization, poliomyelitis was the most common cause of slowed growth in an affected extremity and was highly probable in a child developing paralysis in the limb before 10 years of age.[91] The pathogenesis is obscure, and premature epiphyseal closure is rare. Experimentally induced paralysis of an extremity will diminish both epiphyseal growth (causes shortening) and appositional growth (causes reduction of diameter and thinning of cortex and trabeculae).[89]

Following development of paralysis, the amount of shortening that ultimately results at the time that skeletal growth ceases does not appear to bear an exact correlation with the age at onset or the extent of paralysis,[103,145] although severe paralysis generally, but not invariably, causes greater shortening, so that as much as 3½ inches discrepancy may result. The rate of paralytic shortening and its pattern of progression are highly variable.[137] The major amount of shortening may develop within the first few years and then progresses slowly until maturity; or it may be nonprogressive, developing some shortening early, and then resuming growth at a normal rate, so that the discrepancy remains constant; or the rate of slow growth may continue at a steady pace. Exceptionally, a mild acceleration of growth may occur within the first 2 years, but this is temporary.

These facts indicate that the rate of growth and the pattern of growth in the paralyzed limb are highly unpredictable.

Treatment for Correction. ***Principles.*** Planning the correction of limb length inequality in the growing child requires a basic understanding of the fundamentals of growth and maturation. Before the cessation of growth, and while sufficient growth remains in the unaffected lower extremity, epiphyseal arrest is the procedure of choice. After growth has ceased, bone shortening operations are preferable. Since bone lengthening procedures are fraught with considerable risk, it should only be attempted under exceptional circumstances (*e.g.*, marked shortness of stature) and then only when anatomical conditions are suitable.

Longitudinal growth during infancy is rapid and then gradually decreases until adolescence when an acceleration in the rate of growth, designated as the "adolescent growth spurt," develops. This temporary surge in the rate of growth takes place between 10 and 12 years of age in girls and between 12 and 14 years of age in boys, with the rate often doubling. Before the adolescent growth spurt, the lower limbs grow at a more rapid rate than the trunk; following the spurt, the trunk grows more rapidly than the lower limbs as the rate of growth of the limbs gradually tapers off to zero at maturity. The average age at which the distal femoral and proximal tibial epiphyses close is 15¼ years of age in the female and 17¼ years of age in the male. After growth in the long bones has ceased, the vertebral column continues to grow in length for about 2 years. It should be emphasized that the adolescent growth spurt and cessation of longitudinal growth in long bones takes place in girls 2 years ahead of that in boys, so that growth of the lower limbs ceases at approximately 14 years of age in the female and 16 years of age in the male. Moreover, these times are considered as average, since the epiphyses close 1 year later, and, furthermore, many factors influence growth so as to cause either acceleration or deceleration and the date of skeletal maturity.

Between 4 years of age and maturity, the femur increases its total length by about 2 cm per year, and the tibia by about 1.6 cm per year; 65% of growth of the lower extremity takes place about the knee.[101] In the femur, 70% of its growth occurs at the distal epiphysis and 30% at its proximal. In the tibia, 60% of its growth occurs at its proximal epiphysis and 40% at its distal.[104]

Factors Influencing Normal Growth. Under normal conditions, the rate of growth is modified by many inherent factors in each individual. Preeminent among these factors are genetic traits. A child who appears destined to become a tall adult, as suggested by the extraordinary height of his parents and other siblings, should have greater increments of growth, and the ultimate leg length discrepancy should be greater.

Age of Maturation. The remaining years of growth until maturation are determined by the skeletal age rather than by the chronologial age. The skeletal age at any given time can be determined from skeletal maturation charts standardized from the roentgenographic appearance of the bones of the hands and wrists.[105,148]

Growth Prediction Chart. Permanent or temporary epiphyseal arrest should be carried out at a time determined by the remaining amount of growth in the normal distal femoral and proximal tibial growth plates. First, the skeletal age is established from the skeletal maturation charts as applied to current roentgenographic views of the hands and wrists. The skeletal age is then applied to the growth prediction chart which provides a *range* of growth remaining in 95% of normal growing individuals. For example, by reference to the growth prediction chart, a boy with a skeletal age of 12 can expect additional growth in the lower femoral epiphyseal growth plate that lies within the range of 3 cm to 7 cm. Using this as a guide, adjustments are made using upper values for the tall child and lower values for the short child (Fig. 14-54).[88]

Other Considerations. The obvious weaknesses of using the growth prediction chart are that it anticipates the ultimate height of the individual and presumes that the shortening of the affected limb proceeds at a constant rate.

When shortening is mainly limited to either the femur or the tibia, epiphyseal arrest, if possible, should be limited to the corresponding bone in the normal extremity, for otherwise the knee joints will come to lie at different levels.

When limb length inequality is excessive, and the patient is already short of stature, growth arrest is inadvisable. Leg lengthening and prosthetic devices present alternatives.

If an above-knee orthosis must be worn on a paralytic lower extremity, slight residual shortening is desirable for the swing-through phase of gait.

Orthoroentgenography. The length of each femur and tibia is determined by taking individual views of each joint while a radiopaque ruler is laid alongside the limb. By directing the central ray at a target-to-film distance of 6 feet, the distortion caused by divergent rays is eliminated; the field of exposure and amount of radiation is reduced by using a collimator.

The lengths of the femurs and tibiae are compared by serial examinations, and the progressive increase of discrepancy within a specified period of time is then translated to the anticipated discrepancy at the termination of growth. This determines the time when epi-

FIG. 14-54. Anderson and Green growth prediction chart. The amount of growth potential in the normal distal femoral and proximal tibial epiphyses is shown at various skeletal ages from 10 years and 3 months to 17 years and 3 months. Values for five percentile levels, as well as for the means and standard deviations for each skeletal age, are shown. The broken lines indicate the range of growth between the 10th and 90th percentiles; in other words, 80% of patients are included within this range. Adjustments must be made in the individual patient when predicting the correction to be derived from epiphyseal arrest. (Anderson M, Green WT, Messner MB: Growth and predictions of growth in the lower extremities. J Bone Joint Surg 45A:1, 1963)

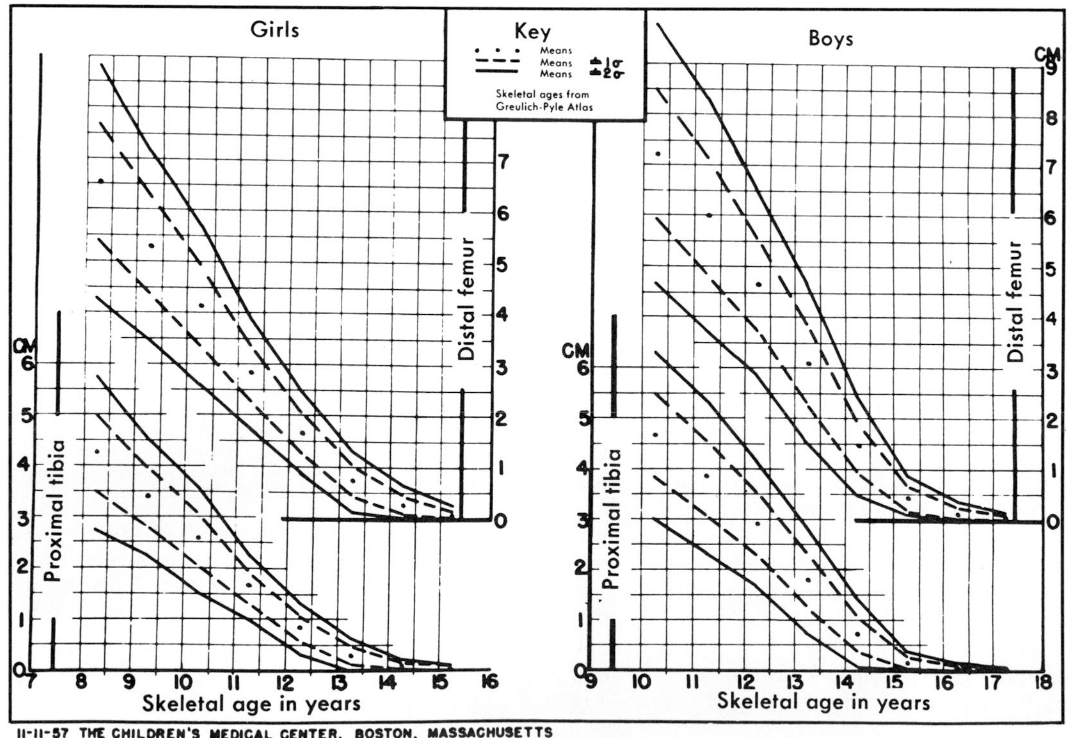

physeal arrest is carried out and whether one or both epiphyseal plates should be inhibited.

Although the rates of growth of a normal limb can be predicted within a certain range with a high degree of accuracy, the rate of growth in the affected limb, particularly when shortening is the result of paralysis, does not follow a definite pattern. For these reasons, the use of temporary arrest as against permanent epiphyseal arrest remains controversial and the prerogative of the orthopaedic surgeon.

Procedure.[104] To accurately prognosticate bone growth and the result of contemplated operations, serial records of growth of the long bones are necessary to determine the individual pattern of progressing discrepancy and the bone age. Observations are carried out at 6-month intervals and include orthoroentgenographic measurements of the femurs and tibiae (the films visualizing the epiphyses) and wrist films, which, when compared with skeletal maturation atlases, denote the skeletal age and the time of skeletal maturity.

The increasing discrepancy until the cessation of growth can be calculated as follows: the ultimate length of both femur and tibia of the short limb is estimated by noting their annual increase in length and by projecting these figures until the age of skeletal maturity. For the unaffected longer normal limb, the ultimate length of femur and tibia is derived from the growth prediction chart at any given skeletal age. It is the combined lengths of both femur and tibia in each limb at maturity that determines the discrepancy that must be corrected.

The growth prediction chart determines the time of epiphyseal arrest to inhibit growth by a predetermined amount. At any skeletal age, corrections of values within the range of predicted growth must be made. When skeletal age is advanced much beyond the chronological age, cessation of skeletal growth should occur at a shorter time, inhibition of normal growth will take place over a shorter period of time, and therefore the lower values on the growth prediction chart for a specified age should be used. When skeletal age is less than the chronological age, cessation of growth occurs later than average and growth should be inhibited over a longer time interval. The upper values must be used. Other evidence of earlier maturity, such as early development of secondary sexual characteristics, should alert one to premature cessation of growth and therefore a shorter period available for equalization of limb lengths.

When uncertainties arise as to predicting skeletal maturity, particularly if the degree of inhibition of growth of the shorter limb is difficult to evaluate, it is preferable to perform a temporary epiphyseal arrest by stapling rather than an epiphysiodesis. Since the latter operation produces final irretrievable stoppage of growth, overcorrection may result from errors in calculation. Stapling permits resumption of growth after the staples are removed. If limb length discrepancy is excessive, a permanent arrest may be performed on one epiphysis and stapling on the other or the second portion of the procedure may be postponed, thereby minimizing errors in prediction. In selecting a single epiphyseal plate for permanent arrest, the femur is preferred in the female to preserve tibial length, since possible complications are fewer and the final appearance is more acceptable.

Alternative Procedure.[152] At the initial visit, accurate lengths of both femurs and tibiae are determined by orthoroentgenographic measurement. The measurements are made from the top of the femoral heads to the lower end of the tibae, and the discrepancy is recorded. Similar studies are conducted at 6-month intervals over the next 2 years. The increased discrepancy indicates the rate of lost growth per year. This wrongly assumes that the patterns and rates of growth proceed unchanged until cessation of growth, both in the short and the normal limb. Recognizing that growth halts at 14 years of age in girls and 16 years of age in boys, the yearly decrement in the remaining growth years is added to the already existing shortening to calculate the final anticipated discrepancy. Next, one must determine the appropriate time for epiphyseal arrest. The lower femoral epiphysis contributes three eighths of an inch growth per year. The upper tibial epiphysis contributes one fourth of an inch per year. One or two epiphyses may then be closed at a time sufficiently in advance of maturity to make up for the eventual shortening.

This method fails to consider the variable patterns of growth in the short limb and the adolescent growth spurt in the normal limb. Moreover, skeletal age more accurately defines the termination of growth than does the chronological age; and shifting patterns of skeletal age also alter the time when skeletal maturity is reached. The many variables result in errors of prediction and correction, which may be obviated by early stapling procedures, since the staples can be removed and growth is resumed when the desired amount of correction has been achieved. The use of the growth prediction chart and skeletal maturity atlas should result in a high degree of satisfactory corrections.

Example. At 8 years of age, the female patient has 1 inch of shortening. At age 10, shortening is 1½ inches. Therefore, the decrement is ¼ inch per year. Eventual discrepancy at age 14 will be 2½ inches. Closure of the lower femoral epiphysis will restrict growth ⅜ inch per year over the next 4 years, or 1½ inches. Closure of the upper tibial and fibular epiphyses at 10 will result in a loss of ¼ inch per year over the next 4 years, or 1 inch. Together, total loss following both epiphyseal arrests will equal 2½ inches, thereby balancing the shorter extremity. The actual skeletal age should always be checked by Todd's maturation chart before proceeding. This is a more nearly accurate way of determining the time of maturation.

Permanent Epiphyseal Arrest. The lower femoral epiphyseal plate is exposed on the lateral side in the interval between the vastus lateralis and the lateral intermuscular septum (Fig. 14-55). The lateral geniculate

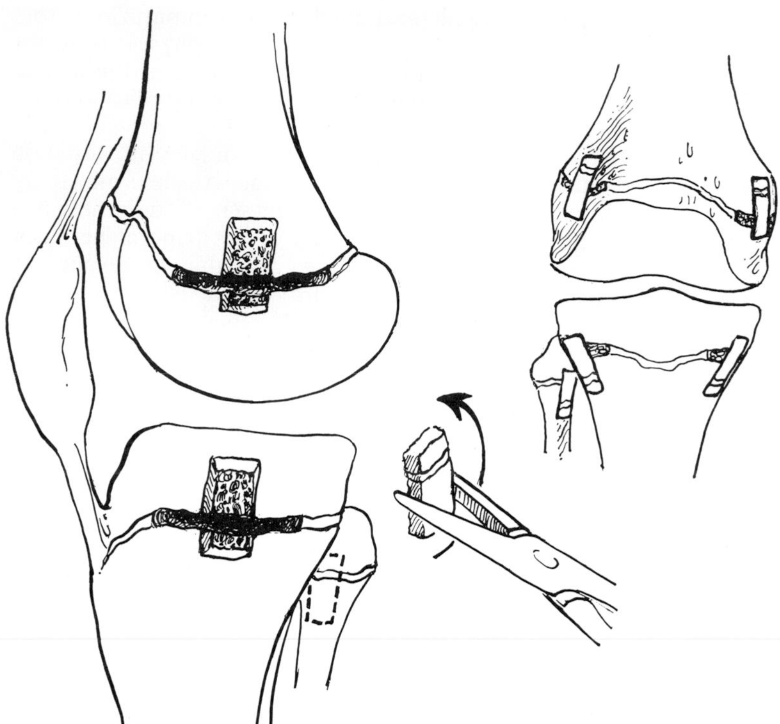

FIG. 14-55. Permanent epiphyseal arrest. The rectangular segment of cortex is removed (*left*) and reversed so that solid bone bridges the epiphyseal line (*right*).

vessels are ligated, cut, and retracted. The cartilaginous plate presents as a white line that passes obliquely from above posteriorly to downward and forward anteriorly. A rectangular block of bone is removed midlaterally, crossing the plate, and includes 1 cm of epiphysis and 2 cm of diaphysis. The disk is cureted or chiseled out anteriorly and posteriorly to a depth of several centimeters. Finally, the block of bone is reversed, reinserted, and held by firm closure of the overlying soft tissues.[134] On the medial side exposure is made by an incision centered over the adductor tubercle and developed between the vastus medialis and the medial intermuscular septum. The medial geniculate vessels are ligated, divided, and retracted. The same procedure is followed as on the lateral side. It must be remembered that the plate is saucer shaped, its peripheral edges lying proximal to the center. The relationship becomes less pronounced with advancing age.

The upper fibular epiphysis is exposed by an incision over the head of the fibula. The common peroneal nerve should be isolated and protected. The cartilaginous disk is completely cureted out, and the defect is filled with small bone chips. Through the same exposure, the upper tibial epiphysis is exposed by elevating the origin of the extensor muscles. Medially, the approach is along the anterior margin of the sartorius tendon. After removal of the rectangular block of bone from both sides of the tibia, the cartilaginous plate, which is in the form of an inverted saucer or V, is cureted out. Each block is reversed and reinserted.

Postoperatively, immobilization for 3 weeks is required. If removal of the plate is inadequate in any one portion, growth may continue therein, with consequent deformity.

Temporary Epiphyseal Arrest. Haas found that by encircling the epiphyseal plate with a loop of wire, epiphyseal growth is arrested.[108] When the wire is removed, normal growth is resumed. Blount confirmed this work but used staples instead of wires.[93] When sufficient staples are inserted so as to bridge the epiphyseal plate, cessation of growth is immediate and complete (Figs. 14-56 and 14-57). Growth pressure is tremendous, so that one or two staples usually prove to be inadequate and will bend or break. To halt growth completely, three staples are inserted on each side of the epiphyseal plate. After sufficient shortening has been attained and limb lengths equalized, the staples are removed, and normal growth is resumed. This method dispenses with the necessity of calculating the appropriate time for epiphyseal closure and the uncertainties of factors of growth and maturation. Premature epiphyseal closure is a rare complication. Stapling can be used to correct deformity. For example, a knock-knee can be overcome by temporarily restricting the medial end of the lower femoral epiphyseal plate.

Lower Extremity Inequality After Cessation of Growth. After the epiphyses have fused, surgical shortening of the femur or the tibia is indicated. Femoral

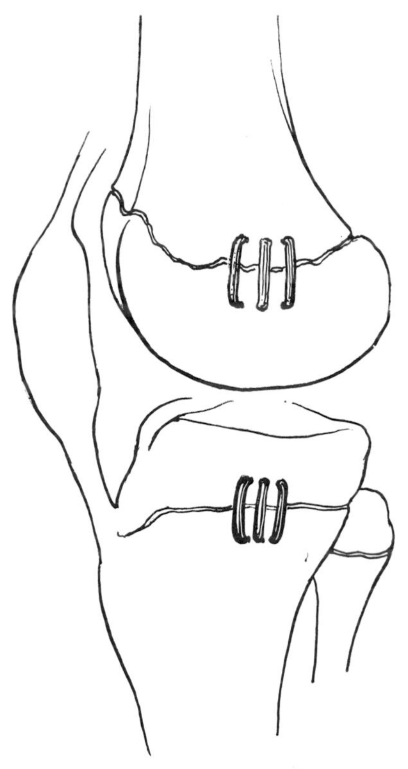

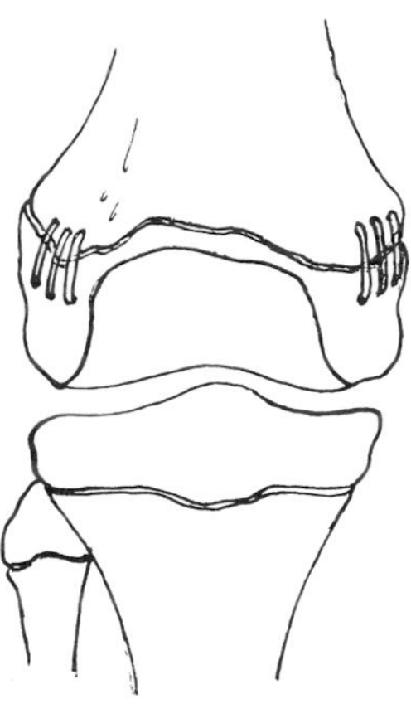

FIG. 14-56. Temporary epiphyseal arrest. To avoid damaging the epiphyseal plate, the staples are inserted so that the major portion of the transverse bar of the staple lies beyond the epiphyseal line of the femur and proximal to the epiphyseal line of the tibia. The staples must not be placed too far anteriorly or posteriorly for fear of creating flexion or recurvatum deformity.

FIG. 14-57. Temporary epiphyseal arrest by stapling. Note the direction of placement of the legs of the staples to correspond with the contour of the growth plate. The cross-arm of the staple is kept extraperiosteal. Accurate positioning will prevent damage to the growth plate and deformity resulting from asymmetrical inhibition of growth. (Courtesy of Dr. Walter P. Blount)

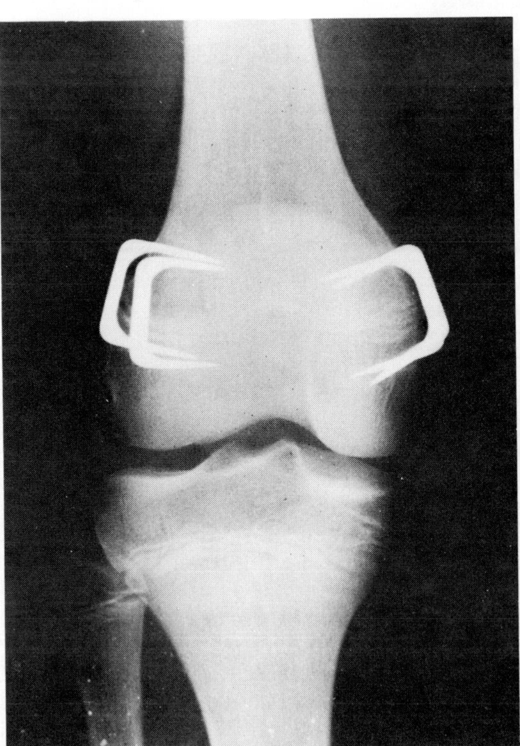

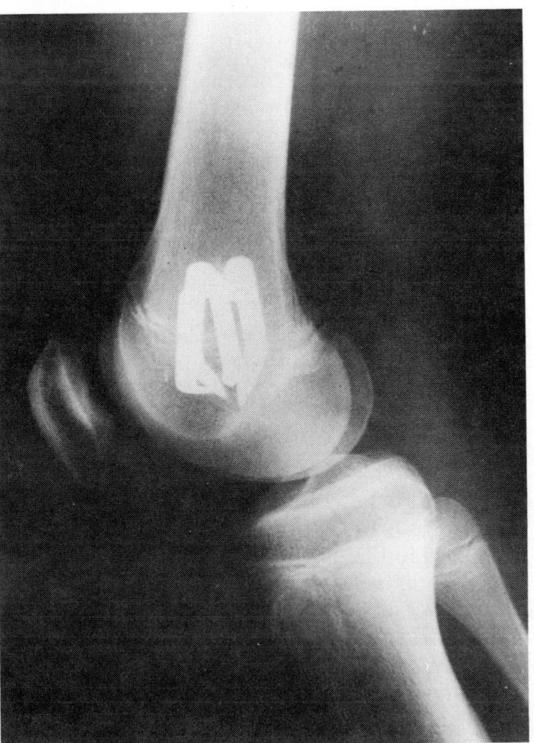

shortening is preferable because the bone is deeply situated beneath the musculature where deformity due to the bone graft and overlap of fragments is not visible, delayed union or nonunion is rare, and thigh muscles quickly recover their strength. The femur may be osteotomized obliquely, overlapped, and held by screws. A bone graft ensures union. If loss of length is obviously confined to the tibia, shortening of the tibia may be preferable. A step-cut osteotomy of the tibia is performed. The removed segment of bone is used as a bone graft about the osteotomy site. A comparable segment of fibula is also removed.

Section IV
Cerebral Palsy

Cerebral palsy is a state of muscular dysfunction that results from injury or disease of the upper motor neurons at the level of the cerebral cortex or throughout the course of their fibers within the brain. The loss of inhibitory control results in excessive impulses emanating from lower motor neurons. Lesions of the cerebellum are included, causing symptoms of ataxia and incoordination.

ETIOLOGY

The chief factors include the following:

Brain Injury at Birth. Mechanical causes are poorly applied forceps, excessive uterine contractions, excessive traction on the neck (ruptured vein causing intracranial hemorrhage), and sudden pressure change caused by precipitous extrusion of the fetus. Prematurity is a contributing factor because the delicate vessels beneath the anterior fontanelle are easily ruptured and the leg areas of the motor cortex are damaged by hemorrhage, with consequent spastic hemiplegia. Prolonged anoxia may be due to excessive use of analgesics and anesthetics, the umbilical cord wrapped around the neck of the fetus, or tracheal obstruction. The nerve cells are highly susceptible to anoxia.

Congenital Brain Defects. Disease in mothers during the first 3 months of pregnancy is associated with a high incidence of congenital anomalies. Diffuse and symmetrical brain involvement produces a clinical syndrome characterized by ataxia and athetosis.

Inborn errors of metabolism, mainly related to metabolism of certain amino acids and glucose, produce widespread brain damage, resulting in mental retardation as well as symptoms of cerebral palsy.

Rh factor. The severe jaundice of erythroblastosis fetalis damages the basal ganglia, resulting in athetosis.

Postnatal causes. These include encephalitis, convulsions, and head trauma.

CLINICAL PICTURE

A history is often obtained of a difficult birth or of illness during the early months of pregnancy. The infant is late in sitting up, standing, walking, and talking. The face is expressionless and may exhibit grimacing and drooling. Speech is difficult. Motion is clumsy, slow, jerky, and uncoordinated. The shoulder is adducted and rotated internally, the elbow flexed, the forearm pronated, the wrist flexed and deviated ulnarward, the fingers flexed, and the thumb adducted into the palm. The hip may be flexed, adducted, and rotated internally; the knees flexed; the ankle plantar flexed; the foot in equinovarus; and the toes flexed. The child must be supported under the armpits when standing. The lower extremities are held tightly pressed together or crossed in scissorslike fashion, and the heels cannot be brought down to the floor when standing. The gait is uncoordinated. Mass movements occur (*i.e.*, attempts to move one portion of an extremity throws all the other muscles into a state of spasm). Passive attempts to move a joint are resisted by a spastic group of muscles that may respond reflexly by a strong sustained contraction. Clonus is often seen. The deep reflexes are hyperactive, and pathologic reflex response is obtained. Athetosis may gradually appear within the first 2 years. Mental retardation becomes evident during the second and the third years. The clinical picture varies with the location and extent of the lesion.

EVALUATION OF MENTAL STATUS

About 70% of cerebral palsy patients have a mentality within normal limits. The speech difficulty should not be interpreted as a sign of mental deficiency. Rather, the response to tests made on several occasions should determine the degree of intelligence. Often a child becomes aware of his physical handicap and inability to play with other children, and so development of mental faculties is retarded.

CLINICOPATHOLOGIC TYPES

The location of the lesion determines the predominating clinical symptoms and findings. Although the following specific types are identified, a mixture of types is usual, but the most outstanding symptoms generally classify the offending lesion.

Cerebral Cortex Lesion

Premotor Area. Spasticity results and is evidenced by increased muscle tone, exaggerated deep tendon reflexes, clonus, pathologic reflexes, and the stretch reflex. The stretch reflex is elicited by stretching that muscle by [illegible]

[illegible] involuntary movements, the patient increases muscle tension, which should not be confused with spasticity. The stretch reflex is absent. Athetosis when controlled in one region by braces or surgical fixation will reappear in another area of the extremity.

Cerebellar Lesion. Characteristic signs of cerebellar dysfunction include ataxia, loss of sense of balance, muscle incoordination, adiadochokinesia, nystagmus, and dizziness. The usual cause is a congenital defect or, less commonly, a hemorrhage at birth. Often the ataxia improves spontaneously as the patient learns voluntary control of balance.

Diffuse Brain Damage (Prolonged Anoxia, Multiple Petechial Hemorrhages, Encephalitis). Generalized rigidity of muscles results and is manifest by loss of muscle elasticity and a "lead pipe" resistance to passive flexion and extension of a joint. The degree of rigidity varies from time to time. No true stretch reflex is present, nor are the deep reflexes hyperactive. Usually the mentality is deficient. Neurectomy is valuable for true spasticity but is of no value for rigidity.

TREATMENT

REHABILITATION PROGRAM

About one third of patients are feeble-minded, and another third are crippled severely and irremediably. These latter patients require institutional care. The remainder can be rehabilitated by reeducation, which includes training in balance and posture, locomotion, relaxation, rhythmic exercises, and speech.

At first only fundamental active motion is taught. This means acquiring the earliest primitive motion of the infant, who at first reaches out with one hand to grasp an object and later uses both hands. First, one leg is kicked, later, both legs. These voluntary rudimentary exercises are performed before more complicated motions. The aim should be toward developing the weak antagonists of spastic muscles. At the same time the spastic muscles are stretched repeatedly but gently to avoid exciting the stretch reflex. Exercises are performed rhythmically and with increased speed to develop coordination. This can be effected by having the child relax on the floor and perform movements to the accompaniment of music. Constant repetition enables the patient eventually to develop these actions without interference by the stretch reflex.

TEMPLE FAY METHOD

The Temple Fay method is aimed at the development and the organization of automatic spinal reflexes, as observed by Sherrington and Babinski in the decerebrate animal, and the ultimate coordination of these reflexes with what remains of higher cortical control.[177] At first, the patient is considered an amphibian (*i.e.*, one who because of partial or complete loss of cortical control must depend on the midbrain). It is usually simple to teach the fundamental motion excited at this level.The child is laced prone with the chin forward on a polished floor. First, the arm and the leg of one side is made to flex, the extended thumb pointing toward the face, which is turned toward the hand. As the limbs are extended outward and downward, the limbs of the opposite side flex, the head rotating toward that side. A regular rhythm of alternating movement is kept up to the accompaniment of music until a definite pattern is developed. The original jerky movements become replaced by a smooth series of regular muscular contractions. Once this homolateral or amphibian pattern is well developed, the child progresses to the reptilian or next stage of evolution, characterized by the crossed or contralateral pattern of movements. As the right arm flexes and the head rotates toward that side, the opposite leg flexes. Eventually, these crossed movements can be performed without passive assistance. After these motions are established, further advanced patterns are developed through stages of creeping and crawling to independent walking, feeding, and writing.

Contractures develop early in the presence of spasticity. Foot equinus is common and can be prevented by repeated stretching of the Achilles tendon and wearing a night brace to maintain dorsiflexion. The brace must be worn throughout the growth period because the taut calf muscles do not keep pace with the growth in length of the tibia. Also, the hips and the knees must be stretched to prevent contracture. Full-length braces for the lower extremity must be avoided, since they prevent motion and development of weakened and stretched antagonists. Occasionally, braces may be used as a temporary measure to enable the patient to gain a sense of balance. The arm is stretched to prevent and overcome adduction contracture. Wrist and fingers are stretched and put through a full range of motion. Contractures do not develop in the athetoid because of constant motion. Because purposeless movements do not appear during sleep, treatment is aimed at relaxation, not repetitive exercises. Braces can be used to control athetosis of the lower extremities. Unfortunately, surgical obliteration of a joint affected by athetoid motion will result only in the appearance of involuntary motion elsewhere in the extremity.

The treatment of the ataxic is by training in balance, gait, and eye-to-hand skill, but it is difficult and often unrewarding. The patient with generalized rigidity and mental impairment requires institutional care.

The most valuable nonsurgical procedures in cerebral palsy are bracing, which enables the spastic or the athetoid to walk between parallel bars and later with crutches; coordination exercises (*e.g.*, building blocks, modeling clay, ladder climbing, bicycle riding); diversion exercises, by which exercises are performed rhythmically to the accompaniment of music; and repetitious unaided individual efforts.[171]

Drugs. Many drugs continue to be evaluated for their effect on convulsive seizures, muscle spasm, athetosis, and behavioral disturbances. Major motor (generalized) seizures are frequently encountered, and are effectively controlled by phenytoin, primidone, or phenobarbital. For akinetic or myoclonic seizures, which are common in cerebral palsy, phensuximide, dextroamphetamine sulfate, or amphetamine sulfate, or methsuximide are helpful. When seizures cannot be controlled by these drugs, phenacemide, a potentially toxic drug may be tried, but it requires constant monitoring of its effect on the hemopoietic system. Phenobarbital is an excellent anticonvulsant, but it adversely affects behavior problems. A whole host of drugs continue under investigation, but the most effective ones have potentially serious side-effects. This subject is beyond the province of this text, but the orthopaedic surgeon should be familiar with the commonly used drugs.

Hyoscine is used especially in postencephalitic cases. It lessens athetosis and favors restoration of previously learned automatic motions. It is of no use to the child handicapped from birth, because he has not learned these automatic movements. For example, hyoscine is administered prior to an attempt at redeveloping reciprocal motion of the legs in walking.

Diazepam (Valium) decreases muscle spasm and allows an increased range of motion. It facilitates correction of contracture by braces or wedging casts and aids in obtaining reciprocation by antagonist muscles by lessening the stretch reflex. Speech difficulty is aided by reducing tongue spasticity.

The *hydantoin group of drugs* (*e.g.*, phenytoin) are relaxants useful for tension athetosis and generalized seizures.

The *amphetamines* are highly specific for behavior disturbances associated with hyperkinesis when these are due to organic rather than environmental influences.

Curare, when administered intramuscularly in a dosage of 0.9 to 3.5 units/kg, will effect muscle relaxation lasting approximately 4 days.[166] During this period, no dangerous or toxic effects are noted and the response to muscle training and reeducation is accelerated. However, the potential toxicity of this drug prohibits its use in the average case.

The following drugs may be useful to some minor extent and are considered safe for general usage:

Mephenesin group (Tolserol, Flexin) for spasticity: Dosage 0.5 g three times a day
Meprobamate (Miltown, Equanil) for athetosis and rigidity: Dosage 0.4 g three times a day
Motion-sickness drugs (Dramamine, Marezine) for ataxia and imbalance: Dosage 0.02 g to 0.05 g three times a day

ORTHOPAEDIC MANAGEMENT

Orthopaedic treatment of cerebral palsy constitutes one phase of a team approach in which the combined efforts of orthopaedic surgeon, physical therapist, pediatrician, speech therapist, and social worker are used. With few exceptions, only the purely spastic case can be functionally improved by orthopaedic treatment and physical therapy. It is therefore necessary at the outset to define the type of case under consideration before embarking on a therapeutic program.

Deformity is caused by muscle imbalance. As a general rule, spastic muscles overpower, stretch, and weaken their antagonists. Less commonly, the antagonists are paretic or flaccid. At an early stage, relief of spasm, whether by medication (*e.g.*, diazepam) or by general or local anesthesia injected directly into the muscle, reduces the deformity. With prolonged persistent spasm, myostatic contracture takes place with secondary adaptive shortening of capsular and ligamentous structures, and the deformity becomes "fixed." Continuing stresses of muscle imbalance acting on the growing skeleton result in structural bony deformity, most notably about the hip joint.

The aim of orthopaedic treatment is to restore prehension and reach to the upper extremity and stability for stance and gait to the lower extremity. This is accomplished by stretching the spastic muscles and associated soft tissue contractures, by exercising and developing coordination of the stretched and weakened antagonist muscles, by applying splints to maintain correction, and by dynamic bracing to secure additional correction. Muscle imbalance must be overcome.

When it is apparent that progressive deformity is developing in spite of conservative treatment, surgery is indicated. The spastic, contracted, deforming structures are released, the antagonist muscles are tightened (*e.g.*, distal transfer of the greater trochanter), or reinforced by tendon transfer. Bony structual deformity is corrected (*e.g.*, subtrochanteric osteotomy).

Preoperatively, bracing the part on which surgery is contemplated will determine the benefit that one may reasonably anticipate by operative means. Surgery is contraindicated in the athetoid and mental defective. If athetoid muscles are sectioned or transferred, the involuntary motions will shift to other muscles of similar function.

During the growth period, deformities develop progressively because the spastic muscles do not keep pace with skeletal growth. Therefore, when stretching, exercising, and splinting are insufficient to prevent deformity, early surgery is indicated. Operative treatment is particularly urgent to prevent severe bony deformity about the hip. If at all possible, surgery should be postponed until 5 to 7 years of age. The child should be evaluated repeatedly during the period of longitudinal growth.

THE LOWER EXTREMITY

With early regular stretching of tightened structures, reeducation and exercising weak antagonists, and proper bracing, most patients never require surgery and achieve good balance and an independent gait.

The objectives are to stabilize for weight bearing, prevent deformity, overcome deformity and establish muscle balance.[156] Severe spasticity, particularly of the iliopsoas and thigh adductors, in the rapidly growing child will cause skeletal structural deformities (*e.g.*, femoral neck anteversion, coxa valga, acetabular dysplasia, subluxation, and dislocation). The adducted internally rotated flexed hips, flexed knees, and ankle equinus must be overcome early to ensure normal development of the hip joint. The more rapid the rate of growth of the limb, the more rapidly does deformity develop.

Progressive limitation of abduction at the hip is an ominous sign. If the range of abduction becomes less than 20°, paralytic dislocation of the hip is likely to ensue.[180] Displacement of the femoral head is more likely to take place in the nonambulatory patient with excessive femoral neck anteversion.

Muscle balance must be restored early, if not by conservative means then certainly by surgery. Early correction of deformity may prevent or correct secondary postural deformities. For example, early correction of hip and ankle deformities will lessen the occurrence of fixed knee flexion deformity. When deformity is fixed at various levels, surgery should embrace the hips, knees, and ankles.

The Hip

A child with muscle imbalance about the hip will eventually develop structural deformities with adaptive shortening of muscles, ligaments, capsule, and tendons associated with spasticity. The hip should be studied by serial radiograms at 6- to 12-month intervals for early evidence of incipient subluxation, such as widening of the joint interval and partial uncovering of the femoral head. Femoral antetorsion and coxa valga gradually develop, leading to failure of acetabular development (shallowness, increased obliquity of the roof), eccentric positioning of the femoral head, and subluxation of the head (Fig. 14-58). The primary distorting force is the unopposed pull of the hip flexors, adductors, and internal rotators. Compounding the problem is delayed weight bearing and persistent positional attitudes of the child who sits on his knees with the thighs internally rotated. The most common deformities about the hip are flexion-adduction and flexion–internal rotation.

The main causes of hip flexion deformity are shortness of the iliopsoas, rectus femoris, and tensor fascia latae. The Thomas test reveals the presence of a hip flexion contracture. When flexion deformity is due to the rectus femoris, it is increased when the knee is flexed; when it is not increased it is due to iliopsoas tightness.

With hip flexion deformity, anterior inclination of the pelvis in conjunction with spasticity of the rectus femoris; the lumbar spine becomes lordotic, but the knees remain straight. If, with hip flexion deformity, the hamstring muscles are spastic and shortened, and cause posterior pelvic inclination, the knees are flexed to maintain the erect posture. When hip flexion deformity is severe, the main deforming force is the iliopsoas.

Adduction deformity of the hip is caused by spasticity of the adductors often combined with spasticity of the gracilis and of the internal rotators. The antagonist abductors are overstretched and weak or flaccid.

Correction of adduction deformity requires adductor release and anterior obturator neurectomy (Fig. 14-59).[159] In addition to the adductor longus and brevis, the medial hamstrings, particularly the gracilis and semitendinosus, are important adductors and when released will also correct associated flexion deformity of the knee.[157] Sufficient abductor power is a necessary prerequisite for adductor tenotomy. Otherwise, the child loses the only means of stabilizing the hip (close approximation of the knees) and a severe disability results. The status of the hip abductors should be evaluated with care whenever adductor release is considered.

In cases of pure adductor spasticity, the limbs will be closely approximated but will not cross unless the hip flexors are involved. A scissors gait in which the limbs cross each other results from a hip flexion–internal rotation deformity in which the tensor fascia latae is the major deforming factor, superimposed on adductor spasticity. To determine this, the child is placed in the supine

(Text continues on p. 566.)

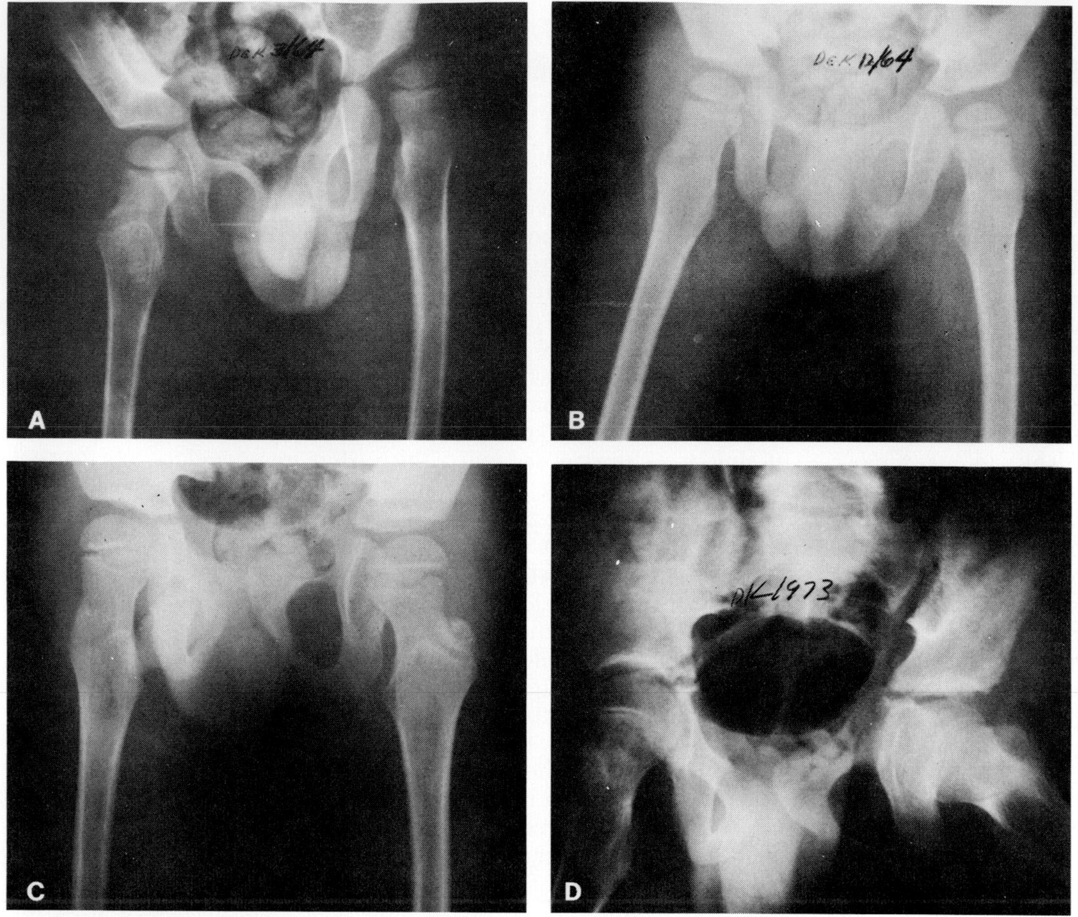

FIG. 14-58. Subluxation of the hip in cerebral palsy. The patient is 3 years old with spastic quadriplegia and has a bad prognosis for ambulation. (*A*) Impending dislocation of left hip. Marked valgus of femoral neck is a reflection of marked anteversion. There is marked adduction deformity. At this juncture, bilateral adductor myotomy, anterior branch obturator neurectomy and bilateral iliopsoas tenotomy were performed. No cast was used. (*B*) Appearance 9 months postoperative, showing relocation of the hip; (*C*) 4 years postoperative; (*D*) 9 years postoperative, showing maintance of reduction. (Courtesy of Dr. E. E. Bleck)

FIG. 14-59. Banks and Green procedure for adductor myotomy and obturator neurectomy. (*A*) A longitudinal incision is made over the course of the adductor longus, starting 1 fingerbreadth distal to the pubis. The adductor longus is defined, and the interval between it and the adductor brevis is developed. (*Continued on facing page.*)

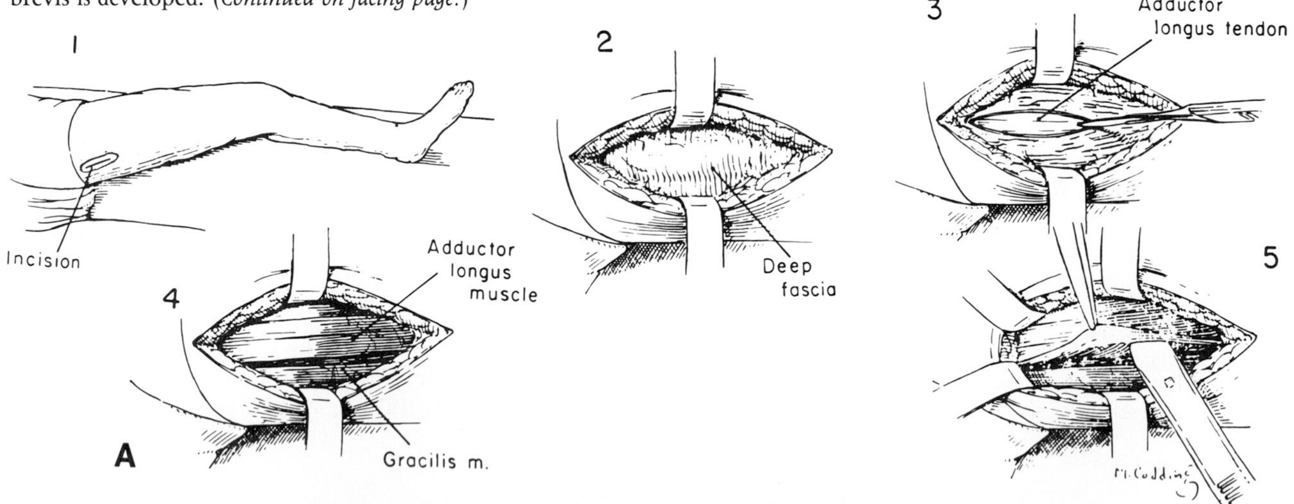

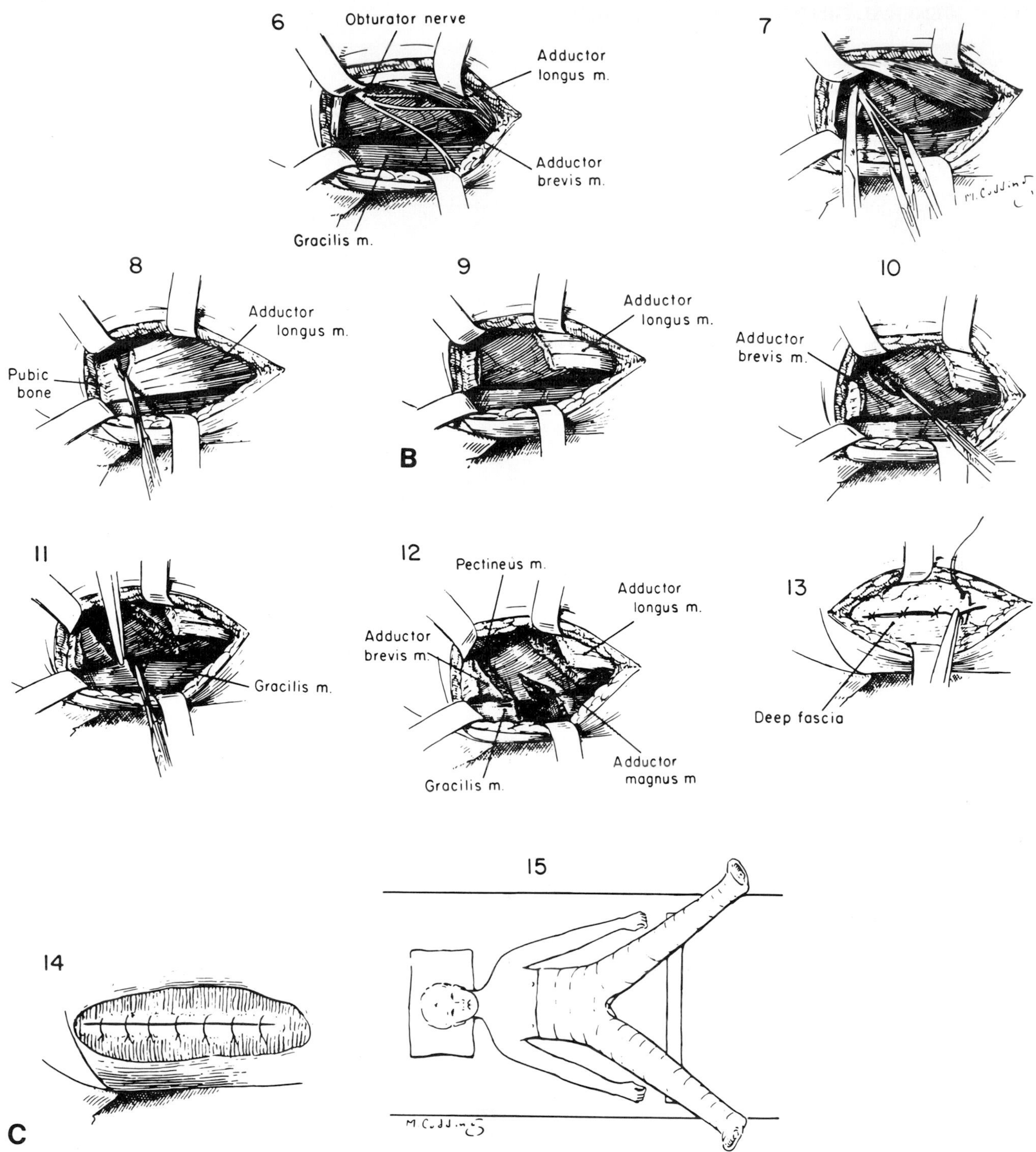

FIG. 14-59. (*Continued*) (*B*) The branches of the anterior obturator nerve to the adductor longus and brevis and the gracilis are defined and sectioned. The gracilis is sectioned, and the adductor longus and brevis are then sectioned. (*C*) When tightness persists, the adductor magnus is partially but never completely divided. The skin and subcutaneous tissues are closed. The patient is immobilized in a plaster hip spica, with the legs widely abducted. (Banks HH, Green WT: Adductor myotomy and obturator neurectomy for the correction of adductor contracture of the hip in cerebral palsy. J Bone Joint Surg 42A:111, 1960)

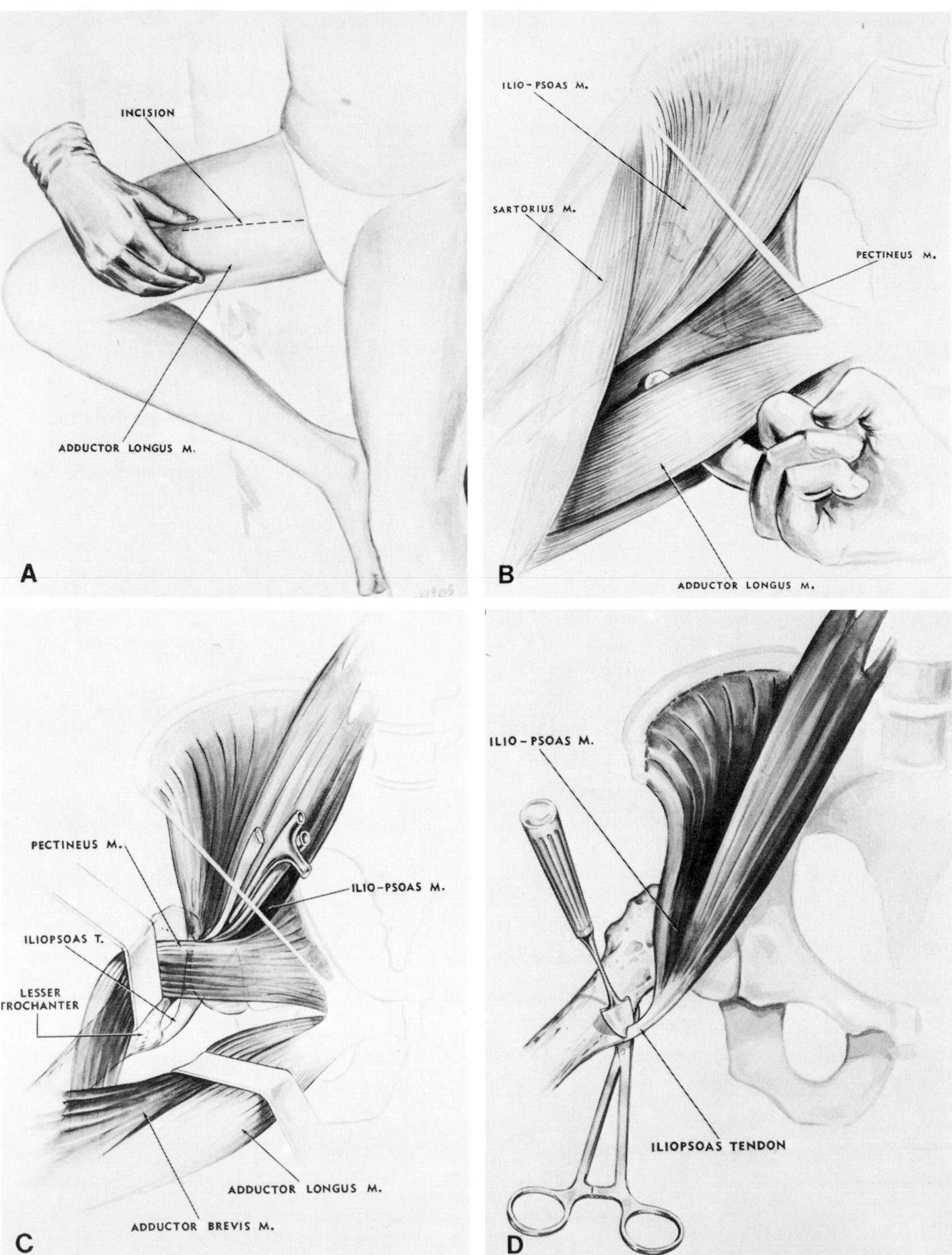

FIG. 14-60. Release of iliopsoas tendon through anteromedial approach to lesser trochanter. (*A*) The limb is fully flexed, fully abducted, and externally rotated. The tense adductor longus is palpated. A longitudinal incision is made along the lateral margin of the adductor longus for 4 to 6 inches. (*B*) Deep fascia is incised and the adductor longus sling is separated from the adductor brevis by blunt dissection and is retracted medially. The anterior division of the obturator nerve is identified as it spreads over the surface of the adductor brevis muscle. (*C*) The interval between the adductor brevis and the pectineus is exposed and widened by blunt dissection. The adductor brevis and proximal fibers of the adductor longus are retracted medially, the pectineus laterally.

(*Caption continues on facing page*)

position and one notes that the limbs internally rotate when they are forcibly brought together. Again, it should be definitely established whether the scissors deformity is an attempt by the patient with weak or flaccid abductors to stabilize the lower extremities.

Operative Technique of Iliopsoas Release (Keats). The patient is placed supine with both hips maximally flexed, abducted, and externally rotated (Fig. 14-60). This position renders the adductor longus prominent. The skin incision is made on the anteromedial aspect of the thigh, beginning at the level of the pubis and extending distally along the line of the adductor longus. Sharrard recommended an oblique incision over the adductor longus, paralleling the inguinal ligament, providing a cosmetically acceptable scar. A longitudinal incision is then made through the fascia overlying the adductor longus muscle. The muscle is severed close to its attachment to the pubis and is drawn aside, exposing the adductor brevis muscle. This exposes the anterior branch of the obturator nerve as it extends over the surface of the adductor brevis. The nerve is grasped and transected and its distal branches avulsed from the muscles. The adductor brevis is then separated from the adductor magnus, transected, and retracted anteriorly. The posterior division of the obturator nerve may now be identified on the surface of the adductor magnus and should be spared. The origin of the gracilis is now transected.

Release of the iliopsoas tendon is added in the patient whose hip cannot be abducted more than 20° with the knees extended. The interval between the adductor brevis and the pectineus muscle is widened by blunt dissection, exposing the lesser trochanter and the broad tendinous attachment of the iliopsoas, which is now transected. When the pectineus is not contracted, it may be mobilized and retracted medially for a wide exposure of the lesser trochanter. The incision is closed.

Postoperatively, the infant's limbs are maintained in abduction with a Richards plastic abduction splint reinforced with a metal crossbar. For older patients, the extremities are fixed in abduction at night with long leg braces with an adjustable thigh-spreader bar. The use of these braces should be continued until maximal improvement of skeletal abnormalities about the hip joint is demonstrable radiographically. A vigorous exercise program is aimed at strengthening the abductors.

Medial Hamstring Adduction Deformity. Spasm and contracture of the medial hamstrings, particularly the gracilis and semitendinosus, can be the major deforming force. It is essential to define their role, because their release alone may be sufficient to overcome adduction at the hip while at the same time relieving flexion of the knee.

Modified Phelps Test. The patient is placed supine, knees fully flexed, both hips at 90° flexion and maximal abduction, stabilizing the patient.[157] The knee on the side to be tested is extended as much as possible or to the point at which it is necessary to adduct the hip to allow further extension of the knee. If the gracilis or one of the medial hamstrings prevents extension of the knee unless the hip is adducted, the tendon of the muscle most involved in the hip deformity will stand out as a taut band. If to extend the knee, it is necessary to extend but not to adduct the hip, the test is not considered positive for gracilis-hamstring contracture. Normally, it should be possible, without undue force, to extend the knee fully without loss of abduction. In performing the test, the examiner should keep the index and long fingers on the tendons as they become taut. The muscle which comes under undue tension first is the major offender. Inability to extend the knee fully without adduction of the hip taking place is an indication that one, usually the gracilis, or several of the medial hamstrings is the major cause of hip adduction, rather than the adductors, and these should be released.

Technique. When tenotomy is performed, it is preferable that the stretch reflex be maintained during the operation. Tenotomy of the gracilis or the semitendinosus, when done alone, can be carried out under mild sedation with local anesthesia, or with light anesthesia. The patient is placed in the position described for the gracilis-hamstring test and held firmly by two assistants, one on each side of the table. With one assistant holding the opposite side, the surgeon or the second assistant attempts to extend the knee of the extremity being operated upon. The tendons are identified and a 3-cm vertical incision is made in the interval between the gracilis and the semitendinosus tendons. The sheath of the tendon to be released is incised vertically and the tendon is divided without cross sectioning the sheath. If need be, one or more tendons are sectioned. Full extension of the knee without loss of abduction at the hip is used as a guide to the extent of surgery. The procedure can be combined with proximal tenotomy of the adductor longus and anterior obturator neurectomy. In a patient with severe spasticity of the quadriceps, the medial hamstring muscles should be released cautiously. If release is too extensive, the spastic quadriceps may become more active and

This exposes the lesser trochanter. By blunt dissection, the taut iliopsoas tendon is brought into view as it attaches to the lesser trochanter and along the proximal and lateral aspects of the trochanter area. (*D*) A curved hemostat or periosteal elevator dissects under the tendon, which is then cut. The tendon is felt to retract proximally 1 to 2 inches as the hip is placed in hyperextension. Postoperatively, hyperextension is maintained by a pillow strapped to the buttocks. Hyperextension exercises to stretch the iliopsoas and abdominal exercises are started on the tenth day. (Keats S, Morgese A: A simple anteromedial approach to the lesser trochanter of the femur for the release of the iliopsoas tendon. J Bone Joint Surg 49A:632, 1967) undesirable genu recurvatum ensues. Sometimes the semimembranosus is an additional offender and requires tenotomy.

Following surgery, bilateral toe-to-groin casts are applied, holding the knees extended and the hips abducted by means of a spreader bar and immobilized for 2 to 6 weeks.

Correction of Flexion Deformity. The deformity arises from overactivity of hip flexors, particularly the iliopsoas, or from secondary postural deformity in response to flexion deformity of the knee.

Clinical estimates of the degree of hip flexion deformity are accomplished by the Thomas test. More accurate methods are described below.

Milch Method. A line is drawn between the anterior-superior iliac spines and the ischial tuberosities; a second line is drawn along the lateral aspect of the thigh over the femoral shaft, and the angle of intersection of these two lines represents the pelvic-femoral angle. The normal angle is 55°.

Bleck Method. While the patient is in his usual standing posture, lateral roentgenograms of the lumbar spine, pelvis, and proximal parts of the femora are made (Fig. 14-61). On the roentgenogram, one line is drawn along the top of the sacrum and a second line parallel to the shaft of the femur. The intersection of these lines is termed the *sacrofemoral angle.* In normal children, this angle ranges from 45° to 65°. If the patient has a hip flexion deformity, the sacrofemoral angle is less than 45°. If the patient with a hip flexion deformity stands with the knees flexed, the femoral shaft moves toward the horizontal and tends to become parallel to the top of the sacrum. If he stands with the knees extended, both the femoral shaft and the top of the sacrum tend to become more vertical.

Hip flexion deformity is almost always accompanied by increased femoral anteversion. This causes an internal rotation (pigeon-toe) gait, an apparent increased inclination (valgus) of the femoral neck seen in the anteroposterior roentgenogram, increased passive internal rotation, and decreased external rotation of the hip. These are gradually improved following release of the flexors, particularly the iliopsoas. To prevent postoperative hip flexion weakness, the iliopsoas tendon should be fixed to the capsule (iliopsoas recession procedure of Bleck).

FIG. 14-61. Standing lateral roentgenogram used to determine the sacrofemoral angle (method of Bleck). The lines are drawn along the superior endplate of the first sacral segment and the long axis of the femur defining the sacrofemoral angle. The normal range for this angle is 45° to 65°. An angle of less than 45° indicates a flexion deformity. (*A*) Standing lateral roentgenogram of the lumbar spine, pelvis, and femora with the measurement of the sacrofemoral angle in a normal child 12 years of age. (*B*) Sacrofemoral angle of 13° in a 12-year-old child with spastic diplegia and a flexion deformity of the hip with a flexed knee posture, showing that the top of the sacrum becomes horizontally parallel with the femur in this type of posture. (*C*) Sacrofemoral angle of 10° in a flexion contracture of the hip in a cerebral palsied child 7 years of age with spastic quadriceps and an extended knee posture, showing that the sacrum becomes more vertically parallel with the femur in this posture. Note increased lumbar lordosis.

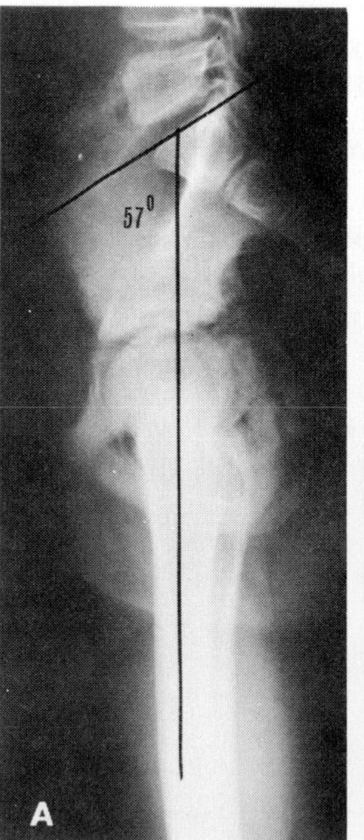

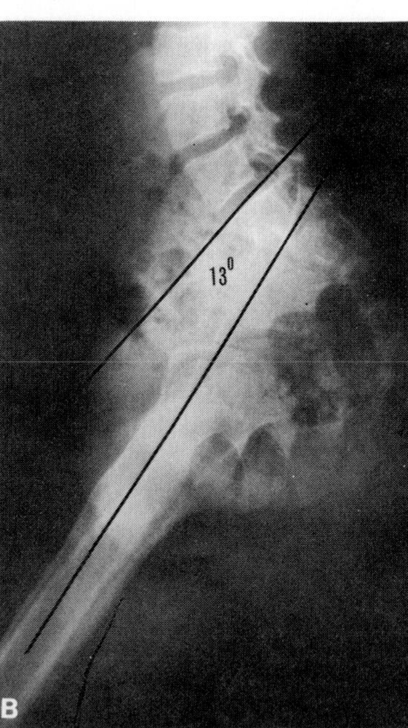

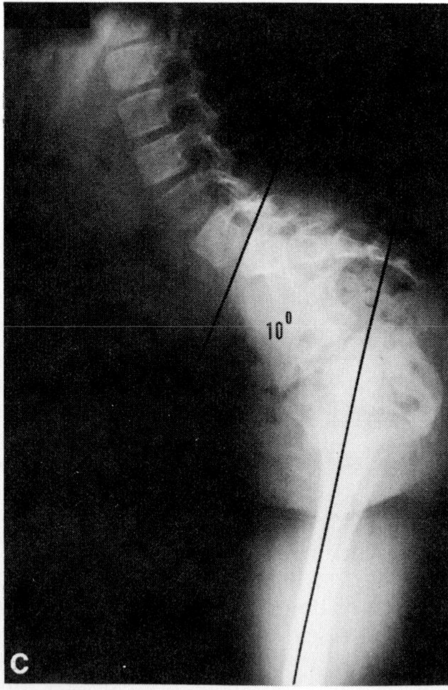

Persistent hip flexion deformity and excessive femoral neck anteversion encourages subluxation and dislocation of the hip joint, particularly in the nonambulatory child.

Flexor Release. Iliopsoas tenotomy may be sufficient. The tendon should be attached to the anterior capsule to prevent postoperative hip flexion weakness. Whether determined preoperatively or at the time of operation, other overactive flexors should be released, and the pelvic origin of the rectus femoris, tensor fascia latae, and sartorius are severed (Soutter). In addition, a tight pectineus may be released.

Operative Technique of Iliopsoas Recession.[160] An anterior iliofemoral incision begins 1.3 cm distal to the anterior-superior iliac spine and courses downward and medially for 10 cm to 15 cm. The sartorius is retracted laterally. The femoral nerve is separated from the iliacus muscle, the borders of which are defined medially and laterally. The femoral nerve is retracted laterally. The iliacus muscle fibers overlap the broad psoas tendon which hugs the anteromedial aspect of the hip capsule. The iliacus muscle is cut through transversely and as far distally as possible, and the psoas tendon is sectioned close to the lesser trochanter. The psoas tendon is brought upward and sutured to the anterior capsule of the hip near the base of the femoral neck, and the iliacus fibers are sutured to the capsule. This preserves active flexion of the hip.

Correction of Internal Rotation Deformity. This contracture, often associated with hip flexion, involves the tensor fascia latae, gluteus minimus and anterior portion of the gluteus medius.[170] These are important stabilizers of the hip laterally and should not be released if possible.

Mild to moderate internal rotation contracture is treated by:

Iliopsoas tenotomy followed by application of torsion-tension cables. Occasionally adductor-gracilis release is added.

Transfer of medial hamstrings to anterolateral aspect of shaft of femur (''barber pole stripe transfer'')

Severe internal rotation deformity is associated with femoral neck anteversion. It is corrected by osteotomy at either the supracondylar of subtrochanteric level, preferably done near the end of the growth period between 12 and 15 years of age. Before this time, iliopsoas tenotomy and its reattachment to the capsule of the hip joint (iliopsoas recession) is effective.[161]

Bone Deformity. Relentless, unopposed pull of the flexors, adductors, and internal rotators on the growing skeleton causes femoral neck anteversion, coxa valga, eccentric position of the femoral head, failure of acetabular development, subluxation, and finally frank dislocation. When the hip is dislocated and antetorsion is less than 45°, closed reduction and stable positioning of the hip in abduction and neutral rotation is possible. When anteversion is more than 45°, abduction and internal rotation (Lange position) is necessary to gain stability. Therefore, anterversion of more than 45° requires surgical correction to prevent redislocation. Release of deforming muscle forces must include the gracilis and iliopsoas also. A valgus neck of more than 140° indicates an incipient subluxation, and one should immediately be alerted to perform radiographic studies for antetorsion. (see Table 14-3).

Hip Subluxation and Dislocation. Progressive limitation of abduction, often in association with flexion deformity, is an indication of early instability of the hip. Such a hip is at risk of subluxation of dislocation.[178,181] A hip showing roentgenographic evidence of subluxation or dislocation invariably has a range of abduction less than 45°, although a few with such limited abduction may never display signs of instability. Hips with a range of abduction greater than 45° almost never proceed to subluxation or dislocation.

The mechanism that causes subluxation is the action of strong adductor and flexor muscles in the presence of weak gluteal abductors and extensors.[176,178,190] The gracilis is an important factor in limiting abduction in spastic hips. Increased valgus and anteversion of the femoral neck are contributory bone deformities, but only when abduction is markedly limited is the hip at risk.

In the very young patient, subtle roentgenographic findings suggesting preluxation should be sought (*e.g.*, increased obliquity of the acetabular roof, partial uncovering of the femoral head, excessive antetorsion). These are indications for immediate adductor-gracilis release, anterior obturator neurectomy, and iliopsoas tenotomy. Postoperatively, splinting the hips in abduction will encourage normal development of the acetabulum (Fig. 14-62).

In older patients, subtrochanteric varus-derotational osteotomy of the femur is done. Internal fixation is essential. Any required soft tissue release must precede bone surgery.

If the socket is not well developed and the roof is inadequate, a Chiari procedure will ensure firm seating of the femoral head.

TABLE 14-3 Normal Degrees of Anteversion*

Age	Anteversion (degrees)
Birth to 1 yr	30–50
2	30
3–5	25
6–12	20
12–15	17
16–20	11
20 and above	8

* Shows progression with age. (After Lusted and Keats)

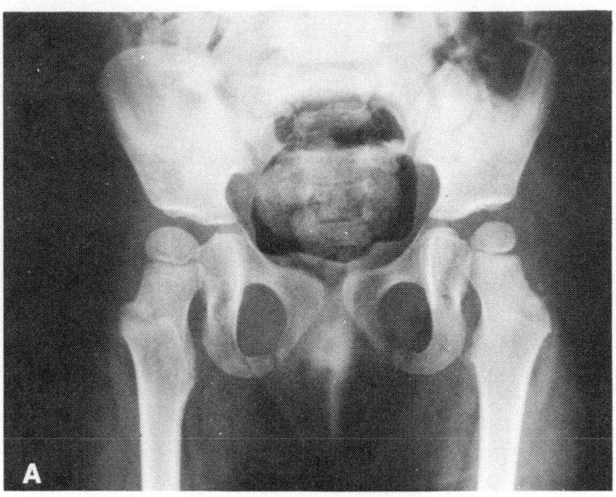

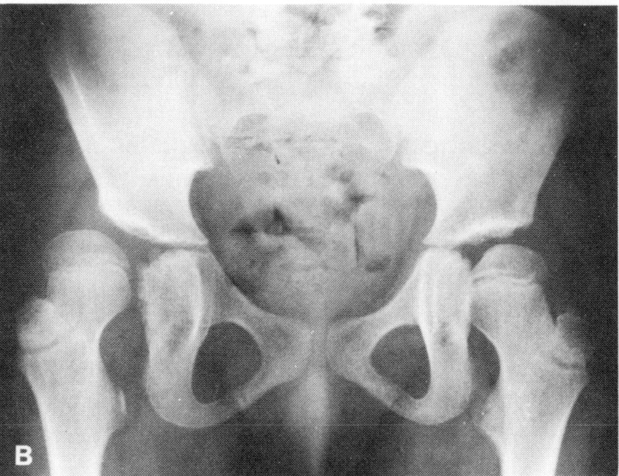

FIG. 14-62. Cerebral palsy hip progressing to subluxation. (*A*) Appearance in a 2½-year-old child with cerebral palsy spastic quadriplegia who was not ambulatory. The hips appear to be normal. (*B*) Appearance at 7 years of age. The patient is ambulatory with a walker and has developed subluxation of the right hip. She has a 30° flexion deformity of the right hip. Flexion deformity as well as adduction deformity must be treated to prevent dislocation, particularly in the nonambulatory patient with marked femoral neck anteversion. (Courtesy of Dr. E. E. Bleck)

The Knee

The most common deformity of the knee is flexion deformity. It is either primary, due to deforming forces about the knee, or secondary, a compensatory deformity that develops in response to flexion deformity at the hip and equinus deformity at the ankle. A third type may be classified as postural, in which the patient assumes a flexed knee position to gain better balance. *Primary knee flexion deformity* is due to muscle imbalance. Spastic hamstrings overpower normal or weakened quadriceps, mainly the rectus femoris. It is rarely due to normal hamstrings acting against weak or flaccid quadriceps. In *secondary knee flexion deformity,* the knee flexes to maintain upright position when hip flexion deformity and ankle equinus develop. If allowed to persist, contracture takes place.

Treatment of Flexion Deformity of the Knee. Secondary flexion deformity in its early stages is a passively correctable deformity which will automatically correct when hip and ankle deformities are overcome. Later it requires a vigorous regimen of stretching the posterior structures and exercises to strengthen the extensors, as well as appropriate splinting and bracing.

Primary spastic flexion contracture requires weakening of the knee flexors and strengthening of the extensors. Initially, this is attempted by stretching, exercises, and bracing. This may be sufficient to correct the deformity, especially when muscle imbalance and deformity about the hip are corrected early.

Surgical treatment is indicated when conservative treatment fails. It is directed toward restoring muscle balance, by reducing flexor power, and, when necessary, increasing extensor power. It is essential to preserve enough flexor power to provide knee flexion against gravity. A normal gait demands reciprocal hip and knee flexion and dorsiflexion of the ankle.

Excessive weakening of the hamstrings can result in genu recurvatum, too much loss of flexor power, reduction of posterior pelvic stability, and increased lumbar lordosis. For these reasons, such various techniques have been advocated as:

Eggers method. Complete hamstring tenotomies are performed; tendons are then fixed to the posterior aspect of the femoral condyles; patellar retinacula are severed (Figs. 14-63 through 14-67).

Green method. Fractional lengthening of all hamstrings is done, with division of iliotibial band.

Keats method. Medial hamstrings are transferred to medial femoral condyle; biceps femoris tendon is lengthened.

The Eggers procedure is the most widely used and most effective procedure. When one is concerned about the possible excessive loss of flexor power, one hamstring may be left untouched.

Patellar Advancement. Patellar advancement is indicated when the patellar tendon is elongated, as evidenced by a high-riding patella, and then only when knee extension is insufficient. Before this is attempted, the quadriceps should be strengthened by graduated exercises. This is often possible in the young child following early release of contractures and correction of muscle imbalance about the hip joint. In the older adolescent or adult, patellar advancement is usually necessary.

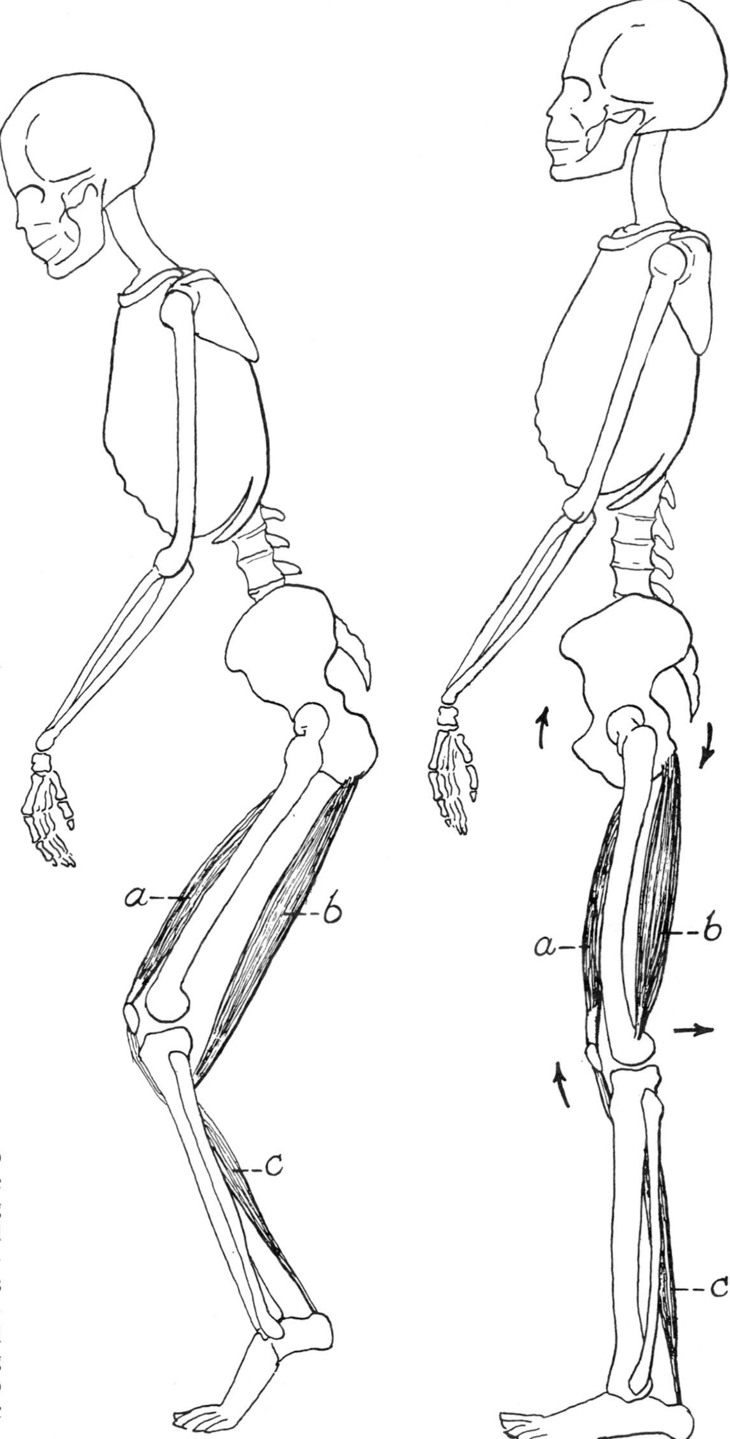

FIG. 14-63. The Eggers procedure for combined hip and knee flexion deformity. (*Left*) The effect of the overacting hamstrings on the tibia in the dynamic walking gait. (*Right*) The hamstrings, transplanted to the femoral condyles, no longer flex the knee and permit the quadriceps to extend the knee. The quadriceps action is rendered more effective by dividing the patellar retinaculum. With the knee extended, the hamstrings extend the hip. (Eggers GWN: Transplantation of hamstring tendons to femoral condyles in order to improve hip extension and decrease knee flexion in cerebral spastic paralysis. J Bone Joint Surg 34A:827, 1952)

Distal Transposition of Tibial Tubercle. This procedure should be avoided in the growing child because of danger of premature anterior epiphyseal closure leading to recurvatum.

Distal Transfer of Patellar Tendon (Baker). The tendinous insertion of the patellar tendon is severed and fixed distally and medially beneath an osteoperiosteal flap with a screw.[179]

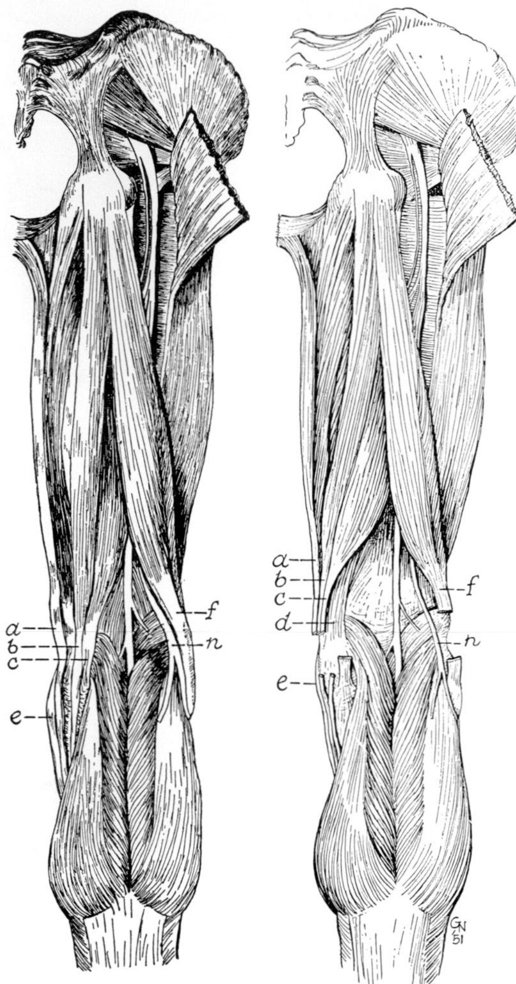

FIG. 14-64. The Eggers procedure for combined hip and knee flexion deformity. (*Left*) Anatomy involved in transplantation of hamstrings: gracilis (*a*); semitendinosus (*b*); semimembranosus (*c*); sartorius (*e*); biceps femoris (*f*); common peroneal nerve (*n*). (*Right*) Division of tendons. Not divided are adductor magnus (*d*) and sartorius (*e*). (Eggers GWN: Transplantation of hamstring tendons to femoral condyles in order to improve hip extension and decrease knee flexion in cerebral spastic paralysis. J Bone Joint Surg 34A:827, 1952)

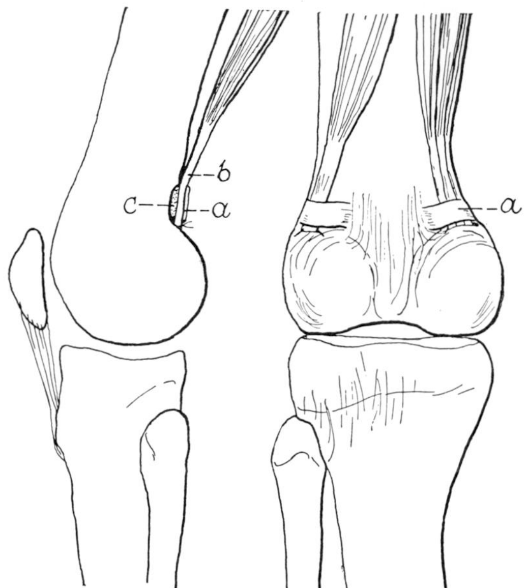

FIG. 14-65. The Eggers procedure for combined hip and knee flexion deformity, showing subperiosteal placing of tendons. The tendons are buried in an osseous groove: periosteal flap (*a*); tendon (*b*); osseous groove (*c*). (Eggers GWN: Surgical division of the patellar retinaculum to improve extension of the knee joint in cerebral spastic paralysis. J Bone Joint Surg 32A:80, 1952).

Plication of Patellar Tendon (Chandler). The patellar tendon is drawn distally and held with braided wire, which passes transversely through the quadriceps aponeurosis immediately above the bone (Fig. 14-68). The two strands are threaded distally in the capsule alongside the patella, emerging through the skin beyond the knee, and are pulled taut and tied over a dressing. A pull-out wire is attached proximally. The patellar tendon is plicated and sutured, Postoperatively, the knee is splinted in extension for several weeks, after which the wire is extracted and gentle motion is begun.[164]

When flexion deformity is rarely due to normal hamstrings overpowering a weak or flaccid quadriceps, the biceps and semitendinosus may be transferred to the patella.

Occasionally, a spastic tensor fascia latae may be a deforming force through the iliotibial band. Resection of the iliotibial band and, medial to it, the intermuscular septum is necessary. Sometimes it is also necessary to cut the heads of origin of the gastrocnemius, permitting further extension of the knee and dorsiflexion of the ankle.

Partial Sciatic Neurectomy. Weakening of the hamstrings by partial neurectomy produces unpredictable results. The nerve is exposed through a longitudinal incision, which starts immediately below the gluteal crease, continues midway between the greater trochanter and the ischial tuberosity, and extends distally several inches. The long head of the biceps, which originates at the ischial tuberosity and crosses the nerve obliquely, is retracted medially. A large branch from the medial side of the sciatic nerve divides into three branches, passing to the long head of the biceps, the semitendinosus, and the semimembranosus. The selected nerve or nerves are avulsed from the muscles, and the parent branch is resected at its point of emergence from the main nerve. Below this level emerges the branch to the short head

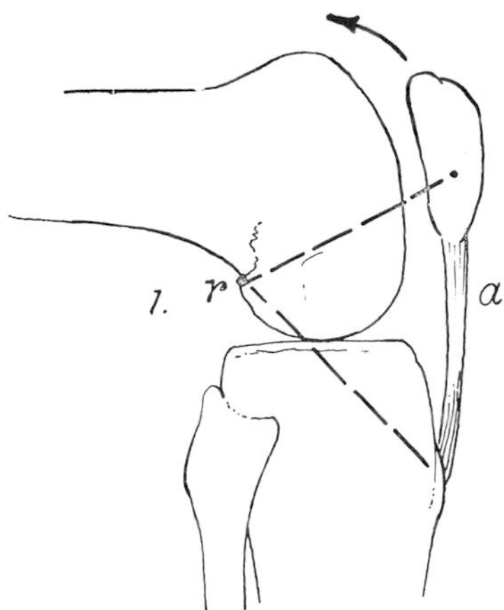

1. When the knee is flexed, the stretching is greatest at the patellar ligament and decreases as the radial center is approached.

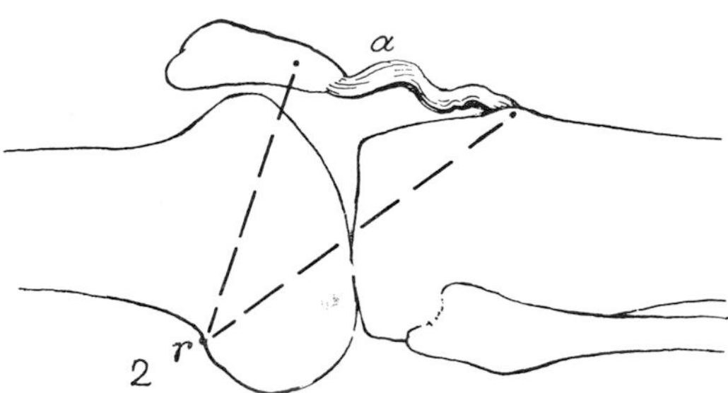

2. When the knee is extended, the structures near radial center are taut. The patellar ligament and adjacent structures are not taut.

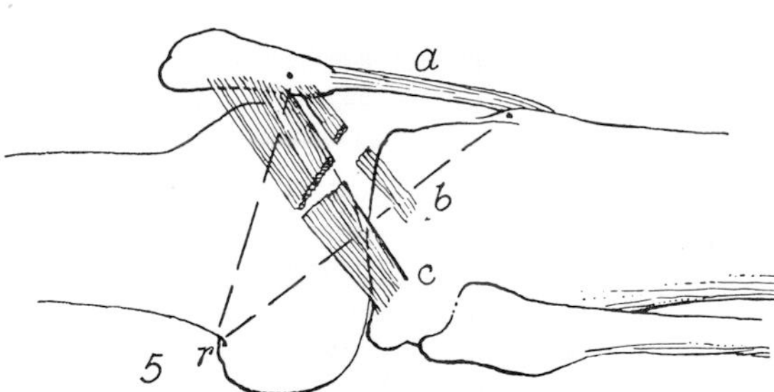

5. The fascial and muscular retinacula are divided. Remove restriction and allow quadriceps extensor force to be applied to tibia by patellar ligament.

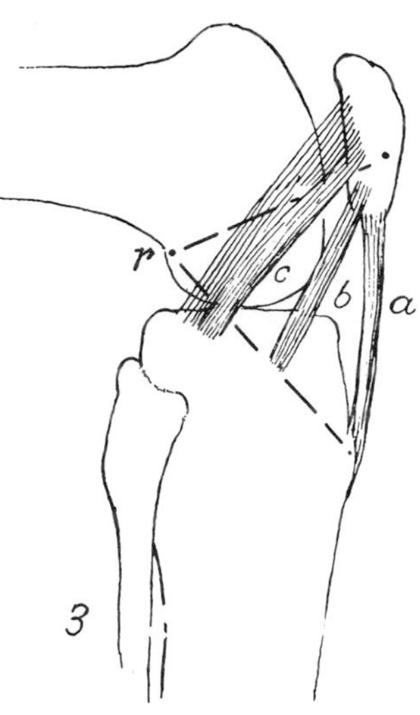

3. The structures near radial center that are less-stretched are fascial retinaculum as well as the lateral and medial portions of muscular retinacula.

a.-Patellar ligament
b.-Muscular retinaculum
c.-Fascial
r.-Radial center

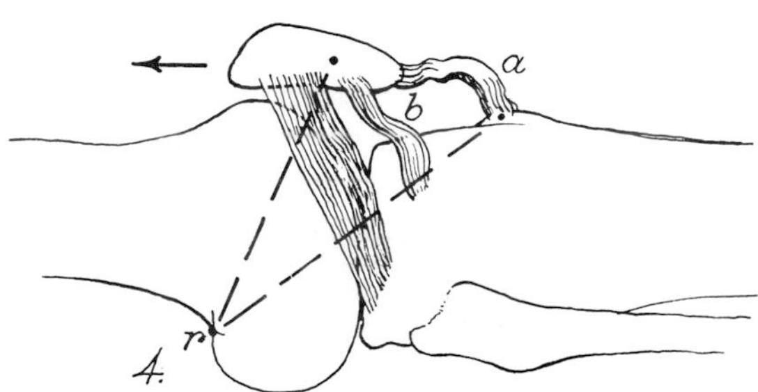

4. When the knee is extended, the quadriceps force is limited by less-stretched muscular and fascial retinacula which are not placed for efficient function. Therefore, extension is incomplete owing to the loss of transmission of quadriceps force to the tibia by the stretched patellar ligament.

FIG. 14-66. The Eggers procedure for combined hip and knee flexion deformity: diagrammatic representation of patellar extension and the restrictive structures (patellar retinaculum). (Eggers GWN: Surgical division of the patellar retinaculum to improve extension of the knee joint in cerebral spastic paralysis. J Bone Joint Surg 32A:80, 1950)

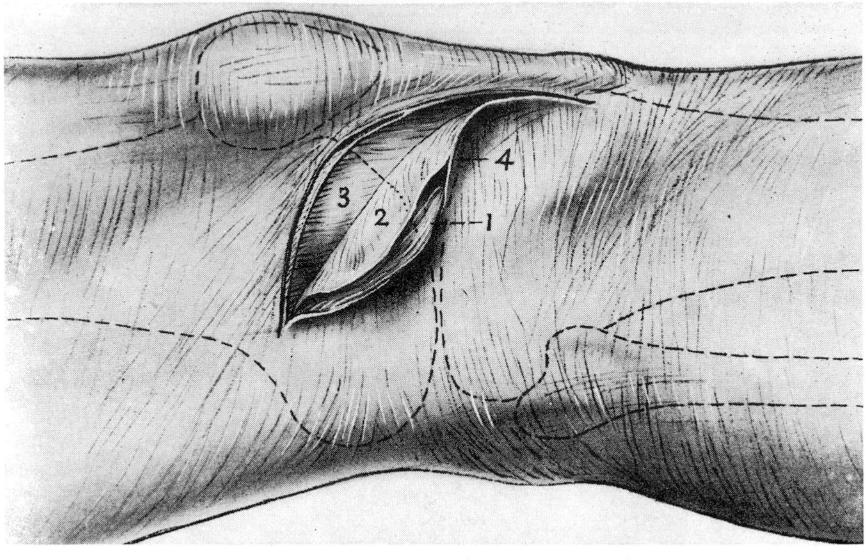

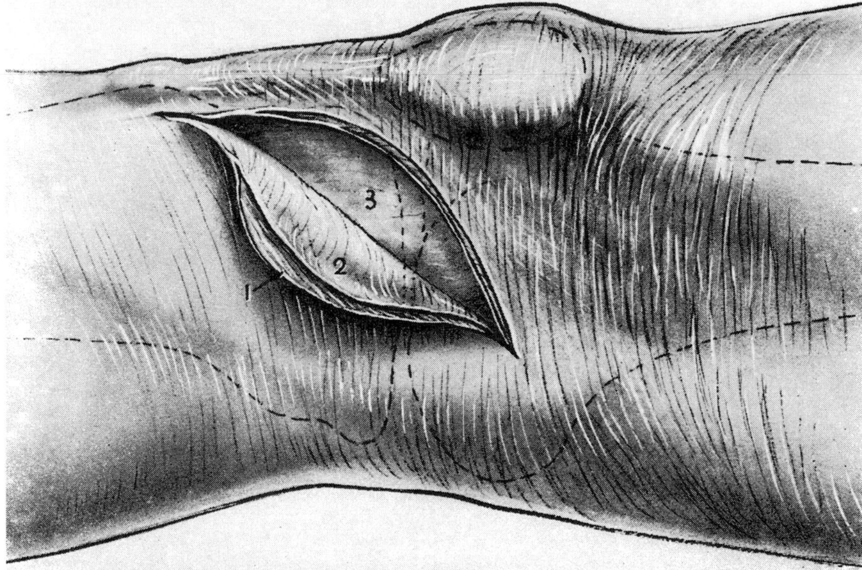

FIG. 14-67 The Eggers procedure for combined hip and knee flexion deformity; (*Top*) Division of patellar retinaculum, exposure on lateral aspect of knee. Incision must reach level of anterior margin of fibular collateral ligament. (*1,* Fascial retinaculum; *2,* muscular retinaculum; *3,* capsule; *4,* fusion margin of musculofascial retinaculum.) (*Bottom*) Division of patellar retinaculum, exposure on medial aspect of knee. Incision must reach level of anterior margin of tibial collateral liagment. (*1,* Fascial retinaculum; *2,* muscular retinaculum; *3,* capsule.) (Eggers GWN: Surgical division of the patellar retinaculum to improve extension of the knee joint in cerebral spastic paralysis. J Bone Joint Surg 32A:80, 1950)

of the biceps. This nerve may be left intact to preserve some flexor power.

Hyperextension Deformity. Hyperextension deformity is due to a spastic quadriceps in the presence of normal or weak flexors, an equinus deformity at the ankle, and an excessive hamstring lengthening or ill-advised tenotomies. The first is treated by tenotomy of the direct head of origin of the rectus femoris; the second, by correcting the equinus; and the third, by shortening or reattaching the hamstring tendons. Prolonged hyperextension deformity leads to structural bony deformity at the upper end of the tibia, which becomes bowed backward and slants downward and forward. A wedge osteotomy of the tibia and fibula corrects this deformity.

Spastic contracture of the quadriceps involves chiefly the rectus femoris, which can be defined by the Ely test. The child lies in the prone position with the hips and knees in full extension. The examiner then passively flexes the knee, thereby tightening the rectus femoris, which in turn, because of the pelvic origin of its direct head, flexes the hip; the pelvis is elevated off the table.

The Ankle and Foot

The spastic patient exhibits various deformities, including equinus, varus,valgus, calcaneus, and flexion contracture of the toes. Since muscle imbalance is the underlying cause of deformity, the status of deforming muscles and their antagonists must be established before treatment can be determined.

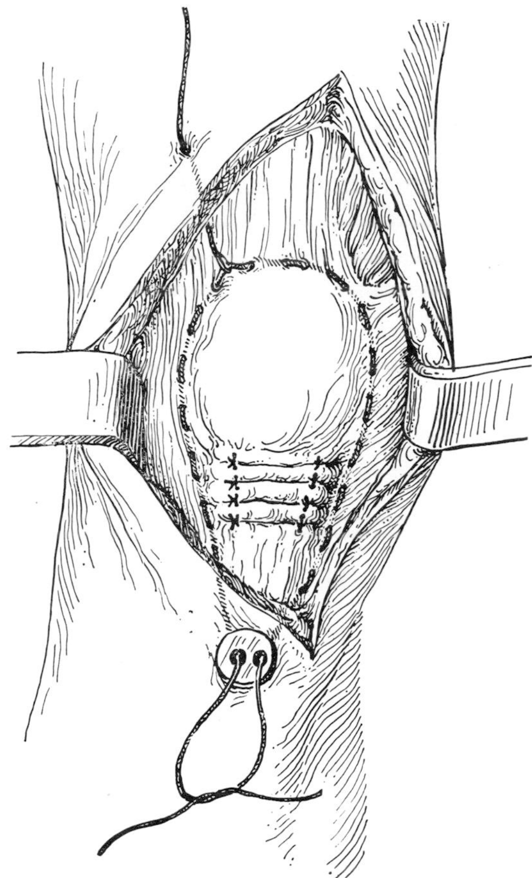

FIG. 14-68. The patellar advancement operation. The tension on the plicated patellar tendon is relieved by an encircling suture of braided stainless steel wire, which holds the patella distally. When the patellar tendon has consolidated, the tension suture is removed by a pull-out wire.

The objectives of treatment are to correct the deformity and provide a well-developed longitudinal arch, to balance muscle function, to obtain a heel-toe gait with adequate push-off, and to secure a brace-free, painless foot. In most cases these aims can be realized by proper splinting and bracing, by stretching contracted muscles, and by muscle strengthening exercises, especially ones directed toward the dorsiflexors. However, in resistant cases, surgery should be done at an early stage, even during the period of active growth, to prevent serious, fixed structural deformities.

Equinus Deformity. Spastic equinus of the foot and ankle is the most common deformity. Usually, it is due to a spastic, shortened triceps surae. The pathologic components include:

Contracture of the gastrocnemius alone, in which the equinus corrects spontaneously when the knee is flexed

Contracture of both gastrocnemius and soleus, in which the equinus does not correct when the knee is flexed

Posterior capsular contracture of the ankle

Thickening of the anterior portion of the body of the talus in longstanding cases, preventing engagement in the ankle mortise on dorsiflexion. A late finding is flattening of the articular surface.

Treatment. In most cases the deformity can be corrected by repeated stretching of the triceps surae, by exercises to strengthen the dorsiflexors, especially the anterior tibial, and by application of a dynamic brace, which gradually obtains complete dorsiflexion by a spring, a control dial at the ankle, or by bending an upright lateral bar at intervals. This is worn during the entire growth period, at first day and night until the foot can be brought flat on the floor. Thereafter, the brace is worn only at night for the duration of the growth period. Otherwise, recurrence is inevitable, because growth in length of the tibia bowstrings the calf muscles and the foot naturally assumes the equinus position during sleep.

Refractory or progressive deformity must be recognized and surgical measures undertaken at an early date to prevent structural bone changes. The type of surgical procedure depends on the type of muscle imbalance.

Spastic Calf Muscles—Spastic Dorsiflexors. The deformity is overcome by braces. Neurectomy or Achilles tendon lengthening is contraindicated, because a reverse deformity would ensue.

Spastic Calf Muscles—Normal Dorsiflexors. Achilles tendon lengthening is preferred because it does not impair the strength of the triceps surae group as much as procedures on muscles (*e.g.*, gastrocnemius muscle recession).

Partial neurectomy to the gastrocnemius or the soleus, depending on which is spastic, may be effective. Spastic involvement of either muscle is determined by exciting the stretch reflex or clonus while the knee is flexed and again while extended. The gastrocnemius, which attaches above the knee, exhibits a stretch reflex and clonus while the knee is extended but not when it is relaxed by knee flexion. The soleus, which originates below the knee, reacts in the same manner regardless of changes in knee position. Partial neurectomy is commonly peformed as an accompaniment to gastrocnemius-muscle recession at the knee.

Spastic Calf Muscles—Flaccid Dorsiflexors. A Lambrinudi type of tarsal stabilization or posterior ankle bone block overcomes the equinus. Partial neurectomy in addition is necessary only for troublesome clonus or extreme spasticity.

Normal Calf Muscles—Flaccid Dorsiflexors. The Lambrinudi procedure is indicated. Normal calf muscles are necessary to the success of the operation.

Flaccid Calf Muscles—Flaccid Dorsiflexors. Panastragalar

arthrodesis corrects the equinus and stabilizes the foot and the ankle.

Achilles Tendon Lengthening. This procedure is the one of choice for equinus deformity. It has the advantages of minimal reduction of calf muscle power so that adequate push-off is retained; it can be repeated during the growth period, and the tendon can be shortened when lengthening is excessive. The tendon is lengthened only to allow sufficient but not excessive dorsiflexion.

Before tendon lengthening is considered to correct equinus, it is necessary to determine whether calf muscle contractions are due to local spasm and contracture or to overflow:

1. *Spasm and Contracture.* Early mild or moderate involvement of the calf muscles needs only Achilles tendon legthening. Severe spasm and contracture require partial weakening of the calf muscles, which is accomplished by gastrocnemius recession.
2. *Overflow.* Active contraction of other regional muscle groups, particularly the adductors, will produce excessive spasm of calf muscles. In such cases, when the extremity is at rest, the equinus deformity disappears. *The stretch reflex is absent.* Treatment is therefore directed to the offending muscle groups.

White Method. Near the insertion, the anterior two thirds of the tendon is divided; 2 to 3 inches proximally, while force is applied to dorsiflex the foot, the medial two thirds is divided distally.[193]

Z-Plasty Method. Two flaps of tendon are fashioned by severing the tendon longitudinally in the frontal plane.[165] The knife is inserted so that the flat surfaces face anterior and posterior and are drawn proximally and distally. Proximally, the division is completed as the posterior half is divided, and distally the anterior half is divided. Thus the posterior flap is left attached to the calcaneus and the anterior flap attached to the triceps surae. The foot is then forcibly dorsiflexed. As the flaps are reapposed and sutured, the only exposed raw surface of tendon lies proximal where it is covered by a thick subcutaneous layer.

In late cases, the posterior capsule of the ankle is contracted and dorsiflexion is still restricted after tendon lengthening. The posterior capsule must be released. It is exposed by retracting medialward the flexor hallucis longus tendon, which passes obliquely across the capsule on the medial side. The nerves, vessels, and tendons are protected where they pass posterior to the medial malleolus.

In older children, the plantaris tendon is extremely hypertrophied and must be resected.

Lengthening is done to the point where the foot is brought up to 90° with the knee fully extended. A cast is applied for 6 weeks and is followed with a night brace until tibial growth is complete.

In the presence of varus or valgus deformity of the heel, Achilles tendon lengthening may be modified. For a varus heel, the distal portion of the tendon is severed medially, removing a possible deforming force. Similarly, for a valgus deformity, the distal tendon is severed laterally. Proximally, the opposite side of the tendon is severed.

Gastrocnemius Muscle Recession. Weakening of the calf muscles should be limited to the gastrocnemius. Soleus power must be preserved for adequate push-off of the forepart of the foot. The benefit of the operation comes from weakening of the muscle and modifying the proprioceptive, or stretch, reflex. By converting the gastrocnemius from a two joint muscle to a one joint, the probability of recurrence is lessened. Good power of dorsiflexion of the foot is a necessary prerequisite to a satisfactory result. One may elect to weaken the muscle further by adding partial neurectomy to the procedure.

When spastic equinus is due chiefly to contracture of the gastrocnemius, the deformity disappears when the muscle is relaxed by flexing the knee. This is the usual type of involvement. Recession of the gastrocnemius is indicated.

When spastic equinus is caused by contracture of both the gastrocnemius and soleus, the deformity remains unchanged whether the knee is flexed or not. Lengthening of the Achilles tendon is indicated.

Recession at the Knee. The heads of origin of the gastrocnemius are released from their attachments at the femoral condyles and displaced below the level of the knee joint.[182,184] Neurectomy of some branches of the tibial nerve, usually those to the medial head, may be added. When hamstring release at the knee is contemplated, preservation of knee flexor power by the gastrocnemius is necessary. Recession is better done at the distal level.

Distal Recession. The aponeurotic tendon of the gastrocnemius is divided transversely just proximal to the point where it joins with the soleus fibers.[156,186,191] The muscle is then separated from the underlying soleus by blunt dissection. The foot is forcibly dorsiflexed to the neutral position, and the retracted aponeurotic tendon is sutured to the underlying soleus. Recurrence of the equinus deformity is rare following this procedure (Figs. 14-69 and 14-70).

Neurectomy. Theoretically, resection of a portion of the nerve fibers innervating a spastic muscle weakens that muscle to a degree proportionate to the extent of denervation (Fig. 14-71).[185] Ideally, the residual muscle power should balance the strength of the antagonist. If the antagonist is flaccid, neurectomy of calf muscles is contraindicated. The antagonist muscles weakened by stretching and disuse should be strengthened by appropriate exercises before determining the extent of neurectomy. Muscle balance must be restored. The original Stöffel operation consisted of exposing the main nerve trunk which sends branches to the spastic muscle; the motor nerve tract, which supplies the muscle is isolated by electric stimulation and is resected. A simpler procedure is to expose the nerve branches at their point of

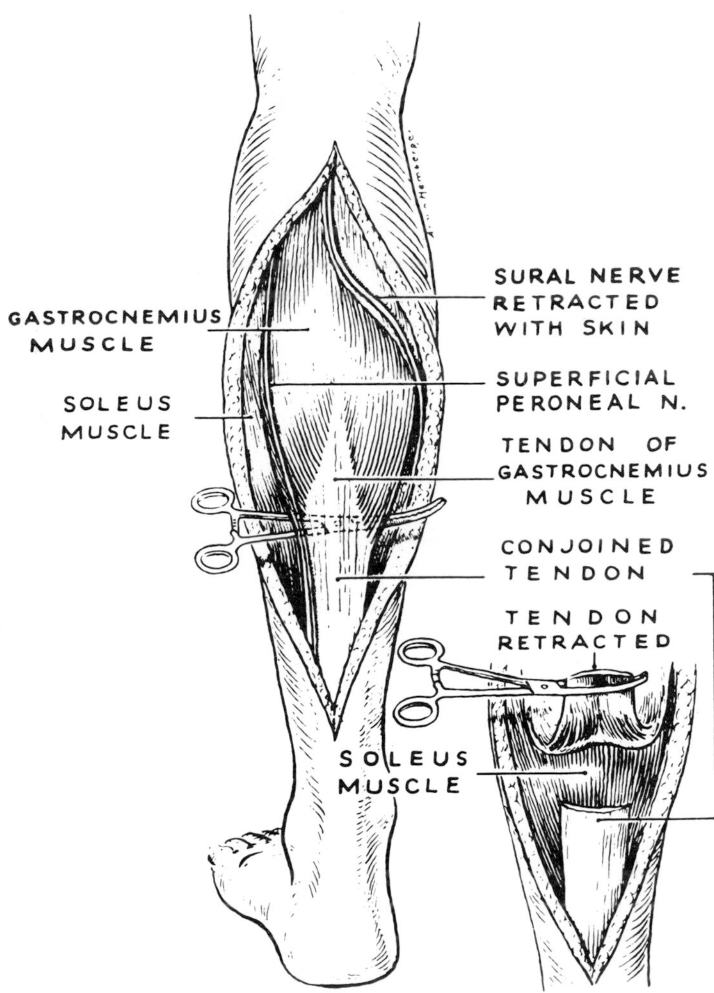

FIG. 14-69. Gastrocnemius muscle recession. (Strayer LM Jr: Recession of the gastrocnemius. J Bone Joint Surg 32A:671, 1950)

emergence from the nerve trunk or at their entrance into the muscle. Before neurectomy, a complete study is made of the muscle and its antagonists before deciding on the extent and the method of correction.

Calcaneus Deformity. Deformity of the calcaneus results from excessive Achilles tendon lengthening or after neurectomy of the calf muscles in the presence of spastic dorsiflexors. Treatment alternatives include shortening the Achilles tendon, tendon transfer (*e.g.*, flexor hallucis longus to Achilles tendon), talectomy, or pan-astragalar arthrodesis.

Calcaneal deformity may occur in the atonic child. Bracing is sufficient with a retraining program of exercise to restore muscle balance. The deformity disappears as the atonic muscle acquires greater tonicity.

Varus and Valgus Deformities. Varus and valgus deformities are the result of muscle imbalance between invertors and evertors. Early cases without myostatic contracture can be corrected by stretching, casts, and splinting to maintain the corrected position, and exercises to strengthen weak antagonists. Advanced cases with myostatic contracture require surgery, which is directed toward removing the deforming muscle force and, if possible, converting it to a corrective force. Late cases with structural bony deformity require osteotomy of the calcaneus.

Tendon transfer of a spastic muscle should be avoided because the results are unpredictable. The spastic muscle may not function sufficiently to restore muscle balance, or its overactivity may produce the reverse deformity. Tendon transfer may be attempted only when the deforming muscle is normal and its antagonist is nonfunctioning. When the foot is in varus, a spastic anterior tibial tendon may be transferred laterally to the base of the second or third metatarsal but not beyond this point. When the peroneus longus is transferred, the distal stump should be sutured to the peroneus brevis. When the anterior tibial is nonfunctioning, the extensor hallucis

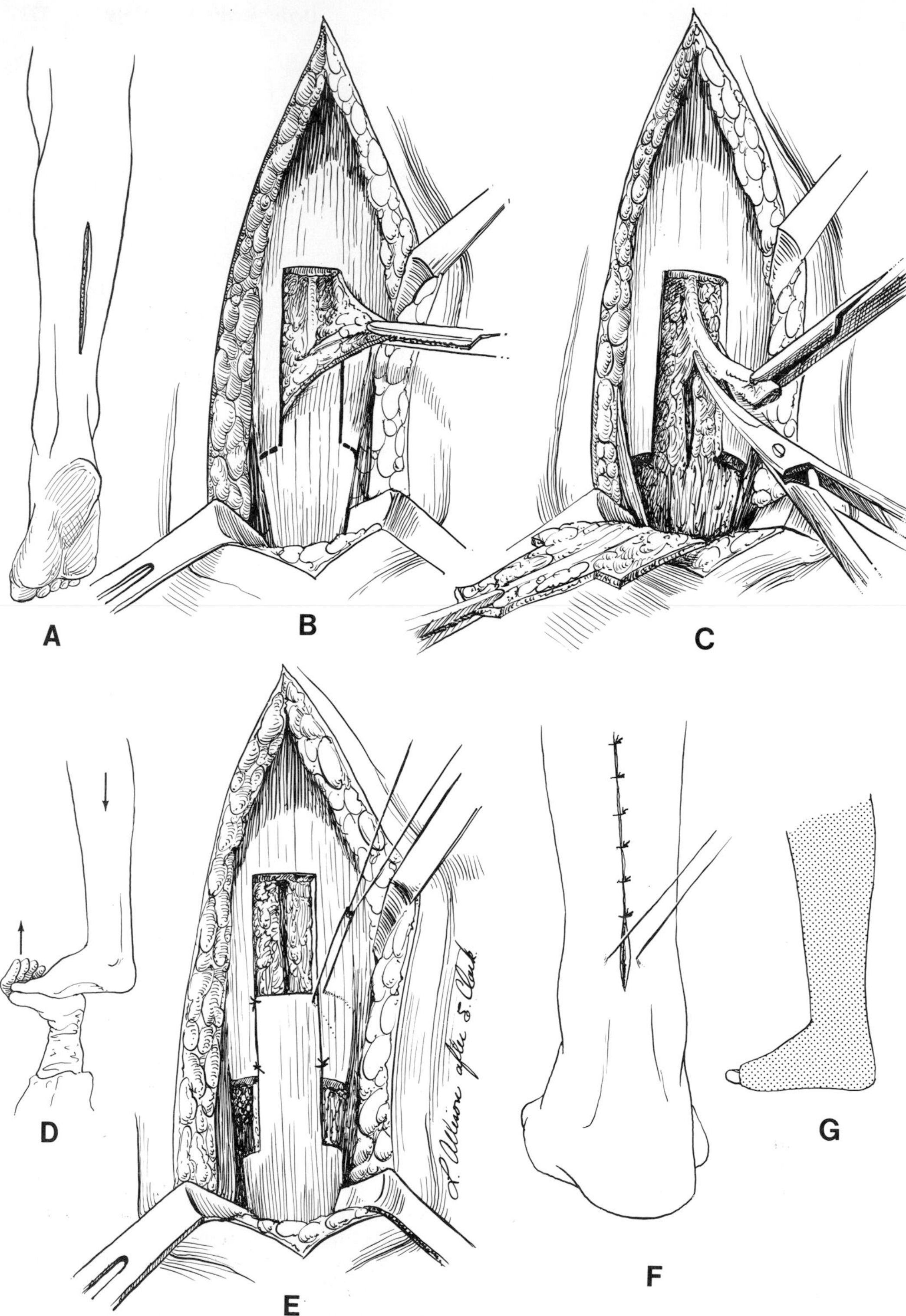

FIG. 14-70. Baker technique for lengthening aponeurosis of gastrocnemius muscle. (*A*) The incision is made from the lower border of the belly of the gastrocnemius to the proximal end of the Achilles tendon. (*B*) An inverted-U incision is made in an aponeurosis; lateral and medial portions remain intact with underlying soleus. Middle portion, or tongue, is dissected from soleus, with care being taken that no muscle fibers remain attached to this portion of the

(*Caption continues on facing page.*)

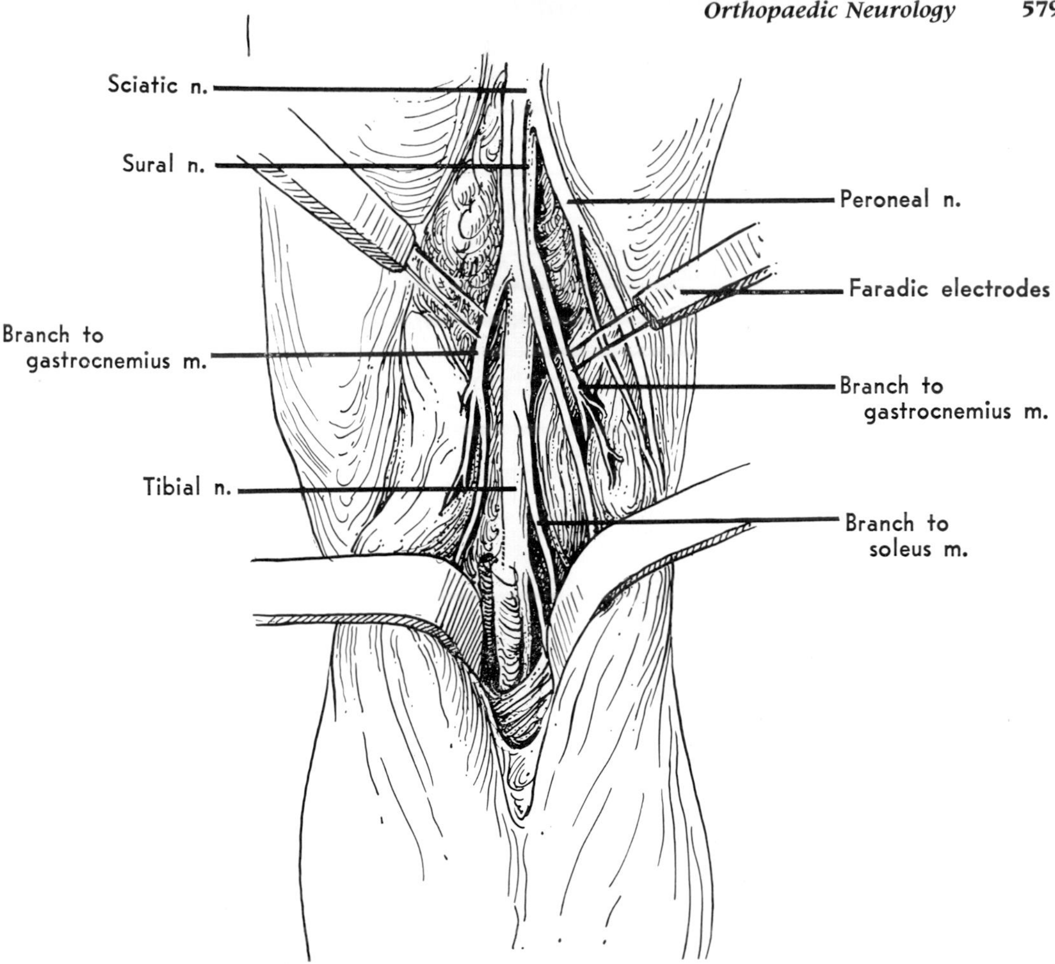

FIG. 14-71. Stöffel's operation for spastic equinus. The branches of supply to the heads of the gastrocnemius are shown being identified by electric stimulation. Only nerve branches sufficient for weakening the gastrocnemius and balancing the foot dorsiflexors are removed.

longus may be transferred to the base of the first metatarsal.

In correcting bone deformity, the integrity of the talocalcaneal joint in the growing child must be preserved. The calcaneus must be positioned beneath the talus in slight valgus with the axis of the talus and calcaneus, forming an angle of 15°. This is accomplished by extra-articular talocalcaneal fusion or by a wedge osteotomy of the posterior articulating portion of the calcaneus.

A spastic posterior tibial muscle causes varus and internal rotation deformity of the foot. By rerouting the tendon anterior to the medial malleolus, the deformity is immediately corrected. To convert the deforming force of the posterior tibial into a corrective force, the tendon and muscle may be rerouted through the interosseous membrane or brought about the medial side of the tibia and fixed to the anterolateral aspect of the foot.

With the patient under local anesthesia, two small incisions are made over the tendon, one below and distal

---

aponeurosis or to the Achilles tendon. (*C*) Dissection of central aponeurosis of bipenniform soleus muscle, carried out sufficiently to allow full dorsiflexion of ankle (*D*). (*E*) Distal attachments of the lateral and medial portions of the aponeurosis are freed from the tendon; the four corners of the overlapping portions of the aponeurosis are held with one black silk suture each. (*F*) Following closure of deep fascia and subcutaneous fascia, the skin is closed with intracutaneous sutures. (*G*) The extremity is incorporated in a toe-to-groin cast with the foot placed in slight dorsiflexion. (Baker LD: A rational approach to the surgical needs of the cerebral palsy patient. J Bone Joint Surg 38A:313, 1956)

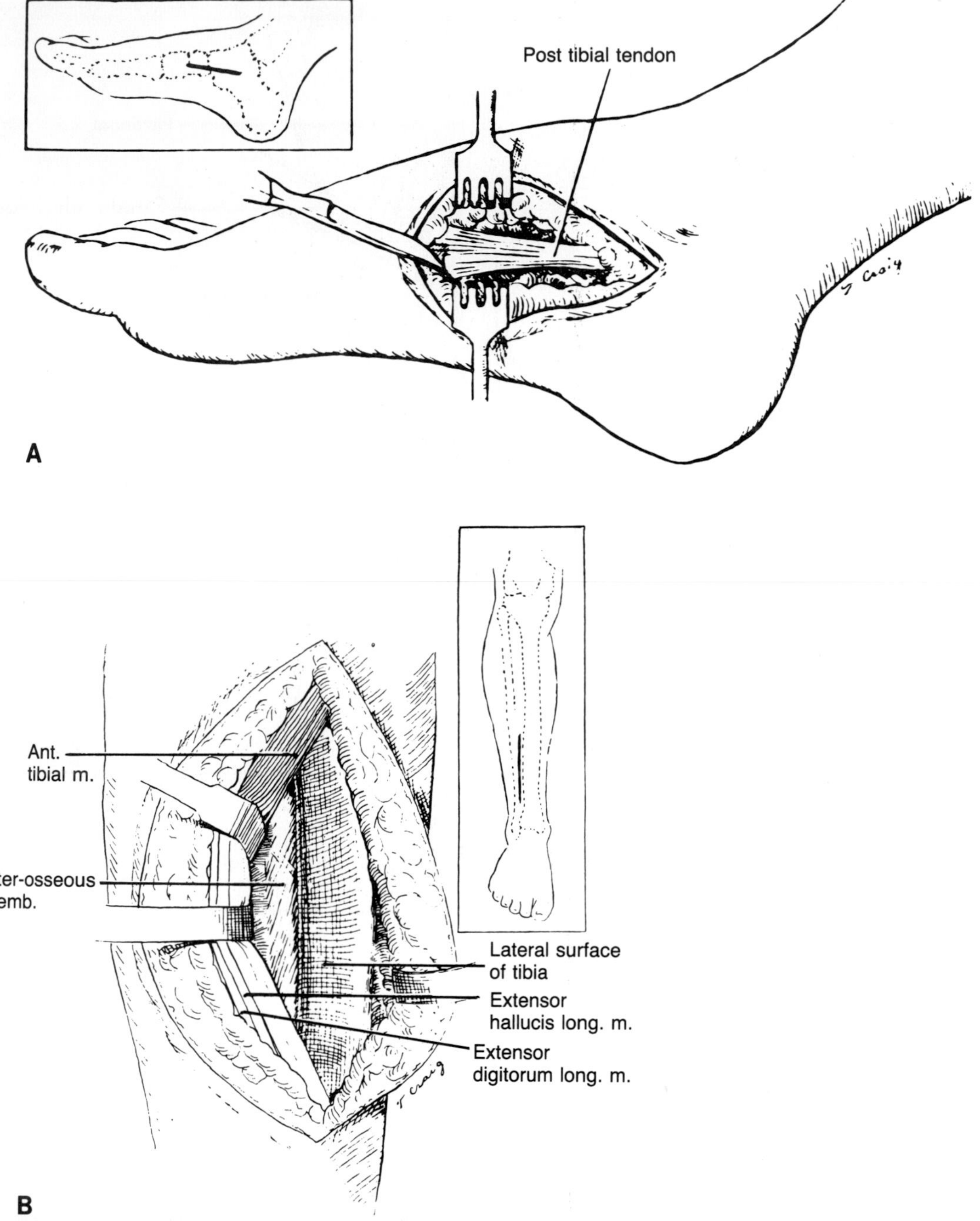

FIG. 14-72. Technique of interosseous rerouting of posterior tibial tendon. (*A*) The first incision is made along the course of the posterior tibial tendon. The tenson is released distally to its primary insertion into the tuberosity of the navicular to gain as much length as possible. (*B*) The second incision is made parallel to and lateral to the lower third of the crest of the tibia. Exposure of the interosseous membrane is accomplished by retracting the anterior tibial muscle from the lateral surface of the tibia. (*C*) The interosseous membrane is opened extensively, so that the underlying posterior tibial muscle is exposed. The tendon is pulled out and the muscle fills the interosseous space. (*D*) The posterior tibial muscle is passed beneath the anterior tibial subcutaneously to the site of its new insertion on the dorsum. (Watkins MB et al: Transplantation of posterior tibial tendon. J Bone Joint Surg 36A:1181, 1954)

(*Illustration continues on facing page*)

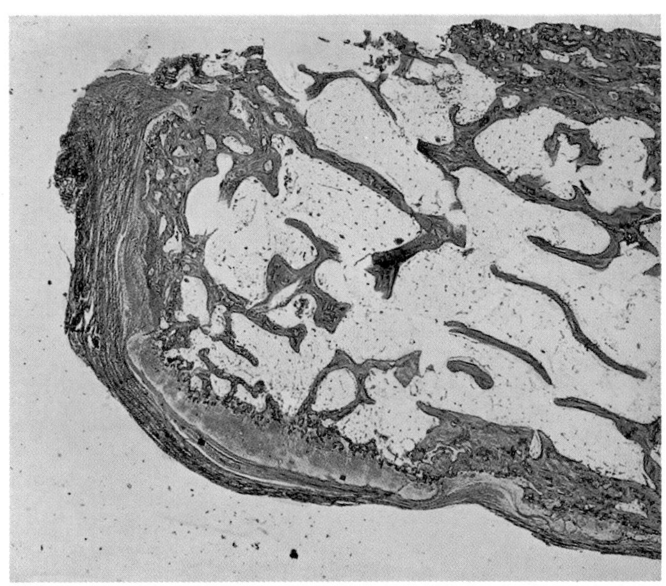

PLATE 15-1. Osteochondroma. Note the cartilaginous cap and enveloping capsule. (×6) (See p. 598.)

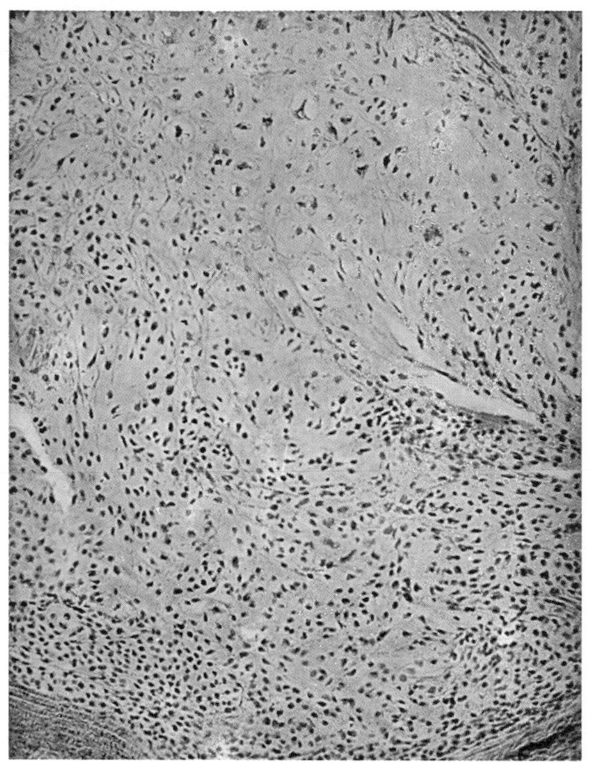

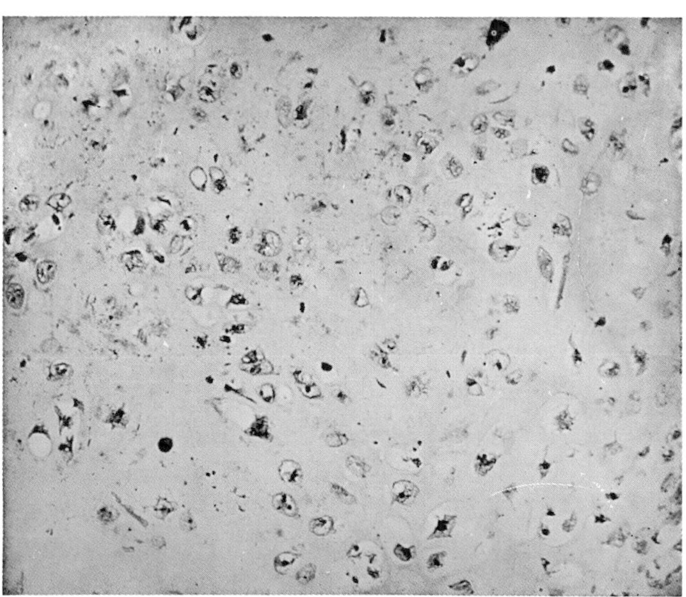

PLATE 15-2. Chondrosarcoma. (*Top* ×85) The typical transition from the embryonic tissue below to the wild-looking atypical cartilage above is well displayed. (*Bottom* ×135) The features indicating malignancy include pleomorphism, irregularity of arrangement, and plump, pyknotic, often multiple nuclei. The matrix characteristically stains poorly. Hypercellularity and presence of binucleate cells are important indications of malignancy. (See p. 604.)

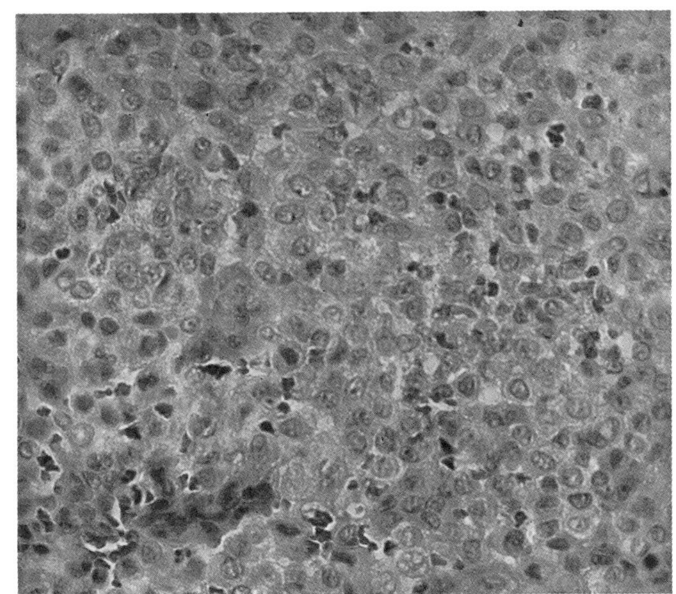

PLATE 15-3. Chondroblastoma. Large sheets of compact round and polyhedral cells with large vesicular nuclei, marked vascularity, and giant cells. Transformation into cartilage is not seen in this area. Reticulin fibers and calcium deposits are not demonstrable except by special staining (*e.g.*, Rio Hortega stain; ×310). (See p. 615.)

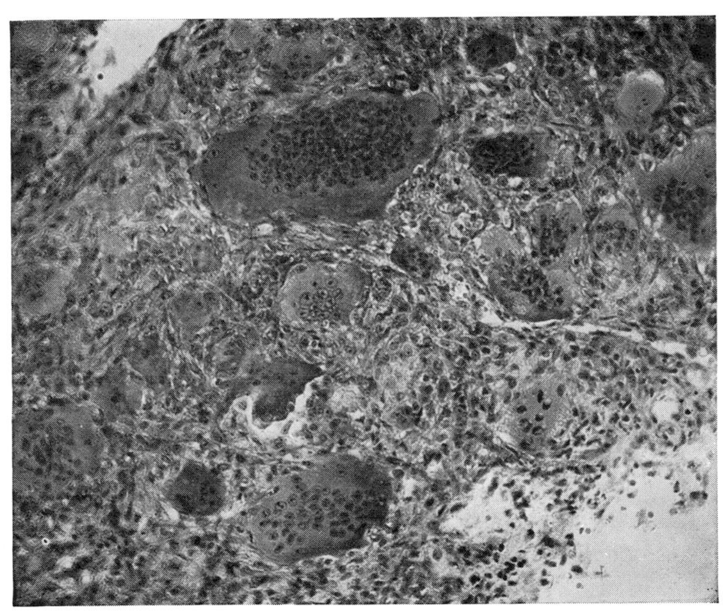

PLATE 15-4. Giant-cell tumor. The tumor giant cell is very large and contains a tremendous number of centrally placed and uniform nuclei. The stroma is fibrous, vascular, and loose and contains spindle cells possessing large heavily chromatinized nuclei. Any tendency toward aggressiveness and malignancy should be sought in the fibroblasts, which become more numerous, plumper, polymorphic, and contain darker nuclei and many mitoses. (×240) (See p. 616.)

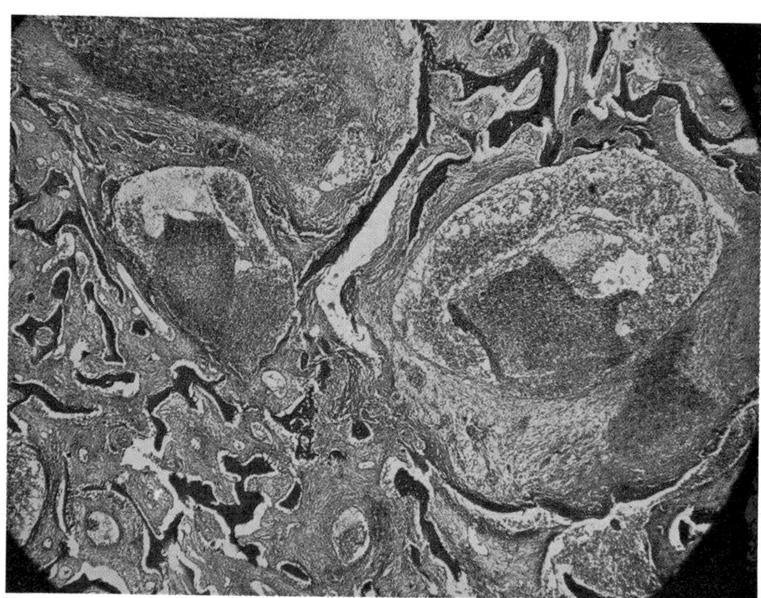

PLATE 15-5. Aneurysmal bone cyst. Characteristic blood-filled lakes are surrounded by reactive bone which forms by metaplasia of the fibrous stroma. (×30) (See p. 622).

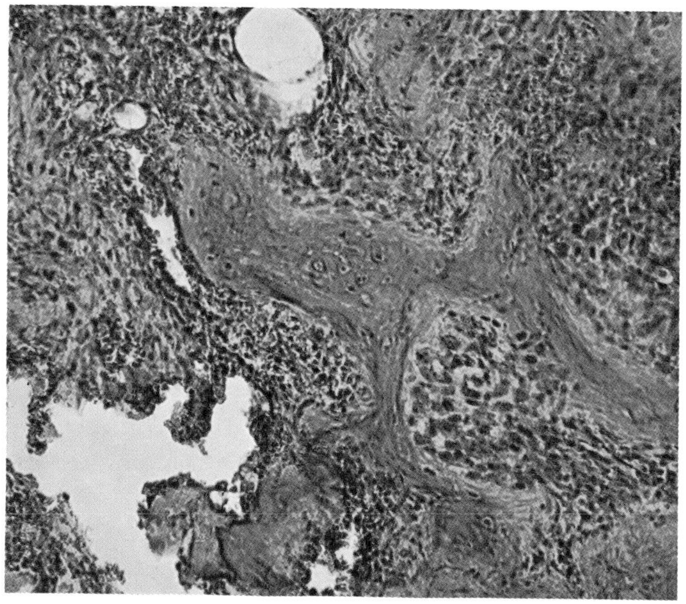

PLATE 15-6. Osteogenic sarcoma. Note the marked cellularity, pleomorphism, mitoses, poorly organized trabeculations, and hypercellular disorganized cartilage. (×140) (See p. 627.)

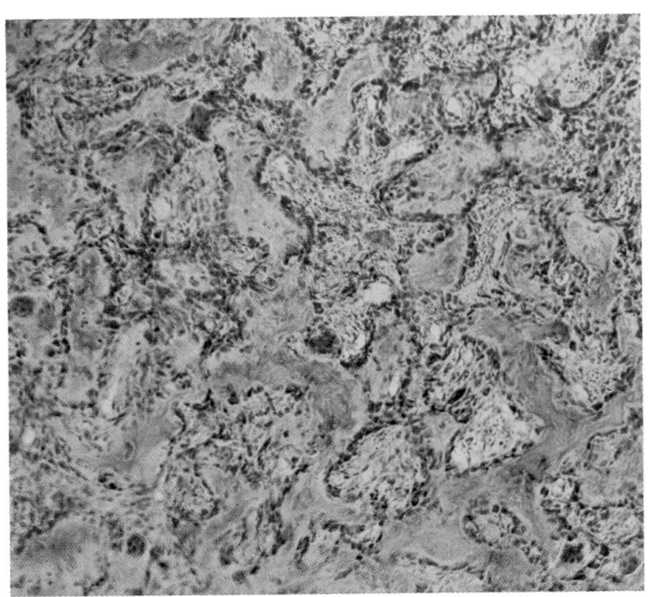

PLATE 15-7. Osteoid osteoma. Abundant pink-staining osteoid tissue surrounded by a vascular mesenchymal stroma containing proliferating fibroblasts and osteoblasts. (×110) (See p. 638.)

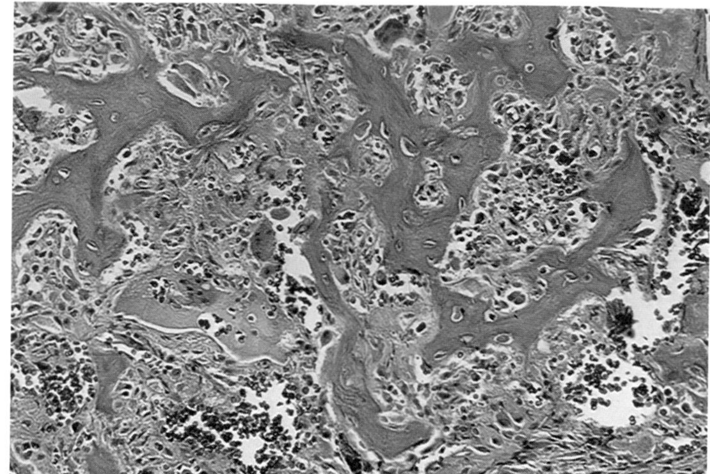

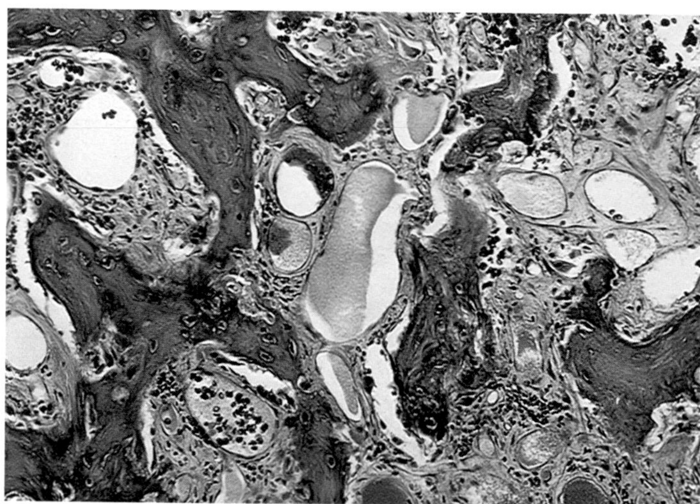

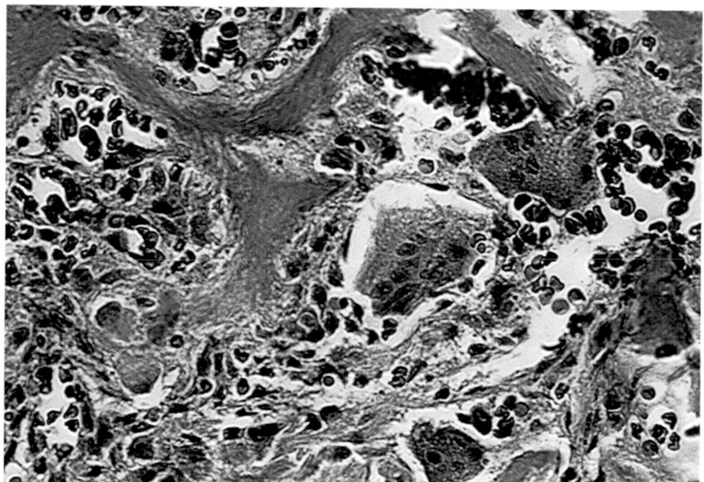

PLATE 15-8. Microscopic findings of benign osteoblastoma. (*Top*) Patches of osteoid are undergoing irregular calcification and conversion to bone. Loose, fibrillar intervening connective tissue are shown. (×100) (*Center*) Between the irregular primitive trabeculae, the osteoblastic connective tissue reveals a rich vascularity. (×250) (*Bottom*) Osteoblasts, multinucleated macrophages including osteoclasts are in evidence among the osteoid deposits. (×810) (Courtesy of Dr. E. R. Ross) (See p. 638.)

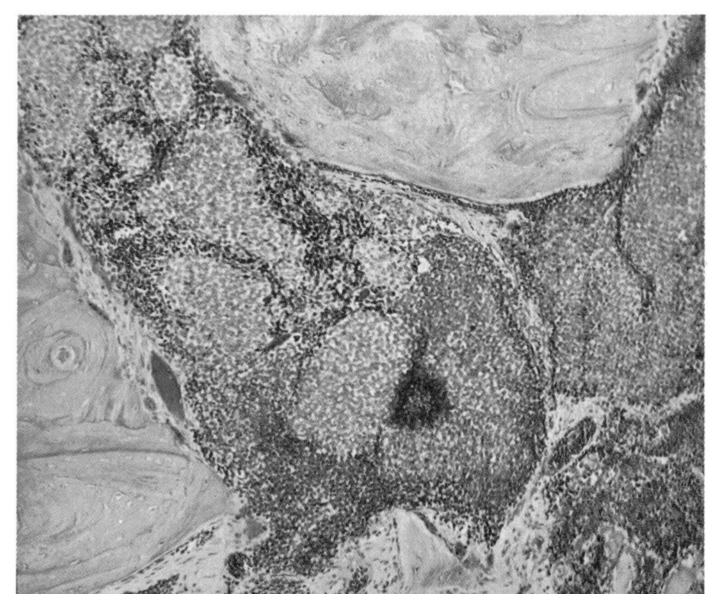

PLATE 15-9. Ewing's tumor. The sheets of cells tend to be grouped in lobules. A characteristic pseudorosette formation is well displayed. The bone is necrotic in some areas because vessels are choked off by tumor cells. (×95) (See p. 644.)

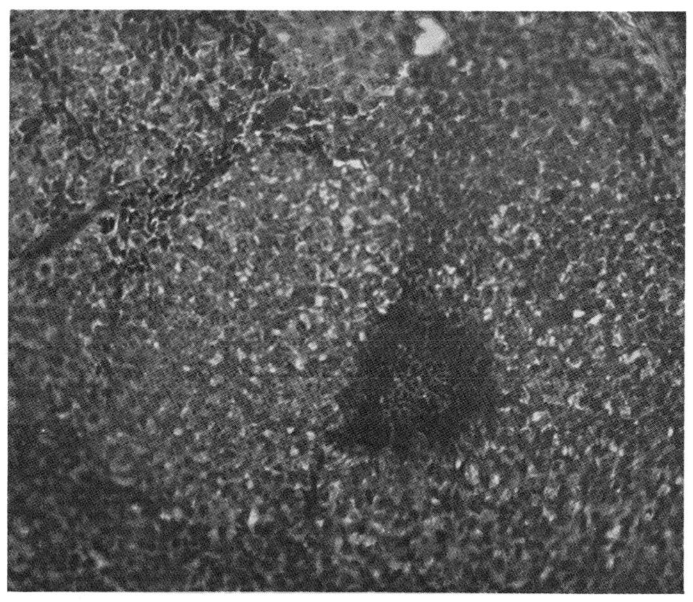

PLATE 15-10. Higher magnification of Ewing's tumor. The tumor consists of small polyhedral cells with ill-defined borders, meager cytoplasm, and nuclei which are large, uniform, prominent, round or oval, and contain powdery blue-staining chromatin. The nucleus is more than twice as large as that of a lymphocyte. No interstitial stroma is seen. The dark-staining ring-shaped accumulation of cells envelopes a center of necrotic cells and therefore is termed a pseudorosette in contradistinction to the rosette of a neuroblastoma whose center contains neurofibrils. (×240) (See p. 644.)

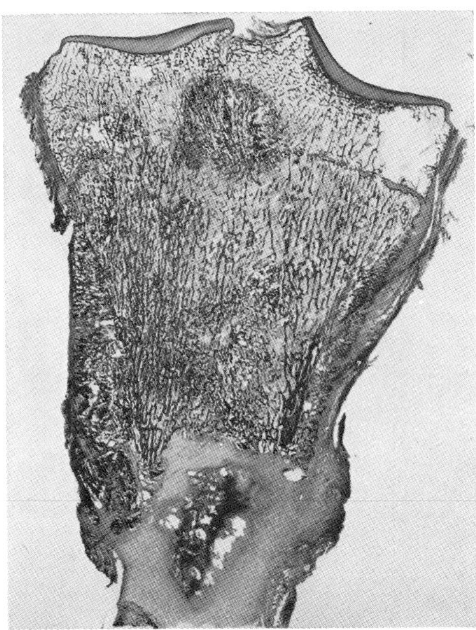

PLATE 15-11. Ewing's tumor of the tibia. The necrotic tissue in the diaphysis represents the remains of the tumor after irradiation. Freshly removed tumor tissue which has not been exposed to x-rays will stain blue. Note elevation of periosteum by reactive new bone. (See p. 644.)

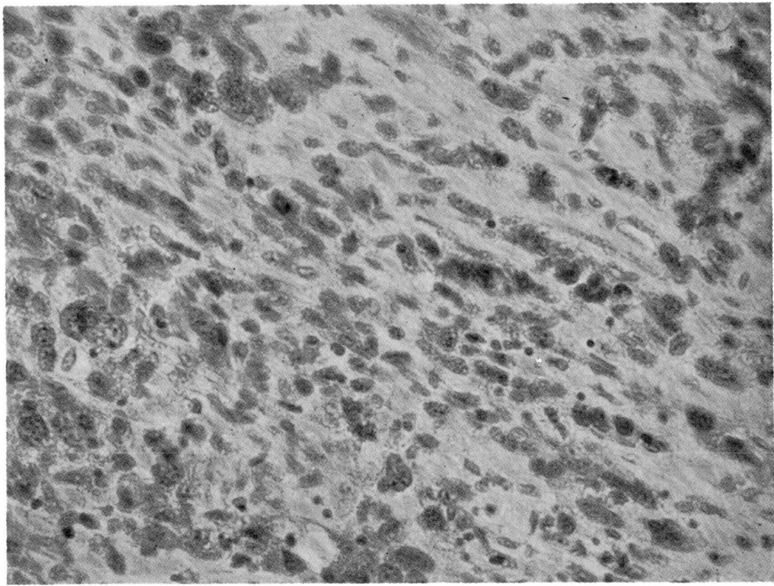

PLATE 15-12. Fibrosarcoma. The cells are grossly irregular in size and shape, are mainly composed of spindle cells, and contain occasional dark-staining nuclei. Mitoses are frequent and intercellular material is sparse. The presence of tumor giant cells differentiates this from a nerve sheath sarcoma. (×360) (See p. 646.)

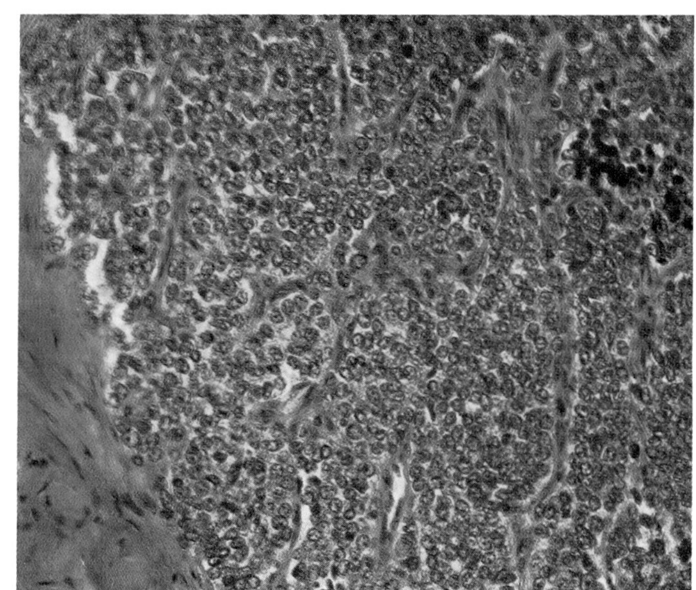

PLATE 15-13. Histiocytic lymphoma (reticulum cell sarcoma). The cellular appearance strongly resembles that of Ewing's sarcoma, but intercellular stroma is very much in evidence and reticulin fibers can be demonstrated by specific stains. (×220) (See p. 647.)

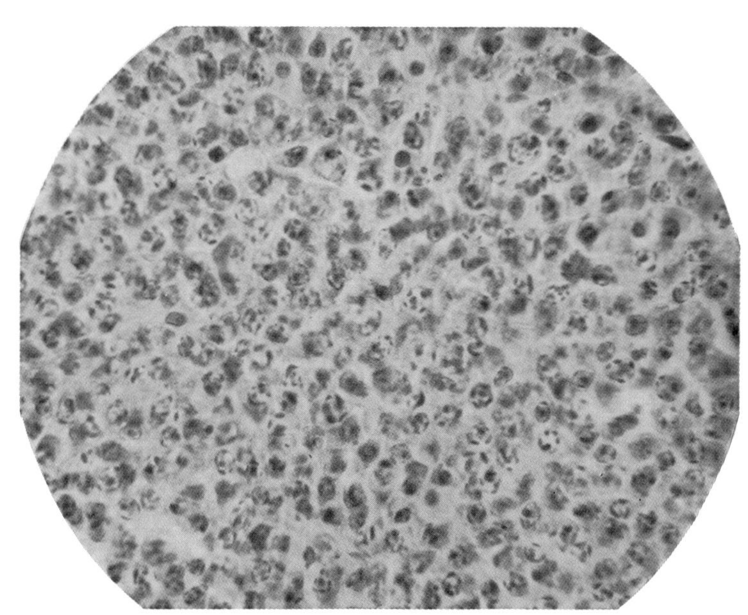

PLATE 15-14. Multiple myeloma exhibiting closely packed typical myeloma cells with rounded eccentrically placed nuclei and spokewheel arrangement of chromatin. (×490, oil immersion) (See p. 651.)

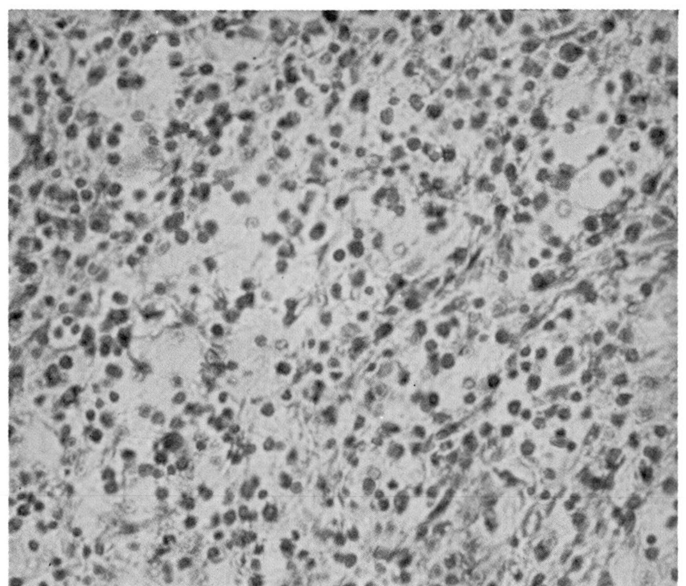

PLATE 15-15. Liposarcoma. This section shows a profusion of lipoblasts. Under higher magnification, features to be sought include signet-ring cells, giant-sized cells containing lipoid vacuoles and abundant pink granules, and areas of malignant fibroblasts. (×415) (See p. 652.)

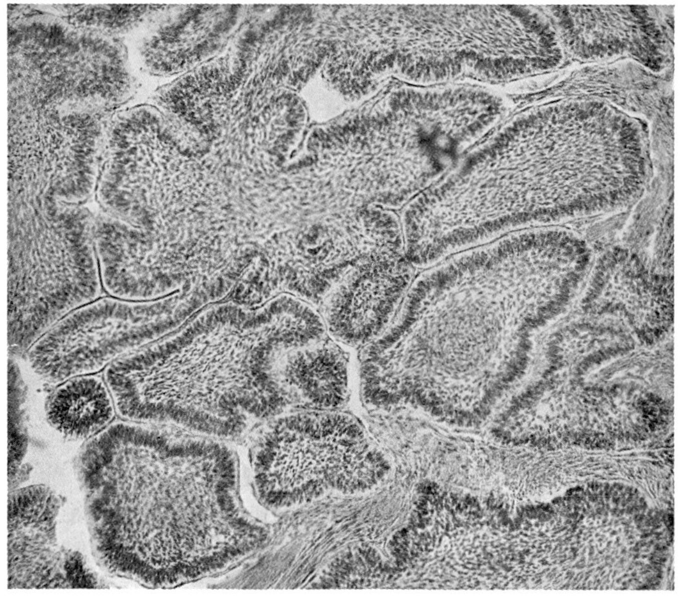

PLATE 15-16. Adamantinoma. This shows one basic pattern of epithelial islands with peripheral columnar cells in palisade fashion and central reticulum formation. The stroma is fibrous. (×84) (See p. 653.)

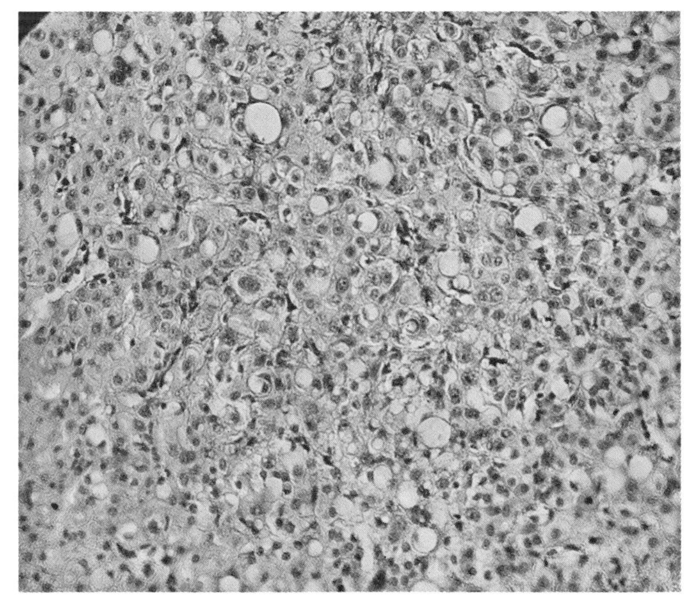

PLATE 15-17. Chordoma. (×160) (See p. 654.)

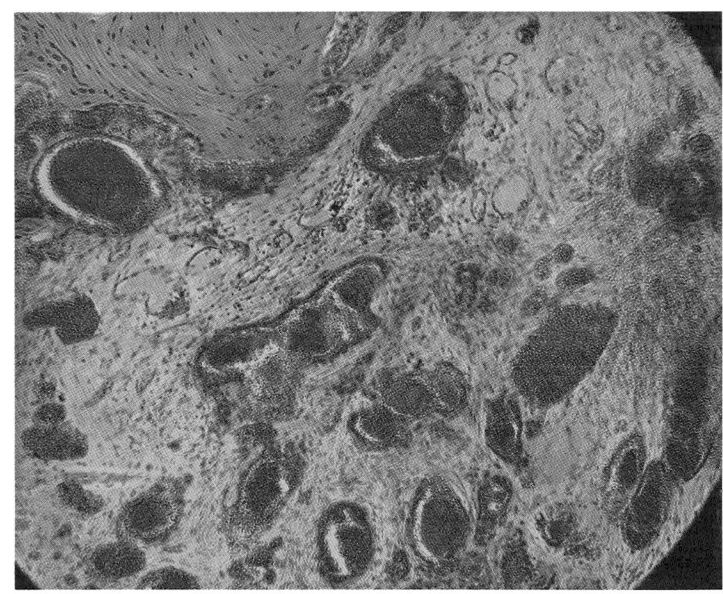

PLATE 15-18. Hemangioma of bone. The vessels appear as blood spaces lined by a single layer of flattened endothelial cells. Vessel walls lack elastic fibers and smooth muscle. Connective tissue between vessels is sparse. At the upper edge of this section, bone is being eroded by pressure of adjacent vessels, whereas in other areas active bone formation is taking place. (×70) (See p. 655.)

CLINICAL PICTURE

In the adolescent or young adult, the tumor causes mild or no pain, slowly increasing local swelling, and a palpable, tender tumor mass fixed to underlying bone. It never metastasizes and sarcomatoud degeneration is extremely rare.

When the tumor develops in people younger than 10, the symptoms are more pronounced and the course is rapid.[50]

ROENTGENOGRAPHIC FINDINGS

Usually a lower limb bone is involved in chrondromyxoid fibroma (Fig. 15-16). The lesion is a translucent mass of variable size located eccentrically in the metaphysis. On the medullary aspect of the lesion, the margin is scalloped and sclerosed. Over its outer aspect, the cortex is expanded and thinned, and may appear interrupted. In a child, at the edge of the base of the tumor, triangular periosteal bone formation, not unlike Codman's triangle, often forms. Within the tumor, a faint trabecular pattern is apparent, but the pseudoloculation represents ridges and corrugations of the inner sclerotic wall.

When the tumor involves a narrow tubular bone (*e.g.*, the fibula) or a small tubular bone (*e.g.*, a phalanx or metatarsal), it generally occupies the entire width of the bone, producing fusiform expansion and thinning of both cortices.

FIG. 15-16. Chondromyxoid fibroma of bone. (Ralph LL: Chondromyxoid fibroma of bone. J Bone Joint Surg 44B:7, 1962)

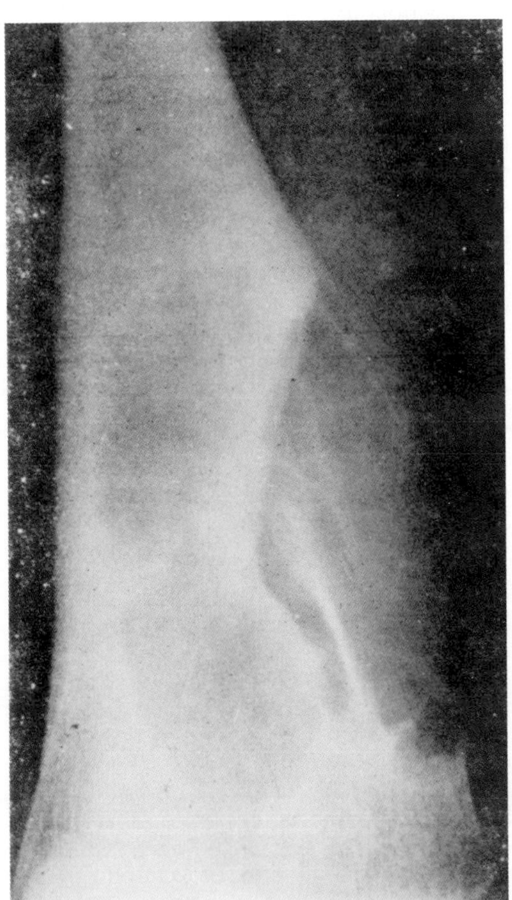

PATHOLOGY

Gross Appearance

When the tumor is excised *in toto*, the outer surface is covered by a thin shell of newly formed periosteal bone or the periosteum itself. Its location in a large tubular bone is eccentric, but within a small tubular bone, it sometimes occupies the entire width, producing a fusiform swelling.

The cut surface reveals a solid tumor mass of greyish white or bluish grey color, somewhat translucent, resembling cartilage, and sometimes containing small cavities with mucoid tissue. The consistency is usually firm. In areas that are predominantly myxoid, the tissue is gray and dull, never having the glary consistency of myxomatous tissue. Calcified areas are unusual. The surface of the tumor mass toward the spongiosa is sharply demarcated, lobulated, and surrounded by a thin, often scalloped, border of dense bone. No bony septa traverse the tumor.

Microscopic Appearance

The tumor is composed of lobulated or pseudolobulated areas of stellate cells with indistinct cytoplasmic borders, lying within the central portion of the lobule and widely separated by intercellular mucinlike material (Fig. 15-17). The cells send out long, branching cytoplasmic

FIG. 15-17. Chondromyxoid fibroma of bone, demonstrating lobules of pale-staining myxoid tissue with some areas of blue-staining chondroid differentiation, usually toward the center of the lobules, and increasing cellularity toward their periphery. Vascular fibrous tissue separates the lobules and contains multinucleated giant cells. (Courtesy of L. L. Ralph)

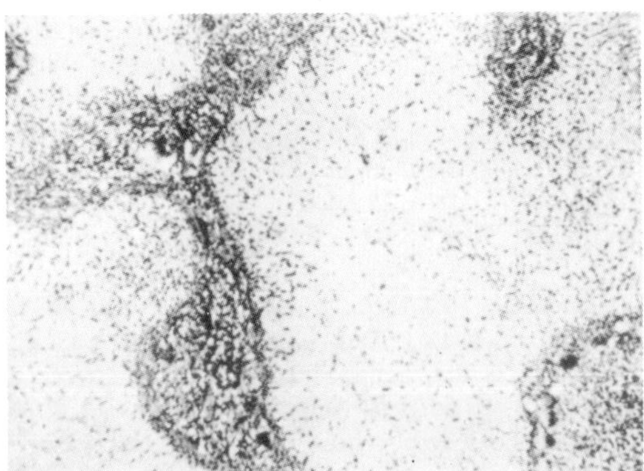

processes. Their nuclei are single, ovoid, and of moderate size, although a few cells have large and multiple nuclei. Sparse collagen fibers form a widespread reticulum at the center of the lobule.

At the periphery of the lobule, the appearance is more cellular and more collagenous. The hypercellularity, pleomorphism, bizarre shaped, hyperchromatic, and often multiple nuclei are characteristics that strongly suggest malignancy.

Both myxoid and chondroid areas stain metachromatically with toluidine blue, and this reaction is absent after hyaluronidase digestion. This is evidence of its cartilage origin.[50]

Malignant transformation is highly unusual.[44]

DIFFERENTIAL DIAGNOSIS

The ominous cellular features at the periphery of the lobules suggest the presence of a chondrosarcoma from which a chondromyxoid fibroma must be differentiated.[50,51]

In chondrosarcomas, the cell population is predominantly chondroid, the nuclei characteristically are deeply indented and lobulated, and prominent nucleoli are evident. Under electron microscopy, large lipid droplets are found in both cytoplasm and matrix.[42] These findings are absent in chondromyxoid fibromas. A distinctive feature of chondromyxoid fibromas, as observed under the electron microscope, is the presence of an electron-dense band 700 A in width between the inner and outer nuclear membranes. Normally the membranes are 120 A to 140 A apart. Throughout the matrix of chondromyxoid fibromas are collagen fibers having an average major banding periodicity of 970 A in contrast with the normal periodicity of mature collagen. In chondrosarcomas the collagen fibers are sparse, whereas they are found in abundance in chondromyxoid fibromas.

TREATMENT

Treatment consists of local excision and filling the cavity with autogenous bone. Curettage is not sufficient because the tumor may recur,[48] especially in children.[49] Wide *en bloc* excision extending well into the surrounding normal bone will result in a high rate of cure.[50] If, despite wide excision, the tumor recurs, additional studies should be done to determine whether malignant transformation has occurred, and the appropriate treatment, local excision or amputation, carried out.

CHONDROBLASTOMA

A chondroblastoma is a cellular, vascular, and cartilaginous tumor of young adults, occurring about the epiphyseal line, destroying cancellous bone, and characteristically containing multiple calcium deposits. Jaffe and Lichtenstein and the majority of reports consider the tumor benign.[52–57]

CLINICAL PICTURE

Age. Onset occurs before obliteration of the epiphyseal line, from 10 to 20 years of age

Sex. Males predominate

Area of Predilection. Ends of long bones about the knee and upper humerus

Position. About one side of the epiphyseal line, chiefly in the metaphysis; it may extend to the epiphysis

Symptoms and Findings. Trauma, pain, tenderness, swelling in most cases; occasionally, limp, joint effusion

Course. Rapid, from 1 month to 2 years

ROENTGENOGRAPHIC FINDINGS

Roentgenograms show a characteristic well-delineated area of rarefaction of cancellous bone extending over and beyond the epiphyseal line quite early. The main mass of tumor is either in the metaphysis or the epiphysis. The position is often eccentric. The cortex may be thinned but rarely penetrated. The tumor borders are irregular, fuzzy, and vague. This is in contrast with a giant-cell tumor, which shows well-defined margins, and the cortex, although thinned, is elevated. Mottled areas of increased density throughout the tumor represent calcium deposits.

PATHOLOGY

Gross Appearance

At first glance the tumor appears as a dark-red, hemorrhagic, and friable tissue within which are scattered small yellow zones of calcification, bluish white translucent nodules of cartilage, and a few spicules of necrotic bone. On closer inspection a soft grayish pink tissue is discovered within the friable tissue representing the basic tumor tissue. When the tumor is less vascular and less necrotic, it is firm and grayish pink and contains a variable amount of cartilage. White or yellow areas of calcium salts are found within the cartilage and in the tumor tissue. The tumor extends irregularly through the metaphysis, destroys the epiphyseal line at one side, and occasionally invades the subperiosteal space. The necrosis and hemorrhage may suggest a giant-cell tumor or malignant aneurysm of bone, but the chondromatous material, absence of new bone, and fusion with the epiphyseal line should clarify the diagnosis.

Microscopic Appearance

Large sheets of compact round or polyhedral cells similar to mesenchymal tissue form the basic tumor tissue. These cells are of moderate size and contain a relatively large nucleus, occasionally two nuclei. Focal areas of calcification distributed throughout the cellular tumor tissue are typical. A scattering of giant cells lies adjacent to areas of hemorrhage and necrosis. When calcification is unusualy heavy, the tumor cells swell and undergo degeneration and necrosis, similar to cartilage tissue undergoing calcification preparatory to ossification, but osseous transformation does not occur. In some areas tumor cells can be seen undergoing transformation to cartilage cells. About necrotic zones, a reparative process occurs by resorption of calcific detritus and organization of hemorrhage (Color Plate 15-3 and Fig. 15-18).

The Rio Hortega stain will reveal calcium deposits and reticulin fibers about the tumor cells. Where the chondroblasts differentiate into cartilage, reticulum formation is rare. This indicates that the basic cell of this tumor is a reticulohistiocytic cell with a tendency to differentiate into chondroblastic tissue and then into cartilage.

Many blood spaces with and without a single layer of endothelium occur throughout the tumor.

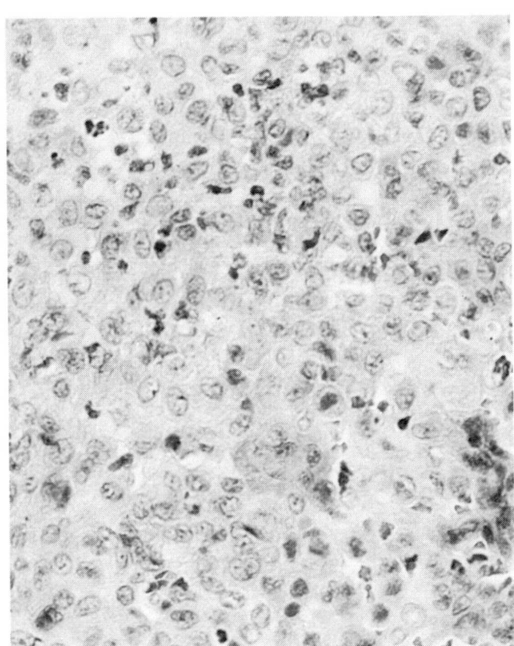

FIG. 15-18. Chondroblastoma. Microscopic appearance demonstrates sheets of closely packed cells with large vesicular nuclei.

TREATMENT

The majority of observers feel that chondroblastomas are benign. Geschickter and Copeland believed that about 50% became malignant. Cases have been reported in which postoperative irradiation has been followed by malignant degeneration.

Conservative surgical treatment consists of curettage and obliteration of the cavity by bone grafts. In view of the possible untoward effects of irradiation, this form of therapy should be avoided.

BENIGN GIANT-CELL TUMOR

A benign giant-cell tumor is an osteolytic tumor (osteoclastoma) occurring in young adults at the epiphysis and typified by an abundance of characteristic large giant cells.[2,59,64,70]

CLINICAL PICTURE

Age. This tumor occurs in young adults after the epiphyseal plate has ossified and longitudinal bone growth is completed. It appears most commonly between 15 and 35 years of age.

Area of predilection. An asymmetric position of the epiphysis of a long bone. The lower femur, the distal radius, and the upper tibia are the common sites.

Course. Chronic, a few months to several years

Sequence. Trauma, pain, tumor, and pathologic fracture

Pain. Chronic, constant, in region of a joint progressively more severe, worse at night, and increases with activity

Swelling. The end of the bone expands to one side, and overlying skin is stretched. In contrast with osteosarcoma, the skin displays no dilated vessels. Pressure over the swelling produces audible and palpable crackling as the cortex is ruptured. Tenderness is moderate or absent.

Limitation of joint motion. Not observed until late as the tumor expands and distorts the end of the bone. There is no increase of joint fluid. The joint is not invaded.

Pathologic fracture. Occurs later in the course as a large extent of cancellous and cortical bone is destroyed.

ROENTGENOGRAPHIC FINDINGS

The tumor is revealed by a large, sharply circumscribed area of reduced density asymmetrically located in the epiphysis, beginning subcortically and extending toward the metaphysis. The cortex is expanded outward and is thinned. No periosteal new bone formation is apparent. Multiple septae of bone and soft tissue traverse the interior and produce a characteristic loculated "soap bubble" appearance. As the tumor enlarges, the septae disappear. The cortex may be disrupted as the tumor invades and thickens the surrounding soft tissues. Extension into the joint is rare (Fig. 15-19).

PATHOLOGY

Gross Appearance

The tumor is composed of ragged, very friable, readily bleeding tissue containing variously sized cavitations and small cysts. These cavities may be filled with old or fresh blood, detritus of degenerated tissue, or a mucinouslike material. The color of the tumor varies from a reddish or chocolate brown, in which the vascular tissue predominates, to grayish or mottled, wherein the connective tissue is the major component. The epiphyseal end of the bone is distorted and enlarged to one side. It is invested by periosteum and cortex, which is thinned and fragile, being easily broken by handling. The underlying bloody tissue imparts a blue color through the transparent thin cortex. No periosteal new bone formation can be discerned grossly. The inner wall of the tumor is lined by a fibrous capsule from which septae extend inward to partition the tumor.

FIG. 15-19. Giant-cell tumor. Characteristics of this tumor include loculus, osteolysis, expansile distention, and thinning, but it does not penetrate the overlying cortex or epiphyseal location.

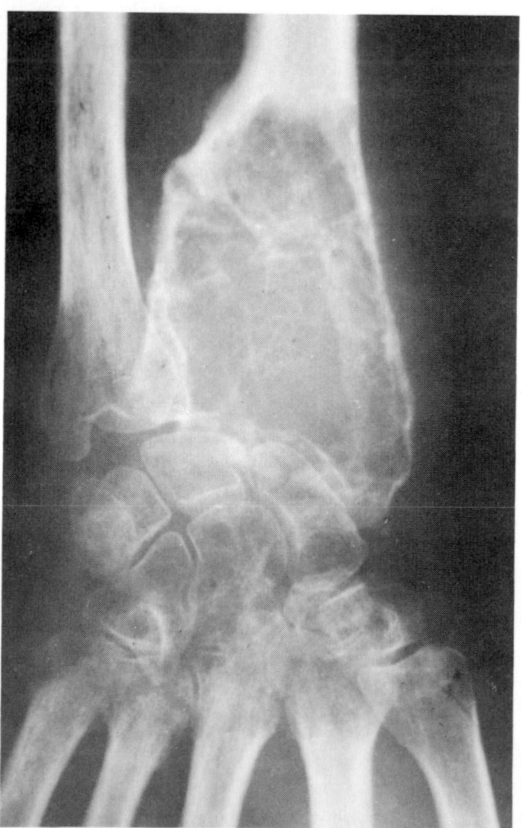

Microscopic Appearance

At the periphery, a fibrous capsule envelops the tumor (Color Plate 15-4). Beyond this, a thin layer of new imperfectly formed bone is seen. The capsule of fibrous tissue and new thin bone explain why the tumor is sharply demarcated and expands rather than infiltrates. The characteristic finding in the tumor tissue is the presence of an abundance of tumor giant cells. These large cells measure from 10 μ to 100 μ and contain many centrally placed uniformly sized nuclei. The number of nuclei varies from fifteen upward, some estimates being as high as 150. The giant cells are numerous about areas of hemorrhage, spicules of old bone, and walls of small cysts. By comparison, the Langhans giant cells characteristic of tuberculosis contain a smaller number of peripherally placed nuclei; foreign body giant cells are smaller, and contain a lesser number, usually less than fifteen, of variously sized, centrally placed, nuclei. The stroma consists of a vascularized loose network of spindle shaped and ovoid cells heavily interspersed with tumor giant cells. The spindle cells are oval, elongate, and contain a relatively large, heavy chromatinized nucleus and a small amount of acidophilic cytoplasm. Fibrils about these cells suggest their fibroblastic function. The appearance of the spindle cells indicates the malignant potential of the tumor. The tumor aggressiveness is proportionate to the increase and the crowding of the stromal cells and the plumping up of these cells, the increase of chromatin in the nuclei, variation in the sizes and the shapes, and the presence of many mitotic figures. The more the atypism, the greater the tendency to metastasize. A benign giant cell tumor displays uniformity of cells. At the periphery of the tumor, spicules of old ragged bone with giant cells closely applied to their surface are seen.

DIFFERENTIAL DIAGNOSIS

Giant cells are frequently found in other lesions, the so-called variants of giant cell tumors. These lesions include nonossifying fibroma, unicameral bone cyst, localized osteitis fibrosa, aneurysmal bone cyst, chondromyxoid fibroma, benign chondroblastoma, and the "brown tumors" sometimes found in hyperparathyroidism. The typical characteristics of a giant-cell tumor are:[60]

1. The patients are nearly all young adults.
2. The majority of giant-cell tumors originate in the

end of long bones in the portion which during the growth years was the epiphysis.
3. Pain, often present at night as well as during activity, is common. By contrast, pain is almost never associated with a solitary bone cyst, fibrous dysplasia, or nonossifying fibroma.
4. Tumefaction is present early and is palpable and tender.
5. The expanded cortex is paper thin and may crackle when palpated.
6. Roentgenograms show a circumscribed osteolytic but expansile tumor, and not uncommonly the thin expanded cortex of bone is perforated. The larger giant cell tumors may appear multilocular and resemble soap bubbles.
7. Periosteal new bone formation is not apparent on roentgenograms.
8. The stromal cells in a giant-cell tumor show greater growth and multiplication and a variety of morphology than do the stromal cells of other lesions which commonly contain giant cells.
9. Stromal and giant cells in a giant-cell tumor contain acid phosphatase but no alkaline phosphatase.
10. In other lesions, giant cells are fewer in number. The stromal cells of lesions that are not true giant-cell tumors contain only alkaline phosphatase and never acid phosphatase.

TREATMENT

Principles

Most giant-cell tumors are invasive and aggressive in their behavior.[58,66] They often recur and may become malignant after unsuccessful surgical removal.[63] A benign giant-cell tumor is at first confined by an overlying attenuated shell of cortex, and the articular cartilage constitutes a barrier to advance of the tumor into the joint. Growth of the tumor generally extends beyond the limits of the osteolytic defect which is apparent on the roentgenogram. It is therefore not surprising that, following attempted surgical removal by curettage, the tumor growth recurs, usually within the first two years, becomes aggressive, destroys a greater extent of bone, and invades the soft tissues. The most likely cause of recurrence is inadequate removal of the tumor tissue.[62] In the event of recurrence, reoperation is indicated, and an *en bloc* excision which extends the resection into normal bone is best. At that time, a thorough microscopic search should be made for foci of malignant change. Amputation is indicated for a malignant giant-cell tumor.

Presently, there is no reliable cytological guide to predict the behavior of a benign giant-cell tumor. The tumor may display benign histologic features and yet behave in an aggressive manner; occasionally it may metastasize.[67] Following adequate primary surgical treatment, preferably resection rather than curettage plus bone grafting, the recurrence rate is low and malignant transformation is rare. *En bloc* excision is especially indicated as the initial procedure if the tumor has already eroded the cortex and broken into the surrounding soft tissues. When local invasion of the tumor is widespread, it is best to proceed with amputation.[71]

Curettment and Bone Grafting

Curettment alone has a recurrence rate of 85%, and the addition of bone grafts reduces recurrence to approximately 40%.[61,62] Curettment of tissue should extend into normal bone so that there is less chance of leaving tumor tissue behind, and the exposure of a normal vascular bed provides a ready source of osteogenesis. Optionally, the walls of the surgical defect may be cauterized, but this has not been shown to reduce the rate of recurrence. Curettage and bone grafting are unsuitable when the tumor has destroyed both condyles and extended through the subchondral bone with imminent collapse of the articular support. For such tumors, *en bloc* resection or amputation is appropriate.

Resection

Because of the proclivity of the tumor to recur and its potential for malignant transformation, especially when the tumor behaves aggressively and displays atypical cytological characteristics, the initial procedure of choice is a widespread resection. An *en bloc* resection should if possible preserve a portion of the uninvolved cortex, provide additional support with cortical bone struts, and the defect filled with autogenous cancellous bone. The tumor is removed with its surrounding bone shell and periosteum and a variable amount of soft tissue. A large lesion at the epiphysis of the femur, tibia, or radius following resection requires arthrodesis, substitution with a freeze-dried allograft,[68] or replacement with a prosthesis. Where the location of the tumor will permit (*e.g.*, distal ulna, proximal fibula, scapula, and small bone of the hand or foot), total excision can be carried out.

Curettage and Acrylic Cementation

When the tumor is large and encroaches on the subchondral bone plate, thorough curettage and filling the cavity with acrylic cement will preserve the articular cartilage, provide stability, allow full and early mobility, and use the residual cortical bone to its fullest for structural stability.[74,76] The well-known lack of methyl methacrylate shear strength does not appear to weaken the resistance of the bone-cement composite to vertical loading stresses. Follow-up periods as long as 7 years indicate a low rate of recurrence. Nevertheless, should recurrence ensue, this method will not compromise other alternatives. It has been suggested that the heat of polymerization may destroy residual stromal cells and giant cells. Complications are rare, and include osteoarthritic degeneration of the articular cartilage, pathologic fractures, and infection.

Curettage and Cryosurgery

Thorough curettage should, if possible, avoid extensive sacrifice of surrounding normal bone tissue needed for preservation of joint function and possible subsequent reconstruction. The minute foci of tumor tissue beyond the periphery of the main tumor mass can be eradicated by cryosurgery.[66,67] Thorough curettage of the tumor followed by instillation of liquid nitrogen appears to greatly reduce the rate of local tumor recurrence, and the formerly reported rate of malignant transformation (15%) is significantly reduced (1.9%). The rationale is to destroy any residual tumor at the margins of curettage by a process of repetitive freezing and thawing.

Technique. Liquid nitrogen is poured into the tumor cavity after thorough curettage. Either a double lumen probe with circulating liquid nitrogen is used, or the liquid nitrogen is poured directly into the curetted cavity through a funnel. The funnel method is preferred because the irregularly shaped cavity is reliably filled and its walls frozen throughout. Thermocouples placed in the bone at varying distances from the freezing source will monitor the extent of freezing. Within the cavity edge the temperature is lowered either to −60° C once, or to −21° C three times to ensure adequate cryonecrosis.

During cryosurgery care must be taken to prevent skin necrosis. This is achieved by using a long skin incision and wide retraction of all soft tissues, particularly the neurovascular structures, and by bathing with lukewarm water. The funnel must be surrounded by a moist Gelfoam sponge which is carefully cut to fit the spout, sealing the medullary canal. As the liquid nitrogen runs in through the funnel, slowly at first, the Gelfoam freezes and seals the funnel to the bone, forming a water-tight cavity. The level of nitrogen in the funnel can then be kept high, ensuring that the cavity is completely filled without spillage. After each freezing and thawing, the residual blood in the cavity must be removed by suction to avoid blocking a portion of the cavity. It is advisable to use a tourniquet when possible. Otherwise, bleeding can be controlled by a Gelfoam pack.

The cavity is then filled with autogenous or homogenous cancellous bone and fibular strut grafts, or methyl methacrylate may be used to fill the cavity and a corticocancellous onlay graft is applied to prevent a pathologic fracture.

Despite negative roentgenograms, a second stage procedure for rebiopsy is carried out 3 to 6 months later. A recurrent tumor usually has a reddish brown or yellow appearance, and if the frozen section is confirmatory, cryosurgery is repeated. The focal recurrence sometimes is situated at a distance from the original tumor. If malignant change is detected, amputation is performed at once.

Complications include infection (rare), skin blistering and necrosis, neurapraxia (usually subsides after several weeks), and pathologic fractures (rare since the use of methyl methacrylate and onlay grafts). After cryosurgery, the healing time is prolonged, especially when the tumor is large, the shell of surrounding bone is thin, and an extensive area of surrounding osteonecrosis must be repaired. Consequently, the extremity must be protected by an orthosis for months, even several years, until bone healing and consolidation has occurred as indicated by serial roentgenograms and bone scans. Scintigraphy is useful for detecting recurrent lesions.

Massive Allograft Replacement

Wide *en bloc* local resection for locally aggressive or limited malignant tumors can provide effective control of such lesions as a giant-cell tumor, low-grade chondrosarcoma, adamantinoma, low-grade fibrosarcoma, and parosteal osteosarcoma.[65,72,73,77] A large defect is created which corresponds to a resected segment of a long bone (intercalary defect), or is the result of removal of a major portion of the end of a long bone which includes the adjacent articular surface [osteoarticular defect] (Figs 15-20 and 15-21). Such limb-sparing extensive local resections require replacement by massive bone grafts that, of necessity, must be procured from cadavers very shortly after death, processed to reduce their antigenicity, and stored in bone banks for ready availability.

Harvesting Massive Allografts. The technique is described in the section on Allografts-Cadaver Bone-Bone Banks. Because many such grafts are osteoarticular and cellular viability of the articular cartilage must be preserved, at least partially, the following principles must be observed. Grafts are completely stripped of periosteum. All tendinous and ligamentous insertions are retained and left at least 2 cm long. The entire shoulder capsule and posterior capsule of the knee are retained for subsequent use in repair. Glycerolization of articular cartilage will maintain viability of at least 50% of the chondrocytes during freezing and thawing by preventing ice-crystal formation. The articular surface of the harvested segment is immersed in 10% glycerol solution for 1 hour immediately following procurement. Aerobic and anaerobic cultures are taken. The allografts are wrapped in sterile plastic bags and x-rayed in two planes. Then they are refrigerated at −4° C for 18 hours (to allow the glycerol to penetrate the cartilage matrix and cells), then frozen to −70° C and stored in the deep-freeze unit until needed. At surgery, the allograft is rapidly brought to ambient temperature by immersion in Ringer's solution at 50° C. This scheme is termed "slow freeze—rapid thaw" which provides the highest rate of survival of the articular cartilage cells.[69]

Surgical Procedure. Prior to surgery[65] the patient is

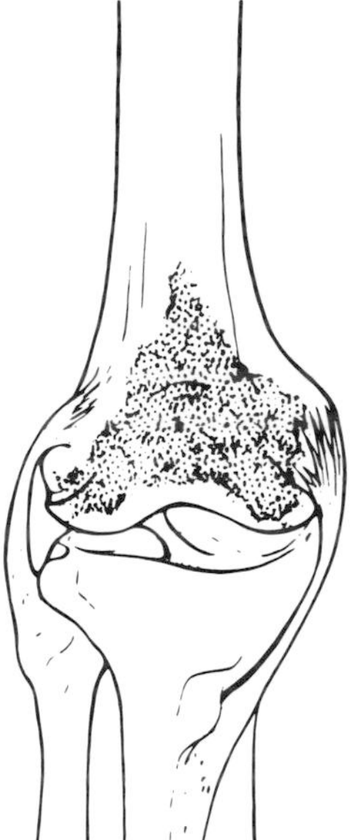
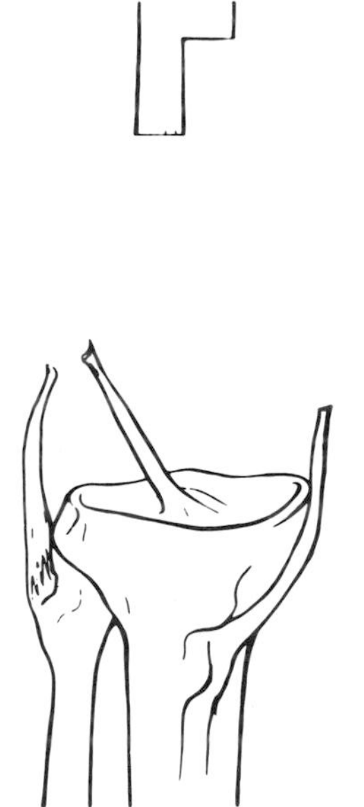
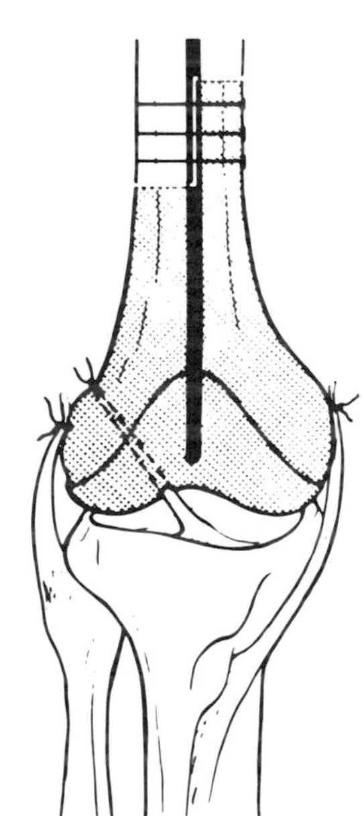

FIG. 15-20. Major distal femoral resection of a giant-cell tumor with alloimplant replacement. Note that the level of resection extends well beyond the apparent proximal extent of the tumor. The capsuloligamentous structures are preserved and sutured to the allograft to provide stability. (Parrish FF: Total resection of giant cell tumors of the extremities. In Management of Primary Bone and Soft Tissue Tumors. Chicago, Year Book Medical Publishers, 1977)

studied to assess the presence of distal metastases, and the local site is carefully examined by roentgenograms, tomograms, xeroradiograms, technetium Tc 99m diphosphonate bone scan, angiograms, and computerized tomography to delineate the extent of the lesion in order to properly plan the surgical procedure. When a total "en bloc" eradication of the lesion is considered feasible, it must include the adjacent periosteum, muscle, and a portion of normal proximal and distal bone. The skin and soft tissues from a previous biopsy site are also excised.

After resection of the lesion, the allograft bone is trimmed to fit and fixed in place by an intramedullary rod or compression plating. Host muscles and ligaments are reattached at appropriate tension to anatomical insertion sites on the allograft with nonabsorbable synthetic sutures. Postoperatively, suction drainage is continued for 2 or 3 days, and external immobilization is carried out for 3 months for the lower extremity and 2 months for the upper extremity. Antibiotics are administered intravenously intra-operatively and postoperatively for at least 1 week, then orally for 6 months. For lower extremity surgery, anticoagulation therapy is used. Immunosuppressive therapy poses a hazard for malignant tumors because of increased risk of infection and, therefore, must be avoided.

After immobilization is discontinued, supervised exercise is carried out. Unrestricted weight bearing is not permitted until roentgenograms disclose solid union at the anastomosis site. For at least 6 to 8 months, the patient must wear a plastic brace and the degree of partial weight bearing using a walker or crutches is dependent on the sufficiency of bone architecture as reflected on roentgenograms.

Follow-up visits are required at regular intervals to carry out various studies by x-rays, bone scans, sedimentation rate, and special tests such as anti-HL-A antibodies, to determine evidence of "rejection" as well as to ascertain the absence of distant metastasis or local recurrence.

Modifications. Depending on the site and extent of resection, the surgical procedure and the type of allograft may be altered to fit the need.

Hemi-Joint Allograft Replacement. Resection does not include entire expanse of the bone. Replacement consists of a segment which does not include the entire cartilaginous surface.

Intercalary Allograft Replacement. A segmental bone graft which does not include an articular surface.

Segmental Graft Plus Endoprosthesis. Used at the hip, a segmental graft is held in place by a long-stem Austin Moore endoprosthesis.

Complications. The two main complications are deep seated infection (in almost 15%) and fracture of the allograft (in 10%).

Deep-seated infection is the most serious complication that often requires removal of the allograft and hardware, and sometimes eventuates in amputation. Appropriate bacteriological controls, proper patient selection (*e.g.*, avoiding those on chemotherapy or immunosuppressive drugs, and those with a history of recent infection), and proper surgical technique (*e.g.*, limiting undermining of skin) should reduce the incidence of infection.

Fracture of the allograft requires further surgery to restore continuity. Weight-bearing subchondral bone may collapse and yet the articular cartilage is found to be viable. Because such fractures occur with greater frequency in rapidly healing allografts, the complication

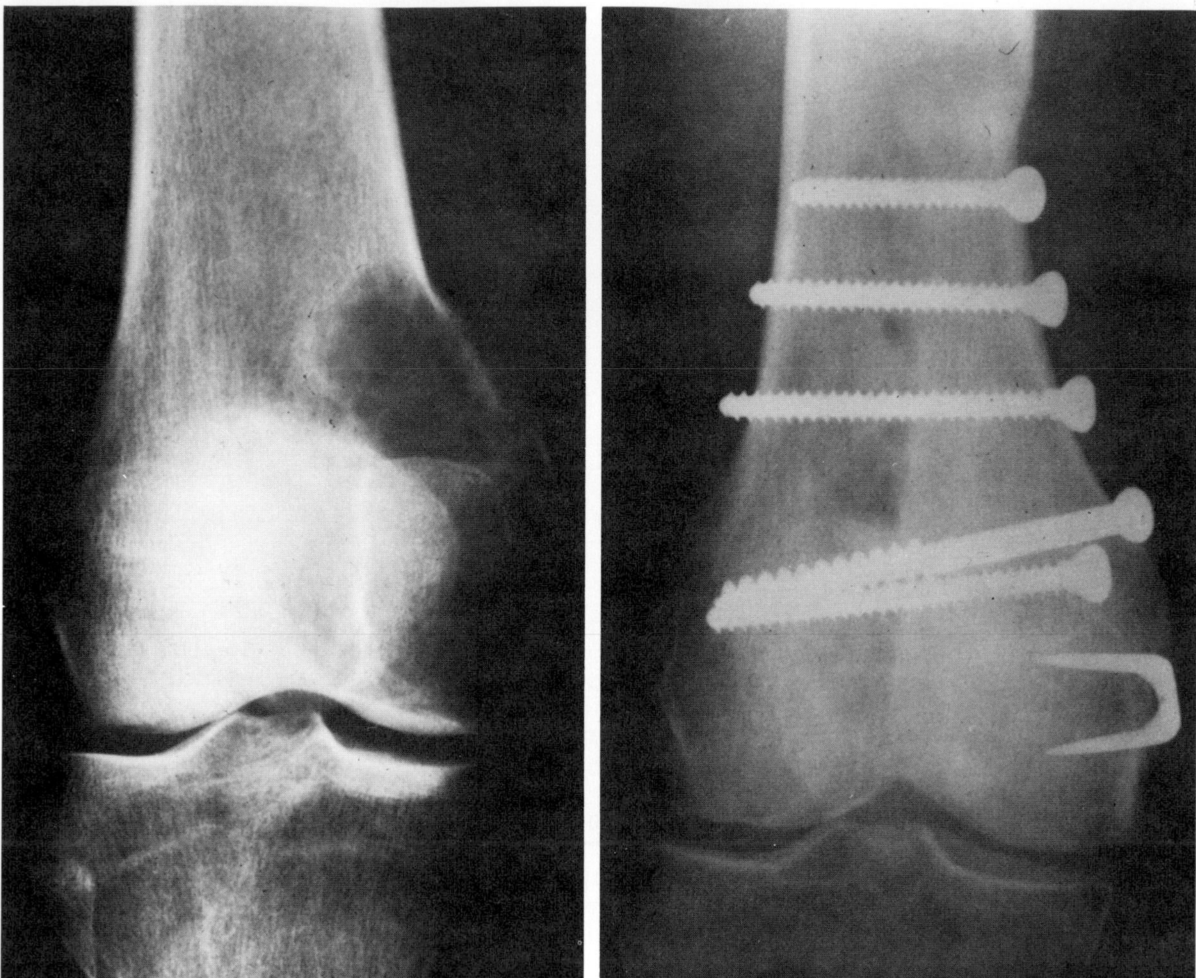

FIG. 15-21. Osteoarticular allograft for a giant-cell tumor of the distal end of the femur. The hemigraft is processed by the slow freeze and rapid thaw method. The viability of the cartilage is preserved by glycerolization of the cartilage prior to freezing. The freeze-drying technique was not used because it was felt that drying alters the physical characteristics of the bone, rendering it more fragile and susceptible to fracture, and impairing the viability of the cartilage. (Mankin HJ,: Osteoarticular and intercalary allograft transplantation in the management of malignant tumors of bone. Cancer, 50:613, 1982)

may arise during active revascularization of the graft, a period when the bone is mechanically unable to withstand excessive stresses.

Delayed union or nonunion at the anastomosis site is relatively common. Insertion of autogenous bone and reimplanting the hardware is necessary. Electrical stimulation, particularly by noninvasive methods, may be considered.

Irradiation Therapy

Radiation therapy for a giant-cell tumor has been shown to increase the incidence of malignant transformation.[61,62,75] After a number of years following irradiation, fibrosarcomatous changes are the usual malignant features observed. Less commonly an osteosarcoma will arise.

Megavoltage therapy is permissible only for inaccessible lesions located in the spine, sacrum, and pelvis. The dosage range varies from 1500r to 5000r given over a 5 to 6 week period.

Amputation

Amputation is indicated for a widespread aggressive tumor with invasion of the soft tissues, for repeated recurrences, and for a malignant tumor. Occasionally, advanced age, ominous cytology and behavior of the tumor, and concurrent unrelated disease may dictate the need for amputation for expediency.

Pulmonary Metastasis

Even a histologically benign giant-cell tumor can behave aggressively locally, invade the regional veins, and produce metastatic lesions in the lung. Ordinarily a "benign" appearing tumor, a primary malignant tumor, or one that has evolved from a benign tumor either spontaneously or as a result of irradiation, which has metastasized to the lung, carries a poor prognosis. Nevertheless, when a solitary lung lesion is discovered, and is accessible, it should be removed because long-term survival is yet possible.

SUBPERIOSTEAL GIANT-CELL TUMOR

A subperiosteal giant-cell tumor is a peculiar variant characterized by rapid development after trauma of an osteolytic lesion containing blood. The tissue consists of giant cells in an ossifying stroma of fibrous tissue. No expansion of cortex occurs. Reossification and healing are spontaneous. This tumor is described under Aneurysmal Bone Cyst.

ANEURYSMAL BONE CYST

An aneurysmal bone cyst is a benign bone lesion (ossifying subperiosteal hematoma, subperiosteal giant-cell tumor) consisting of a mass of vascular spaces enclosed in a shell of periosteal new bone growing outward from a bone and displacing the soft tissues.[78,79]

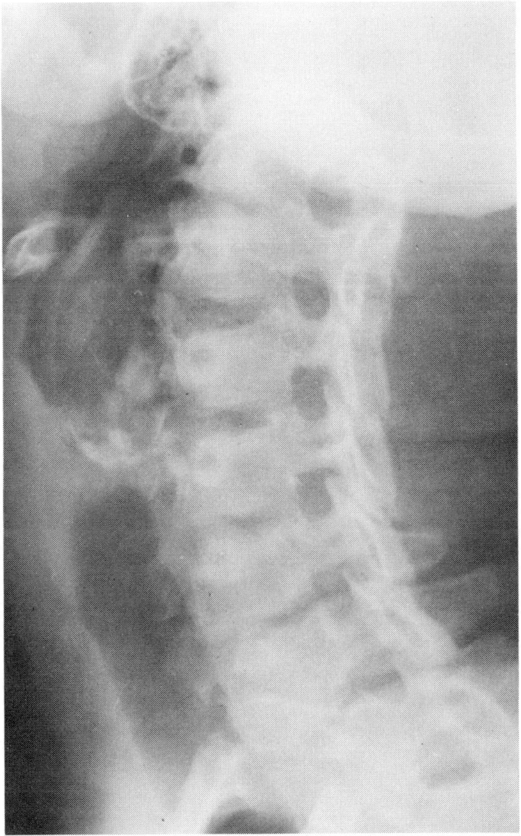

FIG. 15-22. Aneurysmal bone cyst of the cervical spine. The roentgenogram reveals the soft tissue mass (hemorrhage) along the anterior aspect of C3, C4, and C5 and the osteolytic lesion of origin in the anterior-inferior angle of the body of the C4. The mass is just beginning to ossify. Clinically, the onset is sudden and produces pain, torticollis, restriction of neck motion, and dysphagia. Examination reveals a tender, fixed, ligneous mass which is not visible in roentgenograms until ossification develops.

CLINICAL PICTURE

Age. Occurs most commonly between 10 and 30 years of age

Sex. Males predominate

Area of Predilection. The metaphyseal region of long bones; less often, flat bones and vertebrae; in a vertebra, arch usually affected; the body, infrequently

Symptoms and Findings. A history of trauma often antedates pain accentuated by movement, bony swelling, and limitation of joint motion. When a vertebra is involved, signs of spinal cord or nerve root pressure can develop.

ROENTGENOGRAPHIC FINDINGS

The affected bone is expanded, cystic, and ballooned outward. The mass is roughly ovoid, displays a slightly increased soft tissue density, extends outward eccentrically from the bone, destroys the original cortex, and is surrounded by a faint outline representing periosteal new bone (Fig. 15-22). The radiolucent tumor gradually becomes mottled and coarsely trabeculated and eventually may completely ossify. Although the underlying cortex is destroyed and the medullary canal exposed, the shaft is not expanded. When the tumor involves a vertebra, the arch is usually affected. However, when situated within the vertebral body, it must be differentiated from a hemangioma. The vertical striations peculiar to hemangioma are never observed in an aneurysmal bone cyst.

PATHOLOGY

Gross Appearance

The large mass is attached by a broad base to the shaft of a long bone growing outward and displacing the soft

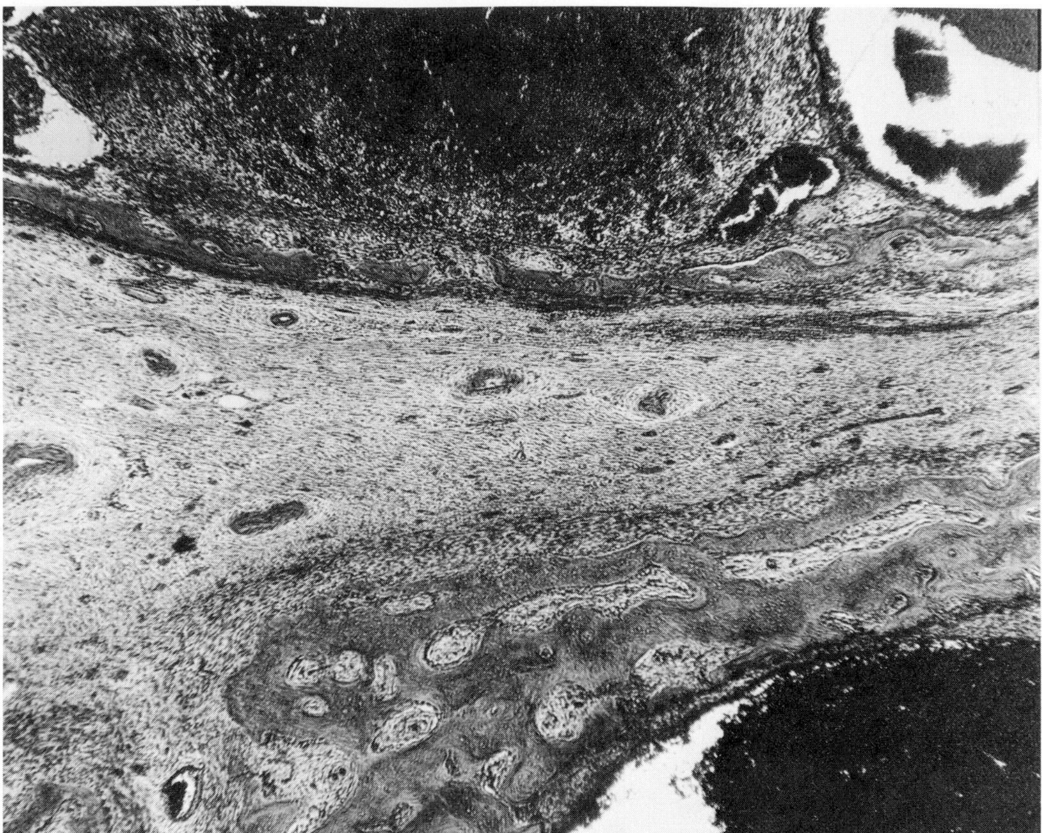

FIG. 15-23. Aneurysmal bone cyst. The walls of connective tissue display new bone formation and giant cells which are smaller than the tumor-type of giant cells.

tissues. It is surrounded by a thin shell of bone enclosing cystic blood-filled spaces. The thin bony shell is easily penetrated, and a reddish brown, liverlike friable mass interspersed with gritty particles of bone is encountered. A semiliquid substance having the appearance of partially organized blood clot lies in the center. Occasionally, the soft center may be continuous with the medullary canal. The highly vascular tumor bleeds profusely but slowly on attempted removal. Fibro-osseous septae extend throughout the tumor.

Microscopic Appearance

The spongy bone and marrow are replaced by small and large pools of blood enclosed in fibro-osseous septae (Color Plate 15-5 and Fig. 15-23). The supportive connective tissue bordering the vascular spaces contains multinuclear giant cells, new bone formation, and calcium deposits. The giant cells are small and contain small nuclei in contrast with large tumor giant cells. The peripheral shell displays active periosteal new bone formation.

TREATMENT

These lesions may regress spontaneously and ossify. Irradiation therapy hastens the process. Before the tumor becomes extensive, it is advisable to curet the lesion, fill the defect with bone grafts, and follow with irradiation therapy.

UNICAMERAL BONE CYST

The unicameral (Latin: *unus* = one; *camera* = vault) bone cyst was initially described by Jaffe and Lichtenstein in 1942.[87] It is an uncommon but not rare non-neoplastic lesion usually seen during the first two decades of life, although not necessarily limited to these age groups. It is characterized pathologically by a thin-walled cavity developing most often within the metaphysis of a long tubular bone closely adjacent to the growth plate, and appearing to migrate away from the growth plate as it matures. It is subject to pathologic fracture, and may occasionally affect the epiphyseal growth plate so as to disturb longitudinal growth. Jaffe stated that a solitary unicameral bone cyst persists indefinitely unless obliterated by surgery.[86] However, the rarity of this lesion in adults suggests that spontaneous healing occurs.

PREDISPOSING FACTORS

Age. A lesion at the proximal end of the humerus occurs predominantly in childhood between the ages of 5 and 15. It is rarely seen after age 20. A lesion at the proximal end of the femur occurs predominantly in adolescents and adults with a mean age of 20.[90] More than 50% of all lesions occur in persons younger than age 10, and about 40% occur between ages 10 to 20.[81]

Sex. Males are favored 2:1.

Location.[82] Upper end of the humerus in about 55% of all lesions. Seventy percent of active lesions at this site appear to remain adjacent to the epiphysis when observed over a period of years.[90] Lesions appear in the upper end of femur in about 26% of cases. The calcar is generally preserved. Less common sites are the ilium, lower humerus and femur, tibia, calcaneus, talus, radius, ulna, and ribs.

PATHOLOGY

Gross Appearance

The bone displays an area of fusiform expansion. The periosteum lifts away easily, and the underlying bone is "egg-shell" thin, semitranslucent, bluish, and easily penetrated. The cavity is a single chamber containing yellow fluid. Recent trauma may cause the fluid to become serosanguinous or hemorrhagic. Following a healed fracture, the cavity may become divided by fibro-osseous septa. A thin layer of grey connective tissue lines the inner surface of the cyst wall, which displays multiple scroll-like ridges that account for the pseudoloculated appearance on roentgenograms. A thin layer of cancellous bone is almost invariably interposed between the cyst wall and the adjacent epiphyseal growth plate;[86,90] rarely, the epiphyseal plate may abut directly on the cyst cavity, or the cyst may very rarely extend through the plate into the epiphysis.

Microscopic Appearance

The connective tissue is composed of layers of flattened cells (fibroblasts) lying on vascular collagenous or myxomatous tissue containing multinucleated giant cells, foam cells containing hemosiderin and lipids, and cholesterol crystals imbedded in fibrin masses. The cortical wall is composed of loosely trabeculated osseous tissue, and many thin-walled vessels. Following fracture, periosteal new bone apposition may be evident.

Jaffe and Lichtenstein regard the bone cyst as "active" and continuously enlarging when it is situated closely adjacent to the growth plate, and the cyst become "latent" as it moves away from the growth plate, becoming separated from the latter by newly formed bone.[86] However, histologic studies show that a layer of spongiosa is almost invariably present when the cyst appears to be closely approximated to the plate.

Johnson and Kindred have described a glistening, white, firm, rubbery "nubbin" of tissue resembling cartilage, which either projected into the cyst cavity or extended outward into the surrounding spongiosa. They theorized that failure to sufficiently excise the surrounding cancellous bone when resecting the cyst so as to remove this "angiomyxofibrillar lipoma" accounted for regeneration of the cyst.[88]

CLINICAL PICTURE

The lesion remains asymptomatic until attention is drawn to it when trauma induces local aching pain which often is found to be due to a fracture through the cyst wall. When pain appears to develop spontaneously, close inquiry will usually disclose a trivial traumatic episode (*e.g.*, the act of throwing), and symptoms can be attributed to an "infraction" which may or may not be visible on the roentgenogram. A fracture may produce local swelling and tenderness. Recurring fractures are not unusual. In a weight-bearing bone, intermittent limp may be the initial complaint.

A unicameral bone cyst causes local loss of bone structure and susceptibility to pathologic fracture. The fracture heals rapidly, usually within a few weeks. As the fracture unites, spontaneous obliteration of the cyst may take place, occurring in approximately 15% of cases. In approximately 30% of cases, as a consequence of continuing bone growth and remodeling of the metaphysis, the cyst becomes displaced at a variable distance down the shaft. In most instances, the cyst appears to remain in its juxta-epiphyseal location.[90]

A cyst that is situated adjacent to the epiphyseal growth plate may induce growth disturbances. Growth retardation and deformity in the upper extremity is rarely significant. However, a cyst at the proximal portion of the femur may produce a coxa vara deformity, but rarely coxa valga. Shortening or overgrowth may occur.[82]

ROENTGENOGRAPHIC FINDINGS

The lesion in a long tubular bone is usually situated in the juxta-epiphyseal portion of the metaphysis, but it is sometimes already several centimeters removed from the growth plate (Fig. 15-24). It is a large, well-localized radiolucent, expansile defect that is sharply delimited from the diaphysis. The diameter of the affected region is expanded. The regional cortex is attenuated, the

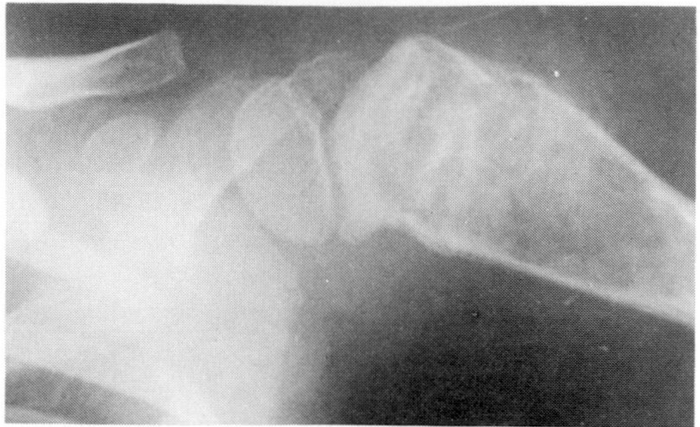

FIG. 15-24. Unicameral bone cyst with pathologic fracture.

thinning occurring from its medullary aspect which is scalloped, whereas the periosteal surface is smooth. A loculated appearance is due to the presence of ridges over the inner surface of the cyst rather than bony partitions, but following the healing of a fracture fibro-osseous septa may actually form. The initial infraction or fracture occurs without displacement and is usually situated in the proximal half of the cystic area.

In the upper portion of the femur, the cyst is usually situated in the subcapital area of the femoral neck, generally extending toward the lesser trochanter, but the calcar is preserved. The cyst may also develop at the base of the neck adjacent to the growth plate of the greater trochanter.

DIFFERENTIAL DIAGNOSIS

The diagnosis of unicameral bone cyst is established by aspiration, injection of a radiopaque substance, and direct operative exposure including biopsy.

TABLE 15-1 Differential Diagnosis

	Primary Histiocytic Lymphoma	Ewing's Sarcoma
Age	20 to 50 years	5 to 16 years
Site	Epiphysis or metaphysis	Metaphysis and diaphysis
Roentgenograms	Osteolytic, no reactive bone, no tumor bone	Initial bone condensation Later osteolytic Onion-peel periosteal bone
General Condition	Usually little altered	Seriously affected
Fever	Absent	Frequent
Metastases	Rare and distant	Frequent and early
Course	Slow	Rapid
Prognosis	High number of cures	Fatal in nearly all

Eosinophilic Granuloma. This circumscribed osteolytic defect is more likely to be situated toward the middle of the shaft, is generally smaller when first seen, and is more painful. Periosteal new bone formation is considerable and extends beyond the radiolucent defect. Biopsy reveals numerous eosinophiles and histiocytes.

Enchondroma. The favored site is the shaft of a short tubular bone (*e.g.*, metacarpal and metatarsal), the rarest site for a unicameral bone cyst. Radiopacities within the radiolucent defect represent calcifications within the solid cartilaginous tumor. In a unicameral bone cyst, opacities representing newly formed osseous foci may develop following a fracture.

Fibrous Dysplasia. The predominantly fibrous lesion forms a radiolucent defect which is situated in an eccentric location, usually within the diaphysis, and is multilocular. Greater amounts of trabeculated bone impart a "ground-glass" appearance on roentgenograms. Biopsy is diagnostic.

Giant-Cell Tumor. The osteolytic defect of a long bone involves the epiphysis in an adult and is eccentric. A unicameral bone cyst extends through the epiphyseal plate into the epiphysis very rarely. Biopsy of the giant-cell tumor discloses plump spindle-shaped or ovoid stromal cells with a profusion of highly multinucleated giant cells.

Aneurysmal Bone Cyst. The radiolucent defect is eccentric although it may occupy the entire center of the bone, eroding and distending the cortex to one side ("blowout"), and often extending beyond the bone where it produces a radiologically evident soft tissue density. Confusion may exist when, following a fracture, the unicameral bone cyst contains large blood-filled spaces. Biopsy is diagnostic.

TREATMENT

The cyst does not disappear spontaneously except rarely after a fracture. The threat of pathologic fracture and growth disturbances always remains. Consequently, prolonged periods of restricted activity are unjustified. Early operative treatment is indicated in spite of the known risks of recurrence and possible additional damage to the epiphyseal growth plate. A period of watchful waiting, particularly while a fracture is healing, is permissible to allow additional new bone to form between the growth plate and the cyst and to provide additional structural strength to preserve length and alignment following surgery. It should be recognized that 70% of "active" cysts remain adjacent to the plate for lengthy periods of time.[89] After operation, using former conservative procedures, which consist essentially of curettage and insertion of bone grafts through a small cortical opening, recurrences are frequent, necessitating repeated procedures. Recently introduced radical operations, which consist of extensive subtotal or total resection and bone grafts, appear to have a highly successful rate of cure.

In a true recurrence, the cavity reappears and enlarges causing expansion of the bone again. The cortex is thinned and fracture is threatened. Incomplete obliteration should not be considered as a true recurrence. When the original defect has been partially obliterated, the small residual defect will ultimately disappear within a few years.[90]

The principles of surgical treatment are as follows:

- Recurrence is more probable when the patient is younger than 10 years of age, particularly when the lesion is in the upper humerus, and closely adjacent to the growth plate.[84]
- Allow the fracture to heal to preserve length and stability.
- Adequate opening in cortex
- Break down cyst wall to permit rapid revascularization
- Curet membranous lining
- Avoid injury to growth plate
- Fill cavity with bone grafts. Autogenous cancellous grafts preferred. Thick cortical bone struts to preserve length. In the very young immature patient, freeze-dried cancellous bone[92] or cortical bone allografts[91,93] may be used.
- Adequate subperiosteal resection. Periosteum preserved for replacement osteogenesis.

Types of Operation

Curettage and Bone Grafts. The membranous lining is removed through a small window in the cortex and cavity thoroughly filled with autogenous or bank bone. There is an unacceptable high rate of recurrence.

Sub-Total Resection and Bone Grafts.[83] The periosteum is incised longitudinally and the affected bone is exposed extending to normal bone at both ends of the cyst. Transverse cuts are made 1 cm proximal and distal to the cyst, approximately three fourths of the way through the shaft. Longitudinal cuts are made to connect the transverse cuts and two thirds to four fifths of the cyst wall is removed in this manner. In the active cyst, the proximal transverse cut is made 1 cm distal to the epiphyseal plate. A portion of the cyst wall is preserved to maintain length and alignment, and cortical bone struts are placed longitudinally within the area for stability and length, and autogenous cancellous bone chips are placed about the struts. The periosteum is closed over the grafts. Postoperatively a Velpeau bandage provides immobilization. Obliteration of the cyst is successful in a high percentage of cases.

Total Resection (Diaphysectomy) and Bone Grafts.[80,85] The periosteum is split longitudinally and elevated circumferentially, freeing it to the levels of normal bone. Metal markers are placed above and below the suspected lesion and a roentgenogram localizes the levels of resection. A malleable band retractor is slipped between the periosteum and bone. The portion of the bone containing the cyst is then excised leaving the periosteal sleeve. The periosteum is then partially closed, and cancellous chips and matchstick-sized grafts are packed into the periosteal tube. Closure of the periosteal sleeve is then completed. Postoperatively, limb length and alignment are maintained by skeletal traction through the olecranon or by a hanging cast. Within a few weeks osteogenesis is sufficiently advanced to provide stability and allow full activity, especially in the young immature child, within 6 to 8 weeks. The tubular bone appears to be completely reconstituted, although retardation of longtidinal growth is unaffected.

Intracystic Injection of Corticosteroids.[94] When a slowly absorbed microcrystalline corticosteroid is injected into a unicameral bone cyst, particularly during the rapid growth period, the cyst will heal in most cases by new trabecular bone formation.

Method. Two needles are introduced into the cavity to allow for free escape of cystic fluid. Attempts at forced aspiration through a single needle should not be attempted since it may provoke profuse venous bleeding. Removal of fluid should be thorough so that the injected suspension of prednisolone acetate crystals can reach and cover the whole wall of the cyst. For small cysts and young patients, 40 mg to 80 mg are injected; for larger cysts, up to 200 mg are injected. Radiographic followup is carried out at 2 to 3 month intervals. For areas which appear to show scanty osteogenesis, the injection is repeated. Up to 5 or 6 repeat injections may be required in some instances before complete repair is achieved. As a general rule, when the treatment is carried out at a very early age or during growth spurt periods, repair is usually rapid and complete. The relief of pain is swift. The injection does not appear to impair the growth of the epiphyseal plate, and no biochemical disturbances have been noted.

Pathologic studies of specimens obtained 2 months after the initial injection show edematous fibroblastic tissue filling the cystic cavity, and active osteogenesis laying down new trabecular bone from the cyst wall toward the cavity. By 3 years after treatment is initiated, complete obliteration of the lesion and replacement by normally structured bone is achieved.

OSTEOGENIC SARCOMA

Osteogenic sarcoma, often called osteosarcoma, is a highly malignant bone tumor characterized by the invariable formation of neoplastic osteoid and tumor tissue. Since it arises from a common multipotential mesenchymal tissue, fibrosarcomatous and chondrosarcomatous tissues are also components of the tumor. In any individual tumor, the osteoblastic, fibroblastic, and chondroblastic components vary in amount, but neoplastic osteoid tissue and bone, even when scarce, is always present and can be traced to originate directly from primitive mesenchymal tissue. A tumor that may initially appear to be either a fibrosarcoma or a chondrosarcoma, tumors of a lesser degree of malignancy, may on diligent search reveal isolated foci of neoplastic bone and the typical hypercellular osteoblastic sarcomatous stroma which defines it as an osteosarcoma with an extremely ominous prognosis.

When osteogenic sarcoma forms abundant tumor bone, it is designated sclerosing sarcoma; when forming relatively little bone, it is called osteolytic. These are only descriptive terms, but regardless of its histiologic variability, an osteogenic sarcoma of any type generally follows a typical clinical course. Usually one half of tumors show heavy ossification, one fourth a moderate degree of ossification and one fourth relatively little ossification reflected roentgenographically.[135] Osteolytic tumors, in addition to having mottled foci of new bone, show prominent secondary features such as necrosis, cystic softening, hemorrhage, and telangiectasis.

ETIOLOGY

Predisposing Factors

Age. Peak incidence during second decade; rare below 10 years

Sex. Slight preponderance in males

Anatomical Site. More than 90% in the metaphysis of major tubular bones; predilection for bones about the knee; less common at upper humerus; jaws a favorite site in the aged; sites other than long bones exceedingly rare in children

Exciting Factors

Virus.[117] Osteosarcoma can be produced in experimental animals by oncogenic viruses introduced either systematically[116,153] or locally.[124] Oncogenic viruses are generally classified as those containing either RNA or DNA. RNA viruses which induce bone tumors include the Harvey and Moloney mouse sarcoma viruses.[118,152] Certain DNA viruses also produce osteosarcoma (*e.g.*, the polyoma virus[156] and the SV40 virus).[111]

When murine sarcoma virus (Moloney) is injected into the tibia of rats, palpable tumors develop, progress, and metastasize to the lungs. The sarcoma is more likely to develop in neonatal animals because the virus is highly antigenic in adult animals. The experimentally produced tumor does not consistently resemble human osteosarcoma in terms of morphology and spread.[100,131]

Presently there is no epidemiological evidence that viruses are responsible for human osteosarcoma.

Radiation[165] Actively proliferating cells which are barely differentiated toward osteoblasts ("osteoprogenitor cells") are most sensitive to radiation. These cells are predominantly situated about areas of active growth in the metaphysis adjacent to the growth plate and over the extensive surfaces of the trabeculae. The greater the inherent growth potential of a bone exposed to external irradiation, the more severe the radiation effect. Osteosarcoma can result from localized radiation at a dose above 2000 rads. Experimental production of both osteosarcoma and fibrosarcoma has been accomplished by external radiation.[99] The latent period before the tumor appears is prolonged, as much as 3 to 4 years or more.

Nearly all radionuclides that localize in bone can produce bone tumors. Radionuclide α-emitters are more oncogenic than β-emitters; strong β particles are more oncogenic than weak β particles; radionuclides with a long biologic half life are more oncogenic than those with short half-lives. Young growing bone retains more bone-seeking radionuclides than does adult bone.[115] Large bones are more responsive to radionuclides, and females are more susceptible.

Chemicals. Induction of osteosarcoma has been accomplished by many agents such as 20-methylcholanthrene,[104] cupric-chelated N-hydroxy-2-acetylaminofluorene[155] and beryllium compounds.[129,163] With beryllium, splenic atrophy occurs. After splenectomy, osteosarcoma develops in all experimental animals receiving beryllium. In unsplenectomized animals, only 50% develop osteosarcoma.

PATHOLOGY

Osteogenic sarcoma assumes a wide variety of histologic patterns which can be typed according to the predominating tissue as osteoblastic, chondroblastic, or fibroblastic;[110,119,130,135] or according to the gross appearance as sclerosing or osteolytic.[119] Such classifications have no prognostic significance. For the purpose of understanding and recognizing the variable nature of this ominous tumor, the following description will attempt to detail the general characteristics of osteosarcoma; this will be followed by a description of the two extreme types, osteoblastic (sclerosing) and the osteolytic tumors. It is important to understand that the most common tumor will possess characteristics of both an osteogenic and a sclerosing sarcoma to an extremely variable degree.

Osteosarcomas have several characteristics.

Gross Appearance

The tumor is most often situated in the metaphysis of a large long bone, usually at the lower end of the femur, upper end of the tibia, and upper end of the humerus,

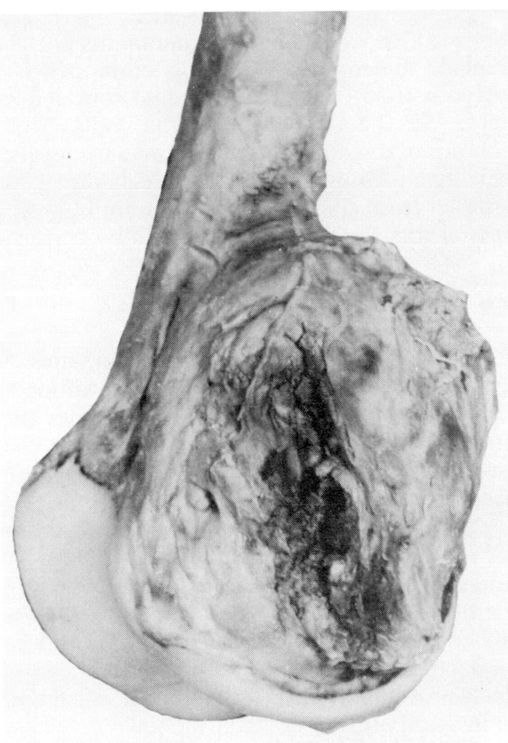

FIG. 15-25. Gross specimen of osteogenic sarcoma.

in descending order of frequency. Less often it occurs at the upper end of the fibula, the iliac bone, vertebrae, jaw bone, and rarely at other sites. In the large long bone, it may occasionally originate in the midshaft.

In the typical metaphyseal location, it appears as a large tumor with destruction of the inner cortex as it extends into the subperiosteal space (Fig. 15-25). Its consistency varies from stony hard to soft and gritty. Its color reflects its components: fibrous, white; osseous, yellowish white; and cartilaginous, bluish white. Some tumors contain large vascular channels and hemorrhage. Necrotic foci and areas of disintegration causing cysticlike cavitations are most pronounced in rapidly growing tumors. Extension of the tumor through the medullary canal is greater than is reflected on roentgenograms. The most cellular and least differentiated portion of the tumor is within the advancing core in the medullary cavity and beneath the elevated periosteum. This soft, whitish, cellular, extending tumor tissue contains streaks of irregular, delicate tumor bone.

Within the subperiosteal space, the newly formed neoplastic bone becomes oriented perpendicular to the surface of the cortex, producing the characteristic sunburst appearance seen on the roentgenogram. The periosteum acts as a barrier and is lifted away from the parent bone as the tumor tissue accumulates in large amounts beneath the periosteal envelope, sometimes completely encircling the bone. Reactive subperiosteal bone is laid down, and this is most pronounced at the proximal and distal osteoperiosteal attachments, producing Codman's angles seen on roentgenograms. Rarely, multiple layers of subperiosteal reactive bone produce a lamellated appearance, but this is not distinctive of osteosarcoma. Eventually the periosteum is penetrated as the tumor extends into the surrounding soft tissues.

During the active growth period while the epiphyseal plate is still intact, it acts as a barrier to extension of the tumor into the epiphysis. After epiphyseal closure, the tumor may extend into the epiphysis but the articular cartilage bars further extension into the joint.

Metastasis is early and hematogenous, producing pulmonary deposits. Rarely, early metastases to other bones may suggest a multifocal origin of the sarcoma.

Microscopic Appearance

Although the histologic picture is quite variable, the absolute criteria for diagnosis are sarcomatous stroma and direct formation of tumor osteoid and bone by the malignant connective tissue (Color Plate 15-6). Therefore, the tumor must always contain directly formed neoplastic osteoblastic areas to qualify as an osteogenic sarcoma. The tumor also contains malignant cartilage and fibrous tissue in variable amounts. The latter may dominate the histologic picture so that a chondrosarcoma or a fibrosarcoma is suggested, but the finding of minute foci of neoplastic osteoid and bone directly formed from the anaplastic cellular stroma categorizes the tumor as an osteosarcoma.

The stromal cells are large, resemble osteoblasts, and their malignant characteristics include anisocytosis, poikilocytosis, nuclear pyknosis, pleomorphism, polyhedral contours tending toward a spindly shape, and frequent mitosis. The best evidence of malignancy is seen at the advancing borders of the tumor where a profusion of anaplastic cells destroy the normal trabeculae and produce neoplastic osteoid in disordered sheets between and along remnants of normal trabeculae. Sometimes randomly strewn collagen fibers are observed among the cells and appear to undergo transition to peculiar osteoidlike tissue.

The central portions of the tumor are routinely the most sclerotic where the formation of neoplastic bone is most pronounced. As the anaplastic cells become enclosed in new bone, they become smaller and rounded and thus may be unsuitable for diagnosis. Therefore, the peripheral zones are the most satisfactory for diagnosis.

The highly malignant, more cellular tumors are very soft and fragile, and contain extensive zones of necrosis and hemorrhage. Such rapidly growing tumors undergo disintegration, producing a cystlike appearance and vascular lakes and channels often containing tumor emboli.

Malignant tumor cartilage may undergo calcification and osseous transformation as it does in true chondrosarcoma. This finding in itself is not diagnostic, and only the detection of osteoid and bone directly formed from anaplastic stromal cells will define the tumor as a true osteosarcoma, a tumor with a much greater degree of malignancy than chondrosarcoma.

Benign multinucleated cells are observed in some osteogenic sarcomas.

Of great prognostic significance is the differentiation of the primary bone sarcomas: osteogenic (osteoid-producing) sarcoma, fibrosarcoma, chondrosarcoma, and parosteal (juxtacortical) sarcoma. Chondrosarcomas and fibrosarcomas have a much better outlook after resection. Parosteal sarcomas uniformly have low-grade malignant characteristics and a good prognosis.[164]

The 5-year survival rate of fibrosarcoma is twice that of osteosarcoma,[120,137] and chondrosarcoma three times that of osteosarcoma.[122]

Dahlin has subtyped osteogenic sarcomas into osteoblastic, chondroblastic, and fibroblastic variants, depending on the predominating tissue.[110] Geschickter and Copeland subtyped osteogenic sarcomas as sclerosing or osteolytic.[119] Such subtyping has not proved to be of prognostic value.

Paget's sarcoma, a secondary osteosarcoma superimposed on a Paget's lesion, usually in a case with widespread Paget's disease, has an almost uniformly dismal prognosis.

SCLEROSING OSTEOSARCOMA

A sclerosing osteosarcoma is a greyish white tumor with a consistency varying between that of fibrous tissue and bone. The central older portion of the tumor is composed of dense, often streaked, neoplastic bone. The most recently formed lobulated advancing tissue is softer and gritty to the feel. Typically, the tumor first develops in the metaphysis where the epiphyseal growth plate restricts the spread of the tumor toward the epiphysis. Instead, the tumor extends distally in the medullary space, the soft cellular advancing tissue destroying the trabeculae in its path. The medullary spread is generally greater than is evident on roentgenogram. After disappearance of the epiphyseal plate, the tumor proceeds into the epiphysis. The joint is practically never invaded.

The tumor partially erodes the inner cortex as it appears to infiltrate and merge with the cortex as a dense, mottled bony mass invading the subperiosteal space. The latter most recently formed tissue is more cellular and softer. Within this new advancing tissue, new bone formation is visible as grains or streaks which generally run outward at right angles to the shaft. As the periosteum is elevated from the shaft, it excites new bone formation from the inner osteogenic layer of the periosteum. The reactive new bone is best seen at the upper and lower angles of the subperiosteal space.

At a late stage, the tumor penetrates the periosteum and invades the surrounding soft tissues.

Metastases occur early, are hematogenous, and as microemboli form small pulmonary deposits which at first cannot be detected on roentgenograms.

Microscopically, the histopathologic picture is dominated by extensive irregular sheets of new osteoid and bone which extend between remnants of trabeculae and replace the marrow. The cells entrapped by neoplastic osseous tissue become small and rounded, and do not resemble the anaplastic stromal cells. The peripheral lobules of the most recently formed tumor tissue contain the hypercellular stroma in which direct formation of osteoid from the anaplastic cells are best observed, and it is at this site that biopsy should be performed.

OSTEOLYTIC OSTEOSARCOMA

The osteolytic tumor (malignant bone aneurysm, telangiectatic sarcoma) is a destructive tumor which, like other types of osteogenic sarcoma, arises in the central metaphyseal region of a large long bone. It is a rapidly growing tumor with an unusual tendency to pathologic fracture that does not heal.

Grossly, this is a vascular tumor exhibiting evidence of recent hemorrhage. It is a soft, friable, bloody tissue interspersed with fibrous tissue that encloses necrotic, hemorrhagic cavities. The main mass of tissue is found subcortically. The inner aspect of the cortex is motheaten and penetrated so that the tumor comes to lie subperiosteally. Finally, the surrounding soft tissues are infiltrated and present a ragged, bloody mass of tissue. Within the shaft, the tumor extends distally in the medullary cavity, and, after epiphyseal closure, into the epiphysis. The bone usually fractures transversely in the metaphysis.

Microscopically, blood-containing spaces without endothelial linings lie within tissue composed mainly of abundant, plump spindle cells and anaplastic osteoblasts with vesicular hyperchromatic nuclei and frequent mitoses. A variable amount of osteoid is scattered throughout, but actual osseous tissue is sparse or nonexistent. Giant cells are present but are few in number, small, and contain less than fifteen nuclei. The foreign-body type of giant cell is more common in slow-growing tumors. The rapidly growing more malignant growths display the multinucleated tumor giant cells which may simulate those of a malignant giant-cell tumor. In such a diagnostic problem, the detection of extremely anaplastic osteoblastic cells directly forming neoplastic osteoid establishes the diagnosis of osteosarcoma.

DIFFERENTIAL DIAGNOSTIC FINDINGS

Osteosarcoma, as mentioned earlier, is a rapidly growing, extremely malignant tumor possessing the invariable characteristic of producing neoplastic osteoid directly from anaplastic, osteoblastlike cells. It is important to identify this directly developing osteoid tissue which implies an extremely serious outlook. The tumor may be histologically similar to fibrosarcoma or chondrosarcoma, each of which has a relatively less malignant prognosis.

Osteosarcoma contains any one or all the elements of osteogenesis, including osteoblasts, osteoid, bone, and calcifying cartilage which eventually is replaced by bone. In addition to anaplastic osteoblastlike cells, fibroblasts and chondroblasts are likewise subject to anaplastic changes inasmuch as these are derived from a common stem cell.

Osteosarcoma varies in appearance depending on the predominating component. At one extreme, the neoplasm is soft and vascular, mesenchymelike tissue is abundant, and a profusion of anaplastic polyhedral osteoblasts occupies the main mass. Anaplasia of osteoblasts is evidenced by their large size, large, hyperchromatic nuclei, and frequent mitoses. Growth proceeds so rapidly that it seldom reaches beyond the point of osteoid formation, and then in small foci which must be diligently sought out before the diagnosis is established. This soft highly vascular tumor constitutes the rapidly growing osteolytic type of osteosarcoma.

At the other end of the spectrum, the tumor is strongly osteogenic. Anaplastic osteoblasts form in an irregular manner osteoid and bone which become intermingled with the remnants of partially resorbed bone trabeculae and cortical lamellae. As the tumor bone encloses the anaplastic cells, the latter lose their malignant characteristics, becoming small and rounded. Therefore, the central portion of the tumor containing the dense bone is unsuitable for diagnostic biopsy. Specimens of tissue should be taken from the peripheral, most recently formed lobules which are highly cellular.

Between the two extremes of tumor types lies the more common type of tumor possessing characteristics of both. This tumor presents the often described roentgenographic picture of mottled areas of increased and decreased densities in the metaphyseal region of a large long bone, obliterating the lines of normal bone trabeculation, eroding and intermingling with the cortex which loses its definition and producing the sunburst appearance caused by radial streaks of neoplastic bone outside the cortex. These pictures are quite variable depending on the degree of osteogenesis and the rate of growth of the tumor at the time of the initial examination of the patient.

Lichtenstein[135] and others state that the main criteria identifying osteosarcoma are a sarcomatous stroma, and direct formation of neoplastic osteoid and bone by the sarcomatous stroma. Cartilage always has the potential for calcifying and transforming to bone by metaplasia. When this type of ossification is exhibited by malignant cartilage tissue, and the above criteria cannot be met, the tumor is properly labelled a chondrosarcoma, a tumor which has a lesser degree of malignity than osteosarcoma. Similarly, in a tumor which appears to be fibrosarcoma, an exhaustive search for foci of osteoid formation directly from the sarcomatous stroma must be carried out before the proper label with its implied prognosis can be ascertained (Fig. 15-26).

CLINICAL PICTURE

Age. Osteosarcomas are commonly found in childhood, adolescence, and young adulthood. Its peak of incidence

FIG. 15-26. Problem: Is this a chondrosarcoma or an osteogenic sarcoma? By Geschickter and Copeland's classification, because of the presence of neoplastic new bone, it is called chondrosarcoma-type of osteogenic sarcoma. However, true osteogenic sarcoma develops new bone in the sarcomatous stroma and carries a grave prognosis. By Lichtenstein's classification, because the new bone is developing by metaplasia from cartilage, a potential of any cartilaginous tissue, the tumor is rightfully termed a chondrosarcoma. This has a lesser degree of malignity.

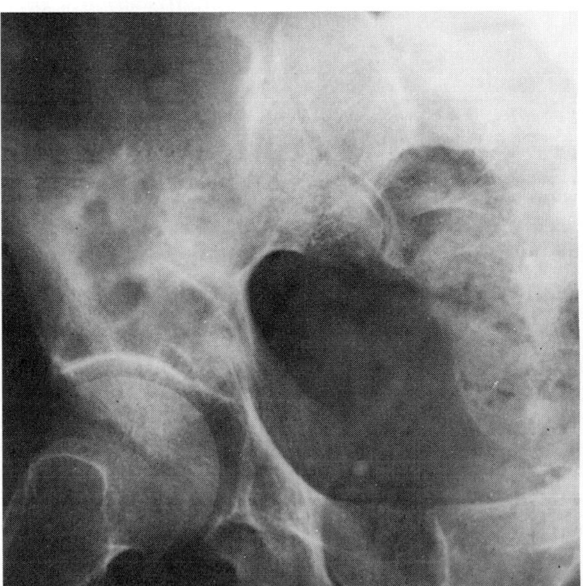

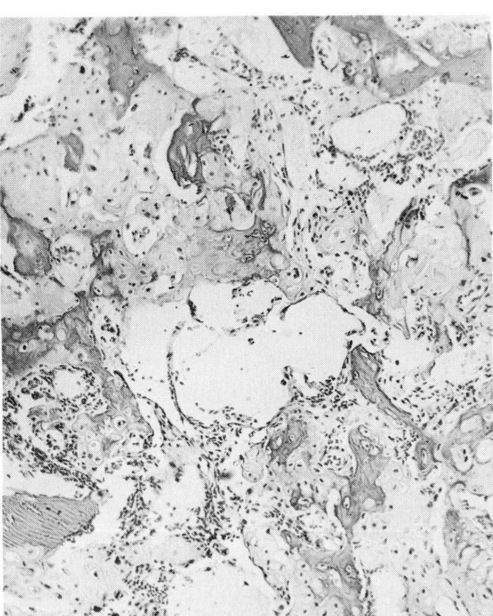

is in the second decade, its incidence decreasing with advancing age.

Location. It is found predominantly in the metaphyseal region of a large long bone, occasionally in the midshaft region. The lower end of the femur, upper end of the tibia, and upper end of the humerus are most often involved in decreasing order of frequency. Rarely, it may be found in other sites.

Sex. It is slightly more common in males.

Onset. The onset is gradual and spontaneous. Occasionally, trauma precipitates symptoms, and infrequently a pathologic fracture occurs through an osteolytic process near the end of a long bone.

Symptoms. Pain is intermittent at first but eventually becomes continuous and incapacitating. The pain usually antedates other symptoms, although swelling may have been present for several months.

Findings. When the case is first seen at an early stage, the painful, palpable mass is small and the overlying tissues appear normal. The swelling develops near the end of a long bone, and its consistency varies from very soft, almost fluctuant, to firm and indurated, to bony hard. As its size increases and extends toward the surface, the soft tissues becoming infiltrated by the tumor are immobile. The overlying skin may become stretched, thin and glossy, and may exhibit distended veins, but never ulcerates. Local inflammatory signs and general constitutional symptoms are absent. Motion of the adjacent joint is unimpaired until the muscles acting on the joint become incarcerated by the infiltrating tumor.

When a soft, rapid-growing tumor develops, a peculiar boggy or lobulated mass is palpable as the tumor extends toward the surface. The overlying skin becomes tense, is not inflamed, often contains dilated veins, and occasionally the presence of pulsations may suggest an aneurysm. Invasion of the soft tissues and the epiphysis results in limitation of joint motion. Abnormal mobility and crepitus indicate the presence of a fracture.

Course. In at least 80% of cases, progressive pulmonary metastases develop at a very early stage but are not roentgenographically detectable much before 5 months. Sometimes the metastases extend to other sites including the skeleton. The process is usually fatal within 2 years. In a small percentage, the course is chronic over 3 to 5 years with eventual demise. These figures apply to cases treated by ablation alone, but have been considerably improved by recent advances in chemotherapy, irradiation with megavoltage, and surgical resection of pulmonary lesions.

In children with rapidly growing untreated sarcomas, particularly about the knee, appreciable weight loss and moderate anemia develop especially after a pathologic fracture. Such a tumor may attain considerable size before the patient seeks medical advice, and treatment is delayed. Occasionally, the patient may have been aware of the tumor for a number of months before the pain or a fracture causes him to seek aid.

Laboratory Findings. The alkaline phosphatase is significantly increased when the tumor and its metastases are highly osteogenic. After removal of the primary tumor, the alkaline phosphatase declines, but rises again as the metastatic disease becomes extensive.

ROENTGENOGRAPHIC FINDINGS

The roentgenographic findings of osteosarcoma are characterized by a variable mixture of radiopacities of osteogenesis and the radiolucencies due to destructive changes and replacement with osteoid tissue. One or the other may dominate the picture so that there is great variation in the radiographic shadows (Figs. 15-27 and 15-28).

The tumor and therefore the radiographic changes are initially noted in the metaphysis of a long bone situated eccentrically, infrequently the tumor develops in the midshaft. The destructive changes are represented by irregular, poorly defined areas of radiolucency. The inner margin of the cortex is soon lost, since it is irregularly eroded and appears motheaten. Interspersed among the osteolytic defects are radiodensities which vary from mottled or streaked areas to more extensive extreme radiopacities, representing mineralized osteoblastic areas. Osteoid substance itself produces no radiopacity if it is unmineralized.

As the tumor shadow extends along the medullary canal, radiolucencies with loss of trabecular markings are observed at the periphery of the advancing margin. These represent the most recently formed neoplastic and as yet unmineralized tissue.

As the tumor invades the cortex, the latter loses its definition as it becomes destroyed and intermingled with the tumor shadow. In an extremely osteogenic, markedly radiopaque tumor, the cortical markings may be completely lost.

The most recently formed tumor tissue is that which has not reached its full osteogenetic potential, and therefore appears less radiopaque as it extends beyond the cortex and raises the periosteum. Fine lines of increased density, representing newly formed spicules of bone, radiate laterally from and at right angles to the surface of the shaft, giving the typical "sunburst" appearance (Fig. 15-29). As the periosteum is elevated, a triangle of reactive periosteal ossification produces a triangular radiopacity at the upper and lower angles (Codman's triangle). Non-neoplastic bone may also be deposited in layers by the periosteum, producing a lamellated appearance. These periosteal reactive signs are not characteristic of neoplasm alone. Any process (*e.g.*, infection) that elevates the periosteum can produce this effect. It has been observed in Ewing's sarcoma.

If the tumor extends beyond the periosteum, a shadow

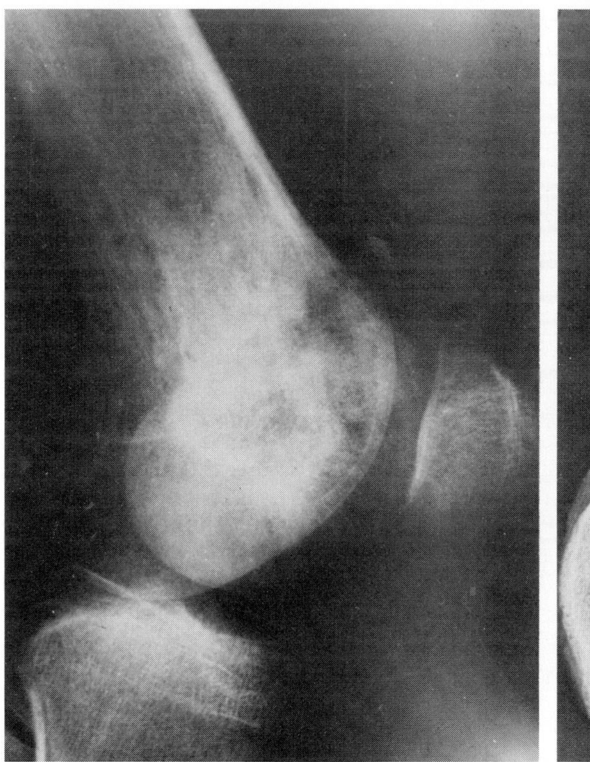

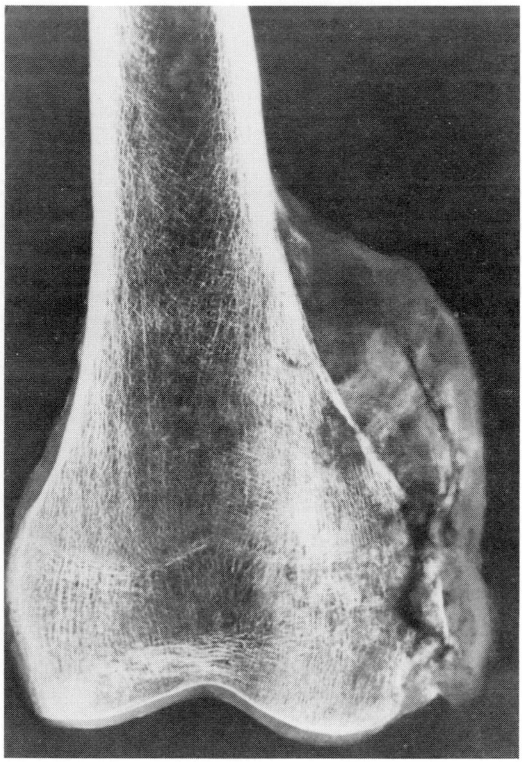

FIG. 15-27. Roentgenographic appearance of osteogenic sarcoma. (*Left*) Lateral view. Destruction, sclerosis, and mottled appearance. The location is typical. (*Right*) Roentgenogram of specimen from which soft tissue has been removed. Subperiosteal extension of the tumor and radiating rays of new bone are amply demonstrated.

containing mottled densities may be detected in the soft tissues.

Fracture through the metaphysis, particularly in markedly osteolytic areas, may be noted.

Additional roentgenographic studies should include:

1. *Tomograms* of the entire bone to define more accurately the extent of the tumor. It may reveal a fracture.
2. *Complete skeletal survey* to determine metastatic lesions
3. *Chest x-ray and tomogram* to define metastatic disease

However, shadows of early pulmonary metastases, although these lesions are invariably present as microemboli, are rarely demonstrable when the patient is initially seen.

Additional laboratory studies should include a bone scan of the entire bone to help establish the extent of the osteogenic tumor and liver function tests to determine whether hepatic metastases are present.

PROGNOSIS

Following early amputation alone (without adjunctive therapy), 50% of cases show evidence of metastatic disease, usually pulmonary, by 5 months. Considering

FIG. 15-28. Roentgenographic appearance of the anteroposterior view of osteogenic sarcoma. At the epiphysis and metaphysis of the femur note the loss of trabeculations, mottled effect of destruction and sclerosis, and sun-ray extending from the medial aspect of the epiphysis.

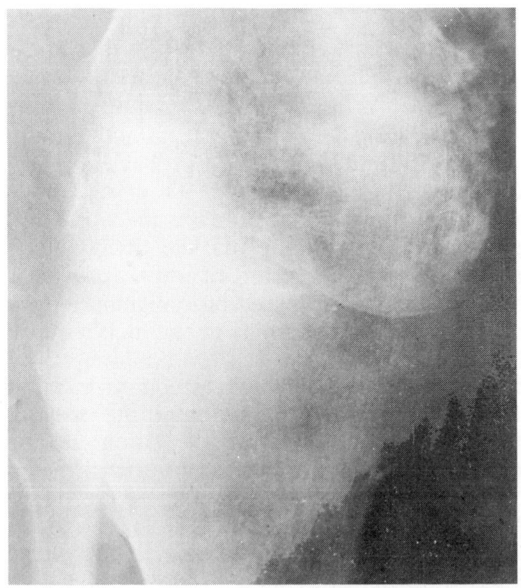

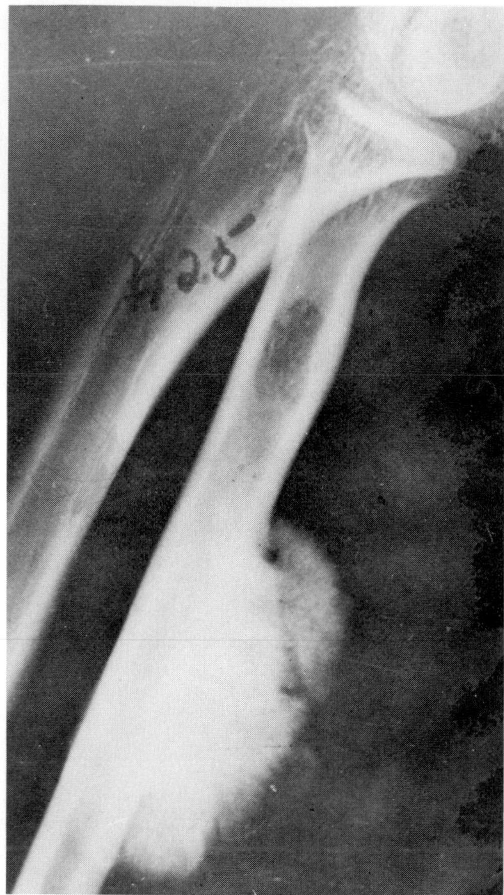

FIG. 15-29. Osteogenic sarcoma demonstrating the characteristic sun-ray appearance.

all cases, the median time for pulmonary metastases to become evident is approximately 8.5 months, and the average period between the discovery of pulmonary metastases and death is 6 months.[158,162] Studies show that 90% of patients who are free of disease at 1 year remain disease-free. If no metastases can be detected by 2½ years, subsequent spread is highly unusual, invasion of vital organs a rarity, and a cure is very probable.[138,143,144] The 5-year survival rate, with and without metastatic disease, is variously quoted at between 5% and 23%.[125,135] It seems quite probable that the marked discrepancies are accounted for by the inclusion of improperly diagnosed tumors with a lower degree of malignancy (*e.g.*, fibrosarcoma and chondrosarcoma) in the high survival groups.

In untreated cases (*i.e.*, without ablation or other therapy) the median time for survival after the onset of pulmonary metastases is 2.9 months.[139] Tumors at the proximal rather than distal portions of an extremity and of the axial skeleton are said to have poorer prognoses.[109,136]

Adjunctive therapy by chemotherapy, high-voltage irradiation, and pulmonary resection of large tumor deposits has increased the 5-year survival rates to more than 60%.

Chemotherapy appears to delay the eventual appearance of lung disease, and caution should be exercised when interpreting the results after 1 year. A 5-year study is more accurate.

TREATMENT

Osteosarcoma, because of its extremely grave outlook, demands early, radical amputation. When true osteosarcoma is defined by rigid histologic criteria (thereby eliminating tumors of less malignity: fibrosarcoma, chondrosarcoma), a 95% fatal termination is expected within 1 year when ablation alone is done. Recently, the prognosis has been vastly improved by a regimen which encompasses ablation, megavoltage irradiation, chemotherapy, and aggressive pulmonary resection.[140]

Whereas chemotherapy has previously been used in the treatment of end-stage disease, it is now directed toward treating newly diagnosed disease in an attempt to forestall or prevent metastases. Many agents have been tried, and the primary chemotherapeutic agents in use are either methotrexate in massive doses[127] or Adriamycin,[108] or a combination of both.[145,158] This chemotherapeutic approach assumes that at least 80% of patients, at the time of the initial diagnosis, already have microscopic foci of disease in the lungs, which by present methods are undetectable.[128] There is a latent period between the time of recognition of the primary tumor and the roentgenographic appearance of pulmonary lesions which does not represent new disease but rather the growth of lesions already present. Chemotherapy is used early, as soon as the diagnosis is established, to destroy microscopic areas of tumor at a stage when these malignant cells are most susceptible to the action of chemotherapeutic agents.[151] Chemotherapy given in this manner has greatly increased the 5-year survival rate of osteosarcoma.[159]

Chemotherapy prevents metastases in about 60% of cases. Many of the remaining 40% ultimately become disease-free as a result of an aggressive attack on their metastases by pulmonary resection (single or repeated), chemotherapy and radiation therapy, in addition to amputation and ablation.[140] After metastases appear, chemotherapy decreases their size and number, rendering them more suitable for resection.

Chemotherapeutic agents are potent drugs which are very toxic and require frequent monitoring. High-dose methotrexate with citrovorum-factor "rescue" (CFR) has a mortality rate of approximately 6%,[128] although this figure varies among different institutions. Adriamycin can cause fatal myocardiopathy. Chemotherapy should be administered only in special centers and by those with considerable experience in their use.

When the patient refuses amputation but accepts local

resection and insertion of an implant, chemotherapy may be used to reduce the bulk of the tumor while awaiting fabrication of the implant.[147] When immediate amputation is done, chemotherapy should be delayed until healing of the stump is secure, because the agents may interfere with soft tissue healing.

The following regimens are being studied:

1. Treatment of primary lesion: amputation followed by high-dose megavoltage therapy; or a full course irradiation followed, after several months to exclude irremediable cases, by amputation.
2. Total lung irradiation (1700 rads in 10 fractions over 2 weeks)[157]
3. Adriamycin, methotrexate and CFR, or multidrug, multicycle: methotrexate, vincristine, actinomycin D, cyclophosphamide, and Adriamycin.[166]

The foregoing facts indicate that the treatment of an osteosarcoma requires a coordinated team approach that includes the orthopaedic surgeon, medical oncologist, pediatrician, roentgenologist, radiotherapist, and the thoracic surgeon.

Surgical

The essential first principle of a curative regimen must be complete control of the primary tumor. This means early and radical ablation. The second principle is the prevention of metastases, or their control once they are established. This is accomplished locally by preoperative irradiation and by chemotherapy as soon as possible after ablation of the primary tumor. Moreover, large pulmonary lesions may be resected.

By the time the patient seeks medical attention, local tumor extension and hematogenous metastatic spread, usually to the lung, have already occurred in most instances. At this early date, tumor microemboli are not demonstrable, but must be considered in the treatment protocol.

The first consideration is to establish the diagnosis which can only be ascertained by biopsy. Since the trauma of securing a specimen may appear to provoke further metastases, the biopsy, a frozen section, and the ablative surgery carried out at the same time seem logical. Such a precaution has not been shown to be of any advantage. Moreover, performing the amputation between two tourniquets so as to preclude hematogenous spread has never been proved to change the clinical course. To obtain the most representative area for immediate pathologic diagnosis, the tissue specimen should be removed from the softer peripheral portion of the tumor. This is the most recently formed tumor whose malignant characteristics are not yet concealed by the formation of osteoid and new bone.

The second consideration is to determine the level of amputation. Theoretically extensive resection including the entire affected bone would appear to offer the greatest chance for eliminating the disease. However, the 5-year survival rate is not affected, regardless of the level of amputation.[134,139]

A third consideration is the timing of the surgical procedures in relation to adjuvant therapy. It has been stated that, "There is no significant difference in the outlook whether amputation is the primary treatment, or whether it is delayed and carried out selectively after irradiation."[105] This philosophy of a waiting period to determine those who might benefit from ablative therapy as opposed to those who would be subjected to unnecessary surgery is practiced chiefly in England.[161] On the other hand, with the newer regimens incorporating a chemotherapeutic attack, aggressive surgery to remove the primary tumor at the earliest moment is mandatory. Moreover, when such treatment fails and with the approach of the terminal state, amputation mercifully prevents the severe morbidity of pain, pathologic fracture, and fungation.

Level of Amputation. In every case, the foregoing facts must be considered in determining the level of amputation. For a tumor at the upper end of the tibia, an amputation through the thigh is carried out. For a tumor at the distal end of the femur, the site of amputation remains controversial. In spite of the fact that the eventual outcome is the same, disarticulation of the hip has been recommended to prevent the morbidity of recurrence which is seen in approximately 15% of cases.[160] However, with current regimens which include chemotherapy and megavoltage irradiation, recurrence is less common, the 5-year survival rate has dramatically improved, and providing a functional stump is a distinct advantage. The more radical ablative surgery is indicated only for tumors at the midshaft when a stump of less than 10 cm is useless for prosthetic fitting. Amputation through the femur is done about 7 cm above the most proximal area of increased uptake seen on the bone scan.

For a tumor at the upper end of the femur or of the innominate bone, hindquarter amputation is required. Such mutilating procedures perhaps are best delayed until local growth control has been accomplished by radiotherapy and adjuvant chemotherapy alone, and then only in the rare patient who has remained free of pulmonary metastases for at least 6 months.[161]

For a tumor at the upper end of the humerus, a forequarter amputation is indicated.

Following amputation, chemotherapy, when administered prematurely, slows healing of the soft tissues within the stump, and the bone may protrude. This should not be confused with bone overgrowth frequently seen after amputation in childhood. The complication may be averted by using nonabsorbable sutures, and by awaiting healing of the wound before instituting chemotherapy, usually about 2 weeks postoperatively.

Pulmonary Resection. At the time of the initial diagnosis and removal of the primary tumor, pulmonary microemboli are already present in most cases.[140,154] The opacities of solitary or multiple metastatic lung tumors generally do not become radiologically apparent for several months to a year and even longer when the patient is being treated with chemotherapeutic agents. The rationale for chemotherapy assumes that tumor microemboli are present, and such treatment is initiated very shortly after ablation of the primary tumor.

When large tumor masses develop in the lung, these can be removed by lobectomy or wedge resection. Large lesions often undergo regression under the influence of chemotherapy, and they become amenable to surgical removal.

The lung tumor is asymptomatic. After ablation of the primary tumor, monthly stereoscopic views of the chest and whole-lung tomograms are taken every 3 months. At the earliest appearance of metastasis, pulmonary resection should be done.

Contraindications to pulmonary resection include widespread metastatic disease beyond the lung, extensive pulmonary involvement (three or more foci), and inability of the patient to tolerate such surgery.

Megavoltage Radiotherapy

Osteosarcomas have previously been regarded as "radiation resistant." However, with megavoltage radiotherapy it is now possible to cause destruction of tumor cells with minimal effect on uninvolved parts. High-dose irradiation has become an integral part of current treatment regimens which incorporate surgical ablation and chemotherapy.[133,162] Although irradiation appears to be a useful adjunct in the treatment of primary tumors of the long bones, its efficacy for nonresectable tumors (*e.g.*, of the vertebrae) is questionable.

With megavoltage, high doses are administered in short sessions with minimal tissue damage and no constitutional disturbance. A high tumor dose of 6000 to 7000 rads, and in some cases as high as 8000 rads, is given to the tumor and the whole bone preferably at a rate of approximately 230 rads/day or 1000 rads weekly.

Advocates of irradiation in the immediate preoperative period, when amputation of the primary tumor is to be done early, give about 1000 rads in the hope that this will reduce the viability of cells that may be disseminated into the bloodstream by the surgical trauma. This practice has not changed the outcome.[139] Moreover, after a full course of radiation, areas of active tumor tissue remain.[96]

The proponents of giving a full course of irradiation and delaying amputation for several months state that, "This permits a safe waiting period to determine whether metastases will or will not become evident, thus sparing unnecessary dismemberment in some patients."

When high-dose irradiation is given to the primary tumor, the clinical response is noted within 2 or 3 weeks after initiating treatment. Sometimes there is apparent worsening: sudden increase in pain and size of the tumor. More often there is gradual reduction of pain and swelling, starting after some 2000 rads and continuing for several weeks after the completion of treatment. Radiographically, a favorable response is indicated by a reduction in the size and an increase in the density of the tumor, and reossification in the subperiosteal area.

Preliminary Studies. Tomography and a bone scan give an indication of the extent of the main tumor mass within the bone. "Skip" metastases may be detected. Xerography may delineate the extent of soft tissue infiltration.

Precautions. When diagnostic biopsy is done prior to a full course of irradiation as the exclusive treatment, or to be followed by ablation at a later date, the biopsy scar should be held to less than 2 cm. Larger incisional scars invite radiation necrosis and skin breakdown followed by intractable infection and hemorrhage. Needle biopsy is preferred.

Chemotherapy increases the susceptibility of tissues to irradiation. Therefore, such regimens require lower irradiation dosages. Proper megavoltage techniques reduce the incidence of the fibrotic, atrophic and painful limb.

Principles. Radical dose levels of 7000 rads to 8000 rads are preferable.[157] Distribute the dose in accordance with the probable distribution of tumor cells. Exclude all normal tissue and protect the biopsy scar. Although with proper treatment a painless and nonedematous limb is attained, the treated limb will be vulnerable to injury and should be protected. pathologic fracture can occur. The part should be protected with a light shield and extremes of heat and cold avoided.

Chemotherapy

Formerly osteosarcoma was regarded as refractory to chemotherapy. Dramatic changes in the outlook for this disease were brought about by demonstrations that high-dose methotrexate (HDMTX) with CFR[126] and Adriamycin,[108] and combinations using both these agents,[148] would cause regression of radiologically evident metastatic disease in a high proportion of cases. By using combinations of chemotherapeutic agents in cyclic courses, and appropriate dosages and schedule sequences of the agents in each cycle, the toxic effects of these potent drugs are held to a minimum. Moreover, the addition of an alkylating agent such as cyclophosphamide with a known efficacy of only 15% makes it possible to markedly increase the interval between the administration of an individual drug and the time that it is repeated in the next cycle, thereby reducing its toxicity and maintaining its effectiveness before refractoriness to the drug develops. The application of this chemotherapeutic approach to the regimen of treatment for the primary tumor makes it possible to secure a disease-free state for many months after ablation of the primary tumor in a large percentage of cases. When treatment is instituted before metastatic disease is apparent, more than 60% of 5-year survivals can be secured. Moreover, at this early ongoing period of investigation, freedom from disease appears to persist in many cases after chemotherapy has been discontinued. To achieve such results, an essential part of the regimen is early diagnosis and radical ablation of the primary tumor. Chemotherapeutic agents are most effective when the body burden of tumor cells is lowest.

Chemotherapy should be administered only by those proficient in use of the agents and only in centers where the effects can be closely monitored.

The orthopaedic surgeon should familiarize himself with the principles of chemotherapy, particularly as they apply to surgical decisions. As an introduction to this subject, the characteristics and use of Adriamycin and methotrexate, the most effective drugs against osteosarcoma, are described. Continuing research will no doubt modify their use to reduce their toxicity and increase their efficacy, and other chemotherapeutic agents will become available.

Types of Chemotherapeutic Agents. Chemotherapeutic agents[107] are compounds which are cytotoxic and produce their destructive effects on cells undergoing processes concerned with mitosis and reproduction. The agents which have been most effective in osteosarcoma are classified as follows:

Alkylating agents: cyclophosphamide, phenylalanine mustard
Antimetabolites: 5-fluorouracil, methotrexate
Antibiotics: mitomycin C, actinomycin D, Adriamycin

Adriamycin (Doxorubicin).[108] Adriamycin is a glycoside antibiotic derived from *Streptomyces peuceticus var. caesius.* It is an analogue of an earlier clinical compound Daunorubicin. Its probable antineoplastic action at the cellular level is by drug-binding to DNA, thereby inhibiting RNA synthesis. It is rapidly cleared from the plasma and is bound for prolonged periods in the liver, spleen, kidney, lung, and heart. It is metabolized mainly by the liver. Therefore, patients with hepatic dysfunction show prolonged plasma levels. Impaired liver function is an indication for reduced dosage.

Toxic effects are dose-related and reversible: leukemia, transient capital alopecia, nausea and vomiting, stomatitis, and cardiac effects. Transient electrocardiogram (ECG) changes may appear within the first few days after administration, but cause no morbidity, and revert to normal as the drug is withheld. A more serious and potentially lethal myocardiopathy may occur in a small percentage of cases when the cumulative dose exceeds 500 mg/m.[2] It is manifest as a rapidly progressing syndrome of congestive heart failure which may be fatal unless immediately recognized and reversed by conventional medical treatment.

Thrombocytopenia, anemia, and hemorrhages may require platelet or whole blood transfusion. Local tissue necrosis is due to extravasation during intravenous administration.

Dosage and Schedule. Treatment is started when wound healing is complete. The dose is 30 mg/m^2 of body-surface daily for 3 successive days repeated every 4 to 6 weeks for 6 courses.[108] The first course is usually given in the hospital, and subsequent treatments are administered on an ambulatory basis. The drug is most effective when the leukocyte count is below 3000, but a count below 1000 requires lowering the dosage to 20 mg/m^2 day for 3 days.

Hematological, biochemical, and electrocardiographic examinations, stereo chest x-ray and tomogram, and bone survey are conducted before, during, and after treatment to check for tumor recurrence and drug toxicity.[112,113]

Methotrexate (Amethopterin).[112,113] This compound is a folic acid antagonist whose efficacy depends on achieving adequate intracellular concentrations. Its antineoplastic effect is due to the methotrexate tightly binding to an enzyme, dihydrofolate reductase, resulting in cessation of thymidylate synthesis, and ultimately disruption of DNA synthesis.[101] The intracellular accumulation of methotrexate depends on the plasma level and is not time dependent. Its transport or diffusion across the cell membrane is facilitated by vincristine which must be given shortly before administration of the chemotherapeutic agent.[158] The need for a continuous high blood level is not necessary once saturation of the cell occurs and all available enzyme is bound. The cell succumbs when entering a sensitive stage (DNA synthesis). This explains the continuing regression of tumor cells well beyond the disappearance of methotrexate from the plasma. Provided that the drug is administered over a short period of time, many bone marrow cells are invulnerable to methotrexate.[103] Citrovorum factor is given immediately after each dose of methotrexate. This bypasses the block in folate reduction and encourages the recovery of rapidly proliferating normal cells, thereby reducing or eliminating the cytotoxic effects on normal tissues. When the duration of exposure of methotrexate is lengthy (*i.e.*, 24 to 48 hours) serious hematological and gastrointestinal toxic effects are probable.

Toxic effects[121] are directly related to the duration of exposure to the drug rather than to the dose itself. Hematopoietic depression and severe oral mucositis are common and require prolonged cardiac failure (CF) therapy. Superinfection with *Candida albicans* requires nystatin or amphotericin B. Other common toxic effects are nausea and vomiting, transient elevation of bilirubin and serum glutamic-oxaloacetic transaminase (SGOT), transient ECG changes, increased sensitivity to irradiation which requires reduction of dose, and hyperuricemia.

Dose and Schedule. Vincristine, 2 mg/m^2 is given IV half an hour before each methotrexate infusion on the basis that it might promote methotrexate uptake by tumor cells. Methotrexate is given by IV infusion over a 6-hour period; the initial dose is 1500 mg/m^2. Treatment is given at 2-week intervals, the dose being gradually increased to a maximum of 7500 mg/m^2 of body-surface area. Thereafter, treatment is given at 3-week intervals and continued for 2 years. Citrovorum factor is started 2 hours after each methotrexate infusion is completed, and is given either orally or IV at 9 to 15 mg/m^2 every 6 hours × 12. Toxicity requires an upward adjustment of dosage and longer administration. Citrovorum factor is a reduced folate that bypasses the methotrexate-enzyme block and allows for the use of large doses of methotrexate. Throughout this treatment, a continuous infusion of 5% dextrose in water insures adequate hydration, and the urine is kept alkalinized.

Multiple Drug, Multicycle Chemotherapy.[146] This involves the use of multiple drugs given in a definite sequence constituting a single cycle of treatment. The cycle is repeated at specified intervals. In its simplest form, high-dose methotrexate (HDMTX) followed by CFR and Adriamycin, the two most effective agents, form the constituent agents of each cycle. The rationale is to use multiple drugs in order to provide continuous treatment, each cycle consuming a specific period of time (2 to 5 weeks depending on the number and types of agents used), and recycled over an extended period of time without the development of cumulative toxicity or tumor resistance which might be anticipated if any single agent were administered alone at intervals frequent enough to suppress tumor growth.

The application of this regimen is initiated immediately after diagnosis and primary treatment of "nonmetastatic" osteosarcoma.

Multiple Drug Protocol. Vincristine 1.5 mg/m^2 on day 1, high-dose methotrexate 200 mg to 300 mg/kg IV on day 2, with CFR 9 mg every 6 hours × 12, followed by cyclophosphamide 40 mg/kg IV; then 2 weeks later Adriamycin 15 mg/kg day × 2; in 2 weeks cyclophosphamide is repeated. After a 2-week rest, the 56-day cycle is repeated. Treatment is continued for a period of 1 year. The most frequent severe gastrointestinal manifestation of toxicity is oropharyngeal mucositis. Hematologic depression is mild to severe.

The efficacy of this program in osteosarcoma with metastatic disease has encouraged its use as a primary treatment after ablation of the primary tumor and has resulted in a dramatic increase in the 5-year survival rate and the disease-free state.

Treatment should await complete healing of the operative wound. Preliminary studies conducted to determine the extent of the disease should include stereo chest roentgenograms or full chest tomography, skeletal survey, bone scan with ^{18}F or ^{99}Tc-diphosphonate, complete biochemical profile, intravenous pyelogram (IVP) and creatinine clearance to determine adequacy of renal function. Follow-up studies include biweekly or monthly roentgenograms of the chest, a survey of bones known to have metastases, and a complete bone survey every 3 to 6 months.

SECONDARY OSTEOSARCOMA

Osteosarcoma frequently develops in patients whose skeletal system is affected by benign tumors or general skeletal disease. As such it is termed "secondary osteosarcoma." When pain develops or increases in an osseous site occupied by a benign and relatively asymptomatic process, whether neoplastic or not, the orthopaedic surgeon should be alerted to the possibility of malignant transformation. Immediate investigation is mandatory, particularly by roentgenograms, tomograms, bone scans, and, if necessary, by biopsy. Secondary osteosarcoma generally is highly malignant, even more so than primary osteogenic sarcoma.

PAGET'S SARCOMA

Secondary osteosarcoma most often arises from malignant transformation in Paget's disease. In controlled population studies, the probabilities of development of osteosarcoma in Paget's disease are less than 1%.[110,142] Since the great majority of cases of Paget's disease are symptomless and go unrecognized, this may account for the reported high estimates of malignant degeneration.[102,132] The incidence of this complication increases with advancing age, and the risk of its development is greater at the site of a pathologic fracture.[141] This malignant tumor is almost invariably fatal within a mean survival time of 3 years, although rare cases of "cure" have been reported.[149]

Paget's sarcoma is most often found in the femur, humerus, pelvis, skull and tibia, in that order of frequency. It may be multicentric, although it is difficult to distinguish bone metastases from the primary tumor.

Clinical Picture

Severe pain developing at a previously asymptomatic site is the chief complaint. When the pain radiates distally, involvement of the peripheral nerves is the cause. A tumor mass is palpable in every instance. Occasionally, associated findings include dilated veins surmounting the tumor and swelling of the extremity. The tumor may develop weeks or months later at the site of a previous pathologic fracture through bone affected by Paget's disease. Failure of the fracture to unite or the development of pain and swelling at the region of the old fracture should be regarded with alarm.

Roentgenographic Findings

The only single valuable finding is destructive change in the cortex. However, in such a disease characterized by mixed areas of increased density and absorption, interpretation is difficult and unreliable. Metastatic lesions of the chest and other bones may be detected.

Pathology

The tumor is predominantly osteoblastic or fibroblastic. The extremely hypercellular stroma shows highly malignant characteristics such as many hyperchromatic nuclei, marked pleomorphism, numerous mitoses, and plump spindle cells. Benign multinucleated giant cells of the osteoclast type are frequently seen.

Prognosis and Treatment

The tumor is extremely malignant and rapidly fatal. Treatment consists of ablation and amputation as palliative measures. When resection is not feasible, irradiation may be considered. The effect of chemotherapy has not been established.

RADIATION-INDUCED OSTEOSARCOMA

Osteosarcoma as well as a whole spectrum of neoplastic growths can be induced in bone by irradiation.[98] This radiation can be in the form of internal radiation (*e.g.*, radium) or external radiation, either orthovoltage or megavoltage. Radiation-induced cases of osteosarcoma which have been described are uncommon, are directly traceable to radiation therapy, and a long latent period (induction time) from a few to many years is typical.

Very often benign osseous growths preexist. In many instances, osseous, soft part, and visceral neoplasms were treated by a radiation beam which passes through the eventually involved bone. The most common antecedent benign bone growth is a benign giant-cell tumor.

The relationship to the dosage and its concentration is not clear, but most cases in man have been treated by dosages exceeding 3000 rads. In animal experiments, induction of bone tumors by radiation is less likely when the radiation is given in divided doses over a period of time.

The type of osteosarcoma produced by radiation is a highly osteogenic, sclerosing tumor characterized by profuse osteoid and new bone formation. Extraskeletal postirradiation osteosarcomas can also develop.[95,97]

Within the bone immediately adjacent to the tumor, typical radiation-induced osseous changes are seen: coarse trabeculae, areas of rarefaction, necrotic and disintegrated trabeculae and marrow necrosis and fibrosis.

Treatment consists of ablation. Additional radiotherapy is indicated for recurrence for reduction in size and pain. Chemotherapy has not been properly evaluated, since this tumor is uncommon.

The 5-year survival rate is approximately 30%.

The described sequence of events is initiated by a specific genetic alteration (somatic mutation).[106] The effect is produced by the direct action of radiation on the genetic apparatus, or indirectly by primary damage to extragenetic sites or activation of a latent virus.

FIBROUS DYSPLASIA

Malignant transformation to osteosarcoma, fibrosarcoma, giant-cell sarcoma, or chondrosarcoma can take place within a lesion of fibrous dysplasia.[123,150] The age peak of incidence is similar to that of primary osteosarcoma (15 years), although neoplastic change can occur at any time. When the sarcoma coexists with, but develops separately from, fibrous dysplasia, the average age is generally higher (35 years).

OSTEOSARCOMA OF SOFT TISSUES[114]

Development of osteosarcoma outside of the skeleton is rare. When they occur in the soft tissues, they are highly malignant, invariably metastasize to the lungs, possess histologic characteristics similar to osteosarcoma of bone, and must be clearly differentiated mainly from myositis ossificans and parosteal osteoma, lesions with much less malignity. It affects an older age group, usually more than 30 years old. Its location corresponds to that of osteosarcoma of bone; the extremities, especially the lower extremities, are favored sites. Some of these rare tumors described in the literature appear to have originated from benign growths that probably were myositis ossificans.

OSTEOID OSTEOMA

Jaffe was the first to give an accurate description and establish this tumor as a definite entity.[169] However, it was Bergstrand in 1930 who published the first description of the pathology.[167] Defined, it is a small rarefying lesion in enchondral bones, composed of vascular fibrous tissue, proliferating fibroblasts, and minute spicules of newly formed osteoid.

CLINICAL PICTURE

Young adults, especially males, from 10 to 25 years of age, are predisposed, although the condition occurs from 5 to 35 years. It has a predilection for the long bones, particularly the tibia and the femur. The small bones of the hands and the feet may be involved. It is a solitary lesion which causes pain, mild at first, then becoming progressively more severe, continuous, agonizing, and worse at night. The person may limp. Gradually, a localized swelling which is palpable as a bony enlargement fusiform in shape becomes manifest. It is tender, sometimes exquisitely so. When the lesion occurs in the spine, acute localized back pain, muscle spasm, secondary scoliosis, and pelvic tilt form the clinical picture. Systemic symptoms are absent. The temperature is normal and blood counts are negative. The overlying skin is not reddened or warm.

ROENTGENOGRAPHIC FINDINGS

A solitary small rarefied lesion, usually less than 2 cm in diameter, is found in the cortex, the subcortical region, or the subperiosteal area, surrounded by thickened and sclerotic bone. The surrounding reactive bone may attain large proportions and is fusiform in shape. It may even obscure the nidus. Occasionally, a small dense center of ossification may be seen in the nidus. When sciatica is the presenting complaint, the femur should be x-rayed routinely. An incidence of as high as 5% of osteoid osteoma lesions may be found.

When the clinical picture is suggestive of an osteoid osteoma, but ordinary roentgenograms do not reflect typical bone structural changes (*e.g.*, at a subperiosteal site) radionuclide imaging is useful as a screening procedure that will point to the site of a reactive bone lesion.[168,172] Then high-resolution axial tomography will define the area of sclerotic bone and its central nidus. This method is especially valuable for identifying and accurately localizing a lesion within the spine or about juxta-articular bone structures.[171]

PATHOLOGY

A vascular mesenchymal type of connective tissue stroma with proliferating fibroblasts and osteoblasts surrounds abundant pink-staining osteoid tissue. The osteoid forms an irregular branching network.[2,170] At the center of the lesion, a minute amount of poorly formed osseous tissue sometimes is found, but this may be entirely lacking. Surrounding this tissue is marked bony proliferation which is more marked when the lesion is intracortical. The marrow is somewhat fibrous. No leukocytes can be found, suggesting the noninflammatory nature of the lesion. Cartilage is never found (Color Plate 15-7).

DIFFERENTIAL DIAGNOSIS

Osteoid osteoma should be differentiated from sclerosing nonsuppurative osteomyelitis of Garré, benign bone cyst, Brodie's abscess, chronic osteomyelitis with annular sequestrum, syphilitic ossifying periostitis, and eosinophilic granuloma.

TREATMENT

Complete excision of the nidus immediately and effectively relieves the pain. It is not necessary to remove the surrounding sclerotic bone because this recedes after removal of the center.

BENIGN OSTEOBLASTOMA

A benign osteoblastoma[175–177] (osteogenic fibroma of bone[174], giant osteoid osteoma[173]) is an uncommon vascular osteoid and bone-forming tumor. It is slow growing and causes symptoms by encroachment on neighboring structures.

CLINICAL PICTURE

Age and Sex. Young adults, usually less than 20 years of age; males are predisposed in a ratio of 2:1.

Location. The majority occur in the spine affecting the posterior elements, the metaphyseal or diaphyseal areas of the long bones of the lower extremities, and the small bones of the hands and feet.

Symptoms. Dull, aching pain, not nocturnal or relieved by aspirin (contrary to osteoid osteoma). When a cervical or thoracic vertebra is affected, and the tumor encroaches on the spinal cord, weakness and paresthesias develop in the lower limbs. Involvement of a lumbar vertebra causes pains and paresthesias in the lower extremities. Symptoms occur generally from a few months to 2 years before the tumor is discovered.

Findings. A single tender mass is palpable when the tumor is superficial. Neurologic deficit is due to intraspinal compression. Scoliosis develops in many when the tumor arises in the thoracic or lumbar spine or the ribs.

PATHOLOGY

Gross Appearance

The mass is deep red, friable, and gritty. It is richly vascular. The size varies from a pea-sized nodule removed from an intraspinal location to a large mass when situated superficially.

Microscopic Appearance

The tissue is loosely fibrillar and highly vascular, containing numerous dilated thin-walled vascular channels. Within the vascular tissue a profusion of osteoblasts lies between sheets of osteoid and primitive bone trabeculae. The degree of mineralization of osteoid varies. In the more advanced stage, the primitive osseous tissue undergoes osteoclastic resorption and replacement by mature lamellar bone (Color Plate 15-8 and Fig. 15-30).

Giant cells are prominent, represent osteoclasts and macrophages, and are unlike those in giant-cell tumors.

The stromal cells are compact, round, ovoid, or spindly but are distinct, relatively uniform, and mitotic figures are rare.

ROENTGENOGRAPHIC FINDINGS

The tumor presents a variable picture depending on the size, location, and degree of ossificaton.

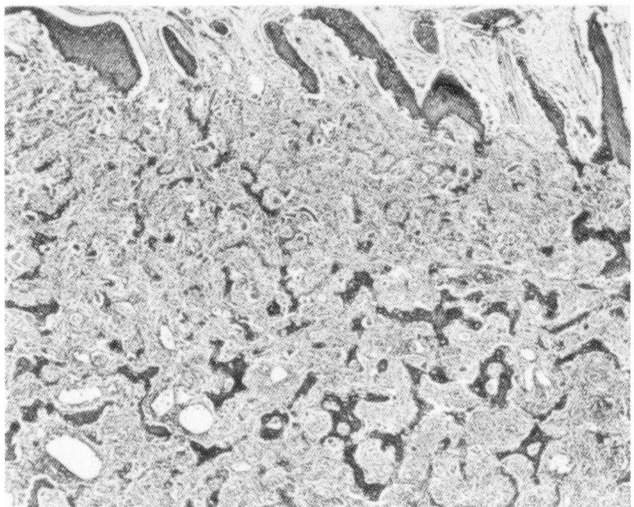

FIG. 15-30. Microscopic appearance of benign osteoblastoma. Shown is extensive formation of sheets of osteoid and primitive osseous tissue between which is loose fibrillar tissue. (Dahlin DC, Johnson EW: J Bone Joint Surg 36A:559, 1954)

A vague mass may develop within the medulla, is essentially radiolucent or mottled, well circumscribed, and as it enlarges, the cortex is gradually attenuated, but the tumor is delimited by a delicate shell of periosteal new bone. Within the main bone of origin, the tumor is surrounded by a thin rim of reactive bone. The extensive dense bone reaction, which characteristically surrounds an osteoid osteoma, is never seen. Within the tumor, faint stippled densities are noted.

When the tumor develops in the posterior element of a vertebra, the affected spinous process, lamina, pedicle, or transverse process appears markedly enlarged, but the true extent is difficult to ascertain. Tomography may be helpful (Figs. 15-31–15-33).

Long-standing tumors become extremely dense, especially after radiation treatment.

FIG. 15-31. Benign osteoblastoma. The tumor has produced expansion of the right transverse process of C7. (Dahlin DC: Bone Tumors. Springfield, Ill, Charles C Thomas, 1957)

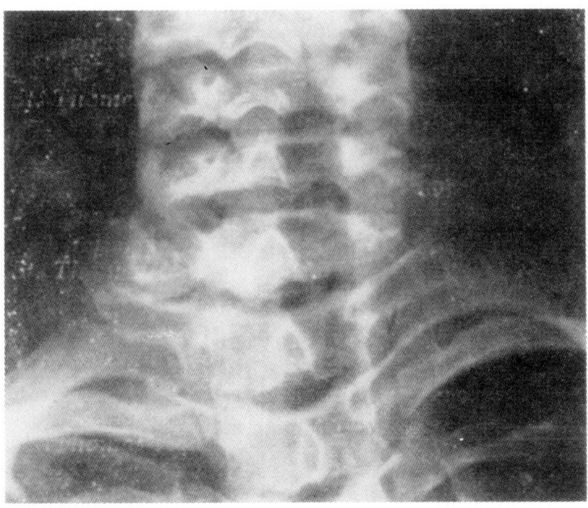

FIG. 15-32. Benign osteoblastoma. Characteristic involvement of posterior vertebral arch. (*A*) The right pedicle of L2 appears to be slightly enlarged, and the margin of the L2 vertebral body is indistinct. (*B*) At a later stage expanding combined osteolytic and ossifying mass involves the right portion of the posterior arch including lamina, pedicle, and transverse process and also the right half of the body of L2. A soft tissue mass extends outward toward the right, is sharply circumscribed by a calcific shell, and contains mottled opacities of new bone. In this location, in addition to back pain, encroachment on the spinal canal produces a neurologic deficit. (Pochaczevsky R et al: The roentgen appearance of benign osteoblastoma. Radiology, 75:429, 1960)

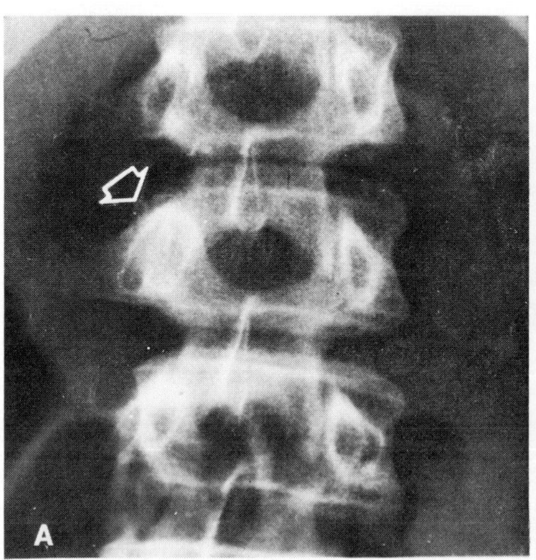

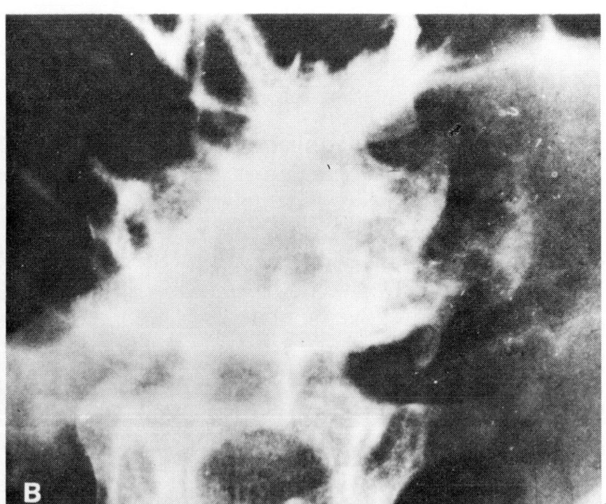

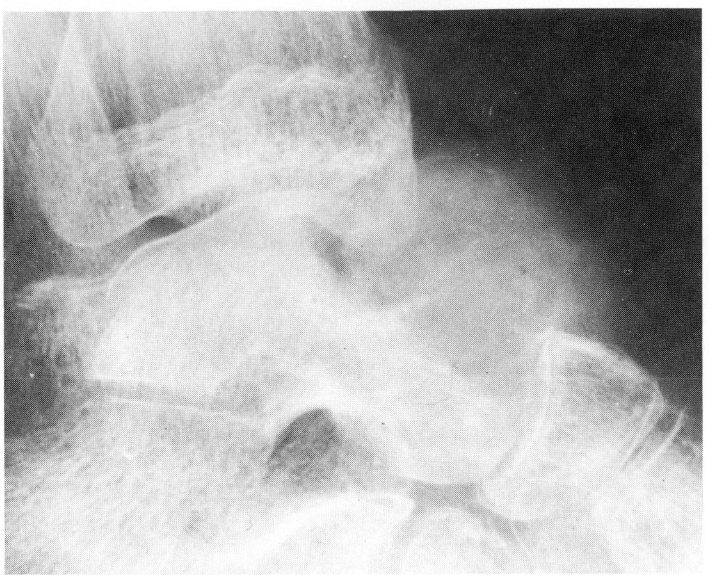

FIG. 15-33. Benign osteoblastoma. An osteolytic, expanding tumor has eroded the cortex of the talus and has extended outward. It is sharply circumscribed by a delimited thin shell of bone. Scattered minute opacities throughout the tumor represent new bone. (Pochaczevsky R et al: The roentgen appearance of benign osteoblastoma. Radiology, 75:429, 1960)

DIFFERENTIAL DIAGNOSIS

Osteoid Osteoma. The osteoblasts are less numerous, the lesion is smaller, reactive surrounding bone is extreme, a central nidus is present, and nocturnal pain relieved by aspirin is characteristic.

Osteogenic Sarcoma. In benign osteoblstoma, the stromal cells are not large but they are relatively uniform. Mitoses are rare, sarcomatous giant cells are absent, and tumor cartilage does not form.

Giant-Cell Tumor. More than half of the giant-cell tumors are located in the epiphyses about the knee or distal part of the radius. Involvement of the spine is rare, and then always in the body. The tumor lacks stippled densities and gritty consistency. A soap-bubble pattern is characteristic.

TREATMENT

Complete excision results in a cure. A resulting large defect in a weight-bearing bone should be filled with bone grafts. A neurologic deficit arising from intraspinal compression requires a decompressive laminectomy.

If inaccessible, the tumor will reossify under the influence of a moderate dose of cobalt therapy. However, radiation should be avoided if possible because it may induce more aggressive behavior.[178]

PAROSTEAL OSTEOGENIC SARCOMA

A parosteal osteogenic sarcoma (juxtacortical osteogenic sarcoma, parosteal osteoma) is a markedly osteogenic neoplasm, usually of low-grade malignant potential, which appears to develop within the periosteum and extend outward where, as it increases in size and surrounds the bone, it remains in intimate relationship to the outer surface of the periosteum. Thus it has been called a periosteal osteogenic sarcoma. Benign and malignant forms are said to occur,[182] but the currently accepted concept holds that all such tumors are malignant and differ only in degree. Moreover, although most such tumors have low grade malignant potential, these may undergo gradually increasing degrees of malignant transformation, particularly when the neoplastic growth recurs after an inadequate excision. Parosteal osteogenic sarcomas have a strong tendency to recur. About one fifth of these tumors are histologically high grade at the outset, have a serious outlook, and should be subjected to early radical surgery.[179,181,183]

This neoplasm should be clearly differentiated from an intramedullary osteogenic sarcoma which generally has a more serious outlook, occurs in a younger age group, causes considerable pain, and complaints are of relatively short duration (*i.e.*, weeks to a few months). In contrast, parosteal osteogenic sarcomas occur most often during the third and fourth decades, are painless, swelling is the major complaint that develops over many months or years, and the outlook is more favorable.[187,184]

PREDISPOSING FACTORS

Age. 14 to 40 years of age

Sex. No predilection for either sex

Location. Metaphyseal region of a long tubular bone; favors posterior aspect of distal end of femur; proximal end of humerus is next most favored site

PATHOLOGY

Gross Appearance

A lobulated, hard, encapsulated mass is firmly attached by a narrow or broad base to the underlying cortex. Nearly all of the tumor is located outside of and closely adjacent to the parent bone, being separated from the latter by the periosteum except at one point where it merges with the cortex. In approximately one half of the tumors, the neoplastic tissue infiltrates the cortex and penetrates a short distance into the spongiosa. The cortex at this point may appear to be eroded or sclerotic.[180] In many cases, the tumor mass comes to encircle the bone (Figs. 15-34 and 15-35).

The cut surface is gray or white. Areas of fibrous tissue are admixed with spicules of bone and rare foci of cartilage. The base of the tumor is more densely ossified than the periphery where the spicules of bone are widely separated by fibrous tissue.

Microscopic Appearance

The tumor is composed of cellular fibrous tissue, mature, organized bone lamellae, newly formed islands of immature, woven bone, and occasional foci of cartilage, all in various stages of dedifferentiation. The level of anaplasia may vary from slight to extreme, but within the individual tumor all components essentially have the same level of malignant characteristics.

Grading of Tumor

Multiple specimens, best obtained from the peripheral actively growing portion of the tumor, are examined and the malignant histologic features of each of the fibrous, osseous, and cartilaginous components (*i.e.*, hypercellularity, pleomorphism, hyperchromatism, woven bone formation, and mitoses) are noted.[180] The highest degree of such changes, perhaps found only in a single specimen, determines the malignant potential: low degree = grade I; medium degree = grade II; high degree = grade III (Fig. 15-36).

CLINICAL PICTURE

The duration of symptoms is generally one to several years. The chief complaint is a localized painless swelling and sometimes mechanical interference with the motion of the neighboring joint. On examination, a circumscribed, bony-hard swelling is found, and is fixed to the underlying bone. Little or no tenderness is perceived. The overlying skin appears normal. In contrast, intramedullary osteogenic sarcoma causes pronounced local pain, duration of symptoms is a matter of weeks or a few months, and the overlying skin often displays redness and engorged veins.

ROENTGENOGRAPHIC FINDINGS

In most cases, a bulky, lobulated, oval or spherical, dense shadow is situated at the metaphyseal region of a long

FIG. 15-34. Grade-I lesion of parosteal osteogenic sarcoma. (*Left*) Roentgenogram shows an irregular ossified mass with prominent lucency indicating a large amount of fibrous and cartilaginous tissue. The subjacent cortex is sclerotic. (*Center*) Typical external appearance. This is the most common location of the tumor on the posterior aspect of the distal end of the femur at the popliteal area. (*Right*) Sagittal section shows that this tumor merges imperceptibly with the cortex along its entire base. The underlying cortical bone is thickened. (Ahuja SC et al: Juxtacortical (parosteal) osteogenic sarcoma. J Bone Joint Surg 59A:632, 1977)

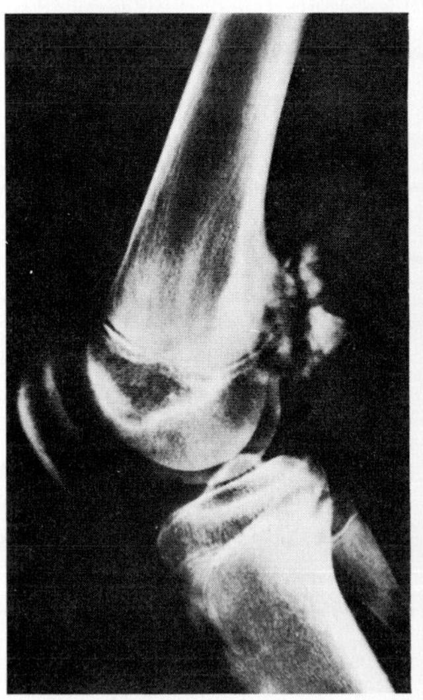

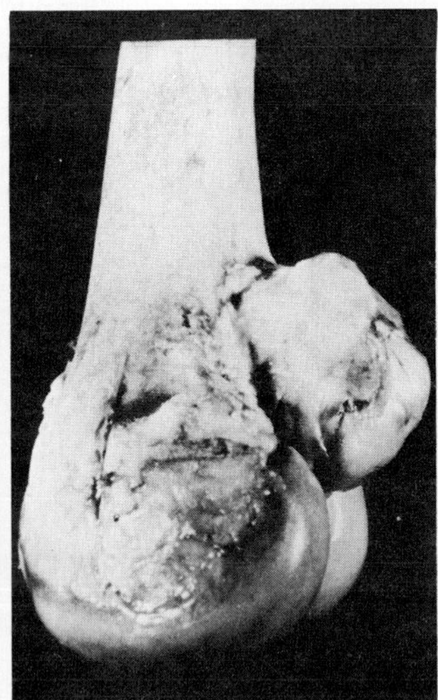

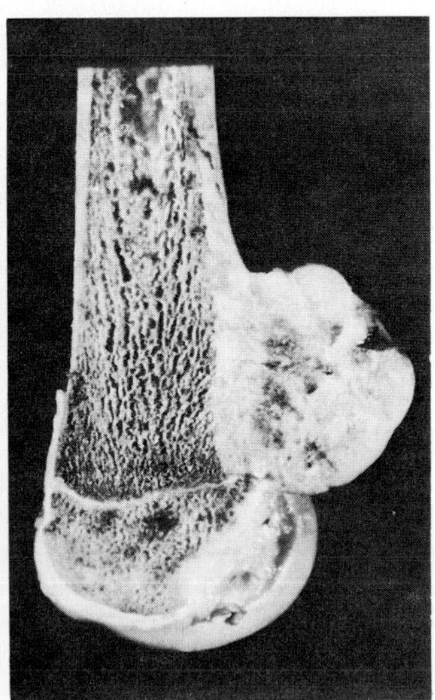

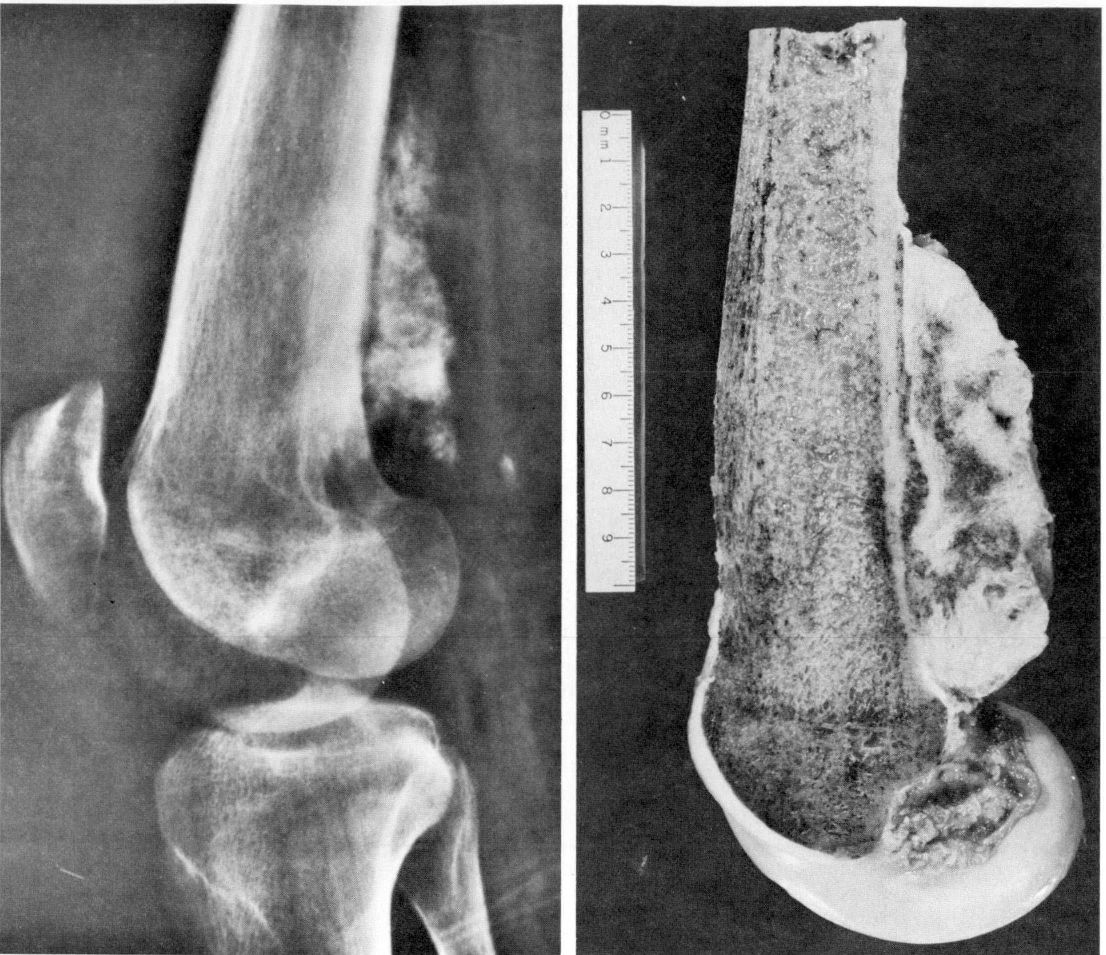

FIG. 15-35. Grade-II lesion of parosteal osteogenic sarcoma. (*Left*) Roentgenogram shows a nonhomogeneous tumor with the highly diagnostic broad linear lucency between the osseous neoplasm and the underlying cortex. Note the spiculated margin. (*Right*) Sagittal section of the gross specimen shows that the tumor is merged only focally to the underlying cortex distally. Elsewhere the tumor is separated from the cortex by a thickened band of periosteal fibrous tissue. (Ahuja SC et al: Juxtacortical (parosteal) osteogenic sarcoma. J Bone Joint Surg 59A:632, 1977)

bone (Figs. 15-34*A* and 15-35*A*)[185]. Its greatest density is at the base of the tumor, where it is continuous with the cortex. At this site, the cortex and adjacent spongiosa may appear eroded or sclerosed, suggesting invasion by the tumor. Elsewhere, the dense tumor opacity is separated from the underlying cortex by a highly diagnostic longitudinally disposed radiolucent line, usually 2 mm or 3 mm in width, which probably represents interposed periosteum.

In the more peripheral parts of the tumor, the degree of ossification varies so that dense linear streaks extend outward. The tumor density characteristically and progressively encircles the shaft.

When the tumor recurs, scattered radiopacities appear to develop outside the main tumor mass. These areas, if not removed with the main mass of bone, may give rise to another recurrence.

PROGNOSIS

For all parosteal osteogenic sarcomas as a group[186], disregarding their malignant grade, simple excision results in at least an 80% rate of recurrence,[187] and *en bloc* excision lowers this to approximately 50%. When such treatment is directed against an established low-grade tumor, the recurrence rate is markedly reduced. Although the probability of recurrence is directly related to the level of malignant histologic features, benign-appearing tumors may metastasize, although rarely, even after

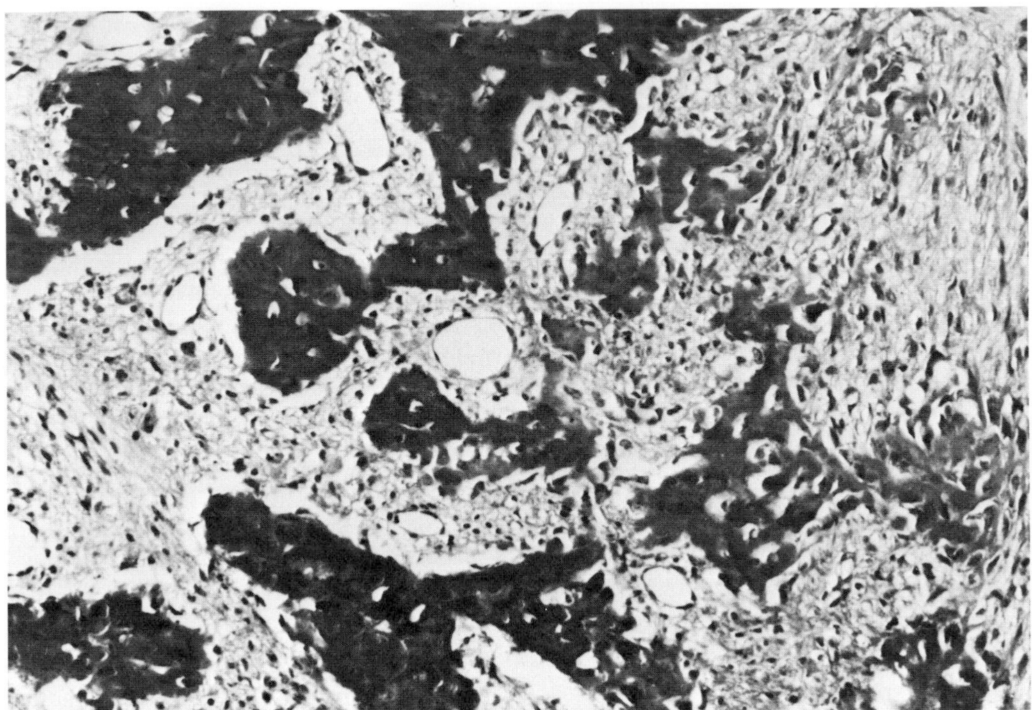

FIG. 15-36. Histologic features of parosteal osteogenic sarcoma, showing Grade-II fibrous and osseous components. An admixture of primitive woven bone and lamellar bone is present. The osteoblasts are plump and hyperchromatic. The fibrous stroma is hypercellular containing fibroblasts with plump, hyperchromatic nuclei and some mitotic figures. A more malignant tumor, Grade-III, would demonstrate a greater proportion of woven bone, marked hypercellularity with frankly sarcomatous osteoblasts and fibroblasts, and, often, an irregular lacework pattern of osteoid that is indistinguishable from that of osteosarcoma. (Ahuja SC et al: Juxtacortical (parosteal) osteogenic sarcoma. J Bone Joint Surg 59A:632, 1977)

amputation.[182] This may suggest that insufficient specimens from the supposedly benign tumor had been scrutinized. Successive recurrences occur at shorter intervals, and the recurring neoplasm is usually more aggressive.[184] Invasion of the regional bone does not necessarily affect the outlook adversely; however, such tumors are often high grade, and amputation is necessary.

Low grade (grade I) and medium grade (grade II) tumors are amenable to *en bloc* resection provided the entire tumor can be removed with a good margin of uninvolved soft tissue and underlying bone. Grade III tumors, on the other hand, have a poor prognosis despite early amputation or disarticulation.[180] When a grade I tumor metastasizes, the pulmonary lesion can often be resected with a good chance for prolonged survival. A tumor with a predominantly fibrosarcomatous component generally has a more favorable outlook.[186]

TREATMENT

The malignant grade of the tumor is the main factor that determines the appropriate treatment.[182]

Excision. *En bloc* excision removes the tumor with a portion of uninvolved soft tissue and bone including the spongiosa. The extent of bone removal can be determined by tomography, xeroradiography, and bone scan. This procedure is permissible only for tumors that are not too large, have low-grade histologic features, are clearly separated from the cortex, and complete removal is technically feasible. If invasion of the shaft is suspected or demonstrated, segmental resection is preferred.[187]

Segmental Resection. This treatment is limited to low-grade tumors with extensive invasion of the bone where a reasonable chance exists for preservation of function. It represents an alternative to amputation. Replacement of the resected bone may be accomplished with an allograft or a custom-made prosthesis.

Amputation or Disarticulation. This treatment is indicated for a high-grade tumor, a low-grade tumor with extensive involvement, and a recurrent tumor, especially when increasing malignant change is evident.

Roentgen Irradiation. Irradiation, including megavoltage therapy, has no effect either for the primary or recurrent tumor. Its use may induce additional malignant change.

EWING'S SARCOMA

Theoretically, two types of tumors may arise from the bone marrow. From the marrow cells themselves arises the myeloma. From the supportive marrow structure composed of reticuloendothelial tissue develops Ewing's tumor, reticulum cell sarcoma, and hemangioendothelioma. The majority of observers believe that the reticulum cell is the stem cell for Ewing's tumor (undifferentiated round cell sarcoma, endothelial myeloma) and reticulum cell sarcoma. Others favor a lymphogenous (Geschickter and Copeland) or a sympathetic tissue origin (Willis).[189–196]

Ewing's tumor is a malignant tumor typified by its occurrence in childhood, clinical findings of fever and leukocytosis, a characteristic onion-peel periosteal shadow in roentgenograms, and extreme radiosensitivity. A fatal outcome is invariable.

CLINICAL PICTURE

Age. 4 to 25 years, Caucasians almost exclusively

Area of Predilection. Long bones, although other bones may be affected

Location. The diaphysis

Symptoms. *Pain,* intermittent, recurring with greater intensity and persistency, worse at night; *tumor,* palpable, indurated, tender, and fixed to underlying bone; skin reddened, edematous, and contains dilated veins; *constitutional reaction,* including fever, leukocytosis, and anemia.

Course. There are periods of remissions with decreased size of tumor, and exacerbations with increased size of tumor, over a period of months to a few years. It metastasizes to other bones particularly the skull, the vertebrae, and the ribs. It metastasizes late to the lungs, causing chest pain and hemoptysis. Metastatic spread occurs through both the lymphatics and the bloodstream.

ROENTGENOGRAPHIC FINDINGS

At the midshaft of a long bone, the cortex first displays increased density, which extends externally as periosteal new bone forming multiple thin layers parallel with the surface of the shaft. This is called the "onion-peel" appearance and is most frequently found in association with this tumor, but occasionally this type of reactive bone formation develops in response to elevation of the periosteum by other tumors and subperiosteal infection. In addition, some of the periosteal new bone may form at right angles to the shaft. Later, a diffusely spreading area of rarefaction develops through the cortex and the medulla as bone destruction becomes apparent (Fig. 15-37).

PATHOLOGY

Gross Appearance

The tumor extends for a greater distance through the medulla than is apparent in roentgenograms. It extends through and replaces the cortex and often forms a large mass beneath the elevated periosteum. Cut section reveals a grayish white tumor which is firm and encapsulated by fibrous tissue, sending septae into the tumor and separating it into lobules. Some cystic and necrotic yellowish areas may be visible. Within the subperiosteal tumor, multiple layers of bone lie parallel with the shaft. Some new bone is also deposited around vessels, extending radially from the periosteum to the shaft. The tumor is usually quite vascular and contains hemorrhagic foci. At first, the tumor infiltrates rather than destroys the cortex, usually spreading through the haversian canals. Later, the cortex is destroyed, and the tumor spreads toward the metaphysis and the epiphysis.

Microscopic Appearance

The tumor consists of compactly arranged sheets of small polyhedral cells with ill-defined borders, meager cytoplasm, and containing nuclei which are large, uniform, prominent, round or oval, and possess scattered chromatin (Color Plates 15-9, 15-10, and 15-11). The nucleus is more than twice as large as that of a lymphocyte. The cytoplasm stains poorly acidophilic. No interstitial stroma can be identified. Many trabeculae of dead bone surrounded by masses of tumor cells almost give the appearance of osteomyelitis. No multinucleated cells are present. The tissue is very vascular. Often, especially in areas of hemorrhage, the tumor cells are clustered about a vessel, and for this reason the tumor has been thought to have an endothelial origin. However, the adventitia of the vessel can be seen interposed between the tumor cells and the endothelium.

Occasionally, a ring of tumor cells form a pseudorosette, which is similar to the rosette frequently observed in neuroblastoma. However, Ewing's tumor cells tend to accumulate about a center of necrosing tumor cells. On the other hand, the rosette of neuroblastoma is composed of an aggregate of tumor cells about a central core of filamentous neurofibrils.

The tumor cells have a pronounced tendency to degenerate if not fixed and examined soon after removal for biopsy. The nuclei usually shrink and appear pyknotic. This explains the discrepancies between Ewing's original description and that of later observers.

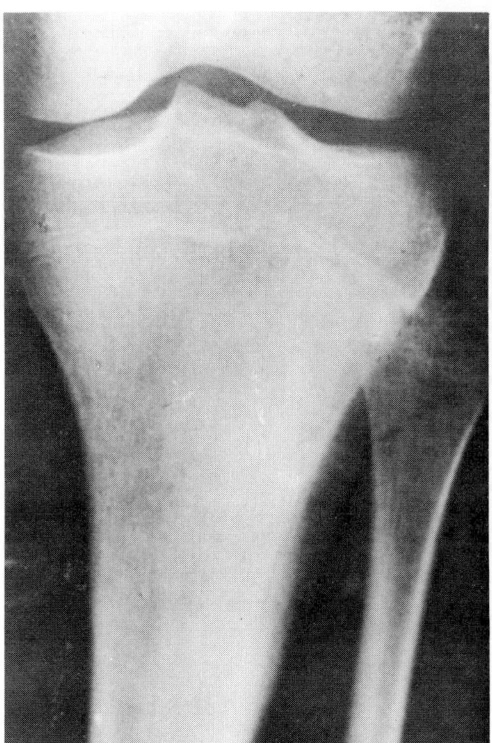
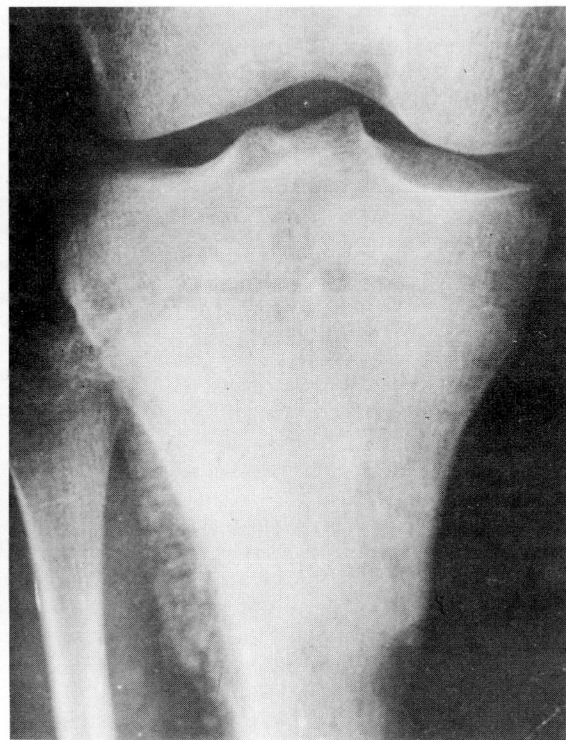

FIG. 15-37. Typical "onion-peel" appearance of Ewing's sarcoma.

The microscopic appearance bears a stong resemblance to that of a reticulum cell sarcoma, but special staining characteristics will serve to differentiate the two. This is especially important in view of a vastly better prognosis of the latter tumor.

A useful method of differentiating Ewing's tumor from reticulum cell sarcoma is by staining for glycogen positivity by PAS, and proving its presence by dissolving the glycogen by diastase. Glycogen is absent in reticulum cell sarcoma. A silver stain for reticulum fibers will demonstrate its presence in reticulum cell sarcoma and its absence in Ewing's sarcoma.

TREATMENT

The tumor is very sensitive to irradiation, melting quickly, but recurring after several months. Succeeding growths are much less responsive. Radical surgery, removing the bulk of the tumor whether by extensive local excision or ablation by amputation prior to megavoltage therapy, will greatly increase the disease-free interval. Nevertheless, the prognosis is grave. Lesions of the pelvic and axial bones tend to have a prognosis worse than that for other anatomical locations.

Currently, chemotherapy added to the treatment regimen of ablative surgery and megavoltage therapy will greatly increase the disease-free interval with apparent cures after 5 years. Intensive multi-drug, multi-course chemotherapy, using such drugs as vincristine, cyclophosphamide, and Adriamycin, has effectively prolonged survival time.[188]

FIBROSARCOMA

A fibrosarcoma of bone is a malignant neoplasm, the basic cell of which is the fibroblast in varying degrees of anaplasia. Histologically, it is identical with a fibrosarcoma which arises from soft tissue structures (*e.g.*, fascia).

CLINICAL PICTURE

Age. Over 30 years of age

Site of Predilection. Long bones, especially the femur; also in ribs, skull, vertebrae, mandible

Position. Subperiosteal area of diaphysis or metaphysis; or originates in medulla and penetrates through to subperiosteal space

Solitary Lesion

Symptoms and Findings. Gradual onset of continuous pain, worse at night; gradual appearance of swelling, which is smooth, firm, rubbery textured, firmly fixed to underlying bone; occasionally, tumor infiltrative, fixes overlying soft tissues, thereby restricting joint motion

Pathologic Fracture Occasionally

Metastases. To lungs; may metastasize to other subperiosteal spaces

ROENTGENOGRAPHIC FINDINGS

A soft tissue shadow slightly denser than muscle is revealed by soft tissue technique. The shadow is usually a single lesion, extra-osseous but immediately adjacent to the cortex of a long bone. Directly beneath the tumor shadow is a saucer-shaped cortical erosion of varying depth. At the upper and the lower corners of the periosteal shadow, slight triangles of reactive bone (Codman's triangles) may be found, particularly in slower growing tumors. Slight calcific densities are sometimes seen within the shadow. The tumor is generally large in contrast with the amount of bone destruction. If the tumor is very malignant and infiltrative, the sharp borders of the shadow are lost (Fig. 15-38).

When the tumor has penetrated the cortex, the latter is riddled with multiple small lytic areas. The medulla is then involved and shows vague areas of rarefaction.

When the tumor rarely originates within the medulla, a central irregular moth-eaten area of rarefaction appears. However, no reactive bone density is seen about it, and the cortex, although rarefied locally, is not expanded. Eventually, it forms a shadow external to the bone.

FIG. 15-38. Fibrosarcoma.

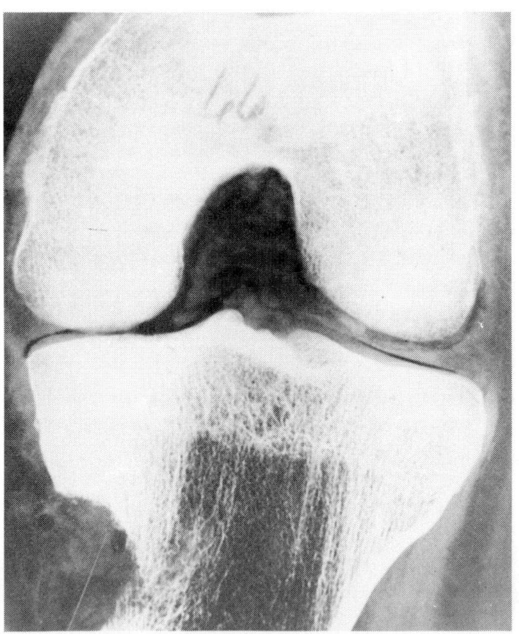

PATHOLOGY

Gross Appearance

The tumor is a well-encapsulated, firm, white, fibrous, glistening mass beneath the elevated periosteum on one side of a long bone. On cut section, strands of fibrous tissue are arranged in striations, or whorls, or are crisscrossed. The cortex may be uninvolved, and the tumor may peel away easily from the bone. If the tumor has invaded the cortex, the tumor is separated with difficulty, and the underlying bone presents a saucer-shaped depression of varying depth. When the tumor is markedly invasive, the cortex is thoroughly destroyed, the medulla infiltrated, and the bone markedly weakened so that a pathologic fracture occurs. Usually, the tumor grows by expansion and penetrates the periosteum at a late stage to enter the surrounding soft tissues. A very malignant tumor is more infiltrative, destroys, and easily spreads through the periosteum, engulfing the overlying structures. The main mass of tumor may occupy the interior of the bone, destroying and replacing both cortex and medulla.

Microscopic Appearance

The most malignant type of fibrosarcoma consists mainly of a very cellular tissue composed of small oat-shaped cells resembling mesenchymal cells. (Color Plate 15-12). These cells have scanty cytoplasm and contain small, dark, rounded nuclei with mitoses very much in evidence. The cells are packed tightly so that very little intercellular substance is seen. They are considered to be the least differentiated form of fibroblasts. A less malignant fibrosarcoma is one in which the cells are more differentiated. The preponderant cell is the spindle cell. This is larger, contains more cytoplasm, and the nucleus is ovoid and vesicular in appearance. These cells, too, are packed tightly, but more intercellular tissue fibers are apparent. Cells and fibers are arranged in fasciculi or bundles, typically in whorls, but may also form palisades and criss-crossings. The least malignant tumor is composed chiefly of fibroblasts and more intercellular material of the eosinophilic collagenous type. It resembles a nerve sheath sarcoma, but tumor giant cells are present. Each tumor frequently contains all three types of cells. The degree of malignity is suggested by the preponderant cells, but this is not absolutely true. No tumor new bone is formed.[199]

ORIGIN

Most authorities agree that fibrosarcomas originate from the fibrous layer of the periosteum, in a fashion identical with fibrosarcomas starting in other fibrous tissues. Because fibrous tissue occurs in the medulla, the tumor is thought by some observers to start also within the bone.[197,198,200] Others believe that fibrosarcoma within the medulla is in reality an osteogenic sarcoma in which ultimate osteogenesis has not occurred. However, a true fibrosarcoma never forms tumor bone at its original site or in its metastases.

TREATMENT

Theoretically, one can differentiate between a benign and a malignant growth. However, a fibroblastic innocent-appearing tumor can be very destructive and metastasize early. Refinements of microscopic diagnosis should not enter into the decision. Amputation offers the only hope of cure. In general, the fibrosarcomas are less malignant than the osteogenic sarcomas.

HISTIOCYTIC LYMPHOMA

All blood-forming tissues have a framework of reticular fibers and cells. These fibers are sheathed by a thin layer of protoplasm in which are scattered pale oval nuclei. These are primitive reticular cells which show no cell limits. They are not actively phagocytic. However, under certain conditions (*e.g.*, toxicity or inflammation) they are capable of transforming into all types of blood and connective tissue cells. They transform into large active phagocytic reticular cells, the fixed macrophages, which have an abundant cytoplasm, a large pale nucleus, are stellate or spindle-shaped and adhere to the reticular fibers. They contain the debris of dead cells and foreign materials and are capable of ingesting certain dyes, such as lithium carmine. They may become free macrophages. Macrophages are often flattened and resemble endothelial cells. However, true endothelial cells are incapable of ingesting dyes. This dye method may be used to distinguish macrophages from true endothelial tissue. Reticular fibers are best displayed by the silver impregnation method of Hortega.

The reticuloendothelial cell thus has a pluropotentiality which explains the formation of several types of tumors, notably Ewing's tumor and histiocytic lymphoma (reticulum cell sarcoma).

Histiocytic lymphoma is a tumor similar in clinical course, pathologic appearance, and radiosensitivity to Ewing's tumor but having a more favorable prognosis.[201,202,204,205]

CLINICAL PICTURE

Age. All ages, usually between 20 and 50 years

Site of Predilection. Long bones chiefly

Position. In the medulla, the epiphysis, or metaphysis

Symptoms. Typically, does not alter the general condition of the patient; pain is usually the initial symptom, mild to moderate, never severe; soft swelling; no fever or leukocytosis; metastases rare, usually to lungs, rarely to other bones

Course. Onset insidious, progression very slow, metastases late

Pathologic fracture. Common

ROENTGENOGRAPHIC FINDINGS

The tumor is osteolytic. The area of decreased density appears in the medulla of the metaphysis or the epiphysis and spreads rapidly to the cortex, then invades the soft tissues. There is notable absence of reactive bone formation either in the cortex or the periosteum. Occasionally, residual bone trabeculae within the area of destruction may give a loculated appearance to the tumor. A large area of the bone is rapidly affected. Surprisingly, symptoms are minimal at this time and the general condition of the patient is good.

PATHOLOGY

Gross Appearance

The tumor is grayish, and its consistency varies between firm and friable. It is vascular and exhibits small areas of hemorrhage. The periosteum is elevated without reactive bone formation. The cortex is thinned, distended, and perforated at several points. The tumor tissue extends over a large area in the medulla, the cortex, and the subperiosteal space.

Microscopic Appearance

The tissue is practically identical with histiocytic lymphoma of lymph nodes (Color Plate 15-13). There is an intense proliferation of the cellular elements. The cells possess slightly basophilic cytoplasm with poorly defined borders, sometimes appearing ameboid, but definitely ramified, throughout the tissue, by cytoplasmic processes. The nuclei are large, oval, lobulated, or reniform and are poor in chromatin. Blood vessels are intimately associated with the tumor cells, which occasionally are seen invading the vessel wall. By staining with Hortega's technique, a characteristic reticular fibrillar network is displayed (Fig. 15-39). Starting at the adventitia of blood vessels as a close mesh, it gradually becomes more open as it spreads throughout the tissue. However, it maintains a constant effect of enclosing small groups of tumor cells simulating areolae.

In contrast, Ewing's tumor exhibits a compact mass of cells of uniform shape, with rounded or oval nuclei and ill-defined and scanty cytoplasm. The reticulum fibers, when exposed by silver impregnation, surround much larger areas of cells, forming lobules within which the fibrillae do not penetrate.

It may be necessary to perform special staining for glycogen in order to distinguish between the two tumors. The presence of abundant glycogen granules in the cytoplasm of tumor cells establishes the tumor in question as a Ewing's tumor; conversely, glycogen granules are absent in the cells of a histiocytic lymphoma. For this special procedure, the specimen must be fixed in 80% alcohol at 5° C. Formalin fixation is unreliable for preserving glycogen.[203]

TREATMENT

Histiocytic lymphoma (reticulum-cell sarcoma) when limited to a single site, such as bone, is curable with wide-field megavoltage radiotherapy (5000 to 5500 rads).[202A] However, because the majority of patients with lymphoma of bone have more extensive disease, which is nonradiation curable, a thorough search should be carried out in collaboration with a medical oncologist or hematologist.[204A] It may be necessary to perform an exploratory laparotomy to detect involvement of viscera or retroperitoneal lymph nodes. Multifocal disease requires chemotherapy in addition to radiotherapy. One-half or more of such cases are curable with combination chemotherapy.[204B] Amputation or *en bloc* resection of the bone tumor is almost never necessary.

MULTIPLE MYELOMA

Multiple myeloma (also known as myelomatosis, multiple myelomatosis, solitary myeloma, plasmocytoma, monoclonal gammopathy) is characterized by the presence of cells resembling plasma cells, which replace bone, and because of the formation of abnormal proteins leads to complications that hasten a fatal termination. It usually, but not exclusively, occurs in older persons.

CLINICAL PICTURE

Age. Occurs in people 40 to 60 years of age; sexes equally affected

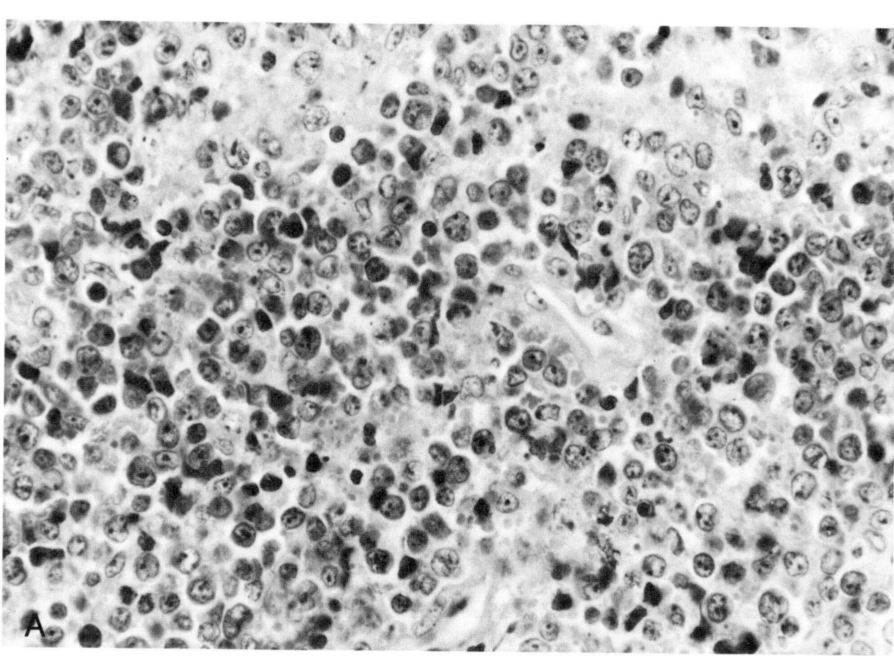

FIG. 15-39. (*Continues on facing page*)

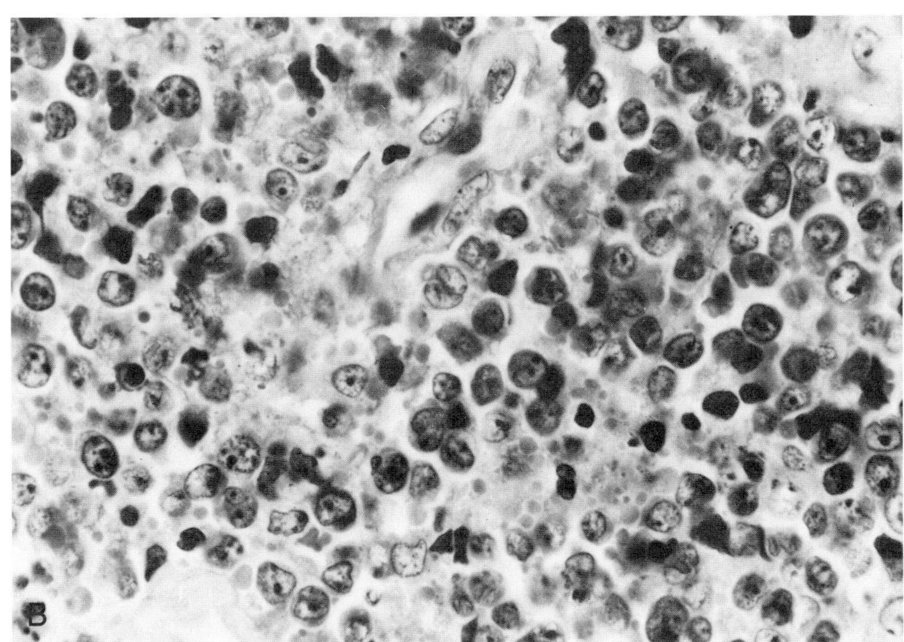

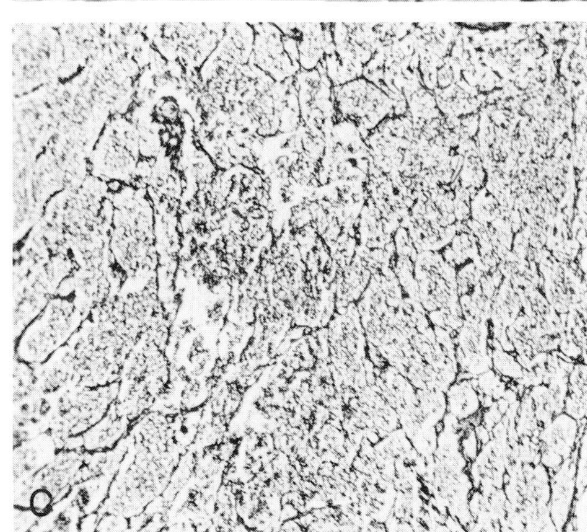

FIG. 15-39. Reticulum cell sarcoma (large cell lymphoma, malignant lymphoma) of bone, cytological features. Lymphoma arising primarily in the skeletal system is composed of a combination of undifferentiated (mesenchymal?) cells, large lymphoblasts or lymphocytes, and histiocytes. The specific tumor is labeled by the predominating cell, the most common osseous type being the large lymphoid cell lymphoma. Histiocytes can be identified by ultramicroscopic and histochemical evidence of heightened intracytoplasmic metabolic activity and engulfed intracellular inclusions. When the lymphoma is localized to a single bone, the outlook is good. The tumor can be differentiated from Ewing's tumor by reticulum fiber staining. (*A*) Microscopic appearance (× 640) and (*B*) showing mixture of large lymphoid cells and histiocytes (× 1000). (Photomicrographs courtesy of Dr. A. G. Huvos). (*C*) Silver impregnation stain for reticulin fibers.

Symptoms. Early, silent; gradual development of pain, at first mild, intermittent and vague; frequently affecting lumbar and sacral areas, chest, and ribs

At intervals a severe attack of sharp pain is superimposed and may be brought on by a sudden movement or exertion, as a lifting strain. It may be neuritic and girdlelike at the level of the chest, representing a fractured rib or dorsal vertebra; or it may occur in the lower back and be referred to a lower extremity, representing either a fracture of a lumbar vertebra or intraspinal compression of the cauda equina by the neoplastic tissue. The sharp pain may gradually lessen and disappear, and such acute attacks may recur with increasing frequency. Often a diffuse, persistent backache develops and may be confused with the pain of senile osteoporosis. This type of pain is constant. When confined to the lower back, and when associated with radicular pain in a lower extremity, it may be confused with the clinical picture of a protruded disk. However, the pain of myelomatous disease is continuous rather than episodic.

Pain in an upper extremity may represent local disease, most often at the upper end of the humerus; or it may be referred from involvement of a cervical or upper dorsal vertebra. At times, progressive weakness and eventual paralysis of the lower extremities may develop as a consequence of intraspinal compression.

Findings. Early, none. The signs of a pathologic fracture may be the earliest manifestations of the disease. Vertebral collapse results in flattening of the lumbar spine and increased rounding of the dorsal spine. Superficial bone structures, particularly the sternum and ribs, may gradually develop diffuse, palpable, tender swellings. Painful, restricted motion of the cervical, dorsal, or lumbar areas of the back associated with local tenderness and occasionally with a neurologic deficit reflect spinal involvement.

Course. The onset is insidious with rheumaticlike pains, usually in the back and loins, intermittent and progressive over several years, then persistent. Eventually, a fatal termination is the result of extensive marrow replacement, severe anemia, thrombocytopenia, and hemorrhages. Also, renal failure commonly occurs as a result of tubular blockage by protein casts (myeloma kidney).

Complications. Pathologic fractures, particularly of the ribs, are frequent and union is delayed. Other complications are spinal cord or nerve root compression,[135,207] progressive, severe anemia; leukopenia in late stages; renal failure; and immunological deficiency with frequent severe bacterial infections.

Laboratory Findings. Bence Jones protein is found in the urine, in 30% of patients. On boiling the urine, a white precipitate appears at about 50°C, then dissolves at the boiling point, especially after acidifying the urine. On cooling, a precipitate reappears. If serum albumin is present, the albumin is filtered off at the boiling point, and the procedure is repeated. The protein is found intermittently in early stages of the disease, and repeated examinations are often necessary. It is found sooner or later in about one third of the patients.

The serum globulin is increased, and the albumin-globulin ratio is reversed in most cases. In some cases the serum globulin may be normal by chemical methods. Therefore, electrophoretic analyses must be done to detect the specific abnormal globulin in the serum and urine. Further, it must be recognized that gamma globulins are increased in some infections and conditions in which immunization processes are active. Hyperglobulinemia is also present in a large number of diseases (*e.g.*, liver disease, collagen disease, and various malignant tumors). Paper electrophoresis of serum and urine proteins is mandatory. Usually a single spike is found in the α-2, β, or γ regions. The nature of the spike can be resolved by immunoelectrophoresis.

Hypercalcemia is common and is often associated with renal involvement.

Red cell sedimentation rate is raised in almost all cases. Anemia is normocytic and normochromic, but with bleeding may become hypochromic, and is partly responsible for fatigue and lassitude in generalized disease. The red cells typically show a tendency to rouleaux formation.

An important diagnostic point is the finding of a *low* normal alkaline phosphatase despite the presence of extensive bone destruction.

Marrow biopsy is the most readily performed diagnostic test. Samples of marrow are taken from the sternum and ilium, and plasma cells seen to be proliferating in sheets of contiguous cells may be considered significant.

ROENTGENOGRAPHIC FINDINGS

Bone involvement is represented either as diffuse osteoporosis or lytic lesions (Fig. 15-40). Early, the roentgenograms are negative. With diffuse generalized disease the bone changes are subtle and not diagnostic. With extensive involvement of the spine, the picture is typical of generalized osteoporosis, with biconcave vertebral bodies and vertebral collapse. Characteristic punched-out circular areas of rarefaction eventually develop in most cases and are best seen in the skull and pelvis. The typical lesion is an osteolytic defect which develops within the interior of the bone and extends outward to erode and penetrate the cortex. The cortex is not expanded, and no reactive bone is seen, either about the lesions or in the subperiosteal space. The osteolytic defect is rarely observed in the vertebral body because the bone collapses before the defect becomes visible. The picture closely resembles that more often seen in idiopathic osteoporosis of the spine. When rarefaction of the vertebra progresses, complete dissolution may extend throughout the vertebra producing the picture of "the disappearing vertebra."

PATHOLOGY

Gross Appearance

The tumor tissue is a grayish red, or dark red, soft gelatinous mass which bleeds freely. It lies chiefly within the medullary portion of the bone and where the cortex

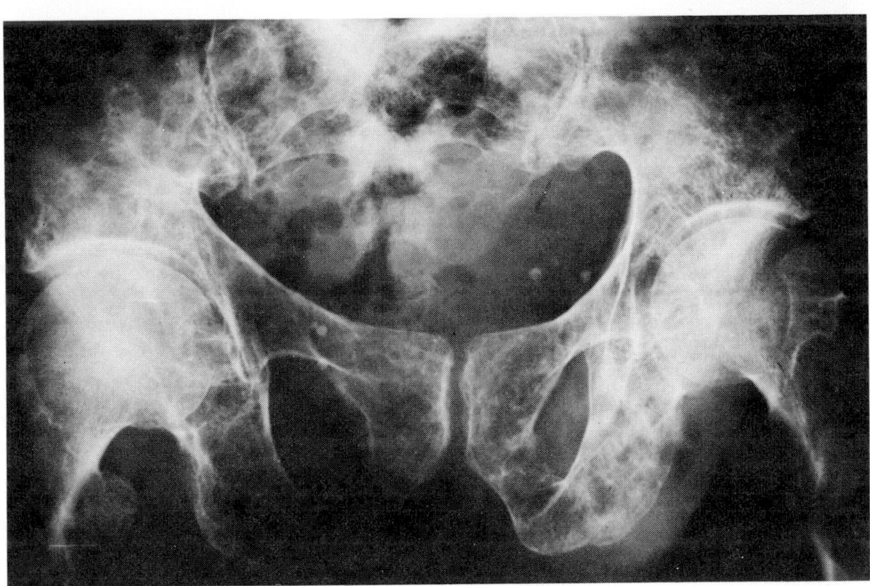

FIG. 15-40. Multiple myeloma showing multiple round osteolytic defects without alteration in the contour of the bone.

has been eaten away. The overlying cortex is thin and easily broken. No bone trabeculae exist within the tumor tissue. The neoplasm erodes and extends beyond the cortex. In the spinal canal it compresses the spinal cord and the nerve roots.

Microscopic Appearance

The typical cells are round and contain an eccentrically placed nucleus with a nucleolus (Color Plate 15-14). The chromatin is sparse and arranged in spokes-of-wheel fashion. The nuclear membrane is well defined. The cytoplasm is eosinophilic. However, the perinuclear halo typical of plasma cells is not seen; and the plasma cell stain, polychrome methylene blue, is not well taken. The tumor cell may represent lack of complete differentiation. Other cells resembling lymphocytes and myelocytes may represent stages in differentiation from the stem cell to the plasma cell. The cells are closely packed, and no supporting stroma is visible. Thin-walled blood vessels pervade the tumor. Fat cells, megalokaryocytes and eosinophils are present. The tumor cells surround and directly eat away spicules of bone.[208,210,211]

Associated Pathology

Pathognomonic changes in the kidneys consist of plugs of protein within the tubules, surrounded by foreign body giant cells. This leads to tubular atrophy, interstitial scarring, and renal insufficiency. Generalized bone resorption results in metastatic calcium deposits in kidneys, lungs, and other tissues. Amyloidosis occurs in parenchymatous organs and within the neoplastic tissue. Neurologic manifestations ensue from compression of the cord and the nerve roots. Nodules in the lungs produce such pulmonary complications as bronchitis and emphysema.

PROGNOSIS

Myelomatosis is invariably fatal. The interval from onset of symptoms to termination varies from a few months to several years. Long survival is exceptional. In the vast majority of cases, death occurs within 3 years and in almost all within 5 years. A solitary lesion in which there is no evidence of generalized disease for at least 3 years offers a better prognosis, and survival for 10 years or more is possible.

TREATMENT

Widespread dissemination and an eventual fatal outcome make treatment essentially palliative. The tumor is radiosensitive. This relieves pain, but the tumor eventually loses its susceptibility. Individual foci may be treated in this manner, but progression of generalized disease is not significantly retarded. Temporary relief of bone pain may be attained in some cases by use of chemotherapeutic agents, such as melphalan (Alkeran), a nitrogen-mustard compound,[213] urethane (ethyl carbamate), cyclophosphamide (Cytoxan) and steroids.

Compression of intraspinal nerve structures is treated by laminectomy, removal of myelomatous tissue from the spinal canal and postoperative irradiation.[206] In addition, instability may require a spine fusion, although this is seldom necessary.

Intramedullary fixation of a pathologic fracture of a long bone is seldom possible because the soft bone retains the metal badly. A solitary focus, when it occurs in an accessible bone and there is no evidence of disseminated disease, should be surgically removed and followed by radiotherapy. When this single focus is situated in a vertebral body, irradiation alone may suffice.

SOLITARY MYELOMA

A single osteolytic myelomatous lesion[212] without evidence of generalized disease usually represents the initial manifestation of disseminated disease which may not become obvious for several years, and possibly for as long as 10 to 15 years. As a general rule, although not invariable, the course is slow and long survival is usual. Like multiple myeloma, the vertebral column is the most common site. However, unlike the generalized disease, in which the bone architecture of the spine is reduced only to an osteoporotic state within the time limited by the fatal outcome, a localized lesion slowly proceeds to complete destruction of a single vertebra. The vertebral body may collapse before the osteolytic feature is evident. The entire vertebra including the posterior arch may be dissolved producing the x-ray picture of "the disappearing vertebra." The osteolytic process may extend across the disk space to involve an adjacent vertebra, and the roentgenogram may simulate tuberculosis. The myelomatous tissue may extend backward to encroach on the intraspinal neural structures producing a neurologic deficit corresponding to the level of compression. It does not appear to penetrate the dura. Other sites of involvement such as the greater trochanter may remain asymptomatic until revealed by routine x-ray examination or fracture.

True solitary myeloma is considered "benign" and may be eradicated by excision and x-ray therapy. Regardless of possible future extension of disease, the course is so slow that a single lesion should be treated in this manner. When intraspinal compression occurs, laminectomy, removal of the tumor tissue from within the spinal canal, and x-ray treatment will usually effect marked improvement of the neurologic deficit. The need for spine fusion is dictated by the degree of instability of the affected vertebra. If the myeloma is confined to the vertebral body, x-ray treatment alone may suffice.

A single focus which remains solitary without eventual further involvement is extremely rare, and such a diagnosis rarely is upheld in the face of thorough investigation, particularly adequate study of the sternal marrow, the iliac marrow, and the plasma proteins.

LIPOSARCOMA

A liposarcoma is a rare neoplasm of bone resembling a fibrosarcoma in appearance but displaying histologic evidence of origin from fat cells. It is characterized clinically by osteolytic destruction, predilection for the extremities of long bones, destruction of the cortex with spread into contiguous soft parts, a slow course with eventual spread to other bones, and finally visceral metastases. It is radiosensitive.

PATHOLOGY

Gross Appearance

The tumor is soft, grayish yellow, lobulated, and coarsely fascicular, resembling a fibrosarcoma.[214] It replaces bony substance, perforates the cortex, and a lobulated tumor mushrooms out into the surrounding tissues. It displays islands of glistening, opaque mucoidlike tissue.

Microscopic Appearance

Interlacing spindle cells resemble those of medullary fibrosarcoma but are more blunt and the cytoplasm more acidophilic (Color Plate 15-15). Its malignant character is revealed in central nuclei, which display bizarre sizes and shapes, abundant mitoses, and hyperchromatism. No fat droplets are contained in these cells which make up the bulk of the tumor.

The irregular islands of mucoidlike tissue contain fat cells. These consist of large adult fat cells with the usual peripheral position of the nucleus; smaller young fat cells with nuclei, either central or peripheral, small, rounded and dark, or very large and occupying most of the cell; fusiform cells with hyperchromatic ovoid nucleus and cytoplasm vacuolated like fat cells. This last type of cell seems to become more atypical, loses its fat content, and assumes the appearance of the main tumor cells.

The existence of a liposarcoma primary in bone is controversial, but the histologic appearance and the distinctive clinical course seem to point it out as a distinct entity.

ADAMANTINOMA

Adamantinoma is a rare but distinctive primary bone tumor. The designation *adamantinoma* was originally given[217] because of its histologic resemblance to the benign but locally invasive tumor of proliferating odontogenic epithelium embedded in a fibrous stroma, now generally called *ameloblastoma.* The components were supposedly derived from enamel-producing cells. However, this derivation has recently been challenged, and the various hypotheses include an angioblastic neoplasm,[218] and a dermal inclusion tumor.[219]

The number of cases reported (approximately 100) is inadequate for determining its etiological characteristics. The greatest age incidence seems to be between 10 and 35 years, and blacks are predisposed. In the appendicular skeleton, the tibia is the favored location.[215]

CLINICAL PICTURE

The tumor develops insidiously over a period of years. At first it may be asymptomatic and discovered on roentgenograms, or the first indication may be a pathologic fracture. The initial symptom varies, and includes pain, swelling, tenderness, and the acute development of symptoms associated with pathologic fracture. The tumor is locally invasive, spreading slowly but progressively without metastasizing even after unsuccessful removal. Despite a protracted local invasion which suggests that the tumor is benign, metastases have been recorded: regional lymph nodes (inguinal,[215,220] axillary[218]), lungs,[222] abdominal viscera,[215] ribs,[221] and tibia to humerus.[218]

ROENTGENOGRAPHIC FINDINGS

A sharply defined rarefaction in a medullary location and eccentrically involving the overlying cortex is the main finding. The lesion is small at first, but with growth the cortex becomes attenuated, often eroded in a characteristic saw-toothed fashion, and expanded. A honeycombed or loculated appearance is typical. Almost no periosteal reaction is noted. The lytic lesion may ultimately attain large size, is often multicentric, more so than is apparent on the roentgenogram,[216] and, although slow-growing, comes to occupy a major portion of the shaft. The shaft becomes widened and deformed and eventually the cortex is penetrated with extension into the contiguous soft tissues.

Following a pathologic fracture, intensive periosteal new bone formation may produce a large spindle-shaped deformity of the bone.

PATHOLOGY

Gross Appearance

The appearance varies, but most often the tumor is yellow,[218] gray or grayish white, and fleshy or firm in consistency.

Microscopic Appearance

Three basic patterns are observed (Color Plate 15-16).

1. Elongated anastomosing masses of stellate epithelial cells are seen. The peripheral cells are columnar and arranged in palisade fashion. The central cells of these masses are stellate and produce a reticulum appearance. A characteristic epithelial ameloblastic pattern is produced with convoluted and infolded double layered structures and scanty intervening stroma. (See colored photomicrograph)
2. Discrete islands of basal cells with peripheral palisading and central cystic degeneration. This is a follicular ameloblastic pattern
3. Islands of squamous epithelium and pearl formation. The stroma is fibrous. Islands of spindle cells may be a feature.

Sometimes a vascular pattern with hyperplastic endothelial lined vascular channels is seen adjacent to the processes of solid tumor cells. This suggests an angioblastic origin of the tumor.[218]

TREATMENT

The tumor is slow-growing and highly radioresistant, and recurs frequently after attempts at local excision. Since the tumor is more extensive than is apparent on roentgenograms, curettage is unreliable as a treatment. When roentgenograms and CT scans suggest that the tumor is limited in extent and confined to the bone, *en bloc* excision may be attempted. Because the lesion is often multifocal within the same bone, the resection should extend well beyond the apparent limits of the tumor. Resection of the diaphysis should include the periosteum and transection should pass through the metaphyses. Such massive segmental resection requires, in the case of the tibia, an autogenous fibular transplant (Fig. 15-41). The fibula, retaining its blood supply, should be reinforced with an intramedullary pin. It is detached at each end and implanted into the remaining epiphyseometaphyseal segments of the tibia. Additional fixation is needed. Firm plaster or orthotic supports are necessary for several years until union is secure and the transplanted fibula is hypertrophied. Instead of the fibula, a large allograft may be implanted, supplanted by autogenous cancellous bone (composite graft), and the cortical allograft reinforced with a Steinmann nail. *En bloc* excision should always be accompanied by removal of suspiciously enlarged regional lymph nodes. If *en bloc* excision is followed by recurrence, amputation is indicated.

Amputation is generally curative, and should be performed when the tumor has extended beyond the limits of the bone, particularly when multifocal involvement is pronounced and widespread. It is indicated when local recurrence is evident. The possibility of metastatic disease should be investigated prior to treatment.

CHORDOMA

A chordoma is a rare neoplasm of the cranium and the spine apparently derived from embryonic remnants of the notochord. The notochord originates from the entoderm and persists as small remnants in the nucleus pulposus of the intervertebral disks. The majority of chordomas arise in the skull about the spheno-occipital region and in the sacrococcygeal region. Their location

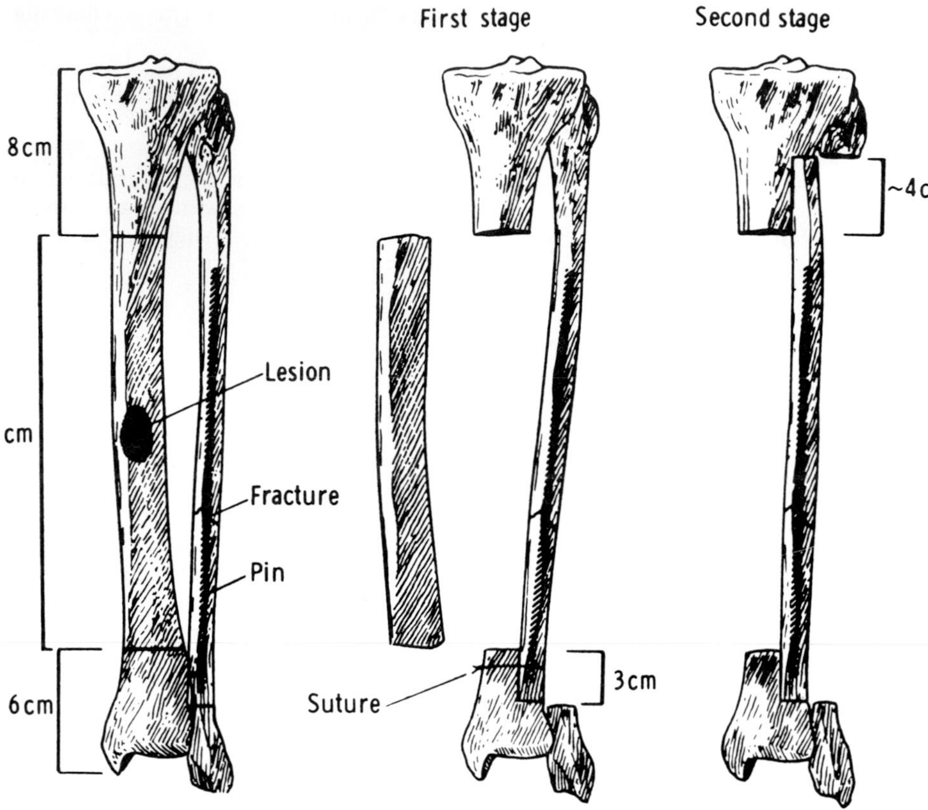

FIG. 15-41. Adamantinoma of the tibia. Treatment is by en bloc resection including diaphysis, periosteum, and scar of biopsy incision; two stage transfer of fibula, first imbedded at one end into the highly vascularized metaphysis, and later fixing the other end into the other metaphysis. An intramedullary pin inserted into the fibula through a fracture or osteotomy increases the strength of the bone against fracture. The nutrient artery is preserved so that the transplant remains viable, readily unites with the tibial metaphyses, and hypertrophies with functional stresses. When this procedure is performed before skeletal maturity, premature epiphyseal closure may occur. (Wilson PD Jr: Clin Orthop 87:81, 1972)

in other areas of the spine is exceedingly rare. Spheno-occipital tumors favor young adults, and sacrococcygeal tumors most often develop after 40 years of age.[225] However, no age is immune.

CLINICAL PICTURE

The following relates only to sacrococcygeal chordoma.

Symptoms are due to expansion and bone destruction. At first, pain occurs in the rectal and anal regions and is mild and intermittent. Obstinate constipation and urinary difficulty develop. Later, incontinence is followed by motor and sensory disturbances of the lower extremities, the gluteal region, and the external genitalia. Finally, pain becomes intractable, the lower extremities display muscle weakness and fecal and urinary incontinence is severe. The course is slow but progressive.

Examination reveals a tender, soft, smooth, fixed mass over the posterior or anterior aspect of the sacrum.

PATHOLOGY

Gross Appearance

The tumor is a large, round, smooth, soft gelatinous mass firmly fixed to the bone and locally invaded tissues. The bone is destroyed and replaced by the tumor and, at first, the cortices are thinned and expanded outward. The lower half of the sacrum is usually involved by sacrococcygeal tumors. Growth and extension of the tumor are slow, bulging the sacrum posteriorly and anteriorly before penetrating the cortex and extending into the soft tissues. Within the pelvis, the tumor involves the lumbosacral plexus, the rectum, the bladder and the genital organs. Metastases to the regional lymph nodes occur very late, usually after a period of years.

Cranial chordomas likewise develop slowly, destroy and replace bone and invade intracranial structures.

Vertebral chordomas develop first within the body and extend to the arch, with eventual collapse of the vertebra. Several adjacent vertebrae may be destroyed.[226]

Microscopic Appearance

The tissue consists of large, polyhedral cells with small nuclei and characteristic intracellular and extracellular vacuoles of mucin (Color Plate 15-17). The cells resemble bladder epithelium and are arranged in cords, columns, or clusters.[224]

ROENTGENOGRAPHIC FINDINGS

A well-circumscribed osteolytic expansile defect is observed in the lower sacrum. A rounded soft tissue shadow extends anteriorly and posteriorly. In the case of rare vertebral involvement, one or several adjacent vertebral bodies and their arches are destroyed and collapsed.

DIFFERENTIAL DIAGNOSIS

Chordomas of the sacrococcygeal region must be differentiated from chondrosarcomas, tuberculosis, tumors of the female pelvic organs, sacrococcygeal teratoma, and rectal carcinoma.

TREATMENT

Although generally regarded as radioresistant, the tumor has been eradicated successfully by special rotation techniques employing extremely high voltages.[223] Chordomas in children are more radiosensitive than in adults. Otherwise, complete surgical excision should be attempted, but recurrence is almost inevitable.

HEMANGIOMA OF BONE

Hemangiomas of bone (angioma of bone) are slow-growing benign tumors composed of masses of fully developed adult blood vessels. They occur frequently as silent lesions in any portion of the skeletal system and other organs. About 12% of spines contain the lesion. However, seldom does it become symptomatic and then only because of pressure effects. A hemangioma has often been thought to cause spontaneous hemorrhage, the resultant hematoma antedating the development of a bone cyst.[233]

ETIOLOGY

Two theories are held:

Congenital Hamartoma.[234] A vast plexus of primitive vascular channels exists in the embryo. Those not forming part of the circulatory system are obliterated. If they persist, they constitute congenital malformations.

Neoplasm.[232,235] Congenital rests, by a process of endothelial proliferation, differentiate into blood vessels.

PATHOLOGY

Gross Appearance

The tumor consists of masses of blood vessels in a fibrous stroma. The adjacent bone is resorbed by expanding pressure, and new reactive bony trabeculae form. The periosteum is not perforated. There is a tendency to extensive thrombosis, organization, regression of the lesion, and healing. When a vertebra is involved, particularly in the normally narrow dorsal area, enlargement of the vertebra or extension into the vertebral canal causes compression myelitis and radiculitis.

Microscopic Appearance

Two types of tumors are identified. The *capillary type* consists of closely packed small blood vessels lined by a single layer of nearly cuboidal endothelial cells.

The *cavernous type* is more common. It is composed of a multitude of large blood-filled spaces lined by a single layer of flattened endothelial cells. No elastic fibers or smooth muscle can be observed in vessel walls. Connective tissue between vessels is sparse and may be compressed thin. Adjacent bony trabeculae are resorbed, possibly because of vascular tension. In other areas, new reactive bone formation is active (Color Plate 15-18 and Fig. 15-42).[229,235]

CLINICAL PICTURE

Most lesions are silent and are discovered accidentally. Symptoms are produced by pressure on surrounding structures and may develop at any age. The site of predilection is a vertebra, often between T4 and L4. The next favored site is the skull, where the lesion usually originates in the meninges and the scalp. Infrequently, the long bones are involved. Pain constitutes the main local symptom. Hemangioma of a vertebra, especially when midthoracic in location, will produce neurologic manifestations, depending on the site and the degree of narrowing of the spinal canal. The tumor increases in size very slowly, then may persist or undergo spontaneous regression and healing.

ROENTGENOGRAPHIC FINDINGS

Roentgenographic findings depend on the type of bone involved.

Flat Bone

Trabeculae of new bone radiate outward from a central focal point producing a characteristic "sunburst" appearance (plexiform angioma).

Vertebra

Coarse, dense, vertical striations in the body may extend into the vertebral arch. The body becomes ballooned, with rounding of the concave borders.

Tubular Bone

The lesion is usually metaphyseal and eccentric. Multilocular cystic cavities of various sizes and irregular shapes resemble the soap-bubble appearance of a giant cell tumor, but the loculi are smaller. A fine

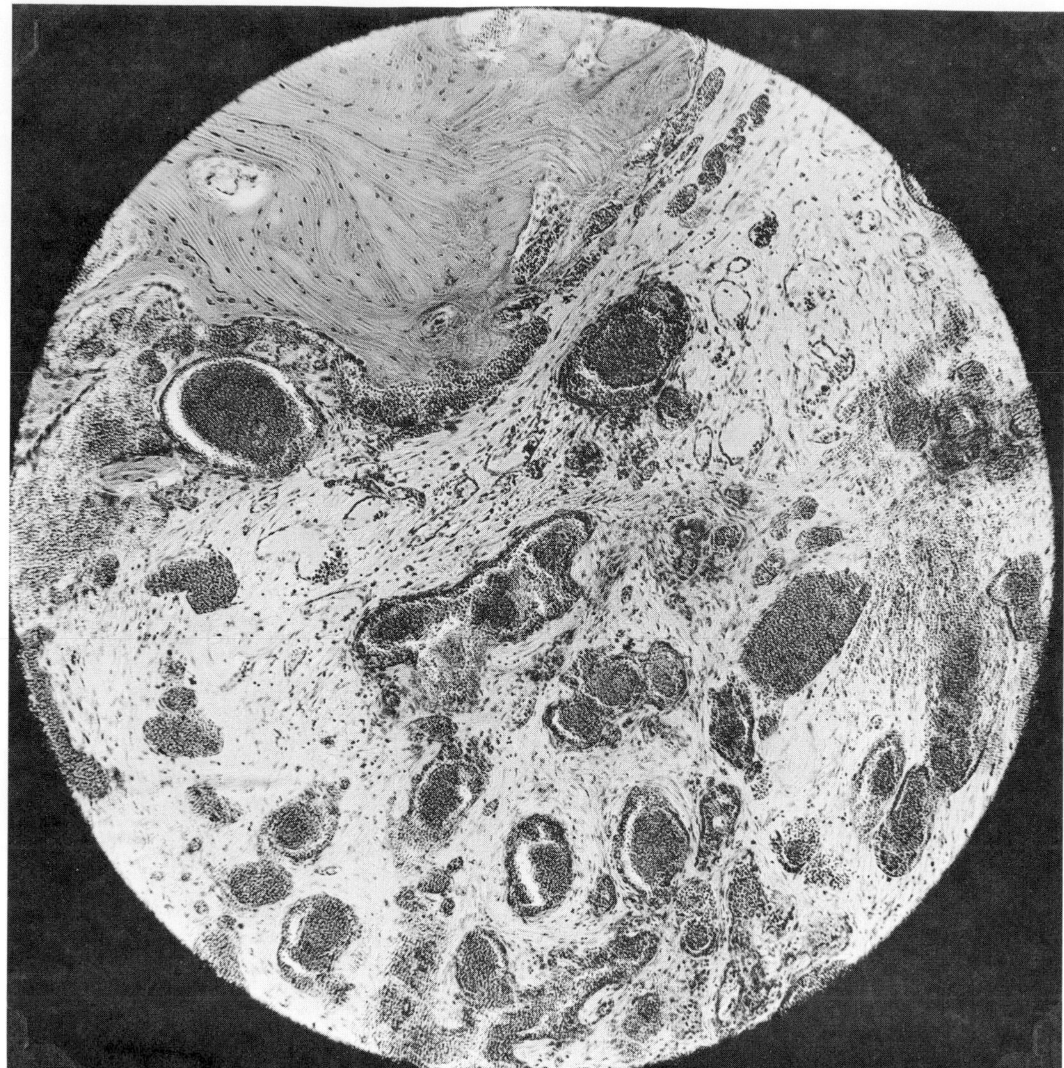

FIG. 15-42. Hemangioma of bone. The vessels appear as blood vessel spaces lined by a single layer of flattened endothelial cells. Vessel walls lack elastic fibers and smooth muscle. Connective tissue between vessels is sparse. At the upper edge of this section, bone is being eroded in some areas by vessels, and in others active bone formation is taking place. This is the cavernous type of hemangioma.

fibrillary network is contained within each locule. A local or general uniform spindle-shaped expansion of the shaft occurs. The cortex is thinned but intact.

The spinal cord may be compressed by ballooning of the vertebral body and posterior arch encroaching on the spinal canal, or by actual invasion of the peridural space by tumor tissue. The level of compression is usually in the dorsal spine, most often at T4, and rarely in the cervical spine. Clinically, the initial symptom may be local pain, the signs of cord compression developing slowly; or gradually developing motor and sensory loss in the lower extremities may be the first signs of an intraspinal tumor.

Diagnosis of a hemangioma of a thoracic vertebra may be difficult and may require tomograms to define the typical vertical striations and ballooning of the vertebral body. The myelogram reveals the block.

TREATMENT

Surgery is fraught with the danger of uncontrollable hemorrhage. These tumors may regress and heal under the influence of x-rays given at regular intervals over a number of months.[230]

An asymptomatic vertebral hemangioma requires no treatment,[227,231] but should be observed by roentgenograms for changes in appearance, and clinically for developing neurologic signs. When the lesion appears to be enlarging, or when a neurologic deficit develops, cobalt therapy is the treatment of choice. Surgery is considered only if response to x-ray treatment is poor or if the rate of progression of the neurologic deficit is threatening. A thorough decompressive laminectomy is performed and followed by radiation therapy. Preoperative preparation for blood replacement is mandatory. Any attempts at removing a portion of the tumor for biopsy will cause profuse bleeding which is difficult to control. In some situations, tumor tissue may be destroyed by cauterization.[229] If vertebral collapse and displacement seem imminent, spine fusion is necessary.

Megavoltage therapy is fraught with the danger of damage to the spinal cord, and should be avoided when surgical excision is feasible.

HEMANGIOENDOTHELIOMA

A hemangioendothelioma[236,241] is a very rare tumor (also known as angioendothelioma, hemangiosarcoma) of which the basic cell is endotheliomatous in appearance; therefore, it might be classified as a variant of a Ewing's tumor. It represents an extremely malignant tumor which often has extended by hematogenous spread before it is recognized.

CLINICAL PICTURE

Age. Adults exclusively

Area of Predilection. Reported in long bones and ilium; more common near surface of the body as soft bluish red tumors with satellite nodules

Symptoms. Pain varies from ache to sharp shooting

Findings. Deep-seated swelling, soft, tender, pulsating; if extends to surface, bluish color apparent; bruit on auscultation

Pathologic Fracture

ROENTGENOGRAPHIC FINDINGS

Single or multiple osteolytic areas without reactive bone. Moth-eaten appearance.

PATHOLOGY

Gross Appearance

The tumor may appear benign and similar to an ordinary bluish red hemangioma of bone. The interior is composed of a mass of bleeding vessels.

Microscopic Appearance

This bulky, cystic tumor is composed of a mass of anastomosing vascular channels. The vascular walls are formed by the tumor cells, which are large polyhedral cells with a well-defined cell membrane and pale vesicular nuclei with dusty chromatin. The cells are several layers thick in contrast with the benign angiomatous tumors in which a single cell thickness is found. When many vessels are seen in cross section, an alveolar appearance results and may be confused with metastatic hypernephroma. However, the latter's cells are large, cylindrical, have small nuclei and the lumens are empty. Hemangioendothelioma tumor cells often freely invade blood vessels and flourish as intravascular tumor thrombi.

Occasionally, the tumor is densely cellular and almost fibrosarcomatous in appearance. However, many small blood vessel spaces lined by and surrounded by multiple layers of endothelial cells can be identified.

The histologic picture varies even in the same case from time to time, depending on the rapidity of cellular growth and differentiation into vasoformative elements. The diagnostic feature is always the formation of new blood vessels. Typical endothelial cells should be identified.

TREATMENT

The tumor is only slightly radiosensitive. After radiation therapy, a malignant tumor displaying hypercellularity, pleomorphism, mitoses and disorderly appearance may revert to a benign appearance resembling a capillary hemangioma. The change is temporary, and malignant characteristics reappear. Radical surgical excision by amputation is recommended, but the outlook is poor.

IDENTIFICATION OF ENDOTHELIAL TISSUES

The literature is replete with the term endothelioma, which has caused confusion in classifying various tumors. A tumor labeled endothelioma should contain a considerable number of cells which can be identified positively as endothelial cells. These cells possess certain histologic characteristics,[242] and definite evidence of their vasoformative potential should be present.

During embryonic development, the squamous endothelial cells arise through flattening of mesenchymal cells. Mesenchymal cells are smaller than fibroblasts but have the same general appearance. They are outstretched, stellate cells with large, oval, pale, vesicular nuclei containing dustlike chromatin particles. The endothelium of blood vessels may have identical potencies with mesenchymal cells (*i.e.*, they are capable of differentiating into various blood and macrophagic elements). Also, the endothelium has the potential of reverting to mesenchymal cells and vice versa.

When connective tissue fibrils appear between mesenchymal cells, the tissue becomes connective tissue. The appearance of fibroblasts is almost identical in appearance with mesenchymal cells. Therefore, undifferentiated mesenchymal cells may be considered to be present at all times within connective tissue. These are observed particularly about capillaries.

Endothelial cells are structurally similar to fibroblasts and mesenchymal cells. The elongate oval nucleus is flattened and contains fine dustlike chromatin particles. However, it lacks the large nucleoli. Its membranes often show longitudinal folds. The flat endothelial cells are usually stretched along the axis of the capillary and have tapering ends. In wider capillaries they are shorter and broader. In a silver nitrate stain, sharply stained black boundaries of cells are demonstrable.

Great numbers of capillaries are collapsed and not visible when the organ is at rest. They open up and are made visible when blood flows through them.

Benign vascular tumors may constitute distention of preexisting channels or an increased vasoformative potential of undifferentiated mesenchymal cells. Malignant vascular tumors may represent a wild, disorderly, rapid exhibition of vasopotential of mesenchymal tissue. Growth may be so rapid that the tissue is very cellular and does not have time to differentiate into clearly vascular structures; or typical endothelial cells are formed in profusion and tend to arrange themselves in tubules or alveoli whose lumens contain blood. The one feature which identifies an endothelioma is a recognizable vasoformative tendency.[243]

REFERENCES

Classification

1. Ewing J: A review and classification of bone sarcomas. Arch Surg 4:485, 1922
2. Geshickter CF, Copeland MM: Tumors of Bone. Philadelphia, JB Lippincott, 1949

Osteoma

3. Lichtenstein L: Bone Tumors. St Louis, CV Mosby, 1952

Osteochondroma

4. Jaffe HL: Hereditary multiple exostoses. Arch Pathol 36:335, 1943
5. Schramm G: Pathogenesis of cartilaginous exostoses and enchondromas. Arch Orthop 27:421, 1929

Chondroma

6. Coley BL, Higinbotham NL: Significance of cartilage in abnormal locations. Cancer 2:777, 1949
7. Jaffe HL: Juxtacortical chondroma. Bull Hosp Joint Dis 17:20, 1956
8. Lichtenstein L, Hall JE: Periosteal chondroma: A distinctive benign cartilaginous tumor. J Bone Joint Surg 34A:691, 1952
9. Rockwell MA, Saiter ET, Enneking WF: Periosteal chondroma. J Bone Joint Surg 54A:102, 1972

Chondrosarcoma

10. Aegerter E, Kirkpatrick JA: Orthopaedic Diseases. Philadelphia, WB Saunders, 1958
11. Arlen M, et al: Radiation-induced sarcoma of bone. Cancer 28:1087, 1971
12. Barnes R, Catto M: Chondrosarcoma of bone. J Bone Joint Surg 48B:729, 1966
13. Bingold AC: Prosthetic replacement of a chondrosarcoma of the upper end of the femur. J Bone Joint Surg 54B:139, 1972
14. Burrows HJ, Wilson JN, Scales JT: Excision of tumours of humerus and femur, with restoration by internal prosthesis. J Bone Joint Surg 57B:148, 1975
15. Coley BL, Higinbotham NL: Secondary chondrosarcoma. Ann Surg 139:547, 1954
16. Dahlin DC, Henderson ED: Chondrosarcoma, a surgical and pathological problem. J Bone Joint Surg 38A:1025, 1956
17. Dahlin DC, Salvador AH: Chondrosarcomas of bones of the hands and feet: A study of 30 cases. Cancer 34:755, 1974
18. Evans HL, Ayala AG, Romsdahl MM: Prognostic factors in chondrosarcoma of bone. Cancer 40:818, 1977
19. Gilmer WS, Higley GB, Kilgore WE: Atlas of Bone Tumors. St Louis, CV Mosby, 1963
20. Henderson ED, Dahlin DC: Chondrosarcoma of bone: A study of 288 cases. J Bone Joint Surg 45A:1450, 1963
21. Jaffe HL: Tumors and Tumorous Conditions of the Bones and Joints. Philadelphia, Lea & Febiger, 1958
22. Keiller VH: Cartilaginous tumors of bone. Surg Gynecol Obstet 40:510, 1925
23. Lettin AWF: Fibular replacement of the upper humerus after segmental resection for chondrosarcoma. Proc Soc Med 57:90, 1964
24. Lichtenstein L, Goldman RL: Cartilage tumors in soft tissues, particularly in the hand and foot. Cancer 17:1203, 1964
25. Lichtenstein L, Jaffe HL: Chondrosarcoma of bone. Am J Pathol 19:553, 1943
26. Linberg BE: Interscapulo-thoracic resection for malignant tumors of the shoulder joint region. J Bone Joint Surg 10:344, 1928
27. Marcove RC: Chondrosarcoma: Diagnosis and treatment. Orthop Clin North Am 8:811, 1977
28. Marcove RC, Huvos AG: Cartilaginous tumors of the ribs. Cancer 27:794, 1971
29. Marcove RC, et al: Chondrosarcoma of the pelvis and upper end of the femur: An analysis of factors influencing survival time in 113 cases. J Bone Joint Surg 54A:561, 1972
30. O'Neal LW, Ackerman LV: Chondrosarcoma of bone. Cancer 5:551, 1952
31. Pack GT, Baldwin JC: The Tikhor–Linberg resection of shoulder girdle. Surgery 38:753, 1955
32. Peimer CA, Yuan HA, Sagerman RH: Postradiation chondrosarcoma. J Bone Joint Surg 58A:1033, 1976
33. Phemister DB: Chondrosarcoma of bone. Surg Gynecol Obstet 50:216, 1930

34. Roberts PH, Price CHG: Chondrosarcoma of the bones of the hand. J Bone Joint Surg 59B:213, 1977
35. Sanerkin NG: The diagnosis and grading of chondrosarcoma of bone—A combined cytological and histological approach. Cancer 44:1375, 1979
36. Sanerkin NG, Gallagher D: A review of the behaviour of chondrosarcoma of bone. J. Bone Joint Surg 61B:395, 1979
37. Schajowicz F et al: Ultrastructure of chondrosarcoma. Clin Orthop 100:378, 1974
38. Sim FH, Cupps RE, Dahlin DC et al: Postradiation sarcoma of bone. J Bone Joint Surg 54A:1479, 1972
39. Steiner GC: Postradiation sarcoma of bone. Cancer 18:603, 1965
40. Tikhor PT: Tumor Studies. Russia, 1900
41. Unni KK, et al: Chondrosarcoma: Clear-cell variant. J Bone Joint Surg 58A:676, 1976

Chondromyxoid Fibroma

42. Anderson CE, et al: Ultrastructural and chemical composition of chondrosarcoma. J Bone Joint Surg 45A:753, 1963
43. Dahlin DC: Chondromyxoid fibroma of bone. Cancer 9:195, 1956
44. Iwata S, Coley BL: Report of six cases of chondromyxoid fibroma of bone. Surg Gynecol Obstet 101:571, 1958
45. Jaffe HL: Tumors and Tumorous Conditions of the Bones and Joints. Philadelphia, Lea & Febiger, 1958
46. Jaffe HL, Lichtenstein L: Chondromyxoid fibroma of bone: A distinctive benign tumor likely to be mistaken especially for chondrosarcoma. Arch Pathol 45:541, 1948
47. Lichtenstein L: Bone tumors. St Louis, CV Mosby, 1965
48. Ralph LI: Chondromyxoid fibroma of bone. J Bone Joint Surg 44B:7, 1962
49. Scaglietti O, Stringa G: Myxoma of bone in children. J Bone Joint Surg 43A:67, 1961
50. Schajowicz F, Gallardo H: Chondromyxoid fibroma (fibromyxoid chondroma) of bone. J Bone Joint Surg 53B:198, 1971
51. Tornberg DN, et al: The ultrastructure of chondromyxoid fibroma: Its biologic and diagnostic implications. Clin Orthop 95:295, 1973

Chondroblastoma

52. Codman EA: Epiphyseal chondromatous tumors of the upper end of the humerus. Surg Gynecol Obstet 52:543, 1931
53. Coley BL, Santora AJ: Benign central cartilaginous tumor of bone. Surgery 22:411, 1947
54. Copeland MM, Geschickter CF: Chondroblastic tumors of bone, benign and malignant. Am J Surg 129:724, 1949
55. Jaffe HL, Lichtenstein L: Benign chondroblastoma of bone. Am J Pathol 18:969, 1942
56. Kolodny A: Bone sarcoma. Surg Gynecol Obstet (Suppl 1) 44, 1927
57. Valls J, Ottolenghi CE, Schajowicz F: Epiphyseal chondroblastoma of bone. J Bone Joint Surg 33A:997, 1951

Benign Giant-Cell Tumor

58. Barnes R: Giant-cell tumor of bone. J Bone Joint Surg 54B:213, 1972
59. Bloodgood JC: Benign giant cell tumor of bone; its diagnosis and conservative treatment. Am J Surg 37:105, 1923
60. Compere EL: The diagnosis and treatment of giant-cell tumors of bone. J Bone Joint Surg 35A:822, 1953
61. Dahlin DC, Cupps EE, Johnson EW Jr: Giant-cell tumor: A study of 195 cases. Cancer 25:106, 1970
62. Goldenberg RR, Campbell CJ, Bonfiglio M: Giant-cell tumor of bone: An analysis of 218 cases. J Bone Joint Surg 52A:619, 1970
63. Goldenberg RR, Campbell CJ, Bonfiglio M: Giant cell tumor of bone. J Bone Joint Surg 52B:775, 1970
64. Jaffe HL, Lichtenstein L, Portis RB: Giant cell tumor of bone: Its pathologic appearance, grading, supposed variants and treatment. Arch Pathol 30:993, 1940
65. Mankin HJ, Doppelt SH, Sullivan TR et al: Osteoarticular and intercalary allograft transplantation in the management of malignant tumors of bone.
66. Marcove R, et al: Giant-cell tumors treated by cryosurgery. J Bone Joint Surg 55A:1633, 1973
67. Marcove R, et al: Cryosurgery in the treatment of giant-cell tumors of bone: A report of 52 consecutive cases. Cancer 41:957, 1978
68. McGrath PJ: Giant-cell tumor of bone: An analysis of 52 cases. J Bone Joint Surg 54B:216, 1972
69. Meyers MH, Chatterjee SN: Osteochondral transplantation. Surg Clin North Am 58:429, 1978
70. Meyerding HW: Treatment of benign giant cell tumor by resection or excision and bone grafting. J Bone Joint Surg 27:196, 1945
71. Murphy WP, Ackerman LV: Benign and malignant giant-cell tumor of bone: A clinical-pathological evaluation of thirty-one cases. Cancer 9:317, 1956
72. Ottoleghi CE: Massive osteo and osteoarticular bone grafts: Technique and results of 62 cases. Clin Orthop 87:156, 1972
73. Parrish FF: Allograft replacement of all or part of the end of a long bone following excision of a tumor: Report of twenty-one cases. J Bone Joint Surg 55A:1, 1973
74. Persson BM, Wouters HW: Curettage and acrylic cementation in surgery of giant cell tumors of bone. Clin Orthop 120:125, 1976
75. Riley LH, Hartmann WH, Robinson RA: Soft tissue recurrence of giant-cell tumor of bone after irradiation and excision. J Bone Joint Surg 49A:365, 1967
76. Vidal I, et al: Plastie de comblement par métacrylate de méthyl traitement de certaines tumeurs osseusses bénignes. Montpellier Chirurgical Tome XV, No. 4, 1969
77. Volkov MV, Immaliyev AS: Use of allogenous articular bone implants as substitutes for autotransplants in adult patients. Clin Orthop 114:192, 1976

Aneurysmal Bone Cyst

78. Lichtenstein L: Aneurysmal bone cyst. Cancer 3:279, 1950
79. Thompson PC: Subperiosteal giant cell tumor. J Bone Joint Surg 36A:281, 1954

Unicameral Bone Cyst

80. Agerholm JC, Goodfellow JW: Simple cysts of the humerus treated by radical excision. J Bone Joint Surg 47B:714, 1965
81. Campanacci M, DeSessa L, Bellando–Randone P: Bone cysts: Review of 275 cases. Results of surgical treatment and early results of treatment by methylprednisolone acetate injections. Chir Organi Mov 62:471, 1976
82. Cohen J: Unicameral bone cysts: A current synthesis of reported cases. Orthop Clin North Am 8:715, 1977

83. Fahey JJ, O'Brien ET: Subtotal resection and grafting in selected cases of solitary unicameral bone cyst. J Bone Joint Surg 55A:59, 1973
84. Garceau GJ, Gregory CF: Solitary unicameral bone cysts. J Bone Joint Surg 36A:267, 1954
85. Gartland JJ, Cole EL: Modern concepts in the treatment of unicameral bone cysts of the proximal humerus. Orthop Clin North Am 6:487, 1975
86. Jaffe HL: Tumors and Tumorous Conditions of the Bones and Joints, p 63. Philadelphia, Lea & Febiger, 1958
87. Jaffe HL, Lichtenstein L: Solitary unicameral bone cyst with emphasis on the roentgen picture, the pathologic appearance, and the pathogenesis. Arch Surg 44:1004, 1942
88. Johnson LC, Kindred RC: The anatomy of bone cysts. J Bone Joint Surg 40A:1440, 1958
89. Neer CS III, Francis KC, Johnston AD et al: Current concepts on the treatment of solitary unicameral bone cysts. Clin Orthop 97:40, 1973
90. Neer CS III, Francis KC, Marcove RC et al: Treatment of unicameral bone cysts: A follow-up study of one hundred and seventy-five cases. J Bone Joint Surg 48A:731, 1966
91. Spence KF, Bright RW, Fitzgerald SP et al: Solitary unicameral bone cysts: Treatment with freeze-dried crushed cortical-bone allograft. J Bone Joint Surg 58A:636, 1976
92. Spence KF, Sell KW, Brown RH: Solitary bone cysts: Treatment with freeze-dried cancellous bone allograft. J Bone Joint Surg 51A:87, 1969
93. Spence KF, Sell KW, Harris B et al: A comparative evaluation of freeze-dried cancellous and cortical bone allografts in dogs. Proc Am Acad Orthop Surg J Bone Joint Surg 54A:1350, 1972
94. Scaglietti O, Marchetti G, Bartolozzi P: Effects of methyl prednisolone acetate in treatment of bone cysts. J Bone Joint Surg 61B:200, 1979

Osteogenic Sarcoma

95. Allan C, Soule E: Osteogenic sarcoma of the somatic soft tissues. Cancer 27:1121, 1971
96. Allen CV, Stevens KR: Preoperative irradiation for osteogenic sarcoma. Cancer 31:1364, 1973
97. Alpert LI, Abaci IF, Werthamer S: Radiation-induced extraskeletal osteosarcoma. Cancer 31:1359, 1973
98. Arlen M, et al: Radiation-induced sarcoma of bone. Cancer 28:1087, 1971
99. Baserga R, et al: The delayed effects of external gamma irradiation on the bones of rats. Am J Pathol 39:455, 1961
100. Berman LD: Comparative morphology study of the virus-induced solid tumors of Syrian hamsters. JNCI 39:847, 1967
101. Bertino JR, Cashmore AR, Hillcoat BL: "Induction" of dihydrofolate reductase. Farification and properties of the "induced" human erythrocyte and leukocyte enzyme and normal bone marrow enzyme. Cancer Res 30:2372, 1970
102. Bird CE: Sarcoma complicating Paget's disease of bone. Arch Surg 14:1187, 1927
103. Bruce WR, Meeker BE, Valeriote FA: Comparison of the sensitivity of normal haemopoietic and transplanted lymphoma colony-forming cells to chemotherapeutic agents administered in vivo. JNCI 37:233, 1966
104. Brunschwig A: Production of primary bone tumors (fibrosarcoma of bone) by intramedullary injection of methylcholanthrene, Am J Cancer 34:540, 1938
105. Cade S: Osteogenic sarcoma. J R Coll Surg Edinb 1:79, 1955
106. Cole LT, Nowell PC: Radiation carcinogenesis: Sequence of events. Science 150:1782, 1965
107. Cortes EP, Holland JF, Wang JJ et al: Chemotherapy of advanced osteosarcoma: Colston paper No. 24, Bonn. In Price CHG, Ross FGM (eds): Certain Aspects of Neoplasia, p 265. London, Butterworth, 1972
108. Cortes EP, et al: Amputation and Adriamycin in primary osteosarcoma. N Engl J Med 291:998, 1974
109. Coventry MB, Dahlin DC: Osteogenic sarcoma: A critical analysis of 430 cases. J Bone Joint Surg 39A:741, 1957
110. Dahlin DC, Coventry MB: Osteogenic sarcoma: A study of 600 cases. J Bone Joint Surg 49B:101, 1967
111. Diamandopoulas GT: Induction of lymphocytic leukemia, lymphosarcoma, reticulum cell sarcoma, and osteogenic sarcoma in the Syrian golden hamster by oncogenic DNA simian virus 40. JNCI 50:1347, 1973
112. Djerassi I: Methotrexate infusions and intensive supportive care in the management of children with acute lymphocytic leukemia: Follow-up report. Cancer Res 27:256, 1967
113. Djerassi I, et al: Long-term remissions in childhood leukemia. Use of infrequent infusions of methotrexate. Supportive role of platelet transfusions and citrovorum factor. Clin Pediatr 5:502, 1966
114. Fine G, Stout AP: Osteogenic sarcoma of the extra-skeletal soft tissues. Cancer 9:1027, 1956
115. Finkel MP, Biskis BO, Farrell C: Nonmalignant and malignant changes in hamsters inoculated with extracts of human osteosarcomas. Radiology 92:1546, 1969
116. Finkel MP, Biskis BO, Jinkins PB: Virus induction of osteosarcomas in mice. Science 151:698, 1966
117. Friedlaender GE, Mitchell MS: A virally induced osteosarcoma in rats. J Bone Joint Surg 58A:295, 1970
118. Fujinaga S, et al: Light and electron microscopic studies of osteosarcomas induced in rats and hamsters by Harvey and Moloney sarcoma viruses. Cancer Res 30:1698, 1970
119. Geschickter CF, Copeland MM: Osteogenic sarcoma. In Tumors of Bone and Soft Tissues (8th Annual Clinical Conference on Cancer, 1963), p 299. Chicago, Year Book, 1965
120. Gilmer WS, MacEwen GD: Central (medullary) fibrosarcoma of bone. J Bone Joint Surg 40A:121, 1958
121. Goldie JW, Price LA, Harrap KR: Methotrexate toxicity and correlation with duration of administration, plasma levels, dose and excretion patterns. Eur J Cancer 8409, 1972
122. Henderson ED, Dahlin DC: Chondrosarcoma of bone. J Bone Joint Surg 45A:1450, 1963
123. Huvos AG, Higinbotham NL, Miller TR: Bone sarcomas arising in fibrous dysplasia. J Bone Joint Surg 54A:1047, 1972
124. Ikemoto K, Yamamoto T: Induction of rat osteosarcoma by inoculation of murine sarcoma virus into bone marrow. Gan 63:141, 1972
125. Jaffe JL: Tumors and Tumorous Conditions of the Bones and Joints. Philadelphia, Lea & Febiger, 1958
126. Jaffe N: Recent advances in the chemotherapy of metastatic osteogenic sarcoma. Cancer 30:1627, 1972
127. Jaffe N, Frei E III, Traggis D et al: Adjuvant methotrexate and citrovorum-factor in osteogenic sarcoma. N Engl J Med 291:994, 1974
128. Jaffe N, Watts HG: Multidrug chemotherapy in primary treatment of osteosarcoma. J Bone Joint Surg 58A:634, 1976
129. Janes JM, Higgins GM, Herrick JF: Beryllium-induced osteogenic sarcoma in rabbits. J Bone Joint Surg 38A:809, 1956
130. Johnson RJ, Bonfiglio M, Cooper RR: Osteosarcoma. Clin Orthop 78:314, 1971
131. Kano–Tanaka K, et al: Different neoplastic response of mice

and rats to infection by murine sarcoma virus (Moloney). Gan 63:445, 1972
132. Kolodny A: Bone sarcoma. Surg Gynecol Obstet (Suppl) 1:71, 1927
133. Lee ES, MacKenzie DH: A study of the value of preoperative megavoltage radiotherapy. Br J Surg 51:252, 1964
134. Lewis RJ, Lotz MJ: Medullary extension of osteosarcoma: Implications for rational therapy. Cancer 33:271, 1974
135. Lichtenstein L: Bone Tumors, 3rd ed. St Louis, CV Mosby, 1965
136. Lockshin MD, Higgins TT: Prognosis in osteosarcoma. Clin Orthop 58:85, 1968
137. McLeod JJ, Dahlin DC, Ivins JC: Fibrosarcoma of bone. Am J Surg 94:431, 1957
138. Marcove RC, et al: Osteogenic sarcoma under the age of 21: A review of 145 operative cases. J Bone Joint Surg 52A:411, 1970
139. Marcove RC, et al: Osteogenic sarcoma in childhood. NY State J Med 71:855, 1971
140. Marcove RC, Martini N, Rosen G: The treatment of pulmonary metastasis in osteogenic sarcoma. Clin Orthop 111:65, 1975
141. Poretta CA, Dahlin DC, Janes JM: Sarcoma in Paget's disease of bone. J Bone Joint Surg 39A:1314, 1957
142. Price CHG: The incidence of osteogenic sarcoma in Southwest England and its relationship to Paget's disease of bone. J Bone Joint Surg 44B:366, 1962
143. Price CHG, Jeffree GM: Metastatic spread of osteosarcoma. Br J Cancer 28:515, 1973
144. Price CHG, et al: Osteosarcoma in children. J Bone Joint Surg 57B:141, 1975
145. Rosen G, et al: High-dose methotrexate with citrovorum-factor rescue and adriamycin in childhood osteogenic sarcoma. Cancer 33:1151, 1974
146. Rosen G, et al: The rationale for multiple drug chemotherapy in the treatment of osteogenic sarcoma. Cancer 35:936, 1975
147. Rosen G, et al: Chemotherapy, en bloc resection, and prosthetic bone replacement in the treatment of osteogenic sarcoma. Cancer 37:1, 1976
148. Rosen G, Tan C, et al: Vincristine, high dose methotrexate with citrovorum factor rescue, cyclophosphamide, and adriamycin cyclic therapy following surgery in childhood osteogenic sarcoma. Proc Am Assoc Clin Oncol 15:172, 1974
149. Schatzki SC, Dudley HR: Bone sarcoma complicating Paget's disease: A report of 3 cases with long survival. Cancer 14:517, 1961
150. Schwartz T, Alpert M: The malignant transformation of fibrous dysplasia. Am J Med Sci 247:1, 1964
151. Skipper HE, Schabel FM Jr, Wilcox WS: Experimental evaluation of potential anticancer agents. XIII. On the criteria and kinetics associated with "curability" of experimental leukemia. Cancer Chemother Rep (Part 1) 35:1, 1964
152. Soehner RL, Dmochowski L: Induction of bone tumors in rats and hamsters with murine sarcoma virus and their cell-free transmission. Nature 224:191, 1969
153. Soehner RL, Fujinaga S, Dmochowski L: Neoplastic bone lesions induced in rats and hamsters by Moloney and Harvey murine sarcoma viruses. In Dutcher RM (ed): Comparative Leukemia Research, 1969, p 593. New York, Karger, 1970
154. Spanos RK, et al: Pulmonary resection for metastatic osteogenic sarcoma. J Bone Joint Surg 58A:624, 1976
155. Stanton MF: Primary tumors of bone and lung in rats following local deposition of cupric-chelated N-hydroxy-2-acetylaminofluorene. Cancer Res 27:1000, 1967
156. Stewart SE, Eddy BE, Irwin M, et al: Development of resistance in mice to tumor induction by SE polyoma virus. Nature 186:615, 1960
157. Suit HD: Radiotherapy in osteosarcoma. Clin Orthop 111:71, 1975
158. Sutow WW, et al: Evaluation of chemotherapy with metastatic Ewing's sarcoma and osteogenic sarcoma. Cancer Chemother Rep 55:67, 1971
159. Sutow WW, et al: Multidrug chemotherapy in primary treatment of osteosarcoma. J Bone Joint Surg 58A:629, 1976
160. Sweetnam R: Amputation in osteosarcoma. J Bone Joint Surg 55B:189, 1973
161. Sweetnam R: The surgical management of primary osteosarcoma. Clin Orthop 111:57, 1975
162. Sweetnam R, Knowelden J, Seddon H: Bone sarcoma: Treatment by irradiation, amputation or a combination of the two. Br Med J 2:363, 1971
163. Tapp E: Beryllium induced sarcomas of the rabbit tibia. Br J Cancer 20:778, 1966
164. van der Heul RO, von Ronnen JR: Juxtacortical osteosarcoma: Diagnosis, differential diagnosis, treatment and an analysis of 80 cases. J Bone Joint Surg 49A:415, 1967
165. Vaughan J: The effects of radiation on bone. In Bourne GH (ed): The Biochemistry and Physiology of Bone, p 485. New York, Academic Press, 1971
166. Zager RF, Frieby SA, Oliviero VT: The effects of antibiotics and cancer chemotherapeutic agents on the cellular transport and antitumor activity of methotrexate in L1210 murine leukemia. Cancer Res 33:1670, 1973

Osteoid Osteoma

167. Bergstrand H: Über eine eigenartige, warscheinlich bisher nicht beschreibene osteoblastiche Krankheit in den langen Knochen der Hand und des Fusses. Acta Radiol 11:597, 1930
168. Gore DP, Mueller HA: Osteoid osteoma of the spine with localization aided by 99mTc-polyphosphate bone scan: Case report. Clin Orthop 113:132, 1975
169. Jaffe HL: Osteoid osteoma: A benign osteoblastic tumor composed of osteoid and atypical bone. Arch Surg 31:709, 1935
170. Sherman MS: Osteoid osteoma. J Bone Joint Surg 29:918, 1947
171. Reis ND, et al: High-resolution computerized tomography in clinical orthopaedics. J Bone Joint Surg 64B:20, 1982
172. Winter PF, et al: Scintigraphic detection of osteoid osteoma. Radiology 122:177, 1977

Benign Osteoblastoma

173. Dahlin DC, Johnson EW: Giant osteoid osteoma. J Bone Joint Surg 36A:509, 1954
174. Golding JSR, Sissons HA: Osteogenic fibroma of bone. J Bone Joint Surg 36B:428, 1954
175. Jaffe HL: Benign osteoblastoma. Bull Hosp Joint Dis 17:141, 1956
176. Lichtenstein L: Benign osteoblastoma. Cancer 9:1044, 1956
177. Marsh BW, et al: Benign osteoblastoma: Range of manifestations. J Bone Joint Surg 57A:1, 1975
178. Schajowicz F, Lemos C: Osteoid-osteoma and osteoblastoma. Acta Orthop Scand 41:272, 1970

Parosteal Osteogenic Sarcoma

179 Ackerman LV, Spjut HJ:Tumors of bone and cartilage. In Atlas of Tumor Pathology, Sec II, Fascicle 4, p 91. Washington, DC, Armed Forces Institute of Pathology, 1962
180. Ahuja SC, et al: Juxtacortical (parosteal) osteogenic sarcoma: Histologic grading and prognosis. J Bone Joint Surg 59A:632, 1977
181. Dahlin DC: Bone Tumors: General Aspects and an Analysis of 2,276 Cases. Springfield, IL, Charles C Thomas, 1957
182. Geschickter CF, Copeland MM: Parosteal osteoma of bone: A new entity. Ann Surg 133:790, 1951
183. Jaffe HL: Tumors and Tumorous Conditions of the Bones and Joints. Philadelphia, Lea & Febiger, 1958
184. Scaglietti O, Calandriello B: Ossifying parosteal sarcoma, parosteal osteoma or juxtacortical osteogenic sarcoma. J Bone Joint Surg 44A:635, 1962
185. Stevens GM, Pugh DG, Dahlin DC: Roentgenographic recognition and differentiation of parosteal osteogenic sarcoma. Am J Roentgenol 78:1, 1957
186. van der Heul RO: Het periostale ossificerende fibrosarcoom en de gradering van osteosarcomen. Thesis, Leiden, 1962
187. van der Heul RO, von Ronnen JR: Juxtacortical osteosarcoma. J Bone Joint Surg 49A:415, 1967

Ewing's Sarcoma

188. Bacci G, et al: The treatment of localized Ewing's sarcoma. Cancer 49:1561, 1982
189. Campbell WC, Hamilton JF: Gradation of Ewing's tumor. J Bone Joint Surg 23:869, 1941
190. Coley WB: Endothelial myeloma or Ewing's sarcoma. Am J Surg 27:7, 1935
191. Ewing J: Endothelial myeloma of bone. Proc New York Pathol Soc 24:93, 1924
192. Geschickter CF, Copeland MM, Maseritz IH: Ewing's sarcoma. J Bone Joint Surg 21:26, 1939
193. Jaffe HL: Pathology, problem of Ewing's sarcoma. Bull Hosp Joint Dis 6:82, 1945
194. Kolodny A: Bone sarcoma. Surg Gynecol Obstet 44:126, 1927
195. Suit HD et al: Radiation therapy and multi-drug chemotherapy. In Price CHG, Ross FGM (eds): Bone—Certain Aspects of Neoplasia. London, Butterworth, 1973
196. Willis RA: Metastatic neuroblastoma of bone presenting the Ewing's syndrome, with a discussion of Ewing's sarcoma. Am J Pathol 16:317, 1940

Fibrosarcoma

197. Budd JW, MacDonald I: Osteogenic sarcoma: A modified nomenclature and review of 118 five-year cures. Surg Gynecol Obstet 77:413, 1943
198. Coley BL: Neoplasms of Bone and Related Conditions, New York, Hoeber, 1949
199. Ewing J: A review of the classification of bone tumors. Surg Gynecol Obstet 68:971, 1939
200. Phemister DB: Cancer of bone and joint. JAMA 136:545, 1948

Histiocytic Lymphoma

201. Khanolkar VR: Reticulum cell sarcoma of bone. Arch Pathol 46:467, 1948
202. Parker F Jr, Jackson H Jr: Primary reticulum cell sarcoma of bone. Surg Gynecol Obstet 68:45, 1939
202A. Reimer RR, Chabner BA, Young RC et al: Lymphoma presenting in bone. Results of histopathology, staging and therapy. Ann Int Med 87:50, 1977
203. Schajowicz F: Ewing's sarcoma and reticulum cell sarcoma of bone. J Bone Joint Surg 41A:349, 1959
204. Sherman RS, Snyder RE: The roentgen appearance of primary reticulum cell sarcoma of bone. Am J Roentgenol 58:291, 1947
204A. Sweet DL, Golcomb HM: Treatment of histiocytic lymphoma. Sem Oncol 7:302, 1980
204B. Sweet DL, Mass DP, Simon MA et al: Histiocytic lymphoma (reticulum-cell sarcoma) of bone. J Bone Joint Surg 63A:79, 1981
205. Valls J, Muscolo D, Schajowicz F: Reticulum-cell sarcoma of bone. J Bone Joint Surg 34B:588, 1952

Multiple Myeloma

206. Cohen IM, Svien HJ, Dahlin DC: Long term survival of patients with myeloma of the vertebral column. JAMA 187:914, 1964
207. Davison C, Baker BH: Myeloma and its neural complications. Arch Surg 35:913, 1937
208. Geschickter CF, Copeland MM: Multiple myeloma. Arch Surg 16:807, 1928
209. Griffiths DL: Orthopaedic aspects of myelomatosis. J Bone Joint Surg 48B:703, 1966
210. Kolodny A: Bone sarcoma. Surg Gynecol Obstet 44:126, 1927
211. Rosenthal N, Vogel P: Value of sternal puncture in multiple myeloma. J Mt Sinai Hosp 4:1001, 1938
212. Valderrama JAF, Bullough PG: Solitary myeloma of the spine. J Bone Joint Surg 50:82, 1968
213. Waldenstrom J: Melphalan therapy in myelomatosis. Br Med J 1:859, 1964

Liposarcoma

214. Stewart FW: Primary liposarcoma of bone. Am J Pathol 14:621, 1938

Adamantinoma

215. Baker PL, Dockerty MB, Coventry MB: Adamantinoma (so-called) of the long bones. J Bone Joint Surg 36A:704, 1954
216. Bullough PG, Goldberg VM: Multicentric origin of adamantinoma of the tibia: A case report. Rev Hosp Spec Surg 1:71, 1971
217. Fischer B: Über ein primäres Adamantinomm der Tibia. Frankfurt Zeitschr f Pathol 12:422, 1913
218. Huves AG, Marcove RC: Adamantinoma of long bones. J Bone Joint Surg 57A:148, 1975
219. Lichtenstein L: Dermal inclusion tumors in bone (so-called adamantinoma of limb bones). In Bone Tumors, 4th ed. St Louis, CV Mosby, 1972
220. Mangalik VS, Mehrotra RMI: Adamantinoma of the tibia: Report of a case. Br J Surg 39:429, 1952
221 Morgan AD, Mackenzie DH: A metastasizing adamantinoma of the tibia. J Bone Joint Surg 38B:892, 1956
222. Naji AF, et al: So-called adamantinoma of long bones: Report of a case with massive pulmonary metastasis. J Bone Joint Surg 46A:151, 1964

Chordoma

223. Friedman M, Hine GJ, Dresner J: Principles of supervoltage rotation therapy, illustrated by treatment of a chordoma of a vertebra. Radiology 64:1, 1955
224. Gentil F, Coley BL: Sacrococcygeal chordoma. Ann Surg 127:432, 1948
225. Mabrey RE: Chordoma: A study of 150 cases. Am J Cancer 25:501, 1935
226. Wood EH Jr, Himadi GM: Chordoma: Roentgenologic study. Radiology 54:706, 1950

Hemangioma of Bone

227. Bell RL: Hemangioma of a dorsal vertebra with collapse and compression myelopathy. J Neurosurg 12:570, 1955
228. Bucy PC: Hemangioma of bone. Am J Pathol 5:381, 1929
229. Bucy PC, Capp CS: Primary hemangioma of bone. Am J Roentgenol 22:1, 1930
230. Meyerding HW: Hemangioma of bone. J Bone Joint Surg 18:617, 1936
231. Reeves DL: Vertebral hemangioma with compression of the spinal cord. J Neurosurg 21:710, 1964.
232. Ribbert H: Geschurulstlehre, p 201. Bonn, Friedrich Cohen, 1914
233. Ritchie G, Zeier FG: Hemangiomatosis of the skeleton and spleen. J Bone Joint Surg 38A:115, 1956
234. Schafer PW: Pathology in General Surgery, pp 26, 120. Chicago, University of Chicago Press, 1950
235. Thomas A: Vascular tumors of bone. Surg Gynecol Obstet 74:777, 1942;

Hemangioendothelioma

236. Allen EV, Barker NW, Hines EA: Peripheral Vascular Diseases. Philadelphia, WB Saunders, 1946
237. Copeland MM, Geschickter CF: Tumors of Bone. Philadelphia, JB Lippincott, 1949
238. Gordon–Taylor G, Wiles P: Pulsating angio-endothelioma of the innominate bone treated by hindquarter amputation. J Bone Joint Surg 31B:410, 1949
239. Luck JV: Bone and Joint Diseases. Springfield, IL, Charles C Thomas, 1950
240. Resink JEJ: Case of skeletal hemangioendothelioma. Fortschr Geb Röntgenstr 80:732, 1954
241. Thomas A: Vascular tumors of bone. Surg Gynecol Obstet 74:777, 1942

Identification of Endothelial Tissues

242. Maximow AA, Bloom W: Textbook of Histology. Philadelphia, WB Saunders, 1958
243. Thomas A: Vascular tumors of bone. Surg Gynecol Obstet 74:777, 1942

16

Secondary Tumors of Bones

CHARACTERISTICS

Secondary neoplastic growths of bones, as the name implies, are cancerous tumors, originating in other organs and involving the skeletal structures of the body.

Bones may become involved by secondary tumors by direct invasion from contiguous growths, and by blood-borne metastases. According to Willis' definition, metastasis is a secondary growth originating from a detached tumor fragment.[6] Thus, invasion by a contiguous growth cannot be considered a true metastasis. It should also be mentioned that some authors have suggested the possibility of bone metastases by the lymphatic channels.[4] However, the following circumstances are against the possibility of lymph-borne metastases.[6]

Evidence Against Lymph-Borne Metastases

1. Lymphatics have not been demonstrated in bone marrow.
2. Cancerous permeation of the lymphatics of the periosteum is found rarely, and solely at the level of the foramina.
3. Metastases in bones and in adjacent lymph nodes coexist in only a minority of cases and such coexistence is often clearly accidental.
4. There is indubitable evidence that the distribution of metastatic growths in bones depends on the normal or pathologic distribution of the red bone marrow and the peculiarities of the venous system[1,2,5] and is unrelated to the location of the primary growth.

Therefore, it is generally accepted today that the true embolic bone metastases are blood borne; furthermore, that "the distribution of metastases in the bones depends almost exclusively on the arrangement of the blood vessels into which tumor emboli are released and by means of which they gain entrance to the capillary beds."[3]

DIRECT NONMETASTATIC INVASION FROM CONTIGUOUS GROWTHS

Meningiomas and craniopharyngiomas, although considered essentially benign tumors, may erode and invade the bones of the skull. The facial bones, the mandible, the hyoid bone, and occasionally the base of the skull and the cervical vertebrae may be invaded by ulcerating cutaneous, oral, or pharyngeal carcinomas or by their cervical lymph node metastases. Carcinoma of the nasal mucosa, especially of the antrum, may result in extensive

* Original tables, microphotographs, and photographs of gross specimens are from the Museum of Pathology, Presbyterian St. Luke's Hospital, Chicago.

destruction and perforation of the adjacent bones. More unusual cases include carcinoma of the ethmoid invading the cranial bones, and melanoma of the eye invading the orbital bones. The thoracic skeleton may suffer direct invasion from mammary, pulmonary, or esophageal carcinomas. Mammary carcinoma mainly spreads into the adjacent ribs, whereas carcinoma of the esophagus often invades the vertebral bodies. In these cases, ulceration and secondary infection of the cancerous growths markedly accelerate bone destruction (Fig. 16-1). In noninfected tumors, the periosteum or perichondrium constitute a most effective barrier to tumor extension. Pelvic bones may be invaded by carcinomas of the urinary bladder or of the uterine cervix. Rarely, an ovarian carcinoma or a carcinoma of the rectum may invade the sacrum and the coccyx by contiguity. Other tumors reported in the literature as invading the bones are carcinoma of the salivary glands invading the mandible; chordoma invading the sacrum, the vertebrae, or the base of the skull; and sarcoma of adjacent soft tissues, chondrosarcoma, and synovioma invading the long bones.

Direct bone invasion from contiguous growths has little clinical importance. As a rule, these tumors do not present difficult diagnostic problems, and their spread is usually beyond the reach of therapeutic measures. The symptoms depend on the location of the primary growth, its extension, and the structures involved.

FIG. 16-1. Metastatic carcinoma of the lumbar vertebrae with secondary infection (primary in the urinary bladder). Note extension into the intervertebral disk.

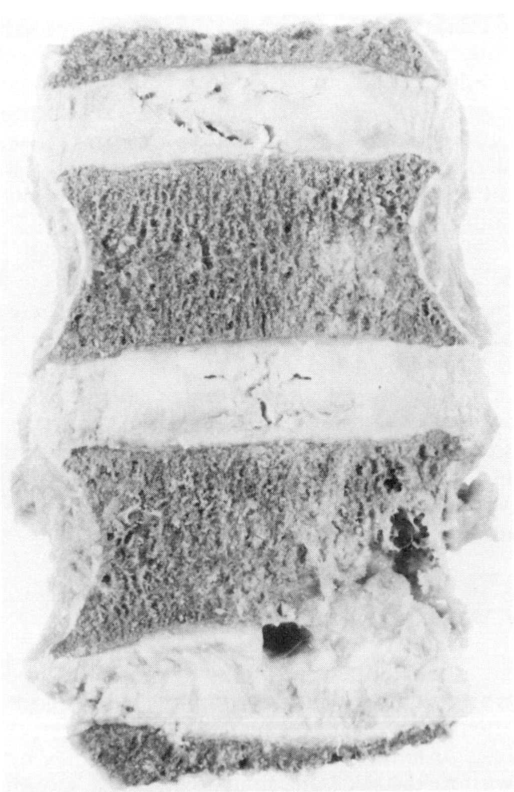

BONE METASTASES

Blood-borne metastases to the bone greatly outnumber primary bone tumors to such an extent that after 40 years of age every bone tumor must be considered metastatic unless proven otherwise.[57] Moreover, the actual incidence of metastatic disease is greatly underestimated. In 1000 autopsies of known carcinoma, an incidence of 27% was reported,[7] and recent studies have shown that approximately 35% of malignant disease is associated with dissemination to the skeleton.[36,67] Since the usual autopsy provides limited access to the bone, even greater percentages are probable. Jaffe stated that if all the bones were sampled adequately, the chance of finding skeletal metastases in patients dying of malignant neoplasm is 70% and in those patients with carcinomas that commonly metastasize to the bone, the overall chance of metastasis would approximate 85%.[33] It is of considerable importance to note that histologic sections of material obtained by needle aspiration of the marrow at autopsy revealed carcinoma in only 10%.

In Table 16-1, the tendency "percentagewise" of various tumors to metastasize to bone is demonstrated. More recent studies from the Armed Forces Institute of Pathology quote the following figures: 73% of carcinoma of the breast, 32% of carcinoma of the lung, 24% of carcinoma of the kidney, 13% of carcinoma of the rectum, and 11% with carcinoma of the stomach have histologic evidence of metastasis to the bone at autopsy.[65] No figures on prostatic carcinoma were available.

The mechanism by which destruction or production of bone is brought about by a metastatic tumor is unexplained. It is theorized that bone is destroyed by two mechanisms: the mechanical effect of expansion of the tumor and a destructive substance elaborated by the tumor. Bone production mechanisms are postulated as being effected by bone being reactively stimulated to effect repair and by diffusible products from the tumor cells (Willis).

Metastatic growths may appear in any part of the skeleton and even in heterotopic bone. However, von Recklinghausen's conclusions[69] regarding the most probable sites for localization of skeletal metastases are still valid. These sites are the vertebrae, ribs, pelvis, proximal ends of the femur and humerus, sternum, and skull vault.[70] These are the regions where red marrow is found in the adult. It is unusual for metastatic neoplasms to involve bones distal to the elbows and knees, but exceptions do occur, and metastases to the small bones of the hand and foot are being reported with increasing frequency.[28,29,62]

The propensity of a miscellaneous group of malignancies to metastasize to various sites is illustrated by Table 16-2.

TABLE 16-1 Incidence of Skeletal Metastases According to the Location of the Primary Growth*†

Site of Primary Growth	Number of Cases	Number of Cases with Skeletal Metastases	Percentage
Mammary gland	85	40	47.0
Prostate	42	19	45.2
Kidney	31	9	29.0
Lung	187	43	22.9
Thyroid	9	2	22.2
Liver	21	4	19.0
Urinary bladder	45	7	15.5
Uterine cervix	34	5	14.7
Pancreas	42	4	9.5
Stomach	108	8	7.4
Large bowel	166	10	6.0
Other sites	225	25	11.1

* Excluding lymphomas

† This material, collected at autopsy at St. Luke's Hospital, Chicago, in a 15-year period (1940–1954) consisted of a total of 1237 cancerous growths. From this group were excluded 42 cases of leukemia and multiple myeloma and 137 cases of brain tumors, which do not metastasize. Among the remaining 1058 cases, 213 had metastases in the bones for an incidence of 20.1%.

TABLE 16-2 Distribution and Incidence of Bone Metastases in 176 Cases of Malignancy (Excluding Lymphomas)

Sites	Number of Cases with Metastases
Spine	122
Ribs	88
Skull	21
Pelvis	18
Sternum	18
Femur	13
Humerus	8
Others	12

Ordinarily, metastases are uncommon below the knees or the elbows, but numerous exceptions do occur (Fig. 16-2).[27] Cases have been reported of metastatic epidermoid carcinoma of the lung in a terminal phalanx, carcinoma of the breast in small bones of the feet, carcinoma of the cervix in the lower end of the tibia, and carcinoma of the colon in the bones of the hands and feet.

CLINICAL PICTURE

Clinically, pain, pathologic fractures, and anemia are important features. The location, the frequency, the radiation, and other characteristics of the pain depend on the bone involved. When the skull is involved, headache may result. Metastatic growths of the spine, by compressing the nerve roots or the spinal cord, cause girdle pains and neurologic manifestations. Numbness of the legs or the arms, objective loss of sensation, spastic paralysis or weakness of the extremities, loss of vesical control, and weakness of the rectal sphincter are observed. Metastatic deposits in the bones of the extremities produce pain, swelling, and tenderness. Metastases in the ribs and the sternum, on the whole, are frequently silent. Small growths may be asymptomatic or may produce mild and transient pain which attracts little notice. Such cases are often discovered fortuitously during roentgenographic study for other diseases. Conversely, when metastases are voluminous or located in an area which is subject to pressure, the onset may be sudden and characterized by intense pain.

Pathologic fractures are frequent especially, it is stated, when the femur is involved, but pathologic fractures of the ribs are equally frequent. As the disease progresses and skeletal involvement becomes more widespread, destruction of the vertebral bodies produces impaction and collapse of the vertebrae. However, osteoplastic metastases progress more slowly than the unossified forms, and pathologic fractures are less frequent. In the terminal stages of the disease, emaciation, anemia, and pathologic fractures, often with considerable pain, predominate the picture.

LABORATORY DIAGNOSIS

Metastatic bone marrow involvement may be associated with a perfectly normal complete blood count. However, anemia, thrombocytopenia or thrombocytosis, leukocytosis or leukopenia, and eosinophilia may be associated with metastatic bone marrow deposits. Occasionally, the

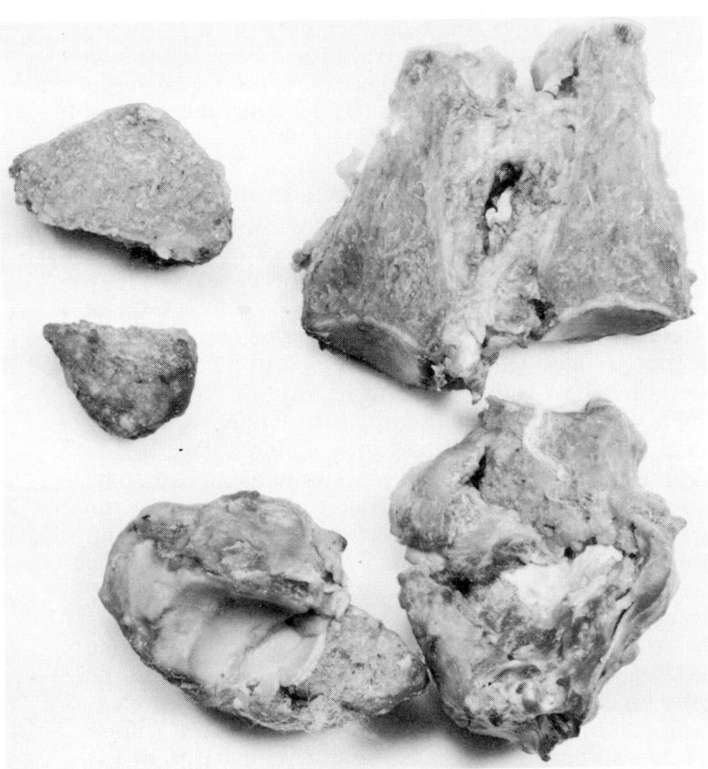

FIG. 16-2. Metastatic carcinoma of the lower epiphysis of the radius and of the small bones of the hand (primary in the lung).

anemia may be associated with a leukoerythroblastic peripheral blood exhibiting immature granulocytes and nucleated red blood cells.[56] A syndrome characterized by severe hemolytic anemia with irregularly contracted red blood cells, thrombocytopenia, and fibrinogenopenia can be seen with carcinomas of the stomach, pancreas, breast, or lung.[63,64] Metastases in this syndrome are often microscopic and associated with tumor thrombi in small vessels. In such instances the bone marrow and lung show the most extensive metastases.[34] The importance of the microangiopathy for the hemolytic anemia in this syndrome was stressed by Brain and associates.[17] This syndrome is an example of a consumptive coagulopathy caused by disseminated intravascular coagulation.[43]

Other laboratory studies helpful in the diagnosis of metastatic bone marrow disease include an elevated serum calcium and alkaline phosphatase. An elevated serum or bone marrow acid phosphatase is helpful for the diagnosis of metastatic prostatic carcinoma. Skeletal scans with radionuclides are also helpful.

In cases of anemia due to cancerous replacement of the bone marrow, compensatory heterotopic myeloid hemopoiesis has been observed in the spleen and in the liver.

Open needle biopsy and aspiration biopsy offer valuable aids to diagnosis and are actually the only procedures that can be depended on in determining conclusively the type of growth. However, even open biopsies often present difficult diagnostic problems, especially in locating the primary focus, and some cases must await a thorough postmortem examination for solution.[31]

Marrow aspiration has been used in the diagnosis of metastatic bone cancer.[35,47] Sites of marrow aspiration are selected by preference in areas of bone pains, tenderness, and roentgenographic or bone scan abnormality. Marrow sections are much preferable to marrow spreads.[9] Tumor implants are found in about one half of the patients with malignant disease—most frequently in patients with carcinoma of the lung, prostate, or breast. Such procedure has been recommended to establish the diagnosis of widespread cancer, especially in cases in which extensive surgery is being contemplated.

ROENTGENOGRAPHIC FINDINGS

The great majority of skeletal metastases are not demonstrable roentgenographically.[57,70] In a minority of cases, they bring about grossly visible bone lesions, of which two types are recognized: the osteolytic, which is more frequent, and the osteoplastic. The latter is not uncommon in metastases from carcinoma of the prostate. Osteolytic lesions appear as irregular or sharply circumscribed areas of reduced density with little evidence of repair. There is practically no periosteal reaction. Mottling with increased density of the bone occurs within the area of destruction, and thickening of the cortex appears above or below the site of metastasis. This reaction is often marked after roentgen therapy over the affected bone. When mottling occurs within an area of destruction in the bone, it favors the presence of metastatic processes as opposed to the more definitely punched-out areas of destruction seen in multiple myeloma.

Osteoplastic metastases appear as areas of increased density, often accompanied by periosteal reaction. The bones assume a mottled or marbled appearance.

A solitary area of metastatic carcinoma must be differentiated from a latent cyst of the bone, a solitary focus of multiple myeloma, and the osteolytic form of osteogenic sarcoma. A latent cyst of bone occurs usually in the younger age group, is confined to the interior of the bone, has distinct signs of ossification in the bone shell, and usually symptoms are minimal. A solitary focus of multiple myeloma can be differentiated by the abnormal pattern of the plasma proteins and in some cases by the presence of Bence-Jones protein in the urine. Pulmonary metastases, when present, rule out multiple myeloma. The osteolytic form of osteogenic sarcoma has a greater tendency to be asymmetrically located in the bone, and there is evidence of more rapid destruction and periosteal reaction. If the single bone metastasis is from a renal carcinoma, which is often the case, an examination of the patient will disclose hematuria and other evidence of kidney involvement. Diffuse osteoplastic metastases must be differentiated from Paget's disease. In the latter the serum alkaline phosphatase is markedly elevated, but the serum acid phosphatase is within normal limits.

PATHOLOGY

In most instances of bone metastases the primary tumor is known, but even if we restrict bone lesions of metastatic nature to those in which the diagnosis is obscure, metastatic tumors are still the most common of all malignant bone neoplasms.[8] Metastatic growths in bones being blood borne, they are situated initially in the bone marrow.[60] Metastatic growths in the spine are situated almost invariably in the vertebral bodies, rarely in the arches or the processes. Blood-borne periosteal metastases without medullary growths are very rare and then are found only at the level of the foramina. Grossly, bone metastases appear as bone-destroying or bone-producing lesions or a mixture of these two. In the osteoclastic or osteolytic type, metastases appear as well-defined nodules of gray tumor tissue occupying and replacing the cancellous bone and bone marrow (Fig. 16-3). Cartilage constitutes an effective barrier against tumor invasion. Pathologic fractures are not infrequent, but they may heal by osseous union in a normal fashion even without treatment. In the ribs and in advanced stages, the metastatic tumor may produce a fusiform swelling, involving and replacing an entire segment of bone (Fig. 16-4). In the osteoplastic type, the affected bone is heavier and denser than normal. Marrow spaces are obliterated by the deposition of new bone, whose structure may be spongy or eburnated (Fig. 16-5). Thickenings and deformities of the bone due to subperiosteal deposition are present and may result in a diffuse nodular enlargement of the bone. Pathologic fractures rarely occur. It should be noted that carcinoma metastases, particularly from the prostate, may be of the osteoplastic type in early stages of the disease, while those developing in the same person later, and especially in the terminal stages, may be entirely of the osteolytic type.

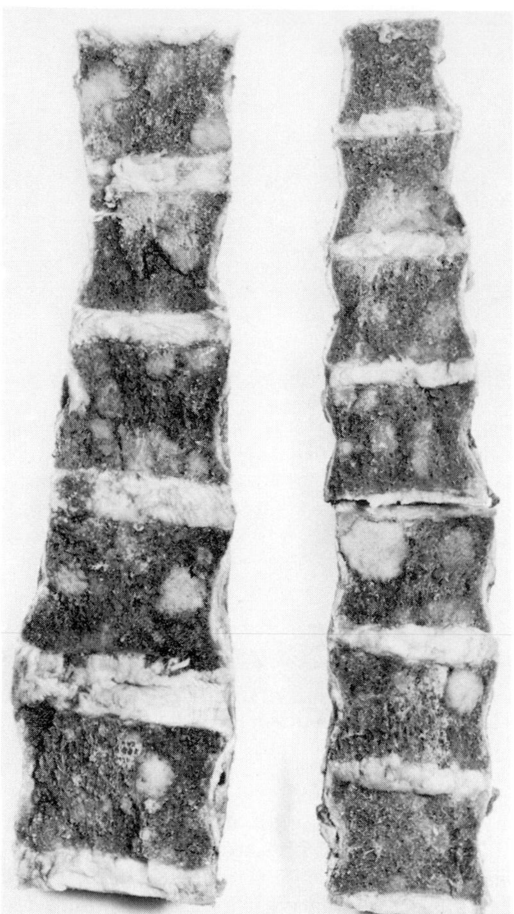

FIG. 16-3. Osteolytic metastases of the thoracic and lumbar vertebrae.

It should be emphasized that both osteoclastic and osteoblastic metastatic processes may be seen in the same histologic section, and attempts to grade the response of bone to tumor invasion[50] can be regarded as pure intellectual curiosity. In osteoclastic metastases, the cancerous growth is accompanied by proliferation of connective tissue. (Fig. 16-6), which may exceed that of the growths themselves. The margins of the tumor are surrounded by a wide zone of myelofibrosis.

Osteoplastic metastases stimulate osteogenesis on the part of the local bone, especially in the metastatic,

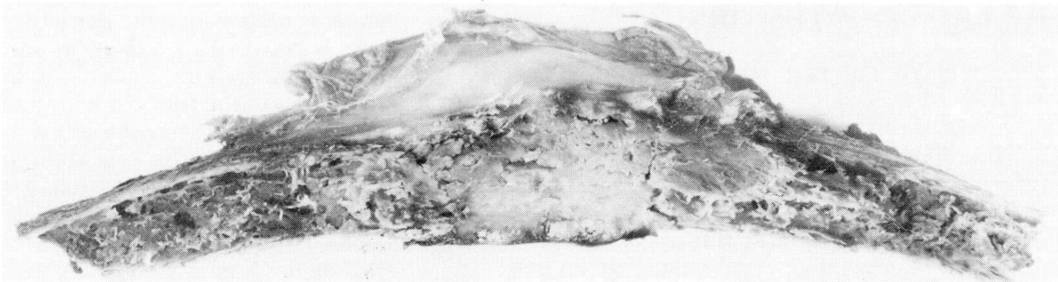

FIG. 16-4. Metastatic carcinoma of the rib (surgical specimen).

FIG. 16-5. Osteoplastic metastases of the lumbar vertebrae (primary in the prostate). The dark areas are the residues of marrow spaces.

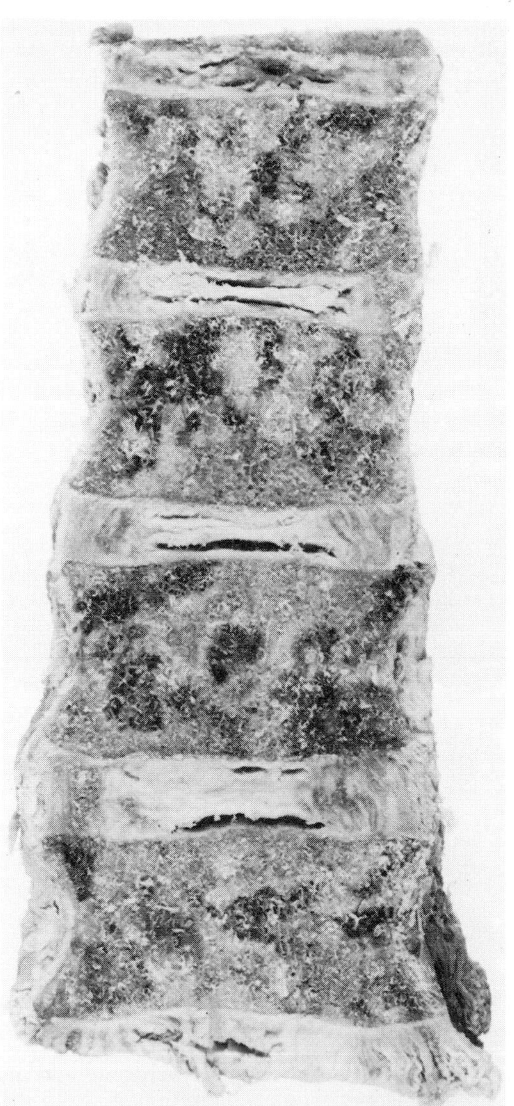

FIG. 16-6. Proliferation of connective tissue in metastatic carcinoma of bone (primary in the mammary gland). (×390)

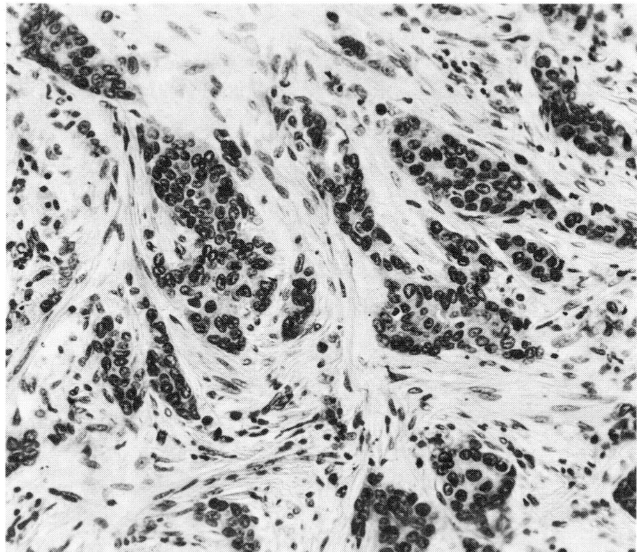

sclerosing lesions from the prostate. They are accompanied by an intense periosteal bone proliferation. The tumor cells may become enclosed in the bone, and bony tissue may be most abundant in very cellular areas of tumor cells. Extensive resorption of new bone by osteoclasts may follow the plastic process. There has been much speculation concerning the nature of the new bone formation in osteoplastic metastases, the number of theories being only slightly less than the number of investigators. According to Willis,[6] the proliferation of bone accompanying metastatic lesions is similar to the proliferation of the connective tissue stroma in desmoplastic growths or to the glial reaction to tumors invading the central nervous system. Osteoplasia, desmoplasia, and glial proliferation are similar expressions of different stromal reactions to neoplastic invasions. In fact, many osteoplastic carcinomas are also desmoplastic. Osteoplastic mammary carcinomas (always) and osteoplastic carcinomas of the prostate (often) are slow, infiltrative growths showing scirrhous characters in soft tissues.

THE PRIMARY TUMORS

CARCINOMA OF THE BREAST

Carcinoma of the breast (mammary gland) leads the list with a frequency of bone metastases of about one half of the fatal cases. The bones most frequently involved are the spine, pelvis, femur (upper third), skull, ribs, and humerus (at the junction of the upper and the middle thirds). The interval between radical mastectomy and actual roentgenographic demonstration of bone metastases is between 15 and 30 months, with an average of 19.8 months. Bone metastases are often preceded by metastases to the regional lymph nodes, and in one third of cases they are accompanied by pulmonary metastases.[47] Clinically, the appearance of metastases is characterized by severe pain that varies according to the location of the metastases. Pathologic fractures occur in almost half of the cases, more often in the vertebrae, the ribs, or the femur. Roentgenographically, from 80% to

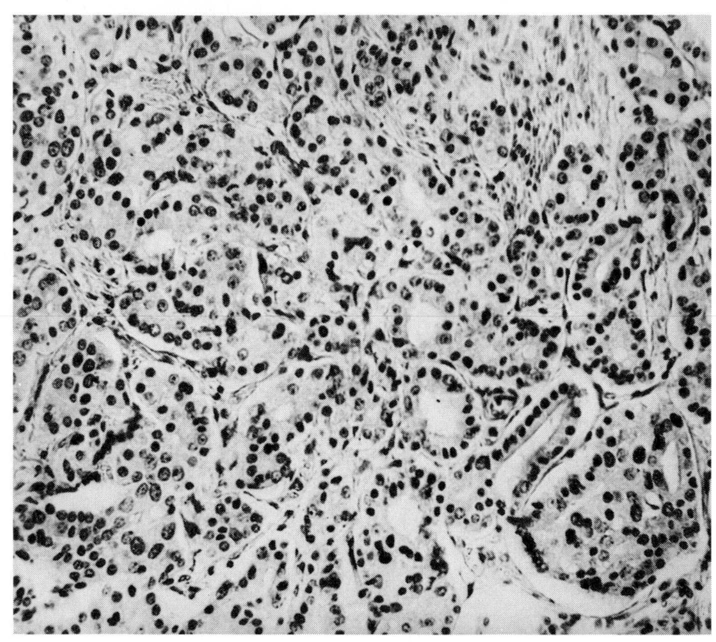

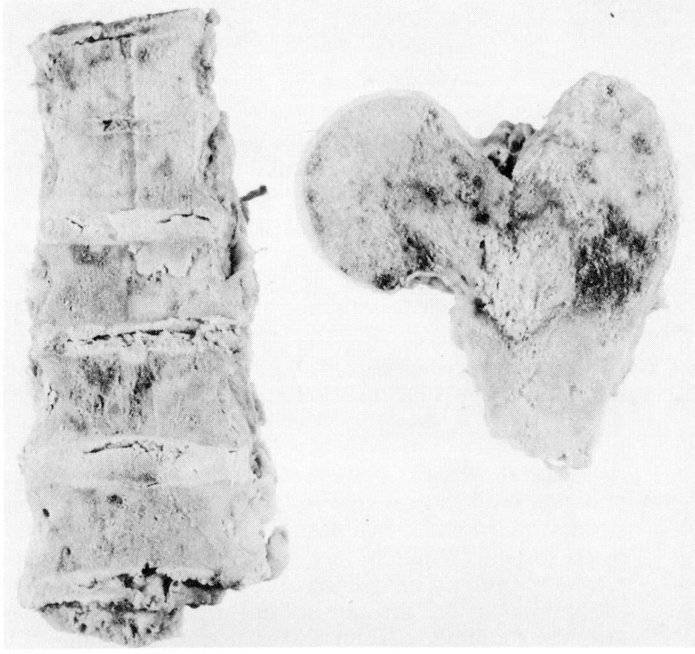

FIG. 16-7. (*Top*) Histologic appearance of carcinoma of the prostate. (×390) (*Bottom*) Extensive osteoplastic metastases of the lumbar vertebrae and upper third of the femur (primary in prostate). Note the pathologic fracture of the neck of the femur.

90% of the metastatic deposits are of the osteolytic type.[66] The diagnosis is confirmed by laboratory tests. The copper-resistant serum acid phosphatase is not only of diagnostic importance[55] but it is also an indication of the effectiveness of treatment.[42] Regressions or remissions of bone lesions are accompanied by a decrease of the serum level of the acid phosphatase and by a decreased calciuria.

CARCINOMA OF THE PROSTATE

Carcinoma of the prostate produces skeletal metastases in about 50% of cases. The bones most frequently affected are the vertebrae, femur, pelvis, skull, ribs, and sternum (Fig. 16-7). Clinically, metastatic carcinoma of the prostate is accompanied by progressive emaciation, anemia, and excruciating pains in the affected bone. Roentgenographically, the lesions are of the osteoplastic type. There is a marked increase in the density of bone with light mottling which suggests some destruction. Such metastases are accompanied by an increase of the serum acid phosphatase. As in the case of metastatic mammary carcinoma, copper-resistant acid phosphatase has a better diagnostic and prognostic value than the usual acid phosphatase.[55]

CARCINOMA OF THE KIDNEY

Bone metastases in carcinoma of the kidney occur in probably 30% to 50% of the cases (Color Plate 16-1).[28] Bones most frequently involved are the humerus, spine, femur, pelvis, ribs, foot, skull, and sternum. Pain and pathologic fractures are the main symptoms. In more than one half of the cases the secondary deposits are found as a single focus. In such cases it is imperative that the metastatic lesion be biopsied (Fig. 16-8) so that it will not be mistaken for a benign process or treated as a primary malignant bone tumor. Late bone metastases occurring up to 10 years after the removal of the primary growth are also recorded. The lesions are usually of the osteolytic type, and if the tumor extends through the bone into the soft tissue, pulsatile masses may be present.

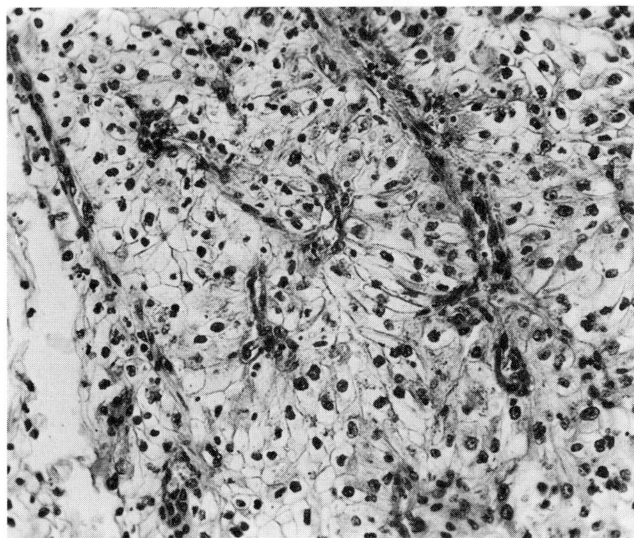

FIG. 16-8. Histologic appearance of a bone metastasis from a primary carcinoma of the kidney. (×390)

FIG. 16-9. Metastatic carcinoma of the tibia (primary in the thyroid). (×390)

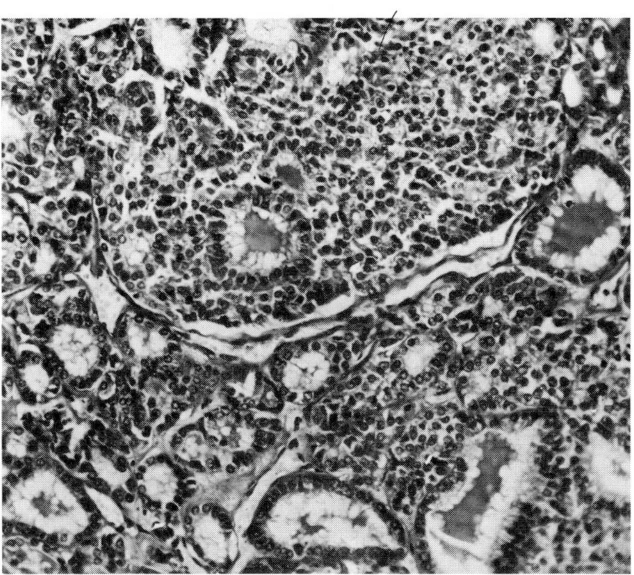

CARCINOMA OF THE THYROID

Malignant thyroid tumors have a frequency of skeletal metastases of 25% to 30%[20,25] but is much lower when well-differentiated carcinomas are included. The bones most frequently affected are the skull, ribs, sternum spine, and humerus. The metastatic growths appear at epiphyses or along sutures. As in carcinoma of the kidney, carcinoma of the thyroid may develop only a single bone metastasis, sometimes before the primary growth is detected. Conversely, a single skeletal metastasis may appear many years after removal of the primary neoplasm. As a rule, the lesions are of the osteolytic type or of the cystic type, with encrusting bony shell.[61] Diagnosis is made by biopsy (Fig. 16-9). Radioactive iodine may be used in certain instances to confirm the diagnosis.[41]

CARCINOMA OF THE LUNG

Carcinoma of the lung metastasizes to the bones with a frequency of about 40% of cases. Both bronchogenic and alveolar cell carcinomas may give rise to skeletal metas-

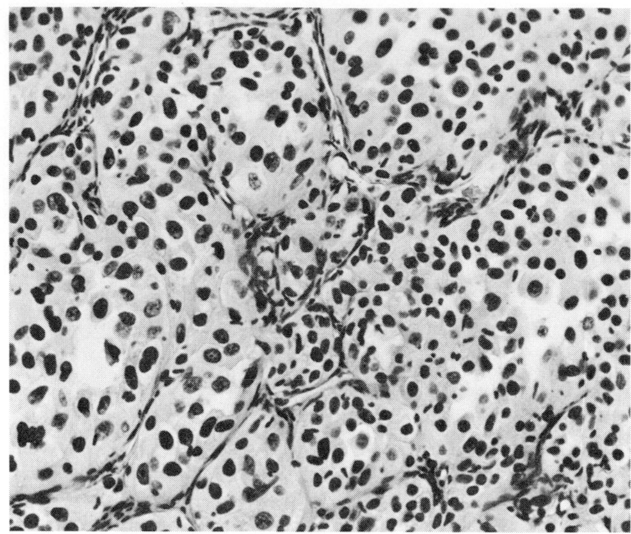

FIG. 16-10. Metastatic carcinoma of the spine (primary in the lung).

tases.[54] Such metastases are often accompanied by metastases to other organs. They are preferably located in the thoracic spine and in the ribs; less frequently in other bones. In Geschickter's series[28] the metastases involved the vertebral column in every case. Not infrequently, a small carcinoma of the lung may first reveal itself with a metastatic lesion. In such instances the microscopic pattern of the biopsy material will be the only available means to determine the diagnosis (Figs. 16-10 and 16-11). The roentgenogram is characterized by osteolytic lesions.

FIG. 16-11. Metastatic carcinoma of the tibia in a 9-year-old girl. The primary tumor was found only at autopsy, and it was located in the lung. (×390)

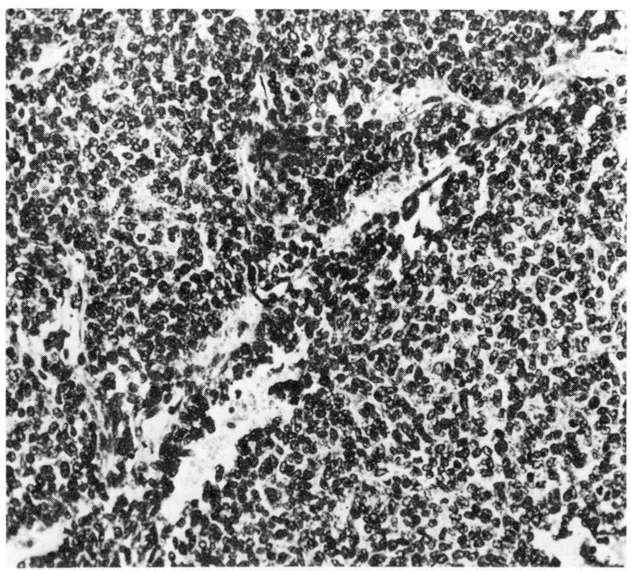

OTHER TUMORS

Skeletal metastases from other tumors are of minor clinical importance because they are usually accompanied by widespread metastases in other organs. However, there are cases of carcinoma of the stomach in which the primary growth is a small symptomless one. The bones may be the principal or only site of metastases, and the patient's illness may closely simulate pernicious anemia.[28] Metastatic carcinoma from the rectum and the pancreas (Fig. 16-12) may simulate a primary bone lesion.[13] Carcinoma of the liver[11,24] and of the urinary bladder[39] metastasizes to the bone frequently. Carcinoma of the uterus metastasizes to the bones in 5% of the cases, but the diagnosis is usually established before skeletal metastases appear. The skeleton, especially the skull with the typical brushlike appearance of the skull vault, is the favorite site of metastases from neuroblastomas. Other tumors metastasize less frequently, although the literature reports metastases from practically every primary growth, including carcinoma of the esophagus, the large intestine, the mouth or the pharynx, seminoma of the testis (particularly of the spine), retinoblastoma, chorionepithelioma, melanotic tumors,[59] carcinoma of the ovary, retroperitoneal carcinoma, salivary mixed tumor, carcinoma of the ureter, Ewing's sarcoma,[4] and even osteogenic sarcomas.[22]

Sarcomas of soft tissue origin do not as frequently involve bone. Hodgkin's disease of the lymphocytic depletion type frequently implicates bone but only in

FIG. 16-12. Metastatic carcinoma of the pelvic bones (primary in the pancreas). (×390)

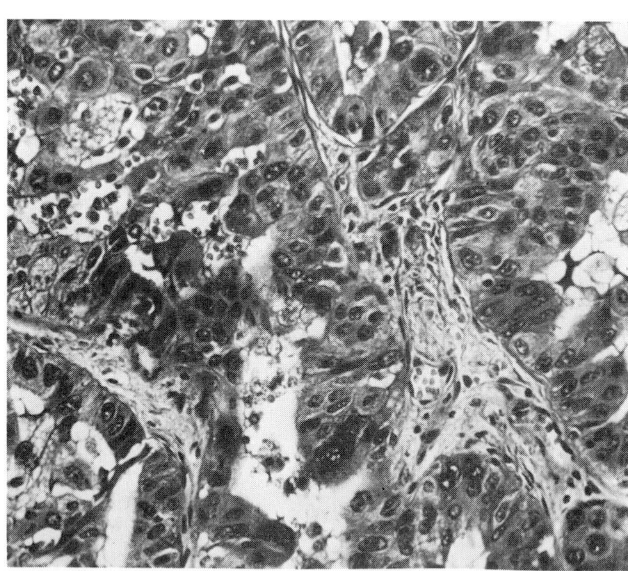

advanced cases. Lymphosarcomas may involve bone, usually as an osteolytic process, but invariably the lymphosarcoma has been noted previously and diagnosed. Metastases of many lymphosarcomas into bones, especially the small lymphocytic, but also forms of reticulum cell sarcomas, do not cause appreciable destruction of the bone structure but markedly replace the basic marrow tissue.[31]

TREATMENT

Metastatic growths in the skeleton are nearly always multiple, and when a single isolated lesion is found, it should be regarded as part of disseminated disease. In most instances, metastatic bone disease represents the advanced stage of malignant disease with little or no hope of eradication, and treatment is aimed at retarding its progression while relieving pain and preventing pathologic fractures. With the advent of megavoltage radiation and chemotherapy, the outlook for achieving these objectives while improving the survival rate has improved. The orthopaedic surgeon, because he is a member of a coordinated team effort, should become acquainted with the principles of treatment by the various disciplines.

Radiotherapy

An understanding of the basic principles is essential to a rational approach to planning external radiation therapy[14] of metastatic disease of bone (see Effects of Ionizing Radiation on Bone). The use of high energy radiation, such as derived from a cobalt-60 unit or a linear accelerator, has reduced the incidence of aseptic necrosis, pathologic fracture, and soft tissue complications. Since the tumor cannot be cured, the dosage administered is that which will reduce the rate of its growth, thereby alleviating pain and preventing fracture. It must never be pushed to the point at which it induces aseptic necrosis. In a large weight-bearing bone, a higher dose is necessary, generally about 3000 rads to 4000 rads over a period of 3 to 4 weeks. In general, although the effects of external radiation are distinctly worthwhile, the results are unpredictable.[44]

When internal fixation is planned, whether for treatment of a fracture or for prophylaxis of an impending fracture, about 1500 rads are given prior to surgery. Postoperatively, a waiting period to allow the radiation reaction to subside is advisable. Then the course of radiotherapy is completed.

A bone scan will define the field for radiotherapy since the actual extent of involvement is not apparent on roentgenograms. However, lytic lesions do not provide sufficient reactive bone for adequate uptake of the radionuclide.

Following external radiation, increasing radiopacity may develop within the radiated area. This should not be construed as increasing ossification and strengthening of the bone. Therefore, continuing protection and support, especially for a weight-bearing bone, is mandatory.

In multiple myeloma, the true extent of bone involvement is impossible to detect because little or no reactive bone forms. Consequently, an extended area of radiation therapy is advisable. When the spine is involved, 1500 rads are given over the entire spine over a period of 7 to 10 days. For a localized destructive process, 2500 rads to 3000 rads are required.

When a radiosensitive tumor causes intraspinal compression, a low dose of radiation is initially given, then gradually built up to a full dose. Tissue edema and worsening of the neurologic signs is an infrequent adverse effect. Surgical decompression may be necessary.

Surgical Management

Pathologic fracture of a major long bone most often results from metastatic disease from the breast or bronchus (Figs. 16-13 and 16-14). A fracture through an area of malignancy will heal, although with minimal callus formation, and radiotherapy will reduce the amount of callus. A patient with widely disseminated disease and deteriorating functional capacity should not be subjected to unwieldy external splintage and a bedfast state. Instead, immediate internal fixation of the humerus will permit instant use of the arm, and internal fixation of the femur or tibia will allow prompt resumption of weight bearing[18,46] If bone loss is excessive, additional stability is achieved by acrylic cement anchoring both main fragments. Postoperatively, assuming that the internal fixation is secure, pain is relieved and active use of the extremity is encouraged. Postoperatively, radiation therapy is initiated.[38]

Prophylactic internal fixation is done for "impending" fracture, especially in a weight-bearing bone, as at the upper end of the femur.[10,26,30]

A progressive neurologic deficit due to spread from a vertebral lesion requires a decompressive laminectomy. This should be done at the earliest moment and should be immediately followed by radiotherapy.

Endocrine surgery is most often performed for metastatic carcinoma of the breast. Oophorectomy benefits 45% of premenopausal cases[37] and bilateral adrenalectomy produces a remission in 55%[71] Combined oophorectomy and adrenalectomy has produced long survival in many.[19] For prostatic cancer, orchiectomy combined with estrogen therapy is effective. Surgical hypophysectomy followed by implantation of radioactive materials is said to result in a high rremission rate in breast carcinoma.[23,51]

Hormone Therapy

The following are the main metastatic tumors treated with hormones.[32,49,53]

Prostatic Carcinoma. Orchiectomy and administration

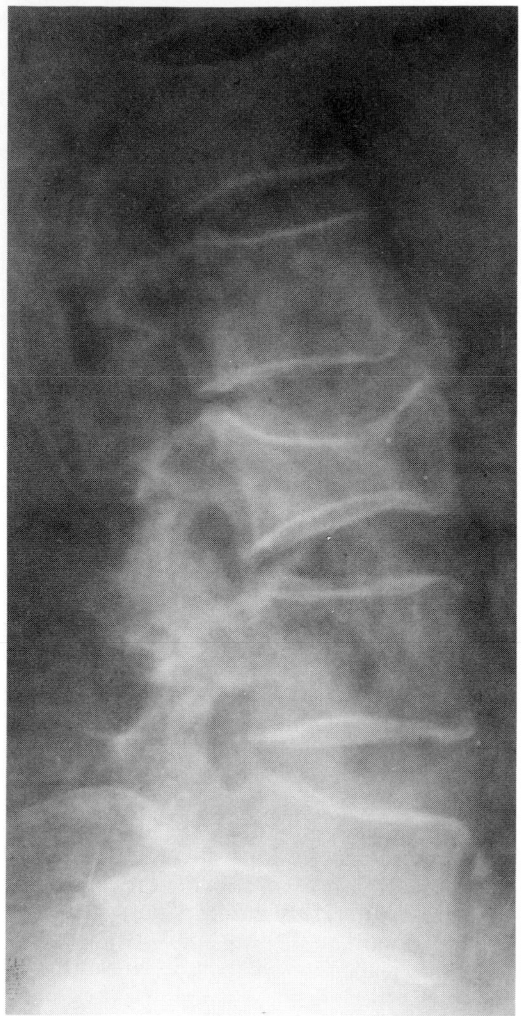

FIG. 16-13. Pathologic fracture of the spine. Compression fractures of the vertebral body ordinarily are wedge shaped, the apex being anterior and the wedge smooth. In this case the maximum compression occurs centrally at a point of weakened resistance due to the neoplastic lesion. Such a fracture is often the first sign of metastases.

of estrogenic hormone often provide dramatic relief of bone pain. The degree and duration of relief is variable, but prolonged survival is not unusual. Adrenalectomy has been disappointing, but oral adrenal corticosteroids (prednisone 20 to 30 mg daily) can decrease bone pain.

Breast Carcinoma. Estrogenic hormone in physiologic amounts stimulates growth of mammary tissue. Thus the beneficial effects of oophorectomy, adrenalectomy, and hypophysectomy. Massive doses of estrogen have the opposite effect.[27] Diethylstilbestrol, 5 mg three times a day or four times a day, or ethinyl estradiol (Estinyl), 0.5 mg to 1.0 mg three times a day, or conjugated estrogens (Premarin), 20 mg to 30 mg daily.

Androgen is less effective, but will produce a remission in the postmenopausal patient. An oral androgen fluoxymesterone (Halotestin, Ora-Testryl) in a dose of 20 mg to 30 mg daily is comparable to injectable androgens.

Corticosteroids suppress adrenal function and reduce the output of estrogens. They may be used for recrudescent disease after oophorectomy and estrogenic hormone have failed. Less than 30 mg of prednisone daily will reduce bone pain.

Thyroid Carcinoma. The malignant cells retain the dependence of the thyroid gland on thyroid-stimulating hormone (TSH) of the pituitary. TSH is suppressed by administering thyroid hormone which in turn causes regression of thyroid carcinoma; 1-triiodothyronine (T_3) is superior for suppressing the pituitary, and bone pain is relieved. The dosage is 200 μg daily. If this treatment fails, ^{131}I is given.

Renal Carcinoma. This is reported to be responsive to various hormones.[16]

Radioisotope Therapy

Radioactive phosphorus has an affinity for bone, concentrating within the reactive bone about a metastatic lesion,[40] Its usefulness is limited by its damaging effect on the bone marrow.

When metastatic carcinoma of the thyroid can be shown to have an affinity for radioactive iodine, this agent can effectively control the disseminated lesions.[58] The remaining normal thyroid tissue must first be ablated

FIG. 16-14. Carcinomatous metastases of the hip.

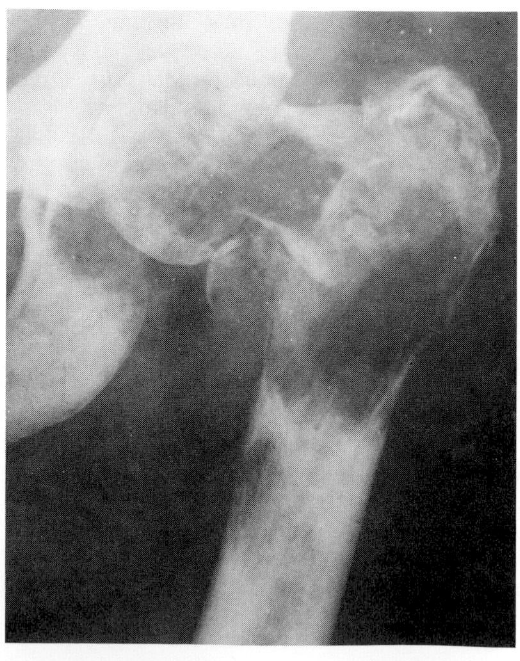

surgically or by ^{131}I. The tumor tissue is then "stimulated" with TSH, a tracer dose of radioactive iodine is given, and bone scans and retention studies are carried out to determine whether uptake by the metastatic lesions is sufficient for treatment with this isotope. The disease can then be controlled for years with ^{131}I. After a specified period of treatment, the effect of treatment can be evaluated by administering a dose of ^{131}I and scanning the skeleton.

Chemotherapy

Temporary remissions of disseminated malignant disease can be achieved by chemotherapeutic agents.[21] Each drug has potential serious side-effects, and their administration must be carried out by oncologists proficient in their use and within centers where adequate monitoring is available. The following are the classes of cytotoxic agents in current use.

Alkylating agents act by alkylating nucleic acids, thereby disrupting the nuclear material. Examples include cyclophosphamide (Cytoxan), melphalan (Alkeran), and chlorambucil (Leukeran).

Antimetabolites act by interfering with a specific metabolic pathway. Examples include methotrexate, a folic acid analogue which completely inhibits folate reductase, an essential enzyme for the metabolism of folic acid; 5-fluorouracil (5-FU, Fluorouracil); and azathioprine (Imuran).

Antibiotics act by binding deoxyribonucleic acid (DNA) and preventing nucleic acid synthesis. An example is doxorubicin (Adriamycin).

For plant alkaloids the mode of action is unknown, but cell division is prevented by interference with the organization of the mitotic apparatus. Vincristine (Oncovin) is an example.

Management of Spinal Metastases

Spinal metastases[14,68] may be silent but eventually severe intractable pain develops and may be initiated by collapse of a vertebral body. When a compression fracture occurs with insufficient trauma or apparently without cause, especially when the roentgenogram discloses collapse through the center of the vertebral body, underlying neoplastic disease must be suspected. Unless widespread involvement of the spine or other metastatic disease becomes known, biopsy is mandatory to confirm the presence of a neoplasm, its origin and its characteristics.

When vertebral destruction results in instability, particularly in the cervical spine, the patient should be immobilized on a Stryker frame and skull tong traction applied. Sandbags about the sides of the head provide additional immobilization while radiotherapy is carried out. Pelvic or femoral traction may be added when neoplastic destruction affects multiple areas.

Radiosensitive tumors are treated with megavoltage radiation. If the tumor can be controlled and stability assured, the patient can then be made ambulatory with appropriate bracing.

Surgical decompression is indicated for progressive neurologic involvement. Metastatic tumors are very vascular, and provision must be made for adequate blood replacement at surgery. Postoperatively, a sensory deficit recovers more readily than motor weakness. Sphincter involvement and rapid progression are ominous prognostic signs. The thoracic segments between T1 and T4 are most vulnerable to compression of the vascular structures, and improvement by laminectomy is highly unlikely.

Radiotherapy remains the main modality for spinal metastases. Tumors from the breast, lung, and thyroid are most responsive. On an average, 4000 rads to 5000 rads are given over a wide area within a period of 1 week.

Management of Prostatic Carcinoma

The endocrine treatment of prostatic cancer consists of anti-andogenic measures, both orchiectomy and administration of estrogens.[48] When the response to castration or estrogen therapy is favorable, patients can live comfortably for years. When the response is poor, or when recrudescence of disease occurs, ^{32}P with testosterone propionate may be effective. Bilateral adrenalectomy may rarely effect a remission.

Management of Mammary Carcinoma

Ninety percent of breast cancer metastases[15] involve the femur and are usually associated with other bone metastases. Since almost half of femoral lesions sustain pathologic fractures, internal fixation as a prophylactic measure is often carried out. Following fracture, internal fixation, preceded by a short course of megavoltage therapy, should be done, ambulation should be started early, and the radiation treatment continued.

In premenopausal patients, 45% will respond to bilateral oophorectomy.[37] Bilateral adrenalectomy has also induced profound remissions. Oophorectomy and adrenalectomy are usually carried out at the same time, effecting a remission in 55%.[71] The estrogen from the adrenals is removed, and substitution therapy with corticosteroids is necessary, and this too may have a favorable effect on metastases.[12] When adrenalectomy is not done, the adrenals can be suppressed with prednisone.

Massive doses of estrogens will often cause profound regression of tumor growth.

Another endocrine approach to therapy is hypophysectomy, which can be accomplished surgically or by external radiation.[32]

Chemotherapy is the last resort at suppressing tumor growth. The agent of choice is 5-fluorouracil.[21]

Testosterone can induce temporary improvement,[45] but can accelerate tumor growth. This latter phenomenon has been explained by the theoretical conversion of testosterone to estrone or estradiol.[52,57]

REFERENCES

Characteristics

1. Batson OV: The role of the vertebral veins in metastatic processes. Ann Intern Med 16:38, 1942
2. Coman DR, deLong RP: The role of the vertebral venous system in the metastasis of cancer to the spinal column. Cancer 4:610, 1951
3. Coman DR, deLong RP, McCutcheon M: Studies on the mechanisms of metastasis; the distribution of tumors in various organs in relation to the distribution of arterial emboli. Cancer Res 11:648, 1951
4. Hodges PC, Phemister DB, Brunschwig A: The roentgen-ray diagnosis of diseases of bone. In Ross Golden's Diagnostic Roentgenology. New York, Nelson, 1941
5. Prinzmetal M, Ornitz EM, Simkin B et al: Arteriovenous anastomoses in liver, spleen and lungs. Am J Physiol 152:48, 1948
6. Willis RA: The Spread of Tumors in the Human Body. St. Louis, CV Mosby, 1952

Bone Matastases

7. Abrams HD, Spiro R, Goldstein N: Metastases in carcinoma: Analysis of 1,000 autopsied cases. Cancer 3:74, 1950
8. Ackerman LV: Surgical Pathology. St Louis, CV Mosby, 1953
9. Agress H: Comparative study of spreads and sections of bone marrow. Am J Clin Pathol 27:282, 1957
10. Altman H: Intramedullary nailing for pathological impending and actual fractures of long bones. Bull Hosp Joint Dis 13, No. 2:239, 1952
11. Auerbach O, Trubowitz S: Primary carcinoma of the liver, with extensive skeletal metastases and panmyelophthisis. Cancer 3:837, 1950
12. Baserga R, Shubik P: Action of cortisone on disseminated tumor cells after removal of the primary growth. Science 121:100, 1955
13. Bertin EJ: Metastases to bone as the first symptom of cancer of the gastrointestinal tract; report of 3 cases. Am J Roentgenol 51:614, 1944
14. Bhalla SK: Metastatic disease of the spine. Clin Orthop 73:52, 1970
15. Blake DD: Radiation treatment of metastatic bone disease. Clin Orthop 73:89, 1970
16. Bloom JJG et al: Sex hormones and renal neoplasia. Cancer 20:2118, 1967
17. Brain MC, Dacie JV, Howrihane OB: Microangiopathic haemolytic anemia: The possible role of vascular lesions in pathogenesis. Br J Haematol 8:358, 1962
18. Brenner RA, Jelliffe AM: The management of pathologic fracture of the major long bones from metastatic cancer. J Bone Joint Surg 40B:652, 1958
19. Cade S: Adrenalectomy for disseminated breast cancer. Br Med J 2:613, 1966
20. Dinsmore RS, Hicken NF: Metastases from malignant tumors of thyroid. Am J Surg 24:202, 1934
21. Donaldson MH, Horsley JS: Nonhormonal chemotherapy of tumors metastatic to bone. Clin Orthop 73:64, 1970
22. Dresser R, Dumas C: Osteogenic sarcoma. Am J Roentgenol 23:65, 1930
23. Edelstyn GA et al: Hypophysectomy and breast cancer. Lancet 1:1211, 1966
24. Edmondson HA, Steiner PE: Primary carcinoma of the liver. Cancer 7:462, 1954
25. Erhardt O: Zur Anatomie und Klinik der Struma maligna. Beitr Klin Chir 35:343, 1902
26. Francis KC: Prophylactic internal fixation of metastatic osseous lesions. Cancer 13:75, 1960
27. Gardner WU: Inhibition of mammary growth by large amounts of estrogen. Endocrinology 28:53, 1941
28. Geschickter CF, Copeland MM: Tumors of Bone. Philadelphia, JB Lippincott, 1949
29. Gold GL, Reefe WE: Carcinoma and metastases to the bones of the hand. JAMA 184:237, 1963
30. Higinbotham NL, Marcove RC: The management of pathological fractures. J Trauma 5, No. 6:792, 1965
31. Hirsch EF: Pathology in Surgery. Baltimore, Williams & Wilkins, 1953
32. Huggins C: Control of cancers of man by endocrinologic methods; a review. Cancer Res 16:825, 1956
33. Jaffe HL: Tumors metastatic to the skeleton. In Tumors and Tumorous Conditions of the Bones and Joints. Philadelphia, Lea & Febiger, 1958
34. Jarcho S: Diffusely infiltrative carcinoma. Arch Pathol 22:674, 1936
35. Jonsson U, Rundles RW: Tumor metastases in bone marrow. Blood 6:16, 1951
36. Johnston AD: Pathology of metastatic tumors in bone. Clin Orthop 73:8, 1970
37. Kennedy BJ, Fortung IE: Therapeutic castration in the treatment of advanced breast cancer. Cancer 17:1197, 1964
38. Knutson CO, Spratt JS Jr: The natural history and management of mammary cancer metastatic to the femur. Cancer 26:1199, 1970
39. Kretschmer HL: Carcinoma of the bladder with bone metastases. Surg Gynecol Obstet 34:241, 1922
40. Lawrence JS, Mahoney EB: Thrombopenic purpura associated with carcinoma of the stomach with extensive metastases. Am J Pathol 10:383, 1934
41. Lawrence JH, Tobias CA: Radioactive isotopes and nuclear radiations in the treatment of cancer. Cancer Res 16:185, 1956
42. Lemon HM, Reynolds MD: Regression of mammary cancer metastases following decline of serum acid phosphatase induced by antiestrogen therapy. Proc Am Assoc Cancer Res 2:129, 1956
43. Ley AB: Mechanisms of anemia in cancer. Med Clin North Am 40:857, 1956
44. Lichtenstein L: Bone Tumors. St Louis, CV Mosby, 1952
45. Loeser AA: Mammary carcinoma response to implantation of male hormone and progesterone. Lancet 2:698, 1941
46. MacAusland WR Jr, Wyman ET Jr: Management of metastatic pathological fractures. Clin Orthop 73:39, 1970
47. Mallett L: Hibernation de la cellule cancereuse. Acta Intern Union Against Cancer 6:993, 1950
48. Mayfield JR Jr et al: The use of radioactive phosphorus and testosterone in metastatic bone lesions from breast and prostate. South Med J 51:320, 1958
49. Mellette SJ: Management of malignant disease metastatic to bone by hormonal alterations. Clin Orthop 73:73, 1970
50. Milch RA, Changus CW: Response of bone to tumor invasion. Cancer 9:340, 1956
51. Moore FD et al: Carcinoma of the breast. N Engl J Med 277:460, 1967
52. Myers WPL, West CD, Pearson OH et al: Androgen-induced exacerbation of breast cancer measured by calcium excretion; conversion of androgen to estrogen as a possible underlying mechanism. JAMA 161:127, 1956

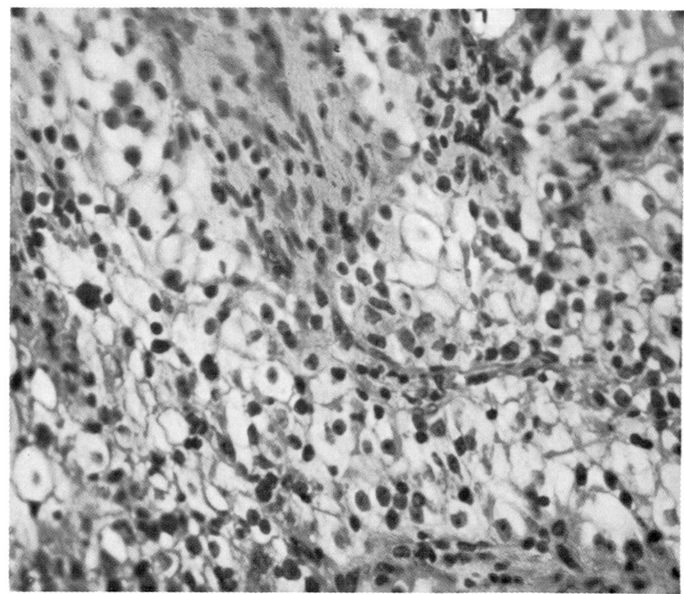

PLATE 16-1. Metastatic hypernephroma. (×360) (See p. 671.)

m WC: Endocrine control of prostatic carci-
nd statistical survey of 1,818 cases. JAMA

affiotti U: Il carcinoma bronchiolare. Arch
20:1, 1953

HM, Byrnes WW: Copper-resistant
I. Method and values in health and
3, 1956

of the Bone Marrow. Boston, Little,

dl E et al: Roentgen-Diagnostics
New York, Grune, 1952

et al: Radioiodine therapy of
thyroid: A six-year progress
949

roentgen study of bone
67:224, 1956

f bone to metastases
rostate. Arch Pathol

arance of thyroid
, 1950

with metastatic

63. Smith WI, Whitfield AGW: Intravascular microembolic carcinomatosis as a cause of purpura. Br J Cancer 8:97, 1954
64. Sohier WD Jr, Juranies E, Aub JC: Hemolytic anemia, a host response to malignancy. Cancer Res 17:767, 1957
65. Spjut HJ et al: Tumors of bone and cartilage. In Atlas of Tumor Pathology, 2nd series, Fascicle 5. Washington, DC, Armed Forces Institute of Pathology, 1971
66. Staley CJ: Skeletal metastases in cancer of the breast. Surg Gynecol Obstet 102:683, 1956
67. Suprun H, Rywlin AM: Metastatic carcinoma in histologic sections of aspirated bone marrow: A comparative autopsy study. South Med J 69:438, 1976
68. Vieth RG, Odom GL: Extradural spinal metastases and their neurosurgical treatment. J Neurosurg 23:501, 1965
69. von Recklinghausen F: Die Fibrose oder deformierende Ostitis, die Osteomalacie und die osteoplastiche Carcinose in ihren gegenseitigen Beziehungen. Festschrift zu Rudolph Virchow's 71 Geburtstage, p 17, 1903
70. Walther HE; Krebsmetastasen. Basel, Schwabe, 1948
71. Wilson RE, Moore FD: Biochemical and Clinical Factors in the Selection of Patients for Endocrine Surgery. Baltimore, Williams & Wilkins, 1968

17

Diseases of Muscle

HISTOPATHOLOGY OF SKELETAL MUSCLE

Skeletal muscle is subject to degeneration (due to i
tion or trauma) and to necrosis (due to ischem
trauma).[1,2] The ensuing process is similar to that i
tissues. First, the debris is removed by mononucle
and macrophages. Then repair is effected by regen
of muscle from surrounding normal muscle fi
by ingrowth of granulation tissue and fibrosis. R
of the mode of destruction, whether by trauma,
or toxic degeneration, regeneration of muscle

Microscopically, necrosed muscle fibers un
mentation and stain irregularly, and the s
nuclei become shrunken and pyknotic. The
undamaged muscle is prevented from retra
connective tissue. Within a few days,
inflammatory cells and macrophages inva
zone and remove the debris. After abo
rounding muscle fibers send deeply ba
nucleated, protoplasmic processes into
ulation tissue invades at the same tim
the slender straps are prolific and pe
gaps quickly, especially where sarcole
persisted. When sarcolemmic tubes ar
of multinucleated sarcoplasm is dela
replacement is pronounced. After 2 w
acquire sarcolemmic sheaths, cross s
fibers enlarge, basophilic staining i
appearance is acquired. The new m
ularly woven together. After 6 w
and microscopically appears norm
small areas of fibrosis.

This sequence of events indica
should be protected for a mini
allowing activity.

Zenker's Degeneration or hyaline (glasslike) degenerati
In a severe form, it is found
pneumonia, and is observe
the rectus abdominis. Othe
tious disease, it occurs t
muscle. Microscopically,
(owing to increased osm
without striations, and s
ically, such muscle is ea
cular hemorrhage. The
after a severe febrile il

Histology of Dene goes progressive at
peripheral fibers i
though sarcolemmi
cross striations per
by 3 weeks wal
fibrosis replaces

muscle is traumatized, it regenerates exactly as the normal muscle does.

Identification of Striated Muscle Tumors. Certain neoplasms that stem from skeletal muscle present such a pleomorphic appearance that their origin is difficult to ascertain. Strands of acidophilic tissue are suspected of being muscle fibers. Their cross striations can be displayed best by staining with phosphotungstic acid.[12]

TUMORS OF SKELETAL MUSCLE

RHABDOMYOMA

Rhabdomyoma, a benign tumor arising in striated muscle, is extremely rare. It tends to form an infiltrative, nonencapsulated nodule.

Microscopically, the tumor is composed chiefly of interlacing bundles of long straplike cells with single nuclei, myofibrils, and, occasionally, cross striations. The cytoplasm is acidophilic but not granular. Mitoses are not seen.

RHABDOMYOSARCOMA

PATHOLOGY

Rhabdomyosarcoma is a rare malignant tumor derived from mesenchymal cells that bear cytologic characteristics similar to those of striated muscle. It can occur at any age from infancy to old age, but its greatest incidence is between 30 and 60 years of age. It usually develops within or adjacent to skeletal muscle, but it may also be found where striated muscle does not exist (*e.g.*, urogenital tract, orbit, respiratory passages).[7] Its orthopaedic importance is its early detection within the musculature of the extremities and pelvic and shoulder girdles.

Gross Appearance. The tumor mass varies from a few centimeters in diameter to as large as 15 or 20 cm in its greatest dimension.[4] It is usually located within an individual muscle or between muscles where, by gradual enlargement, it compresses the surrounding tissue and forms a pseudocapsule. The tumor tends to be lobulated and extends along fascial planes. Superficial tumors are less encapsulated, infiltrating into the subcutaneous tissue and breaking through the skin to form a red, fungating mass, especially after an incomplete local excision. It can also invade and destroy the adjacent bone.

Microscopic Appearance. A wide variety of pleomorphic cells are observed.[6] The nuclei are large, the cytoplasm is deeply acidophilic, and many cells contain longitudinal fibrils and cross striations characteristic of skeletal muscle (Color Plate 17-1). Four types of cells can be identified:

Strap Cell
Most common type; long, meandering cytoplasmic process containing two or more nuclei ("tandem nuclei")

Racket Cell
Nucleus bulges at one end; tapering tail of cytoplasm resembles handle of tennis racket

Tumor Giant Cell
Cytoplasm vacuolated, resembles spider web; nuclei extremely large and anaplastic; vacuoles contain glycogen

Embryonal Myoblast
Small, dense nuclei, scanty cytoplasm

CLINICAL PICTURE

A palpable, painless, soft mass within or adjacent to muscles appears deceptively benign. Occasionally, local discomfort follows minor trauma. Radicular pain and paresthesia develop when the tumor infiltrates about nerve structures. Most often, the patient does not seek medical attention for the gradually enlarging painless mass until many months after it is first noticed.

ROENTGENOGRAPHIC FINDINGS

A soft tissue density may be seen. A superficial erosive defect or reactive periosteal bone formation may occasionally be found in the adjacent bone.

TREATMENT

Treatment consists in amputation or a radical en bloc excision, postoperative irradiation in adequate dosage (*e.g.*, 6000 rads over 6 weeks), and intensive multiple-drug chemotherapy over an extended period (*i.e.*, 2 years).[3] When this program can be instituted while the lesions are apparently localized, 2-year survival rates of 80% to 90% can be achieved. The overall survival rate is approximately 50%.

CAVERNOUS HEMANGIOMA OF STRIATED MUSCLE

Cavernous hemangioma is a benign tumor that is not uncommon; it is composed of many thin-walled blood vessel spaces within a densely fibrous tissue.[8,10–12] The cause is unknown. Young people are affected most often.

The majority of hemangiomas are located intramuscularly, and usually a single tumor is confined to a single muscle. The quadriceps is involved most frequently. Rarely, the cavernous hemangioma involves a group of muscles or forms part of extensive angiomatosis of an entire extremity.

PATHOLOGY

Gross Appearance

The muscle appears swollen, and its color and consistency vary, depending on the relative proportion of cavernous sinuses to fibrous tissue replacing the muscle substance. On cut section, the muscle locally contains dense interlacing fibrous strands extending in all directions and gradually merging with surrounding normal muscle fibers. The fibrous strands enclose numerous thin-walled bleeding sinuses, many of which contain thrombi. Characteristically, the tumor contains multiple minute, grayish white, round, hard nodules representing calcified thrombi.

Histologic Appearance

A large number of vascular spaces lined with a single layer of endothelium are observed. Surrounding these is a dense fibrous matrix within which may be seen degenerating muscle fibers. The walls of arterioles display fibrous thickening. The cavernous spaces contain thrombi in various stages of organization and calcification.

CLINICAL PICTURE

A sensation of tenseness or actual pain, particularly on contraction of the muscle, is the usual complaint. The muscle appears diffusely swollen. On palpation, a poorly delimited mass is perceived. It is tender, and its consistency varies from soft to hard, depending on the relative amounts of vascular spaces to fibrous stroma. Multiple pea-sized nodules are often palpable. The tumor grows slowly. It is often confined to one muscle, commonly the quadriceps, and it moves and becomes prominent with contraction of the muscle. The mass may be rendered tense and more easily palpated by applying a tourniquet, compressing the veins above it. On releasing the tourniquet, the swelling once again becomes soft and boggy. Elevation and dependency of the extremity produce similar changes. Aspiration yields blood.

ROENTGENOGRAPHIC FINDINGS

A soft tissue density is observed within the swollen muscle. Opacities of phleboliths lie within the tumor shadow. These are differentiated from similar opacities of trichinosis, which are much smaller, and cysticerci, which are elongated and less dense. Periosteal reactive ossification is observed in adjacent bone.

Arteriography discloses an intricate arterial ramification entering a mass that usually is lightly radiopaque and beyond which the venous phase shows small loculations of dye due to multiple ectasias. The increased soft density of the hemangioma persists after the dye has disappeared from the efferent venules.[5,9]

COMPLICATIONS

Rupture of the muscle has been observed.

TREATMENT

Complete surgical excision is advisable. Other more conservative therapeutic measures are uncertain and often are followed by recurrence. If the defect created by removal is large, fascial replacement or muscle transfer may be necessary.

TRAUMATIC CONDITIONS OF MUSCLE

Muscle can be injured by direct trauma, such as a forceful blow, or indirect trauma, which stretches and tears the muscle fibers.

DIRECT TRAUMA

Crushing of nerve fibers and connective tissue sheaths causes a variable amount of necrosis which to a great extent is proportionate to the degree of vascular damage. The biceps and the anterior tibial muscles are especially prone to extensive post-traumatic necrosis because of a solitary blood supply. When the traumatic force is applied to large areas of muscle, parenchymal necrosis and subsequent scar-tissue replacement is extensive. A muscle injury localized to a small area can be followed by complete muscle regeneration with a minimum of scar.

MUSCLE RUPTURE AND FASCIAL TEARS

The mechanism of indirect injury is either prolonged exercise in an untrained person, or a violent contraction of certain muscles. Muscle fibers rupture, hemorrhage and edema follow, and the muscle herniates through a rent in the overlying fascia or epimysium. A soft elastic tumor that is not adherent to the skin presents itself. It becomes tense and painful on contraction of the muscle. It can be reduced by compression while the muscle itself is relaxed. The biceps, the rectus femoris, and the gastrocnemius are involved most often. With passage of time, the hernia becomes fibrosed. Rarely does it necrose.

Complete rupture of a muscle takes place most often through the muscle belly, less often at the musculotendinous or tendo-osseous junctions. Its occurrence in certain muscles is favored by muscle action peculiar to certain occupations. For example, the biceps and the triceps are frequently ruptured in baseball pitchers; the calf muscles, in boxers; and the thigh adductors, in horseback riders. Rupture may occur also in severe tetanus or in electric shock injuries, which cause violent concurrent contractions of antagonist muscles. Clinically, the sequence of events is an audible snap, associated with severe pain, occurring during a strong contraction; swelling or bulge of retracted muscle; and weakness or paralysis. A partial muscle rupture exhibits only localized pain and tenderness and is often diagnosed as a sprain or a charley horse. The degree of weakening of muscle power is proportionate to the extent of disruption. Often an incomplete rupture may become complete the following day.

Pathologic rupture may occur in certain conditions characterized by parenchymatous degeneration (*e.g.*, trichinosis, typhoid fever, tuberculosis, and other infections).

MUSCLE HEMORRHAGE

Hemorrhage occurs in muscle from the following:

Trauma

The exposed limb muscles are predisposed.

Severe Infectious Diseases

Generalized Zenker's waxy degeneration of sarcoplasm renders all muscle quite fragile. A thin exposed muscle, such as the rectus abdominis, is predisposed. Streaks of extravasated blood develop between the muscle fibers, or a discrete hematoma may form. The muscle is diffusely tender and painful.

Hemorrhagic Diseases

Scurvy and thrombocytopenic purpura are examples.

If hemorrhage is small, it may be absorbed; if it is large, the clot may become encapsulated or organized or converted to cartilage or bone. Muscle fibers about a hemorrhage may be destroyed or undergo hyaline degeneration. Later, regeneration occurs by accumulation of sarcoplasm about multiplying nuclei, forming giant cells of muscle reconstruction.

TRAUMATIC MYOSITIS OSSIFICANS

Traumatic myositis ossificans (localized myositis ossificans, extraosseous localized non-neoplastic bone and cartilage formation, myositis ossificans traumatica, myoosteosis, myositis ossificans circumscripta, traumatic ossifying myositis, ossifying hematoma) is a reactive lesion occurring in soft tissues and at times near bone and periosteum. It is characterized by fibrous, osseous, and cartilaginous proliferation and by metaplasia.[17] Any term that includes *itis* and *myo* is a misnomer because skeletal muscle is often not involved and inflammatory changes are rarely evident. In the early phase of its evolution, formation of bone may not be observed, so the term *ossificans* is not always applicable.

Most, if not all, patients with myositis ossificans have a history of trauma, a simple severe blow or a series of repeated minor traumas. The condition may be classified according to its location as extraosseous, periosteal, or parosteal.

A hematoma seems to be a necessary prerequisite. The muscles most often involved are the brachialis anticus, quadriceps femoris, and adductor muscles of the thigh. It is significant that these muscles gain attachment to the bone over a wide surface area, suggesting that the periosteum participates to some extent in the process.

Young, athletic men are predisposed. The region of the elbow is a favorite site, and when the process appears to restrict elbow motion progressively, ill-advised forcible manipulation will cause a widespread involvement.

PATHOGENESIS

Muscle is commonly, but not invariably, involved, and fascia, tendon, and periosteum can also be the locale. The process basically is a peculiar alteration within the ground substance of connective tissue, almost always associated with a striking proliferation of undifferentiated mesenchymal cells.[13,14]

Initially there is degeneration and necrosis of the tissue, and, in the case of muscle, disrupted muscle fibers retract. There follows histiocytic invasion for removal of necrotic debris. Within 3 or 4 days, fibroblasts from the endomysium invade the damaged area and rapidly form broad sheets of immature fibroblasts. At the same time, primitive mesenchymal cells proliferate within the injured connective tissue. The intense cellular proliferation of fibroblasts and mesenchymal cells produces a histologic picture that may be erroneously diagnosed as a fibrosarcoma or myosarcoma.

Simultaneously, sarcolemmic nuclei at the ends of the damaged muscle fibers begin to proliferate, and chains and columns of plump polyhedral cells appear, followed by production of sarcoplasm, which extends as buds, straps, or clublike projections from preexisting fibers. The sarcolemmic nuclei cluster within the center of these sarcoplasmic masses. It is these large areas of multinucleated buds that prompt the diagnosis of giant cell tumor or myosarcoma.

Within the proliferating mesenchyme, significant changes occur in the ground substance. This material becomes homogeneous or glassy or waxy, suggesting

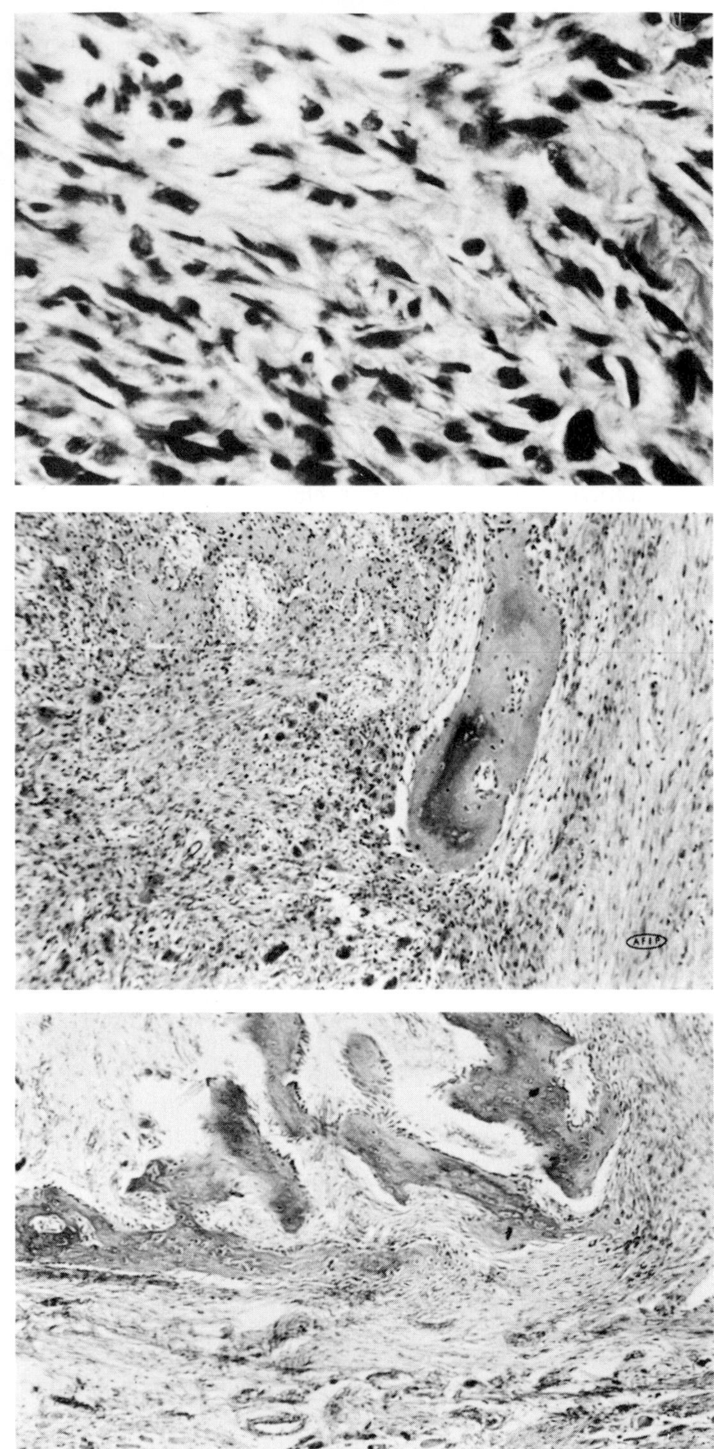

FIG. 17-1. Myositis ossificans, microscopic features. (*Top*) The cellular inner zone illustrates numerous cells with occasional atypical mitotic figures and variations in size and shape of the cells. The histologic appearance is sarcomatous. (*Center*) The middle zone shows osteoid formation with a fibrovascular background. The cellular pattern is uniform. (*Bottom*) The outer zone illustrates mature, fairly well oriented peripheral bone. The fibrous stroma appears more mature than at the center of the lesion. (Courtesy of Dr. William Bacon)

some type of edema.[16] This colorless or faintly eosinophilic material contains indistinct, delicate fibrils. The ground substance increases in amount and encloses some of the mesenchymal cells, which then assume the morphological characteristics of osteoblasts. Mineralization follows, and bone is formed.

This sequence of events typically takes place first within that portion of the tissue that is least damaged (*i.e.*, at the periphery).[15] As the process of osteoid formation and mineralization eventuating in mature bone evolves, it progressively extends toward the central, more severely damaged area. Consequently, myositis ossificans in the midst of its evolution and progression from periphery to the center toward complete ossification will show an extremely cellular area in its central area and mature, well-delimited bone at its periphery. If tissue is taken for biopsy from the central area alone, especially during the first 3 to 4 weeks, when there has not yet been time for orientation or new bone formation to occur, microscopic evaluation will be impossible. The extreme variation in the size and shape of cells and mitotic activity would make for a plausible diagnosis of sarcoma (Fig. 17-1).

Of great diagnostic importance is the study of all areas and the observation of zone phenomena.[13] The central, highly cellular region is surrounded by a second zone of fibroblastic tissue, and this in turn is enveloped by a third zone of mature, well-oriented new bone. This zonal phenomenon, which is not present in soft tissue sarcomas, classifies the lesion as benign and obviates the need for radical measures. When ossification has developed, the "tumor" is at least 3 to 4 weeks old and is best differentiated at the periphery.

If there has been considerable hemorrhage in the central portion, large lakes of blood may form, surrounded by foreign body giant cells. In some cases, the invasion of regenerating multinucleated muscle fibers exaggerates the giant cell picture, thereby imitating a giant cell tumor.

Some ossifications completely disappear, and probably the smaller ones regress because of osteoclastic resorption within the muscle belly. There is complete restoration of muscle contour, but muscle function is never normal.[18]

When the process is confined to fascia, the changes are identical except that muscle does not participate (Fig. 17-2). When the process involves tendon, it is observed at points of attachment to bone, eventuating in the formation of an exostosis.

Periosteal ossification can be said to represent the same process. Any trauma that produces a hematoma beneath the periosteum, or damages it sufficiently to elevate it, will produce highly cellular proliferation in the space between the periosteum and bone; osteoid develops, and this is rapidly converted to bone.

When myositis ossificans is not removed and is allowed to mature, it usually becomes oriented and covered by a cartilaginous cap, probably because of the muscle action over the lesion. This has been called a post-traumatic osteochondroma and is common in the region of the knee joint.

CLINICAL PICTURE

The condition occurs as a result of a single or repeated trauma. The brachialis anticus is a favorite site after a posterior dislocation of the elbow. During development of the extraosseous mass, the elbow area is quite swollen and tender and active and passive motion is greatly restricted. Gradually, as the pain and the general swelling are reduced, a circumscribed, indurated, later hard tumor mass is palpable over the anterior aspect of the elbow. Active extension of the joint is limited by virtue of inelasticity of the muscle, and flexion is prevented by obstruction offered by the mass.

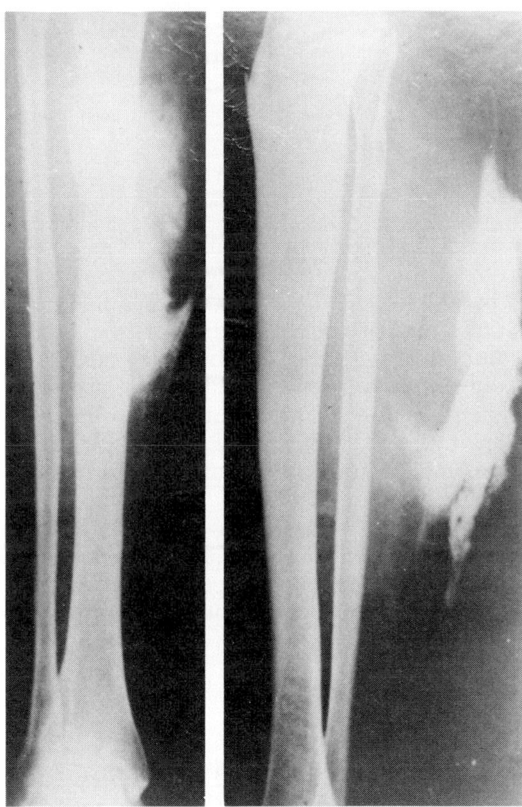

FIG. 17-2. Heterotopic ossification.

Ossification in the deltoid is common in foot soldiers due to the trauma caused by carrying a rifle. The constant pressure of the saddle against the adductors in riders causes ossification in that muscle. The syndrome is known as Prussian disease.

Subperiosteal hemorrhage followed by formation of bone may be included in this category, although not occurring in muscle. The pathogenesis is similar. The ossification in the quadriceps area occurring in football players is an example.

Myositis ossificans is self-limited in that it undergoes maturation and may persist as a hard ossified mass, usually within a muscle or fixed to the adjacent long bone. In some cases, it undergoes almost complete regression.

Lesions that are designated as post-traumatic osteochondromas have in all probability developed on the basis of localized myositis ossificans. It generally forms at the region of the knee and becomes covered with a cartilaginous cap.

DIAGNOSIS

A totally excised lesion or a biopsy that extends deeply will demonstrate the zoning effect characterized by a central area in which there are numerous cells of various sizes and shapes and occasional mitotic figures. As the lesion is examined toward the periphery, the next zone shows osteoid formation with a fibrovascular background. This is the more advanced stage, in which the cells are more uniform, indicating a benign lesion. In the outer zone, trabeculae of well-formed bone and more mature fibrous stroma are observed.

Osteosarcoma is the main tumor that must be excluded. In the latter tumor, the zoning effect is not seen, and malignant cellular characteristics extend throughout the lesion, most pronounced at the periphery.

TREATMENT

The growth should not be removed in the premature stage. The result of such ill-advised attempts is disastrous. The ossification becomes exuberant, infiltrates beyond the original site, and compromises the soft tissues about the joint beyond hope of repair. Restraint is the watchword. When by serial roentgenograms the mass is dense, well delineated, and at a standstill, it may safely be removed. One may ensure against recurrence by waiting until a very late date. It may be possible to prevent myostitis ossificans by aspirating the original hematoma.

MYOSITIS OSSIFICANS PROGRESSIVA

Myositis ossificans progressiva is a congenital condition that starts without antecedent trauma before or shortly after birth. It consists of frequently repeated episodes of sudden extension of ossification in the muscles, the fasciae, the tendons, and the aponeuroses. The only laboratory finding is an elevated eosinophil count. The blood chemistry is normal. Other congenital deformities, such as microdactyly, brachydactyly, and Klippel-Feil syndrome, are frequently associated. The ossification usually starts with the upper back muscles, particularly the trapezius and the latissimus dorsi, and spreads distalward and eventually involves soft tissue structures throughout the body. The interphalangeal joints of the thumb, the large toe, and the spine are liable to fuse. All joint motion is finally lost, and the patient dies of intercurrent infection. The condition is very rare.

TREATMENT

There is no known effective treatment. The administration of corticotropin seems to have a deterrent effect on the heterotopic bone formation. The eosinophil count drops, and joint motion may even increase.[19,20]

COMPARTMENT SYNDROME

The compartment syndrome may be defined as a condition of muscles and associated structures contained within an osseofascial compartment of the forearm or leg. It is characterized etiologically by impaired blood perfusion of diverse origin, resulting in ischemia, swelling, and rising interstitial fluid pressures. Pathologically, there is edema followed by necrosis of muscle fibers and, finally, by variable amounts of muscle regeneration or fibrous tissue replacement, eventuating in a contracture deformity. At the onset there is local pain, tenderness, tenseness, and stretch pain over the affected compartment; preservation, at least in the early stages, of peripheral pulses, or progressive loss of peripheral pulses when a main artery is involved; and partial sensory nerve dysfunction, causing paresthesias and hypoesthesia in an autonomous zone supplied by the nerve coursing through that compartment and, if severe and left untreated, resulting in a resistant deformity due to both muscle fibrous contracture and neurologic deficit. Although multiple compartments may be affected, those predominantly involved are the volar compartment of the forearm (often referred to as Volkmann's ischemia and Volkmann's contracture) and the anterior compartment of the leg (anterior tibial syndrome).

PATHOPHYSIOLOGY

Muscle is highly vulnerable to changes in oxygen tension within the tissue. Partial reduction of oxygen tension (plus changes in the constituents of the interstitial fluid) cause muscle fibers to undergo degeneration of its sarcoplasm and its organelles and, should the relative anoxia persist, causes disintegration of the sarcolemmic sheath itself, followed by absorption of its constituent substances into the general circulation (*e.g.*, potassium, myoglobin). Although the level of oxygenation is insufficient for muscle survival, it is adequate for the growth of collagen, which proceeds unhampered.

Oxygen tension within muscle tissue is directly related to the adequacy of tissue perfusion. The volume and rate of blood flow through the intracompartmental tissues are affected by many factors, chiefly by local tissue pressure and also by vascular occlusion, whether locally, as a result of compression or arteriolar spasm, or at a proximal level, by spasm, laceration, compression, or intravascular obstruction of a main artery.

Ischemia will damage the microcirculation within the muscle, leading to progressive swelling of muscles and nerves and producing increased pressures within the unyielding fascial compartment. This can best be understood by a study of the following facts.

Normally, fluid exchange through the capillary wall is effected by a filtration force of the capillary blood pressure forcing fluid and crystalloids out into the tissue fluid. Counteracting this is the osmotic differential of the plasma proteins drawing fluid back into the capillary. At the arterial end of the capillary the filtration force exceeds the osmotic force and so the fluid leaves the capillary. At the venous end the position is reversed and the fluid returns.[27]

After tourniquet-induced ischemia there is a reactive hyperemia, so the filtration force increases. Moreover, there is anoxic damage to the capillary wall, so the plasma colloids leak out and the osmotic differential increases. Much more fluid leaves the capillaries than returns, and there is an increase in the tissue fluids. Where the tissues are confined within compartments, this increase in volume will cause a rise in pressure in the tissues. As the pressure rises, the venous end of the capillary will become occluded, and eventually the whole capillary and even the arterioles may become occluded. A stage will be reached where almost no fluid returns to the capillary. As the microcirculation in the soft tissues becomes occluded, the ischemia becomes increasingly severe and a vicious circle develops. Once this is established, the circle can be broken only by a prompt and generous fasciotomy.[39]

Experimentally, it has been shown that a tourniquet-induced ischemia will make the muscles swell after release of the tourniquet.[36] After 2 hours of tourniquet-induced ischemia, the muscles increase in weight 35%, and after 3 hours the muscles increase by 50%; the swelling is completely reversible. After 4 hours of ischemia, although the swelling is no greater than after 3 hours, the ischemia is perpetuated and a permanent contracture develops.[37] Ischemia therefore induces progressive intramuscular edema. Since expansion of muscle is limited by its fascial envelope, the intracompartmental pressure increases and reflexly causes spasm of the proximal artery and the arterioles.[24] This too constitutes a vicious circle in which a self-perpetuating reflex arterial spasm continues until the intracompartmental pressure is released.

Normal resting muscle tissue pressure is reported to be approximately 4 mm Hg (±4).[41,74] External pressure will increase the interstitial fluid pressure in the local area of compression. Muscle contraction will cause a temporary increase in pressure. Diverse precipitating insults, whether local (prolonged compression, external or internal) or proximal (main arterial spasm, laceration, compression, thrombosis), will cause the muscles to swell within an unyielding compartment, and pressure within it builds up progressively while causing a corresponding diminution in tissue perfusion.[22,40,44] It should be emphasized that regardless of the type or site of the initiating insult, whether above or below the knee, the ischemia is "selective," involving the muscles and nerves within the compartments distal to the elbow or knee, whereas the peripheral parts, the hand and foot, are unaffected. Furthermore, the phenomenon of intracompartmental muscle swelling and pressure may be precipitated by an injury at a distance. For example, by injecting a volume of fluid under pressure into the front of the upper arm and the front of the thigh, a dramatic increase occurs in intracompartmental pressure of the forearm and leg.[39]

There is no agreement as to the exact level that tissue pressure must reach before tissue perfusion ceases altogether, but blood flow ceases in the microcirculation when local tissue pressure is equal to the diastolic pressure.[22,23,30] Experimentally, a precipitous drop in local blood flow occurs when tissue compression is increased to within 30 mm Hg of intravascular pressure at normotensive blood pressure levels. The critical arteriolar closing pressure is reached when tissue pressure is in the range of 40 mm Hg to 50 mm Hg. At this point, the arteriolar pressure approximates the diastolic, and the arterioles collapse.

The transmural pressure within an arteriole is its intravascular pressure minus the surrounding tissue pressure. Impaired perfusion occurs when active closure of small arterioles under vasomotor tone results from lowered intramural pressure, either by fall in intravascular pressure or by rise in tissue pressure. Passive collapse of soft-walled capillaries results when tissue pressure rises above the capillary pressure.

Arteriolar spasm is a reflex phenomenon that reduces blood flow, resulting in anoxia and capillary stasis, which in turn cause increased capillary permeability, transudation of plasma, tissue edema, and marked swelling of muscles. Since the expansion of muscle is limited by its fascial envelope, the intracompartmental pressure increases and reflexly causes spasm of the proximal artery and arterioles.[24] Locally, increased intracompartmental pressure will reflexly induce vasospasm. Proximally, injury to a main artery, by compression, contusion, or angulation over a bone fragment, will reflexly cause generalized arteriolar spasm. Partial ischemia results. It should be duly noted that whereas the small arterioles that furnish blood flow to the vascular beds are chiefly affected, the large main vessels remain intact until a later stage. Thus, the preservation of the peripheral pulses does not truly reflect ongoing ischemic necrosis. An exception to this rule is the case of a severe injury to a large-caliber artery. The artery may undergo persisting spasm, narrowing it to a mere fraction of its original size, or it may suffer an intimal injury followed by thrombotic occlusion; beyond the point of obstruction, the artery collapses. In either case, distal perfusion is reduced and peripheral pulses are markedly diminished or absent.

Histologically, tissue pressures at 50 mm Hg to 60 mm Hg cause venous congestion, edema, and inflammatory exudate followed by degeneration of muscle fibers, provided that these pressures are applied over a sufficiently long period. At high pressures, 70 mm Hg or more, ischemic necrosis occurs. The nuclei become pyknotic, severe degeneration of sarcoplasmic elements takes place, and, ultimately, the sarcolemmic cylinders disintegrate. Hypotensive patients with low intravascular pressure will have inadequate tissue perfusion when tissue pressure rises slightly. Conversely, hypertensive patients with high intravascular pressure can withstand higher tissue pressures. Consequently, an interpretation of adverse effects of rising tissue pressure must consider the relationship between intravascular and tissue pressures.

Nerves are particularly vulnerable to pressure and anoxia. As litte as 70 mm Hg pressure applied to a nerve trunk will diminish its conductive capacity.[63]

TEMPORAL-PRESSURE RELATIONSHIP

The effects of rising tissue pressure are directly related to the duration of exertion of such pressure. In experimental animals, it can be shown that there exists a threshold pressure level (30 mm Hg) and duration (8 hours) at which significant muscle necrosis occurs at normal blood pressure.[36] Inversely proportionate pressure-duration relationships exert similar adverse effects.

Experimentally, the same inversely proportionate relationship can be demonstrated.[37] Severe intracompartmental pressure causes a gradual decline of nerve conduction and decrease of muscle action potentials. At pressure between 80 and 120 mm Hg, nerve conduction is completely blocked in less than 2 hours. Similarly, a complete block can be obtained at a pressure as low as 50 mm Hg over a 5-hour period. The conduction block is incomplete at 30 mm Hg after 6 to 8 hours of pressurization. Therefore, it is reasonable to assume that 30 mm Hg at 6 to 8 hours is a critical level of pressure at which fasciotomy should be performed in the patient threatened with a compartment syndrome.

CLINICAL PICTURE

The most common sites of involvement are the volar compartment of the forearm, the anterior tibial compartment, the deep posterior compartment of the leg, and the peroneal compartment.

Following trauma, either directly about the compartment or at a proximal level (*e.g.*, a supracondylar fracture of the humerus in a child), pain develops that is deep, intractable, and poorly localized. Rarely, pain may be minimal or absent, and attention is drawn to the area rather late. Paresthesias and numbness of the distal parts are frequent complaints.

Findings include progressive swelling and tenseness or induration over the affected compartment. These objective findings are not apparent when the deep posterior compartment of the leg is involved. Stretch pain is highly characteristic; this consists of inability to perform any movement of the foot or hand that stretches the affected muscles without provoking severe pain. For example, extending the fingers is limited and painful when the flexor compartment of the forearm is involved. Hypoesthesia, especially to two-point discrimination and light touch rather than pinprick, can be demonstrated in an autonomous zone of the affected peripheral nerve. As an example, when the anterior tibial nerve is involved, a wedge-shaped area of diminished sensation will be detected on the dorsum of the foot proximal to the base of the first and second toes. For the volar compartment of the forearm, a median nerve deficit is usual, and ulnar nerve deficits are common. As a general rule, during the early acute phase, the peripheral pulses are intact but may steadily decrease in volume.

DIAGNOSIS

Early diagnosis is essential and requires an awareness of potentially injurious factors that can produce a compartment syndrome. Moreover, once the possibility exists, it is exceedingly important to detect increased intracompartmental pressures and to perform a decompressive procedure before muscle necrosis and a neurologic deficit have developed. When paralysis is established before the fasciotomy is done, recovery of nerve function is incomplete and occurs only in a few cases.[15] The diagnosis should, if possible, be made and immediate treatment rendered while palpable pulses are still present. Irreversible changes are already taking place long before peripheral pulses are lost.

The causative factors may be classified into two main types: type I, which might involve a major artery and which occurs proximal to the site at which ischemia subsequently develops (above the elbow or above the knee), and type II, in which direct trauma to the limb produces ischemia at the same site (below the elbow or below the knee).[40]

In the upper extremity, the most common type I injury producing Volkmann's ischemia is an extensor-type supracondylar fracture of the humerus, usually treated by closed reduction and immobilization with the elbow flexed more than 90°. The brachial artery is injured by a direct blow that causes an intimal tear exposing the raw surface on which a thrombus may form. The thrombus occludes not only the main artery but also the collateral vessels. Distal to the point of occlusion, the artery collapses to a fraction of its original size. Such post-thrombotic narrowing must be differentiated from arterial spasm. During manipulative reduction or at the time that the bone is broken, the artery may be injured by traction. Stretching the arterial muscular media results in severe arterial spasm, and the vessel beyond this point will collapse. Arterial spasm can be detected and overcome by injecting a bolus of fluid through the narrow segment.[57] Time-honored procedures such as sympathetic block, local infiltration with papaverine, or periarterial stripping are of no value.[41] If the maneuver fails to reexpand the artery, the narrowed caliber of the artery represents collapse of the vessel distal to the point of obstruction by a thrombus, which must be removed. Injury to the brachial artery and Volkmann's ischemia are rare when this fracture is treated by Dunlop's traction, overhead pin traction, or percutaneous pinning.[29,31,35]

Type II injury of the forearm most commonly is due to both bone fractures and prolonged limb compression (*e.g.*, that produced by pressure of the head or torso in drug overdose victims). External compression will produce local tamponade and temporary increase in intracompartmental pressures sufficient to cause localized muscle and capillary ischemia and necrosis.[59,60]

In the lower extremity, a common type I injury is fracture of the femoral shaft, especially in children under 2 years of age treated by Bryant's traction. The same may be said of any femoral shaft fracture treated by Buck's traction while the knee is fully extended and the extremity elevated. Forcible distraction of femoral shaft fractures can induce arterial spasm and decreased perfusion of leg compartments.[40] The relative avascularity of the leg is aggravated by elevation of the extremity and compression of the leg by firm bandaging.

Below the knee, common type II injuries involve the tibia, for example, by fracture, rotational osteotomy, and so forth. External limb compression when prolonged is also a prominent cause.

The crush syndrome is characterized by prolonged severe compression of one or several compartments (*e.g.*, the torso compressing several limbs in drug overdose victims, compression by rocks and debris in mine cave-ins). As a consequence of multiple compartment involvement and extensive myonecrosis, there occurs a massive outpouring of myoglobin and potassium into the systemic circulation, producing hyperkalemia, cardiac arrhythmia, shock, and myoglobinuric renal failure and death. The loss of intravascular fluids into the muscle interstitial tissues produces hypovolemic shock. This potentially lethal situation may be averted by prompt fasciotomies and restoration of intravascular fluids.

Exercise will increase muscle volume by 20% and therefore will increase the pressure within the affected compartment. In certain predisposed people, in whom it can be shown that a slight increase in intracompartmental pressure exists in the resting state, the additional pressure brought on by swelling of the exercised muscle may be sufficient to produce the critical closing arteriolar pressure. The anterior tibial compartment syndrome is typical of this problem, which can be relieved by fasciotomy.

Statistically, tibial fractures constitute the most com-

FIG. 17-3. Measurement of intracompartmental pressure. The tissue pressure is measured by determining the amount of pressure within the closed system that is required to overcome the pressure within the closed compartment when injecting a minute quantity of fluid. (Whitesides TE et al: Tissue pressure measurements as a determinant for the need of fasciotomy. Clin Orthop 113:43, 1975)

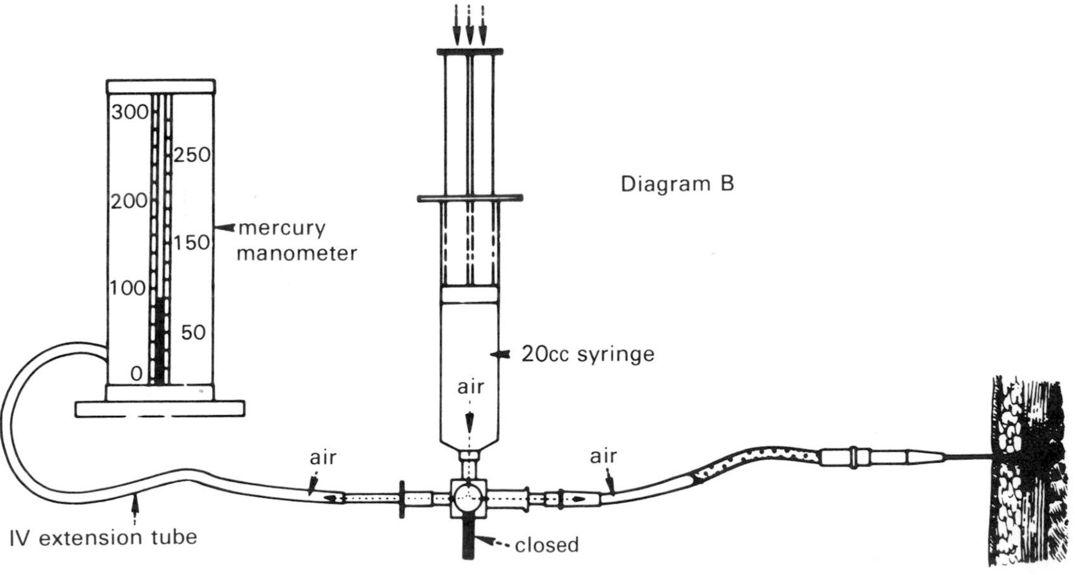

mon cause of a compartment syndrome, and the anterior compartment of the leg is the most frequently involved.

MEASUREMENT OF INTRACOMPARTMENTAL PRESSURE

When a high index of suspicion exists, direct measurement of the pressure within the compartment is necessary to determine whether the muscle contents are threatened. Various methods have been devised for measuring the interstitial tissue pressure.[56,73] Basically they consist of inserting a large-bore needle or cannula into the compartment, connecting the needle through a fluid-filled assembly with a manometer, and noting the millimeters of mercury pressure necessary to overcome the resistance within the compartment when attempting to inject fluid into it (Figs. 17-3 and 17-4). If the tissue pressure approaches the range within 10 mm Hg to 20 mm Hg of the diastolic pressure, cessation of blood flow is imminent. When tissue pressure reaches 40 mm Hg to 50 mm Hg, muscle-threatening compression and ischemia are present. A pressure of 30 mm Hg or greater may be used as a criterion for performing a fasciotomy. Immediate fasciotomy with débridement of obviously necrotic muscle is important not only to prevent further damage to remaining viable muscle but also to decrease the systemic effects of myonecrosis (see Crush Syndrome).

TREATMENT

Surgical decompression is urgent. The entire fascial envelope must be split over a wide area sufficient to allow all muscles within the compartment to protrude. In addition, each muscle must be released by splitting its epimyseal sheath over its entire length.[32] This must be done with caution to avoid the nerve structures. When this procedure is done at an early stage, the pale, gray, lifeless muscle bulges through and at once blushes with a reactive hyperemia and considerable oozing of blood. Failure of this phenomenon to develop is ominous because it denotes poor perfusion. Following fasciotomy and epimysiotomy, if distal pulses are not restored, the main artery proximally must be inspected. Marked narrowing of the vessel may be the result of persistent spasm. Infiltration of papaverine about the vessel will often relax the arterial muscle wall, but this effect requires about 15 to 20 minutes to become apparent.[46] If this maneuver fails to restore the original diameter of the artery, the spasm may be relieved by injecting a bolus of fluid into the proximal segment of the artery.[57] If the artery, despite these measures, fails to expand, the narrowing may represent collapse of the vessel immediately distal to the point of obstruction by a thrombus. An arteriotomy and thrombectomy are necessary. If the artery is compressed by a fragment of bone, this must be corrected and soft tissue release carried out.

The need to explore and decompress major nerves will depend on the degree of the neurologic deficit. Within the forearm, the median nerve may need to be freed where it passes between the heads of origin of the pronator teres and through the tendinous arch of the flexor superficialis.

In the forearm, the deep muscle group, composed of the flexor digitorum profundus and the flexor pollicis longus, is frequently involved, and, unless they are sought beneath the superficial muscles and decompressed, necrosis and contractures are inevitable.

The fascia is left open. The marked swelling will not permit primary skin closure, and secondary suture, probably aided by skin grafts, is done after swelling has subsided.

The paralyzed parts must be splinted in an overcorrected position, but care must be taken to avoid overstretching the swollen muscles. A functional position must be sought in the event that some contracture develops. Gently performed range of motion exercises maintain mobility and prevent deformity. Later, active exercises and dynamic splinting are added.

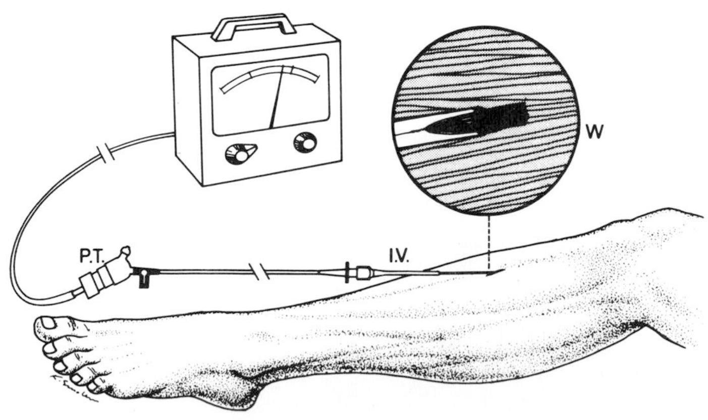

FIG. 17-4. Wick catheter measurement of intracompartmental pressures in the leg. (Owen CA et al: Intramuscular pressures with limb compression. N Engl J Med 300:1169, 1979)

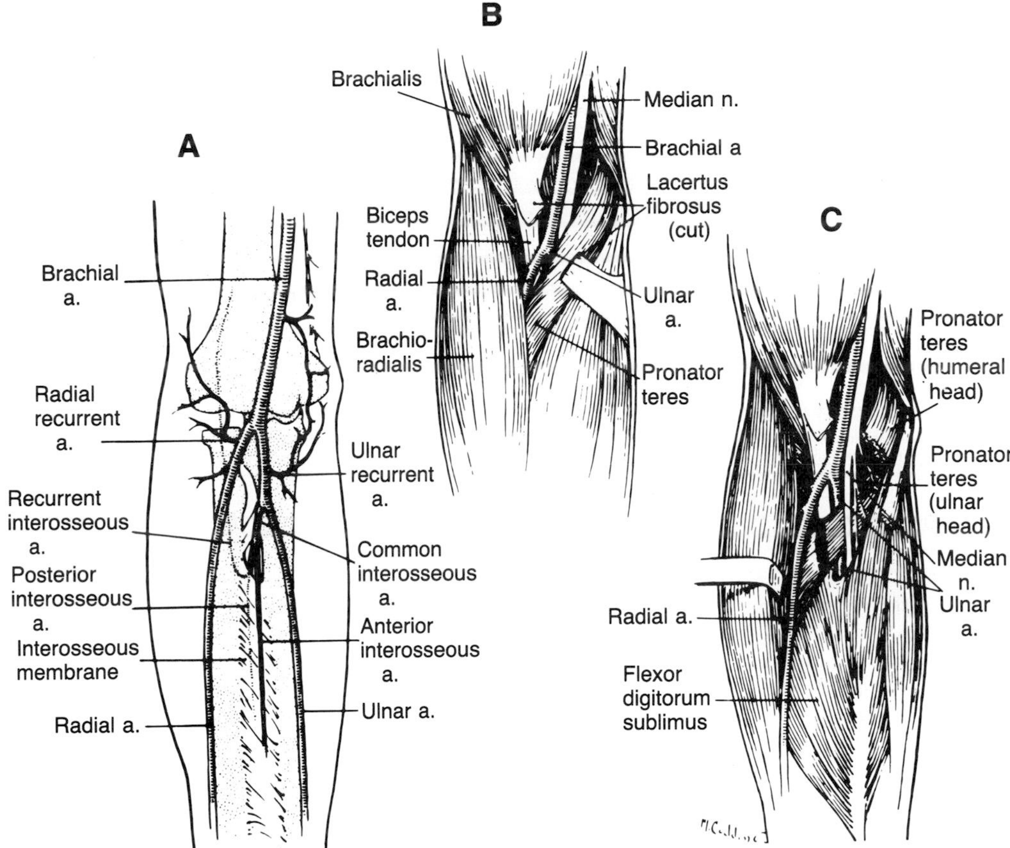

FIG. 17-5. Anatomy of Volkmann's ischemia. (*A*) Collaterals about the elbow do not communicate with vessels within the volar compartment. Their connections to brachial, radial, and ulnar arteries are proximal to the pronator teres. (*B*) The brachial artery and median nerve enter the forearm through a narrow interval formed by biceps tendon insertion laterally and pronator teres medially and roofed over by lacertus fibrosus; at this point they may be compressed by muscle swelling or hematoma. (*C*) The radial artery, arising from the brachial artery, passes superficially to the wrist. It is not crossed by any structure. The ulnar artery passes beneath pronator teres and lies in deepest portion of the compartment. The median nerve usually passes between the humeral and ulnar heads of the pronator teres, where it may be compressed, and again by the firm arcuate tendinous band of origin of the superficialis. (Eaton RG, Green WT: Epimysiotomy and fasciotomy in the treatment of Volkmann's ischemic contracture. Orthop Clin North Am 3:175, 1972)

VOLKMANN'S ISCHEMIC CONTRACTURE

As originally described by Volkmann in 1881, this condition is characterized by ischemic necrosis of the structures contained within the volar compartment of the forearm, usually following a severe injury about the elbow or directly to the forearm, eventuating in crippling contractures often associated with varying degrees of a neurologic deficit.[71] Although the classic type of Volkmann's ischemic contracture is described here, the term is often applied to compartmental syndromes elsewhere. A more appropriate designation is *anterior compartmental syndrome of the forearm.* The pathogenesis producing the vicious circle of edema-compression-ischemia, described in the previous sections, is identical in all compartment syndromes.

ANATOMICAL CONSIDERATIONS

At the entrance to the flexor compartment of the forearm, the lacertus fibrosus fans medially from the biceps tendon. Beneath the lacertus fibrosus, the bulky pronator teres muscle creates a V-shaped sphincter beneath which the brachial artery and median nerve pass to enter the flexor compartment (Fig. 17-5). These structures may be compressed at this site by edema or hemorrhage. The brachialis artery may be impaled on the sharp edge of the proximal fragment of a supracondylar fracture against which it is held by the lacertus fibrosus. Beyond this point, the brachial artery divides into the radial and ulnar arteries. The radial artery then courses superficially and is not crossed by any structure in the forearm. On the other hand, the ulnar artery passes deep to the pronator teres and with its major branch, the interosseous artery, provides the major blood supply to the forearm muscles. The common interosseous artery arises from the ulnar artery beneath the pronator teres and immediately divides into the anterior and posterior interosseous arteries. The anterior or volar interosseous artery passes distally on the interosseous membrane and is the sole blood supply to the flexor digitorum profundus and flexor pollicis longus muscles.

The median nerve accompanies the brachial artery beneath the lacertus fibrosus arch and enters the substance of the pronator teres, usually passing between the humeral and ulnar heads. As it proceeds distally, it passes beneath the fibrous arch created by the radial and ulnar origins of the flexor superficialis muscle. It is therefore possible for the nerve to be compressed by a swollen pronator teres or the sharp unyielding edge of the conjoined tendon of the flexor superficialis muscle.

In severe Volkmann's ischemia, arterial spasm affects all branches of the common interosseous artery. The extensive collateral circulation about the elbow does not communicate with vessels within the flexor compartment.[32]

ETIOLOGY

In the child under 10 years of age, an injury about the elbow, particularly a supracondylar fracture of the humerus, is the most common precipitating injury and generally produces the more severe types of ischemic necrosis and contracture. Mild cases are usually due to a contusion or a crush injury of the forearm, sometimes associated with fractures of the forearm, and occurring in people 20 to 25 years of age.

CLINICAL PICTURE

Following the precipitating trauma, an interval of hours elapses before the onset of symptoms. At first, severe, deep, unrelenting, poorly localized pain develops in the forearm. The volar aspect of the forearm is swollen, red, and warm, is exquisitely tender, and is tense to palpation. The fingers are held in flexion, and attempts to extend the fingers intensifies the pain (stretch pain). The peripheral pulses are present at least during the initial stages while muscle necrosis is already taking place, but they may diminish in volume and entirely disappear; by then severe irretrievable damage will already have occurred. Initial nerve involvement is evidenced by diminished sensation in the autonomous sensory zone of the affected nerve, most commonly the median nerve, less often the ulnar nerve. Two-point discrimination and light touch are more reliable than pinprick. Complete glove anesthesia during the early stages implies extreme ischemia and an ominous prognosis.[69] Active finger flexion is weak, progressing, if left untreated and compounded by nerve damage. to paralysis. Advanced nerve deficit results in paralysis of not only the flexor muscles but also the intrinsic muscles of the hand.

Within a few days the pain and swelling subside and the volar aspect of the forearm develops a wooden induration. The resulting deformity represents contractural plus paralytic origin. When it is mild, the deep flexor muscles are partially involved, particularly the flexor digitorum profundus, producing a flexion contracture deformity of one or more fingers: the long finger alone; the long and ring fingers; the long, ring, and little fingers; or all fingers except the thumb. The thumb may be partially affected. When the wrist is hyperflexed, the fingers can be extended. Resistant pronation contracture deformity is caused by cicatrization of either the pronator teres (induration palpable in proximal forearm) or the pronator quadratus (induration palpable in distal forearm).

A moderate contracture involves most of the flexor digitorum profundus and flexor pollicis longus and part of the flexor digitorum superficialis. Nearly always, a neurologic deficit exists, and the median nerve is more severely affected than the ulnar nerve. The deformity is an intrinsic-minus hand, a flexion contracture of all of the digits, and diminished sensation in the distribution of the median and ulnar nerves.

Severe Volkmann's contracture involves all the flexor muscles and occasionally some of the extensor muscles. The neurologic deficit is severe, joint contractures are marked, and skin scarring and bone deformity may be added (Fig. 17-6).

Certain diagnostic signs regarded as classic and typical of the acute compartment syndrome of the forearm (impending Volkmann's ischemic contracture) have been described. These classical "Ps" will vary depending on whether the cause is local compression or a major arterial injury, or both. When local compression is the cause, the five Ps in the hand are pulses intact (at least during the early phase), paresis, stretch pain, paresthesia, and pink coloring (good capillary filling). With major arterial injury, the signs are pain on stretch, paresthesias, pulselessness, pallor (or cyanosis), and paresis. A sensory deficit can usually be mapped out that will define a specific neurapraxia pointing to involvement of the compartment through which the nerve courses. In the chronic contracted phase of Volkmann's ischemic contracture resulting from local compression, the pulses in most cases are intact and there is usually little or no pain.

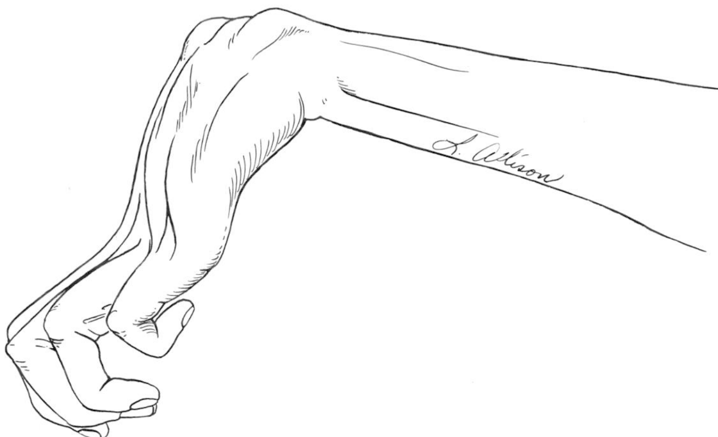

FIG. 17-6. Volkmann's ischemic contracture showing the typical severe deformity.

When injury is sustained in childhood and ischemic necrosis is mild, the complication may be overlooked. The contracture at first may not be apparent, but progressive deformity develops with advancing skeletal growth. Consequently, continuing watchfulness after a supracondylar fracture is mandatory.

TREATMENT

Acute Stage. Impending Volkmann's contracture should be recognized and treated at the earliest moment as a surgical emergency.[33,34] If possible, surgical decompression should be performed long before the peripheral pulsations are lost. The need for surgical intervention can be determined by direct measurement of the intracompartmental pressures. When tissue pressure approaches the level of the diastolic blood pressure, severe irretrievable muscle necrosis is imminent and the compartment should be widely opened by fasciotomy. Epimysiotomy of each muscle must be added. Surgical exploration must extend deeply to the flexor digitorum profundus, which sustains the maximum degree of necrosis, and the flexor pollicis longus. Grayish necrotic muscle tissue must be excised. The median nerve should be freed where it passes beneath the lacertus fibrosus, through the pronator quadratus, through the arcade formed by the flexor digitorum superficialis origins, and at the carpal tunnel. The ulnar nerve likewise should be freed and, if necessary, transplanted anteriorly. Caution must be exercised to protect both neural and vascular structures.

If peripheral pulses are not restored, the brachial artery must be inspected and decompressed. The vessel may be found in spasm especially distal to the site of a supracondylar fracture. A laceration of the artery is repaired. Injection of 2.5% papaverine or a local anesthetic about the artery may relieve spasm. Stripping of the adventitia, in effect a periarterial sympathectomy, may be required. Complete occlusion by a thrombus requires a thrombectomy. The surgical wound is left open until swelling subsides, and secondary closure is done later. The extremity is supported with a splint in the functional position, and care must be exercised to avoid stretching the friable muscles. Later, dynamic splinting and exercises prevent deformity.

Established Deformity. Deformities, for planning a program of treatment, can be categorized into mild, moderate, and severe types.[62,68,70]

Mild Type. One or more fingers are affected, and when the wrist is hyperflexed, the fingers can be fully extended. Treatment consists in dynamic splinting, physical therapy, and functional training. When contracture is limited to two fingers, the extent of muscle fibrosis is limited, and excision of the affected area will suffice. When contracture is more extensive, involving three or four fingers, a muscle sliding operation is indicated.[62]

The sliding operation consists in releasing the flexor muscles from their origins. The flexor muscles that gain attachment to the interosseous membrane are also released. Excision is carried out while the fingers are passively extended to note whether adequate release has been achieved. The anterior interosseous artery and nerve must be protected, especially where the dorsal interosseous artery and vein pass to the dorsum. Neurolysis is effected, and, if necessary, anterior transposition of the ulnar nerve is carried out. Postoperatively, the forearm is immobilized in supination with the wrist extended, the metacarpophalangeal joints in slight flexion, and the fingers extended for several weeks. Then a dynamic splint is worn to prevent recurrence, and exercises are begun.

Less often, the contracture chiefly involves the pronator teres, producing a pronation contracture and involvement of the median nerve. The induration is palpated over the proximal portion of the forearm. Treatment consists in freeing the attachments of the muscle, excising the scar, and, effecting neurolysis. The same deformity is produced by contracture of the pronator quadratus in the distal portion of the forearm where the induration is palpable. Treatment requires dissecting out the muscle, tenolysis, and neurolysis. In all of the mild types, the outlook following treatment is favorable.

Moderate Type. When nearly all of the flexor profundus and flexor pollicis longus are affected and a neurologic deficit exists in which the median is more severely affected than the ulnar nerve, the following deformity is produced: intrinsic–minus clawhand, flexion contracture of all digits, and diminished sensation of median and, to a lesser degree, ulnar distribution.

A muscle sliding procedure, excision of cicatrix, and neurolysis are done. Extensive release of both superficial and deep muscles must include the detachment of the insertions of the pronator teres and the origin of the flexor pollicis longus from the radius. This is approached through an incision between the brachioradialis and the flexor pollicis longus and pronator teres. Usually good return of sensation and intrinsic function can be expected, although with some reduction of grip strength. If necessary, approximately 5 to 6 months later, after the extensors regain their strength, tendon transfers of extensors to the flexor pollicis longus and flexor digitorum profundus may be done.

Severe Type. All flexor muscles are fibrotic, the neurologic deficit is severe, joints are markedly contracted, the skin is scarred, and bone deformities are often associated. Treatment is difficult and results are poor. Often a pedicle skin graft is required. If the extensors are preserved, the brachioradialis and wrist extensors are transferred to the flexor pollicis longus and the profundus of the fingers. The superficialis tendons are excised at the same time. Where no muscle is available for transfer, a flexor tenodesis and an intermetacarpal fusion, placing the thumb in opposition, may be considered.

ANTERIOR COMPARTMENT SYNDROME OF THE LEG

The anterior compartment syndrome of the leg (also known as anterior tibial syndrome and traumatic necrosis of pretibial muscles) is characterized pathologically by progressive necrosis of the muscles within the anterior tibial compartment brought about by increased pressure within that space; if left untreated it leads to paralysis and contracture.[49,67]

FIG. 17-7. Cross section at the junction of the middle and distal thirds of the leg illustrates the four compartments and their respective nerves. Beyond this point, the sural nerve courses outside of the fascia. (Mubarak SJ, Owen CA: Double-incision fasciotomy of the leg for decompression in compartment syndromes. J Bone Joint Surg 59A:184, 1977)

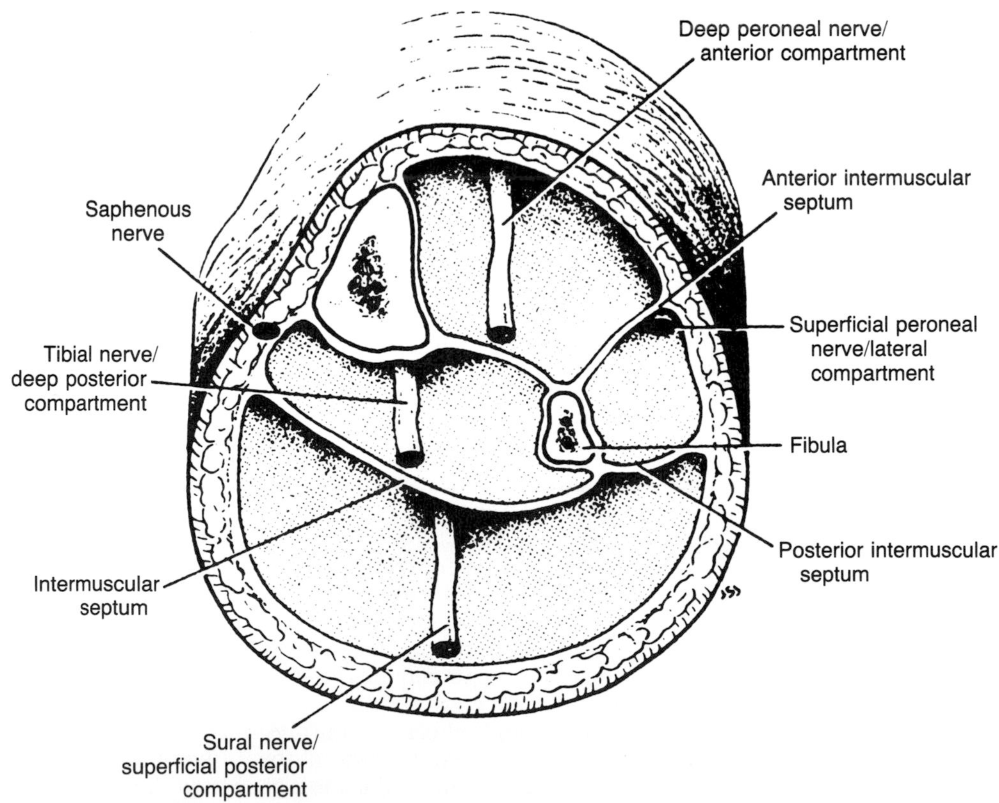

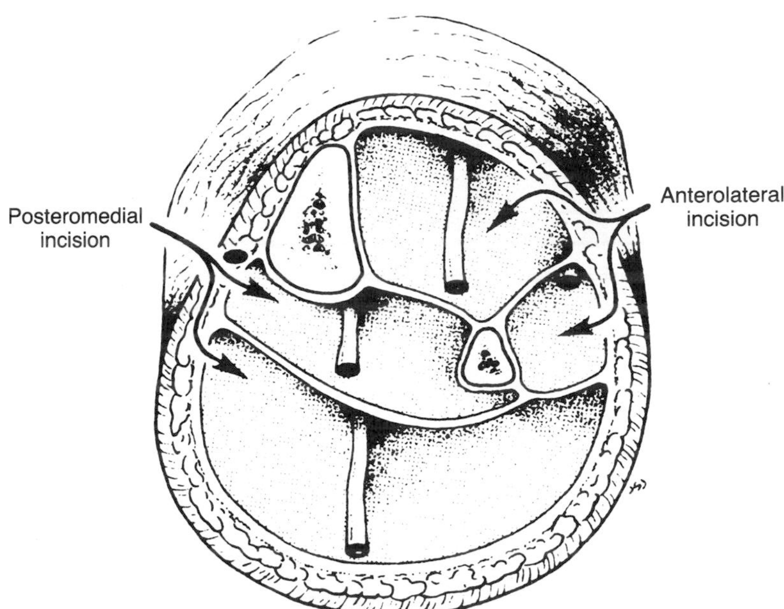

FIG. 17-8. Illustration of four-compartment decompression using a double-incision method. (Mubarak SJ, Owen CA: Double-incision fasciotomy of the leg for decompression in compartment syndromes. J Bone Joint Surg 59A:184, 1977)

ANATOMICAL CONSIDERATIONS

The osseofascial enclosure is bounded posteriorly by the tibia, fibula, and interosseous membrane and anteriorly by the anterior crural fascia. Its contents include the anterior tibial, extensor hallucis longus, and extensor digitorum longus muscles; the anterior tibial artery and vein; and the deep peroneal nerve, which supplies these muscles and whose autonomous sensory zone is a triangular area on the dorsum of the foot proximal to the web between the first and the second toes (Figs. 17-7 through 17-9).

ETIOLOGY AND THEORY OF PATHOGENESIS

The main pathogenetic factor is increased intracompartmental pressure, which by compressing the minute vessels of the vascular bed and reflexly inducing spasm of the arterioles produces relative anoxia that results in muscle necrosis and fibrous tissue replacement.[43,48] The most common precipitating cause is a vigorous period of exercise, usually in a young person unaccustomed to such physical exertion.

Normally, when muscle contracts repeatedly during exercise, its bulk is increased by 20%, and pressure within the closed compartment rises. Hyperemia develops, and increased filtration of fluid out of the capillaries and into the interstitial tissues takes place. This phenomenon presumably is caused by increased capillary pressure and increased capillary surface area. The increase of muscular volume and mechanical factors during muscular contraction produce an increase in total intramuscular pressure that remains elevated after exercise has been discontinued. After a rest period of 5 to 10 minutes, the interstitial fluid volume lessens and the intramuscular pressure is restored to normal levels.

In an abnormal situation, the resting pressure is generally higher than normal (0 mm Hg – 4 mm Hg) and rises to a greater height with exercise, and recovery is slow and incomplete. Presumably, increased capillary permeability, which allows excessive transudation of fluid, is the result of anoxia, which is perpetuated by increasing intracompartmental pressure.

Less frequently the cause is closed fracture of the tibia. Rarely, about 12 to 36 hours after vascular occlusion of a large artery has been surgically relieved and blood flow restored, an anterior compartment syndrome may develop. Blockage of the anterior tibial artery itself does not produce the syndrome, because collateral circulation through the posterior tibial and peroneal arteries is adequate. A soft tissue injury that causes an intracompartmental hemorrhage can produce excessive tissue pressure that can initiate the vicious circle.

In certain centers for acute trauma, the causes of the compartment syndrome of the leg may vary in frequency. For example, a closed tibial fracture may be the leading initiating factor, and other common causes may include a severe contusion of the leg, a major arterial injury or the postoperative sequela of vascular reconstruction, improper traction procedures (especially in a child), and postural limb compression in drug overdose victims. A leg compartment syndrome provoked by an acute unaccustomed vigorous exercise may prove the exception, and chronic exertional activity may more often initiate the syndrome.[53] Despite these variations in frequency, the orthopaedic surgeon should develop an awareness of the diverse factors that can produce increased inter-

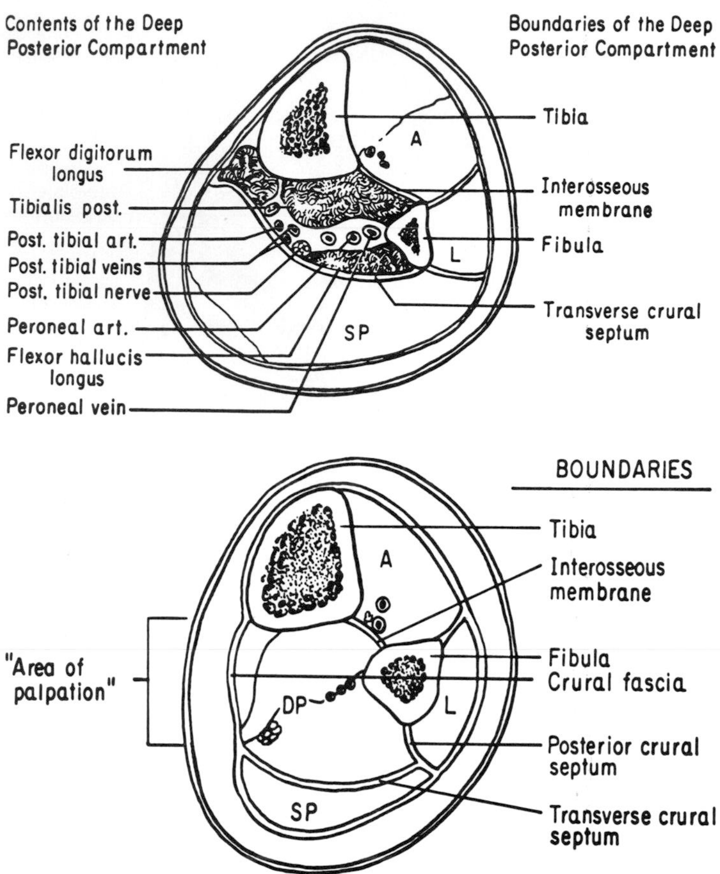

FIG. 17-9. (*Top*) Coss section through the midportion of the leg, showing contents and boundaries of the deep posterior compartment as well as the location of the anterior (*A*), lateral (*L*), and superficial posterior (*SP*) compartments. (*Bottom*) Cross section at the junction of the middle and distal thirds of the leg showing the boundaries of the deep posterior compartment (*DP*), including the posterior crural septum and the crural fascia. The "area of palpation" is the site where tenseness of the compartment may be palpated. (Matsen FA III, Clawson DK: The deep posterior compartmental syndrome of the leg. J Bone Joint Surg 57A:34, 1975)

stitial tissue fluid pressure and muscle ischemia within one or several closed osseofascial compartments of the leg.

CLINICAL PICTURE

The syndrome is precipitated by any one of diverse known local or proximal factors; the orthopaedic surgeon should be aware of these and have a high index of suspicion to recognize and treat this complication at the earliest moment. As an example, following a period of unaccustomed exercise, and after an interval of 10 to 12 hours, the patient, often a young adult male, develops aching pain in the anterior aspect of one or both legs. The intensity of the pain varies and may be severe and unremitting; however, the pain may be entirely lacking. A tense, tender swelling is perceived over the entire anterior compartment. Active and passive movement of the foot, particularly plantar flexion of the ankle and toes, which stretches the affected muscles, intensifies the pain (stretch pain). Weakness of the pretibial muscles, especially the anterior tibial and extensor hallucis longus, develops quickly and may progress to complete paralysis. The resulting footdrop is less pronounced than that associated with nerve lesions because of developing contracture in the affected muscles. These muscles lack electric excitability, failing to respond to either faradic or galvanic current, and electromyography shows complete silence on attempted voluntary contraction. The overlying skin is erythematous, glossy, edematous, and warm. Mild systemic symptoms, such as a low-grade fever, leukocytosis, and albuminuria, and sometimes myoglobinuria, are not uncommon.

In the initial phase of muscle weakness, the extensor digitorum brevis is included, reflecting involvement of the deep peroneal nerve. In an incomplete compartment syndrome, the extensor digitorum longus is less involved than the other muscles.

Hypoesthesia is detected in the autonomous zone of the deep peroneal nerve: a triangular area over the dorsum of the foot just proximal to the web of the first and second toes.

The dorsalis pedis pulse is generally palpable, unless the vessel is absent as an anatomical variation.

The pain, dermal erythema, and systemic symptoms subside within a few days. However, the paralysis may persist, and fibrous contracture develops and plantar flexion of the foot is limited by the contracture.

DIAGNOSIS

Measurement of total intracompartmental pressure should detect an excessive pressure that threatens to produce muscle necrosis and irretrievable damage.[64] In the acute case, tissue pressures will be inordinately high, generally approaching the level of disastolic pressure. Repeated measurements may be necessary to determine the progressiveness of the condition. When correlated with progressively developing clinical signs, a presumptive diagnosis is sufficient grounds for performing a decompression surgical procedure. Procrastination and awaiting the development of definite signs such as paralysis have permitted irretrievable damage to take place.

Certain patients who develop symptoms after exercise, causing the patient to discontinue performance of strenuous endeavors such as athletics, may have milder but nevertheless disabling manifestations of the same condition. This syndrome may be designated as the chronic compartmental syndrome. It can be defined by measurements of intracompartmental pressures after a short period of exercise. Such people at rest have higher than normal intracompartmental pressure; following exercise, the pressure rises to abnormally great heights; after rest, the pressure subsides slowly but never reaches normal resting levels. A useful tool is the phlebogram. After exercise, the high intramuscular pressure will prevent adequate venous filling.

TREATMENT

The crural fascia should be incised immediately over a wide area sufficient to allow the swollen muscles to protrude. The epimysium of each muscle should likewise be incised. Necrotic tissue should be excised to reduce the amount of fibrous replacement. The skin and fascial wounds are left open, and after swelling has subsided, generally within a week to 10 days, secondary skin closure is done. Foot and ankle motion must be prevented by splinting to protect the muscles from tearing, until regeneration and fibrous replacement have occurred. If necrosis is not too extensive, and decompression has been performed early before the development of paralysis, recovery of muscle function may be anticipated. During the acute stage, manipulation of the paralyzed legs is prohibited, because sudden severe destruction of muscle fibers may lead to myoglobinuria, lower nephron nephrosis, and death.[66]

DEEP POSTERIOR COMPARTMENT SYNDROME OF THE LEG

The deep posterior compartment of the leg contains the flexor hallucis longus, flexor digitorum longus, and posterior tibial muscles, the posterior tibial and peroneal arteries, and the posterior tibial nerve. The compartment is bounded anteriorly by the tibia and fibula and interosseous membrane and posteriorly by the posterior crural fascia and its medial and lateral extensions. The posterior tibial artery enters the tibia at the junction of its upper and middle thirds, where it is tethered and subjected to injury. Bleeding from a laceration of the posterior tibial or peroneal artery associated with fractures may increase intracompartmental pressure. The posterior tibial nerve runs adjacent to the posterior tibial artery. It innervates all of the intrinsic muscles of the foot except the extensor digitorum brevis; its autonomous sensory zone includes the plantar surface of the toes and the sole of the foot except the instep.

The syndrome most commonly follows, after a latent period of hours to several days, fractures of the tibia and fibula, less often soft tissue injury, and intracompartmental pressure may be compounded by poorly fitted encircling casts or dressings. Its characteristics include pain, which may vary from slight to severe and boring and is intensified by passive extension of the toes, plantar hypoesthesia (posterior tibial nerve), weakness of toe flexion, and tenseness and tenderness perceived in the distal medial part of the leg between the tibia and the triceps surae.[51,61]

Decompression within 12 hours of onset will prevent permanent sequelae: clawtoes, posterior tibial neuropathy, and weakness or contracture of long toe flexors and the posterior tibial.

PERONEAL COMPARTMENT SYNDROME

The peroneal compartment syndrome is an uncommon condition that involves the peroneal muscles and the common peroneal nerve or the superficial peroneal nerve alone within the peroneal myofascial compartment of the leg.[26,50,65] Like the anterior tibial syndrome with which it is sometimes associated, there is no history of injury, although the condition occurs in young healthy men and follows unusual strenuous activity. The onset is gradual, the condition developing some hours after cessation of the activity. There is increasingly severe pain over the lateral aspect of the leg which usually awakens the patient at night. The outer side of the leg becomes swollen and tender, and the overlying skin becomes red and warm. Any active movement of the foot provokes severe pain in the peroneal area, and passive inversion of the foot, which stretches the peronei, causes intense pain. Palpation over the peroneal muscles reveals a wooden or firm rubbery resistance, and the lightest touch causes discomfort. Involvement of the common peroneal nerve, which courses through the compartment before dividing into superficial and deep peroneal (anterior tibial) branches, is manifested by a sensory deficit over the distal portion of the lateral aspect of the leg, the dorsum of the foot, and an autonomous zone of the deep peroneal nerve at the dorsum of the foot proximal to the first interdigital cleft. As the nerve deficit worsens, active eversion is impossible, and paralysis of the extensor digitorum brevis attests to involvement of the deep peroneal nerve. Peripheral pulses are unaffected.

If the condition remains untreated, the pain, tenderness, redness, and swelling gradually subside over several days. The affected muscles within the lateral compartment are then felt to be wooden hard. As a contracture develops, active and passive inversion of the foot are restricted, and active eversion is weak or lacking. During the acute phase, the peroneal muscles are unresponsive to electrical stimulation and may remain so thereafter.

TREATMENT

Extensive unroofing of the peroneal compartment is considered a surgical emergency. In addition, the epimysium of each muscle should be split to permit the muscle belly to bulge outward. A necrotic muscle is gray and friable and should be excised to reduce the possibility of infection and fibrous tissue replacement. Otherwise, the muscle should be covered with sterile dressings and secondary skin closure effected after the swelling subsides.

Because the anterior tibial compartment is often involved at the same time, it too should be decompressed by fasciotomy and its contents inspected. An alternative procedure, a transfibular approach, will decompress both compartments as well as the deep posterior compartment. This latter operation is particularly useful for decompressing all compartments to relieve the generalized muscle edema that occurs after restoration of circulation following temporary arterial occlusion.[34,45]

Technique of Transfibular Approach.[66a] All compartments are approached through a long lateral incision made directly over the fibula extending from just below the fibular neck to a point 3 cm to 4 cm above the lateral malleolus. The incision is deepened to incise the fascia overlying the lateral compartment which is opened throughout its length. The anterior flap is retracted to expose the fascia overlying the anterior compartment, and a second long incision is made through the fascia decompressing the long extensor muscles. Care is taken to avoid the superficial peroneal nerve that exits from the fascia in the distal third of the leg near the septum between the anterior and lateral compartment and then courses anteriorly. Then the posterior flap is retracted to uncover the superficial posterior compartment fascia that is incised the full length of the gastrocnemius and soleus. Next, the attachments of the soleus to the fibula are separated so that the gastroc-soleus can be retracted backward to visualize the fascia overlying the deep posterior compartment encasing the tibialis posterior, flexor hallucis longus, and flexor digitorum. The fascia is incised. Care is taken to avoid injury to the peroneal and posterior tibial vascular bundles. Epimysiotomy of individual muscle bellies within each compartment may be carried out if necessary. The wound is left open and packed with fine-mesh gauze. Wound closure can be accomplished by primary suture in 1 to 2 weeks or by split thickness grafts after the swelling has subsided.

SUPERFICIAL POSTERIOR COMPARTMENT SYNDROME OF THE LEG

The superficial posterior compartment of the leg is the osseofascial compartment that contains the gastrocnemius and soleus muscles and the sural nerve. The enclosure is formed by the deep fascia posteriorly and an intermuscular septum (deep transverse fascia) anteriorly, the latter constituting the roof of the deep posterior compartment. Normally the lateral portion of the fascial covering is quite thin and allows the muscles to expand, but in exceptional instances it is thick and unyielding. At the lateral side, the posterior layer and the intermuscular septum join to attach to the fibula. Therefore, removal of the fibula will provide ready access to both posterior compartments. On the medial side, the deep fascia and intermuscular septum join to attach to the posteromedial aspect of the tibia. The sural nerve, which arises from the posterior tibial nerve, courses beneath the posterior layer of deep fascia until the midportion of the leg, where it penetrates the fascia and continues its course outside the fascia adjacent to the short saphenous vein en route to the outer aspect of the foot. It supplies sensation to the lateral border and adjacent dorsal surface of the foot and the lateral aspect of the little toe.

Acute involvement of this compartment alone is exceedingly rare, and when this occurs it appears to be due to the intramuscular tearing and hemorrhage that follow a period of vigorous unaccustomed exercise.[55] More commonly it shares with one or more compartments of the leg the effects of local causes (closed tibial fracture, crush syndrome, vigorous unaccustomed exercise) or proximal causes (arterial injury, traction for femoral fracture).

Certain etiologic factors, despite provoking multiple compartment involvement, appear to chiefly affect the posterior superficial compartment, and the end result of the neglected untreated case is a fibrous contracture of the gastrocnemius and soleus muscles and a resistant equinus deformity.

Improperly applied Bryant's traction, especially in a child over 2 years of age, is especially prone to produce multiple intracompartmental ischemia of the leg, leading to fibrous replacement of the gastroc-soleus group.[58] Unfortunately, this complication generally goes unrecognized until a resistant ankle equinus contracture has developed.[54] Multiple compartment involvement may also result from Buck's traction applied for femoral fractures when the leg is elevated and fully extended.

The ischemia and eventual contracture likewise appear to favor the posterior superficial compartment, but the complication is less severe than that associated with Bryant's traction.[54]

Vigorous repeated exercises to which the patient is not accustomed may produce unusual swelling of the gastroc-soleus group and excessive intracompartmental pressures that ultimately lead to ischemic necrosis and contracture.[47,55] In these subjects, the extent of exercise-induced interstitial edema and pressure is found to be greater than normal. Furthermore, their resting intracompartmental pressure is often found to be greater than normal (4 mm Hg ± 4).

Clinically, the acute involvement of the superficial posterior compartment is characterized by local calf pain intensified by dorsiflexing the foot and a tense, tender calf often surmounted by erythematous skin. A sensory deficit occurs late and involves the outer side of the foot and small toe. The pulses are preserved unless arterial injury is the precipitating cause.

Preventative treatment refers to identifying the causative factor and avoiding it. Bryant's traction should not be used in a child over 2 years of age and weighing more than 30 lb.[58] Fracture of the femur treated by Buck's traction should be monitored at least during the early days for increasing intracompartmental pressure within the leg. Instead of straight-leg traction, split Russell's traction is preferable. Excessive distraction of the femoral fragments may induce arterial spasm and should be avoided. Extreme elevation of the leg will greatly reduce arterial flow at the ankle and may contribute to compartment ischemia. When unaccustomed repeated exercise (*e.g.*, forced marches, jogging) induces leg pain despite preserved foot pulses and the period of rest required to relieve the pain becomes progressively longer, such exertional activity must be suspended.

When the acute episode persists despite elimination of the probable causes and intracompartmental pressure reaches 30 mm Hg, a decompression fasciotomy is indicated.

CRUSH SYNDROME

Prolonged direct compression of muscles in widespread areas, particularly those confined within tight fascial compartments, produces extensive muscle necrosis with outpouring of large quantities of myoglobin and potassium into the systemic circulation; this results in serious and possibly life-threatening visceral impairment. The syndrome is characterized etiologically by compression of several limbs for more than several hours; pathologically by severe and extensive swelling and necrosis of muscles, high intracompartmental pressures, and renal tubular changes that develop rapidly, leading to kidney failure which is often fatal; and clinically by massively swollen, tense limbs, hypovolemic shock, myoglobinuria, and renal failure. The first descriptions of this condition were those of earthquake victims in Messina, Italy, in 1909, and it was notable during the bombardments of World War I and II and the Vietnam Conflict, when extremities were crushed by falling debris.[28] It is now recognized as a hazard in many situations involving massive compression, such as coal mine cave-ins, abnormal postures of drug overdose, and the knee-chest position for lumbar spine surgery.[21,25,42]

PATHOLOGY

The descriptions of ischemic and necrotic muscles within closed fascial compartments have been presented in previous sections. All such muscles, including those outside such compartments, are blanched, friable, and necrotic, resembling fish flesh. The kidneys are enlarged and swollen. Microscopically, tubular necrosis is pronounced. If the patient dies within the first week from kidney failure, the renal tissue is edematous and there are large hyaline casts and brown pigment material within the distal convoluted tubules. The proximal convoluted tubules show cloudy swelling and desquamation. Areas of necrosis are seen in the boundary zone and distal convoluted tubules.[28]

Theories of renal failure include blockage of distal convoluted tubules by precipitated myoglobin, tubular anoxia due to hypotension, and tubular anoxia due to reflex vasoconstriction.

Other organs are also involved, notably the lung, which may exhibit findings typical of contusion or blast lung.

CLINICAL PICTURE

The patient has been subjected to massive crush injury that has been prolonged for several hours or longer. It is only after release of the compressive force that the clinical picture evolves. Initially, sudden masssive swelling of the involved areas develops because of the marked edema and a variable degree of local hemorrhage. This is the result of the anoxia during the period of compression that causes increased capillary permeability with massive transudation and extravasation of plasma and electrolyte-bearing fluid. This leads to the first phase of shock, which is well compensated for by peripheral vasoconstriction, producing pale, cold, moist skin while maintaining a normal level of blood pressure. Eventually the compensatory mechanism is unable to keep up with the fluid loss, the blood pressure falls, and the second stage of shock develops. At this point, the life-threatening situation requires giving large volumes of plasma and crystalloid solutions to restore an adequate blood pressure.

After the blood pressure is stabilized, the condition of the patient may cause no concern until urine specimens reveal pigment resembling hemoglobin and giving a positive benzidine reaction. The urine also contains albumin, creatinine, and pigmented granular casts. The urine is highly acid because the extensive breakdown of tissue liberates large amounts of lactic and phosphoric acids.

Meanwhile, the damaged limb becomes increasingly swollen and hard over 4 or 5 days and becomes covered with vesicles, bullae, and petechiae. The degree of patchy anesthesia is highly variable. The degree and extent of paralysis are related to the involved muscles. Peripheral pulses are usually absent but may be preserved and are misleading as to the extent of muscle involvement. The limb may be pale and cold, and damage to the main arterial supply may be associated.

LABORATORY FINDINGS

Myoglobinuria is demonstrated by a positive benzidine test in the absence of red blood cells. Myoglobinuric renal failure (crush kidney) is evidenced by rising blood urea nitrogen (BUN) and phosphate concentrations and decreased carbon dioxide combining power. The blood myoglobin content is extremely high. Serum potassium levels rise and produce a hyperkalemic metabolic acidosis. The creatine phosphokinase is markedly elevated, often as high as 14,000 I. U. (normal = up to 130 I. U.). Intracompartmental pressure is two to three times the normal diastolic pressure.[30] When these laboratory values are progressive and accompanied by reduced urinary output, the prognosis is extremely grave.

SUBSEQUENT COURSE

The patient often experiences pain in the loin about the fourth or fifth day, presumably due to swelling of the kidney which distends the renal capsule. The end of the first week is the critical period. In those patients who recover, a sudden diuresis is seen, and the blood findings revert to normal.

In severe involvement with progressive renal failure, a hyperkalemic-induced cardiac irregularity is noted, and the patient may suddenly die.

TREATMENT

The treatment of massive crush injury demands emergent medical and surgical measures.

Initial Period of Shock. Hypovolemic shock requires the replacement of lost intravascular fluids with crystalloid solutions, preferably alkaline to prevent precipitation of myoglobin crystals in the kidney tubules. An intravenous infusion of isotonic sodium citrate or sodium lactate one sixth molar is given along with plasma. Alternatively, 30 g to 40 g bicarbonate is given orally or a lesser amount intravenously. If tetany is induced, calcium gluconate is given intramuscularly. Potassium salts should not be used. Whole blood should not be used because the patient is already suffering from hemoconcentration.

Compartment Decompression. Decompression should include epimysiotomy of all muscles and neurolysis where the nerves pass through narrow passageways. All necrotic muscle should be excised.[52]

Infection. Infection is a major cause of death. The infection may develop deeply within the necrotic muscle and lead to septicemia and death. This requires prompt incision and drainage and excision of necrotic muscle. Appropriate antibiotics are administered.

Renal Failure. Acute kidney necrosis and renal failure is the single most important factor that determines the outlook for survival. Treatment includes the administration of large quantities of alkaline fluids intravenously or by mouth to prevent precipitation of myoglobin crystals.[72]

The infusion of mannitol solution, 250 mg/kg, followed by a continuous intravenous drip of mannitol will effectively prevent renal failure and distal tubular necrosis.

When there is a marked increase in serum potassium and BUN, hemodialysis is most effective when given during the first few days. Since decreased sodium levels accentuate the hyperpotassemia, sodium should be administered but should be kept at normal levels. The dialysis may need to be repeated at 2- to 4-day intervals if the period of reduced urine output is extended. The need for hemodialysis is determined by frequent monitoring of serum potassium and BUN levels.

ISCHEMIC NECROSIS OF MUSCLE

Muscle tissue has such rich collateral circulation that infarction is rare in the absence of peripheral circulatory diseases. The causes of ischemic necrosis of muscle are:

1. Occlusion of a main artery by embolism, thrombosis, or compression
2. Thrombosis of multiple peripheral vessels as in Buerger's disease or atherosclerosis
3. Thrombosis of multiple intramuscular vessels as in polyarteritis nodosa
4. Swelling or hemorrhage in certain muscle groups enclosed within rigid fascial compartments (*e.g.*, the pretibial muscles).

PATHOLOGY

Gross Appearance

Necrotic muscle is friable with patches of yellowish green discoloration. The margins of the infarct where the circulation is preserved are a mottled red and yellow; rose-colored foci appear later. Yellow coloration represents destroyed muscle, and rose color represents the regenerating muscle.

Microscopic Appearance

Necrotic fibers are fragmented and stain irregularly. Sarcolemmic nuclei are shrunken and pyknotic. At the margins of the necrotic zone, fibers undergo degenerative changes such as waxy or hyaline appearance, loss of striations, and pyknosis and disappearance of sarcolemmic nuclei. Next, neutrophilic leukocytes and macrophages infiltrate and remove the damaged fibers. Adjacent to the infarct new fibers are formed. These young fibers are distinguished from old ones by their small size and basophilic coloration in hematoxylin-eosin stains. Finally, vascularized connective tissue replaces the disappearing muscle fibers.

Massive necrosis may not occur, particularly when reduction of circulation is gradual. Instead, there develops a diffuse interstitial fibrosis or multiple foci of necrosis with replacement fibrosis. Under the microscope, interstitial fibrosis is seen as individual healthy muscle fibers or fascicles separated by connective tissue. Scattered collections of lymphocytes and histiocytes infiltrate the perimysium and surround blood vessels. The process suggests vascular congestion and edema causing diffuse alteration of muscle and hyperplasia of connective tissue.

Massive necrosis of an entire muscle is inevitable in the case of certain muscles whose single nutrient artery is compromised by thrombosis, embolism, or injury. Muscles with this peculiarity include the gastrocnemius, the long head of the biceps, and the anterior tibial muscles.

Multiple scattered infarcts throughout a muscle are characteristic of periarteritis nodosa, which causes thrombosis of many minute intramuscular vessels. On the other hand, atherosclerosis or the necrotizing arteriolitis of malignant hypertension rarely occurs in vessels as small as those found in muscle.

Experimental evidence seems to indicate that venous occlusion is more likely to produce a diffuse interstitial fibrosis, whereas arterial occlusion may have no effect whatsoever or may cause multiple foci of necrosis or massive necrosis.[76,80]

RADIOISOTOPE MEASUREMENT OF SKELETAL MUSCLE NECROSIS

Acute skeletal muscle necrosis can be identifed and quantified by using scintigraphy in conjunction with uptake of technetium 99m stannous pyrophosphate (^{99m}Tc-PYP). The accumulation of this pyrophosphate radionuclide is specific for irreversible ischemic injury and later tissue calcification, acting by selective adsorption of pyrophosphate to tissue calcium stores.[77,79] The necrosis is associated with significant accumulation of calcium in mitochondria and sarcoplasmic reticulum, and these sites localize ^{99m}Tc-PYP in proportion to the level of calcium, thus yielding a quantitative correlation between the extent of tissue necrosis and radionuclide uptake.[78] This noninvasive method has been useful for experimental studies of factors involved in the production of the compartment syndrome.[36] It has been found to correlate well with the increased creatine phosphokinase in serum and decreased muscle potassium, both of which occur as a result of skeletal muscle necrosis.

MYOSITIS

The term *myositis* is defined as inflammation of muscle. This implies that an irritative agent, such as bacteria, parasites, virus, produces a reactive vasodilatation, outpouring of serum and cells, and healing by granulation tissue. The inflammatory process takes place in the interstitial tissue, whereas the muscle fibers are destroyed by toxins, compression of accumulating exudate, or ischemia secondary to focal thrombosis. Subsidence of inflammation is followed by attempted regeneration of muscle fibers. True inflammatory myositis should be distinguished from parenchymatous degeneration, which occurs in the course of a systemic infectious disease and displays no inflammatory phenomena.

BACTERIAL (ACUTE SUPPURATIVE)

Abscess formation in muscle is rare. It usually arises by spread from an adjacent focus, such as osteomyelitis, or by a puncture wound; rarely, it is hematogenous. The common causative organisms are staphylococci and streptococci.

PATHOLOGY

Early, edema and cellular infiltration occur in the interstitial tissue. Muscle fibers are intact but display parenchymatous changes, such as swelling, obscuring of cross striations, and granularity or vacuolization. The process may subside with complete restoration of normal histology. It may extend and cause a diffuse interstitial cellular infiltration with vascular thromboses, producing an indurated phlegmonous mass of tissue. An exudate accumulates from continued outpouring of cells, serum, and liquefaction of necrotic tissue. Muscle fibers are destroyed by compression, toxic degeneration, ischemic necrosis, and liquefaction. When the muscle is enclosed in a rigid fascial compartment, the intrafascial tension mounts rapidly, and destruction of muscle fibers develops quickly. Abscesses may become encapsulated by fibroblastic granulation tissue and, after resolution or evacuation, are transformed into fibrous tissue. Extensive destruction of muscle is followed by replacement by dense cicatrix, leading to contracture.

CLINICAL PICTURE

Constitutional symptoms of chills, fever, and sweats are followed shortly by local pain in the affected muscle. Initially, the overlying skin may be reddened and warm. The muscle is swollen, indurated, and very tender, but these findings may be masked when the muscle, such as the anterior tibial, is enclosed in a rigid fascial compartment. Softening and fluctuation may become apparent, and spontaneous drainage may occur. At first, muscle power is reduced, and electric excitability is diminished, but reaction of degeneration never does develop. As destruction progresses, loss of muscle function is complete.

Healing in the early stage permits complete restoration of muscle function and power. A slight amount of residual fibrosis may be manifest only in easier fatigue following extreme activity demanding strong muscular contractions. Excessive fibrosis produces contractural deformity. Severe muscle tissue loss with minimal fibrous replacement in effect produces permanent paralysis and deformity due to unopposed pull of the antagonist.

TREATMENT

Diagnosis and treatment are urgent. A small amount of exudate, which under other circumstances is relatively benign, can effect rapidly mounting tension within a fascial compartment enough to destroy the entire muscle. Immediate incision and drainage, even before signs of fluctuation, are mandatory. Antibiotics of several kinds are given while awaiting bacterial culture and sensitivity tests. Hot, moist compresses are applied, and blood transfusions are given. The extremity is elevated and splinted in the position of function to counteract contracture and provide rest to the muscle.

CLOSTRIDIAL OR ANAEROBIC

Gas gangrene, or clostridial myonecrosis, is caused in 70% of cases by *Clostridium perfringens;* the remaining 30% of infections are due to *Clostridium novyi* and *Clostridium septicum.*[81–83] These organisms produce many lethal toxins, the most important of which is the powerful lecithinase, an exotoxin responsible for the severe toxemia. Healthy muscle ordinarily is resistant to clostridia, but trauma renders it susceptible. The tissue undergoes toxic degeneration and necrosis, followed by disintegration and liquefaction as gas bubbles (carbon dioxide from muscle glycogen) form and penetrate the subcutaneous and fascial compartments. Unless the condition is recognized early and aggressively treated, severe toxic effects become manifest: hypotension, tachycardia, renal necrosis, anuria, hemolysis, and cardiovascular collapse.

PATHOLOGY

The muscle appears red, friable, and, in places, semitranslucent. Microscopically, all tissue elements (endomysial connective tissues, sarcolemma, vascular, neural) about the wound are necrotic. The muscle fibers undergo coagulation necrosis with loss of striations, and nuclei are pale staining or disappear. Dead fibers become thin and disappear or they fuse and liquefy. Large numbers of gram-positive bacilli are prominent in both the muscle fibers and the interstitial tissues. Exudation of fibrin is profuse. Beyond the necrotic zone, newly involved tissue displays intense congestion, hemorrhages, leukocytic infiltration, edema separating muscle fibers, obscuring of striations, pyknosis and pallor of sarcolemmic nuclei, and granular destruction of interstitial connective tissue.

If infection is controlled, the necrotic muscle is removed, muscle regeneration is sporadic and inadequate, and fibrosis with marked diminution of muscle size is the usual result.

CLINICAL PICTURE

Gas gangrene usually follows a deep puncture wound, as is common with compound fractures. The onset is acute, with an abrupt fever, chills, and prostration. Pulse and respiratory rates rise; blood pressure falls. The wound is severely painful, swollen, and red. The surrounding skin is grossly edematous and red at first, then develops a bronze or copper-colored appearance. Serosanguineous exudate drains profusely from the wound. The swollen tissues may mask the crepitus of gas bubble accumulations, which gradually spreads in the subcutaneous tissues along fascial planes. A characteristic acid odor is noted. Rarely, septicemia may develop, with jaundice, hemoglobinemia, hemoglobinuria, and death.

TREATMENT

The clostridia cannot survive in the presence of oxygen. By using the hyperbaric chamber, high concentrations of plasma oxygen can be achieved; 100% oxygen is administered by mask while 3 atmospheres absolute pressure is maintained over a period of 2 hours. Blood is given to combat the hemolytic effect of the exotoxin. Penicillin and the tetracyclines are the antibiotics of choice. Two hyperbaric oxygen treatments are given daily, and usually two to four such treatments will effect dramatic clinical improvement.[82,83] The wound should be widely opened and peroxide of hydrogen or zinc instilled. Necrotic tissue is débrided. Early amputation is no longer necessary and should be deferred until systemic toxicity is relieved and demarcation between necrotic and viable tissue is established. If amputation becomes necessary, it should be of an open type, to be closed later when infection has been overcome. Polyvalent antitoxin is of questionable value.

TUBERCULOUS

Striated muscle is never involved by a primary tuberculous lesion except, rarely, by accidental inoculation with an infected needle. More common forms are included here.

Extension from Neighboring Focus. A cold abscess erodes the epimysium and spreads along the sheaths. Muscle fibers and connective tissue are destroyed by caseation necrosis. An example is the common psoas abscess.

Hematogenous Spread (Miliary Tuberculosis). The lesion is usually small and confined to one muscle. It forms an abscess and a sinus tract or a nodular sclerosis with eventual calcifications. Tubercles form in the interstitial connective tissue in relation to intermuscular vessels. Muscle fibers adjacent to the tubercle are destroyed. Only when an abscess forms do muscle fibers at a distance undergo pressure atrophy. Damaged muscle fibers may regenerate. Muscle lesions, as a rule, are asymptomatic.

Polymyositis. Multiple involvement with tubercles (which may be difficult to differentiate from Boeck's sarcoid) is manifested clinically by progressive weakness, atrophy, reflex loss, and pronounced contractures, causing severe disability. Microscopically, muscle fibers undergo granular or fatty degeneration and are replaced by fibroblastic connective tissue.

SYPHILITIC

Syphilitic myositis is rare. The lesion consists of a gumma, a solitary circumscribed focus of yellowish gray tissue enveloped by dense connective tissue. The sternocleidomastoid and the biceps are involved most often. Another type of involvement is a diffuse interstitial myositis in which large amounts of fibrous connective tissue replace degenerated muscle fibers in many muscles. These muscles are unusually hard and painless. Contractures are frequent.

PARASITIC

TRICHINOSIS

Trichinosis is the most frequent parasitic infection in muscle. About 17% of the adult population in the United States is said to be infected. Other parasites include *Cysticercus cellulosae,* the larval parasite of the pork tapeworm *Taenia solium;* the embryo parasite of the tapeworm *Echinococcus granulosus:* the *Sarcosporidia* parasite, which occurs in the striped muscle of most domestic animals; and *Toxoplasma* and *Trypanosoma.* From the orthopaedic standpoint, trichinosis is most important, because it produces muscle symptoms, findings, and sequelae. The tendency of other parasites to localize in skeletal muscle is without symptoms, but muscle biopsy is often used for diagnosis.

The cause of trichinosis is *Trichinella spiralis,* a nematode infecting humans by ingestion of raw or poorly cooked pork. The encysted trichinae escape in the intestinal tract as the pork muscle is digested, and the larvae penetrate the duodenal mucosa. The fertilized female deposits batches of embryos, which enter the lymphatics and emigrate through the bloodstream to various tissues. Only in striated muscle are conditions favorable for their growth.

Pathology

When infestation is heavy, the muscle tissue is pale, soft, and granular. Small elongated grayish streaks appear as connective tissue proliferates and the muscle becomes firm. After 6 to 18 months, whitish specks of calcification, which are ovoid, are formed throughout the muscle. Initially, the young trichina lies within the muscle fiber, curls up, and evokes an eosinophilic response and granular degeneration with loss of cross striations of the adjacent sarcoplasm. The sarcoplasm undergoes hyaline degeneration, fragmentation, or vacuolization, but the sarcolemmic sheath remains intact and sarcolemmic nuclei rapidly enlarge and multiply. The sarcoplasm of the intact portion of the fiber becomes basophilic, and the nuclei migrate centrally, congregating about the parasite. Cellular infiltrations consist of both mononuclear and polymorphonuclear cells, but eosinophils are prominent. When neighboring muscle fibers adjacent to the one harboring the parasite undergo hyaline degeneration and fragmentation, it is considered an effect of toxin elaborated by the parasite. When any part of an invaded fiber is destroyed, the remaining portion is stimulated to regenerate. This is evidenced by basophilia and granularity of the sarcoplasm, hyperplasia of sarcolemmic nuclei, and re-forming of cross striations. After the fifth or sixth week, the parasites gradually become encapsulated. Calcification requires from 6 months to 2 years. The larvae may remain viable in the encysted form for many years.

Muscles most susceptible to invasion are, in order of frequency, the diaphragm, extraoculars, tongue, laryngeals, jaw, intercostals, neck, back, abdominals, and limbs.

Muscle fiber degeneration and infiltration with inflammatory cells can occur in apparent absence of parasites. This suggests that many parasites are destroyed by the inflammatory reaction.

Clinical Picture

Three stages are recognized:

1. *The intestinal stage* is characterized by symptoms of gastroenteritis during the first week.
2. *The stage of muscular invasion* lasts about 5 weeks. Symptoms include chilliness, irregular low-grade fever, pains in the trunk and the extremities, muscular tenderness, edema of the conjunctivae and the periorbital tissues, fatigue, and, rarely, prostration. Muscle weakness may appear and when severe may be associated with loss of tendon reflexes. Muscle weakness may be generalized, or it may be limited to certain groups of muscles (*e.g.*, ocular muscles).

   The muscles are tender, often swollen, and painful on movement. These symptoms are pronounced in the muscles of respiration, mastication, and swallowing. Heavy infestations of the central nervous system causes such symptoms as delirium, somnolence, and coma. Myocardial involvement manifested by tachycardia and electrocardiographic changes is common.
3. *The stage of convalescence* starts during the second month as the symptoms slowly subside. Occasionally, rheumatic pains and stiffness will persist. Trichinosis is seldom fatal.

It is unusual to detect all three stages. Many cases remain asymptomatic and are discovered at autopsy.

Laboratory Findings

Muscle biopsy may reveal the trichinae. A negative finding does not rule out trichinosis, and biopsy should be repeated. Complement fixation and intradermal tests, using an antigen prepared from larvae, are of questionable value, because many people have become sensitized from previous infection.

Treatment

Prophylaxis demands thorough cooking of pork. Otherwise, symptomatic treatment is given. The prognosis is good.

CYSTICERCOSIS

Cysticercosis is common in Eastern Europe and India. It is caused by ingestion of eggs of the pork tapeworm *Taenia solium*. Larval parasites, the *Cysticercus cellulosae*, like trichinae, invade the intestine and reach the muscles, where they cause muscle weakness and tenderness, fever, and eosinophilia. Nodules may be palpable in the tongue and other muscles. The encapsulated parasites are situated in the interstitial tissue of the muscle, where they assume a spindle shape and ultimately become calcified. Characteristic shadows of elongated blunt rods are seen on roentgenograms. The diaphragm, the proximal limb muscles, and the tongue are preferred sites. Chronic brain lesions causing epilepsy may be the main clinical feature.

INFLAMMATORY MYOSITIS OF UNKNOWN ETIOLOGY

POLYMYOSITIS

CLINICAL PICTURE

Polymyositis is the term applied to a group of idiopathic disorders characterized pathologically by degenerative and inflammatory changes of skeletal muscle and clinically by severe muscle weakness chiefly affecting the proximal muscle groups about the pelvic and shoulder girdles, the anterior neck muscles, and often the muscles of deglutition. Polymyositis, when it is associated with a collagen vascular disorder with a highly characteristic rash, is called dermatomyositis (Fig. 17-10). All ages are affected, with two peaks of incidence, in late childhood and in the fifth and sixth decades. It is more common in females in a ratio of 2.5:1.

The clinical picture is quite variable. The onset may be acute or insidious and the course fulminating and short or chronic and prolonged over years.

In contrast to the muscular dystrophies, the disease generally progresses over weeks to months, rather than years, and is said to show periods of spontaneous exacerbation and remission.[93] Dysphagia and respiratory muscle weakness may occur. Distal strength is well maintained. Facial muscles are typically uninvolved.

FIG. 17-10. Dermatomyositis, microscopic appearance.

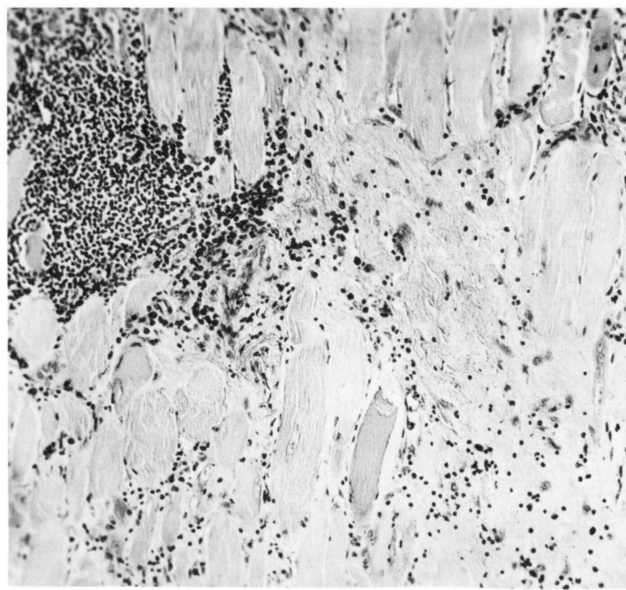

Deep tendon reflexes are maintained, and muscle atrophy does not occur until very late in the course of the illness. Early in the disease, muscle strength is decreased out of proportion to the degree of atrophy. Occasionally, muscle destruction may be very rapid, with diffuse and profound muscle weakness, pain, tenderness, and swelling.

In collagen vascular associated disease, Raynaud's phenomenon may occasionally be observed. Although arthralgia is common, the presence of frank arthritis should alert one to the presence of collagen disease, which when associated with polymyositis is considered an "overlap" disorder, which carries an adverse outlook. Such a combination introduces widespread necrotizing vasculitis, and visceral involvement is manifested, for example, cardiac arrhythmias, heart block, esophageal hypomotility, and interstitial pneumonitis.

The presence of dermatologic features (dermatomyositis) is more likely to be associated with rapid and progressive myositis and with neoplasia, especially in a man over 50 years of age.[88,92] However, the true incidence of this association is unknown.

Proximal muscle weakness of the upper and lower extremities is the most frequent complaint at the outset. Rarely distal weakness may occur but is mild. Muscle pain, bilateral and symmetrical, involving the shoulder and upper arms, is present in most patients. Dysphagia is a prominent feature at the onset in about one fourth of patients but seems more common with collagen vascular disease of dermatomyositis.[86]

In most cases examination reveals bilateral and symmetrical weakness in the proximal limb muscles. Distal muscle weakness occurs in about one third of patients and is generally mild. The neck flexors are commonly weak. Upper-limb contractures occur in about 10% of patients, are bilateral and symmetrical, and involve the elbows, fingers, knees, ankles, and, uncommonly, hips. Rarely ptosis and weakness of the orbicularis oculi are found. Respiratory impairment due to intercostal muscle weakness is infrequently observed at the onset. However, with progression, severe weakness can cause respiratory failure.

The characteristic rash of dermatomyositis is often observed at the onset.

DIAGNOSIS

Accurate diagnosis is essential because this is one of the few treatable myopathic disorders and when untreated results in significant morbidity and mortality. Not all criteria may be present, but in the absence of the rash of dermatomyositis, a greater number of criteria, such as the following, make the diagnosis more probable.[85]

1. *Symmetrical weakness of the limb-girdle muscles and anterior neck flexors,* progressing over weeks to months, with or without dysphagia or respiratory muscle involvement
2. *Muscle biopsy:* Necrosis of type I and II fibers; phagocytosis; regenerative activity evidenced by basophilia, large vesicular sarcolemmic nuclei with prominent nucleoli, internal migration of nuclei; perifascicular atrophy and degeneration; variation in fiber size; mononuclear, perivascular, inflammatory exudate; increase in endomysial and later perimysial connective tissue
3. *Elevation of serum skeletal muscle enzymes,* particularly creatine phosphokinase, most of which resides within the skeletal muscle. Other enzymes, originating also from other sites, such as the liver, may also be elevated: aldolase, serum glutamic oxaloacetic and glutamic-pyruvic transaminases, and lactic dehydrogenase (LDH)
4. *Electromyographic changes:* The triad: polyphasic, short, small motor-unit potentials; fibrillation, positive sharp waves, increased insertional irritability; bizarre, high-frequency, repetitive discharges
5. *Dermatologic features:* Lilac discoloration of eyelids (heliotrope) with periorbital edema; scaly, erythematous dermatitis over the dorsum of metacarpophalangeal and proximal interphalangeal joints (Gottron's sign), and involvement of the knees, elbows, and medial malleoli, as well as the face, neck, and upper torso. (This type of distribution is said to be pathognomonic of dermatomyositis.)

Childhood dermatomyositis (or polymyositis) associated with necrotizing vasculitis, a condition in which the small blood vessels are affected by intimal proliferation and thrombosis leading to multiple infarcts, is a special category. The widespread vasculitis involves the viscera as well as the skin, and soft tissue contractures, muscle atrophy, and subcutaneous calcification are common.

When polymyositis or dermatomyositis is associated with a collagen vascular disorder, there is an overlap of symptoms, so that arthralgia, arthritis, muscle weakness, or Raynaud's phenomenon may reflect the presence of systemic sclerosis, systemic lupus erythematosus, or rheumatoid arthritis. The concomitant connective tissue disorder adversely influences the outlook. Serologic abnormalities such as the antinuclear antibody and the rheumatoid factor are often seen in this overlap group.

PROGNOSIS

Improvement occurs in two thirds of patients and is greatest during the first 3 years, remaining relatively constant thereafter.[86] The average grade of disability after 4 years is a minimal degree of atrophy or weakness with little or no functional loss. About one third of patients have significant disability after 3 years.

The average disability at the onset is severe, with a waddling gait, inability to run, and, in most cases, inability to climb stairs without support.

The disease burns itself out in almost all cases by 10 to 15 years. The mortality rate is approximately 30% and is highest in those with malignant disease and those with well-defined collagen disorder (*e.g.*, rheumatoid arthritis). Any delay in treatment carries a worse prognosis.

TREATMENT

Corticosteroids. High-dose corticosteroids have reduced the mortality and residual disability.[89,91] The initial dose should be 60 mg to 80 mg prednisone per day, and doses as high as 100 mg may be required if muscle weakness is severe. Within 1 month, the serum enzymes should decrease, but continued elevations suggest the need for larger doses. The initial corticosteroid dosage should not be reduced until the serum enzymes have returned to normal. Then the steroid dosage is gradually decreased in decrements of 5 mg prednisone at monthly intervals until the maintenance dose of 5 mg to 15 mg/day is reached, depending on the clinical response. Patients who respond poorly are those receiving an inadequate dose, those with an accompanying collagen vascular disorder, and those with malignant disease. Steroid-resistant cases should have a trial with immunosuppressive drugs.

Immunosuppressive Agents. The rationale for immunosuppressive therapy is the hypothesis that polymyositis is an immunologically mediated disease. It is indicated for steroid-resistant cases or when steroid side-effects are life-threatening. Chemotherapy is generally given concomitantly with small doses of steroids. The following drugs are currently being studied:

Intravenous methotrexate. This is said to be very effective.[87,90]

Azathioprine. This appears to be the drug of choice.[84] The dose is 1.5 mg to 2 mg/kg/day, and the dose is adjusted upward until mild depression of the white blood cell count is obtained. Cyclophosphamide, 6-mercaptopurine, and chlorambucil have also been employed with variable success.

Orthopaedic Treatment. During the early stage of severe pain and muscle weakness, warm, moist packs are applied. Gentle passive range of motion exercises should not be carried out to the point of stretching fragile muscle structures. Splints are applied to prevent deformity. After the acute phase has passed, as indicated by serum enzyme studies, the exercise program is increased. Contractures are overcome by stretching. Residual muscle imbalance require orthoses, but no corrective surgery (*e.g.*, tendon transfers) should be done until the disease has burned out or at least 4 years have elapsed and the disease is under control.

INTERSTITIAL NODULAR POLYMYOSITIS

Miliary inflammatory nodules develop in the interstitial tissue with destruction of contiguous muscle fibers in skeletal muscles in a group of collagen diseases, including rheumatoid arthritis, rheumatic fever, scleroderma, and lupus erythematosus. In any one muscle are seen multiple foci of cellular aggregations consisting chiefly of lymphocytes with other round cells and histiocytes. The infiltrations most frequently are perivascular in location. Muscle fiber degeneration adjacent to the inflammatory focus is evidenced by hyalinization, vacuolization, a loss of striations, and eosinophilic staining sarcoplasm. Regeneration occurs by formation of muscle giant cells, increase of sarcolemmic nuclei, and formation of basophilic sarcoplasm. Where fibers are extensively destroyed, fibrous tissue replacement occurs.

Clinically, symptoms are minimal or lacking. Perhaps slight and vague muscle aching and tenderness are experienced, and a moderate amount of disuse atrophy is noted.

In rheumatoid arthritis, the muscle fibers are extremely atrophied and thin. In rheumatic fever, the nodules occur in the enveloping muscle sheaths and in tendon bundles near the junction with the fibers rather than in the muscle substance.

FIBROMYOSITIS

This is an inflammation of fibrous tissues, particularly those of muscle sheaths, fascia, and aponeuroses. The cause is unknown, although cold, dampness, and trauma often antedate symptoms. Pain and stiffness about muscles are accentuated by active and passive movement. Firm, tender nodules are often palpable. Pain may be referred to the upper or the lower extremity. The exact histopathology is unknown.

POLYARTERITIS

This collagen disease causes fibrinoid degeneration and mononuclear infiltration in small-caliber blood vessels. As a result, thrombosis and secondary ischemic necrosis ensue. Muscular involvement by multiple lesions is only one part of generalized disease throughout the body. Grossly, the muscles appear normal. Occasionally, small hemorrhages are visible. Microscopically, multiple well-circumscribed areas of necrosis of muscle fibers are seen. the fibers are swollen, striations disappear, sarcoplasm is eosinophilic and hyaline, and sarcolemmic nuclei become pyknotic and smaller. Later, the fibers disintegrate and are removed by macrophages. Replacement takes place by fibrous tissue.

Clinically, the muscles are painful (particularly on motion), tender, and weak. Multiple tender spots can be localized, but the periarteritic nodules are microscopic and not palpable.

EPIDEMIC PLEURODYNIA

This epidemic acute disease (also called Bornholm disease, myalgia epidemica, devil's grip, epidemic myalgia) is probably of viral origin and is characterized by an acute onset of severe paroxysmal pain about the chest, fever, and frontal headache. It has a seasonal occurrence, almost exclusively in the warm months. Children and young adults are predisposed. The severe pain is invariably at the site of attachment of the diaphragm. It is intensified by sneezing, coughing, and deep inspiration. Tenderness is often elicited over the intercostal muscles in the lower thorax. A pleural friction rub may be present. A peculiar characteristic is exacerbation of symptoms at intervals of 1 or 2 days. The condition is benign and subsides in about a week to 10 days. Treatment is symptomatic. An encircling tight bandage about the chest reduces the discomfort. The nature of what appears to be a muscular lesion is unknown.

MUSCULAR DYSTROPHIES

Progressive muscular dystrophy is a primary degenerative disease of skeletal muscles without evidence of regeneration. In contrast with neural and spinal muscular atrophies, the innervation is intact. This group of diseases is characterized by symmetrical distribution of muscular atrophy, preservation of faradic response (proportionate to the residual normal muscle), intact sensation and reflexes, and a heredofamilial incidence.[94,96]

The etiology is unknown but is generally accepted as hereditary.

Degeneration of muscle due to vitamin E deficiency and to the Coxsackie viruses displays not only degeneration but evidence of regeneration and should not be classified in this group.

CLINICAL FORMS

Severe Generalized Familial Muscular Dystrophy (Pseudohypertrophic Muscular Dystrophy of Duchenne). The severe generalized form is a rapidly progressive myopathy that usually begins in early childhood; there is a strong familial disposition, and it occurs predominantly in males, with and without pseudohypertrophy (Figs. 17-11 and Color Plate 17-2). The disease usually begins before the sixth year. At first the child shows a reluctance to walk or run; he stands and walks unsteadily and falls easily. The muscles usually increase in size but occasionally may decrease. Enlargement of calf, infraspinous and deltoid muscles is noticeable early. Occasionally, the

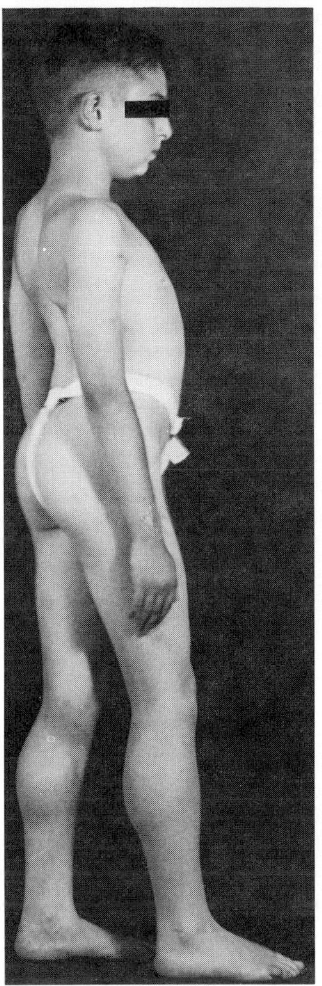

FIG. 17-11. Pseudohypertrophic muscular dystrophy. Note the enlarged calf muscles and posterior displacement of the upper trunk assumed for balance.

triceps, the quadriceps, and the glutei are affected. Rarely does the initial hypertrophy affect all muscles. The enlarged muscles are firm and resilient but are weaker than muscles of comparable size. The size of muscles increases, but later atrophy sets in. Muscles of the pelvis, the lumbosacral spine, and the shoulder girdle are wasted from the onset, causing the characteristic posture and gait. The gait is waddling, the patient standing with the feet spread on a wide base to secure balance. In forward progression, the body inclines from side to side because of gluteus medius weakness. the lumbar spine is extremely lordotic because of weakness of the abdominal wall and the gluteus maximus.

Weakness of hip and knee extensors produce a characteristic movement in arising from a sitting position. The patient pushes his trunk erect by progression, first placing his hands on his legs, then on his knees, and finally on his thighs. Ultimately, all power in hip, knee, ankle, shoulder, and elbow is lost, and atrophy spreads to the periphery of the limbs. Muscles of the hands, the face, and the jaw, and also laryngeal, pharyngeal, and ocular muscles, are relatively spared to the end.

The limbs are flaccid and loose. Shortening and positional contractures appear early. Progression is slow but may be rapid during an intercurrent illness. Eventually, the limbs become thin, and the patient is bedridden.

Mild Restricted Muscular Dystrophy (Facioscapulohumeral Dystrophy of Landouzy and Déjerine). The mild restricted form is less common than the severe generalized type but is not rare.[97] Occasionally, it displays a familial incidence. Both sexes are affected, and the onset occurs at any age but most often between 6 and 20 years. The first complaint is difficulty in raising the arms above the head, often preceded by inability to close the eyes completely because of facial weakness. A myopathic facies, a sphinx-like appearance with looseness and protrusion of the lips, is characteristic. The patient is unable to purse the lips and to whistle. The eyes cannot be closed against resistance. The lower part of the trapezius and the sternal portion of the pectoral are almost invariably affected, resulting in scapular instability and weakened shoulder abduction. The sternocleidomastoid and all periscapular muscles gradually weaken and atrophy, so the shoulders display exaggerated bony prominences. Biceps and triceps atrophy; the upper arm appears thinner than the forearm. The disease is often arrested at this stage. Occasionally, slight weakness of the pelvic girdle develops.

The condition is, by comparison, mild and limited and compatible with life. Pseudohypertrophy is rare, but compensatory physiological hypertrophy may develop in the deltoid and the gluteal musculature.

When muscles of the shoulder girdle and the upper arm are affected without facial weakness, the syndrome is called juvenile muscular dystrophy of Erb.

Dystrophia Myotonica (Myotonic Dystrophy). Dystrophia myotonica is a progressive, familial myopathy of the distal portions of the extremities, the face, and the levators of the eyelids (Fig. 17-12). The condition is characterized by markedly delayed relaxation of a muscle after a voluntary contraction. The prolonged contraction may

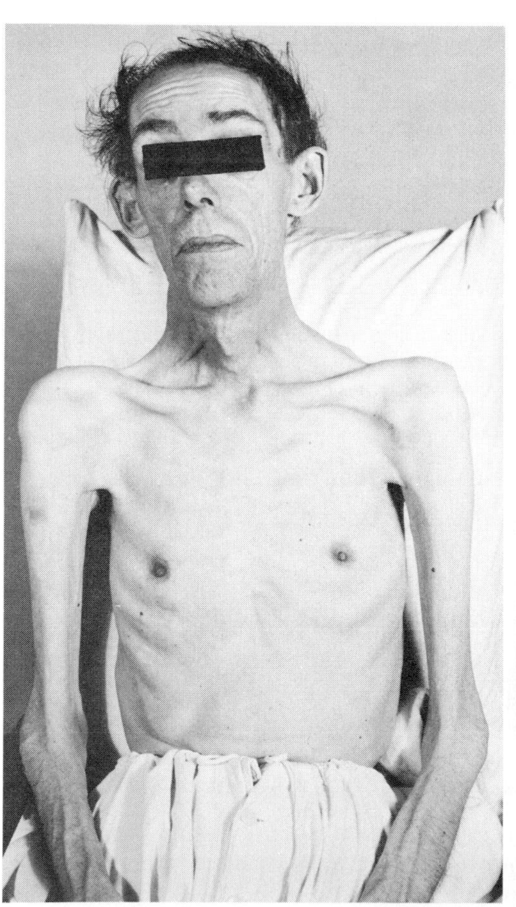

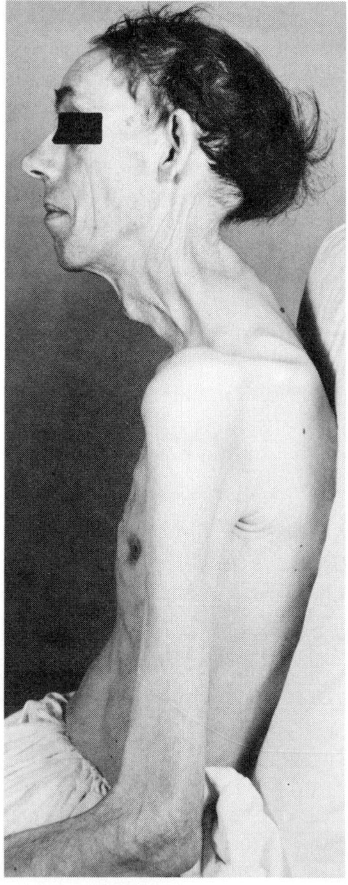

FIG. 17-12. Myotonic dystrophy. (Courtesy of Dr. Alexander T. Ross)

be demonstrated by electrical or mechanical stimulation. This is most pronounced in the hands, the face, and the tongue. Gentle movements, such as blinking of the eyes, do not elicit myotonia. A strong voluntary contraction is necessary. The electromyographic characteristics of myotonia are similar to those of Thomsen's disease except that, contrary to the latter, all muscles are not myotonic.

Often the small muscles of the hands and the forearms are the first to be involved. Muscular wasting usually follows the onset of myotonia by 2 or 3 years. The masseters and the sternocleidomastoids are almost invariably wasted. The peroneals are spared. The disease progresses very slowly. Additional features that typify myotonic dystrophy are endocrine abnormalities, such as testicular atrophy, and cataracts. Muscle wasting causes profound general weakness.

Atrophy of the temporal and masseter muscles produces the characteristic "hatchet face." The lids droop, the cheeks are lax, and the smile is sardonic.

There is no effective treatment.

Progressive Dystrophic Ophthalmoplegia. Progressive ophthalmoplegia is a very slowly progressive myopathy that is limited to the levators of the eyelids and the external ocular muscles. It has no orthopaedic significance but is mentioned for completeness.

LABORATORY FINDINGS

An increased excretion of creatine and decreased creatinine in the urine are characteristic of the dystrophies. Creatine is normally synthesized from glycine and other amino acids, predominantly in liver, and is deposited in muscle. Creatinine probably arises from muscle creatine by loss of phosphate from creatine phosphate. When muscle is destroyed or wasted, it is less capable of storing creatine, which is excreted instead, rather than being converted to creatinine. It is the decreased excretion of creatinine that is pertinent. On the other hand, increased creatine excretion occurs in a number of diseases which do not primarily affect muscles, such as hyperthyroidism.

Normal creatinine excretion is 22 mg/kg/24 hours. Normal creatine excretion is 2 mg to 3 mg/kg/24 hours.

The administration of 12 mg to 18 mg of α-tocopherol (vitamin E) immediately decreases the creatinuria of healthy children and that which occurs after the administration of glycine. This excretion is similarly inhibited in pseudohypertrophic muscular dystrophy, but weakness and atrophy are unaffected.

Serum Enzymes. Elevations of serum aldolase and creatine phosphokinase are diagnostic of myopathy.[100] These enzymes escape from muscle fibers because of the degeneration and increased muscle membrane permeability. Such enzyme elevations are consistently found only in the Duchenne type. The only other common form of primary myopathy, other than progressive muscular dystrophy, is polymyositis, wherein half of the patients have an elevated serum aldolase. The creatine phosphokinase is more specific than the aldolase, because its greatest concentration, in contrast to aldolase, is in skeletal muscle. Aldolase is also found at nonmuscular sites, such as the liver and the blood cells.

When severe muscle degeneration has already occurred, leakage of enzyme is markedly reduced and only a creatine kinase elevation may be detected. Carriers of the disease may often be identified by enzyme studies, because about two thirds of carriers have abnormal elevations of creatine phosphokinase.

24-Hour Urinary Creatine Excretion. This is useful for a quantitative assessment of progression of the disease.

Electromyographic Studies. Individual motor-unit potentials decrease in size during voluntary contraction and the number and rate of unit firings increase.

Muscle Biopsy. Tissue must be obtained from the weakest accessible muscle. A muscle with 50% of strength is more likely to give a positive biopsy than one with end-stage disease. At an early stage, the rectus abdominis is almost invariably involved and is suitable for biopsy.

PATHOLOGY

The findings in all three types of muscular dystrophy are similar.

Gross Appearance

In pseudohypertrophic muscular dystrophy the enlarged gastrocnemii looks like fatty tumors, not like muscle. Other muscles are small, and their color varies from yellowish to pinkish gray. The pale translucent appearance, resembling fish flesh, depends on the relative amounts of fat and fibrous tissue that replace muscle fibers.

Microscopic Appearance

The initial changes consist of swelling and rounding of the muscle fibers, the polygonal contour being lost. Individual fibers become split into daughter fibers, and their interiors become homogenized or hyalinized with loss of striations. Many fibers become smaller than normal. The sarcolemmic nuclei of both swollen and atrophied fibers are increased in number, are larger, and assume various shapes. In the myotonic type of dystrophy, the nuclei tend to line up centrally within the fiber. The muscle fibers atrophy and degenerate by vacuolation or granular degeneration, which breaks up the homogeneous appearance. Fat cells accumulate in large amounts between the muscle fibers. No regeneration is evident anywhere. (This would be demonstrable by accumulation of sarcoplasm about sarcolemmic nuclei and formation of end buds). Bands of connective tissue and large accumulations of fat cells separate atrophic fibers at a late stage. Motor and sensory nerve fibers are not damaged, and the central nervous system is normal. In the heart, myocardial fibrosis is a common finding.

In the mild restricted type of dystrophy (facioscapulohumeral), an increase in collagenous tissue is a prominent feature, thereby explaining liability to contracture. Deposition of fat occurs but not to the degree observed in pseudohypertrophic muscular dystrophy.

TREATMENT

The principles of treatment aim at achieving stabilization and balance so as to enable the patient with muscular dystrophy to ambulate independently or with little support over a longer period than would otherwise be possible.[98,99]

Contractures of the lower extremities frequently develop at an early stage, especially in the calf muscles and tensor fascia lata and iliotibial band, and the equinus deformity of the foot associated with some degree of flexion contracture of the hips and knees and lumbar lordosis all add to the incapacity produced by the muscular dystrophy itself. The contractures must be treated at an early stage by stretching and by splinting at night. Judiciously applied light plaster shells will often prevent contractural deformities. During the day, a strong, steel, long brace with drop-ring locks and a device to keep it from unlocking is worn. Long-lace surgical high shoes are worn.

When the contractures progress, surgical correction may be necessary. Heel cords can be released by subcutaneous tenotomies, and toe-to-groin casts are applied with the knees in extension and the ankles in 10° of dorsiflexion. Following this procedure, the patient no longer can stabilize the knees provided by fixed plantar flexion of the feet. Consequently, long braces must be worn.

Tight iliotibial bands are released by the Yount procedure, in which a large rectangular segment of the band with a corresponding portion of intermuscular septum is removed.

The hips and knees rarely show more than minimal flexion contracture.

The posterior tibial muscles always retain considerable power for long periods. They can be transferred by the interosseous route to the third cuneiform to reinforce the dorsiflexors. Postoperatively, the patient should be encouraged to walk immediately, if necessary with walking casts followed by bracing, because immobilization of these patients rapidly weakens them.

To retard the progression of scoliosis which develops while the patient is in a wheelchair, a corset or plastic jacket is applied. While the patient is walking, a support about the torso is impossible, because of the need for shifting the center of gravity to compensate for weak glutei.

Physical therapy includes instruction on exercises, stretching, and walking with crutches (when possible) and gait training with braces.

With a well-planned program of orthopaedics and rehabilitation, many muscular dystrophy patients can be kept independently ambulatory and self-sufficient for months to years.

MUSCULAR FIBRODYSTROPHY

Fibrodystrophy of muscle is a chronic nonprogressive condition characterized clinically by generalized weakness and lack of extensibility of all skeletal muscules.[95]

ETIOLOGY

The cause is unknown, although a history is often obtained of poliomyelitis or an undiagnosed illness followed by weakness, contractures, and rapid exhaustion on exertion.

PATHOLOGY

The muscles display a varying amount of fibrosis and parenchymatous atrophy.

CLINICAL PICTURE

Symptoms. Severe pain and tiredness in muscles after moderate exercise.

Findings. Loss of normal muscle extensibility is evidenced by flattening and limited forward flexion of the lumbar spine, limited ankle dorsiflexion, limited extension at the knee while the hip is flexed, and inability to touch toes to the floor above the head while lying in the recumbent position. The muscles are soft and lack tone. Tenderness is often found at the musculotendinous junctions. The deep reflexes are diminished. The patient's habitus is asthenic, thin, and stooped; muscle develoment is poor; lumbar lordosis is extreme; and the abdomen is prominent. Rarely, an obese or muscle-bound appearance is noted. All laboratory tests are normal.

TREATMENT

The aim of therapy is to lengthen contracted muscles and strengthen their antagonists in an effort to reduce fatigue and improve posture.

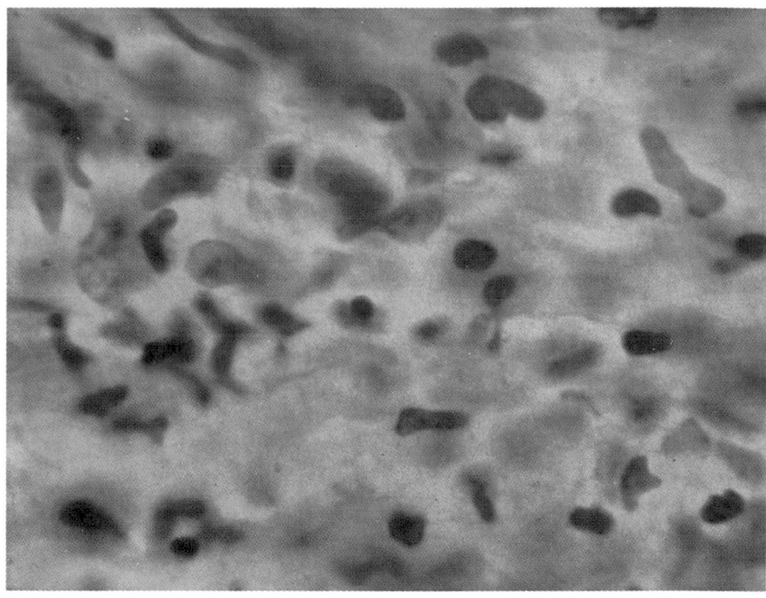

PLATE 17-1. Rhabdomyosarcoma. The typical cells, including the tandem and racquet types, are well displayed. One should seek transverse striations as evidence of origin from muscle. (×1,200, oil immersion) (See p. 679.)

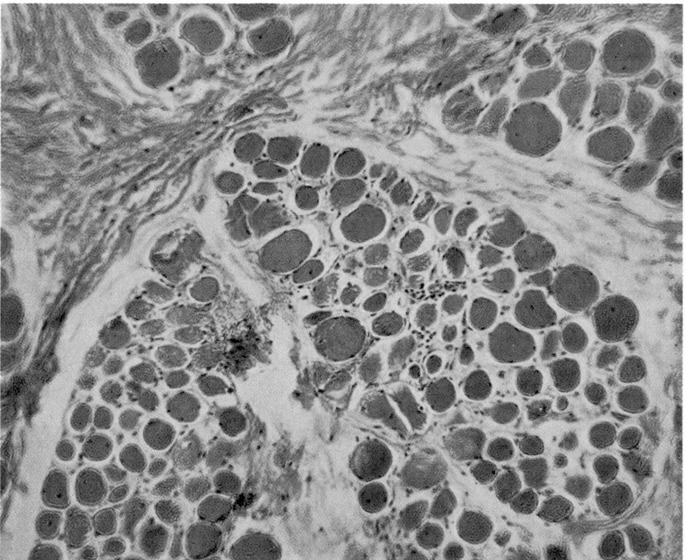

PLATE 17-2. Pseudohypertrophic muscular dystrophy. The muscle fibers are both swollen and atrophic, with loss of polyhedral contour. Collagenous and fatty tissue infiltration of endomysium is shown. (×85) (See p. 705.)

CONGENITAL MYOTONIA

Congenital myotonia (Thomsen's disease) is a rare, occasionally hereditary, familial disease characterized by delayed muscular relaxation after a strong voluntary contraction.[101] The onset can often be traced back to childhood. A child may be late in learning to stand and walk. Difficulty in movement may be noted as early as 6 years of age, but muscle spasms do not become intense until adolescence or early adulthood. Generalized muscular hypertrophy is usually associated, giving a Herculean appearance. The degree of myotonia varies from case to case and is most prominent in the lower limbs.

Characteristically, after a period of rest, the patient has difficulty initiating movements. The first attempt at movement of the lower limbs causes a painless stiffening contraction that is slow in relaxing. With repeated attempts, successive movements become easier to perform until they occur with ease and are followed by natural relaxation. After resting, voluntary movement again provokes muscular spasm. It is generally necessary to make a strong voluntary contraction to initiate spasm. For example, ordinary blinking occurs naturally, but strong closure of the eyelids will make it impossible to reopen the eyes for a minute or so.

Myotonia is also found in dystrophia myotonica and in the very rare paramyotonia congenita, in which the myotonic disease is produced by cold. The three diseases—myotonia congenita, dystrophia myotonica, and paramyotonia congenita—are collectively called the myotonias.

The pathogenesis is unknown, but it is clear that the myotonia is not derived from the nerve of innervation or at the neuromuscular junction, because anesthetizing the nerve and curarizing the motor end-plate does not halt the myotonic response. The muscle itself shows only hypertrophied fibers.[102,103]

DIAGNOSTIC TESTS

Percussion myotonia is a spasm with delayed relaxation set up in a muscle by percussing its surface.

Electric stimulation of brief duration initiates a prolonged contraction, although a single shock fails to do so, and repeated electric stimulation abolishes the phenomenon.

Electromyography will reveal, after a strong voluntary contraction, a burst of large action potentials with relaxation followed by small myotonic action potentials. The latter are similar to those in fibrillation.

Thomsen's disease must be differentiated from dystrophia myotonica. The latter disease exhibits progression, weakness, areflexia, hollowing of muscles (especially the masseter), and often a cataract and an atrophied testicle.

The hypertrophied muscles have a greater ability to store creatine and convert it to creatinine. Hence, congenital myotonia has a high tolerance to creatine (in contrast with the muscular dystrophies). No creatine is excreted in the urine, creatinine excretion is high. The serum calcium is normal.

TREATMENT

Quinine is specific, but it must be continued indefinitely. The dosage is quinine sulfate 300 mg to 600 mg twice a day or three times a day. Procainamide in small doses gradually increased to 4 g to 6 g/day is superior to quinine. Phenytoin 5 mg/kg/day will diminish muscle stiffness and cramping.

FAMILIAL PERIODIC PARALYSIS

THEORY ON PATHOGENESIS

Familial periodic paralysis is in some way related to potassium metabolism. Low serum potassium levels occur during an attack, and the administration of potassium is effective in relieving the attack.

CLINICAL PICTURE

This rare, hereditary, familial type of intermittent paralysis begins in childhood or puberty and recurs for many years. Both sexes are equally affected.[104,105] It is usually inherited as a mendelian dominant trait.

Periodic attacks of flaccid paralysis occur, with loss of reflexes and electric excitability affecting the extremities and the trunk. Each attack lasts from a few hours to several days, with gradual recovery. It begins with weakness in the back and the thighs and gradually spreads downward to involve the legs and upward to involve the shoulder girdle, the neck, and the upper extremities. Muscles supplied by the cranial nerves and muscles of respiration are rarely affected. Premonitory symptoms of excessive perspiration and thirst are common. The attack can be precipitated by excessive cold, carbohydrate ingestion, insulin, ephedrine, and strenuous exercise followed by inactivity. Muscles are normal between attacks. The condition tends to become benign with advancing age.

TREATMENT

Potassium chloride, 5 g to 10 g orally, is given initially, then 5 g three times a day during the acute episode. When respiratory paralysis is life-threatening, 1 g potassium chloride in 50 ml to 60 ml distilled water is given very slowly intravenously. Such treatment should be administered only by those knowledgeable regarding the effects of potassium. Hyperkalemia can interfere with the initiation and conduction of cardiac impulses and can cause cardiac arrest.

ARTHROGRYPOSIS MULTIPLEX CONGENITA

A congenital failure of development of skeletal muscles (amyoplasia congenita), arthrogryposis multiplex congenita results in deforming contractures of joints.[106]

ETIOLOGY

The cause is unknown. Hereditary or familial influences are unproved. It has been suggested that the cause is a congenital defect or antenatal degeneration of anterior horn cells plus the maintenance of a fixed position *in utero*.[94]

PATHOLOGY

In the contractured limb, some muscles are normal in appearance, others are small, and still others are absent or replaced by fat and fibrous tissue.[94] The position of contracture deformity depends on one group of muscles overpowering their antagonists, although both groups may be involved. The more affected muscles have a pale pink color. Microscopically, the fibers are small and retain both longitudinal and transverse striations, which stain indistinctly. Groups of larger, well-striated fibers may be interspersed among the atrophic ones. The endomysial connective tissue is not increased. Fat cells may be numerous.

In the central nervous system, the anterior horn cells may be reduced in number and size. The brain may be underdeveloped.

CLINICAL PICTURE

Involvement may vary from part of one limb to all four extremities. The infant resembles a wooden doll. Fixed deformities occur in any position, but most commonly the arms are rotated internally, the elbows extended, the forearms pronated, the wrists and the fingers flexed, the hips are flexed, abducted, and rotated externally; the knees are flexed or extended; and the feet assume a pronounced equinovarus deformity. Clubhand or clubfoot may be present. Erector spinae involvement causes scoliosis. The head muscles are usually spared.

The affected limbs are small in circumference; by contrast, the joints appear to be large and fusiform. The joints are not completely ankylosed: Some degree of active and passive motion is possible. Muscles are weak, hypotonic, and thin and often are not palpable. They react poorly to electric stimulation, but any evidence of denervation is not demonstrable. Tendon reflexes are absent. The joints may be dislocated or subluxated. Other congenital abnormalities may be associated. As a rule, intelligence is unimpaired.

An isolated muscle involvement may be the explanation for various congenital deformities, such as clubfoot.

TREATMENT

Conservative

Arthrogryposis multiplex congenita is a disease with such a wide spectrum of involvement that certain fundamentals should be stressed so that some degree of improvement can be achieved in most cases. The deformities as found at birth are not due to muscle imbalance and do not progress. Muscle replacement by fibrofatty tissue is quite variable, and in some instances no muscle exists. Strong fibrous bands and deformity of the articulating bones create a deformity that is unyielding. In spite of the severely deforming condition, the intelligence is not impaired, the patients are determined to overcome their handicap, and surprisingly they become adept at functioning within the limits of their disability.[109]

Treatment should be begun early, and once deformities are corrected, a prolonged regimen of stretching and splinting throughout the growth period must be pursued because of a strong tendency to relapse.

Satisfactory upper-extremity prehension is determined by the function of shoulder, elbow, and hand and the manner in which the hands can be placed in a mutually advantageous position by the arms. The lower extremities require stability and good alignment for standing and walking in spite of rigid joints.

Dislocation of the hip is common and should be detected and treated while the femoral head is still radiolucent. Scoliosis may or may not be apparent at birth but certainly develops within 2 years of starting to stand and walk and should, if possible, be controlled with braces throughout the growth period.

Various congenital deformities are often associated. When these involve the central nervous system or spine, the neurologic deficit superimposed on the myopathy presents a complex situation that makes improvement unlikely. A collapsing paralytic type of scoliosis should alert one to the possibility of an intraspinal defect.

In treating the *infant*, the physiotherapist teaches stretching and applying suitable splints. A resistant hip flexion and abduction or adduction deformity may be associated with a dislocation, and manipulation is contraindicated until this can be ruled out. Lower-limb deformities should be corrected before 18 months so that walking will not be delayed. If this cannot be accomplished by stretching, splints, and casts, surgical intervention is indicated. The following are examples of more common deformities and their surgical treatment; these procedures are described in detail elsewhere in this text.[106,108]

Surgical Treatment

Equinovarus. Equinovarus is the most common deformity. The objective is to convert a rigid deformed foot into a rigid plantigrade foot. The procedures available include medial soft tissue release and Achilles tenotomy and tendon transfer of the posterior tibial, which usually retains satisfactory power, by the interosseous route to the third metatarsal; talectomy can be done at an early age when the child cannot await a triple arthrodesis.[110]
Knee Flexion Contracture. The available procedures are supracondylar osteotomy, posterior capsulotomy, and hamstring tenotomies.
Hip Flexion Deformity. Hip Flexion deformity often spontaneously corrects after the knee is straightened; adductor tenotomy is the procedure. At skeletal maturity, an osteotomy is done.
Dislocation of the Hip. Dislocation of the hip is treated aggressively. Closed reduction is attempted; if closed reduction fails, open reduction is done, preferably at 1 year of age. Once reduction is achieved, the hip is stable. Pemberton acetabuloplasty or Salter innominate osteotomy may be needed.
Hands. Function is surprisingly good in spite of flexion deformity at the proximal interphalangel joints and flexion or extension of the metacarpophalangeal joints. No benefit follows soft tissue release.
Wrist. Flexion contracture, with or without ulnar deviation, is often associated with pronation. Capsulotomies are of transient benefit. Transfer of the flexor carpi ulnaris is helpful. Arthrodesis is done at skeletal maturity.
Elbow. Flexor power is essential for lifting the hand to the mouth. After capsulotomy, the pectoralis major is transferred preferably to the ulna or to the tendon of the biceps (if this is present).
Shoulder. Medial rotation and adduction deformity is usual. Derotation osteotomy of the upper third of the humerus is done. This is important for directing flexion of the elbow in the proper plane for self-feeding.
Spine. Mild curves are controlled with a Milwaukee brace.[111] Severe collapsing curves require halofemoral traction followed by spinal fusion and Harrington rods. Capsular thickening and tough fibrous tissue create fixed curves that are relatively resistant to correction prior to surgery.

MYASTHENIA GRAVIS

Myasthenia gravis (Erb-Goldflam disease) is a disease characterized only by muscle weakness.[112,113,115] In its mild form it is extremely common. Frequent involvement of craniopharyngeal and intercostal muscles, or weakness of the back and the lower extremities, causes confusion with poliomyelitis and muscular dystrophy.

ETIOLOGY

Females are predisposed, in the ratio of 2:1. The condition occurs at any age, but people in the fourth decade are favored. Heredity plays no part. A myasthenic mother may give birth to a myasthenic infant. The fact that myasthenia in the infant is of short duration suggests that some causative circulating substance crosses the placental barrier. Infection and injury may precipitate or aggravate the disease. Menstruation usually intensifies symptoms; pregnancy may effect a remission. Because psychic stress often greatly aggravates the muscle weakness, and because thymicolymphatic involvement is seen in certain severe cases, an endocrine etiology in which an adrenal stress mechanism operates is a possibility.

PHYSIOLOGY

Normally, a motor nerve impulse liberates acetylcholine at the myoneural junction. Acetylcholine effects a muscular contraction and then is destroyed by cholinesterase. Therefore, myasthenia gravis may be due to insufficient synthesis of acetylcholine, excess cholinesterase, or a curarelike blocking agent that decreases the receptiveness of muscle to acetylcholine.

The theory of a blocking agent is supported by the following facts:

- The myasthenic resembles the normal curarized person.
- Myasthenics are hypersensitive to curare, from 10 to 50 times normal.
- If in a severe myasthenic an extremity under a tourniquet is exercised and then the tourniquet is removed, general fatigue is aggravated.
- Normal muscle may release a curarelike agent in extreme fatigue.[116]
- The electromyogram of curarized normal muscle is identical with that of a myasthenic.[114]

The thymus is often found to be enlarged, rarely neoplastic. The suggestion that it produces a curarelike agent is unfounded.

PATHOLOGY

The muscles appear normal grossly except for some atrophy of disuse. Microscopically, only small collections of lymphocytes, termed lymphorrhages, are occasionally found in the interstitial tissues.

CLINICAL PICTURE

Abnormal fatigue of voluntary muscles is the one main symptom. It is aggravated by exertion, relieved by rest, worse at the end of the day, and involves a single muscle, group of muscles, or the entire musculature.

The extraocular and lid muscles are the first to be involved in half the cases, causing ptosis, strabismus, and conjunctivitis from incomplete lid closure.

Facial muscle weakness is frequent. It causes a characteristic sad expression.

Fatigue of jaw muscles is noted when masticating tough meats.

Tongue muscle fatigue causes dysarthria. The patient complains that his tongue feels thick, and he talks as though he has his mouth full of hot potatoes.

Dysphagia caused by pharyngeal muscle weakness is worse toward the evening meal. Fluids often regurgitate through the nose or are aspirated. Pneumonic infection is a constant danger.

Neck muscle fatigue may be prominent. The patient is unable to hold his head erect.

Fatigue of the upper extremities is at first noted when attempting upward reaching movements. Women complain of difficulty in caring for their hair. Men may experience tiredness when shaving.

A sense of heaviness in the chest or a feeling of insufficient deep breathing are complaints due to fatigue of respiratory muscles. When these symptoms become severe, respirator care is necessary.

Involvement of the lower extremities is first noted in the complaint of inability to climb stairs, or a sense of collapsing of the knees after a short period of walking.

The spinal and the abdominal muscles are also involved.

DIAGNOSTIC TESTS

Neostigmine Bromide. A parasympathomimetic stimulant, neostigmine bromide is given in doses of 15 mg three times a day. It is important that it be administered after meals, because its absorption from the fasting empty stomach is too rapid. Side-effects of abdominal cramping, diarrhea, or nausea are noted only in mild cases or in normal people and are counteracted by belladonna or atropine. An intramuscular injection of 0.5 mg to 2 mg neostigmine results in prompt relief of the muscular weakness.

If the patient is myasthenic, neostigmine will effect an increase in strength of all affected muscles. It may be necessary to increase the dosage gradually before this effect is noted. If, on the other hand, only side-effects appear, the patient is not a myasthenic.

Myasthenic Reaction of Jolly. When a myasthenic muscle is stimulated by faradic current, the first few contractions will be strong. Subsequent contractions show gradually lessened response. The block in transmission at the neuromuscular junction is seen in the electromyogram as a progressive decline in the voltage of motor-unit potentials.

Provocative Tests. Provocative tests with curare or quinine must be used when a very mild case is suspected or when long-standing cases render the muscles incapable of response to neostigmine. It is important to remember that myasthenics are extremely sensitive to curare. One tenth or less of the minimal curarizing dose for a normal person of the patient's weight is injected slowly intravenously. A transient aggravation of myasthenic symptoms and findings occurs (ptosis of eyelids may be evident). The curare is overcome by intravenous injection of neostigmine, 0.5 mg.

Tensilon Test. Edrophonium chloride (Tensilon) is similar in action to neostigmine. It has the advantage that response to an intravenous injection is instantaneous, and the action is dissipated in a few minutes. Also, severe side-effects are uncommon, making it unnecessary to administer atropine except in patients with asthma or cardiac disease. Tensilon is administered intravenously in a dose of 2 mg to 10 mg. A small dose is given at first and, if no effect is observed, increased doses are given at intervals of 1 minute.

CLINICAL COURSE

The onset may be gradual or sudden. Remissions usually last weeks, months, or years; in most cases the disease is not progressive. Most patients require less neostigmine as time goes on. Occasionally, a patient becomes resistant to neostigmine, weakness worsens, and respiratory failure may occur. Use of a respirator may carry the patient past the crisis. If the disease has been present for 10 years or more, it usually remains benign.

TREATMENT

Medical. Neostigmine bromide, in a syrup base containing 15 mg to the dose, is given four times a day and increased up to 180 mg/day as required for relief. The side-effects of treatment with anticholesterinase drugs (abdominal cramps, nausea, and vomiting) are reduced by simultaneous administration of an atropinelike drug. Only a sufficient amount of neostigmine to control symptoms is necessary. An overdose may cause muscular twitching and excessive weakness due to an excess acetylcholine.

If resistance to neostigmine develops, or if severe side-effects occur, the following drugs may be substituted:

Pyridostigmine bromide (Mestinon): Dosage, 0.6 g to 1.5 g daily

Ambenonium chloride (Mytelase): (Acts twice as long as neostigmine and has fewer side-effects.) Dosage, 5 mg to 25 mg four times a day

Edrophonium chloride (Tensilon): Dosage, 10 mg intravenously gives relief in 20 to 30 seconds; 25 mg to

50 mg intramuscularly relieves myasthenic weakness for hours. During treatment with neostigmine, sudden worsening of weakness is due either to a myasthenic crisis or to overmedication; 2 mg to 3 mg Tensilon intravenously as a test dose will distinguish between a crisis (patient improves) and overtreatment (no change in weakness).

Ephedrine sulfate: Dosage, 12 mg given with each dose of neostigmine; will increase the action of the latter

Under the theoretical assumption that the thymus provides the antibodies for an autoimmune response, thymectomy or irradiation of the thymus has been recommended but is of dubious value.

Corticotropin injections and long-term low doses of corticosteroids will benefit the patient with chronic myasthenia.

A sudden respiratory crisis may develop as a result of weakness of muscles of respiration and accumulation of secretions in the lungs. The patient must be placed in a respirator, a tracheostomy performed, and neostigmine discontinued. In patients who survive a crisis, a remission can occur, sometimes lasting for years.

Orthopaedic. The orthopaedic surgeon may see the patient initially for a supposed orthopaedic complaint and should be acquainted with the early signs and diagnostic procedures. The condition is often misdiagnosed as muscular dystrophy, polymyositis, or poliomyelitis. Weakness of the back muscles causes the patient to assume a swayback habitus to sustain balance, and complaints of pain in the back and lower limbs, always worse toward the end of the day, are common. A peculiar waddle suggestive of hip instability is caused by weakness of the pelvitrochanteric group of muscles. Trendelenburg's test may not be evident until a period of exercise brings on fatigue. Oral neostigmine is diagnostic and therapeutic. When a case is suspect, it should immediately be referred to those proficient in the medical interpretation and treatment of these potentially lethal conditions.

REFERENCES

Histopathology of Skeletal Muscle

1. Clark WE Le Gros: An experimental study of regeneration of mammalian striped muscle. J Anat 80:24, 1946
2. Saunders JH, Sissons HA: Effect of denervation on regeneration of skeletal muscle after injury. J Bone Joint Surg 35B:113, 1953

Tumors of Skeletal Muscle

3. Hays DM et al: Rhabdomyosarcoma: Surgical therapy in extremity lesions in children: From the Intergroup Rhabdomyosarcoma Study Committee. Orthop Clin North Am 8:883, 1977
4. Linscheid RL, Soule EH, Henderson ED: Pleomorphic rhabdomyosarcomata of the extremities and limb girdles. J Bone Joint Surg 47A:715, 1965
5. McNeill TW, Ray RD: Hemangioma of the extremities: Review of 35 cases. Clin Orthop 101:155, 1974
6. Stout AP: Rhabdomyosarcoma of the skeletal muscles. Ann Surg 123:447, 1946
7. Willis RA: Pathology of Tumours, 3rd ed. London, Butterworth & Co, 1960

Cavernous Hemangioma of Striated Muscle

8. Bendeck TE, Lichtenberg F: Cavernous hemangioma. Ann Surg 146:1011, 1957
9. Goidanich IF, Campanacci M: Vascular hamartomata with infantile angiectatic osteohyperplasia of the extremities. J Bone Joint Surg 44A:815, 1962
10. Jones KG: Cavernous hemangioma of striated muscle: A review of the literature. J Bone Joint Surg 35A:717, 1953
11. Selakovitch WG, Sherman MS: Hemangioma of the musculoskeletal system. Ochsner Clin Rep 2:41, 1956
12. Soule EH: Am Acad Orthop Surg Instr Course Lect 14:321, 1957

Traumatic Conditions of Muscle

13. Ackerman LV: Extra-osseous localized non-neoplastic bone and cartilage formation. (So-called myositis ossificans.) J Bone Joint Surg 40A:279, 1958
14. Gilmer WS Jr, Anderson LD: Reaction of soft somatic tissue which may progress to bone formation: Circumscribed (traumatic) myositis ossificans. South Med J 52:1432, 1959
15. Johnson L: Proceedings of seminar of the Southeastern and South Central Region, College of American Pathologists, Miami, 1952
16. Leriche R, Policard A: The Normal and Pathological Physiology of Bone. Moore S, Key JA (trans): St. Louis, CV Mosby, 1928
17. Spjut HJ et al: Tumors of Bone and Cartilage. In Atlas of Tumor Pathology, Fascicle 5. Washington, Armed Forces Institute of Pathology, 1971
18. Thorndike A: Myositis ossificans traumatica. J Bone Joint Surg 22:315, 1940

Myositis Ossificans Progressiva

19. Lockhart JD, Burke FG: Myositis ossificans progressiva. Am J Dis Child 87:626, 1954
20. Robinson GL: Scattered muscle necrosis associated with post-traumatic uremia. Lancet 1:799, 1950

Compartment Syndrome

21. Alexander JP: Problems associated with the knee-chest position for operations on lumbar intervertebral discs. J Bone Joint Surg 55B:279, 1973
22. Ashton H: Critical closure in human limbs. Br Med Bull 19:2:149, 1963
23. Ashton H: The effect of increased tissue pressure on blood flow. Clin Orthop 113:15, 1975
24. Benjamin A: The relief of traumatic arterial spasm in threatened Volkmann's contracture. J Bone Joint Surg 39B:711, 1959

25. Bentley G, Jeffreys TE: The crush syndrome in coal miners. J Bone Joint Surg 50B:588, 1968
26. Blandy JP, Fuller R: March gangrene. J Bone Joint Surg 39B:679, 1957
27. Burton AC: On the physiological equilibrium of small blood vessels. Am J Physiol 164:319, 1951
28. Bywaters EGL, Beall D: Crush injuries with impairment of renal function. Br Med J 1:427, 1941
29. D'Ambrosia RD: Supracondylar fractures of humerus: Prevention of cubitus varus. J Bone Joint Surg 54A:60, 1972
30. Dann I, Lassen A, Westing H: Blood flow in human muscles during external pressure or venous stasis. Clin Sci 32:467, 1967
31. Dodge HS: Displaced supracondylar fractures of the humerus in children: Treatment by Dunlop's traction. J Bone Joint Surg 54A:1408, 1972
32. Eaton RG, Green WT: Epimysiotomy and fasciotomy in the treatment of Volkmann's ischemic contracture. Orthop Clin North Am 3:175, 1972
33. Eaton RG, Green WT: Volkmann's ischemia. Clin Orthop 113:58, 1975
34. Feagin JA, White AA III: Volkmann's ischemia treated by transfibular osteotomy. Milit Med 138:497, 1973
35. Flynn JC, Matthews JG, Benoit RL: Blind pinning of displaced supracondylar fractures of the humerus in children. J Bone Joint Surg 56A:263, 1974
36. Hargens AR et al: Quantitation of skeletal-muscle necrosis in a model compartment syndrome. Presented to the Orthopaedic Research Society, Dallas, Texas, February 21, 1978
37. Hargens AR et al: Peripheral nerve-conduction block by high muscle-compartment pressure. J Bone Joint Surg 61A:192, 1979
38. Harmon JW: Significance of local vascular phenomena in the production of ischemic necrosis in skeletal muscle. Am J Pathol 24:625, 1948
39. Harmon JW, Gwinn RP: Recovery of skeletal muscle fibers from acute ischemia as determined by histologic and chemical methods. Am J Pathol 25:741, 1949
40. Holden CEA: Compartmental syndromes following trauma. Clin Orthop 113:95, 1975
41. Holden CEA: The pathology of prevention of Volkmann's ischaemic contracture. J Bone Joint Surg 61B:296, 1979
42. Howse AJG, Seddon J: Ischemic contracture of muscle associated with carbon monoxide and barbiturate poisoning. Br Med J 1:192, 1966
43. Jacobson S, Kjellmer I: Accumulation of fluid in exercising skeletal muscle. Acta Physiol Scand 60:286, 1964
44. Jennings AMC: Some observations of critical closing pressures in the peripheral circulation of anesthesized patients. Br J Anesthesiol 36:683, 1964
45. Kelly RP, Whitesides TE Jr.: Transfibular route for fasciotomy of the leg. J Bone Joint Surg 49A:1022, 1967
46. Kinmonth JB: The physiology and relief of traumatic arterial spasm. Br Med J 1:59, 1952
47. Kirby NG: Exercise ischaemia in the fascial compartment of the soleus. J Bone Joint Surg 52B:738, 1970
48. Kjellmer I: The effect of exercise on the vascular bed of skeletal muscle. Acta Physiol Scand 62:18, 1964
49. Leach RE, Hammond G, Stryker WS: Anterior tibial compartment syndrome—acute and chronic. J Bone Joint Surg 49A:451, 1967
50. Lunceford EM: The peroneal compartment syndrome. South Med J 58:621, 1965
51. Matsen FA III, Clawson DK: The deep posterior compartmental syndrome of the leg. J Bone Joint Surg 57A:34, 1975
52. Mubarak S, Owen CA: The compartmental syndrome and its relation to the crush syndrome. Clin Orthop 113:81, 1975
53. Mubarak SJ: Etiologies of compartment syndromes. In Mubarak SJ, Hargens AR (eds): Compartment Syndromes and Volkmann's Contracture, chap 5. Philadelphia, WB Saunders, 1980
54. Mubarak SJ, Carroll NC: Volkmann's contracture in children: Etiology and prevention. J Bone Joint Surg 61B:285, 1979
55. Mubarak SJ et al: Acute exertional superficial posterior compartment syndrome. Am J Sports Med 6:287, 1978
56. Mubarak SJ et al: The wick catheter technique for measurement of intramuscular pressure. J Bone Joint Surg 58A:1016, 1976
57. Mustard WT, Bull C: A reliable method for relief of traumatic vascular spasm. Ann Surg 155:339, 1962
58. Nicholson JT et al: Bryant's traction: A provocative cause of circulatory complications. JAMA 157:415, 1955
59. Osborne AH, Dorey LR, Harvey JPJ: Volkmann's contracture associated with prolonged external pressure on the forearm. Arch Surg 104:794, 1972
60. Owen CA et al: Intramuscular pressures with limb compression. N Engl J Med 300:1169, 1979
61. Owen R, Tsimboukis B: Ischaemia complicating closed tibial and fibular shaft fractures. J Bone Joint Surg 49B:268, 1967
62. Page CM: Operation for the relief of flexion-contracture in the forearm. J Bone Joint Surg 5:233, 1923
63. Parkes A: Traumatic ischemia of peripheral nerves. Br J Surg 32:403, 1944–1945
64. Reneman RS: The anterior and the lateral compartment syndrome of the leg due to intensive use of muscles. Clin Orthop 113:69, 1975
65. Reszel PA, Janes J, Spittel JA: Ischemic necrosis of the peroneal musculature, a lateral compartment syndrome: Report of a case. Proc Mayo Clin 38:130, 1963
66. Robinson GL: Scattered muscle necrosis associated with post-traumatic uremia. Lancet 1:799, 1950
66a. Rollins DL, Bernhard VM, Towne JB: Fasciotomy. An appraisal of controversial issues. Arch Surg 116:1474, 1981
67. Rorabeck CH, Macnab I: The pathophysiology of the anterior tibial compartmental syndrome. Clin Orthop 113:52, 1975
68. Scaglietti O: Sindromi cliniche immediate e tardive de lesioni vascolari nelle fratture degli arti. Riforma Med 71:749, 1957
69. Tibbs DJ: Acute ischemia of limbs. Proc R Soc Med 55:593, 1962
70. Tsuge K: Treatment of established Volkmann's contracture. J Bone Joint Surg 57A:925, 1975
71. Volkmann R von: Die ischaemischen Muskellähmungen und Kontrakturen. Zentralbl Chir 8:801, 1881
72. Weeks S: The crush syndrome. Surg Gynecol Obstet 127:369, 1968
73. Whitesides TE et al: Tissue pressure measurements as a determinant for the need of fasciotomy. Clin Orthop 113:43, 1975
74. Widerhelm CA, Weston BV: Microvascular, lymphatic, and tissue pressures in the unanesthesized mammal. Am J Physiol 225:4:992, 1973
75. Willhoite DR, Moll JH: Early recognition and treatment of impending Volkmann's ischemia in the lower extremity. Ann Surg 100:11, 1970

Ischemic Necrosis of Muscle

76. Brooks B: Pathologic stages in muscle as a result of disturbances of circulation: An experimental study of Volkmann's ischemic paralysis. Arch Surg 5:188, 1922

77. Buja LM et al: Sites and mechanisms of localization of technetium-99m phosphorus radiopharmaceuticals in acute myocardial infarcts and other tissues. J Clin Invest 60:724, 1977
78. Oberg MA, Engel WK: Ultrastructural localization of calcium in normal and abnormal skeletal muscle. Lab Invest 36:566, 1977
79. Reimer KA et al: Localization of ^{99m}Tc-labeled pyrophosphate and calcium in myocardial infarcts after temporary coronary occlusion in dogs. Proc Soc Exp Biol Med 156:272, 1977
80. Volkmann R von: Krankenheiten der Bewegungsorgane. Handbuch Chir 2:846, 1872

Myositis

81. Brummelkamp WH, Hoogendijk J, Boerema I: Treatment of anaerobic infections by drenching the atmosphere with oxygen at high atmospheric pressure. Surgery 49:299, 1961
82. Sim FH: Anaerobic infections. Orthop Clin North Am 6, No. 4:1049, 1975
83. Trippel CH, Ruggie AN, Staley CJ et al: Hyperbaric oxygenation in the management of gas gangrene. Surg Clin North Am 47:17, 1967

Inflammatory Myositis of Unknown Etiology

84. Benson MD et al: Azathioprine therapy in polymyositis. Arch Intern Med 132:547, 1973
85. Bohan A, Peter JB: Polymyositis and dermatomyositis. N Engl J Med 292:344, 1975
86. DeVere R, Bradley WC: Prognosis in polymyositis. Brain 98:637, 1975
87. Malaviya AN et al: Treatment of dermatomyositis with methotrexate. Lancet 2:485, 1968
88. Pearson CM: Polymyositis and dermatomyositis. In Hollander JL, McCarty DJ (eds): Arthritis and Allied Conditions. Philadelphia, Lea & Febiger, 1972
89. Sheard C: Dermatomyositis. Arch Intern Med 88:640, 1957
90. Sokoloff MC et al: Treatment of corticosteroid-resistant polymyositis with methotrexate. Lancet 1:14, 1971
91. Vignos PJ, Bowling GF, Watkins MP: Polymyositis: Effect of corticosteroids on the final result. Arch Intern Med 114:263, 1964
92. Williams RC Jr: Dermatomyositis and malignancy: A review of the literature. Ann Intern Med 50:1174, 1959
93. Winkelmann RK, Mulder DW, Lambert EW et al: Course of dermatomyositis-polymyositis: Comparison of untreated and cortisone-treated patients. Mayo Clin Proc 43:545, 1968

Muscular Dystrophies

94. Adams RD, Denny-Brown D, Pearson CM: Diseases of Muscle: A Study in Pathology, 2nd ed. New York, Harper & Row, 1962
95. Bingham R: Muscle fibrodystrophy. J Bone Joint Surg 29:85, 1947
96. Erb WH: Dystrophia Muscularis Progressiva. Klin Pathol Studien Dtsch Z Nervenheilkd 1:13; 173, 1891
97. Landouzy LP, Déjerine J: De la Myopathie Atrophique Progressive (Myopathie Héréditaire) Débutant dans l'Enfance, par la Face, sans Altération du Systéme Nerveux. Comp Rend Acad Sci 98:53, 1884
98. Miller O: Management of muscular dystrophy. J Bone Joint Surg 49A:1205, 1967
99. Spencer GE: Orthopaedic care of progressive muscular dystrophy. J Bone Joint Surg 49A:1201, 1967
100. Vignos PJ: Diagnosis of progressive muscular dystrophy. J Bone Joint Surg 49A:1212, 1967

Congenital Myotonia

101. Thomasen E: Myotonia, Thomsen's Disease, Paramyotonia, Dystrophia Myotonica, p 1. Denmark, Universitetsforlaget i Aarhus, 1948
102. Thomsen J: Tonische Krämpfe. In willkürlich beweglichen Muskeln in Folge von ererbter psychischer disposition. Arch Psychiatry 6:701, 1876
103. Winters JL, Laughlin LA: Myotonia congenita. J Bone Joint Surg 52A:1345, 1970

Familial Periodic Paralysis

104. Gass H, Cherkasky M, Savitsky N: Potassium and periodic paralysis. Medicine 27:105, 1948
105. Talbott JH: Periodic paralysis: A clinical syndrome. Medicine 20:85, 1941

Arthrogryposis Multiplex Congenita

106. Friedlander HL et al: Arthrogryposis multiplex congenita: A review of 45 cases. J Bone Joint Surg 50A:89, 1968
107. Gibson DA et al: Arthrogryposis multiplex congenita. J Bone Joint Surg 52B:483, 1970
108. Lloyd-Roberts GC, Lettin AWF: Arthrogryposis multiplex congenita. J Bone Joint Surg 52B:494, 1970
109. Mead NC, Lithgow WC, Sweeney HJ: Arthrogryposis multiplex congenita. J Bone Joint Surg 40A:1285, 1958
110. Menelaus MB: Talectomy for equinovarus deformity in arthrogryposis and spina bifida. J Bone Joint Surg 53B:468, 1971
111. Siebold RM et al: The treatment of scoliosis in arthrogryposis multiplex congenita. Clin Orthop 103:91, 1974

Myasthenia Gravis

112. Erb W: Zur Casuistik der bulbären Symptomencomplex. Arch Psychiatry Nervenkr 9:336, 1878
113. Goldflam S: Ueber einen scheinbar heilbaren bulbárparalytischen Symptomencomplex mit Betheiligung der Extremitäten. Dtsch Z Nervenheilkd 4:312, 1893
114. Harvey AM, Masland RL: The electromyogram in myasthenia gravis. Bull Johns Hopkins Hosp 69:1, 1941
115. Tether JE: Orthopaedic aspects of myasthenia gravis. Am Acad Orthop Surg Lect 9:171, 1952
116. Torda C: Release of curare-like agent from healthy muscle and its bearing on myasthenia gravis. Proc Soc Exp Biol Med 58:242, 1945

18

Fibrous Diseases

FIBROUS DYSPLASIA OF BONE

Fibrous dysplasia of bone is a relatively rare condition characterized by fibrous tissue replacement of the skeleton.[1–3] It may be monostotic (confined to one bone) or polyostotic (situated in many bones).

ETIOLOGY

The cause of fibrous dysplasia is unknown. The condition begins in childhood, and it may progress beyond puberty and through adulthood. Both sexes are equally affected.

PATHOLOGY

Fibrous dysplasia may implicate one, several, or many bones and often favors one side of the body. Favored locations are the long bones of the lower extremities and the base of the skull. The epiphyses are not involved, so that extensive fibrous replacement of the diaphysis extends to, but not beyond, the epiphyseal growth plates. Basically, the bony structure is replaced to a variable degree by avascular fibrous tissue, within which are formed thin trabeculae of bone.

Gross Appearance

The affected bone is irregular and often bent. The cortex is thin and bulged outward by the underlying abnormal tissue. Removal of the cortex exposes a reddish gray or gray tough fibrous tissue that cuts with a gritty resistance. On passing the finger over the cut surface, the tissue feels like fine sandpaper.

The long bone may be shortened but occasionally may be longer than normal. Pathologic fractures occur, but displacement is prevented by the fibrous tissue, and healing takes place readily but with deformity. Outward bowing of the shaft of the femur and a varus deformity of the neck produces a characteristic "shepherd's crook" deformity of the bone. A characteristic hyperostosis develops at the base of the skull and may obliterate the sinuses and encroach on the foramina.

Microscopic Appearance

The tissue is composed chiefly of dense, mature collagenous tissue in which are embedded evenly spaced fiber bone trabeculae (Color Plate 18-1).[4] The elongated fibroblasts are oriented either in linear fashion or in whorled intersecting bundles. The bone trabeculae are thin, anastomose to form an interlacing network, have no particular orientation, and are characteristic of "woven" bone. In the classic lesion, the bone develops by metaplasia from the collagenous tissue and there is a conspicuous absence of osteoblasts rimming the trabeculae (Lichtenstein). (In contrast, in an osteoblastoma, osteogenesis arises from a highly cellular stroma and a profusion of osteoblasts surround the developing trabeculae.) Giant cells are sparse except in areas of degeneration and hemosiderin deposition. Small islands of cartilage are rare and are present in only about 10% of cases; they are usually found in areas of cystic degeneration or in an area of a previously healed fracture. The fibrous tissue appears to erode and replace the cortex, but a peripheral thin shell of cortex remains.

The histologic evolution of the lesion is derived from a study of serial biopsies performed over the years. No essential change is revealed, except that the tissue may appear to be less cellular, more collagenized, and poor in woven bone.

CLINICAL PICTURE

The dysplasia starts in early childhood but is usually mild and asymptomatic, often being discovered roentgenographically. Onset of symptoms generally occurs before 10 years of age, and the initial complaint may be a limp, pain in a leg, fracture, and, in the female, abnormal vaginal bleeding. At the outset, the extent of the disease is immediately apparent.

A bending deformity may gradually develop or follow a fracture. Pathologic fractures are frequent but unite readily. The involved extremity is usually shorter but occasionally may be longer than its fellow. A "shepherd's crook" deformity of the femur is the most common cause of lower extremity shortening (Fig. 18-1).

In the skull, a hyperostosis frequently develops at the base and causes asymmetry of the head and the face.

Characteristic large, brown, irregular patches of skin pigmentation are usually associated with the polyostotic type of fibrous dysplasia.

Sexual precocity is typical in females and is evidenced by early menstruation, breast development, and epiphyseal closure. The condition is often unilateral in distribution.

Albright's syndrome consists of the combination of unilateral polyostotic fibrous dysplasia, pigmentation, and sexual precocity occurring in a female.

When the disorder is mild and limited in distribution at the outset, it generally does not become widespread. When extensive involvement is immediately apparent, progression is rapid, with the development of new lesions, multiple fractures, and many deformities.

LABORATORY FINDINGS

The serum calcium, phosphorus, and alkaline phosphatase levels are normal. In severe cases, the alkaline phosphatase level may be elevated.

ROENTGENOGRAPHIC FINDINGS

The typical localized lesion is well circumscribed, occupying a portion or all of the shaft of a long bone. It may present a homogeneous, diffuse rarefaction that can be likened to ground glass, or it may appear cystic and multilocular as a result of endosteal scalloped erosion of the cortex. The overlying cortex is thinned and expanded. The appearance is almost identical with that of a unicameral bone cyst, a nonossifying fibroma, or a bone aneurysm. Pathologic fractures cause shortening, bowing, and distortion throughout the lesion. Typical deformities include the "shepherd's crook" deformity of the femur, Harrison's grooves following rib fractures (Figs. 18-1 through 18-8), and intrapelvic protrusion of the acetabulum.

The appearance of the skull is characteristic. A dense

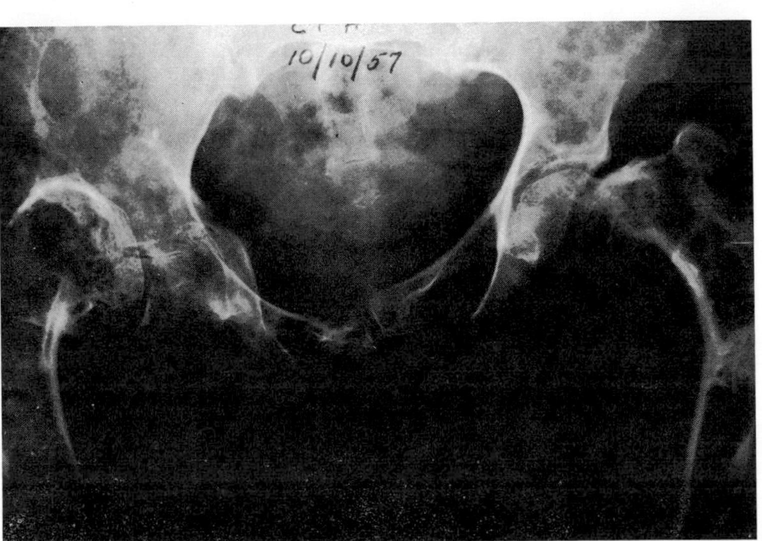

FIG. 18-1. Fibrous dysplasia of bone. The characteristic "shepherd's crook" deformity is shown. (Courtesy of Dr. W. H. Harris)

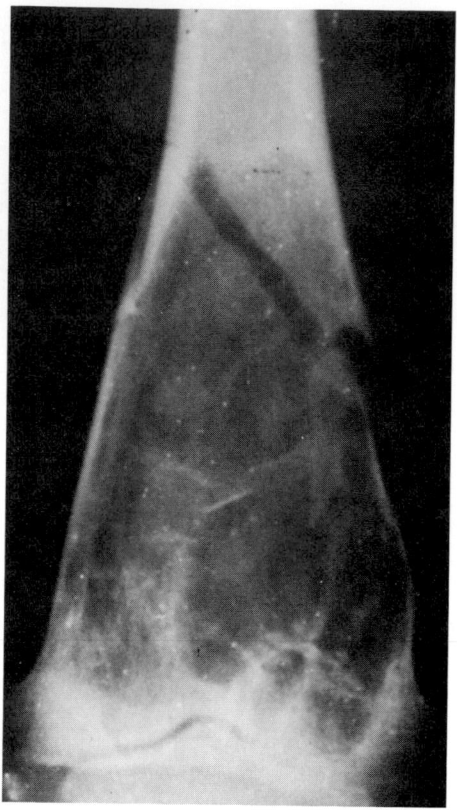

FIG. 18-2. Fibrous dysplasia of bone and a pathologic fracture.

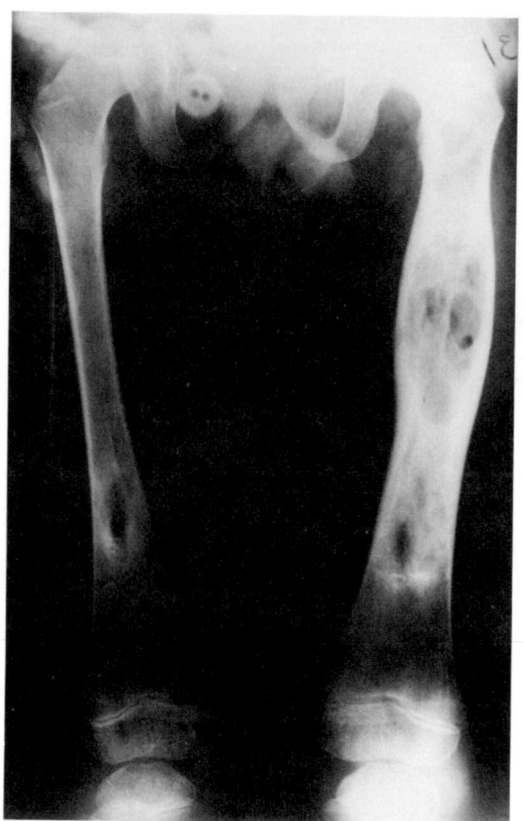

FIG. 18-3. Fibrous dysplasia of bone.

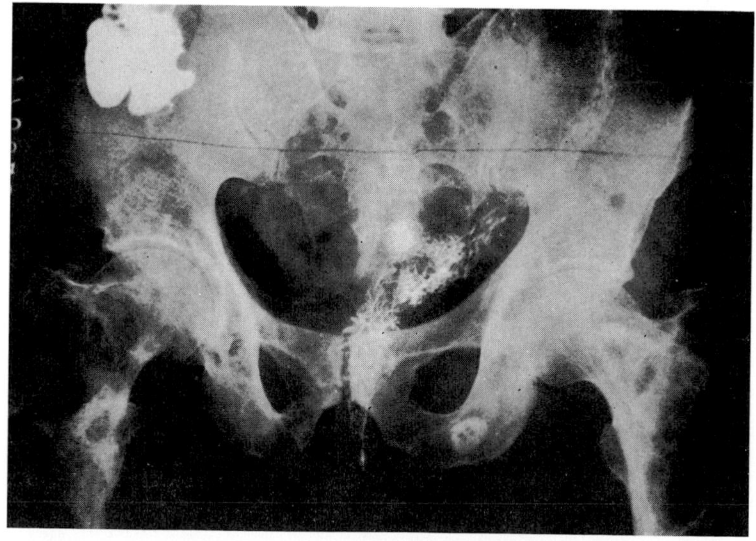

FIG. 18-4. Fibrous dysplasia of bone. (Courtesy of Dr. W. H. Harris)

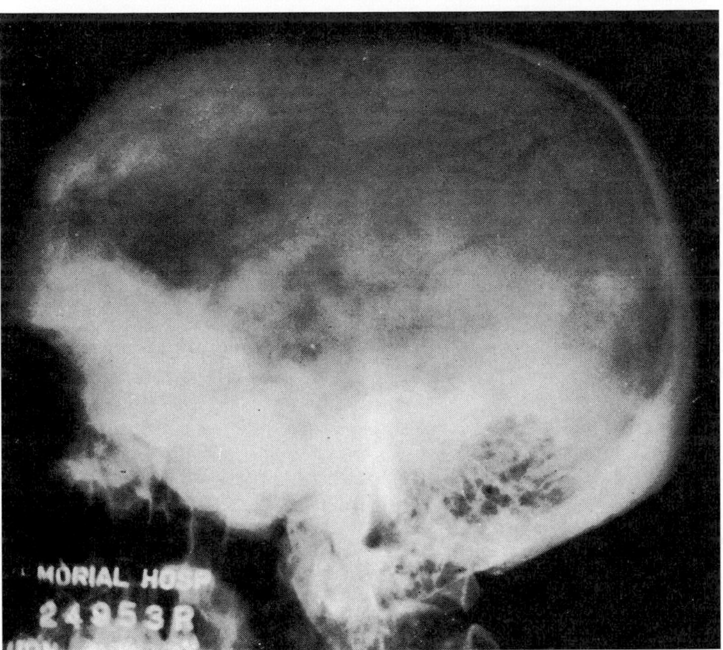

FIG. 18-5. Fibrous dysplasia of bone. A hyperostotic formation at the base of the skull is a feature of this disease. (Courtesy of Dr. W. H. Harris)

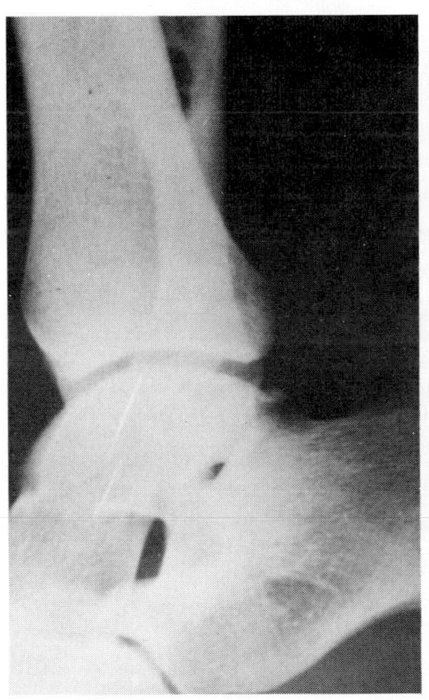

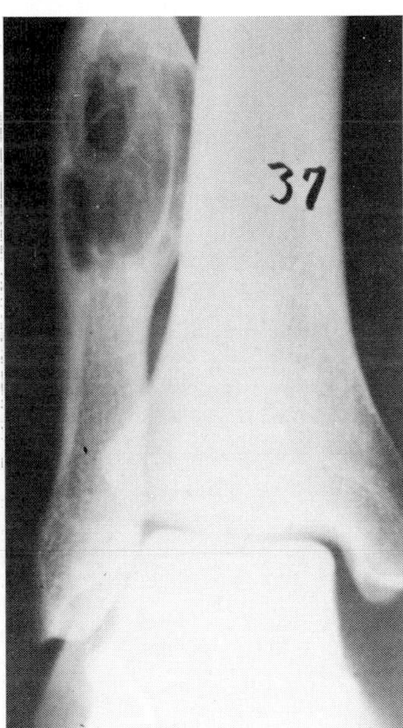

FIG. 18-6. Fibrous "cyst" of fibula.

hyperostotic formation develops and enlarges at the base, obliterating the sinuses and thickening the diploë (Fig. 18-6).

COURSE

The initial bone lesion usually develops in childhood, often before 10 years of age. The condition may remain asymptomatic and unrecognized until a late age. The clinical course is extremely variable. In general, when extensive fibrous dysplasia develops early in life, progression is marked, deformities are severe, and fractures are common. If involvement is localized or sparse, the disease usually progresses slowly and the outlook is favorable. Progression may continue through adult life. Puberty has no effect in preventing the occurrence of new lesions, reducing the incidence of fracture, or re-

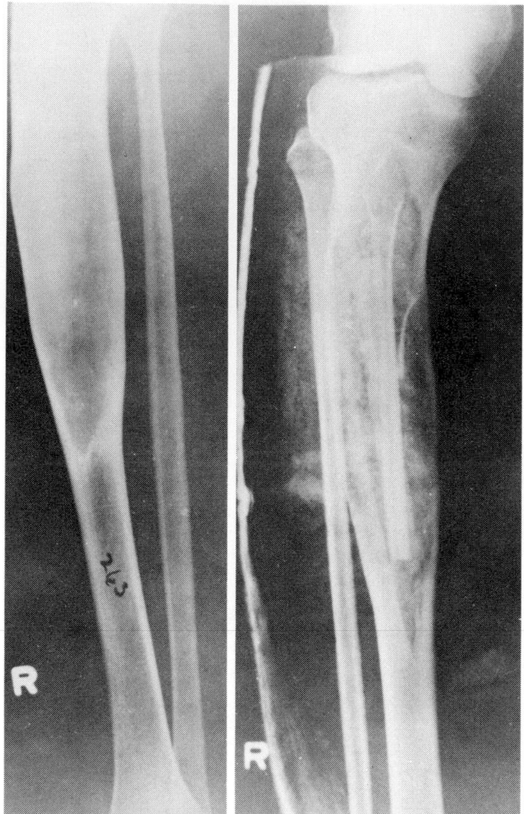

FIG. 18-7. Monostotic form of fibrous dysplasia. Clinically, there is only a local swelling with mild discomfort. Progress is slow. Roentgenograms show a large centrally expanding lesion with a ground-glass appearance. Typically, the lesion is intramedullary and expansile; it erodes, expands, and thins cortex. Grossly, grayish or yellowish fibrous tissue was found and was gritty on cutting. The lesion was cleaned out and replaced with a large cortical graft and multiple cancellous grafts. (N.U. Case No. 220)

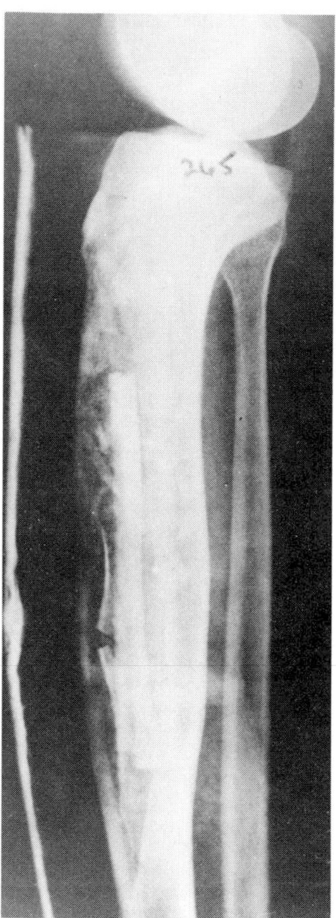

FIG. 18-8. Monostotic fibrous dysplasia. Extensive involvement jeopardized the integrity of the shaft, necessitating resection of the lesion and replacement with bone chips and a long tibial cortical graft.

tarding the progression of existing lesions. Malignant degeneration does not occur unless provoked by radiation therapy. The majority of fractures heal by conservative treatment.

DIAGNOSIS

The diagnosis is established by biopsy.

DIFFERENTIAL DIAGNOSIS

The main conditions to be differentiated are hyperparathyroidism, osteogenesis imperfecta, and neurofibromatosis.

Hyperparathyroidism

In hyperparathyroidism the serum calcium and alkaline phosphatase levels are high and the serum phosphorus level is low. The condition is more generalized and cystic than fibrous dysplasia, and the lamina dura of the teeth is absent. Patients with fibrous dysplasia have normal serum findings (except an elevated alkaline phosphatase level in severe cases) and an earlier onset; osteoporosis is not generalized, the base rather than the vault of the skull is affected, pigmentation is present, and various endocrine disturbances are common.

Osteogenesis Imperfecta

Multiple fractures, blue sclerae, and deafness are characteristic features of osteogenesis imperfecta. The bones are slender in contrast to the widened shafts in fibrous dysplasia. The osteoporosis is generalized. Vertebral bodies are compressed. In fibrous dysplasia, the spine is rarely affected.

Neurofibromatosis

In neurofibromatosis the lesions of bone predominantly involve the lower end of the femur and the upper end of the tibia; there is no tendency to unilateral distribution; the pigmented skin patches are smoother in outline; and multiple nodules in the subcutaneous tissue are often palpable. Microscopically, the tissue when stained by the method of Rio Hortega, displays specific cells, the lemmocytes.[5]

TREATMENT

Although fractures invariably heal, deformity often develops. Fracture of a long bone, especially a weight-bearing bone, should be treated by open reduction, autogenous bone grafts, and internal fixation, preferably by an intramedullary nail. A large lesion that jeopardizes the integrity of the shaft requires curetting and obliteration by bone chips.

After closure of the epiphyseal plate, femoral neck lesions should be treated by curettage, autogenous bone grafts, and nail plate fixation.

Severe coxa vara requires subtrochanteric osteotomy with internal fixation and bone grafts.

Leg length discrepancy is corrected by epiphyseal arrest. One must take into account premature closure of the epiphyseal plate and overgrowth that are characteristic of the disease.

A weight-bearing extremity may require brace protection. When the limb is severely involved, deformed, and shortened, amputation and fitting with a prosthesis may seem to be desirable.

Sarcomatous degeneration has rarely been reported. Persistent pain and rapidly developing changes in roentgenographic examination, particularly with a history of previous radiation therapy, are highly suggestive of malignancy and should be pursued further by biopsy.

NONOSTEOGENIC FIBROMA OF BONE

Nonosteogenic fibroma of bone is a benign, well-circumscribed fibrous growth within a small area of a long bone.[6,7] It is probably a localized form of fibrous dysplasia. It is seen in older children and adolescents, usually between 8 and 16 years of age. Both sexes are equally affected. The lesion occurs in the metaphysis of a long bone, most often in the lower limb. It is found predominantly at the lower end of the femur and occurs at both ends of the tibia and the fibula. Frequently, it is symptomless and is discovered accidentally; pain over a palpable, tender, bony swelling is the original complaint, or a pathologic fracture initiates symptoms.

ROENTGENOGRAPHIC FINDINGS

Roentgenographic findings are distinctive. The lesion is sharply defined, translucent, and loculated and possesses a thin border of increased density. It is oval, about 1 to 1½ inches in length, and its long axis lies in the long axis of the bone. The location is eccentric, the overlying cortex being thin and expanded. In slender bone, the fibroma occupies the entire width of the shaft (Figs. 18-9 and 18-10).

PATHOLOGY

Gross Appearance

A thin cortex encloses soft or tough, rubbery, gray-yellow or reddish brown tissue.

FIG. 18-9. Nonossifying fibroma of bone.

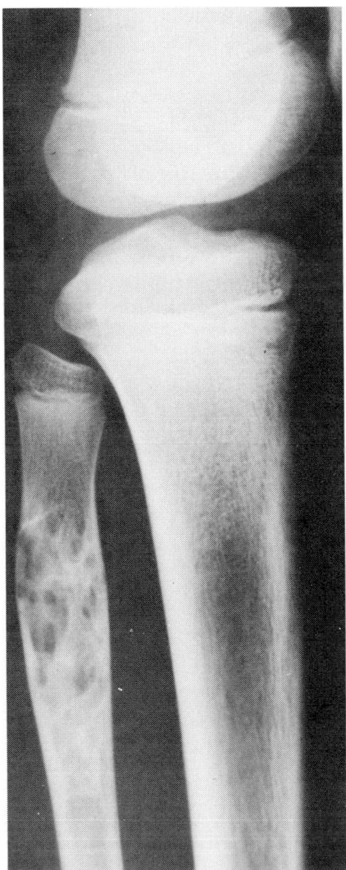

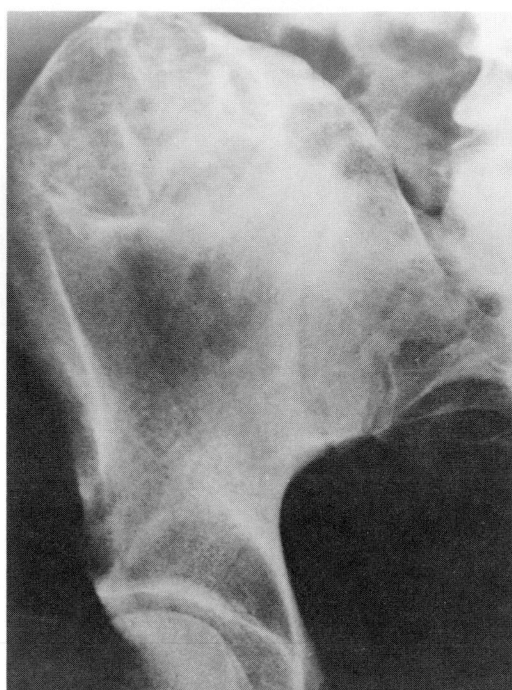

FIG. 18-10. Nonossifying fibroma.

Microscopic Appearance

Fibrous tissue of varying cellularity is seen. A more cellular fibrous tissue contains plump spindle cells and is quite vascular; deposits of hemosiderin produce the reddish brown color. A few giant cells may be seen. Trabeculae are conspicuously absent. When a tissue is more fibrous and in whorls, it is less cellular and less vascular.

HISTORY OF THE LESION

The tendency is for the earliest lesion to appear near the epiphyseal plate, enlarge and move away from the plate, and then gradually become smaller and indistinct and disappear. The lesion is rarely seen in late adult life. Opinion is divided on whether the method of obliteration is metaplasia to bone or ingrowth from surrounding bone.

THEORIES OF ETIOLOGY

Jaffe and Lichtenstein feel that this is a benign tumor.[7] However, spontaneous disappearance of the lesion seems to refute this theory. Hatcher suggests that this "fibrous metaphyseal defect" might be a local disturbance of bone growth originating at the epiphyseal plate.[6]

TREATMENT

The indications for treatment are persistent pain and tenderness and extensive involvement that might jeopardize the integrity of the bone. Treatment consists of complete excision and curetting the lesion down to normal bone and of filling the defect with bone chips. Otherwise, the lesion is considered benign and, given sufficient time, should disappear.

CONGENITAL NEUROFIBROMATOSIS

Congenital neurofibromatosis (also known as von Recklinghausen's neurofibromatosis)[37] is a condition that may be apparent at birth but is usually recognized later in childhood or adolescence. It is characterized by the development, within ectodermal and mesodermal tissues, of one or many neurofibromas, producing skin lesions, enlargement of a limb or portion of a limb, secondary skeletal changes by surface erosion or compression, defective focal osteogenesis of a long bone that may result in a pseudarthrosis, generalized osteoporosis, characteristic and rapidly progressive scoliosis and/or kyphosis, and sometimes a neurologic deficit.

ETIOLOGY

Congenital neurofibromatosis is inherited as an autosomal dominant trait with variable penetrance and a high rate of mutation.[14] It has been found in as many as six generations.

CHARACTERISTIC FEATURES

Skin Lesions. Pigmented café au lait spots are noted. Cutaneous fibromas are flat or raised, soft, and multiple and appear as verrucae or fibroma molluscum.

Multiple Neurofibromas. Multiple neurofibromas consist of connective tissue derived from endoneurium or perineurium that forms whorls of fibrous tissue interspersed with sparse nerve fibers.[26] These lesions can occur wherever a peripheral nerve exists, with the symptoms produced depending on the site.

Subcutaneous. Subcutaneous lesions are tender, painful, palpable nodules, varying from pea sized to a very large tumor occupying almost the entire extremity (Fig. 18-11). Rarely, a plexiform type forms, consisting of tortuous cordlike tumor masses representing enlargement of every nerve filament of an extremity.

Subperiosteal. The tumor by compression causes local bone resorption, then excites the periosteum to produce new bone, which envelops the tumor. A subperiosteal bone cyst results.

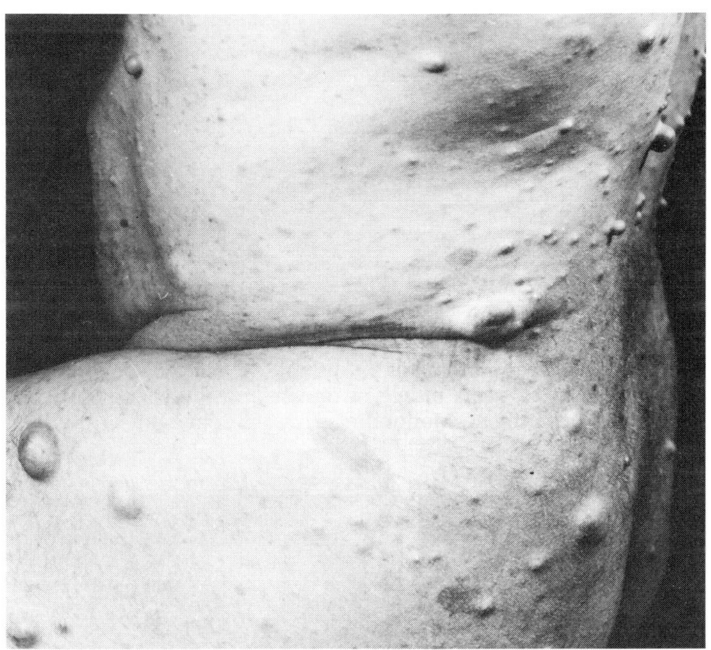

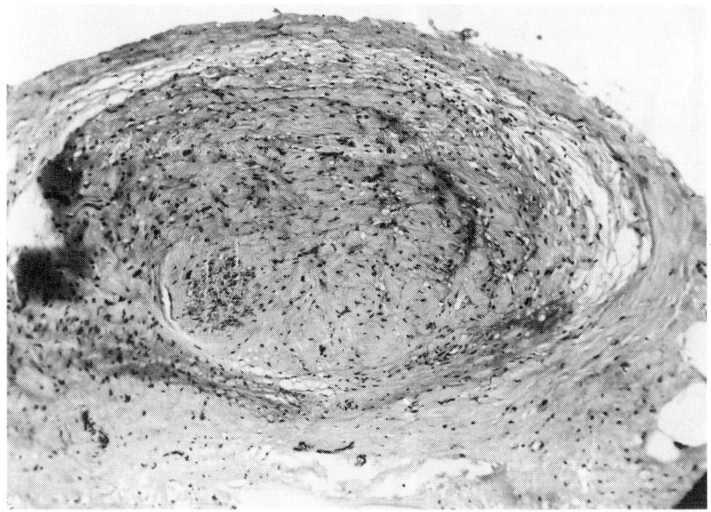

FIG. 18-11. Congenital neurofibromatosis. (*Top*) Typical multiple subcutaneous tumor nodules. These nodules are composed of nerve tissue covered by areolar tissue and skin. (*Bottom*) Low-power magnification of enlarged nerve fiber removed from a plexiform neurofibromatous mass. (McCarroll HR: Clinical manifestations of congenital neurofibromatosis. J Bone Joint Surg 32A:601, 1950)

Endosteal. No typical lesion within the bone has ever been described. However, osseous involvement is suggested by the frequently associated bone changes. The involved bone becomes porous and plastic and increases in length. Rarely, growth is retarded, supposedly by tumor inhibition at the epiphyseal growth plate. Bone cysts and pseudarthrosis, especially of the lower portion of the tibia, may occur.

Intraspinal. An hourglass-shaped, or dumbbell-shaped, tumor of the nerve root may erode and enlarge the spinal canal or an intervertebral foramen (Fig. 18-12). Within the spinal canal, the interpedicle space is widened and the posterior surface of the vertebral bodies displays smooth indentations (scalloping) of erosion. Although neurologic deficits may be produced by the enlarging intraspinal tumors, paraplegia never develops. The cranial nerves may be involved.

Skeletal Changes. Skeletal changes are caused by external pressure and erosion, direct intraosseous involvement by some process as yet not elucidated, and stimulation or inhibition of epiphyseal longitudinal growth. The incidence of skeletal involvement is variously reported to range from 30% to 50%.[21,22]

Long Bones. Increased rate of longitudinal growth is characteristic. At the periosteal surface, a smooth erosion

is found in association with established neurofibromatosis, corrective osteotomy carries a high risk of intractable pseudarthrosis.[10]

Spine. Scoliosis is the most common skeletal lesion.[9,18,24,26] The pathogenesis is unknown. Typically, a single curve involving four to six vertebrae develops in the lower thoracic spine, is sharply angulated, and is progressive.[9,22,24,25,31,35] It is sometimes accompanied by increasing kyphosis. The scoliosis is consistently associated with multiple café au lait spots on the skin.[30] Because it may be rapidly progressive, it demands immediate treatment, sometimes requiring early surgical intervention. Other patterns of spinal deformity may develop.[11] The latter are less severe initially but more often progress and become severe within 3 to 5 years.

Elephantiasis. Enlargement of a portion or all of an extremity is caused by a combination of factors, including diffuse hypertrophy of all soft tissues, edema due to lymphatic involvement, hemangioma formation, a large neurofibroma, and enlargement of a bone (Fig. 18-14).

Two or more of the following four stigmata are considered diagnostic of neurofibromatosis: (1) Five or more café au lait spots, each with a minimum diameter of 1.5 cm; (2) a positive family history of neurofibromatosis; (3) a positive biopsy specimen; and (4) a characteristic bone lesion (pseudarthrosis of the tibia, hemihypertrophy, or characteristic spinal curvature).

PATHOLOGY

Gross Appearance

The neurofibromatous nodule is a firm, dense, fibrous-appearing structure that is usually nonadherent to surrounding structures.

Microscopic Appearance

The tissue is almost identical with that of a fibroma (see Fig. 18-11). The dense strands and whorls of fibrous tissue are seen everywhere and may be easily confused with the picture of fibrous dysplasia when the specimen has been removed from bone. However, in von Recklinghausen's disease, when the tissue has been stained by the method of Rio Hortega, specific cells, the lemmocytes, are identified.[33] These cells are of neural (ectodermal) origin, are elongated, have rodlike nuclei, which often are aligned so as to create a "palisading" appearance, and have scarce cytoplasm that terminates in two or three prolongations, designated by Rio Hortega as "neuritides." Also found are mesodermal cells, the fibroblasts and histiocytes. Electron microscopic studies have shown that cellular elements of a peripheral nerve (*i.e.*, Schwann cells, fibroblasts, and perineurial cells) participate in the tumor formation. A high concentration of mast cells is characteristic of neurofibromas.[19,23]

Neurofibromas, particularly the deep-seated lesions, may undergo sarcomatous degeneration. [32] Metastasis is by the hematogenous route.

CLINICAL PICTURE

The asymmetry of the face, the body, and the limbs is apparent. Symptoms of pain and disturbance of function are related to the particular peripheral nerve involved. The lesions may or may not be progressive when first seen. However, the exception is the kyphoscoliosis, which almost invariably increases and becomes painful, severely deforming, and crippling. It may contribute to a neurologic deficit originating at the intraspinal level, but as a rule the primary cause is the development of enlarging tumors within the spinal canal.

Elephantiasis of a limb or portion of a limb is typical and may be due to a tumor of massive proportions or may be secondary to interference with venous and lymphatic drainage (Fig. 18-14). Inequality of upper or lower limbs becomes apparent with growth. When anterolateral bowing deformity of the lower tibia is detected at an early age, it is prone to pathologic fracture and nonunion (pseudarthrosis).

Less common lesions include the following:[20]

Head lesions. Macrocranium may be noted along with a wide variety of calvarial, facial bone, and dental lesions, which rarely may produce grotesque features.

Optic glioma. This lesion occurs in children. When seemingly discovered as an independent tumor, it is virtually always a manifestation of neurofibromatosis. It produces widening of the optic canal; sometimes it may be an intraocular lesion.

Bilateral acoustic neuroma. This disorder usually occurs in the adult but may rarely occur in children. It produces enlarged auditory canals.

Cervical kyphosis. Kyphosis usually begins in early childhood and may rapidly become severe at an early age.

Vascular lesions. Schwann cell proliferation and secondary fibrosis develops in both small and large arteries in various organs. For example, renal artery stenosis may cause hypertension in the child.[16,29] Peculiarly, pheochromocytoma, which causes hypertension in the adult, is often associated with neurofibromatosis.[36]

DIAGNOSIS

At least two of the following criteria must be identified to establish the diagnosis:[12]

Positive family history
Positive biopsy findings

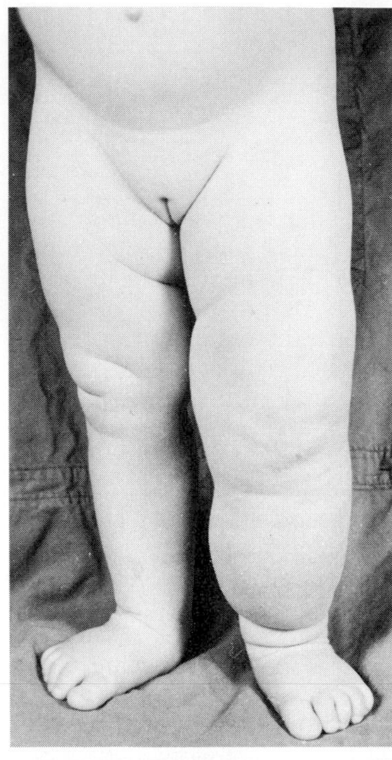

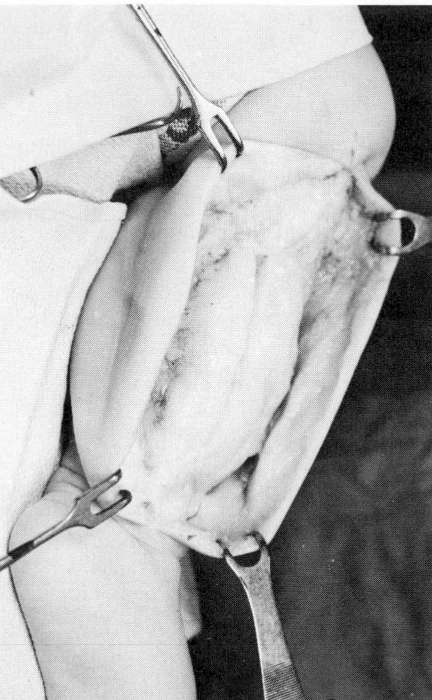

FIG. 18-14. Congenital neurofibromatosis. (*Top*) Diffuse soft tissue hypertrophy and increased length of the lower extremity. At right a typical tumor mass of hypertrophied soft tissue is exposed at operation. It is not encapsulated and is superficial to the deep fascia. (*Bottom*) Hypertrophy of the left thumb and index finger and corresponding portion of the hand. Massive skeletal hypertrophy in the involved segments. (McCarroll HR: Clinical manifestations of congenital neurofibromatosis. J Bone Joint Surg 32A:601, 1950)

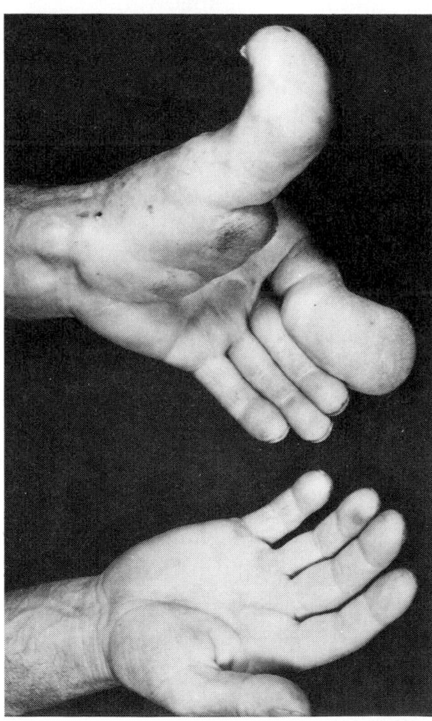

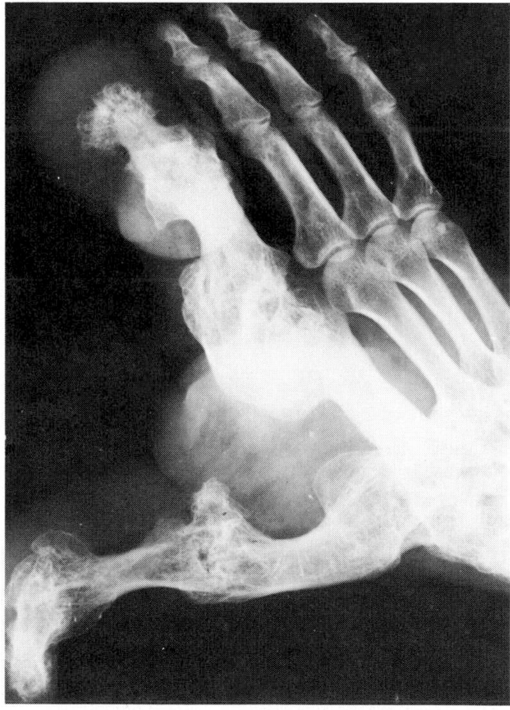

Minimum of six café au lait spots, each at least 1.5 cm in width

Multiple subcutaneous neurofibromas

These diagnostic criteria are mainly applicable to the adult and have been modified for children.[38] Any child with five or more café au lait spots, each 0.5 cm or more in diameter, has neurofibromatosis until proved otherwise. The spots are more apt to be found on the dorsal aspect of the trunk, especially over the buttocks.

Iris nodules, the so-called Lisch spots, are bilateral pigmented or nonpigmented lesions that are detected on ophthalmologic examination and are specific for neurofibromatosis.

ROENTGENOGRAPHIC FINDINGS[20]

Kyphoscoliosis, the most common lesion, usually develops in patients between 11 and 15 years of age. The most common pattern is a sharp, single lower thoracic curve involving fewer than five vertebrae that is highly characteristic of neurofibromatosis.[22,27] There is no standard pattern. The affected vertebrae show anterior, posterior, and lateral scalloping; hypoplasia of the transverse processes or pedicles; and "pencil pointing" of vertebral margins. Posterior scalloping is usually associated with dural dysplasia and meningocele. Adjacent "twisted ribbon" ribs are characteristic. Kyphosis is a bad prognostic sign for progression. (See Neurofibromatosis Scoliosis.)

Myelography and computed axial tomography will define widening of the spinal canal and intervertebral foramina, intraspinal tumors, and associated anomalies, such as diastematomyelia and distal tethering of the cord.

Cervical kyphosis displays the typical anterior and posterior scalloping of the vertebral bodies with marked deformity of a single vertebra. The deformity begins in childhood but may reach full-blown proportions at an early age (Fig. 18-15).

Optic glioma is diagnosed by demonstrating enlargement of one or both optic foramina. Axial tomography is the most accurate method of measuring the optical canal or foramen.[17] Pneumoencephalography and cerebral angiography will detect tumors that have extended into the brain.

Acoustic neuroma is revealed by cerebral angiography and CT scan, which demonstrate widening of the auditory canals.

A CT scan and cerebral angiography reveal intracranial findings of a meningioma, which is said to be pathognomonic of neurofibromatosis.

TREATMENT

Complete excision is the only treatment for the tumor. Because the tumor often infiltrates into the surrounding tissues, the excision must extend beyond the apparent confines of the tumor to prevent recurrence. Elephantiasis is treated by repeated resection of hypertrophied soft tissues as well as of the tumors.

Scoliosis demands early correction and fusion. A curve that is associated with marked dystrophic changes, and especially with kyphosis, is disposed to rapidly progressing and severely crippling deformity. Compression of the spinal cord and cauda equina can result from bony compromise of the anterior aspect of the spinal canal. (See Neurofibromatosis Scoliosis.)

Painful tumors within the spinal canal, which may produce a neurologic deficit, require a laminectomy and removal. In the presence of a short, sharp angular curve, a posterolateral fusion must be added. When kyphosis is present, a laminectomy as an initial procedure is

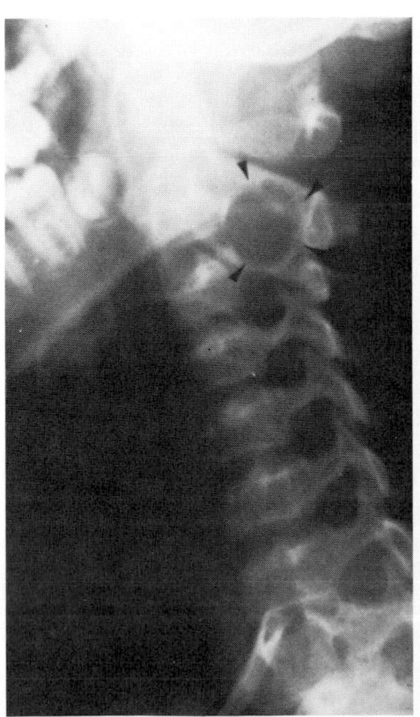

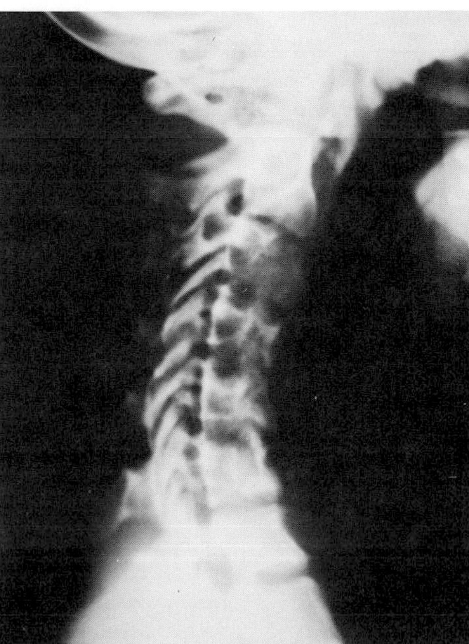

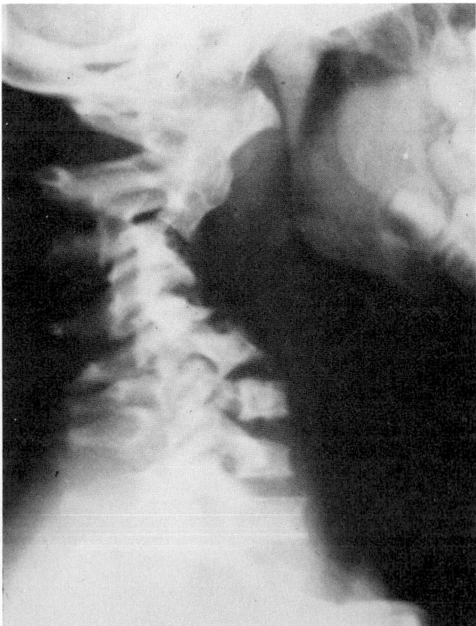

FIG. 18-15. Cervical spine abnormalities in neurofibromatosis. Various deformities can develop in early life and are often asymptomatic at first. They occur more frequently in the patient with scoliosis, especially when the curve is short, sharp and dysplastic and has a kyphotic element. Even in the patient with a severely deformed cervical spine, the changes are generally long standing and fixed and relatively stable, as demonstrated by flexion-extension roentgenograms. This spine may be injured by ill-advised cervical traction or manipulation and handling of the patient during induction of anesthesia or attempted correction of the scoliosis. (*Left*) Enlarged foramina and dysplasia of posterior elements. (*Center*) Fixed reversal of cervical lordosis. (*Right*) Gross cervical kyphosis with subluxation in asymptomatic patient. (Yong-Hing K, Kalamchi A, MacEwen GD: Cervical spine abnormalities in neurofibromatosis. J Bone Joint Surg 61A:695, 1979)

absolutely contraindicated, since it will inevitably exaggerate the kyphosis, which in turn will endanger the cord. Anterior correction of the kyphoscoliotic deformity and an anterior spinal fusion is necessary before the intraspinal tumors can be removed by laminectomy and a posterolateral fusion added.

When the spinal cord or cauda is compressed anteriorly by a progressive kyphotic deformity, anterior decompression is necessary, while at the same time correction of the deformity and anterior stabilization is done. A posterior fusion must be added later.

Anterolateral bowing of the tibia must be protected against pathologic fracture until skeletal maturity is reached. When pseudarthrosis exists, or is the result of a pathologic fracture or ill-advised osteotomy, surgical intervention is necessary. (See Pseudarthrosis of Tibia.)

Surgery in these patients is fraught with the dangers of hemorrhage and shock to which they are peculiarly susceptible.

Warning regarding cervical spine lesions (see Fig. 18-15): There is a frequent association of abnormalities of the cervical spine with scoliosis and kyphoscoliosis, especially when these curves are severe. These cervical deformities usually begin in childhood, are often silently progressive, and require an awareness for their early detection. Early signs of involvement (*e.g.*, foraminal enlargement, scalloping) should be sought. Progressive vertebral deformity, subluxation, and kyphosis generally develop slowly and become fixed, even in the severely deformed spine, with relatively little symptoms. A neurologic deficit, such as progressive spasticity, develops infrequently.

Roentgenographic examination of the cervical spine should be done routinely in patients with neurofibromatosis, especially those about to undergo general anesthesia or traction. An unrecognized deformity of the cervical spine is prone to damage if subjected to stresses of traction and repeated manipulation,[39] and serious neurologic consequences, including paraplegia, can ensue.

COLLAGEN DISEASES

Several conditions are included under the general classifications of collagen diseases because each possesses a common pathologic characteristic. The histologic abnormality is a "fibrinoid change," a degenerative process that is observed in collagenous connective tissue. Specifically, this refers to a homogeneous, eosinophilic staining area seen wherever collagenous fibers are found, either in the wall of blood vessels or in connective tissue proper. In addition, varying degrees of vascular inflammation and necrosis of small- and medium-sized arterioles lead to disseminated granulomas, thromboses, aneurysms, and infarctions. Although collagen diseases are categorized into definite clinical entities, considerable overlap of these disorders is the rule (*e.g.*, the coexistence of systemic lupus erythematosus and rheumatoid arthritis). Because collagen is widely distributed throughout the body, many organs are affected. These multisystem disorders may affect, at their outset, any region of the body, such as a joint, a kidney, or the heart. When many areas are involved, a single organ or system may be affected predominantly, and the symptoms referable to that part form the major portion of the clinical picture.

The initial or outstanding symptoms often point to the musculoskeletal system, and the orthopaedic surgeon is usually the first one to be confronted with the diagnostic problem. Whenever muscle, bone, or joint pain is the presenting complaint, the differential diagnosis must consider collagen diseases.

The picture may be that of a monoarticular arthritis, which may remain confined to one joint or may blossom into a polyarthritic syndrome, often resembling rheumatoid arthritis; peripheral nerve involvement may be manifested as a sciatica or a Morton's toe; or severe recurrent muscle pain and stiffness may be revealed eventually as part of a dermatomyositis. The striking and characteristic feature of collagen diseases is their episodic tendency to produce symptoms in waves of exacerbations and symptom-free remissions.

The following discussion describes only the pertinent points that will enable the orthopaedic surgeon to identify the offending condition. Further intensive study and treatment belong within the realm of the internist. The diseases to be considered include systemic lupus erythematosus, polyarteritis nodosa, scleroderma, and dermatomyositis. Rheumatoid arthritis and rheumatic fever, which possess similar pathologic changes, are discussed elsewhere.

The exciting cause is obscure, but an autoimmune mechanism is suggested by hypergammaglobulinemia, low complement levels, multiple "autoantibodies," accumulation of lymphocytes and plasma cells in damaged tissues, effectiveness of corticosteroid treatment, and frequent coexistence of various antoimmune disorders.

SYSTEMIC (DISSEMINATED) LUPUS ERYTHEMATOSUS

Systemic lupus erythematosus (SLE) is a noninfectious, inflammatory disease that involves the connective and the vascular tissues of many organs.[41,46,56,57] Although the name implies that cutaneous lesions form an essential part of the condition, such external manifestations are often lacking, particularly in the early stages. Instead, the more common and outstanding symptoms at the outset are referable to the musculoskeletal system. Its importance to the orthopaedic surgeon lies in the fact that its arthritic involvement closely resembles and must be differentiated from rheumatoid arthritis.

PATHOLOGY

Fibrinoid changes are observed within the walls of blood vessels and in the connective tissue proper, producing a disseminated arteritis that is situated not only in viscera widely scattered throughout the body but also within synovial tissues. A synovial biopsy taken from an inflamed joint will not only display fibrinoid lesions but occasionally will demonstrate diagnostic "hematoxylin bodies." These homogeneous purple masses of nuclear material are found extracellularly and also as an inclusion body within a polymorphonuclear leukocyte. The latter is the typical LE cell.

CLINICAL PICTURE

Most commonly, the patient is in the third or the fourth decade, but the disease can develop at any age. The onset and the subsequent course are extremely variable. The acute fulminating form, which produces generalized visceral involvement, is fatal within a few weeks.

The more common chronic form poses a diagnostic problem for the orthopaedic surgeon (Table 18-1). The course, encompassing many years, is typified by exacerbations and remissions of apparent good health. Each explosive acute epidose is frequently initiated by arthritic phenomena that either occur alone or, when associated with other symptoms, form a prominent part of the picture. Severe arthralgia is the main complaint. The joint findings may be negative on examination; a migratory polyarthritis akin to rheumatic fever may be seen; or features closely resembling rheumatoid arthritis develop in a third of patients. However, severe deformities and subcutaneous nodules are rarely observed. The arthritis usually involves the wrists, the hands, and the knees. Although visceral involvement is variable and symptoms are protean, the most common clinical manifestations to be sought in establishing the diagnosis include the following:

- Symptoms occurring in episodes
- Cutaneous lesions, particularly the "butterfly rash" of the face
- Generalized lymphadenopathy
- Cardiac involvement, such as endocarditis and pericarditis
- Renal involvement. Glomerulonephritis is a serious feature, causing uremia and hypertension.
- Pleurisy with effusion occurring in over half the patients
- Retinal lesions in more than 25% of patients. These are small white spots in the nerve fiber of the retina known as "cytoid bodies."

LABORATORY DIAGNOSIS

Whenever joint disease is suspected of being a manifestation of lupus erythematosus, the following tests are used to provide confirmatory evidence:

LE Cell Phenomenon

The LE cell is a polymorphonuclear leukocyte largely filled with an inclusion body, a globular mass of homogeneous material appearing like ground glass and staining red-purple with Wright's stain. The same material may be observed extracellularly as free globs, or rosettes, which are globs surrounded by neutrophils. In performing the test, the patient's serum is added to a suspension of red blood cells. The LE factor, which is contained within the γ-globulin of the serum, is complement fixing with the nuclear material of degenerated leukocytes, and the purple-staining globs are deposited.

False-positive results are observed in as high as 15% of patients with other collagen diseases (*e.g.*, rheumatoid arthritis), hepatic conditions, and the hydralazine syndrome, which consists of rheumatoid symptoms developing in patients being treated over long periods of time with hydralazine.

Antinuclear Antibodies

Antinuclear antibodies (ANA) are a heterogeneous collection of antibodies directed against numerous discrete macromolecules that are normal constituents of the cell nucleus. These antibodies belong to the γ-globulin fraction of the serum and cross-react in general with nuclei from different sources, thus lacking tissue or species specificity. These antigen-antibody reactions, together with complement fixing, result in an immune complex mechanism that forms the pathogenetic basis for various diseases, especially those included in collagen disorders.[47]

Immunofluorescence is a currently used screening test that detects any type of ANA without regard to their specificities (total ANA). At least three types of ANA or antinuclear factors (ANF) are of diagnostic importance: antinucleoprotein antibodies (anti-DPN); antideoxyribonucleic acid (anti-DNA); and nonspecific antibodies against non-DNA material. In addition to serums, ANA have been detected in other body fluids (*e.g.*, in synovial fluid where they may represent the source of an autoimmune mechanism for the production of rheumatoid arthritis).[42]

The nonspecific fluoresence test requires conjugating the protein of the test serum with fluoresceine. The conjugate is then mixed with a substrate, a standardized preparation of cells, and various patterns of fluorescence are observed, each one supposedly representative of a particular immune complex. A titer of between 1:10 and 1:30 or higher is considered positive.[48,49]

An enzyme-conjugated (horseradish peroxidase) antiglobulin has been substituted for the fluorochrome-conjugated antiglobulin for the detection of ANA. The electron-dense peroxidase complexes can be observed by electron microscopy.[40]

The total ANA is positive in 100% of cases of SLE, whereas the LE cell is positive only in 60% to 70% of cases. Since other diseases and drug-induced SLE can produce a positive result, a negative result of an im-

TABLE 18-1 American Rheumatism Association: Preliminary Criteria for Classification of SLE

The proposed criteria are based on 14 manifestations that include 21 items as follows. For the purposes of classifying patients in clinical trials, population surveys, and other such studies, a person shall be said to have systemic lupus erythematosus (SLE), if any 4 or more of the following 14 manifestations are present serially or simultaneously, during any interval of observation:

1. *Facial erythema (butterfly rash):* diffuse erythema, flat or raised, over the malar eminence(s) and/or bridge of the nose; may be unilateral
2. *Discoid lupus:* erythematosus raised patches with adherent keratotic scaling and follicular plugging; atrophic scarring may occur in older lesions; may be present anywhere on the body
3. *Raynaud's phenomenon:* requires a two-phase color reaction, by patient's history or physician's observation
4. *Alopecia:* rapid loss of large amount of the scalp hair, by patient's history or physician's observation
5. *Photosensitivity:* unusual skin reaction from exposure to sunlight, by patient's history or physician's observation
6. *Oral or nasopharyngeal ulceration*
7. *Arthritis without deformity:* one or more peripheral joints involved with any of the following in the absence of deformity: (a) pain on motion, (b) tenderness, and (c) effusion or periarticular soft tissue swelling (peripheral joints are defined for this purpose as feet, ankles, knees, hips, shoulders, elbows, wrists, and metacarpophalangeal, proximal, interphalangeal, terminal interphalangeal, and temporomandibular joints)
8. *LE cells:* two or more classic LE cells seen on one occasion, or one cell seen on two or more occasions, using an accepted published method
9. *Chronic false-positive results of serologic test for syphilis:* known to be present at least 6 months and confirmed by TPI or Reiter's tests
10. *Profuse proteinuria:* greater than 3.5 g/day
11. *Cellular casts:* may be red cell, hemoglobin, granular, tubular, or mixed
12. *One or both of the following:* (a) *pleuritis,* good history of pleuritis pain; rub heard by physician; or roentgenographic evidence of pleural thickening and fluid; or (b) *pericarditis,* documented by electrocardiogram or rub
13. *One or both of the following:* (a) *psychosis* and (b) *convulsions,* by patient's history or physician's observation in the absence of uremia and offending drugs
14. *One or more of the following:* (a) *hemolytic anemia,* (b) *leukopenia* (white blood cell count less than 4000/cu mm on two or more occasions), (c) *thrombocytopenia* (platelet count less than 100,000/cu mm)

(Cohen AS, Reynolds WE, Franklin EC et al: Preliminary criteria for the classification of systemic lupus erythematosus. Bull Rheum Dis 21:643, 1971)

munofluorescence test of enzyme-conjugated test is significant, since it makes the possibility of SLE in the untreated patient most unlikely. It should be noted that a significant reduction in titer of ANA occurs during treatment with high doses of corticosteroids or during a remission.

Biopsy

Synovial membrane will exhibit hematoxylin bodies. A punch biopsy of the kidney will show characteristic glomerular lesions.

Rheumatoid Factor

The presence of rheumatoid factor is detected by agglutination tests. However, it is elevated in only about 35% of patients and therefore is not diagnostic.

TREATMENT

Steroids produce dramatic improvement of the acute episode. Salicylates are given in the intervals. The patient should avoid exposure to the sun, which is known to produce an exacerbation.

When a drug that the patient has been taking for more than 3 months is suspected of being the causative agent, it should be discontinued.[51] The disease process will reverse itself, beginning within a few days, on cessation of the drug therapy. The most common offenders are hydralazine and procainamide; less common ones are practolol, D-penicillamine, and isoniazid; and phenytoin, ethosuxamide, the thiouracils, trimethadione, primidone, and chlorpromazine (and other phenothiazines) are incriminated infrequently.

SCLERODERMA (SYSTEMIC SCLEROSIS)

Scleroderma is a chronic condition characterized by fibrous thickening of the dermis and the connective tissue of many viscera.[44,53,54] Vascular lesions of the type encountered in polyarteritis nodosa are frequently associated. In the initial stages, which may last for months and years, complaints are usually confined to the hands and include Raynaud's phenomenon, hyperhidrosis of the palms, and stiffness of the fingers and the hands. Therefore, the orthopaedic surgeon is faced with the early diagnostic problem.

PATHOLOGY

The dermis is thickened by coarse collagen bundles lying parallel with the surface of the skin and extending deeply into the adipose tissue. Eventually, fibrinoid changes appear. Amorphous calcium deposits in the skin are often observed. The fibrosis also occurs in the muscles and many viscera. Vascular lesions involve small arteries and arterioles, occlude their lumens, and produce infarctions, especially in the kidney. Glomerulonephritis is not found.

CLINICAL PICTURE

Middle-aged people are usually affected, and the condition is more prevalent in women. The course is prolonged and slowly progressive over many years. The patient at first presents symptoms and findings identical with Raynaud's disease. Stiffness and hyperhidrosis of the hands are usual. Gradually, over ensuing months and years, a diffuse, nonpitting edema appears about the hands and the feet. The involved skin becomes waxy, taut, hard, thickened, and firmly bound to underlying structures. The normal skin folds disappear, producing a masklike face. The process tends to spread centrally from the distal portions of the extremities, and the entire integument becomes involved. Brown pigmentation and vitiligo are common. The fingers become immobilized in flexion. Ulcers appear over the fingertips and other points of pressure. Both diffuse subcutaneous calcifications (calcinosis universalis) and periarticular calcifications (calcinosis circumscripta) are seen. Recurrent polyarthritis is common but rarely leads to deformities.

Other symptoms, referable to visceral involvement, are protean (*e.g.*, dysphagia is due to esophageal involvement; dyspnea results from sclerodermatous constriction of the thorax; renal involvement with uremia and hypertension is a terminal event).

LABORATORY FINDINGS

Roentgenograms reveal osteoporosis, destruction of the distal phalanges, and subcutaneous or periarticular calcifications. The erythrocyte sedimentation rate is elevated. The albumin-globulin ratio is reversed. Biopsy of the skin is diagnostic.

TREATMENT

Physical therapy may be used to combat contractures and attempt to preserve mobility. Sympathectomy may give some relief from early vasomotor phenomena.

POLYARTERITIS (PERIARTERITIS) NODOSA

In polyarteritis nodosa the medium and the small arteries throughout the body are affected by lesions showing segmental necrosis, fibrinoid change, and leukocytic infiltration.[45,50] Depending on the sites of arterial involvement, various multisystem manifestations arise. The characteristic features that the orthopaedic surgeon is apt to encounter include painful peripheral neuritis, often bilateral, which can be represented as sciatica, Morton's toe, cervical and brachial neuritis; myositis, exhibited as multifocal areas of muscle pain and tenderness; and severe arthralgias without true arthritis. The diagnosis is established by biopsy from a painful area of muscle, nerve, or renal punch biopsy. Arteriographic studies reveal characteristic aneurysms in the renal, celiac, mesenteric, hypogastric and hepatic arteries.

DERMATOMYOSITIS

Dermatomyositis is an ill-defined degenerative and inflammatory condition affecting the skin and the striated muscles.[43,52,55] The proximal muscle groups of the extremities are involved more frequently and severely than the distal ones. The involved muscles are tender and have a doughy consistency. The patient complains of aching, weakness, and stiffness and may by unable to raise the arms or to ambulate. The overlying skin displays swollen erythematous patches, which often desquamate. Characteristically, edema and a purple-red discoloration appear about the face, particularly in the periorbital regions. As the disease progresses, the muscles become firm, atrophic, and fibrotic and contractures develop about the shoulders, the elbows, the hips, and the knees. Disability is progressive.

DIAGNOSIS

The diagnosis is established by muscle or skin biopsy. As in other muscle-destroying conditions, the urinary excretion of creatinine is reduced and that of creatine is increased. The creatine phosphokinase level is elevated. On roentgenographic examination, extensive subcutaneous and periarticular calcifications are noted.

TREATMENT

The orthopaedic surgeon is mainly concerned with prevention of disabling contractures by appropriate splinting and physical therapy.

REFERENCES

Fibrous Dysplasia of Bone

1. Albright F, Butler AM, Hampton AO, Smith D: Syndrome characterized by osteitis fibrosa disseminata, areas of pigmentation, and endocrine dysfunction with precocious puberty in females. N Engl J Med 216:727, 1937
2. Harris WH, Dudley HR Jr, Barry RJ: The natural history of fibrous dysplasia. J Bone Joint Surg 44A:207, 1962
3. Pritchard JE: Fibrous dysplasia of bone. Am J Med Sci 222:313, 1951
4. Spjut H, Dorfman H, Fechner R, Ackerman L: Tumors of Bone and Cartilage, second series. Washington, DC, Armed Forces Institute of Pathology, 1970

5. Valls J, Polak M, Schajowicz F: Fibrous dysplasia of bone. J Bone Joint Surg 32A:311, 1950

Nonosteogenic Fibroma of Bone

6. Hatcher CH: The pathogenesis of localized fibrous lesions in the metaphyses of long bones. Ann Surg 122:1016, 1945
7. Jaffe HL, Lichtenstein L: Non-osteogenic fibroma of bone. Am J Pathol 18:205, 1942

Congenital Neurofibromatosis

8. Aegerter EF: The possible relationship of neurofibromatosis, congenital pseudarthrosis, and fibrous dysplasia. J Bone Joint Surg 32A:618, 1950
9. Allibone EC, Illingworth RS, Wright T: Neurofibromatosis (von Recklinghausen's disease) of the vertebral column. Arch Dis Child 35:153, 1960
10. Andersen KS: Congenital pseudarthrosis of the tibia and neurofibromatosis. Acta Orthop Scand 47:108, 1976
11. Chaglassian JH, Riseborough EJ, Hall JE: Neurofibromatous scoliosis. J Bone Joint Surg 58A:695, 1976
12. Crowe FW, Schull WJ, Neel JV: A Clinical, Pathological, and Genetic Study of Multiple Neurofibromatosis. Springfield, IL, Charles C Thomas, 1956
13. Ducroquet R: A propos des pseudarthroses et inflexions congénitales du tibia. Mém Acad Chir 63:683, 1937
14. Fienman NL, Yacovaks WC: Neurofibromatosis in childhood. J Pediatr 76:339, 1970
15. Green WT, Rudo N: Pseudarthrosis and neurofibromatosis. Arch Surg 46:639, 1943
16. Halpern M, Currarino G: Vascular lesions causing hypertension in neurofibromatosis. N Engl J Med 273:248, 1965
17. Harwood-Nash DC: Axial tomography of the optic canals in children. Radiology 96:367, 1970
18. Heard GE, Holt JF, Naylor B: Cervical vertebral deformity in von Recklinghausen's disease of the nervous system: A review with necropsy findings. J Bone Joint Surg 44B:880, 1962
19. Heine H, Schaeg G, Nasemann T: Licht- und elektronenmikroskopische Untersuchungen zur Pathogenese der Neurofibromatose. Arch Dermatol Res 256:85, 1976
20. Holt JF: Neurofibromatosis in children. The 1977 Edward B. D. Neuhauser Lecture. AJR 130:615, 1978
21. Holt JF, Wright EM: The radiologic features of neurofibromatosis. Radiology 51:647, 1948
22. Hunt JC, Pugh DG: Skeletal lesions in neurofibromatosis. Radiology 76:1, 1961
23. Isaacson P: Mast cells in benign nerve sheath tumours. J Pathol 119:199, 1976
24. James JIP: Scoliosis. Edinburgh, E & S Livingstone, 1967
25. James JIP: The etiology of scoliosis. J Bone Joint Surg 52B:410, 1970
26. McCarroll HR: Clinical manifestations of congenital neurofibromatosis. J Bone Joint Surg 32A:601, 1950
27. Meszaros WT et al: Neurofibromatosis. AJR 98:557, 1966
28. Moore BH: Some orthopaedic relationships of neurofibromatosis. J Bone Joint Surg 23:109, 1941
29. Rosenbusch G et al: Renovasculare Hypertension bei Neurofibromatose. Fortschr Geb Rontgenstr Nuclearmed Erganzungsband 126:218, 1977
30. Scott JC: Scoliosis and neurofibromatosis. J Bone Joint Surg 47B:240, 1965
31. Sharrard WJW: Paediatric Orthopaedics and Fractures. London, Blackwell Scientific Publications, 1971
32. Speed K: Malignant degeneration of neurofibromata of peripheral nerve trunks (von Recklinghausen's disease). Ann Surg 116:81, 1942
33. Valls J, Polak M, Schajowicz F: Fibrous dysplasia of bone. J Bone Joint Surg 32A:311, 1950
34. van Nes CP: Congenital pseudarthrosis of the leg. J Bone Joint Surg 48A:1467, 1966
35. Veliskakis KP, Wilson PD Jr, Levine DB: Neurofibromatosis and scoliosis: Significance of the short angular spinal curve. J Bone Joint Surg 52A:833, 1970
36. Veyne B et al: Association pheochromocytoma-neurofibromatose. Nouv Presse Med 4:2873, 1975
37. von Recklinghausen FD: Uber die multiplen Fibrome der Haut und ihre Beziehung zu den multiplen Neuromen. Berlin, August Hirschwald, 1882
38. Whitehouse D: Diagnostic value of the café-au-lait spot in children. Arch Dis Child 41:316, 1966
39. Yong-Hing K, Kalamchi A, MacEwen GD: Cervical spine abnormalities in neurofibromatosis. J Bone Joint Surg 61A:695, 1979

Collagen Diseases

40. Benson MD, Cohen AS: Antinuclear antibodies in SLE: Detection with horseradish peroxidase-conjugated antibody. Ann Intern Med 73:943, 1970
41. Cohen AS, Reynolds WE, Franklin EC et al: Preliminary criteria for the classification of systemic lupus erythematosus. Bull Rheum Dis 21:643, 1971
42. Cracchiolo A, Barnett EN: The role of immunological tests in routine synovial fluid analysis. J Bone Joint Surg 54A:828, 1972
43. Currie S et al: Immunologic aspects of polymyositis. Q J Med 40:63, 1971
44. D'Angelo WA et al: Pathologic observations in systemic sclerosis (scleroderma): A study of 58 autopsy cases and 58 matched controls. Am J Med 46:428, 1969
45. Dornfield L, Lecky JW, Peter JB: Polyarteritis and internal artery aneurysms. JAMA 215:1950, 1971
46. Estes D, Christian CL: The natural history of systemic lupus erythematosus by prospective analysis. Medicine 50:85, 1971
47. Fernandez-Madrid F, Mattioli M: Antinuclear antibodies (ANA): Immunologic and clinical significance. Semin Arthritis Rheum 6(2):83, 1976
48. Friou GJ: Clinical application of lupus-serum nucleoprotein reaction using fluorescent antibody technique. J Clin Invest 36:890, 1957
49. Friou GJ: The LE cell factor and antinuclear antibodies. In Cohen AS (ed): Laboratory Diagnostic Procedures in the Rheumatic Diseases. Boston, Little, Brown & Co, 1967
50. Fronhert PP, Sheps SG: Long-term follow-up study of periarteritis nodosa. Am J Med 43:8, 1967
51. Lee SL, Chase PH: Drug-induced systemic lupus erythematosus: A critical review. Semin Arthritis Rheum 5:183, 1975
52. Medsger TA Jr, Dawson WW Jr, Masi AT: The epidemiology of polymyositis. Am J Med 48:715, 1970
53. Medsger TA Jr et al: Survival with systemic sclerosis (scleroderma): A life-table analysis of clinical and demographic factors in 309 patients. Ann Intern Med 75:369, 1971
54. Norton WL, Nardo M: Vascular disease in progressive systemic sclerosis (scleroderma). Ann Intern Med 73(4):317, 1970

55. Rose AL, Watson JN: Polymyositis: A survey of 89 cases with particular reference to treatment and prognosis. Brain 89:747, 1966
56. Statsny P, Ziff M: Cold insoluble complexes and complement levels in systemic lupus erythematosus. N Engl J Med 280:1376, 1969
57. Wallace SL, Diamond H, Kaplan D: Recent advances in the rheumatic diseases: The connective tissue diseases other than rheumatoid arthritis—1970 and 1971. Ann Intern Med 77:455, 1972

19

Unclassified Diseases of Bone

PAGET'S DISEASE

Paget's disease (osteitis deformans) is a very common idiopathic chronic condition of the skeleton ocurring in patients past middle age. It is characterized pathologically by partial or complete involvement of a single or multiple bones by exaggerated rates of resorptive and osteogenic activity, leading to bony thickening and deformity and clinically by bone pain, bone deformity, deafness, susceptibility to fractures with trivial trauma, and such complications as secondary osteoarthritis, sarcomatous degeneration, referred pain and nerve entrapment syndromes, and, in extensive disease, high-output cardiac failure.

ETIOLOGY

The actual cause of Paget's disease is unknown. Endocrine and metabolic disturbances are unlikely because, despite extensive involvement, many bones are free of disease. Males are affected more often than females. Occasionally, a hereditary influence is noted. [2,26] Most cases are observed in patients over 50 years of age. Schmorl believed that approximately 3% of everyone over age 40 has osteitis deformans.[38] The disease is more prevalent in those of Anglo-Saxon origin.

Under electron microscopy, nuclear inclusions, which are similar to those observed in certain viral diseases, are found in the highly multinucleated osteoclasts of all patients with Paget's disease.[33,41]

PATHOLOGY

Early, the basic process is one of extensive osteoclastic destruction accompanied by increased vascularity and fibrosis. Trabeculae are thinned, and haversian canals are enlarged. Periosteal new bone and, to a lesser extent, endosteal new bone form and thicken the cortex. This fibrous vascular bone is soft and yields easily to stresses and strains of weight bearing.[14,21]

Next, the stage of repair begins (Color Plate 19-1). Large numbers of osteoblasts are seen laying down thick, coarse trabeculae of new bone, replacing the old cortical lamellae and the recently formed trabeculae beneath the periosteum. Repair and destruction are taking place at the same time. As new bone is being formed in some places, it is destroyed in others. The process is disorderly and disorganized. The new trabeculae are distorted in shape and direction and often are laid down about trabeculae that are old and incompletely absorbed. The new and old fragments of trabeculae are joined by deeply staining cement lines that are arranged in a bizarre fashion and are referred to as the mosaic pattern that is characteristic of the disease. There appears to be no effort at formation of haversian systems. In contrast to the soft fibrous bone, dense mosaic bone is brittle and easily fractured. Osteogenetic processes are stimulated by activity, so that those bones that are subjected repeatedly to loading of weight bearing and stresses of muscular contractions display early and intense new bone formation. Thus, the long bones of the lower extremities and the vertebrae exhibit the dense bone of an active reparative process, which keeps pace with the destructive process. In the skull, where stresses and strains are at a minimum, repair lags considerably behind in the early stages and resorption predominates, as revealed by a sharply demarcated soft, vascular, osteolytic area. The outer skull surface becomes greatly thickened by periosteal fibrous bone. Replacement by mosaic bone is delayed but ultimately occurs. Grossly, the bony surface is thick and hard and has the appearance of finely porous pumice stone.

Periods of remission are thought to occur. At this time, the microscopic appearance is one of thickened, irregularly disposed mosaic bone, acellularity, and marrow spaces occupied by avascular fibrous tissue.

Although any bone may be affected, those involved, in the order of greatest frequency, are pelvis, femur, skull, tibia, and spine. The bones of the hand and the foot are seldom affected (a differential point from polyostotic fibrous dysplasia). The condition may be confined at first to a portion of one bone (usually the tibia or the femur) and spreads gradually to the rest of the bone. At its advancing, a sharply delimited edge may be observed, providing microscopic evidence of early osteoclastic bone resorption. It may remain within that bone for years as a solitary lesion, but, almost invaribly, other bones eventually become affected. Although the condition becomes widespread, many areas escape, and the distribution becomes typically asymmetric.

Grossly, the bones are thickened and display irregular rough surfaces, which on close inspection contain fine pores and resemble pumice stone. The long bones become bowed anterolaterally in response to weight-bearing loading. Over the convex outer cortex are often seen transverse fissures; these fissures represent incomplete fractures, which eventually heal with a minimum of callus. Frequent refracturing and consequent outward bowing cause actual lengthening of the shaft. A complete transverse fracture may take place and likewise heals slowly but with a minimum of callus. The cortex is thickened not only externally but also internally, with encroachment on the medullary cavity. The spongiosa is composed of thickened coarse strands of bone, and the cellular marrow spaces are gradually transformed into fibrous tissue, with diminishing cellularity and reduced vascularity.

Involvement of the skull ranges from one or several areas of osteoporosis circumscripta to pronounced thickening of the calvarium and extreme thickening of the base of the skull. *Osteoporosis circumscripta* of the calvarium represents an early unique phase of skull involvement; it is asymptomatic and is radiolucent. The lesion is composed of loose-meshed diploic bone that extends through the entire thickness of the skull as the inner and outer tables disappear. As the disease progresses, the diploic bone becomes thicker and more closemeshed and develops dense sclerotic foci seen as small radiopacities. The whole area ultimately becomes very dense and thickened by bone deposition on both surfaces, and the thickness involves not only the calvarium but also the base. The inner thickening progressively encroaches on the cranial cavity and compresses the brain. The foramen magnum may be narrowed. Although the foramina for the cranial nerves may be reduced, neurologic deficits are unusual. The cause of progressive deafness so characteristic of the disease is inexplicable. An intermingling of shadows of various densities in the calvarium creates a highly typical roentgenographic appearance described as a "cotton ball" skull.

Although any portion of the vertebral column and pelvis may be involved, the disease has a peculiar predilection for at least some lumbar vertebrae, for parts of the sacrum, and for the innominate bones. Within the vertebra. the changes are more conspicuous in the body than in the processes. At the periphery of the body, the spongy bone is compacted to form a framelike configuration. The centrally placed trabeculae are thick, coarse, vertically disposed pillarlike structures and enclose myeloid and fatty marrow. Severely involved vertebrae may become deformed, usually reduced in height, and increased in their anteroposterior and transverse dimensions through deposition of periosteal new bone, which may encroach on the spinal canal and neural foramina and their contents.[13,39]

The epiphyseal ends of long bones and juxta-articular portions of the innominate bones are often involved, and the adjacent joints develop osteoarthritic changes to a variable degree. At the hip joint, the often associated coxa vara or protrusio deformities compound the mechanical problem.

The aorta and larger arteries are very atheromatous, sclerotic, and extensively calcified.

PATHOPHYSIOLOGY

The fundamental process of Paget's disease is at first a wave of predominantly osteoclastic resorptive activity producing regional osteoporosis. Roentgenographically, this appears as a sharply demarcated focus of radiolucency designated as *osteoporosis circumscripta* in the skull, whereas in a long bone it appears as a "flame shaped" radiolucent expansile lesion that replaces and expands the cortex. After an interval of time, osteoblastic activity becomes more dominant, and an abnormally large amount of bone is produced at the site, increasing the thickness of the parent bone. The histologic sections are generally obtained at an advanced stage of the disease and reflect markedly exaggerated resorptive and oteogenic activity (*i.e.*, greatly increased rate of bone turnover.[1,4] The disease may run a course at any given site of repeated periods of heightened activity ("hot phase") alternating with periods of reduced activity ("cold phase") and ultimately may become quiescent, with the cellular population diminishing to the point of disappearing. In some cases with multifocal disease, the entire disease burns out, leaving only structural abnormalities.

Rarely is it possible to observe the sequence of events, as postulated by Jaffe: initial resorption characterized by an advancing radiolucent lesion, followed in its wake by striking osteogenesis, which replaces the osteolytic lesion and produces dense, thick bone. Instead, with widespread multifocal involvement, continuing disease activity of resorption and osteogenesis at one or several sites is usual. An acute reawakening of markedly heightened disease activity in an involved bone is manifested clinically by pain and increased local heat. While some disease foci demonstrate continuing activity, others display only structural abnormalities as residuals of burnt out disease.[6]

Although active disease may be widespread, and considerable bone resorption takes place, counterbalancing osteogenesis acts to maintain calcium homeostasis. Local reutilization of calcium and phosphorus ions appears to be the homeostatic mechanism. Despite accelerated bone turnover (more than 20-fold over normal in patients with extensive active disease[29]), the loss of calcium ions into the extracellular fluids is negligible. The enormous rates of bone resorption and deposition are balanced. It may be that the increase in bone formation is a homeostatic response to protect against increases in the concentration of calcium of such magnitude that might provoke major alterations in critical cellular function. It can be demonstrated that calcium isotopes persist in involved areas long after other bone-seeking isotopes (*e.g.*, diphosphonate coupled with technetium Tc 99m) have cleared.

Under conditions of fracture, inactivity, and immobilization, the stimulus for bone formation is lessened, while bone resorption continues. Reduction of osteogenesis is reflected in lowered serum levels of heat-labile isoenzyme alkaline phosphatase.[25] Loss of calcium ions into the extracellular fluids may be rapidly cleared by functionally competent kidneys, and hypercalcemia may not be apparent. An excessive negative calcium balance is detected by an increased urinary calcium excretion, often more than 1000 mg/day. It is only when the calcium excretory capacity of the kidneys is exceeded that hypercalcemia develops and often leads to metastatic calcification.

Immobilizing a patient with extensive Paget's disease, especially one who is already ingesting large quantities of milk, invites the threat of "chemical death." Hypercalcemia may lead to the formation of renal calculi and ultimately may cause anuria and a fatal termination. The ominous symptoms of hypercalcemia include dryness of the nose and throat, nausea and vomiting, and difficulty in swallowing. Hypercalcemia must be controlled by a low calcium diet, oral magnesium salts, forcing fluids, and increasing the patient's activity.

Resorption of bone includes degradation of the protein matrix, liberating fragments of peptides containing hydroxyproline, a constituent solely of bone collagen. The large amounts of peptide-bound hydroxyproline excreted in the urine are characteristic of active Paget's disease and serve as an index of the increased bone resorptive activity.

During the active resorptive phase of the disease, intense vascular hyperplasia develops within the diseased bone and increases local blood flow, which together with increased vascularity of the overlying soft tissues is responsible for the extraordinary warmth of the part. Despite the large number of arterioles and venous sinuses that decrease local vascular resistance, arteriovenous shunts have never been demonstrated. When at least one third of skeletal structures are affected by active disease, cardiac output is raised and may ultimately result in high-output cardiac failure.[9,34]

CLINICAL PICTURE

Most commonly the disease exists asymptomatically in one or several bones and is discovered as an incidental finding on roentgenographic evaluation. The innominate bone, a vertebra, or the tibia are favored sites for the early monostotic form of the disease.

When involvement is widespread, the onset is so insidious that the actual beginning of the disease is generally unknown. By the time that the disease is first discovered, the patient is usually of middle or advanced age; males have a predisposition for the disorder (Fig. 19-1). The initial complaint may be pain in the area of bone involvement. This pain varies in type and intensity: it may be a dull ache, a "neuralgic" discomfort, or a sharp stabbing sensation, and it may be intermittent or constant and aggravated by various causes, especially inclement weather. Spontaneous relief of discomfort is not unusual. When pain is felt over the tibia, the bone is often found to be enlarged and bowed in an anterolateral direction, the so-called saber shin. The skin overlying the subcutaneous aspect of the tibia is often unusually warm to the touch, but the bone is not tender. Headache is a common symptom. The head gradually enlarges, necessitating frequent changes of hat size. Progressive deafness is often associated and may be due to otosclerosis, but usually the source of this problem is not discernable.

Gradually, over a number of years, skeletal disease becomes widespread. The enlarging head is in sharp contrast to the relatively small face. One or both legs or thighs become bowed anterolaterally, the enlarged tibiae increasing the circumference of the legs. A diffuse kyphosis develops throughout the thoracic spine, and the lumbar lordotic curve is gradually obliterated. The chest is narrowed in its transverse diameter. As the advanced stage is reached, the posture is highly characteristic. The patient stands in a crouched position with the enlarged head thrust forward, the trunk bent, and the lower extremities widely bowed outward. The gait is slow. Muscle weakness and fatigue are evident.

Backache is a common complaint with involvement of the spine. Radicular pain may encircle the chest or abdomen or may radiate to the lower extremities, where it may be confused with bone pain of local active disease or the pain of osteoarthritis. Rarely, vertebral bodies affected by active disease may deform and enlarge and may encroach on the spinal canal and its contents. A neurologic deficit may develop insidiously.

Although the cranium is thickened, compression of the brain and narrowing of foramina are highly unusual. The mentality is unimpaired except that which results from the severe atherosclerosis that usually accompanies extensive disease.

Although seemingly disabled, the victim of Paget's disease may live out his normal life's expectancy unless he develops sarcomatous degeneration or succumbs to high-output cardiac failure.

COMPLICATIONS

The most common complication is fracture, especially of weight-bearing long bones.[20,24,29] Fracture is thought to be more common in the vascular, soft stage. At this time multiple incomplete transverse fissures are found over the apex of the convexity of the bowed shaft. These fissures heal rapidly. Occasionally, however, a complete transverse fracture can occur and heals readily, although with a minimum of callus. When fracture occurs in the late stage of dense bone, union is delayed.

At least 5% of cases undergo malignant degeneration.[30] The tumor is osteogenic sarcoma, fibrosrcoma, or round cell sarcoma. Its development is often heralded by an increase in pain and rapid increase in size of a bone. It is often multicentric. Osteolytic or sclerotic changes are noted on roentgenograms. The tumor is highly malignant. It is said to arise more commonly in the vascular phase, and its origin is often subperiosteal. Biopsy confirms the diagnosis.

Osteitis deformans of a vertebra can, by bony enlargement or by malignant transformation, cause compression of intraspinal structures, producing a progressive neurologic deficit. The complaints include chronic back pain, with or without radicular involvement, and increasing paraparesis. The thoracic spine is the usual site of the lesion; less often the upper lumbar spine is involved (see Chapter 30).

In extensive widespread active disease, and the extreme osseous vascularity of such involvement, the demands on cardiac function may ultimately lead to high-output cardiac failure. Contributing to this problem, Paget's disease is often associated with advanced degrees of atherosclerosis.

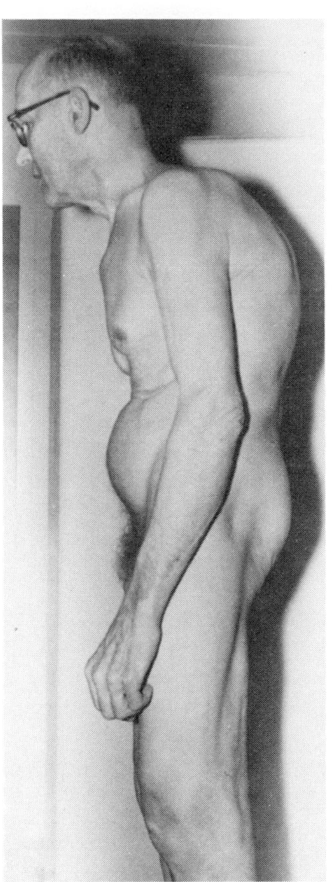

FIG. 19-1. Paget's disease, affecting mainly the spine, the pelvis, and the left femur.

ROENTGENOGRAPHIC FINDINGS

The roentgenographic appearance varies, depending on the relative amount of destruction and reconstruction.[31] Actually, even when the disease is detected early in a long bone, some bony formation is already taking place, especially by periosteal new bone formation thickening of the cortex. Only at the advancing sharp edge of the lesion can one see the rarefaction, the earliest stage of the lesion. Eventually, the cortex is thickened, the medulla is often narrowed, the shaft is bowed, and thick coarse strands of bone develop, which vary from a honeycombed or spongy appearance to large dense strands of bone (Fig. 19-2). Small transverse radiolucent lines often interrupt the cortex over the convexity, representing incomplete fractures or Looser's zones of transformation.

In the pelvis (Fig. 19-3), trabeculation is very coarse

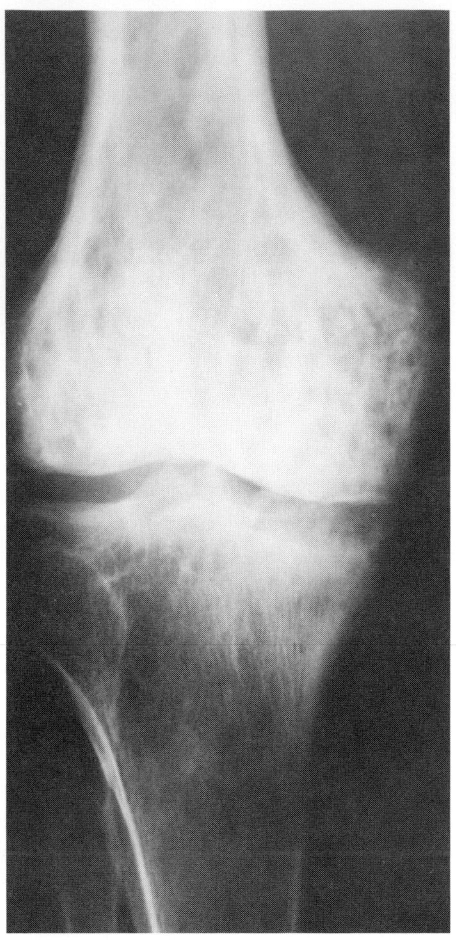

FIG. 19-2. Paget's disease of the femur. The changes at the upper end of the tibia are reactive and degenerative in response to irregularity of the lower surface of the femur.

FIG. 19-3. Paget's disease of the pelvis.

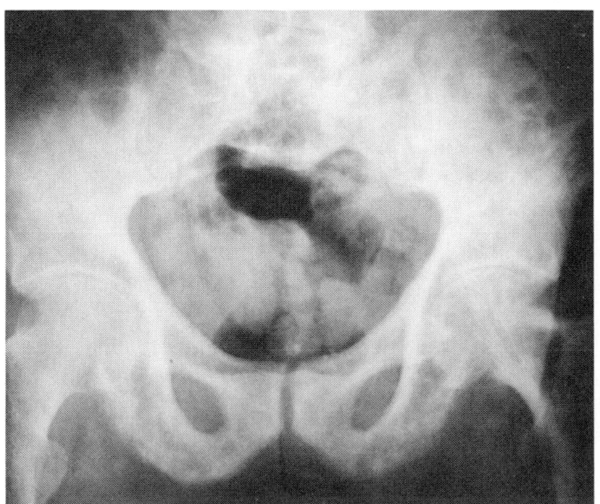

and thick and most conspicuous at the periphery as multiple, parallel, curvilinear lines below the iliac crest. An early finding is exaggerated trabeculae above the acetabulum. Occasionally, the transverse diameter of the pelvis is narrowed by pressure of weight bearing during the "soft period." The pubic and the ischial bones are widened. This finding is especially important when the bone is quite dense and must be differentiated from osteoplastic metastases.

In the spine, one or more vertebrae are affected. Coarse trabeculae form parallel with the periphery and densely outline the vertebral body. The remainder of the body in the early stages appears decalcified and soft and is often compressed and widened in its transverse diameter. However, encroachment on the spinal canal occurs infrequently, usually at the lower thoracic and upper lumbar regions. Ultimately, the body becomes quite dense and devoid of the trabeculated architecture. Its contour often is square.

The best example of the destructive phase is seen in the skull (Fig. 19-4). Early, a well-delineated decalcified lesion is seen affecting chiefly the outer table and is termed *osteoporosis circumscripta.* A thin layer of periosteal bone may overlie the lesion. Eventually, multiple spots of increased bone density develop within the rarefied area. These new bone densities often are round with ill-defined edges and are described as "cotton ball" spots. Ultimately, the densities extend irregularly throughout the skull. The outer table thickens, and the distinction between outer and inner tables is lost.

When a sarcoma develops, it is often revealed by a saucer-shaped erosion of the outer cortex, which usually signifies a fibrosarcoma, or by the usual signs of osteogenic sarcoma, including irregular areas of destruction within the shaft, periosteal new bone, and sun-ray appearance (Fig. 19-5 and 19-6).

LABORATORY FINDINGS

The serum calcium and phosphorus levels are usually normal. The heat-labile alkaline phosphatase value is higher in active Paget's disease than in any other condition. Its level is considered as an index of bone formation. Conversely, the disease is regarded as in a state of remission when the level of serum heat-labile alkaline phosphatase is normal.

During an active phase, the rate of new bone formation is increased, and consequently the rate of collagen synthesis is greater. A portion of collagen that is not used in the formation of osteoid is excreted in the urine. In addition, the high rate of resorption causes large amounts of matrix collagen to undergo degradation, and this, too, must be eliminated, along with peptide fragments derived from other sources of degraded collagen. Consequently, the level of urinary hydroxyproline in active Paget's disease is markedly increased. Normal

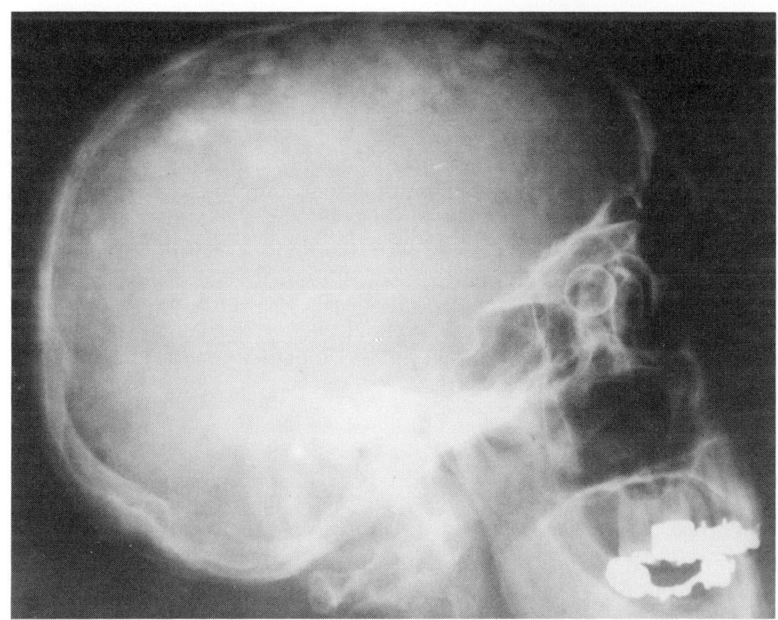

FIG. 19-4. Paget's disease of the skull. Note the woolly or cotton ball spots and loss of distinction between inner and outer tables. Large well-demarcated areas of osteoporosis circumscripta are observed in the frontal and the occipital regions.

urinary hydroxyproline levels of a patient on a constant but not hydroxyproline-free diet are below 50 mg/day. The highest values occur in patients with active Paget's disease and may exceed 1 g/day.[46] As the disease becomes less active, urinary hydroxyproline levels recede.

Measurements of serum heat-labile alkaline phosphatase and urinary hydroxyproline excretion can be used as indexes of disease activity and the efficacy of treatment.

With the use of a bone-seeking radioisotope, intense pickup reflects exaggerated osteogenetic activity and rapid disappearance of the dense radioactivity signifies rapid bone turnover. If the disease responds to a suppressive agent and the local disease process becomes quiescent, the bone scan findings revert to normal.

TREATMENT

Inactive pagetic lesions require no treatment. The treatment of active disease is mainly medical, and the goals are the suppression of active disease; relief of pain; prevention of deformity, especially of large weight-bearing bones; counteracting high-output cardiac dysfunction; reducing the tendency to fracture; preventing and correcting hypercalcemia; and lessening the probability of sarcomatous transformation. Surgical treatment is reserved for management of fractures, correction of bone deformities, total hip replacement or other reconstructive procedures, spinal surgery, and ablative therapy for malignant lesions. Whenever elective procedures are planned, they should always be preceded and followed by suppressive therapy. It has been shown that treatment

FIG. 19-5. Osteogenic sarcoma arising in Paget's disease of the tibia. Sun-ray appearance is evident.

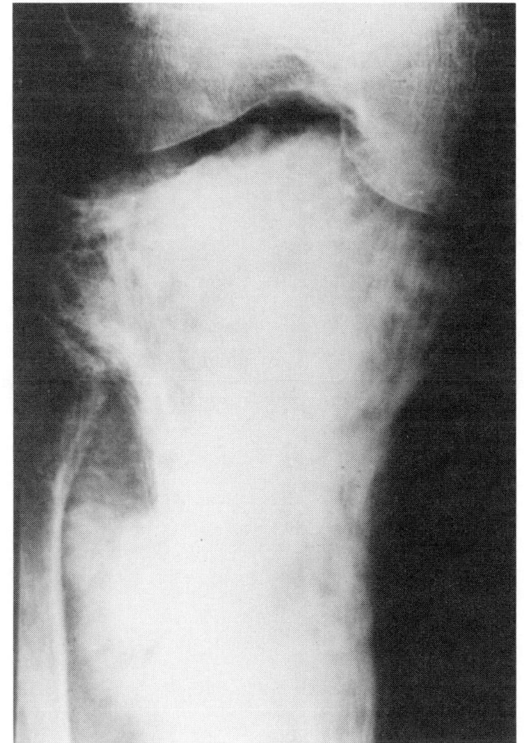

with human calcitonin induces normal remodeling and formation of normal lamellar and trabecular bone.

Medical Management

Pain is the most common symptom requiring treatment, and often can be controlled by simple analgesics such as aspirin. Both aspirin and corticosteroids can suppress active disease, as shown by their ability to reduce serum heat-labile alkaline phosphatase and urine hydroxyproline excretion levels, but long-term use of the amounts required produces serious side-effects. For the same reason, the use of phenylbutazone and indomethacin is not advised.[17,46]

Suppressive Agents

Resorption and formation of bone occur at greatly exaggerated rates, and the increased biochemical activity is reflected in elevation of heat-labile alkaline phosphatase and increased urinary excretion of hydroxyproline, which is liberated by bone collagen undergoing degradation. The levels of these substances serve as convenient parameters of active disease.[29] Therefore, measurement of these substances, as well as relief of symptoms, can be considered parameters of efficacy of various drugs. Mithramycin, calcitonin, and diphosphonate are the chief agents used to suppress the disease, and all act by inhibiting resorption.

FIG. 19-6. Paget's disease, malignant degeneration. The diagnostic features include increased density, local obliteration of the medullary canal, and densities radiating outward beyond the confines of the cortex. The histologic appearance was that of osteogenic sarcoma.

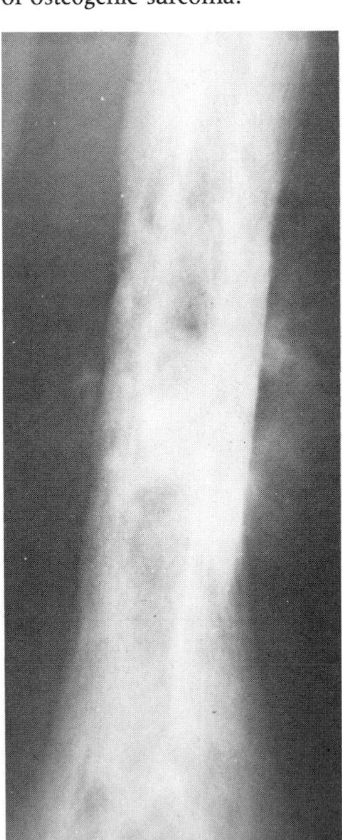

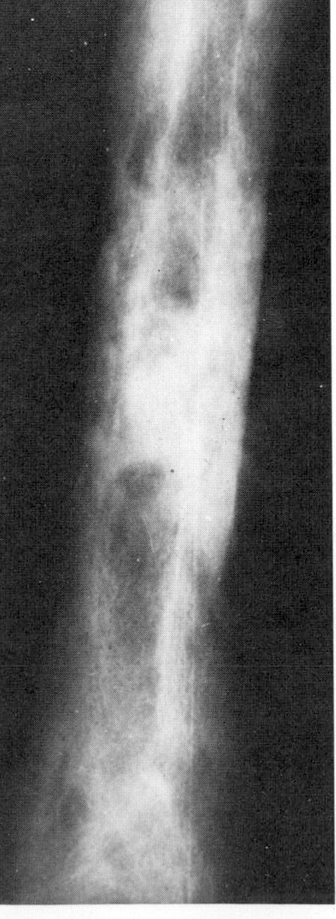

Mithramycin. Mithramycin is a cytotoxic compound which is a deoxyribonucleic acid (DNA)–directed ribonucleic acid (RNA) inhibitor. It lowers serum calcium, relieves bone pain, markedly reduces serum heat-labile alkaline phosphatase and urinary hydroxyproline levels, and improves related congestive heart failure.[35] With the use of small doses to minimize untoward side-effects and with constant monitoring for hepatic and renal toxicity and early signs of bone marrow suppression, especially thrombocytopenia, repeated courses will induce remissions and may enhance the benefit of radiotherapy for localized disease. During treatment with mithramycin, a bone biopsy discloses a decrease of osteoclasts, indicating inhibition of bone resorption.[36] The bone scan often reverts to normal, and sometimes bone remodeling progresses toward a more normal appearance.[35] Complete pain relief can be expected in many patients, with partial relief in a few, but when pain persists, sarcomatous transformation should be suspected.[12]

D actinomycin, another cytotoxic substance that likewise is an inhibitor of DNA–directed RNA synthesis and that has been shown to block the effects of parathyroid hormone and vitamin D on bone,[11] has similar but less pronounced effects.[37]

Calcitonin. Calcitonin, a small polypeptide substance (32 amino acids) secreted in humans by the "C" or parafollicular cells of the thyroid and derived from the ultimobranchial body in lower animals, will inhibit bone resorption. The structure of salmon, porcine, and human calcitonin has been determined, and these hormones can be synthesized and made available for therapeutic use. Salmon calcitonin is about 200 times more potent than either porcine or human calcitonin in its ability to induce hypocalcemia.

Calcitonin will effect improvement in Paget's disease when administered over many weeks.[5] It is given either by subcutaneous or intramuscular injection either daily or three times a week in single or divided doses. Salmon and porcine calcitonin will cause the formation of antibodies and will gradually lose their effect when administered over many months. Human calcitonin does not provoke an antigen-antibody response, nor is its effect nullified by the presence of antibodies to porcine or salmon calcitonin. Long-term calcitonin therapy, because of a chronic parathyroid response that compensates for the hormone-induced hypocalcemia, may sometimes produce permanent hyperparathyroidism.[8] Calcitonin

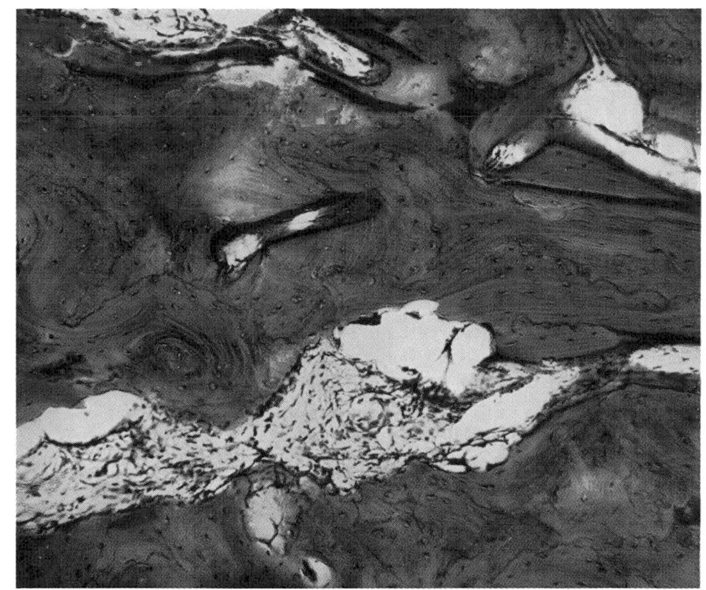

PLATE 19-1. Paget's disease showing the mosaic structure of thick trabeculae, very active bone formation, and vascular fibrous structure of the medullary spaces. (×85) (See p. 734.)

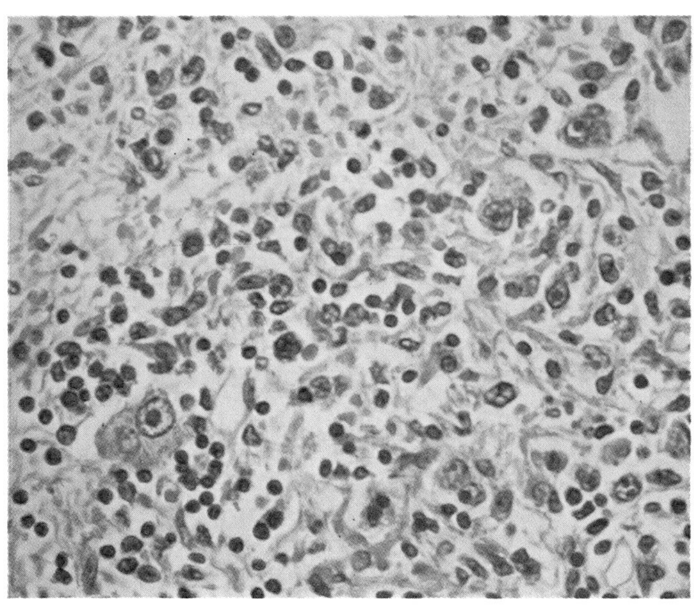

PLATE 19-2. Hodgkin's disease. Typical Reed-Sternberg cells are shown. (×415) (See p. 748.)

an elective procedure is planned, administration of a suppressive agent for several months beforehand is advisable. Not only does the disease become inactive but often the newly formed bone and remodeling assume a semblance of normalcy. This medical regimen must be continued postoperatively.

When disease activity has long been halted, the large weight-bearing bone is thick and prominent over its exterior; the cortex is hard; the marrow is replaced by dense, relatively avascular fibrous tissue; and the contour of the medullary cavity is narrowed and curved. This bone fractures easily and heals poorly. Its curved configuration may be unsuited for intramedullary fixation by a rigid straight rod. Osteotomies should be supplemented by cancellous bone grafts.

Correction of Long Bone Deformity. Calcitonin administered preoperatively decreases the vascularity of the bone and surrounding soft tissues, relieves bone pain, and decreases activity of the disease. It is given as a course over 2 months prior to correcting, for example, a severe tibia vara and internal torsion deformity. The bone pain is relieved within 6 weeks, following which an osteotomy is done.

Procedure. The osteotomy is performed between drill holes made transversely 5 cm or more below the tibial tubercle or at the apex of the deformity. Osteoclasis of the last 0.25 cm of the medial tibial cortex, lateral shift of the distal fragment, and rotation of the distal fragment to correct the torsion are done. Some of the medial periosteum is retained intact, and 0.5 cm to 1 cm of fibula is removed proximally. By manipulation of the distal fragment, the angular and rotatory deformities are corrected so that the planes of the knee and ankle are brought parallel to each other.

At 2 weeks, a well-fitted long walking cast is applied, and 6 weeks after operation, a short cast-brace is fitted and worn until union has occurred. Roentgenographically evident union occurs at from 3 months to 1 year.[28,45]

PAGET'S DISEASE OF THE HIP

Paget's disease may involve either the periacetabular bone or the proximal end of the femur or both, and secondary osteoarthritis develops within the hip joint (coxarthrosis) in most patients. Pagetoid changes about the hip are often accompanied by intrapelvic protrusion of the acetabulum. Involvement at the upper end of the femur may cause enlargement and coxa vara deformity and a high-riding greater trochanter. Pathologic fracture of the femoral neck is a well-recognized complication and often fails to unite despite satisfactory reduction and fixation.[16]

Pelvic and femoral disease about the hip is rarely painful, with such pain being attributed to osteoarthritis. Total hip replacement is necessary for the painful, rigid hip, and, considering the high incidence of nonunion, should be the primary procedure for treatment of fracture of the femoral neck.[44] The operation poses technical difficulties because of hard sclerotic bone. Increased operative bleeding is unusual. A common postoperative sequel is the development of heterotopic bone that causes marked limitation of motion. The incidence and severity of this complication can possibly be lessened by the prior administration of diphosphonates. Because of continuing active disease, late loosening may be a problem, but this can be lessened by therapy with a suppressive agent. Fracture below the stem of the femoral component is a potential hazard.

FRACTURES IN PAGET'S DISEASE

The most common complication of Paget's disease is fracture, especially of weight-bearing long bones. Fracture is thought to be more common in the vascular, soft stage. At this time multiple incomplete transverse fissures are found over the apex of the convexity of the bowed shaft of the femur or tibia during the active phase when osteogenesis predominates. Such fissures may persist, but more often they heal readily. When pain over such a bone develops suddenly and is associated with local tenderness and when roentgenographic changes are absent, a microfracture is the most probable cause and must be treated as a fracture by a period of non–weight bearing.

During the active vascular osteoclastic-osteogenic stage, a complete transverse fracture can occur and heals readily with a minimum of callus. The callus is likewise involved by the pagetic process and exhibits similar roentgenographic and histologic features. Open reduction and internal fixation by compression plates or intramedullary rods is advisable.[16,18] Placement of the rods may be difficult because the bone is bowed. When a complete transverse fracture occurs at a late stage, often with minimal trauma, such bone is dense, hard, and relatively avascular, and delayed union or nonunion is common. In addition to the recommended protocols for the treatment of nonunion, the addition of diphosphonate therapy appears to stimulate union.

Fracture of the femoral neck may not unite, and prosthetic replacement is indicated. Because insertion of the stem of the prosthesis may be impeded, using a shorter small-sized prosthesis may obviate this difficulty. If osteoarthritis is present, total hip replacement is advisable.[44] The femur is highly susceptible to fracture below the stem of the prosthesis.

Before any surgery is undertaken during the acute stage of the disease, preoperative drug treatment is mandatory to reduce activity and vascularity of the disease. To gain this effect rapidly, a course of calcitonin is preferred. Nevertheless, preparations are made for adequate blood replacement at surgery.

PAGET'S DISEASE OF THE SPINE

Osteitis deformans of the spine is highly variable in its pathology and clinical manifestations. A single vertebra may display the framelike configuration of the end-stage, inactive disease and is a common, asymptomatic finding. It rarely produces an increased uptake on bone scans, and pain at this site is usually attributed to secondary osteoarthritis. The active phase of the disease may involve many vertebrae. Bone pain or osteoarthritic pain can be produced, and relatively severe osteopenia may lead to compression fractures. Periosteal bone formation may cause posterior protrusion of the vertebral body into the spinal canal, and, combined with the osteoarthritic enlargement of the posterior articulations, will produce serious encroachment on the spinal canal, resulting in a spinal stenosis syndrome. When this occurs at the level of the lower thoracic spine where the caliber of the spinal canal is normally small, paraparesis or paraplegia may ensue, necessitating a decompressive laminectomy.[18]

When paraplegia or paraparesis develops in Paget's disease, particularly during the acute vascular stage, a course of drug therapy, preferably using the rapidly acting calcitonin, will often improve symptoms, and the need for surgical treatment may be avoided. The inference that the acute bone vascularity has created a "vascular steal syndrome" that produces ischemia of the spinal cord has not been substantiated.

In evaluating back pain, in order to differentiate bone pain of active disease from that due to osteoarthritis or degenerative disk disease, a course of drug therapy is administered. Failure to respond is indicative of a non-pagetoid lesion. (See Osteitis Deformans of the Spine.)

INFANTILE CORTICAL HYPEROSTOSIS

Also known as Caffey's disease infantile cortical hyperostosis is a not uncommon idiopathic condition affecting infants under 6 months of age and characterized clinically by swellings of subperiosteal ossification and constitutional signs of fever, leukocytosis, and an increased sedimentation rate.[49,50]

ETIOLOGY

The cause of infantile cortical hyperostosis is unknown. The condition is often confused with hypervitaminosis A. The constitutional signs suggest an infectious origin.

CLINICAL PICTURE

The onset is acute. The infant is irritable, fretful, and crying. A variable degree of fever is present. Soft tissue swellings appear suddenly over the diaphyses of long bones, particularly the clavicle and the ulna, and over the scapula. Bilateral facial swelling due to involvement of the mandible is common and characteristic. The swelling, although obviously a soft tissue mass, is ligneous, is situated deeply where it apparently is fixed to the underlying bone, and is tender but not warm. These swellings precede roentgenographic changes. When roentgenographic evidence appears, tenderness and fever subside and swellings are already regressing. The course is protracted with remissions and exacerbations.

ROENTGENOGRAPHIC FINDINGS

The diaphyses of long bones, the ribs, the mandible, and the scapula are predisposed. The scapular lesion is often unilateral. The typical lesion is the development of a periosteal elevation by an opacity, often laminated (onion peel) in appearance, representing periosteal new bone formation. The new ossific mass varies in exent, but when it is abundant and extends along the entire shaft it is limited by the attachments of the periosteum to the epiphyseal plate. Periosteal new bone at first exhibits a vague opacity, which gradually increases in density and then blends with and thickens the cortex. Later, remodeling restores bone structure and size to normal (Fig. 19-7).

LABORATORY FINDINGS

Increased sedimentation rate, leukocytosis, increased level of alkaline phosphatase, and anemia, which occasionally may require transfusion, are noted.

PATHOLOGY

Biopsy specimens exhibit periosteal thickening, edema, and subperiosteal new bone formation. No evidence of hemorrhage or inflammation is observed.

DIFFERENTIAL DIAGNOSIS

The importance of infantile cortical hyperostosis lies in differentiating it from the following conditions:

Hypervitaminosis A. This disorder occurs in infants over 12 months of age. The mandible is never involved, fever is absent, a high vitamin A blood level is usual, and discontinuing the vitamin effects a cure in 1 week.

Scurvy. The appearance of subperiosteal ossification is similar. A ground-glass osteoporotic appearance of all bones is characteristic. Dense lines, representing excessive calcified cartilage, are seen in roentgenograms encircling the epiphyseal ossification center (Wimberger's line) and at the diaphyseal side of the epiphyseal plate (Fraenkel's line or Trummerfeld zone).

Osteomyelitis. Fever is high, involvement is often localized to one bone, and destruction of bone accompanies surrounding reactive bone formation. Bacteria can be cultured from the lesion, and antibiotics are frequently effective.

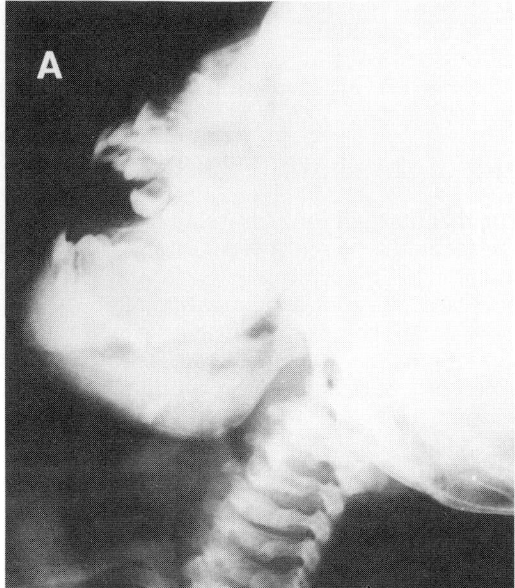

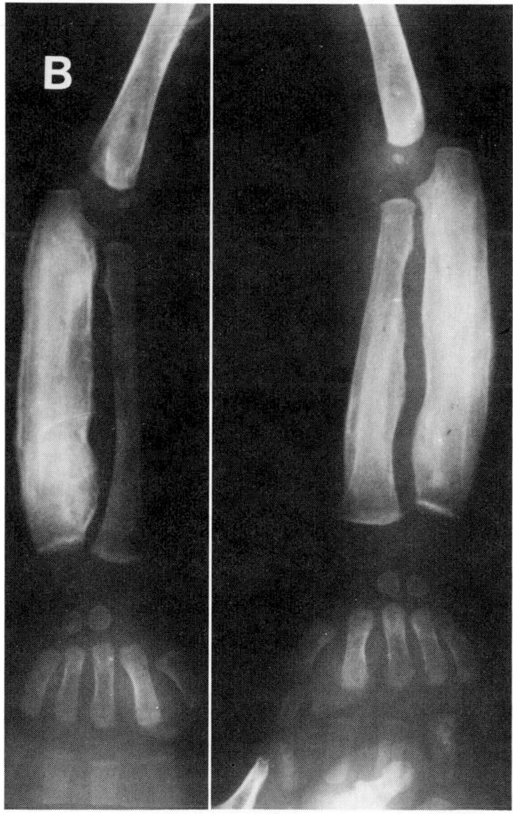

FIG. 19-7. Infantile cortical hyperostosis. The characteristic laminations of subperiosteal new bone are observed (*A*) about the mandible and (*B*) the forearm bones.

Syphilitic hyperostosis

Malignant tumor. Ewing's tumor is similar in appearance because of its typical onion-peel laminations of subperiosteal ossification and accompanying constitutional symptoms. Eventually, central destruction becomes evident, and biopsy reveals the true nature of the lesion.

Trauma. Subperiosteal hemorrhage following a contusion or an incomplete fracture will often ossify. However, the lesion is confined to one bone and resolves without recurrence.

TREATMENT

Treatment is unnecessary, inasmuch as this is a self-limited disease. However, antibiotics should be administered and vitamins are discontinued until the diagnosis can be definitely ascertained.

SARCOIDOSIS

Sarcoidosis (Boeck's sarcoid, pseudotuberculosis, osteitis tuberculosa multiplex cystoides, Jüngling's disease, benign lymphogranulomatosis, Schaumann's disease, uveoparotid fever) is a chronic granulomatous disease of unknown etiology that is characterized pathologically by the formation of noncaseating granulomas in any tissue, a prolonged chronic course with a tendency toward spontaneous healing, and a minimum or absence of symptoms. Although the disorder resembles tuberculosis, acid-fast bacilli are absent, the result of the tuberculin test is negative in a majority of patients, and the outlook for spontaneous cure is good. The importance of this disease to the orthopaedic surgeon lies in its frequent involvement of cancellous bone and synovial tissue of joints, and its differentiation from other osteolytic conditions, particularly tuberculosis and gout, and rarely from osteosclerotic conditions, such as osteogenic tumors of bone.

PATHOLOGY

The basic lesion is the size of a miliary tubercle and consists almost exclusively of large epithelioid cells, which are frequently fused (Fig. 19-8).[55,58,60] Giant cells are infrequent and occasionally resemble the Langhans type. Lymphocytes in the surrounding tissues are sparse and scattered. They are not concentrated about the granuloma (contrary to tuberculosis). Various dark inclusion bodies have been described and may represent the causative factor. The center of the epithelioid lesion never undergoes caseation necrosis, but occasionally clear collections of hyaline or colloid material are observed. Frequently, many epithelioid foci become confluent and form large granulomas that replace large areas of tissue.

Any organ or tissue in the body may be involved, but the sites of predilection are lymph nodes, lung, skin, and

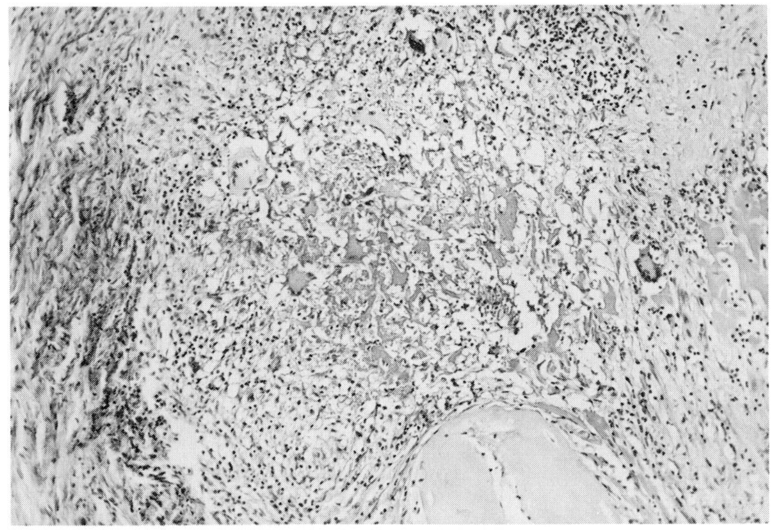

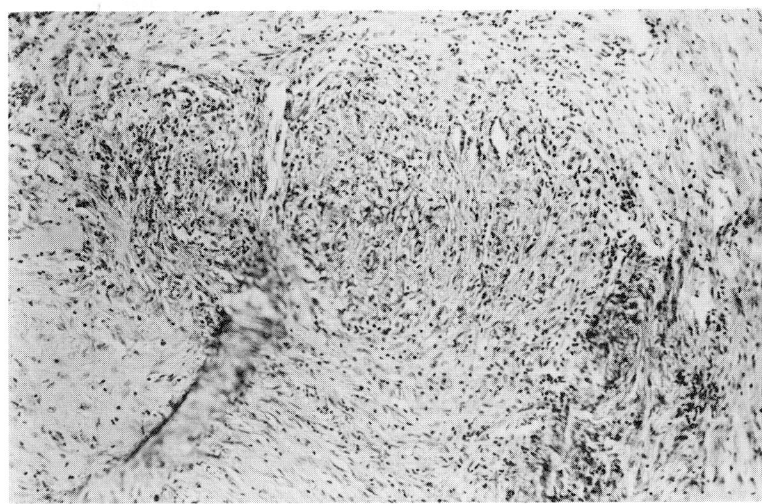

FIG. 19-8. Sarcoid of bone. Note rare giant cells, containing typical densely staining material, especially in the one at the top of the upper section. These are peculiar small accumulations of colloid material; lymphocytes are sparse and diffusely distributed, and epithelioid accumulations and capillary loops of granulation tissue are seen in the lower photomicrograph. (Turek SL: Sarcoid disease of bone at the ankle joint. J Bone Joint Surg *35A*:465, 1953)

bone marrow. Healing takes place either by resorption or by fibrous tissue replacement.

OSSEOUS LESIONS

The incidence of osseous lesions ranges between 13% and 22%.[54,60–62] The bones of the hands and feet are most often involved, and the long bones of the extremities and the vertebrae are infrequently involved.[52]

Sarcoid noncaseating granulomas replace bone trabeculae and cortical bone without evoking reactive bone formation in the surrounding tissues, including the periosteum. The number of small granulomas may be enormous and diffusely scattered throughout the bone, or small foci may coalesce to form large epithelioid aggregations that occupy cystlike punched-out areas of bone. When these sarcoid accumulations occupy large areas within the spongiosa, they erode and thin, but never distend, the cortex. The articular cartilage does not appear to be invaded.[62] However, destruction of the subchondral cortex leads to osteoarthritic changes of the overlying articular cartilage, and, consequently, osteoarthritis is a secondary effect of sarcoidosis of subchondral bone.

Sarcoid lesions of bone heal either by resorption of the granuloma or by fibrous tissue replacement, but in either event reossification is likely. Because osseous repair is a very slow process, a large healed fibrous defect may appear on roentgenograms as a radiolucent cystlike lesion.

When bone transplants are laid into a bed in which sarcoid lesions exist, the sarcoid process does not appear to invade the transplanted bone. Osteogenic induction and replacement of the transplants take place as usual.

When phalanges are involved, bone destruction may be extensive, resulting in pathologic fractures and extension into the surrounding tissues and producing mutilating deformities of the fingers; or the involvement may be limited to localized destruction, producing a cystlike bony resorption of a single phalanx.

Any portion of the spine may be involved, including a single vertebra or multiple vertebrae. Sarcoidosis usually involves the vertebral body, producing an osteolytic defect that occasionally is surrounded by osteosclerotic areas; rarely the vertebral body presents osteosclerotic foci, an exception to sarcoid osseous lesions elsewhere. The disk space is never involved, and, except for sarcoid involvement in the cervical spine, fracture and collapse are unusual.[52,53,63]

CLINICAL PICTURE

Involvement may be extensive throughout the body and yet is generally asymptomatic.[51,56–58] Exceptionally, when symptoms develop, they are generally mild and consist of anorexia, malaise, fatigability, dry cough, chest pain, and slight elevations of temperature. Lungs and lymph nodes often contain extensive infiltrations without symptoms. Skin lesions are common, are often associated with osseous lesions, and characteristically resemble the lesions of erythema nodosum. They are dusky red, slightly elevated, nonulcerating, nonpruritic nodules and are frequently situated about the face (lupus pernio) and hands. Uveoparotitis and iridocyclitis may develop.

Less commonly, the clinical course may resemble pulmonary tuberculosis; the patient presents with a longstanding history of cough, chest pain, dyspnea on exertion, fever, night sweats, weight loss, and cervical adenopathy.

Osseous lesions occur in a high percentage of cases but are usually asymptomatic unless secondary effects arise (*e.g.*, pathologic fracture). The phalanges and metacarpals and metatarsals may contain lesions that are highly variable in extent of bony resorption and destruction. At one extreme, only a single, asymptomatic, cystlike lesion may be discovered within a phalanx on roentgenograms. At the other extreme, the lesions may be extensively distributed throughout many of the phalanges, producing mutilating destruction of the bony structures. The clinical appearance shows massive and marked soft, boggy swelling about the fingers that seems to involve both the joints and soft tissues about the bones. The lesions are nontender, and the overlying skin is normal. There may be markedly limited motion of the interphalangeal joints, but there are no nodules, tophi, or actual extension to the joints themselves.

When subchondral bone is resorbed, the overlying articular cartilage is unable to withstand loading stresses and eventually succumbs to osteoarthritic change.

Sarcoid infiltration of synovial tissues may cause recurring episodes of acute synovitis with effusion, but this condition is benign and heals spontaneously without residual effect. The synovium may be extensively infiltrated with noncaseating granulomas, producing persisting pain, stiffness, and synovial tissue swelling and remaining unresponsive to local treatment; however, this condition is usually benign and eventually recedes without permanent changes.[59] Rarely, osteoarthritic changes supervene.[60] Synovial sarcoidosis can only be identified by arthroscopy and synovial biopsy.

Vertebral involvement is rare. The symptoms vary. Many patients are asymptomatic and others complain of local back pain. After 1 to 2 years, marked symptomatic improvement takes place with or without treatment in most cases. Complicating vertebral collapse and threatening displacement may produce persisting pain that requires surgical stabilization for relief. Neurologic compromise has not been reported.

Although the course of the generalized or local forms of the disease is prolonged, even for years, spontaneous healing is the rule.

ROENTGENOGRAPHIC FINDINGS

Chest roentgenograms show characteristic diffuse reticular interstitial infiltrates and widening of the mediastinal shadow resulting from extensive involvement of the hilar lymph nodes.[54,61]

Osteoporosis and cortical thinning are the most common early detectable signs of sarcoid bone involvement. Localized areas are involved, and a distinctive lacelike reticular pattern is evident. It should be recognized that the bone may be extensively infiltrated with small granulomas without apparent change in bony architecture. It is only when the lesions coalesce and when sufficient local bone resorption occurs that roentgenographic changes appear.

The typical punched-out lesion is formed by localized enlargement or coalescence of adjacent lesions. It appears cystlike and round or ovoid, with smooth edges; the adjacent bone appears normal. No marginal sclerosis develops, except in some cases of vertebral sarcoidosis. The cystlike lesion may be single or multiple and is usually found in the distal ends of the middle phalanges or at either end of the proximal phalanges. The punched-out lesions generally persist for years. These lesions usually heal, but fibrous replacement of the granuloma accounts for the persistent radiolucency. No sequestration or periosteal reaction occurs even when the adjacent cortex is destroyed.

Osteosclerotic lesions are exceptional but may develop, especially within vertebrae or pelvis. Vertebral lesions are usually osteolytic and sometimes surrounded by sclerotic bone. Rarely, the entire lesion appears dense. A single or multiple vertebrae may be involved. Disk space narrowing never occurs.[52,53,63]

LABORATORY FINDINGS

Biopsy of the affected tissue is diagnostic. A liver biopsy or examination of bone marrow aspirate will reveal the characteristic lesions. When a large joint is involved, arthroscopy and synovial tissue biopsy must be done.

Other granuloma-producing diseases that need to be excluded are tuberculosis, blastomycosis, sporotrichosis, coccidiomycosis, and histoplasmosis. A bone biopsy should be cultured for acid-fast bacilli, fungi, and pyogenic organisms. Bronchial washings and lymph node tissue are stained and cultured.

TREATMENT

No definitive treatment is known. Prednisone is presently used, but its efficacy is impossible to determine in view of the spontaneous tendency to healing.

Painful degenerative arthritis may develop in a large weight-bearing joint that is adjacent to extensive sarcoid osseous lesions that impair the strength of the long bone. Consequently, arthrodesis rather than prosthetic replacement is the most expedient means for rehabilitation.

Pathologic fractures may require surgical fixation, but union is markedly delayed. When the spine is involved, spine fusion is indicated only for persisting pain or for threatened displacement. Bone grafts may be inserted without fear of destruction by the sarcoid process.

TUMORS OF HEMATOPOIETIC TISSUES

The basic cells of certain tumors resemble those normally found in the bone marrow or in lymphoid tissues. The supposition is that they arise from a common stem cell and that the ultimate tumor cell represents incomplete differentiation.

GENERAL CHARACTERISTICS

Hemopoietic neoplasms all have the following characteristics in common:

- They involve cancellous bone. Early, roentgenograms are negative, and symptoms consist of vague "rheumatoid" discomfort, with remissions and exacerbations.
- Pain is progressively worse and persistent. It is accentuated by a sudden movement or strain. Involvement of vertebrae causes girdle pain (with or without herpes zoster), lower extremity referred pain, and abdominal pain
- They are osteolytic in hematopoietic tissues, especially of vertebrae (results in compression or collapse of bodies), sternum, ribs, pelvis, skull, and long bones. There are pathologic fractures.
- Leukocytosis and secondary anemia are present. Involvement of marrow results in premature extrusion of immature cells into the bloodstream. With extensive involvement of the blood-forming tissues, leukopenia and severe secondary anemia are typical of the later stage of disease.
- Sternal marrow is frequently infiltrated. Sternal puncture is diagnostic.
- They are sensitive to irradiation. Relief of pain is immediate and dramatic. There is ultimate resistance of the tumor to irradiation.
- Spleen and lymph nodes enlarge.

MALIGNANT LYMPHOMAS

Considered malignant lymphomas, in descending order of frequency, are Hodgkin's disease, lymphosarcoma, histiocytic lymphoma, and giant follicle lymphoma. The skeleton is involved by direct extension from neighboring lymph nodes, by metastatic spread, or independently within the bone. Common characteristics make it advisable to consider this group with the leukemias.

HODGKIN'S DISEASE

The painless progressive involvement of lymph nodes, spleen, liver, and skeletal marrow of Hodgkin's disease is by tissue that is granulomatous in appearance and acts neoplastic.

CLINICAL PICTURE

Age. Young adults, usually males, are affected.

Course. There is early swelling of lymph nodes, particularly in the cervical area. Nodes are at first discrete and painless; later they become greatly enlarged and matted together. There is severe pruritus, weakness, and weight loss. The liver and spleen are enlarged and palpable. Initial bony involvement of the marrow is painless. Slowly, bone pains, at first rheumatic in type and intermittent, become more severe and persistent. Tender swellings appear over the bones, particularly over the ribs and the sternum. Vertebrae are frequently involved, with a high incidence of compression fractures. Compression of intraspinal structures is responsible for referred chest and lower extremity pain. Eventually, compression and direct invasion of vital structures result in death.

Bone Involvement. The disease may occur wherever red bone marrow exists, particularly vertebrae, ribs, sternum, pelvis, skull, scapula, and the metaphyseal area of long bones. Pathologic fractures are rare except for multiple vertebrae compression.

Physical Findings. The superficial lymph nodes are enlarged and discrete early, very large, tender, and matted together late. Late in the course of the disease, the bones are tender and superficial swellings may be palpable. Variable fever is seen.

Laboratory Findings. Leukocytosis, secondary anemia, and eosinophilia are frequently seen. Lymph node biopsy is diagnostic. The alkaline phosphatase level is elevated with bone involvement.

ROENTGENOGRAPHIC FINDINGS

Early the roentgenographic results are negative, later they are osteolytic and diffuse. Occasionally, some medullary reactive bone density about the lesions may be seen if the growth is slow. Superficial cortex indentation represents pressure erosion.

PATHOLOGY

Gross Appearance

The disease frequently starts in the cervical lymph nodes and spreads to axillary, mediastinal, retroperitoneal, mesenteric, and inguinal lymph node groups. The nodes remain discrete at first, even though enlarged. On cut section they are pink, homogeneous, and elastic or firm. Later, the glands are further enlarged, grayish white, firm, and matted together in a mass of fibrous tissue. Where a mass of glands overlies a bone, the latter undergoes localized erosion. Within the bone marrow, the granulomatous tissue is seen in discrete or confluent masses eroding the cortex from within. The tissue may extend to the subperiosteal area, elevating the periosteum with minimal reactive bone. The granulomatous tissue in vertebrae may extensively replace the marrow with consequent collapse of the body and extend to the peridural space with compression of nerve structures. The disks are never involved.

Microscopic Appearance

In a reticular stromal network is seen a variety of cells, including endothelial cells, plasma cells, lymphocytes and eosinophils. The characteristic cell is the Reed-Sternberg, a large endothelial cell with multilobed nuclei (Color Plate 19-2). Where the tumor tissue encroaches on the bone trabeculae, the latter is eroded or absorbed without the benefit of osteoclasts. Early, the tissue is granulomatous. Later, a highly cellular tissue in which the cells are more uniform and round becomes pervaded with fibrous elements.[81,93]

TREATMENT

Palliative treatment consists of wide-field megavoltage radiotherapy using 3,500 to 4,000 rads over 4 weeks. When patients with early stage disease are treated with intensive radiotherapy, and no new manifestations develop within 5 years, they may be regarded as cured. Approximately 30% of patients when seen and treated early have a favorable outlook.[96]

Antitumor chemotherapy using combinations of drugs is reserved for late stages of the disease.[78]

Spinal cord compression is treated with a chemotherapeutic agent, preferably mechlorethamine (nitrogen mustard), 0.4 mg/kg IV, followed in 24 hours by radiation therapy. Bone pain may be similarly relieved.

LYMPHOSARCOMA

Lymphosarcoma of bone is very rare. When it occurs, multiple bone involvement is the rule. The tumor extends diffusely throughout the bone and is centrally destructive without formation of reactive bone. Clinically, pain occurs early and, like other myelomatous lesions, the vertebrae are commonly involved, producing referred girdle chest discomfort and lower extremity pain. Laboratory examinations reveal leukocytosis and relative lymphocytosis, eosinophilia, and secondary anemia. As the marrow is replaced more extensively, severe anemia and leukopenia are late manifestations. Pathologic fractures occur. Eventually, the lymph nodes are involved. The roentgenogram may show a long bone diffusely osteolytic and not surrounded by reactive bone. Vertebrae are partially collapsed. Rarely, the lesion may excite osteogenesis. The tumor is seen to extend diffusely throughout the medulla, eroding the cortex and extending through the haversian canals to the subperiosteal space. The tumor is rubbery and opaque. Microscopically, a diffuse growth of lymphocytes in a reticular tissue stroma is seen. Multinucleated cells are not observed. Treatment consists of irradiation, which promptly relieves pain. The outlook is hopeless, with death occurring within 3 years.[67,75,93]

THE LEUKEMIAS

Leukemia is a condition in which an overproduction of immature forms of lymphocytes (lymphocytic leukemia) or polymorphonuclear leukocytes (myelocytic leukemia) results in extensive replacement of other elements of the hematopoietic and lymphoid tissues. It occurs as an acute or chronic form, the former being most common and predominantly occurring in infancy and childhood. The clinical picture includes fever, anemia, enlarged lymph nodes, splenomegaly, hepatomegaly, tender bones and swollen painful joints, and progressive weight loss. Laboratory examination reveals immature white blood cells in the bloodstream regardless of whether a leukocytosis or a leukopenia (the aleukemic form) exists. Thrombocytopenia leads to increased bleeding time and purpuric tendencies. Symptoms include asthenia and bone and joint pains, thereby simulating acute rheumatic fever. A slightly tender swelling may be palpable over such superficially accessible bones as the ulna. Estimates of bone involvement run as high as 50%; it is usually a late manifestation.[77,79,90,93]

The leukemic tissue infiltrates and replaces the bone

marrow diffusely throughout the bone, resorbing the cancellous bone and later the cortical bone. It reaches and elevates the periosteum, which reacts to form thin laminations of reactive bone parallel with the shaft. Pathologic fracture occurs chiefly in the ribs. Microscopically, the cells of lymphatic leukemia produce a picture similar to lymphosarcoma. The cells of myeloid leukemia are immature myeloblasts and myelocytes.

ROENTGENOGRAPHIC FINDINGS

Roentgenographic findings consist of diffuse osteoporosis, punctate rarefied areas throughout the cortex producing a ragged appearance, a transverse area of increased radiolucency on the metaphyseal side of the epiphyseal line, and thin laminations of periosteal reactive bone. The picture is mainly one of osteolysis, but in chronic leukemia in the adult, osteosclerosis throughout the skeleton is common.

TREATMENT

The principal concern of the orthopaedic surgeon is in differentiating the causes of arthralgia and bone pain. In the growing child, metaphyseal rarefactions observed on roentgenograms represent impaired endochondral ossification due to cellular deposits and marrow replacement. Other conditions such as scurvy can produce a similar picture. Moreover, subperiosteal bony lamellations imitate infection and Ewing's tumor. The orthopaedic surgeon may be called on to perform a bone biopsy.

Irradiation of the bones is effective for relieving bone pain early in the course of the disease. Later, its effectiveness is lost. Leukemic infiltrates in the synovium of joints are common manifestations of the disease, and synovial biopsy may be the earliest diagnostic feature.

The main treatment is carried out by the pediatrician or internist. In acute leukemias, remissions of 1 to 3 years can be achieved by regimens incorporating multiple chemotherapeutic agents. Patients with chronic leukemias have a somewhat longer survival time if chemotherapy plus total body irradiation or radiophosphorus is used. Certain elderly patients with chronic leukemia may remain relatively inactive without treatment for many years.

CHLOROMA

In chloroma, a form of lymphatic or myeloid leukemia, bone manifestations form a prominent feature. Characteristically, the tissue contains a greenish pigment so that the involved tissue, whether bone, lymph gland, or spleen, appears green on cut section. Children near puberty are affected, and the condition is rapidly fatal within 5 months. The greenish tumors most commonly invade the skull and produce symptoms referable to the structures about the head. Typically, the growth extends within the orbital cavities and causes an exophthalmic protrusion and edema of the eyelids. Other bones with much red marrow are also involved, and the tissue may even extend beyond the bone and infiltrate surrounding muscles and tendons. Clinical, roentgenographic, and microscopic pictures are similar to other forms of leukemia. However, the extremely malignant character of the tissue is reflected in the large atypical monocytes; the premature myeloblasts, with numerous mitoses; and the hyperchromatic nuclei. Treatment is confined to small doses of radiation, but the outlook is hopeless.

RETICULOENDOTHELIOSIS

All lymphoid and myeloid tissue contains a mesh of reticular tissue in which are the primitive reticular cells. These cells contain pale oval nuclei and protoplasmic prolongations, which join those of neighboring cells. The reticular fibers are strewn throughout the protoplasmic network. The primitive reticular cells transform into all types of blood and connective tissue cells. They frequently change into similar-appearing but larger cells with abundant cytoplasm; they have large pale nuclei and are spindle shaped.

These are the fixed macrophages that engulf dead cells and debris and are capable of ingesting certain dyes, such as lithium carmine. The inclusions of the macrophages stain deeply with neutral red. These macrophages are flattened and help to form the walls of sinuses or channels through which lymph flows and therefore are thought of as endothelium. However, endothelial cells are incapable of phagocytosis and cannot be stained with lithium carmine. Under certain conditions, as when foreign matter is present, the fixed macrophages transform into free macrophages and float free in the lymph.

The primitive reticular cells also develop into lymphocytes and myelocytes. The lymphocytes vary in size and contain a large darkly staining nucleus and a scanty basophilic cytoplasm, which contains no inclusions.

Eosinophil cells are normally found in the connective tissue in certain sites such as the mammary gland. Under pathologic conditions, they may migrate from the bloodstream and settle in large numbers in the connective tissue.

Plasma cells are transformed from lymphocytes and apparently constitute the ultimate in differentiation, since they are unable to transform into any other cell.

Fat cells are found in variable number in loose connective tissue, particularly about vessels at the site of the primitive reticular cells. In development of the fat cell, multiple small droplets accumulate before fusing into one large drop. The original primitive cell loses its elongated processes and becomes more polyhedral before rounding up.

In formation of foam cells it is tempting to believe that these are transitional fat cells containing certain lipoid substances other than neutral fat.

The foregoing description of reticuloendothelial histogenesis suggests a common denominator for the reticuloendothelioses, which include Hand-Schüller-Christian disease, eosinophilic granuloma, Letterer-Siwe's disease, Gaucher's disease, and Niemann-Pick disease. Many observers refer to them as variants of the same basic disorder.[89,107]

Histologically, the pathology consists of formation of tissue composed of variable amounts of proliferated reticuloendothelial cells, macrophages containing debris and fat, foam cells, eosinophils, lymphocytes, plasma cells and, about areas of necrosis, multinucleated giant cells. Involvement of the skeleton by reticuloendothelial granuloma causes destruction, in single or multiple localized areas, without reactive new bone formation. The tissue is usually soft and friable and varies from reddish (vascular) and yellowish (lipoid) to grayish (fibrous) and firm. Roentgenographic findings consist of areas of rarefaction, multiple or solitary, involving one or more bones. Skull involvement is frequent. Lesions are seen in other flat bones (*e.g.*, pelvis, scapula), and vertebral lesions are rare. The destruction may be large and display sharply scalloped edges. Clinically, lymphadenopathy, splenomegaly, hepatomegaly, and bone lesions are common denominators. The diagnosis is established by biopsy.

The macrophages of certain reticuloendothelioses contain specific lipoid substances. These so-called lipoid histiocytoses include Hand-Schüller-Christian disease, Gaucher's splenomegaly, and Niemann-Pick disease. When lipoid inclusions are not a prominent feature, these nonlipoid histiocytoses are eosinophilic granuloma and Letterer-Siwe disease.

EOSINOPHILIC GRANULOMA

Eosinophilic granuloma, also known as histiocytosis limited to bone, is a solitary, rarely multiple, benign bone-destructive lesion that is characterized by a histiocytic and eosinophilic leukocyte infiltrate of unknown origin. There is no extraskeletal involvement; as a rule the lesion is self-limited and the outlook for healing is good.[83,87,94,106]

CLINICAL PICTURE

Age. Onset is noted between 1 and 15 years of age, with the peak incidence occurring between 5 and 10 years of age.[109]

Distribution. The lesion is usually solitary. Rarely, there are multiple lesions, of which only one is symptomatic. Multiple lesions are more common at a very early age and most commonly involve the skull and femur. Solitary lesions most often affect the ribs, vertebrae, skull, flat bones, and long tubular bones. In the long bones of the extremities, the favored sites are the diaphysis and metaphysis, rarely the epiphysis.

Symptoms. Complaints are limited to local areas of involvement and consist of constant dull aching pain and tenderness. The onset is acute when a pathologic fracture is superimposed.

Findings. Local tenderness, warmth, and swelling over an affected area of the skull or a subcutaneous bone is evident. Vertebral involvement produces local rigidity and muscle spasm.

Pathologic Fracture. Common (Fig. 19-9), along with vertebral collapse.

Course. The course is acute, lasting over a few weeks to several months with a tendency to spontaneous healing.

ROENTGENOGRAPHIC FINDINGS

Lesions of long bones are usually diaphyseal, well localized, and radiotranslucent without surrounding reactive new bone formation (Figs. 19-10 and 19-11). The cortex is eroded from within and expanded as a thin shell. As the cortex is breached, slight periosteal new bone formation creates laminations reminiscent of an "onionskin" appearance of acute osteomyelitis or Ewing's tumor.

Skull and flat bone lesions vary in size, are often confluent, and have a "punched out" appearance with sharply delimited borders. Other than the skull, the supra-acetabular area of the ilium is a common site.

PATHOLOGY

Grossly, the tissue within the defect is soft, friable, and reddish gray or reddish yellow and contains ragged areas of necrosis and hemorrhage. A healing lesion contains firm, gray fibrous tissue with new bone formation.

Microscopically, at an early stage the tissue is very cellular, consisting mainly of histiocytes (macrophages) and eosinophils and sparsely distributed plasma cells, lymphocytes, and neutrophils (Color Plate 19-3). The histiocytes are large and ovoid or polygonal and have a single, pale, indented or reniform nucleus; about areas of hemorrhage, the tissue contains hemosiderin. The Rio Hortega silver stain reveals the reticulin fiber background; a stain for reticuloendothelial elements shows up the histiocytes as possessing an ameboid configuration.[109]

ULTRASTRUCTURAL CHARACTERISTICS OF HISTIOCYTES

Electron microscopic studies reveal highly diagnostic features of eosinophilic granuloma. The histiocytes are

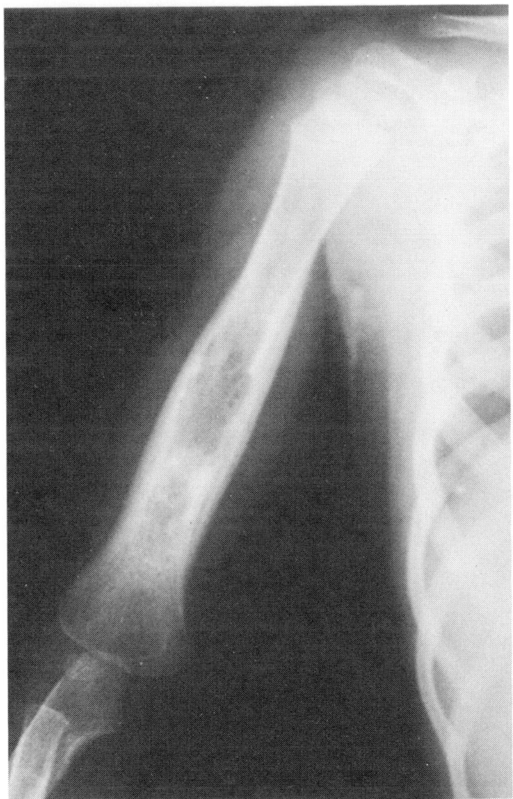

FIG. 19-9. Osseous lesion of histiocytosis and healing of pathologic fracture.

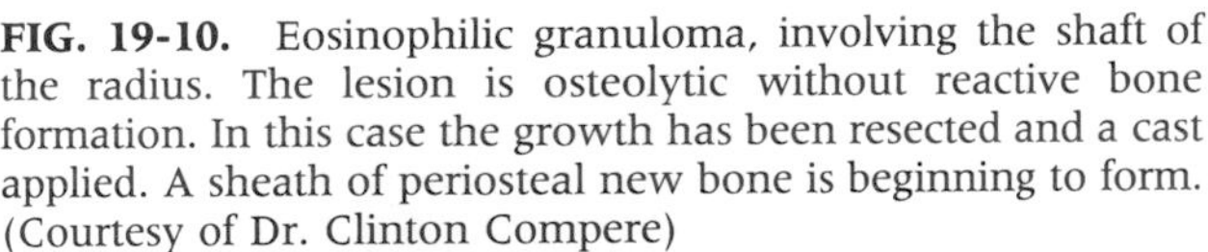

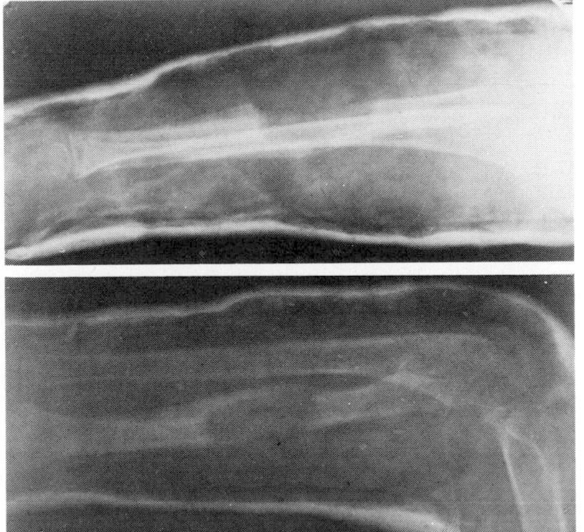

FIG. 19-10. Eosinophilic granuloma, involving the shaft of the radius. The lesion is osteolytic without reactive bone formation. In this case the growth has been resected and a cast applied. A sheath of periosteal new bone is beginning to form. (Courtesy of Dr. Clinton Compere)

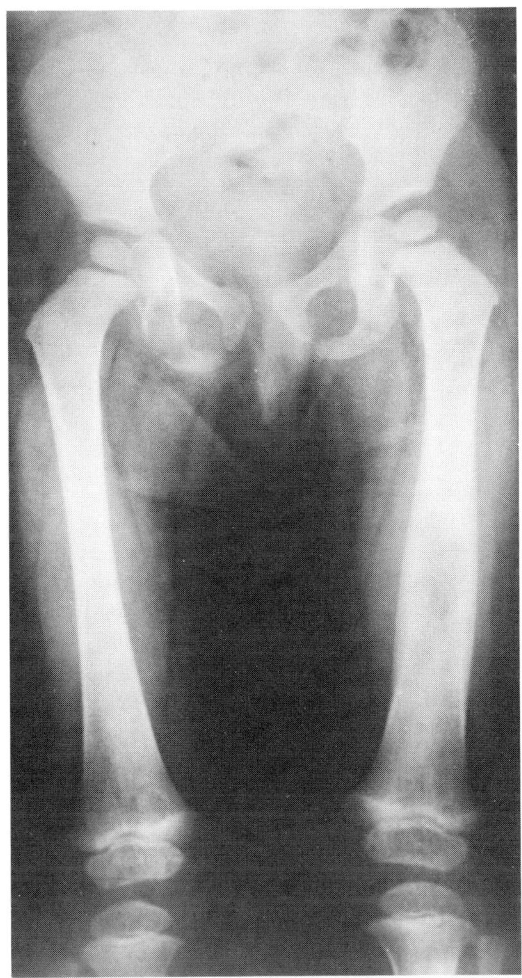

FIG. 19-11. Histiocytosis X in femur and ischium of a 2-year-old. Central destruction also involving cortex and little reactive bone formation, except some periosteal ossification. Punched-out lesions also are seen in skull and rib. Biopsy confirmed the diagnosis. Rapid reossification occurred under the influence of radiation therapy.

small, oval, sometimes irregularly shaped cells with ill-defined borders that are characterized by an eccentric, indented, finely creased large nucleus with fine chromatin surrounded by abundant delicate cytoplasm. The nucleus occupies approximately one third of the cell diameter.

Ultrastructurally, these cells vary in shape and possess long cytoplasmic processes. Within the cytoplasm are pathognomonic Langerhans granules (Birbeck bodies). They are located throughout the cell. In most instances they are tubular-shaped bodies, ranging in length from 150μ to 1500μ, and 400 A to 450 A in width. Running longitudinally through its center is a linear density exhibiting cross striations. These granules are highly characteristic of eosinophilic granuloma, Hand-Schüller-

Christian disease, and Letterer-Siwe disease (see Fig. 19-15 *Bottom*).

As the lesion ages, the histiocytes become more numerous and laden with lipids, which are chemically identical with cholesterol. The eosinophils lessen in number. The sheets or cords of lipid-laden histiocytes are progressively replaced by fibrous tissue and finally by ossification.

DIAGNOSIS

Biopsy is necessary, because the roentgenographic picture resembles that of metastatic lesions, multiple myeloma, and other osteolytic lesions.

TREATMENT

Surgically accessible solitary lesions are managed by biopsy, curettage, and filling the defect with bone grafts.[103] A simple curettage usually effects healing. Rib and clavicle lesions require only subperiosteal segmental resection.

In the presence of multiple lesions, it is necessary to wait and determine whether this represents a transitional stage of Hand-Schüller-Christian disease. If no further lesions develop after 1 year, the case may be classified as multicentric eosinophilic granuloma and the outlook is good. Any symptomatic lesion may be managed as a solitary lesion. The asymptomatic lesions may heal spontaneously or occasionally may be subjected to low dose radiation (300 to 600 rads), provided that the total radiation dosage is not hazardous.

When a transitional form toward Hand-Schüller-Christian disease is suspected, more aggressive treatment may be required. Corticosteroids effect marked resolution of multiple lesions but should be reserved for patients in whom radiation is contraindicated or for lesions that are surgically inaccessible. Chemotherapeutic agents are rarely recommended and then only when multiple lesions do not respond to surgery or radiation therapy.[98,116]

As a general rule, a single lesion that does not jeopardize the function of a part (*e.g.*, long tubular bone) is best left alone, and spontaneous healing can be expected within 1 year.

VERTEBRA PLANA DUE TO EOSINOPHILIC GRANULOMA

Calvé, in 1924, described what he called "osteochondritis of the vertebral body." This consisted of the rapid development, usually in a child, of an osteolytic process in a single vertebral body that resulted in marked flattening and increased density, with the contour appearing like the edge of a coin or disc and not being wedge shaped (Figs. 19-12 and 19-13). Clinically, the onset is gradual or rapid and then there is rapid progression. Back pain, muscle spasm, limited back motion, night cries, and a prominent spinous process or gibbus form the characteristic picture. Spontaneous reossification with variable loss in body height occurs over several years. Several identical cases have been described in which eosinophilic granuloma proved to be the causative condition. Treatment consisted of bed rest, splinting, and radiation therapy.[74]

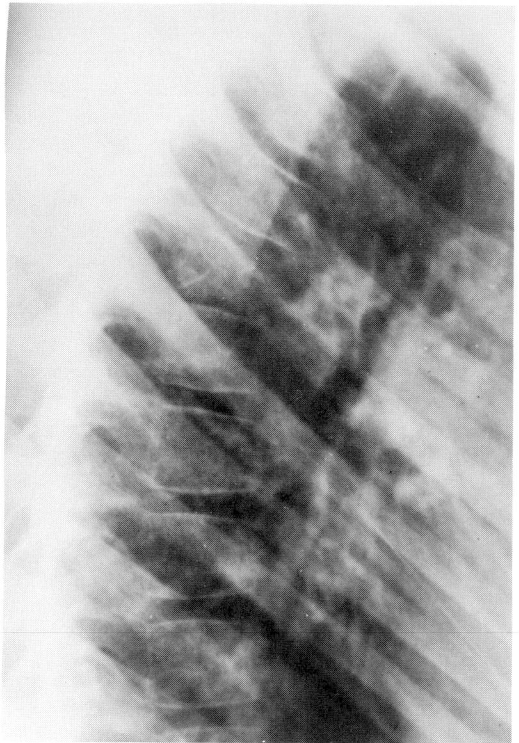

FIG. 19-12. Eosinophilic granuloma of body of T5 vertebra. There is marked deossification and beginning of collapse. Preservation of disk spaces and adjacent vertebrae distinguishes this from tuberculosis.

HAND-SCHÜLLER-CHRISTIAN DISEASE

Hand-Schüller-Christian disease is a subacute or chronic condition of unknown etiology. It is characterized pathologically by widely disseminated (multifocal) granulomatous infiltration of the reticuloendothelial system, including that of bone, by a histiocytic and eosinophilic cellular ingrowth and clinically by the production of large destructive lesions of bone, particularly of the skull, and by involvement of various tissues and organs, typically the pituitary gland and hypothalamus. At a late stage, the histiocytes become the predominant cells, acquiring large amounts of a lipid substance; finally healing takes place by fibrosis. This syndrome constitutes approximately one third of all cases of histiocytoses.[73,85,86,111]

CLINICAL PICTURE

Age. The disease begins in childhood (usually between 5 and 10 years of age) and continues into adulthood.

Areas of Predilection. Most frequently, the lesions develop in the skeletal system, especially the membranous bones and particularly the skull. Less commonly affected are the long bones. Multiple organ systems are involved, including the pituitary, lungs, mucocutaneous surfaces, spleen, liver, and orbit.

Physical Findings. There is a slow, insidious onset. The characteristic triad of defects in skull, diabetes insipidus, and exophthalmos occurs in less than 10% of cases, but the occurrence of one or two of these features is frequent. Hepatomegaly, splenomegaly, enlarged, painless lymph nodes, and endocrine disturbances that result in delay of longitudinal growth and abnormal sexual development are seen. The lesions can frequently be palpated through the scalp.

FIG. 19-13. Eosinophilic granuloma, involving a vertebral body. The body of the T5 vertebra is flattened. Pathology was proved by biopsy. After healing of the lesion, growth of the body is resumed; if a sufficient growth period remains, the body may regain much of its original size. This may explain what has been described as Calve's disease of the spine.

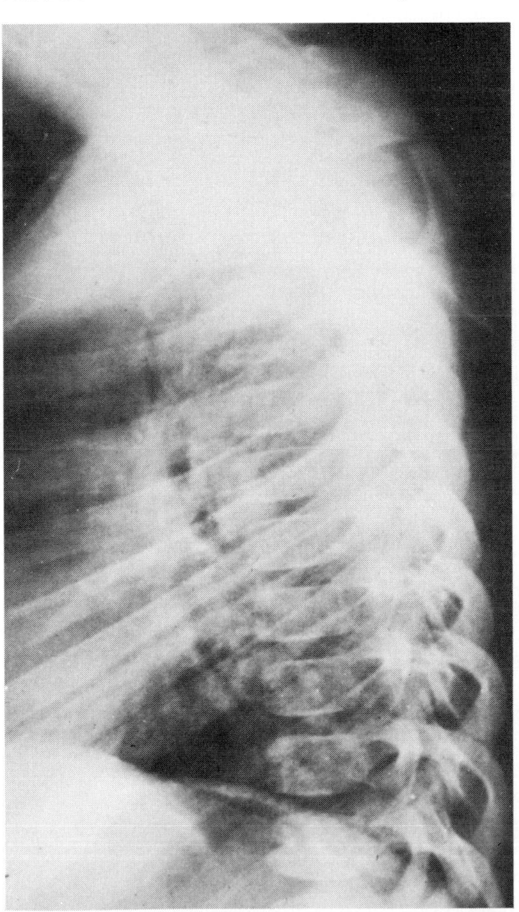

Course. The course is chronic, lasting many years. In the long bones, the lesions progress rapidly and cause marked destruction of the diaphysis or metaphysis.

ROENTGENOGRAPHIC FINDINGS

These roentgenographic findings of Hand-Schüller-Christian disease are similar to those described under eosinophilic granuloma except that the lesions are more numerous. Very large, well-demarcated radiolucent defects occur in the skull (Fig. 19-14), producing the classic "geographic skull," in other flat bones and in long bones; the cortex is thinned; there is no periosteal reaction, and multiple defects may occur.

PATHOLOGY

The infiltrating cellular tissue destroys and replaces bone and extends out into the soft tissue. Within the orbital cavity the enlarging growth pushes the eyeball forward to produce an exophthalmos. In the pituitary fossa the tissue destroys the pituitary gland, causing sexual and growth disturbances (anterior pituitary), and then extends to the posterior pituitary and the hypothalamus to produce diabetes insipidus.

Microscopically, the features and the evolution of the lesion are identical with those of eosinophilic granuloma. Initially, the early lesion shows reticuloendothelial tissue enmeshing great numbers of histiocytes and eosinophils, and a smaller number of neutrophils, lymphocytes, and plasma cells. At first the macrophages contain little or no lipids. As the lesion ages, sheets and columns of histiocytes containing large amounts of lipids predominate and the eosinophils lessen in number. About areas of necrosis and hemorrhage, the histiocytes form multinuclear giant cells containing lipids and hemosiderin. These xanthomatous giant cells are characteristically large; often binucleated; laden with cholesterol, lipoid, and blood pigment; and resemble Reed-Sternberg cells. In the final healing stage, the lesion is composed of masses of collagen fibers, fibroblasts, occasional giant cells, and a few cholesterol crystals.[92]

PROGNOSIS

The overall mortality as reported in the literature approximates 30%. However, with newer chemotherapeutic methods, the chances for prolonged survival appear better. The earlier the onset of disseminated lesions and the greater the number of organ systems involved, the poorer is the prognosis. With advancing age and remis-

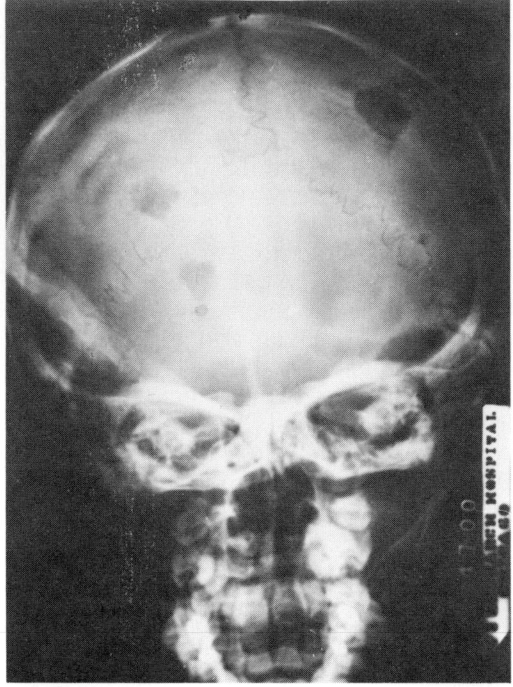

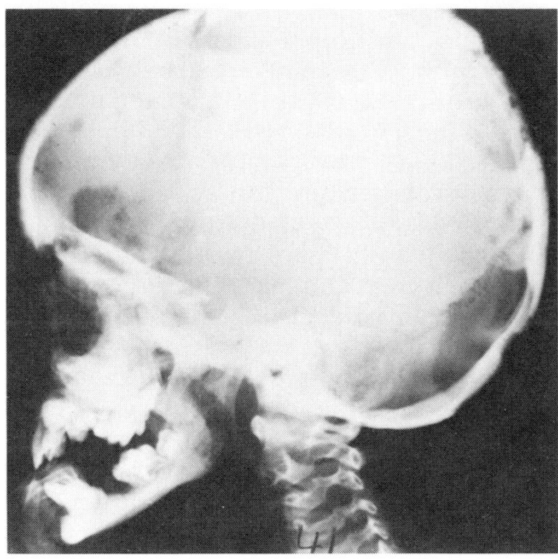

FIG. 19-14. Hand-Schüller-Christian disease, showing sharply demarcated osteolytic skull lesions.

sion of the disease, bone lesions appear to heal spontaneously. The patient may ultimately become short statured.

TREATMENT

Surgical treatment by curettage and bone grafting or by segmental resection (*e.g.*, lesion of rib or clavicle) is limited to symptomatic, surgically accessible lesions.[103] A pathologic fracture requires, in addition, external support as well as medical treatment for the generalized disease. Other sites are controlled by low-dosage radiation. Patients with progressive, disseminated histiocytosis involving organ systems other than the skeletal system require chemotherapy. The cytotoxic agent vinblastine (Velban) presently appears to be the agent of choice in patients whose disease is uncontrolled by surgery, radiotherapy, and corticosteroids.[99,112,116]

LETTERER-SIWE DISEASE

An acute, fulminating, generalized disease, Letterer-Siwe disease is characterized pathologically by widespread histiocytic dissemination affecting many organs and tissues, especially at sites of the reticuloendothelial system. It affects infants and young children, producing markedly destructive lesions, particularly within osseous structures and running a rapid course to an almost invariable fatal termination. The orthopaedic surgeon should have an awareness of this condition when called on to establish the cause of the destructive lesion of bone.

CLINICAL PICTURE

Age. Infants and young children under 3 years of age are affected.

Areas of Predilection. Sites of red marrow (*i.e.*, flat bones, vertebrae, skull) are involved. Nodular lesions occur frequently in lymph nodes, tonsils, thymus, spleen, liver, lymphoid tissue of gastrointestinal tract, and skin. Diffusely disseminated deposits are found in the periosteum of affected bones, lungs, dura, heart, pancreas, renal pelves, and endocrine glands.

Physical Findings. The onset is acute. Characteristic findings include a febrile course; enlargement of spleen, liver, and superficial lymph nodes; cutaneous eruption; seborrheic eczema; hemorrhages; progressive anemia; and one or more destructive lesions in bones, particularly the calvarium, mandible, and sphenoid. Bacterial infection is common, affecting the respiratory, gastrointestinal, and genitourinary systems. Otitis media and mastoiditis may occur. Lung infiltrations, terminal pleural and abdominal effusion, and subcutaneous edema are also found.

Very rarely, the disease becomes chronic and assumes a clinical course similar to that of Hand-Schüller-Christian disease.

PATHOLOGY

Grossly, the bone lesions display grayish yellow nodules that replace cortical and cancellous bone.[91] Microscopically, nodular or diffuse collections of histiocytes are widely dispersed throughout, and eosinophils are present in large numbers as well as smaller numbers of inflammatory cells (*i.e.*, neutrophils, lymphocytes, and plasma cells). The histiocytes are highly vacuolated but contain little or no lipoid; foam cells are rare or nonexistent. The lack of lipids within the histiocytes classifies this disease as a nonlipoid histiocytosis.

In rare cases in patients who survive, one finds considerable fibrous scarring and transformation of histiocytes into lipophagic foam cells.

Many observers believe that Letterer-Siwe disease represents an acute septic expression of the same pathologic process that is manifested in a chronic form by Hand-Schüller-Christian disease.[115] Some authors tend to consider these as isolated entities.[102]

TREATMENT

Although the condition has been regarded as invariably fatal within a few weeks to several months, several reports indicate that prolonged survival and possible cure can be achieved by using various antibiotics, radiation, and steroids.[68] Chemotherapy is being evaluated.

HISTIOCYTOSIS X

Eosinophilic granuloma, Letterer-Siwe disease, and the Hand-Schüller-Christian syndrome are regarded by many observers as manifestations of the same pathologic entity designated as histiocytosis X. The common denominator is an inflammatory histiocytosis.[83,92,101,115]

Opponents of the single nosologic concept cite the marked differences in clinical behavior and the often occurring indefinite histologic features and insist that these are separate entities.[65,102,105]

Nevertheless, this text embraces the unified concept for its prognostic significance and convenience, because this explains why overlap between these conditions does occur.

The histiocyte or free macrophage is a large cell with polyhedral or ragged outstretched outlines. It contains a large, pale, vesicular, oval or reniform or multilobed nucleus, which has coarse chromatin granules and an abundant, finely granular, often vacuolated eosinophilic cytoplasm. Characteristically, the histiocyte will take up acid dyes such as trypan blue and lithium carmine. Under conditions of inflammation, histiocytes become abundant and round.

The histiocytes are designated as such because of the presence in their cytoplasm of phagocytosed cellular debris, hemosiderin granules, lipid material, red blood cells, and granulocytes, particularly in areas of necrosis (Fig. 19-15).

Mature eosinophils vary in number from a few to huge masses of cells. Their nuclei are multilobed and their cytoplasm contains the characteristic coarse eosinophilic granules.

Eosinophilic granuloma, Letterer-Siwe disease, and Hand-Schüller-Christian syndrome are characterized by an intense accumulation of histiocytes. Letterer-Siwe disease represents the acute (or subacute) form and Hand-Schüller-Christian disease is the chronic, disseminated form of the same malady. The accumulation of eosinophils represents a rapidly developing defense to the same etiologic agent, whatever it may be.

The terms *reticuloendotheliosis* and *reticuloendothelial hyperplasia* are regarded as improper designations, because hyperplasia of reticuloendothelial cells may occur in neoplasms, as a response to abnormal lipid storage, and in inflammatory conditions. Further, the typical cells in question are histiocytes, which display phagocytosis.

The localized form of the disease is expressed as an eosinophilic granuloma. One or several, and occasionally many, lesions may be observed; no constitutional illness occurs; and cutaneous, pulmonary, or other extraskeletal involvement is absent. The outcome is favorable. The lesion is destructive, develops rapidly, breaks through the cortex, and heals rapidly after curettement or irradiation. It may heal spontaneously. It represents the most successful defense against the disease.

On the other hand, eosinophilic granuloma may represent a phase of the disease. Dissemination may have already occurred or may become manifest later in other parts of the skeleton or the viscera. Therefore, when an isolated lesion of eosinophilic granuloma is first observed, one should be mindful of the possibility that this may represent the initial stage of widespread disease. Eventually, perhaps after months or years, evidence of dissemination is revealed by fatigability, chronic malnutrition, weight loss, slight fever, predisposition to infection, and other skeletal defects. Then the condition should be reclassified as Hand-Schüller-Christian or Letterer-Siwe disease.

There is great variation in the clinical severity. Even a subacute disseminated histiocytosis may slow its course, become chronic, and undergo clinical remission. The subacute case that terminates fatally is a type that may occur in adults as well as children. The Hand-Schüller-Christian type, although protracted over many years, may prove to be fatal from extensive pituitary disease or serious pulmonary infiltration and secondary right ventricular heart failure.

PATHOLOGIC SIMILARITIES

The typical lesion is characterized initially by an intense inflammatory histiocytosis, with or without an eosinophilic reaction. The influx of eosinophils is more pronounced in the solitary lesion, but it also occurs to some degree in the lesions of the acute (Letterer-Siwe) or chronic (Hand-Schüller-Christian) disseminated histiocytosis. The granulomatous histiocytic proliferation rap-

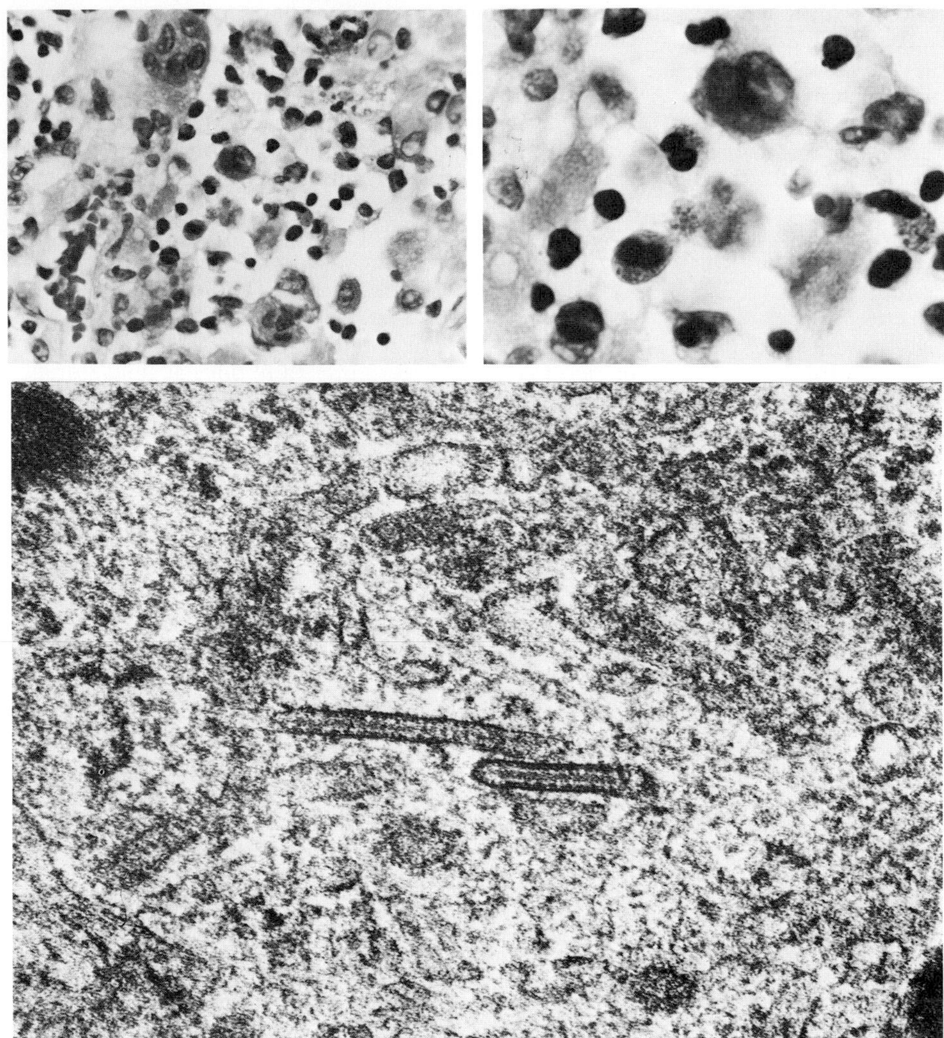

FIG. 19-15. Cytological features of histiocytosis X. (*Top, left*) Smear of aspiration specimen shows an admixture of abundant histiocytes, either containing single or multiple nuclei. These nuclei often contain lipid-filled vacuoles and hemosiderinlike pigment. Also shown are eosinophils, lymphocytes, and neutrophils. (×460) (*Top, right*) Higher magnification. The histiocytes are irregularly shaped with ill-defined outlines, and they contain an eccentric, large, indented, finely creased nucleus with delicate chromatin, surrounded by abundant, delicate pink-staining cytoplasm that contains granular material. The histiocytes sometimes have a loose syncytial appearance, often possess long cytoplasmic processes, and seem to fuse to form giant cells. The granular particulate material within the cytoplasm of histiocytes and giant cells resemble hemosiderin which stains positively with periodic acid-Schiff (PAS). However, it resists digestion by diastase and, therefore, is not glycogen. The histiocytes are present in large numbers in conditions characterized by multisystem and multi-organ involvement, such as disseminated histiocytosis (Letterer-Siwe disease) and malignant histiocytosis. Granulocytes, including eosinophils, are infrequent in these lesions. (×1150) (*Bottom*) Ultramicroscopic features of histiocytosis X shows characteristic Langerhans granules. The electron micrograph shows the tubular inclusions within the cytoplasm of a typical histiocyte of eosinophilic granuloma. These are invariable features of this disease. They may be found in any condition in which the pathologic process is associated with a reactive histiocytosis. (×140,000) (Katz R, Silva EG, de Santos LA et al: Diagnosis of eosinophilic granuloma of bone by cytology, histology, and electron microscopy of transcutaneous bone-aspiration biopsy. J Bone Joint Surg 62A:1284, 1980)

idly destroys the bone. The macrophages engulf small amounts of lipids, hemosiderin, and cellular debris.

Further evolution of the lesion is observed in long-standing cases, with a solitary lesion or multiple lesions (Hand-Schüller-Christian). The histiocytes proliferate, the eosinophils disappear, and the macrophages engulf large amounts of lipids, giving the tissue a distinctly yellow color. With special fat stains, abundant droplets of sudanophilic fat fill the cytoplasm or are displaced toward the periphery of the cell by the nuclei. Multinucleated cells displaying a peripheral ring of dark-staining granules are known as Touton cells. These lipid-laden histiocytes have been differentiated by some observers from true foam cells. The latter are scarce in these lesions and are more common in other inflammatory conditions.[102]

The lesion of histiocytosis X heals by a fibroblastic process while the histiocytes disappear. Complete bone replacement occurs.

In both subacute and chronic forms of the disease, skeletal involvement is diffuse and extraskeletal sites are numerous. The latter are most often recognized as similar to seborrheic eczema or papular eruptions and ulcerations of superficial mucocutaneous surfaces, lymph node enlargements, and pulmonary infiltrations. A pathognomonic finding in chronic disseminated histiocytosis, because of extensive pulmonary infiltrations and fibrosis, is the honeycombing seen on roentgenograms. Episodes of spontaneous pneumothorax are common.

PROGNOSTIC FACTORS

The behavior of the disease in the individual case is highly variable.[72] An adverse prognosis is implied by an early age at onset, particularly within the first 3 years of life; disease involving soft tissues, especially the lungs and liver; and progressive anemia, indicating progressive replacement of the marrow. Histiocytosis confined to the skeleton carries a good prognosis; except for interference with pituitary function in children, resolution can be expected.

GAUCHER'S DISEASE

Gaucher's disease (Gaucher's splenomegaly)[80] is a relatively common familial metabolic disorder characterized by abnormal accumulation of glucocerebrosides in reticuloendothelial cells; the accumulation occurs because of deficiency of an enzyme necessary for the degradation of these glycolipids. The increasing proliferation and masses of the storage cells produce clinical manifestations of the disease, including hepatosplenomegaly, lymph node enlargement, and bone lesions that result from bone marrow replacement, compression of the intraosseous vasculature, and erosion of osseous tissue.[82] The orthopaedic surgeon is concerned mainly with the skeletal manifestations of the disease.

Three syndromes are recognized; (1) a chronic non-neuronopathic or adult form, which is the most common type, becoming evident at any age, and in which bone lesions form a prominent part of the clinical picture; (2) an acute neuronopathic form, manifest in infancy,[64] associated with severe neurologic abnormalities, and usually fatal by 3 years of age; and (3) a subacute or "juvenile" form, which may begin at any age in childhood, combining the features of the chronic adult form with slowly progressive neurologic dysfunction. This last type may present with skeletal involvement, particularly changes about the hip, often erroneously diagnosed as Perthe's disease, and acute periosteal reactions, often mistaken for acute osteomyelitis.

ETIOLOGY

The disease is transmitted by an autosomal recessive gene, rarely by an autosomal dominant gene.[76,84,88,91] The chronic adult type is predominant in Ashkenazi Jews, but the disease has been reported in all races. Both sexes are equally affected.

PATHOGENESIS

A deficiency of a hydrolytic enzyme, termed *glucocerebrosidase,* results in the accumulation of a complex lipid, a sphingolipid designated *glucocerebroside,* in the lysosomes of reticuloendothelial cells.[69,71] These organelles contain numerous enzymes that are responsible for the degradation of many complex lipids, as well as mucopolysaccharides and other metabolic products. Glucocerebrosides arise mainly from the degradation of more complex sphingoglycolipids, the most important source being the normal breakdown of both white and red blood cells. In Gaucher's disease, a specific deficiency of one of the acid hydrolases, glucosylceramide-β-glucosidase (glucocerebrosidase) in the lysosomes results in the accumulation of glucocerebroside, a relatively insoluble compound.

THE GAUCHER CELL

The morphological hallmark of Gaucher's disease is a round or polyhedral pale histiocyte (reticulum cell, macrophage), 20μ to 80μ in diameter, with a small, dark, eccentrically placed nucleus, and a wrinkled cytoplasm, resembling crumpled silk or cigarette paper, that contains an irregular network of fibrils (Fig. 19-16).[108] Under electron microscopy, the fibrils are seen as strands or tubules of glucocerebroside contained within secondary lysosomes having a single limiting membrane. Evidence of phagocytosis is present, and fragments of erythrocytes

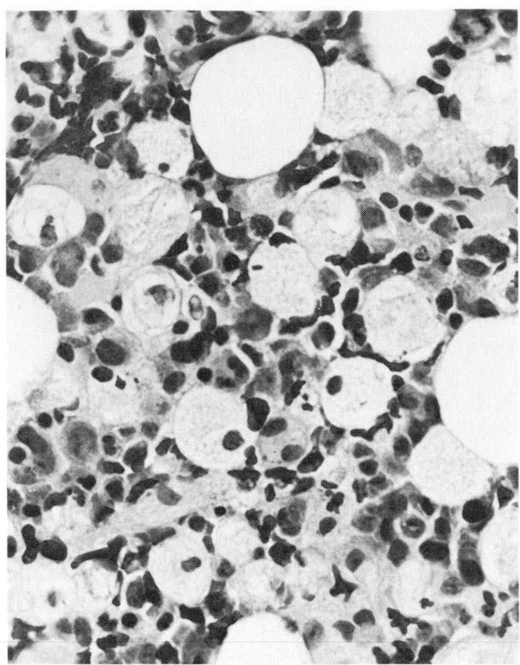

FIG. 19-16. Gaucher's cells, showing granular and fibrillary elements in cytoplasm, and small, dark, eccentrically placed nucleus. (Hematoxylin and eosin, ×494) (Courtesy of Dr. A. M. Rywlin)

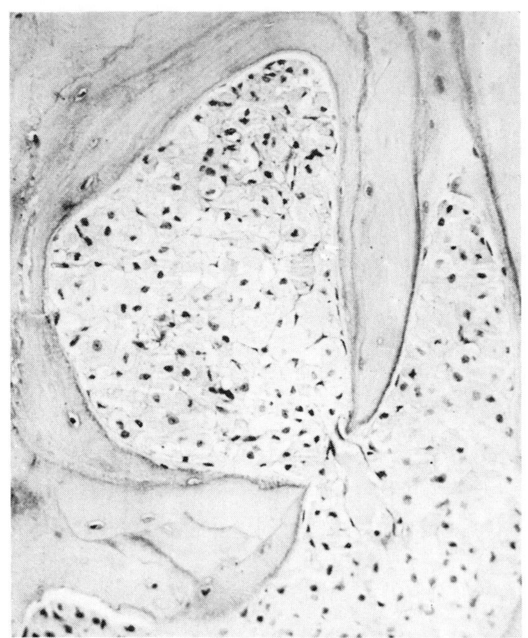

FIG. 19-17. Osseous Gaucher's disease. The bony trabeculae are thick and partially necrotic. The marrow spaces are filled with compact collections of Gaucher's cells, which are large and polyhedral and contain small nuclei and abundant pale, finely granular cytoplasm. (×350) (Gordon GL: Osseous Gaucher's disease. Am J Med 8:332, 1950)

are often visible. The cytoplasm does not stain with fat stains, but the numerous wavy fibrillae are stained deeply with the periodic acid–Schiff reaction or with Mallory's trichrome connective tissue stain. The cytoplasm also demonstrates strong acid phosphatase activity. When stained by prussian blue, a diffuse bluish hue of Gaucher cells is caused by an increased amount of finely dispersed ferritin, a protein-iron complex.

An increased number of plasma cells often coexists with the Gaucher cells and may explain an increased incidence of monoclonal gammopathies in this disease.

The pathognomonic cells are best demonstrated by examination of unstained smears of aspirated bone marrow by phase microscopy.

PATHOLOGY

The intense proliferation of Gaucher cells is responsible for enlargement of the spleen, liver, and intrathoracic and intra-abdominal lymph nodes. The spleen may reach tremendous size.

Within the skeleton, the Gaucher cells are scattered diffusely throughout the marrow, and in some areas tumorlike accumulations erode and expand the cortex (Fig. 19-17).[82,97] Cellular infiltration also involves the lungs, kidneys, thymus, thyroid, and adrenals and wherever lymphoid tissue exists, but, with the exception of the lungs, functional impairment of these organs is unusual.

In children with the acute fatal neuronopathic form of the disease, perivascular foci of Gaucher cells and acute degeneration of neurons is seen.

CLINICAL PICTURE

The chronic nonneuronopathic type is the one usually encountered by the orthopaedic surgeon. Its onset may develop at any age from infancy to old age. The course is extremely variable but tends to be more severe in children. Often, other than an awareness of a progressively enlarging abdominal mass caused by a very large spleen, the patient may be asymptomatic. The second most common presenting complaint is referable to bone lesions. Most patients develop hematologic changes of hypersplenism: thrombocytopenia, secondary anemia, and a bleeding diathesis. The peripheral blood shows immature cellular elements.

The subacute (juvenile) neuronopathic form of Gaucher's disease is rare; few cases have been described, and its clinical features have not been clearly elucidated. It appears to occupy an intermediate position between the early malignant form and the chronic benign form. Its characteristics include hepatosplenomegaly, bone lesions, and neurologic manifestations (*e.g.*, mental retardation, behavioral problems, seizures, choreoathetoid movements.

SKELETAL MANIFESTATIONS

Skeletal changes are more prominent with advancing age.[66,110] The initial presenting complaint is often pain at the hip, knee, shoulder, or spine; occasionally, bone pain is generalized. The onset may be gradual, the course, chronic; and symptoms, episodic; or the onset may be acute, reflecting a pathologic fracture, sudden collapse of a necrotic femoral head, an acute flare-up of degenerative joint disease, or an acute periosteal painful episode.

When initial complaints are nonskeletal (*e.g.*, a massive splenomegaly, bleeding tendencies), skeletal symptoms generally follow at an early age. Patients with widespread skeletal involvement invariably have extensive visceral disease. Skeletal symptoms at an advanced age are more pronounced, since degenerative joint disease is superadded.

The femur is usually the first bone to show pronounced changes. Within the medulla of the diaphysis, typically at its distal region, a circumscribed or diffuse infiltrative growth replaces the marrow and thins, erodes (scallops), and distends the cortex. The entire bone assumes a contour likened to that of an Erlenmeyer flask (Figs. 19-18 and 19-19). Sometimes the proximal portion of the shaft is similarly involved.

The proximal end of the femur at the hip joint is the second most common site of involvement. Necrosis of the femoral head is the most common symptomatic lesion, occurring both in children and adults. In children, such a lesion is often bilateral, and the presenting complaint is pain about the hip, often referred to the knee, and limp. The examination may disclose a flexion-adduction contracture or a muscle spasm that markedly limits passive motion. The roentgenographic findings resemble and are often mistaken for Legg-Calvé-Perthes disease.[114] Symptoms during this growth period may subside by avoiding weight bearing for a prolonged period, with surprising return of normal joint motion and roentgenographic evidence of reconstitution of the femoral head. On the other hand, residual deformity of the femoral head but with relief of symptoms is possible; supervening progressive osteoarthritis is probable with advancing age. Pathologic fracture of the femoral neck may occur in the child but generally heals with internal fixation, usually with residual varus deformity.

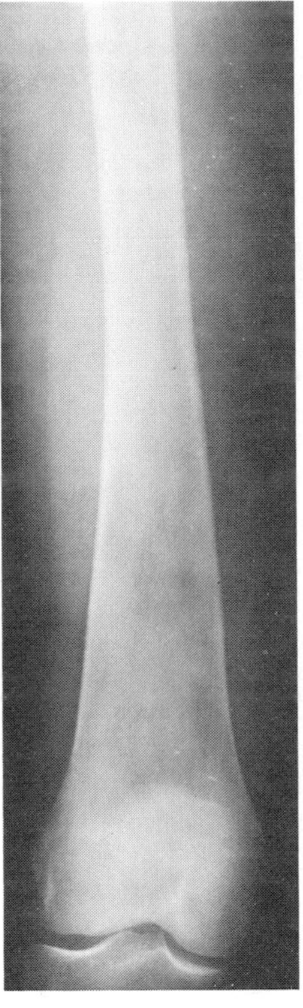

FIG. 19-19. Gaucher's disease, showing the characteristic Erlenmeyer flask appearance (Fischer sign) at the lower end of the femur. Diagnostic findings in roentgenograms include a generalized mottled appearance, increased breadth of the marrow cavity, thinning of cortices, and flaring of the distal part of the femur. (Kroboth FJ Jr, Johnson EW Jr: Osseous Gaucher's disease. Surg Clin North Am 32:1141, 1952)

FIG. 19-18. Gaucher's disease. The cortex of the shaft is thinned, and the medullary cavity is widened because of replacement of cancellous bone by pathologic tissue.

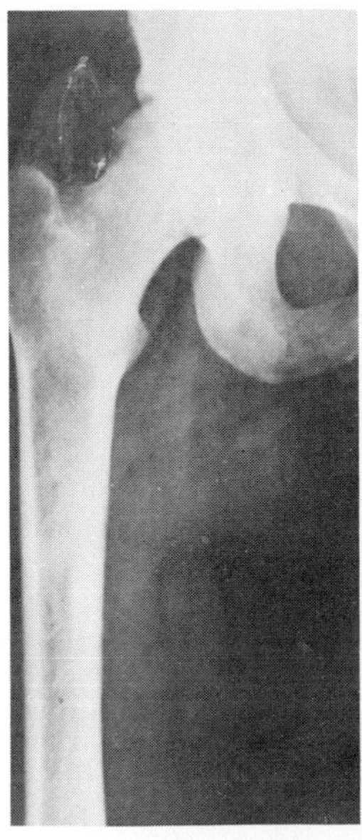

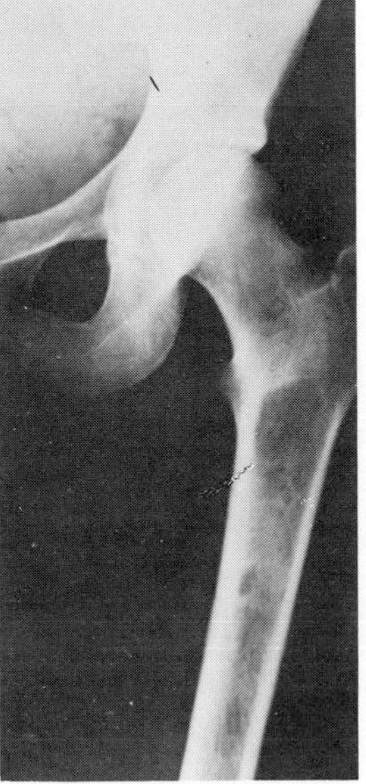

In the adult, repeated episodes of pain, stiffness, and severe limp and of markedly restricted and painful hip motion represent flare-ups of progressive osteoarthritis. Sudden onset of symptoms at the hip may represent collapse of an avascular necrotic femoral head or a pathologic fracture of the femoral neck.

Other long bones and some short tubular bones may be similarly affected. Necrosis and softening of the upper end of the humerus produces marked deformity and degenerative changes about the glenohumeral joint. In the spine, multiple compression fractures produce scoliotic and kyphotic deformities.

Painful, acutely developing periosteal reactions, often following trauma, can produce a clinical syndrome mimicking acute hematogenous osteomyelitis in the child: localized severe pain, tenderness, fever, leukocytosis, and, on roentgenograms, periosteal bone formation and diffuse mottling and motheaten appearance of the subjacent bone. Aspirations are sterile, and the condition is unresponsive to antibiotics. Healing eventually takes place over a prolonged period. The condition, which must be differentiated from acute osteomyelitis to avoid ill-advised surgical invasion of the bone, has been termed *Gaucher's sterile periosteal reaction*[113] or bone crisis.[104]

ROENTGENOGRAPHIC FINDINGS

Skeletal features include localized or diffuse mottled translucencies and thinning and erosion with outward expansion of the cortex. In longstanding cases, coarse trabeculations intermingled with radiolucent foci produce a pseudoloculated appearance.

The lower portion of the femur characteristically is clubbed and expanded, with its contour resembling an Erlenmeyer flask.

The hip joint in the growing child shows mottled translucencies throughout the metaphysis and the neck of the femur, shortening and broadening of the neck, broadening and irregularity of the epiphyseal plate, and often mushrooming deformity of the femoral head. Following fracture of the femoral neck, varus deformity may develop. The deformity and bony architecture closely resemble those of Legg-Calvé-Perthes disease. Regeneration and reconstruction of the femoral head and restoration of congruity sometimes follow prolonged avoidance of weight-bearing pressures. Otherwise, residual deformity eventually results in osteoarthritic changes with advancing age.

In the adult, degenerative changes are superimposed on a deformed femoral head. The disease produces typical changes of avascular necrosis, collapse, crumbling of the head, ultimate involvement of the acetabulum, and fracture of the femoral neck.

The shoulder shows marked irregularity, flattening, and intermingling of coarse trabeculations and radiolucencies throughout the humeral head (Fig. 19-20).

The spine shows marked osteoporosis and numerous collapsed vertebrae.

DIAGNOSIS

Unstained bone marrow smears examined under phase contrast microscopy are ideal for identifying the Gaucher cell. In doubtful cases, the diagnosis may be firmly established by measuring the content of glucocerebrosidase in erythrocytes, which may be one fifth of normal. Needle biopsy of the spleen or liver is seldom needed. Bone biopsy should be avoided, if possible, because of the possibility of inducing a chronically draining sinus.

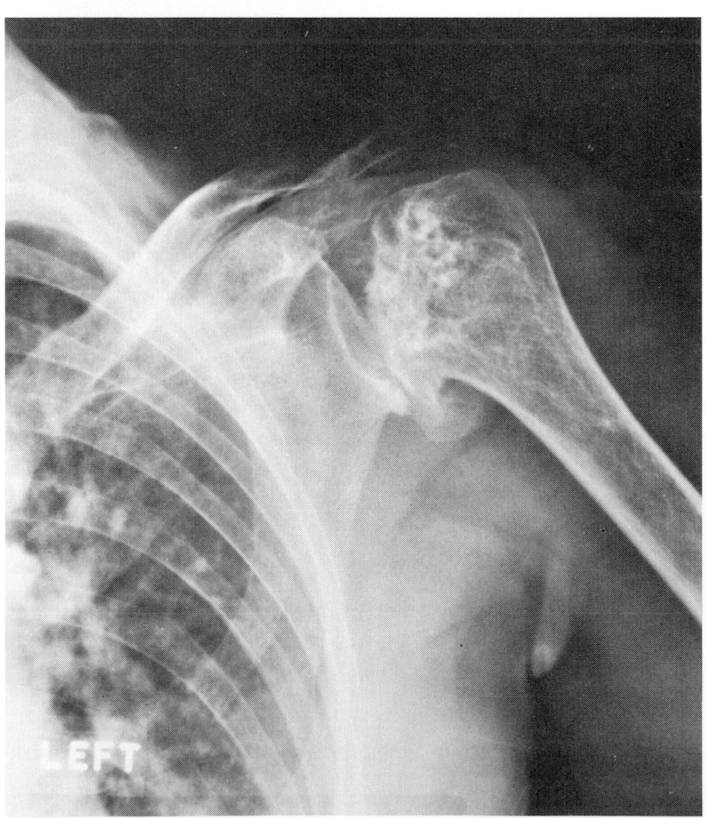

FIG. 19-20. Gaucher's disease of the humeral head. The deformity is the result of osteonecrosis, bony collapse, and supervening osteoarthritic changes. The deformity and architecture of the humeral head are highly characteristic.

The serum acid phosphatase level is markedly increased when measured by the King-Armstrong method but is not elevated when measured by the Bodansky method.

TREATMENT

No specific medical treatment has been devised. Splenectomy will overcome the thrombocytopenia and improve the bleeding tendencies. Brady has demonstrated a definite reduction in the quantity of accumulated glucocerebroside following intravenous infusions of purified glucocerebrosidase derived from the human placenta.[71] The long-range effects of enzyme replacement in certain hereditary diseases appear promising and continue under investigation.[70,95]

Certain principles must be observed before undertaking orthopaedic treatment. A profound susceptibility to infection exists, so that even a minor surgical procedure such as a needle biopsy, can result in a persistently draining sinus. Bleeding tendencies, although diminished by splenectomy, pose the threat of uncontrollable hemorrhage during operation. Preoperative hematologic survey and providing for blood replacement is mandatory. Regardless of the roentgenographic appearance, the structural integrity of the bone is severely compromised by extensive infiltration of the diseased tissue. Fixation devices and implants frequently loosen, settle as further bone resorption takes place, and predispose to fractures. These facts dictate an extremely cautious attitude.

Pathologic fractures of the shaft of a long bone should be treated conservatively if possible. When open reduction is necessary, such as in the aged and infirm, local curettage, intramedullary nailing, additional fixation by acrylic cement, and supplemental bank bone may permit early resumption of activity. When the femoral neck is fractured, internal fixation is indicated in the young patient. In older patients, an endoprosthesis fixed with acrylic cement may be satisfactory. More often osteoarthritis is already present, and total hip replacement should provide a painless, movable joint. Whenever such surgery is performed, walking aids must be used indefinitely thereafter.

Avascular necrosis of the femoral head without an antecedent fracture is the most common symptomatic skeletal lesion. In children it is usually bilateral, and should be treated by a prolonged period of non-weight-bearing. Absolute bed rest is preferable, but an ischial bearing caliper may be worn. Pain generally lessens in time, although with some residual deformity. In the adult, avascular necrosis is usually complicated by partial collapse of the femoral head and degenerative joint disease, which is severely disabling, and temporarily yields to bed rest and traction. Total hip replacement and firm fixation with acrylic cement should correct this problem (Fig. 19-21).

The main complications of total hip replacement arthroplasty in Gaucher's disease are infection, excessive hemorrhage, and a high incidence of loosening.[100] This last-named untoward development can occur despite precautionary measures, such as using components with a low coefficient of friction, performing curettage to ensure close coaptation with cortical bone, plugging the intramedullary canal to ensure pressurized insertion of soft cement, and providing protection agains weight-bearing stresses. Loosening particularly afflicts the younger patient, in whom the procedure should be avoided except as a last resort.

NIEMANN-PICK DISEASE

Niemann-Pick disease is a rare form of lipoid disease seen in the infant. Clinically and pathologically it closely resembles the acute form of Gaucher's disease in infants. However, it is distinguished by storage of the specific lipoid phospholipid, which is also called sphingomyelin. A strongly yellow color is imparted to the enlarged liver, the spleen, the lymph nodes, and the bone marrow. The course is so rapidly fatal that destructive lesions of bone are a rarity. The disease is fatal by lung and central nervous system involvement in the second year.

HISTIOCYTIC LYMPHOMA

Histiocytic lymphoma (reticulum cell sarcoma) is described in Chapter 15 on bone tumors.

TUMORS INVADING BONE FROM OVERLYING STRUCTURES

These tumors include neurogenic sarcoma, myosarcoma, and liposarcoma.

NEUROGENIC SARCOMA

The neurogenic sarcoma (malignant schwannoma, malignant neurinoma) originates from the nerve sheath as shown by the microscopic appearance: wavy nuclei; wirelike fibrillae; palisading, myxomatous intercellular substance; and tumor giant cells. It resembles fibrosarcoma in the fibrillar structure and in the varying degrees of malignity as seen in the spindle cells. Ewing believed that the majority of fibrosarcomas of soft tissue origin are neurogenic in origin. Symptoms of nerve involvement such as pain and tingling are common.

PATHOLOGY

Gross Appearance

The tumor is a soft, beefy red, semitranslucent fleshy tumor, or it may be jellylike and translucent. It extends

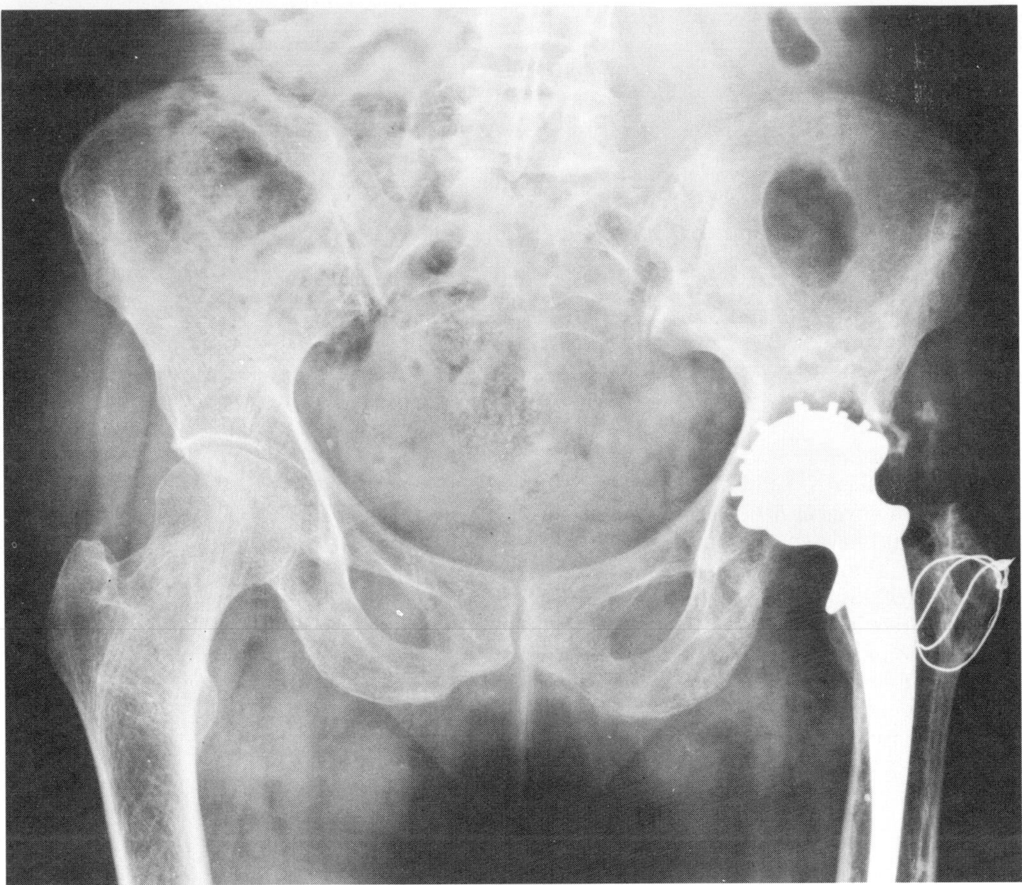

FIG. 19-21. Gaucher's disease of the hip showing total hip replacement which was performed following failure of endoprosthesis without cement fixation. Pain was completely relieved and roentgenographic findings are unchanged after 4 years. (Courtesy of Philip D. Wilson, Jr.)

along a nerve trunk as multiple lobulated tumors and infiltrates as a gray translucent material in the soft tissues. It destroys the adjacent cortex, spreads throughout the medullary cavity, and may even extend into the joint.

Microscopic Appearance

Tightly packed elongated spindle cells are lined up in parallel rows, resembling a fibrosarcoma. However, these spindle cells are longer, are darker, and are rippled or waved. Myxomatous areas containing gliallike elements, and degenerating cells are frequent. Around the myxomatous areas are seen elongated nuclei in cells of the neurilemmoma type in a palisade arrangement, more commonly seen in less malignant tumors. The more malignant tumor displays large pleomorphic nuclei, spindle cells so tightly packed as to crowd out the myxomatous tissue, bizarre tumor giant cells, and relative absence of palisading and whorls.

PROGNOSIS AND TREATMENT

The outlook is very poor. Attempts at local excision are doomed to failure. Even though the tumor microscopically appears benign, radical amputation and deep radiation therapy are justified.

LIPOSARCOMA

Liposarcoma is very rare. It occurs wherever there is fat; consequently, it may originate not only external to the bone but also within the medullary cavity of a bone. It is very malignant and destructive to bone. Therefore, an intraosseous tumor rapidly extends into the soft tissues, and an extraosseous tumor easily invades the bone. Microscopically, the common cells are spindle cells and polyhedral cells, with granular cytoplasm containing fat droplets. These pale swollen polyhedral cells resemble those seen in a hypernephroma. Cells resembling fetal fat cells and tumor giant cells may be present. A common extraosseous location is in the intermuscular tissue about the knee joint. Grossly, the tumor is lobulated and soft and on cut section shows loose, fatty, and myxomatous areas. It metastasizes quickly to the lungs. In the intraosseous type, on the other hand, spread is delayed and metastases occur first to other bones and finally to the lungs. Liposarcoma primary in bone is discussed in Chapter 15 on bone tumors.

RHABDOMYOSARCOMA

Rhabdomyosarcoma is a rare tumor composed of striated muscle. It is very malignant (see Color Plate 17-1). Although its usual sites are the heart, the bladder, the vagina, and the cervix, it may occur in voluntary muscle, in which it secondarily destroys and invades the bone. Grossly, the tumor may be only a few inches in diameter and irregularly ovoid. Although appearing encapsulated, infiltration beyond the capsule is demonstrable. The tumor is generally firm and elastic and on cut section contains small areas of hemorrhage and necrosis. Microscopically, a wide variety of pleomorphic cells including round, spindle, droplet, or "racquet," and tandem cells plus giant cells are seen. The nuclei are large, and the cytoplasm is deeply acidophilic. Many cells contain cross striations characteristic of skeletal muscle. The recommended treatment is wide excision or amputation plus deep radiation therapy. The outlook is very poor.

REFERENCES

Paget's Disease

1. Albright F, Reifenstein EC: The Parathyroid Glands and Metabolic Bone Disease. London, Balliere, Tindall & Cox, 1948
2. Ashley Montagu MF: Paget's disease (osteitis deformans) and heredity. Am J Hum Genet 1:94, 1949
3. Avioli LV, Berman M: Role of magnesium metabolism and the effect of fluoride therapy in Paget's disease of bone. J Clin Endocrinol 28:700, 1968
4. Byers PD: The diagnostic value of bone biopsies. In Avioli LV, Krane SM (eds): Metabolic Bone Disease, vol 1, p 221. New York, Academic Press, 1977
5. Caldwell JG, Avioli LV, Haddad JG: Calcitonin outpatient therapy in Paget's disease of bone (abstr). Clin Res 19:369, 1971
6. Collins DH: Paget's disease of bone: Incidence and subclinical forms. Lancet 2:51, 1956
7. DeRose J et al: Response of Paget's disease to porcine and salmon calcitonins: Effects of long-term treatment. Am J Med 56:858, 1974
8. Dube WJ, Goldsmith RS, Arnaud SB et al: Hyperparathyroidism secondary to long-term therapy of Paget's disease of bone with calcitonin (abstr). Clin Res 19:371, 1971
9. Edholm OG, Howarth S, McMichael J: Heart failure and blood flow in osteitis deformans. Clin Sci 5:249, 1945
10. Editorial: Paget's disease of bone. Br Med J :1427, 1972
11. Eisenstein R, Passavey M: Actinomycin D inhibits parathyroid hormone and vitamin D activity. Proc Soc Exp Biol 117:77, 1964
12. Elias EG, Evans, JT: Mithramycin in the treatment of Paget's disease. J Bone Joint Surg 54A:1730, 1972
13. Feldman F, Seaman WB: The neurologic complications of Paget's disease in the cervical spine. AJR 105:375, 1969
14. Goldenberg RR: The skeleton in Paget's disease. Bull Hosp Joint Dis 12:229, 1951
15. Goodman LS, Gilman A: The Pharmacological Basis of Therapeutics, 3rd ed. New York, Macmillan, 1965
16. Grundy M: Fractures of the femur in Paget's disease of bone: Their etiology and treatment. J Bone Joint Surg 52B:252, 1970
17. Haddad JG: Paget's disease of bone: Problems and management. Orthop Clin North Am 3:775, 1972
18. Hartman JT, Dohm DF: Paget's disease of the spine with cord or nerve root compression. J Bone Joint Surg 48A:1079, 1966
19. Higgins BA: Effect of sodium fluoride on calcium, phosphorus, and nitrogen balance in patients with Paget's disease. Br Med J 1:1159, 1965
20. Jaffe HL: Paget's disease of bone. Arch Pathol 15:83, 1933
21. Jaffe HL: Tumors and Tumorous Conditions of the Bone and Joints. Philadelphia, Lea & Febiger, 1958
22. Jowsey J et al: Treatment of osteoporosis with disodium ethane-1-hydroxy-1, 1-diphosphonate. J Lab Clin Med 78:574, 1971
23. Khairi MRA, Johnston CC Jr: Treatment of Paget's disease of bone (osteitis deformans) with sodium etidronate (EHDP). Clin Orthop 127:34, 1977
24. Lake M: Studies of Paget's disease. J. Bone Joint Surg 33B:323, 1951
25. Marcina RFL: Charakterische Veranderungen de Isozyme der Serumphosphomonoesterasen bei Norbus-Paget-Patienten. Wien Klin Wochenschr 82:255, 1970
26. McKusick VA: Heritable Disorders of Connective Tissue. St. Louis, CV Mosby, 1956
27. Melick RA, Ebeling P, Hjorth RJ: Improvement in paraplegia in vertebral Paget's disease treated with calcitoin. Br Med J 1:627, 1976
28. Meyers MH, Singer FR: Osteotomy for tibia vara in Paget's disease under cover of calcitonin. J Bone Joint Surg 60A:810, 1978
29. Nagant de Deuxchaisnes C, Krane SM: Paget's disease of bone: Clinical and metabolic observations. Medicine 43:233, 1964
30. Price CH, Goldie W: Paget's sarcoma of bone: A study of eighty cases from the Bristol and Leeds bone tumour registries. J Bone Joint Surg 51B:205, 1969
31. Pugh DC: Roentgenologic Diagnosis of Bones. Baltimore, Williams & Wilkins, 1951
32. Purves MJ: Some effects of administering sodium fluoride to patients with Paget's disease. Lancet 2:1188, 1962
33. Rebel A et al: Les inclusions de ostéoclastes dans la maladie osseuse de Paget. Rev Rhum 42:637, 1975
34. Rutishausen E, Veyrat R, Roviller C: La vascularisation de l'os pagetique: Etude anatomopathologique. Presse Méd 62:654, 1954
35. Ryan WG: Treatment of Paget's disease of bone with mithramycin. Clin Orthop 127:106, 1977
36. Ryan WG, Schwartz TG, Northrop G: Further observations on the treatment of Paget's disease of bone with mithramycin (abstr). Ann Intern Med 74:824, 1971

37. Ryan WG, Schwartz TG, Perlia CP: Effects of mithramycin on Paget's disease of bone. Ann Intern Med 70:549, 1969
38. Schmorl G: Über Ostitis deformans Paget. Virchow's Arch 283:694, 1932
39. Siegelman SS, Levine SA, Walpin L: Paget's disease with spinal cord compression. Clin Radiol 19:421, 1968
40. Singer FR: Human calcitonin treatment of Paget's disease of bone. Clin Orthop 127:86, 1977
41. Singer FR, Mills BG: The etiology of Paget's disease of bone. Clin Orthop 127:37, 1977
42. Singer FR et al: An evaluation of antibodies and clinical resistance to salmon calcitonin. J Clin Invest 51:2331, 1972
43. Smith R, Russell RGG, Bishop M: Diphosphonates and Paget's disease of bone. Lancet 1:945, 1971
44. Stauffer RN, Sim FH: Total hip arthroplasty in Paget's disease of the hip. J Bone Joint Surg 58A:476, 1976
45. Wardle EN: Osteotomy of the tibia and fibula. Surg Gynecol Obstet 115:61, 1962
46. Woodhouse NJ: Paget's disease of bone. Clin Endocrinol Metab 1:125, 1972
47. Woodhouse NJ et al: Cardiac output in Paget's disease: Response to long-term salmon calcitonin threapy. Br Med J 4:686, 1975
48. Woodhouse NJ, Bordier P, Fisher M et al: Human calcitonin in the treatment of Paget's bone disease. Lancet 1:1139, 1971

Infantile Cortical Hyperostosis

49. Caffey J, Silverman WA: Infantile cortical hyperostosis. AJR 54:1, 1945
50. Roske G: Eine eigenartige Knochenerkrangung im Sanglingsalter. Monatsschr Kinderheilkd 47:387, 1930

Sarcoidosis

51. Baltzer G et al: Zur Häufigkeit zystischer Knochenveränderungen (Ostitis cystoides multiplex Jüngling) bei der Sarkoidose. Dtsch Med Wochenschr 95:1926, 1970
52. Cutler SS et al: Vertebral sarcoidosis. JAMA 240:557, 1978
53. Goobar JE et al: Vertebral sarcoidosis. JAMA 178:1162, 1961
54. Holt JF, Owens WI: The osseous lesions in sarcoidosis. Radiology 53:11, 1949
55. Lonocope WT, Freiman DG: A study of sarcoidosis: Based on a combined investigation of 160 cases including 30 autopsies from the Johns Hopkins Hospital and Massachusetts General Hospital. Medicine 31:1, 1952
56. Mayock RL et al: Manifestations of sarcoidosis: Analysis of 145 cases with a review of nine series selected from the literature. Am J Med 35:67, 1963
57. McCort JJ et al: Sarcoidosis: A clinical and roentgenologic study of twenty-eight proved cases. Arch Intern Med 80:293, 1947
58. Ricker W, Clark M: Sarcoidosis: A clinicopathologic review of three hundred cases, including twenty-two autopsies. Am J Clin Pathol 19:725, 1949
59. Siltzbach LE, Duberstein JL: Arthritis in sarcoidosis. Clin Orthop 57:31, 1968
60. Sokoloff L, Bunim JJ: Clinical and pathological studies of joint involvement in sarcoidosis. N Engl J Med 260:841, 1959
61. Stein GN, Israel HL, Sones M: A roentgenographic study of skeletal lesions in sarcoidosis. Arch Intern Med 97:532, 1956
62. Turek SL: Sarcoid disease of bone at the ankle joint. J Bone Joint Surg 35A:465, 1953
63. Zener JC, Alport M, Klainer LM: Vertebral sarcoidosis. Arch Intern Med 111:696, 1963

Tumors of Hematopoietic Tissues

64. Aballi AJ, Kato K: Gaucher's disease in early infancy. J Pediatr 13:364, 1938
65. Ackerman LV, Spjut HJ: Tumors of Bone and Cartilage. In Atlas of Tumor Pathology, section II, fascicle 4. Washington, DC, Armed Forces Institute of Pathology, 1962
66. Amstutz HC, Carey EJ: Skeletal Manifestations and treatment of Gaucher's disease. J Bone Joint Surg 48A:670, 1966
67. Baldridge CW, Awe CD: Lymphosarcoma—a study of 150 cases. Arch Intern Med 45:161, 1930
68. Bierman HR: An apparent cure of Letterer-Siwe disease: 17 year survival of identical twins with nonlipoid reticuloendotheliosis. JAMA 196:368, 1966
69. Brady RO, Johnson WG, Uhlendorf BW: Identification of heterozygous carriers of lipid storage diseases. Am J Med 51:423, 1971
70. Brady RO et al: Replacement therapy for inherited enzyme deficiency: Use of purified ceramide trihexosidase in Fabry's disease. N Engl J Med 289:9, 1973
71. Brady RO et al: Replacement therapy for inherited enzyme deficiency (use of purified glucocerebrosidases) in Gaucher's disease. N Engl J Med 291:989, 1974
72. Cheyne C: Histiocytosis X. J Bone Joint Surg 53B:366, 1971
73. Christian HA: Defects in membranous bones, exophthalmos and diabetes insipidus; an unusual syndrome of dyspituitarism; a clinical study. Med Clin North Am 3:849, 1920
74. Compere EL, Johnson WE, Coventry MB: Vertebra plana (Calvé's disease) due to eosinophilic granuloma. J Bone Joint Surg 36A:969, 1954
75. Craver LF, Copeland MM: Lymphosarcoma in bone. Arch Surg 28:809, 1934
76. Crone RI, Bergin JJ: Gaucher's disease in identical twins. Ann Intern Med 49:941, 1958
77. Dale JH Jr: Leukemia in childhood. J Pediatr 34:421, 1949
78. DeVita VT et al: Combination chemotherapy in the treatment of advanced Hodgkins's disease. Ann Intern Med 73:881, 1970
79. Dresner D: Bone and joint lesions in acute leukemia and their response to folic acid antagonists. Q J Med 19:339, 1950
80. Gaucher PCE: De l'Epithelioma Primitif de la Rate. These de Paris, 1882
81. Geschickter CF, Copeland MM: Tumors of Bone. Philadelphia, JB Lippincott, 1949
82. Gordon GL: Osseous Gaucher's disease. Am J Med 8:332, 1950
83. Green WT, Farber S: "Eosinophilic or solitary granuloma" of bone. J Bone Joint Surg 24:499, 1942
84. Groen J: The hereditary mechanism of Gaucher's disease. Blood 3:1238, 1948
85. Hand A: Polyuria and tuberculosis. Arch Pediatr 10:673, 1893
86. Hand A: Defects of membranous bones, exophthalmos and polyuria in childhood: Is it dyspituitarism? Am J Med Sci 162:509, 1921
87. Hatcher CH: Eosinophilic granuloma of bone. Arch Pathol 30:828, 1940
88. Herndon CH, Bender JR: Gaucher's disease: Cases in 5 related Negro sibships. Am J Hum Genet 2:49, 1950
89. Hodgson JR, Kennedy RJL, Camp JD: Reticuloendotheliosis. Radiology 57:642, 1951

90. Hoxie TB: Bone and joint pain in leukemia. N Engl J Med 238:733, 1948
91. Hsia DYY et al: Gaucher's disease. Report of two cases in father and son and review of the literature. N Engl J Med 261:164, 1959
92. Jaffe HL: Metabolic, Degenerative and Inflammatory Diseases of Bones and Joints. Philadelphia, Lea & Febiger, 1972
93. Jaffe HL: Skeletal manifestations of leukemia and malignant lymphomas. Bull Hosp Joint Dis 13:217, 1952
94. Jaffe HL, Lichtenstein L: Eosinophilic granuloma of bone. Arch Pathol 37:99, 1944
95. Johnson WG et al: Intravenous injection of purified hexosaminidase A into a patient with Tay-Sachs disease. Birth Defects 9(2):120, 1973
96. Kaplan HS: Role of intensive radiotherapy in the management of Hodgkin's disease. Cancer 19:356, 1966
97. Kato K: Changes of bone in Gaucher's disease. Trans Am Pediatr Soc 43:43, 1931
98. Katz RL, Silva EG, DeSantos LA et al: Diagnosis of eosinophilic granuloma of bone by cytology, histology, and electron microscopy of transcutaneous bone-aspiration biopsy. J Bone Joint Surg 62A:1284, 1980
99. Kondi ES et al: Diffuse eosinophilic granuloma of bone: A dramatic response to Velban therapy. Cancer 30:1169, 1972
100. Lachiewicz PF, Lane JM, Wilson PD Jr: Total hip replacement in Gaucher's disease. J Bone Joint Surg 63A:602, 1981
101. Lichtenstein L: Histiocytosis X. Arch Pathol 56:84, 1953
102. Lieberman PH et al: A reappraisal of eosinophilic granuloma of bone, Hand-Schüller-Christian syndrome and Letterer-Siwe syndrome. Medicine 48:375, 1969
103. Mickelson MR, Bonfiglio M: Eosinophilic granuloma and its variations. Orthop Clin North Am 8:933, 1977
104. Noyes FR, Smith WS: Bone crises and chronic osteomyelitis in Gaucher's disease. Clin Orthop 79:132, 1971
105. Otani S: A discussion on eosinophilic granuloma of bone, Letterer-Siwe disease and Schüller-Christian disease. J Mt Sinai Hosp 24:1079, 1957
106: Otani S, Ehrlich JC: Solitary granuloma of bone simulating primary neoplasm. Am J Pathol 16:479, 1940
107. Ponseti I: Bone lesions in eosinophilic granuloma, Hand-Schüller-Christian disease, and Letterer-Siwe disease. J Bone Joint Surg 30A:811, 1948
108. Rywlin AM: Histopathology of Bone Marrow. Boston, Little, Brown & Co, 1976
109. Schajowicz F, Slullitel J: Eosinophilic granuloma of bone and its relationship to Hand-Schüller-Christian and Letterer-Siwe syndromes. J Bone Joint Surg 55B:545, 1973
110. Schein AJ, Arkin AM: Hip joint involvement in Gaucher's disease J Bone Joint Surg 24:396, 1942
111. Schüller A: Über eingenartige Schadeldefekte im Jugendalter. Fortschr Roentigenstr 23:12, 1915–1916
112. Siegel S, Coltman CA: Histiocytosis X: Response to vinblastine sulfate. JAMA 197:403, 1966
113. Strickland B: Skeletal manifestations of Gaucher's disease with some unusual findings. Br J Radiol 31:246, 1958
114. Todd RMcL, Keidan SE: Changes in the head of the femur in children suffering from Gaucher's disease. J Bone Joint Surg 34B:447, 1952
115. Wallgren A: Systemic reticuloendothelial granuloma: Nonlipoid reticuloendotheliosis and Hand-Schüller-Christian disease. Am J Dis Child 60:471, 1940
116. West WO: Velban as treatment for diffuse eosinophilic granuloma of bone. J Bone Joint Surg 55A:1755, 1973

20

Peripheral Vascular Disease

THE STUDY of vascular disease overlaps that of many other fields of medicine and surgery. A study of blood vessels of the extremities, although closely allied to the field of orthopaedic surgery, cannot be considered apart from the rest of the body. The state of the heart and the large vessels of the chest and abdomen may have a direct relationship to circulatory disease of the extremities. For example, subacute bacterial endocarditis may be the cause of embolic phenomena, and occlusion at the bifurcation of the aorta results in arterial insufficiency of the lower extremities.

The orthopaedic surgeon must be proficient at identifying and interpreting the state of the circulation in the extremities. Inadequate blood flow must be differentiated from musculoskeletal disease as the source of symptoms. In dealing with complex trauma, the state of the major vessels must be determined and the need for vascular reconstruction considered. When planning an orthopaedic reconstructive procedure of the distal portion of an extremity, the circulatory integrity of the part must be ascertained preoperatively. When progressive arterial occlusion threatens the extremity and angioplastic procedures are contemplated, it is important to establish whether primary amputation below the knee is the preferred operation. Rehabilitation is more feasible following a below-knee amputation, but the possibility of attaining a satisfactory below-knee stump may be compromised by an ill-advised attempt at vascular reconstruction. The ultimate decision should derive from free consultation between the orthopaedic surgeon, internist, and vascular surgeon.

DIAGNOSIS OF VASCULAR DISEASE OF THE EXTREMITIES

The orthopaedic surgeon must have a precise knowledge of symptoms and objective manifestations caused by various vascular disturbances. By following a definite plan of eliciting the history, examining the affected parts, and performing special tests, a comprehensive examination is completed that leads to an intelligent appraisal of the individual case.[1] The following pertinent points must be considered.

PAIN

The most frequent complaint is pain. It is either persistent or intermittent.

Persistent pain may be due to the following:

Rest, Gangrene, and Ulceration

In thromboangiitis obliterans (TAO), ulceration and gangrene cause extremely severe pain. In arteriosclerosis obliterans (ASO), such pain at first may be of less severity but eventually becomes severe, occurring even at rest. Rest pain is an ominous sign denoting extreme occlusive arterial disease and ischemia. This pain is partially relieved by the dependent position and heat; it is intensified by elevation and cold. The patient characteristically sleeps with his legs hanging over the side of the bed. Such severe pain, due to pronounced ischemia, is also known as pretrophic pain because it is the forerunner of ulceration and gangrene.

Sudden Arterial Occlusion.
The onset of excruciating pain may be sudden or gradual, reaching its maximum intensity in several hours, and is associated with color changes. Numbness, coldness, and tingling are frequent subjective complaints.

Ischemic Neuritis
This is severe, diffuse, and spasmodic and does not correspond to the distribution of peripheral nerves. The character of the discomfort is sharp or shooting; pulling, or tearing, or agonizing; burning or throbbing. During paroxysms, the extremity may become mottled, dark, and bluish red owing to excessive vasoconstriction. Between paroxysms, a constant, dull, diffuse, shifting ache is present. Paroxysms occur most often at night and may last for several hours.

Arteritis, Phlebitis, and Lymphangitis
Acute arteritis is extremely rare; it causes mild pain, and the artery is tender. Chronic arteritis is painless. Localized phlebitis causes mild pain and tenderness of the involved vein. When phlebitis is extensive, it may cause extreme pain and is frequently associated with swelling. Lymphangitis is evidenced by a red line, soreness, and tenderness.

Intermittent pain may be due to the following:

Exercise
Exercise produces intermittent claudication and occurs almost exclusively in chronic occlusive arterial disease. Intermittent claudication is caused by deficient blood flow through contracting muscles. It is a severe ache that occurs with exercise. Rest relieves the severe pain, but often a sensation of fatigue and muscle tenderness may persist for a short while. As the occlusion becomes greater in degree and blood flow diminishes further, the amount of exercise required to bring about the pain is correspondingly less. The site of claudication suggests, but is not necessarily related to, the level of occlusion. For example, claudication of the arch of the foot suggests occlusion at or above the ankle. On the other hand, a superficial femoral occlusion in the thigh may cause pain in the calf, foot, or toe. Lessening of intensity and frequency of claudication suggests improving collateral circulation. The presence of arterial pulsations in an extremity affected by intermittent claudication suggests a vasospastic tendency, but vasospasm alone as a cause of intermittent claudication is rare, and organic vascular disease eventually becomes apparent. Intermittent claudication has been explained as an abnormal accumulation of a metabolic substance, "factor P" in the muscle.

For quantitative measurement, the patient walks at the rate of 120 steps per minute. The time elapsing between the beginning of the test and the occurrence of pain is known as the claudication time. This can also be determined by the standard treadmill test: walking at 2 mph on a 12% grade.

Posture
Chronic venous insufficiency causes an ache or a feeling of heaviness after prolonged standing. It is lessened by walking and relieved by recumbency.

Cramps in the legs occurring while in bed are not part of occlusive arterial disease. The cause is unknown. The symptom may arise when stretching the legs or may appear in the course of sleep.

COLOR CHANGES

The skin color reflects the amount of blood and the color of blood in the minute vessels of the skin. The more slowly the blood flows, the more oxygen it gives up and the more cyanotic the skin becomes. Warmth increases the rate of dissociation of oxygen from the blood; cold has the opposite effect.

When blood flow is rapid, minute blood vessel tone will be high and the skin will be warm and pale pink. A warm, deeply colored red skin is due to vasodilatation produced by a vasomotor reflex, drugs, or inflammation.

Typical clinical examples follow.

Raynaud's Disease. Pallor (reduction of blood flow due to vasospasm), cyanosis (stagnation of blood in capillaries resulting in dissociation of oxygen), and rubor (greater local blood distribution) are produced respectively by arteriolar constriction, capillary dilatation, and arteriolar plus capillary dilatation. It is important to note that rubor may occur in a pregangrenous lesion with markedly reduced overall blood flow. This is explained by loss of vasomotor tone due to ischemia.

Thrombophlebitis. Cyanosis (stasis of blood) is due to obstruction to the outflow of blood.

Sudden Arterial Occlusion. Pallor (absence of blood) is due to obstruction of the main vessel and spasm of collaterals.

Erythromelalgia. Red warm skin is due to arteriolar and capillary vasodilatation.

Chronic Occlusive Arterial Disease. Pallor is evident on elevation (insufficient blood); the blood pressure cannot overcome the circulatory obstruction plus the effect of gravity. Cyanosis is noted on dependency (slowed blood flow); the minute blood vessels are chronically dilated as a result of prolonged ischemia.

Normally, elevation of the extremity above the level of the heart may cause a pallor, and the normal color returns within 10 seconds after the part is returned to the dependent position. When arterial circulation is impaired, the pallor is extreme and, if arterial circulation is irregularly distributed, patchy; on lowering the extremity, the color, which is a rubor or a cyanotic redness, returns very slowly and often in an irregular and patchy manner.

Sensitivity to exposure to cold, as detected by placing the part in cold water, is usually manifest by pallor, occasionally by cyanosis, and rarely by rubor. All colors may be present together.

Permanent, uniform, cyanotic discoloration of the skin distal to the wrists and to the ankles usually indicates acrocyanosis. A persistent bluish to bluish red mottling of the skin of the feet and legs, known as livedo reticularis, is particularly noticeable on exposure to cold. Persistent cyanosis of an individual digit is often a manifestation of thrombosis of a digital artery and frequently, but not invariably, precedes gangrene.

A brownish black discoloration at the lower region of the legs is a stasis pigmentation characteristic of chronic venous insufficiency.

ULCERATION, GANGRENE

Gangrene caused by arteriosclerotic occlusive disease usually affects the pedal digits, the first toe being most commonly involved. All digits and the distal parts of the foot, less commonly the hand, may be affected by extensive gangrene. Gangrene or ulceration of more proximal parts, such as the leg or the heel, may follow trauma. Gangrene of the hand is very rare in ASO. It is generally due to severe trauma and may be a complication of arterial catheterization procedures.

In Raynaud's disease, small necrotic ulcerations may develop in the tips of the fingers.

Ulceration of chronic venous insufficiency characteristically affects the inner aspect of the leg just above the ankle. Occasionally it affects the outer side of the ankle.

In sudden arterial occlusion, gangrene may be extensive because of severe concomitant spasm of the collaterals. However, the more distal parts are usually involved.

Ulcerations usually develop in the fingers or toes, rarely in other areas of the extremity, as a result of an arteriovenous fistula and often resemble those due to chronic venous insufficiency. Characteristically, the local skin temperature is elevated.

SWELLING AND EDEMA

The following conditions are of circulatory origin:

Deep Thrombophlebitis

This causes acutely developing edema. Thrombosed veins may be palpable, tender, and painful. Temperature is slightly elevated. Deep venous thrombosis is often silent and detected only by various procedures (*e.g.*, phlebography).

Chronic Venous Insufficiency

Varicose veins, stasis dermatitis or ulceration, and a pitting type of edema are seen.

Lymphedema

There is a gradual progressive extension proximally over a period of weeks, months, or years. If of recent origin, pitting is detected; if extensive and of long duration, the tissues are fibrotic, hypertrophied, and resistant to pitting.

Lipedema

This is a condition in which diffusion of fluid occurs from the small vessels into surrounding tissues when the latter contains excessive fatty deposits. Lipedema of the legs affects women, appearing first during adolescence. The enlargement of the limbs is generalized and symmetrical, and frequently its development is associated with a gradual increase in weight. Often a familial tendency is noted, and the adipose tissue is of a peculiar loose texture. The skin and the subcutaneous tissue are soft and pliable. The enlargement of the extremity is nonpitting, unless edema is extensive and usually at the day's end. Generalized obesity may or may not be present.

Arteriovenous Fistula

This causes edema because of increased pressure in the veins. Increased oxygen content of the venous blood is diagnostic. Engorged veins, which may pulsate and over which a bruit will be heard, are also characteristic.

Chronic Occlusive Arterial Disease

A prolonged, dependent posture is assumed by the patient to get relief from pain, thereby causing edema. Because the veins in TAO are often occluded, resulting in venous statis, edema is more pronounced in this condition than in ASO.

Other causes of swelling of the extremities must be differentiated, including systemic (renal, cardiac, hypoproteinemia) and local (tumor) causes.

TEMPERATURE

Increased blood flow to the skin is perceived by the examiner's hand as warmth, whereas decreased blood flow results in skin coolness. The temperature of the skin *per se* does not indicate the state of the circulation in the entire extremity. Many people with abnormally cool skin have normal blood flow throughout the extremity. The distal portions of the extremities, the digits, show variations in temperature under different conditions, but all digits on any one occasion have temperatures that are almost identical. When one extremity demonstrates a skin temperature lower than than in the opposite extremity, its circulation may be regarded as impaired. An exception to this principle occurs when warmth of a single extremity is the result of vasodilatation from a sympathectomy when the opposite extremity may be normal.

When the examiner's hand is passed over the extremity from the proximal to the distal end, a sudden change in temperature defines the level of circulatory impairment. One may suspect occlusion of a digital artery in a toe whose skin temperature is lower than that in the adjacent toes. When coldness of the skin occurs symmetrically in both extremities, the circulation may be regarded as implicated only if confirmed by other findings (*e.g.*, Doppler readings), and if diminished temperatures are demonstrated repeatedly under basal conditions. Cold skin is associated with chronic occlusive arterial disease and the pallor phase of Raynaud's disease. Warm skin accompanies erythromelalgia.

The subjective sensation of "warmth and burning" is a paresthesia occurring frequently in patients of advanced age and does not necessarily indicate a circulatory disturbance. When associated with warm skin, erythromelalgia must be considered.

ARTERIAL PULSATIONS

The pulsations can be felt in the upper extremity in the subclavian, the radial, and the ulnar arteries; in the lower extremity they can be felt in the femoral, the popliteal, the dorsalis pedis, and the posterior tibial arteries. The degree of expansile force is estimated and recorded. Occasionally, arterial pulsations may be detected in an abnormal location, particularly about the wrist, the knee, and the ankle, and to some degree may reflect the degree of collateral circulation.

In occlusive arterial disease, pulsations in themselves are not sufficient indication of the adequacy of blood flow, either through main arteries or through their vital collaterals. Under the influence of exercise (*e.g.*, the treadmill test), Doppler and plethysmographic readings may show marked reduction of blood flow, and the pulsations at the distal portions of the extremity may even become imperceptible.

Allen's test is used to determine the patency of the palmar or plantar arterial arch distal to the wrist and ankle, respectively, when pulsations at these joints are palpable. When one artery is obstructed, postural color changes and lowered skin temperature may not be apparent, because adequate flow takes place through the uninvolved vessel.

The test is performed as follows: The patient elevates both hands in front of the examiner. If the ulnar artery is suspected of being occluded or absent, the radial artery is manually compressed at the wrist. The patient squeezes the blood out of the hand by clenching the fist tightly for about 10 seconds and then opening it. The return of color is rapid if alternate circulation to the palmar arch is adequate. If the ulnar artery is occluded or absent, pallor is persistent for some time or until the radial artery is released.

The radial, dorsalis pedis, and posterior tibial arteries may be similarly tested. In examining the feet, elevation and dependency are substituted for clenching and opening the hand.

VARICOSE VEINS

Varicose veins are venous channels that have become large and distended by abnormally and chronically increased intraluminal pressure; this results from incompetent venous valves permitting gravitational backflow of blood, from obstruction to blood flow (*e.g.*, thrombophlebitis, tumor compression), or from arteriovenous fistula causing blood to flow directly from the artery into the vein.

Superficial thrombosed veins can be palpated as thickened cords. When thrombophlebitis is acute, a narrow zone of redness overlies the tender palpable vein. Deeply situated veins cannot be palpated, but their patency can be determined by tests of filling and emptying applied to superficial veins.

A vein normally fills within 10 seconds when it is brought to a dependent position after elevation. Delay in filling, assuming competent venous valves, is presumptive evidence of impaired arterial circulation. A vein normally empties when it is elevated above the level of the heart. Failure to empty signifies abnormally increased intravenous back pressure.

Tests to determine incompetency of the saphenous and the communicating veins and occlusion of the deep veins must be performed together. Before removing or obliterating the superficial channels, it is imperative to first establish the patency of the deep channels.

Perthes' Test. While the patient is standing, a tourniquet is applied about the upper thigh sufficient to compress only the long saphenous vein. As the patient walks about briskly, the prominence of the varicose veins is noted (Fig. 20-1). Normally, muscular action should empty blood from the superficial system through the communicating veins into the deep system. Therefore, disappearance of varices indicates that valves in the communicating veins are competent, and varicosities are due soley to incompetent saphenous valves. If varicosities do not disappear while walking, both saphenous and communicating valves are incompetent. If varicosities become distended and prominent and the patient experiences pain while walking, the deep veins are obstructed and

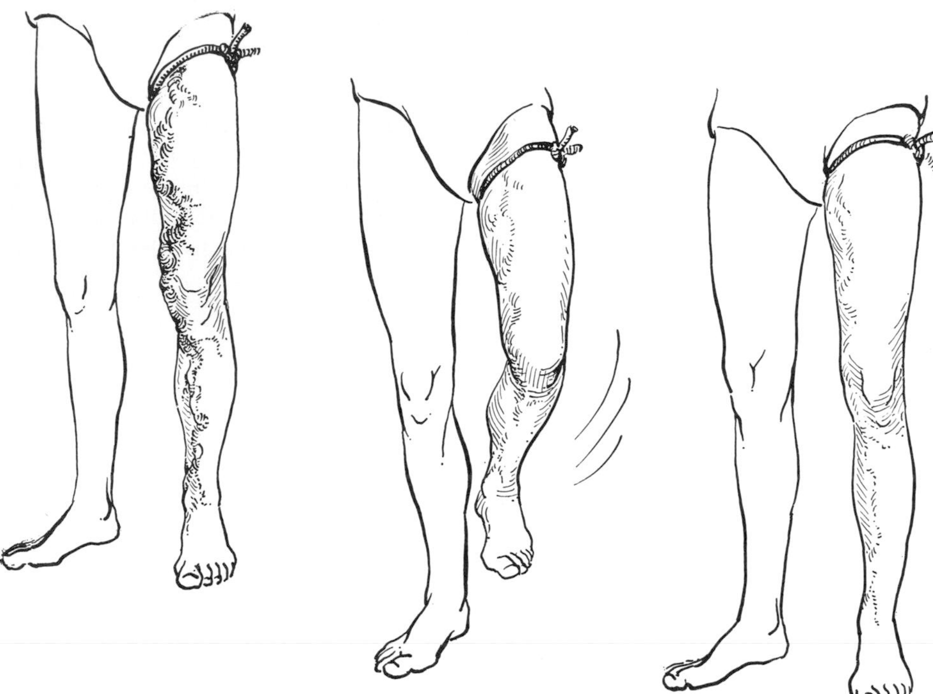

FIG. 20-1. Perthes' test for incompetence of superficial and deep veins. (*Left*) A tourniquet about the thigh compresses the long saphenous vein, preventing reverse flow past this constriction. (*Center*) The patient then exercises this extremity briskly. (*Right*) Normally, blood flow in the venous system is aided by muscular action so that it goes from the superficial to the deep system. If the superficial varices disappear when the leg is exercised, the valves of the communicating veins are competent, and only the saphenous valves are incompetent. If the varices do not disappear with exercise, the valves in the communicating veins as well as those in the saphenous vein are incompetent. If the veins become more prominent with exercise and pain appears, the deep veins are obstructed, and ligation of the superficial system is contraindicated.

the valves of the communicating veins are incompetent. This may also indicate incompetency of communicating veins between the long and the short saphenous veins.

The Pratt Test. The Pratt Test determines the location of the incompetent communicating branches.[2] The recumbent patient elevates the leg and empties the veins. A tourniquet compresses the long saphenous vein at the upper thigh. An elastic bandage is applied from the toes to the level of the tourniquet. The patient stands erect, and the bandage is slowly unwound from above downward. Reflux blood from above is prevented by the tourniquet, so the appearance of a bulge indicates the site of an incompetent communicating vein. This is marked with an indelible pencil. A second bandage is applied from the level of the tourniquet down to and compressing the bulging vein. The first bandage is again unwound downward to the next blowout, which is again marked and compressed by the second bandage. This procedure is continued until all blowouts are identified. Removal of all incompetent communicating veins is necessary to prevent recurrences. While the bandages are applied, severe pain and swelling of the calf indicate occlusion of the deep veins.

SPECIAL TESTS OF PERIPHERAL CIRCULATION

Many procedures have been devised to accurately define the anatomical configuration of and blood flow through vessels in any region in the body. The following tests are of diagnostic value and must supplement direct examination (Fig. 20-2).

ARTERIOGRAPHY

Injection of a radiopaque contrast substance into the lumen of a main artery will permit visualization of the internal anatomical configuration of the artery and its tributaries. The contrast medium is injected into the vessel through a needle that has been introduced into the vessel percutaneously, or a guide wire may be passed through the needle under image amplifier fluoroscopic control, the needle withdrawn, and a catheter inserted over the guide wire to the desired level before the contrast medium is injected (Seldinger technique Fig. 20-3).[5]

Sequential filming makes it possible to visualize remote parts of the vascular tree, including pathologic changes in smaller vessels and individual organs. Refinements of catheter placement technique, the use of new contrast agents, and the development of x-ray equipment and rapid film changers permitting continuous rapid filming from the start of the injection of the medium have created the roentgenologic subspecialty of angiography.

Contrast Media. Contrast media are hypertonic solutions of organic, triiodinated, water-soluble compounds. The ideal contrast medium possesses high iodine concentration, for maximum contrast; low toxicity; and low viscosity, for better flow. Many contrast agents are

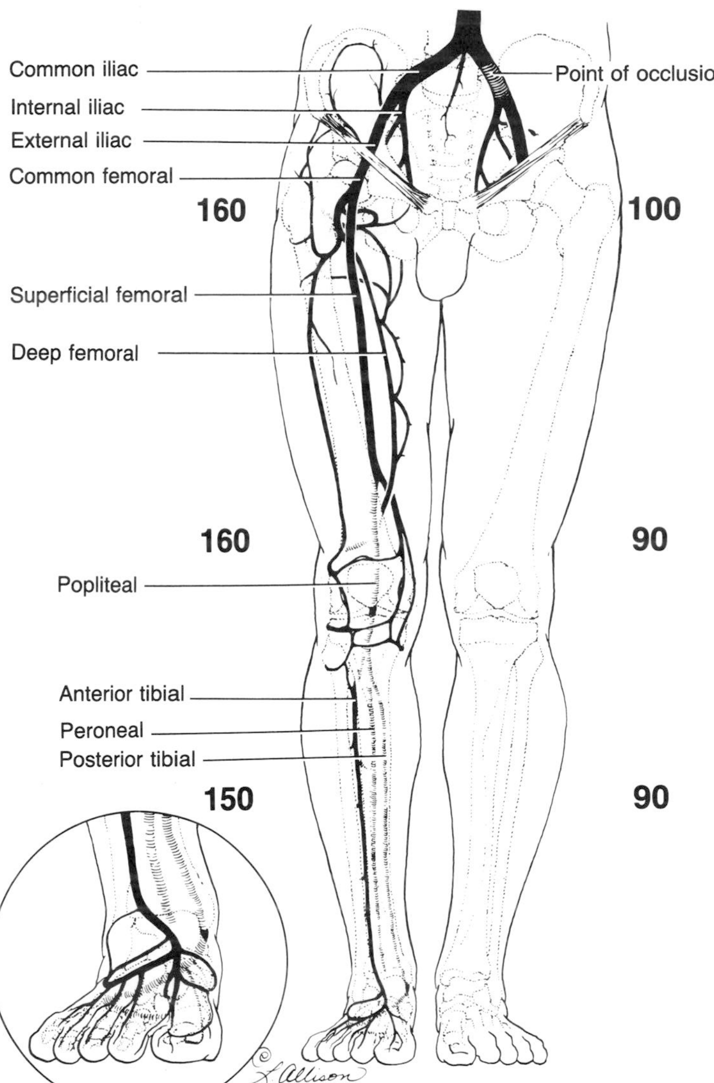

FIG. 20-2. Diagram for recording preoperative assessment of blood flow in the lower extremity as determined by Doppler readings at the ankle, plethysmographic tracings at the toes, and arteriography. Illustrated is an occlusion proximal to the inguinal ligament. Low systolic pressure at the upper thigh establishes the occlusion above this level. Distal to this point, the gradients are normal between successive levels. A reduction of more than 20 mm Hg suggests arterial stenosis or obstruction between two levels and must be confirmed by arteriography. Gradients in the range of 40 mm Hg to 80 mm Hg signify complete segmental occlusion of a main artery.

Below the knee, if either the anterior tibial or posterior tibial artery alone is open, the pressure gradient from below the knee to the ankle is usually normal. When the gradient exceeds 30 mm Hg, both arteries are occluded.

available, varying in their iodine content, which must be adequate for maximum contrast, yet keeping the sodium ion to a minimum for reduced toxicity. Compounds containing methylglucosamine have reduced osmolarity and toxicity but increased the viscosity, thereby impairing the flow rate necessary for peripheral angiography. Meglumine salts of about 28% iodine content are preferable.

Complications. The most common complications of arteriography are the following:

1. *Contrast Agent Toxicity*
   a. Allergy, anaphylaxis. Preliminary skin testing is of no value. One should inquire into allergies, particularly seafoods. Bronchial asthma is a relative contraindication. When allergy is suspected, steroids and antihistamines should be administered before and during the procedure.
   b. Neurotoxicity. This occurs especially during abdominal aortography. The use of a 100% methylglucosamine agent will lessen this problem.
2. *Hematoma Formation*
3. *Dissection of Plaques or Intima.* This is due to penetration by the catheter or the rapid injection of a large volume.
4. *Arterial Spasm.* An intra-arterial vasodilator (*e.g.*, procaine) is injected.
5. *Arterial Thrombosis.* This occurs in 0.5% of transfem-

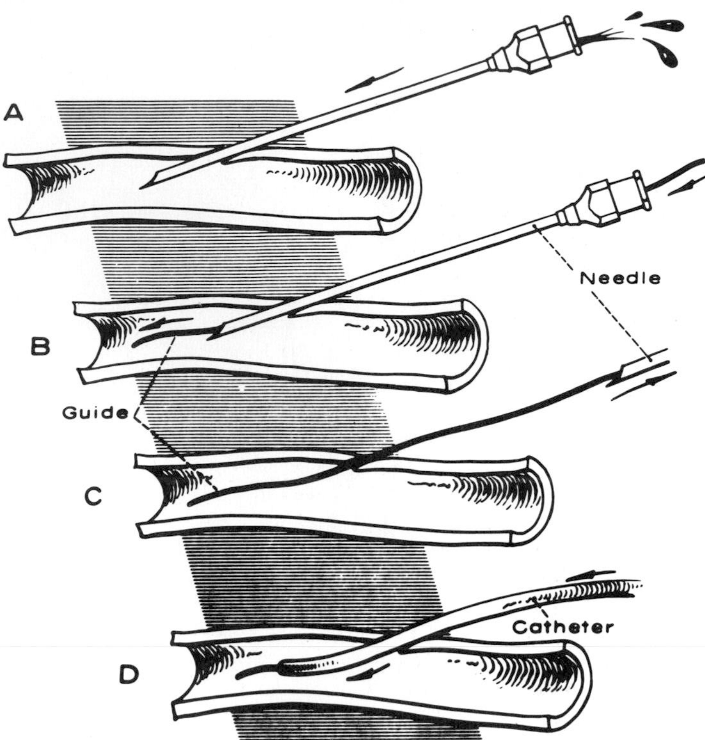

FIG. 20-3. Technique of percutaneous arterial catheterization for aortography or arteriography. (*A*) The artery is punctured. (*B*) A guide wire is inserted. (*C*) The needle is being removed. (*D*) A catheter is passed over the guide wire into the artery. (Kincaid OW, Davis GD: Renal Angiography. Chicago, Year Book Medical Publishers, 1966)

oral or axillary arteriograms.[4] At first, it may not be distinguished from spasm. If, unrelieved by injection of a vasodilator, the pulse remains absent and the extremity remains cold and discolored, early surgical exploration and thrombectomy are indicated; if the vessel is damaged, arterial reconstruction is warranted.

6. *False Aneurysms.* These can occur at the puncture site.

7. *Embolism.* A catheter loosens clots or lifts up plaque. A clot may form on the catheter, from which it is loosened and carried distally as the catheter is withdrawn.

Lower Extremity Studies. When severe atheromatous occlusive disease of the lower extremities is associated with extensive involvement of the large abdominal vessels, it is important to evaluate the inflow proximal to the femoral region, as well as the runoff distal to it.[3] For example, replacement or bypass of an occluded segment of the superficial femoral artery may prove to be ineffectual if flow through the aorto-iliac region is insufficient.

The differential diagnosis of low back pain and pain about the hip or lower extremity often requires precise information about the blood flow of the aorto-iliac complex.

To visualize the abdominal aorta and vessels of the lower extremities, the following two routes are used:

Retrograde Aortoarteriography

The catheter is passed from the femoral artery at the inguinal region backward through the aorto-iliac junction into the abdominal aorta. Locally, complications include hematoma, arterial spasm, thrombosis, and pseudoaneurysm; proximally, injury to the aorta, especially subintimal dissection, is the main complication.

Translumbar Aortoarteriography

The medium is introduced by needle directly into the aorta. If one femoral pulse is palpable, the aorta may be punctured below the renal artery level. When both femoral pulses are absent and extensive involvement of the lower abdominal aorta is likely, puncture at too low a level may be hazardous. Therefore, aortic puncture may be made at the level of the 12th thoracic vertebra. The catheter is introduced retrograde before the injection is made. An alternative route is passage of a catheter by way of the left brachial or axillary artery.

Complications of translumbar aortoarteriography include periaortic bleeding, intramural dissection, visceral damage to organs supplied by the celiac axis and renal or mesenteric arteries, and neurologic sequelae. The latter is possible when a large volume is injected in the presence of obstruction or with injection in the proximity of a lumbar artery. Neurologic complications are rare with the use of meglumine diatrizoate.

Direct femoral arteriography is performed when aortic visualization is unnecessary. Arterial puncture is carried out using a 19- or 20-gauge needle connected to a polyvinyl tubing-stopcock-syringe assembly, the system being prefilled with normal saline solution. The needle tip is directed upstream. Then the saline-containing syringe is replaced with a syringe containing contrast medium, and an injection of approximately 15 ml to 35 ml is made manually. Serial films are exposed during and for a period of time after the injection, the length of such time varying according to the circulation time (several seconds to as long as 50 seconds). Premedication may be used for apprehensive patients, but otherwise no anesthesia or analgesia is necessary.

Upper Extremity Studies. When the subclavian, axillary, and brachial vessels must be visualized, the contrast medium is best introduced into the proximal aorta by retrograde catheterization, preferably through the femoral artery. The catheter is introduced percutaneously into the femoral artery and passed to the desired location in the thoracic aorta or selectively into the brachiocephalic vessels.[5] The method is admirably suited for defining the thoracic outlet syndrome.

Arteries of the arm at a more distal level are visualized by direct puncture of the brachial artery beyond the axillary fold. The dose of medium is usually 20 ml to 25 ml.

Interpretation of Arteriograms of the Extremities. A normal arteriogram is characterized by a smooth, uninterrputed contour of the lumina, a direct course of the vessels, and only a minimum of collateral vessels. A vessel in certain situations normally changes its course, but the change of direction is gradual, not abrupt. Spasm of an artery is characterized by smooth diminution in caliber as the point of occlusion is approached and a gradual resumption of caliber beyond the constriction. The appearance typically varies from film to film.

Collateral arteries become prominent in number and size as main arteries are occluded. These compensatory vessels are identified by an irregular twisting and turning course, variation in size in the same locale, purposeless crossing and recrossing, a transverse course in areas in which they are profuse, and anastomoses. When an artery is partially occluded, an anastomotic branch often forms proximal to the point of occlusion and can be seen running alongside the parent artery, reentering the artery distally. When a digital artery is occluded, numerous minute collateral arteries pass laterally from the companion to the diseased artery. When radial and ulnar arteries are occluded, the interosseous artery, which ordinarily is never visualized beyond the level of the wrist, extends distalward to compensate for loss of blood supply. Complete occlusion of a large artery throughout its course may be compensated by formation of numerous large branches arising above the site of occlusion.

Arteriographic Characteristics. Arteriographic characteristics of peripheral vascular disease are the following (Fig. 20-4):

Thromboangiitis Obliterans (TAO)

Patchy distribution of changes chiefly affecting the peripherally situated small-caliber vessels is characteristic. Adjacent vessels may be affected to a different degree. Involvement is revealed by a moth-eaten, irregular filling of defects, narrowing of the lumen, irregular changes in caliber from segment to segment, and an irregular, rapidly changing course. When occlusion is complete, the point of obstruction is rounded rather than abrupt. Collateral vessels are numerous, more so than in ASO.

Arteriosclerosis Obliterans (ASO)

Typically, the roentgenographic features are extremely irregular lumina, narrow caliber, moth-eaten contour, and a moderate number of collateral vessels.

Aneurysm

The sac often is filled with clotted blood, and the radiopaque material fails to enter the cavity; nevertheless, the shadow of the vessels is interrupted abruptly at the level of the rounded soft tissue density, and the distal vessel is frequently visualized beyond the mass (Fig. 20-5). Occasionally, a thin line of increased density forms a border about the sac.

Arteriovenous Fistula

The arteriographic features are increased size and tortuosity of arteries leading the fistula, pooling of the radiopaque substance in the region of the fistula, absence of filling of the arteries distal to the fistula, and visualization of the veins more rapidly than usual.

Raynaud's Disease

The distal portions of the digital arteries fail to fill, and their caliber is diminished.

Bone Tumors

In benign tumors, the blood vessels may be displaced but are of normal size and number. Malignant tumors often exhibit numerous vascular pedicles and a profuse network of newly formed vessels.

Arterial Occlusion

The site of obstruction can be localized prior to surgical intervention. When no surgery is contemplated, arteriography is contraindicated because it may provoke spasm of the collaterals.

An acute occlusion in a young person without occlusive arterial disease (*e.g.*, entrapment of the brachial artery between the fragments of a supracondylar fracture of the humerus) may require arteriography before surgical exposure of the site of injury. The contrast medium is blocked in an otherwise normal-appearing vessel, and no collaterals are demonstrable.

When acute occlusion occurs in an arterioscle-

(Text continues on page 776.)

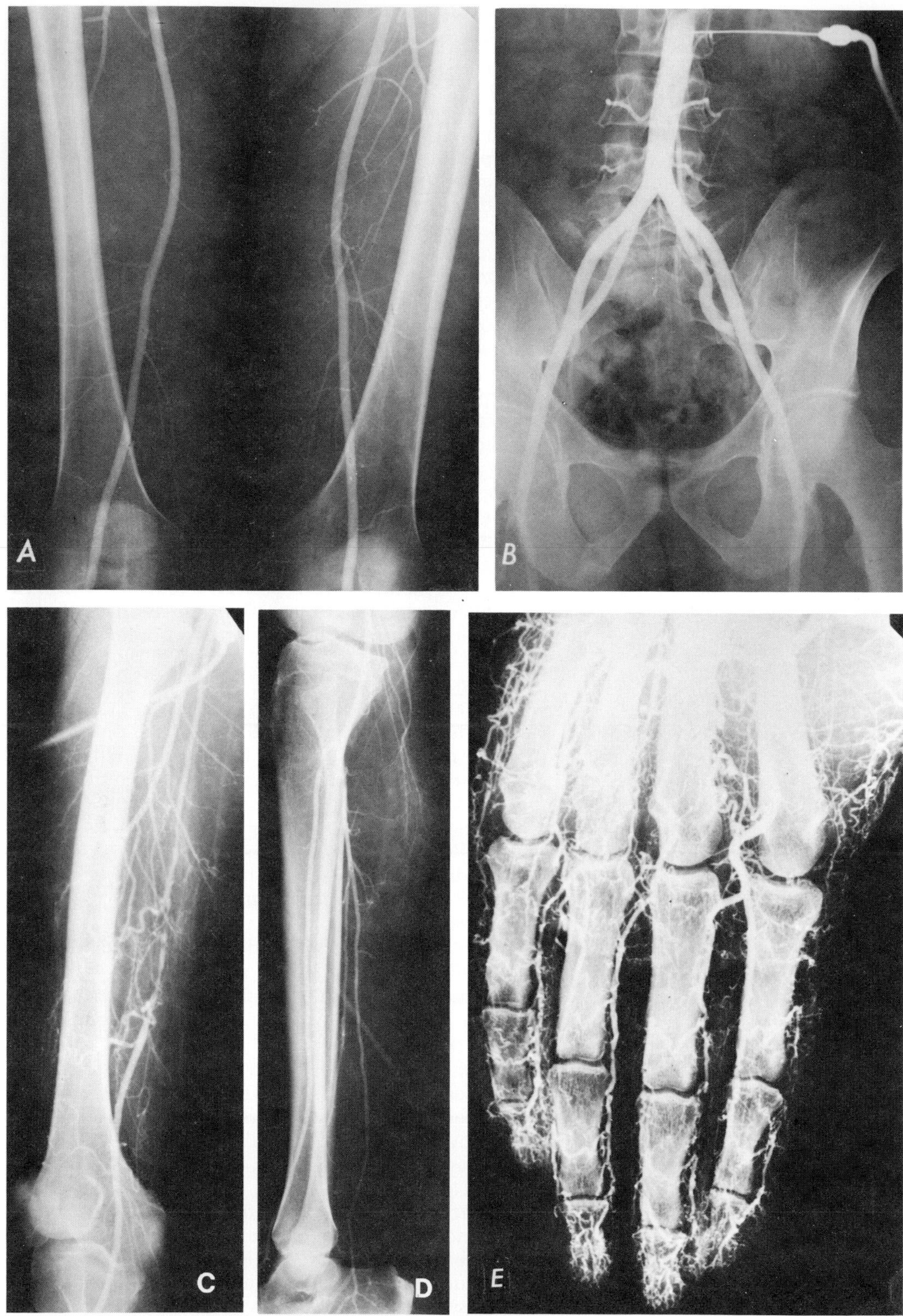
A
B
C
D
E

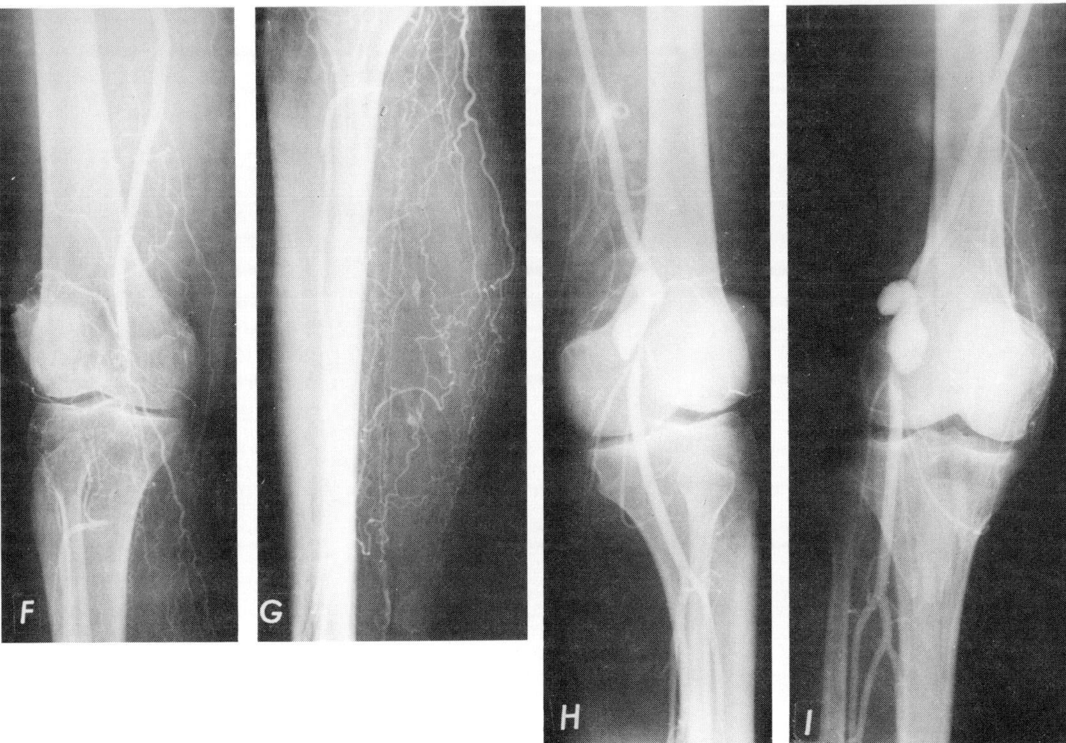

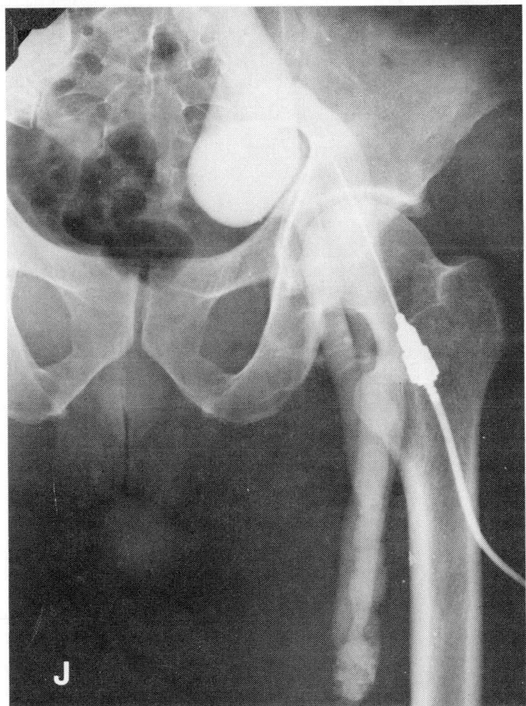

◀ **FIG. 20-4.** Arteriograms, their characteristics in disease. (*A* and *B*) The normal arteriogram. The aorta and the iliac and femoral vessels are of uniform caliber and are smooth and regular in outline. (*C* and *D*) Arteriosclerosis obliterans, showing complete occlusion of the midportion of the superficial femoral artery. There is good distal filling below the obstruction, but all of the vessles show mild irregularities of their lumina, denoting atheromas. (*E*) Thromboangiitis obliterans. This disease has many different characteristics. This arteriogram of an affected hand shows occlusion of most of the digital vessels, with collateral branching, which is nature's way of maintaining adequate circulation. (*F* and *G*) Acute arterial occlusion of the popliteal artery following trauma. Except for the occluded segment, the vessels are fairly normal in appearance. (*H* and *I*) Arteriosclerotic aneurysm of the popliteal artery. The arteriogram demonstrates the channel through the aneurysm. Clinically, the aneurysm is much larger, since most of its interior is filled with clot. (*J*) Traumatic arteriovenous fistula. This is an abnormal communication between the superficial femoral vessels due to a gunshot wound. Note the enormous dilatation of the proximal vein. (Courtesy of John C. Ivins)

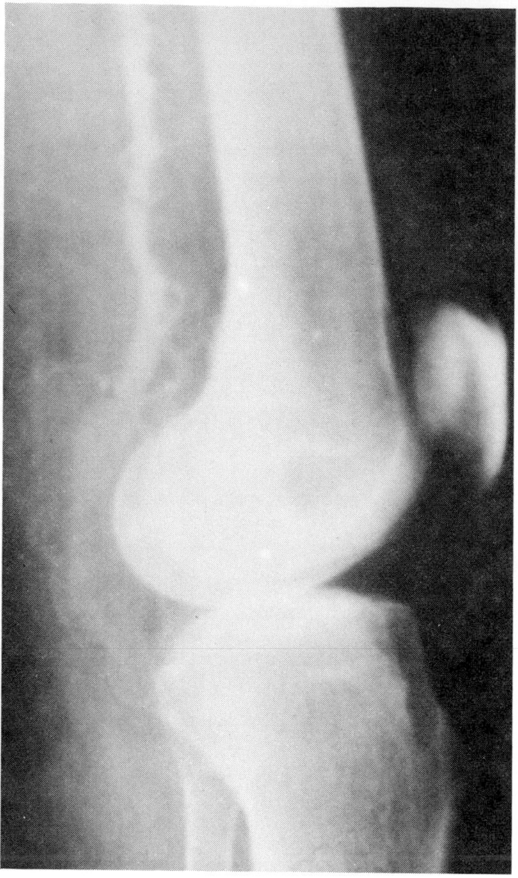

FIG. 20-5. An aneurysm of the popliteal artery is demonstrated by angiography.

rotic vessel, the vessel proximal to the site of obstruction shows the characteristic irregularities of multiple sites of encroachment, and collateral vessels may be visible.

Gradually developing occlusion (chronic occlusion), in addition to presenting the picture of the causative disease, will generally demonstrate evidence of collateral vessels, which are often extensively developed and sufficient for peripheral blood flow.

VENOGRAPHY

The veins are best visualized by injecting Hypaque Sodium 50% into a small vein (Fig. 20-6). For example, the medium is injected into a vein in the foot while a tourniquet occludes the greater saphenous vein above the ankle, thus forcing the dye into the deep venous system. This will localize any clots within the deep venous system and is thus very useful in acute thrombosis and chronic occlusion.[6] By following the course of the dye through the proximal portion of the greater saphenous, incompetent perforating vessels may be demonstrated.

VASCULAR FUNCTION STUDIES

Physiological Principles. Arterial narrowing and occlusion force the blood to follow alternate pathways (collaterals). Since the collaterals are high-resistance conduits, an abnormal pressure gradient develops across the area of involvement. In early disease or segmental localized occlusion with good collaterals, the first change is a reduction of systolic pressure distally. When occlusion occurs at multiple levels, the resistance of the collateral beds is additive and produces a further decrease of distal arterial pressure. As the disease increases in more major arteries, distal pressure may be very low, flow becomes less pulsatile, and distal blood flow is highly dependent on critical collateral pathways. Although the systolic pressure nearly always becomes lowered distal to areas of arterial obstruction, the blood flow level in resting skin and muscle is nearly always normal. At this relatively early stage, abnormalities in flow secondary to arterial obstruction can be brought out by exercise or by 5 minutes of arterial occlusion (reactive hyperemia test).[9]

FIG. 20-6. Normal venogram of the hand. Veins in contrast with arteries pursue an irregular course and communicate freely with one another.

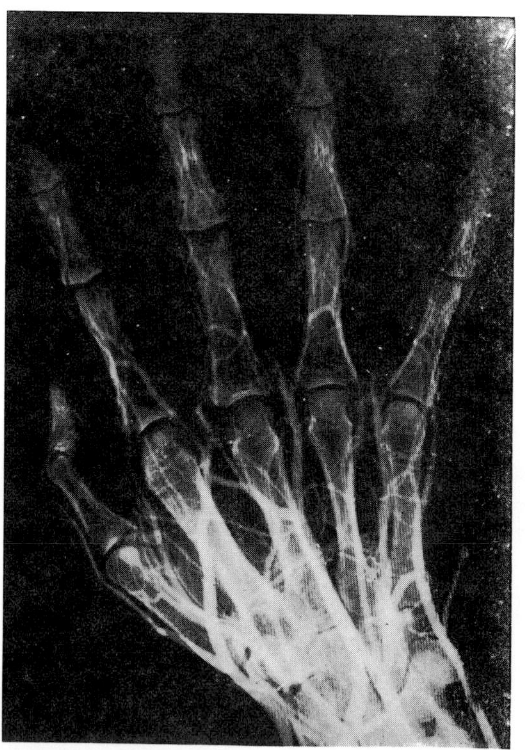

Pressure Measurements. The degree of regional hypotension that develops distal to an area of narrowing or occlusion can be measured by a variety of techniques, the following being representative:

1. Ultrasonic velocity detector[10]
2. Mercury strain gauge plethysmography[9]
3. Capacitance pulse pickups[7]

These instruments are used as sensors to indicate the point at which blood flow is restored to a limb distal to a point of pneumatic compression when the cuff has been deflated from above the regional blood pressure perfusing the limb.

Various techniques have been devised to study the circulation of the extremities. Arteriography has been used and continues to be used to define the anatomical structure of large and medium-sized arteries, but with definite limitations. Instruments using noninvasive methods can now define with precision points of occlusion, the velocity and character of blood flow, and the adequacy of the collaterals. These procedures are particularly useful for evaluating the degree of vascularity of distal areas of the limbs where pulsations are not palpable. For the orthopaedic surgeon, these methods serve to differentiate a vascular from an orthopaedic disorder, to evaluate vascular suitability for a planned orthopaedic procedure, to weigh the risk of a vascular reconstructive procedure against the rehabilitative advantage of immediate amputation, and to determine the level of amputation.

The sensor may be placed over a digit (mercury strain gauge plethysmograph) or dorsalis pedis or posterior tibial artery (ultrasonic velocity detector). The systolic blood pressure is estimated at the level of the upper thigh and lower thigh, below the knee, and at the level of the ankle and then compared to that recorded from the upper arm. At the ankle, the systolic pressure at this level is normally equal to or higher than the brachial systolic pressure.

When arterial occlusion exists at one or more levels, the lowered systolic pressure at the ankle reflects the degree of proximal resistance to blood flow. The ankle-arm pressure can be expressed as a ratio (normal = 1.0 or slightly greater). Although the systemic blood pressure may fluctuate on a day-to-day basis, the ratio is unaffected. Therefore, any change in the ratio permits an estimate of increasing or decreasing blood flow. As additional disease develops, with increasing resistance to blood flow, the ankle-arm pressure ratio will correspondingly decrease. With successful arterial reconstruction, removing areas of abnormally high resistance will restore the ratio toward normal.

The ankle systolic pressure is sensitive to exercise.[8] Measurements are made before and after moderate treadmill exercise (2 mph on 12% grade). Normally, no fall in ankle systolic pressure occurs, and it may actually increase. A patient with intermittent claudication will sustain a drop in ankle pressure with delayed return to baseline levels. This test exposes the individual circulatory response to stress. In arterial occlusion, it tests the ability of the collateral circulation to respond to the increased flow requirements brought on by exercising.

Resting flow determinations in patients with extensive multilevel disease and palpable pedal pulses are of little value, since the results are usually in the normal range. Determinations are best made in the immediate post-exercise period, particularly when claudication can be provoked by the exercise.

DOPPLER ULTRASOUND FLOW VELOCITY METER

An ultrasound beam of 5 or 10 MHz (megacycles per second) emitting from a ceramic crystal, excited by an electric oscillator, is passed through an underlying blood vessel (Fig. 20-7). Ultrasound reflected from red cells is shifted in frequency by an amount proportional to the flow velocity of the red cells. The backscattered sound is detected by another crystal mounted adjacent to the transmitting crystal. This backscattered sound is mixed with the transmitted frequency to produce a signal within the audible range. The pitch of this audio frequency signal is proportional to the blood flow velocity within the vessel. A high velocity of blood movement causes a higher pitched sound than a low-velocity movement. The audible output is amplified and used to drive a loudspeaker or headphones.

By using pulsed ultrasound, based on the same principle of echo-ranging as naval sonar, so that a periodic short burst of ultrasound is produced, the instrument can sample signals from discrete points along the vessel, making it possible to sample blood flow from any selected point (Fig. 20-8).[12,14]

Auscultation. Audible signals are obtained by placing the transducer (flow probe) over an artery. Normal arterial sounds consist of first, second, and third sounds; the pitch rises abruptly to a high peak during systole and falls during diastole. Arterial sounds are recognized by the changes in velocity during each cardiac cycle. Venous sounds, in contrast, are dependent on respiration.

In patients with occlusive or stenotic lesions of proximal arteries and in whom pedal pulses are not palpable, flow signals can usually be obtained over the posterior tibial or dorsalis pedis arteries. Abnormal sounds are heard that result from collateral flow and are of low pitch. Second and third sounds are absent. The flow signal immediately beyond the point of stenosis senses high-velocity flow characterized by a higher pitched sound superimposed on a continuous low-frequency sound. This indicates turbulent flow.

Venous sound, on the other hand, is cyclic with respiration and resembles the noise produced by a windstorm. On holding one's breath or performing the Valsalva maneuver, flow ceases and no sound is heard.

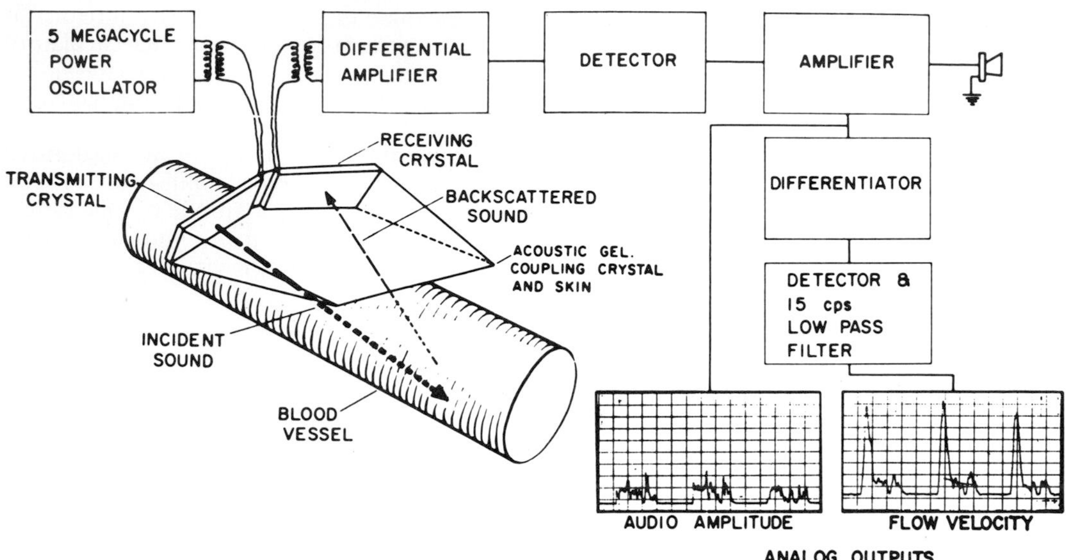

FIG. 20-7. Block diagram of the transcutaneous Doppler flowmeter. (Strandness DE Jr, McCutcheon EP, Rushmer RF: Application of transcutaneous Doppler flowmeter in evaluation of occlusive arterial disease. Surg Gynecol Obstet 122:1039, 1966)

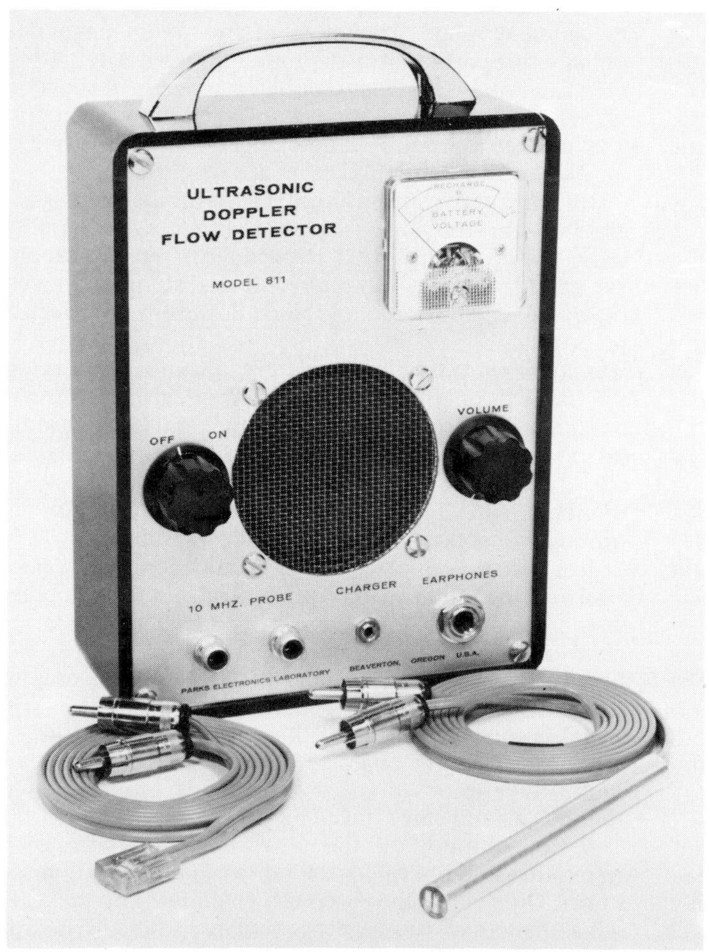

FIG. 20-8. The ultrasonic blood velocity detector. (Courtesy of Parks Electronics Laboratory)

When intra-abdominal pressure is released or inspiration is resumed, rapid venous flow develops, characterized by a loud roaring sound.

Venous flow can be determined proximal or distal to the site of venous occlusion or thrombosis. In total proximal venous occlusion, the sound recorded distal to the site of obstruction is not affected by the respiratory maneuvers. It is continuous and rumbling. The diagnosis of venous occlusion can be made by determining whether venous flow velocity at a proximal level is affected by compression applied at a distal level. In the presence of a normal, patent deep venous system, a surge of blood can be heard in the common femoral vein when the calf muscle is squeezed by the examiner (augmented sound). Absence of an audible or augmented sound suggests an occlusion between the flow probe and the compression site.

Flow Velocity Wave Forms. Audible signals can be converted to analogue output and displayed graphically. Such records are useful for following progression of arterial occlusion or for recording blood flow over a period following arterial reconstruction (Fig. 20-9).

Normal arterial flow velocity is triphasic in pattern, corresponding to audible sounds. The major deflection represents forward flow during systole; the second deflection is caused by reversed flow of low frequency during diastole; the third signal represents return of forward flow.

Distal to an occlusion, the abnormal sound is represented by a monophasic pattern resulting from collateral flow, characterized by slow acceleration during systole, delayed deceleration, low systolic peak velocity, and absence of second and third deflections (Fig. 20-10).

The flow velocity pattern immediately below a stenotic lesion in which high-velocity flow is present is manifested by a rapid rise and fall of systolic flow with absent second and third deflections. The flow pattern becomes irregular when there is a palpable thrill.

Venous flow velocity patterns are characterized by a slow, clear respiratory cycle. During breath holding or the Valsalva maneuver, a flat wave form appears. With resumption of respiration, a high flow rate is seen. With total proximal venous occlusion, respiratory waves are not transmitted and the flow rate is not affected by breath holding or the Valsalva maneuver.

Segmental Pressure Gradients. The transducer is placed over the posterior tibial or dorsalis pedis artery. The blood pressure cuff is placed at the level at which audible

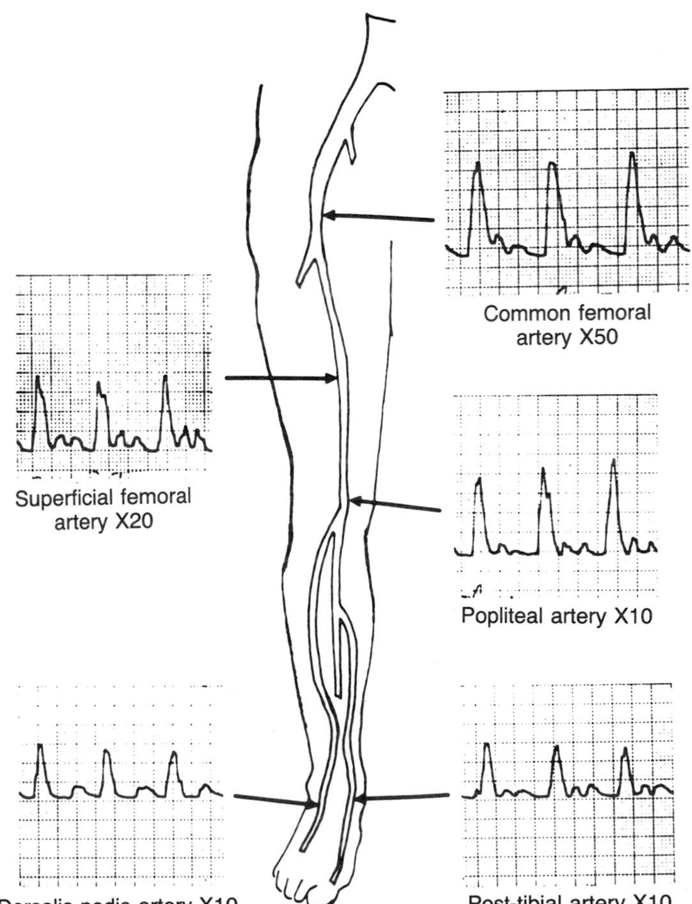

FIG. 20-9. Velocity patterns recorded from the major arteries of the lower extremity. (Strandness DE Jr, McCutcheon EP, Rushmer RF: Application of transcutaneous Doppler flowmeter in evaluation of occlusive arterial disease. Surg Gynecol Obstet 122: 1039, 1966)

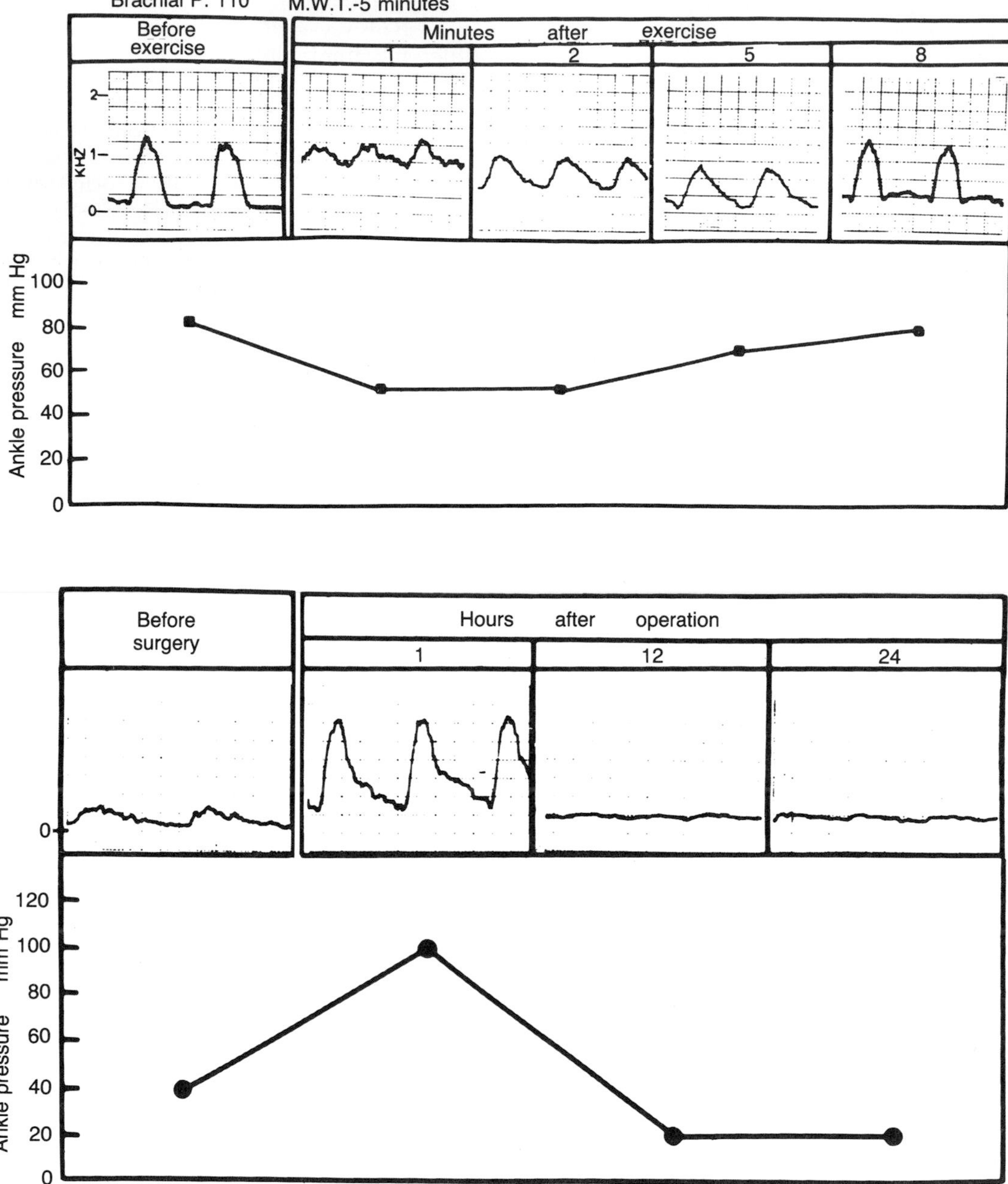

FIG. 20-10. (*Top*) Simultaneous recording of posterior tibial artery flow velocity patterns and ankle pressure before and after exercise in a patient with femoral artery occlusion. Both flow and pressure are decreased after treadmill exercise. (*Bottom*) Monitoring of the flow velocity pattern and ankle systolic pressure in a patient who underwent femoropopliteal artery reconstruction. After initial success, occlusion of the graft was seen at 12 hours postoperatively. (Yao ST, Bergan JJ: Application of ultrasound to arteriol and venous diagnosis. Surg Clin North Am 54:23, 1974)

sound returns while the cuff is deflated. Next, the cuff is placed at the lower thigh, and the systolic pressure is determined. Normally, the pressure drop between the two points is about 10 mm Hg. An excessive differential (*e.g.*, 50 mm Hg) indicates occlusion of the superficial femoral artery. Systolic pressure measurements are also taken just below the knee and at the level of the ankle, and any excessive lowering of pressure is similarly interpreted as representing occlusive disease in the main vessel(s) between the two points (see Fig. 20-2).

In the normal subject, the pressure in the ankle when measured in the supine position is equal to or higher than that in the upper extremity. The ratio of ankle pressure to brachial pressure is a convenient indication of the degree of ischemia. Normally, the pressure index (PI) is greater than 1.0. With intermittent claudication, the average PI is 0.59. With rest pain and impending gangrene, the PI ranges from 0.26 to 0.05, respectively.[13] Even in the presence of arteriographic evidence of poor distal runoff, a reconstructible popliteal artery is assured if the ankle pressure is above 20 mm Hg.

Exercise Test. Using the standard treadmill test, moderate exercise causes a slight increase in ankle blood pressure; cessation of muscle activity allows ankle pressure to return rapidly to normal. With arterial occlusion, a profound drop in ankle pressure develops with exercise, and there is marked delay in return to preexercise levels.

Clinical Applications. For the orthopaedic surgeon, functional studies are essential for the following:

- Evaluating ischemic pain
- Differentiating ischemia from other causes of pain
- Determining the degree of circulatory adequacy for orthopaedic operation
- Determining priorities: vascular reconstruction versus immediate amputation
- Determining the level of amputation

The Doppler device is convenient. Despite impalpable distal pulsations, transcutaneous flow detection using low-intensity ultrasound will reveal flow signals over the posterior tibial or dorsalis pedis artery.

The level of ankle pressure is determined and the ankle-brachial pressure ratio is calculated. Patients with intermittent claudication are thus differentiated from those who develop pain of other causes. In patients with intact peripheral pulses, ischemic pain under conditions of exercise must always be considered. Such differentiation may be difficult, and one may need to rely on graphic patterns. Graphic velocity patterns appear abnormal, ankle pressure becomes less than brachial pressure, and flow is markedly decreased immediately following the standard treadmill exercise.

Measurements of pressure gradients at different levels (*e.g.*, upper thigh, lower thigh, below knee, and ankle) may reveal a marked lowering between two levels, indicating occlusive disease; nevertheless, a normal pressure gradient from below the knee to the ankle indicates adequate collateral flow about the area of obstruction and patency of one or more large vessels beyond the knee.

This testing should supplement angiography to ascertain the status of flow distal to an arterial occlusion. A PI of 0.45 to 0.50 is usually accompanied by a good distal runoff. A reconstructible popliteal artery can be assured if ankle pressure is above 20 mm Hg. When flow or pressure from pedal arteries is not detectable and there is angiographic evidence of poor runoff, angioplastic or bypass procedures are unlikely to succeed. Further, such an inadvisable operation may compromise the chances for success of a below-knee amputation.

Arterial reconstructive procedures are especially not indicated when an abnormal pressure gradient of more than 30 mm Hg is present from below the knee to the ankle. This indicates distal occlusive disease involving all three vessels below the knee, and arterial reconstruction is associated with a high incidence of failure. This is most common in diabetics.

The level of amputation must be determined and if possible carried out distal to the knee. A thigh systolic blood pressure above 80 mm Hg generally assures a successful below-knee amputation.

MERCURY STRAIN GAUGE PLETHYSMOGRAPH

The mercury strain gauge consists of a small-caliber elastic tube filled with mercury and contoured to fit the distal phalanx of a finger or toe (Fig. 20-11). It detects the minute increase in volume of the digit that occurs with each heartbeat. This phasic change in digit volume transmits pressures to the mercury column. The resistance

FIG. 20-11. Placement of the mercury strain gauge on a toe. The nonexpansible portion is over the base of the nail. Digit pulses are normal and are characterized by a sharp systolic peak and a dicrotic wave on the downslope.

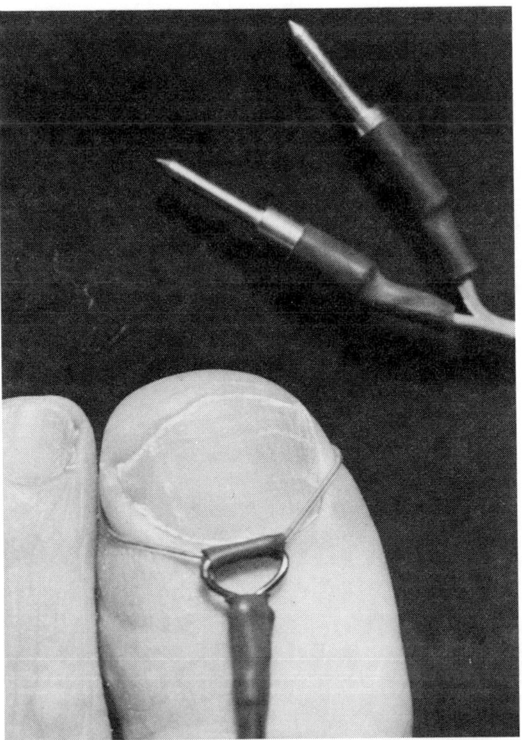

changes in the mercury column, by using an appropriate matching circuit, can be amplified and recorded graphically.[9,11]

Pressure Measurements. Specially contoured pneumatic cuffs are placed at the upper arm and about the lower extremity at the upper thigh and lower thigh, below the knee, and at the ankle (Fig. 20-12). At each level the cuff is inflated above the systolic pressure, then gradually lowered until restoration of digital blood flow, as indicated on the plethysmographic tracing. Normally, the pressure drop between two successive levels proceeding distally is about 10 mm Hg.

FIG. 20-12. Typical normal systolic pressures at the levels at which they are usually determined. A pneumatic cuff is placed at each level and inflated until the pulsations disappear, as shown in the tracing. The cuff is deflated until an upward shift in the baseline occurs, the point of systolic pressure. In plethysmography with the mercury strain gauge, this is the point at which toe blood flow volume increases. (Strandness DE Jr, Radke HM, Bell JW: Use of a new simplified plethysmograph in the clinical evaluation of patients with arteriosclerosis obliterans. Surg Gynecol Obstet 112:751, 1961)

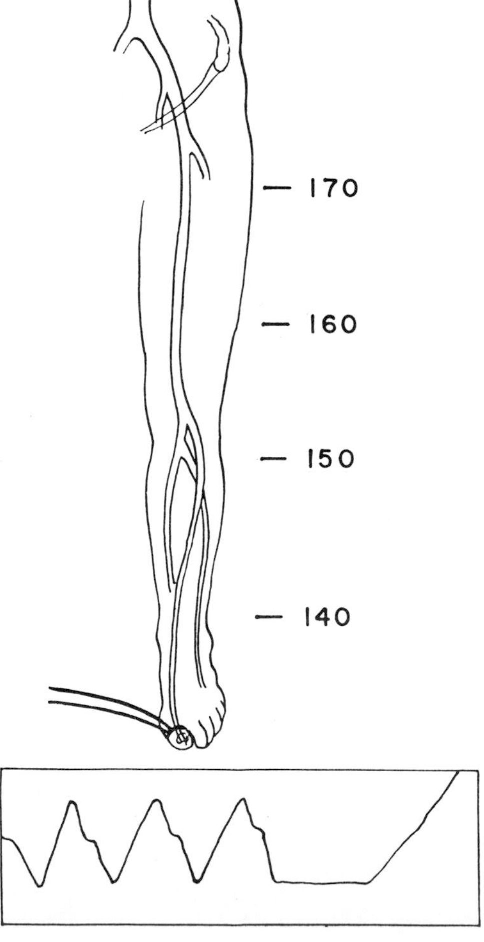

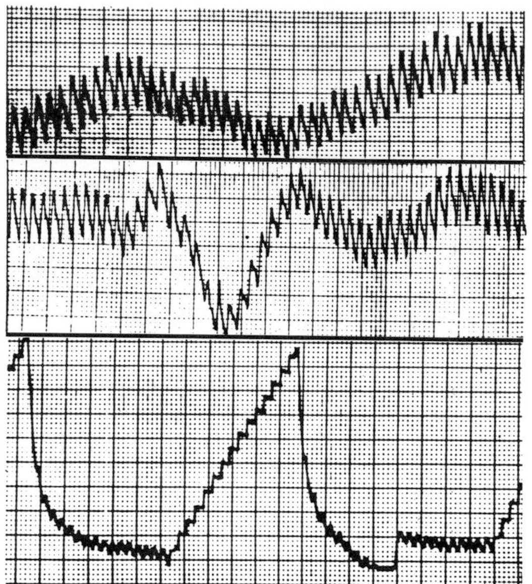

FIG. 20-13. The upper tracing shows the slow waves, the result of rhythmic changes in vasomotor activity. The center tracing shows the sharp decrease in digit volume, the result of a deep inspiration. The lower tracing shows the normal venous congestion test, producing a marked stepwise increase in digit volume. At the peak of the response, the cuff is deflated and digit volume rapidly returns to normal. (Strandness DE Jr, Radke HM, Bell JW: Use of a new simplified plethysmograph in the clinical evaluation of patients with arteriosclerosis obliterans. Surg Gynecol Obstet 112:751, 1961)

Pulse Contour and Volume. The normal peripheral pulse curve has a well-defined systolic peak and a dicrotic wave on the downslope. Anxiety produces vasoconstriction and decrease of pulse amplitude.

Vasomotor Activity and Reflexes. Normally, regular rhythmic changes in vasomotor activity appear as cyclic shifts of the baseline of the plethysmographic pulse curve, termed slow waves (Fig. 20-13). The amplitude of these gradual waves is proportional to sympathetic activity. For example, increased sympathetic function (vasoconstriction) can be provoked by deep inspiration, which causes a sharp decrease in digital volume, the slow wave dropping well below the baseline.

Digital Blood Flow. The rate of flow of arterial blood into the distal portion of the extremity can be demonstrated by temporarily occluding the venous return. By placing a pneumatic cuff about the ankle and inflating it to 50 mm Hg, a stepwise marked increase in digital volume is noted. This sudden upward shift of the baseline of the tracing is the result of arterial inflow.

Mercury strain gauge plethysmography is another method for determining the level of occlusion and adequacy of collateral flow. With short segmental occlusion and good collateral flow, digital pulse volume may be normal. With poor collateral flow, the pulse wave loses its sharp upward inflection and may become flattened.

With far-advanced diffuse occlusive involvement, pulsatile digital flow may be absent.

The method presently is used in certain limited situations, such as for determining the suitability of a patient for sympathectomy. The success of sympathectomy depends on the degree of arterial pressure and the ability of the arterioles to respond to sympathetic denervation. This is determined as follows:

Large pulse waves: indicate good collateral circulation and absence of significant disease in small arteries.

Large slow waves and active inspiratory reflex: indicate active sympathetic function in small arteries.

Reactive hyperemia test: ankle cuff is inflated above systolic pressure, left in place for 5 minutes, then deflated. Normally, potent vasodilatation takes place, and pulse amplitude increases at least 50%, reflecting good arterial inflow.

ANESTHESIA

General anesthesia causes widespread vasodilatation. Spinal anesthesia will effect vasodilatation only in the area of sensory loss. Likewise, injection of an anesthetic into a peripheral nerve will cause a rise of temperature in the anesthetic zone. For practical purposes, the sympathetic block determines maximal vasodilatation of the part. Normally, the lower limit of surface temperature of the great toe after sympathetic block should be approximately 31.5°C. When this reading is lower or a minimal rise of temperature occurs after a sympathetic block, organic occlusive arterial disease is the main cause of impaired circulation. An abrupt rise in skin temperature implicates arterial or arteriolar spasm as the offending factor, and this can be overcome by sympathectomy.

ARTERIOSCLEROSIS OBLITERANS

Arteriosclerosis obliterans (ASO) is characterized by occlusion of large and medium-sized arteries, mainly in the lower extremities, by extensive atheromatous formations and thrombi, causing peripheral ischemia.

ETIOLOGY

The cause of arteriosclerosis is unknown. Theories include the following:

Mechanical cause—a result of continual pulsating trauma of the arteries throughout life. This explains why hypertension is more frequently and earlier associated with arteriosclerosis, why atheromas are commonly found around the orifices of branches of the aorta, and why the more severe lesions are situated in the lower extremities in which blood pressure is higher.

Metabolic disturbances—particularly of cholesterol and lipoids. These explain why lipoids are contained in large amounts in atheromas and correspond in proportions of different constituents to those found in the blood plasma, why the lesion may be reproduced in experimental animals on a diet of cholesterol or animal fat, and why disorders manifested by lipemia are frequently complicated by severe and early atherosclerosis. Diabetes mellitus is a predisposing factor to severe and premature ASO.

PATHOLOGY

The lesions of ASO are situated predominantly in the large arteries (*e.g.*, iliac, femoral, and the popliteal of the lower extremities) and in medium-sized arteries (*e.g.*, anterior tibial and posterior tibial); rarely are the small arteries (*e.g.*, digital and plantar) involved.

Grossly, the arteries are enlarged, irregular, tortuous, and rigid. Sectioning reveals a thin medial coat, calcium deposits in the media or at the base of the atheromas, irregular atheromatous formations extending a considerable distance into the lumen, and partial or complete occlusion of the lumen by gray or red thrombi.

The atheroma is an elevated yellow plaque that consists of connective tissue thickening of the intima and phagocytic cells loaded within fat. These yellow patches tend to develop on one side of the artery and become confluent. As the atheroma enlarges, microscopically one sees large acellular, hyalinelike areas; irregular deposits of fat, fatty acids, and cholesterol; lipophages; fibroblasts; and fibrous tissue. Often a deposit of calcium is situated at the base of the atheroma. The surface is eroded and forms an irregular ulcer upon which a mural thrombus is deposited. Succeeding layers of thrombi are laid down and gradually occlude the artery. The deeper layers of thrombus become organized and merge imperceptibly with the atheroma. Recanalization occurs in some thrombi.

Other pathologic features, the result of ischemia, include atrophy and thinning of the skin, muscle atrophy with fibrofatty replacement, loss of subcutaneous fat, ulceration, and gangrene. Ischemic neuritis is usually associated with extensive arterial occlusion of larger arteries.[1]

PATHOGENESIS

The thrombosis will occur if the atheroma is large and its surface rough and ulcerated. It is more likely to develop in the presence of a blood dyscrasia, particularly polycythemia vera. Increased susceptibility to thrombosis may develop after operations, injuries, and infectious diseases, especially in cases of early atherosclerosis.

PATHOLOGIC PHYSIOLOGY

The obstructive lesions involve large arterial trunks predominantly. The degree of ischemia is proportionate to the extent of occlusion, including obstruction of potential collateral channels, to the height or most proximal point of the occluding process, and to the rapidity of the developing occlusion. Although extensive collateral channels can develop, because the arterial tree is rigid, the potential for formation of collaterals is not as great as in TAO.

Arteriolar constriction can be augmented by cold and tobacco; heat effects vasodilatation. The degree of arteriolar dilatation may be surprisingly great because the small arteries are not much affected by arteriosclerosis.

Arterial pressure is lowered beyond the point of obstruction, as evidenced by lower skin temperature, Doppler readings, and the elevation-dependency test. On elevation, the extremity becomes abnormally pale; on lowering the extremity, there is a delay in the return of color to the skin. Continuing the dependent position, there appears a rubor, the result of capillary atony. The capillaries are atonic because of ischemic malnutrition. Edema of the foot develops not only because of this atony but also because the patient constantly holds the foot in the dependent position to relieve the pain.

The presently accepted theory of the mechanism of production of intermittent claudication is as follows: Because of inadequate blood flow through muscles during exercise, a pain factor, factor P, accumulates and stimulates the sensory nerve endings. The pain disappears when collateral supply becomes adequate or when the affected muscle atrophies and becomes fibrotic.

CLINICAL PICTURE

The symptoms are those due to ischemia, and the findings are those of occlusive arterial disease. They are almost invariably confined to the lower extremity, in which they may come on gradually or abruptly.

The symptoms include the following:

Intermittent Claudication

This is the earliest symptom when arterial occlusion develops slowly. It is usually unilateral at first but eventually becomes bilateral. The extent of arterial occlusion determines the rapidity with which pain appears while walking. The pain is usually situated in the foot or calf when the occlusion is in the superficial femoral or popliteal artery and will appear in the thigh or buttocks when aorto-iliac occlusion is present.

When claudication is confined to the foot, the occlusion extensively involves the vessels distal to the knee. This is more characteristic of TAO.

Rest Pain

In severe degrees of occlusion the ischemia is made worse by the horizontal position. A severe, aching, persistent pain is noted in the toes, the foot, or the leg, especially at night. The patient sits up, rubs his foot, and holds it dependent to relieve the pain. An acute arterial occlusion will cause rest pain. Because this type of pain is frequently the forerunner of ulceration and gangrene, it is often referred to as pretrophic pain.

Pain of Ulceration and Gangrene

A persistent moderate or severe pain is similar to rest pain but is usually confined to the area of ulceration or gangrene.

Pain of Ischemic Neuritis

A paroxysmal, severe lancinating pain extends over the entire extremity and often follows the distribution of the peripheral nerve. Between paroxysms, a steady ache or burning sensation may be noted. This type of pain occurs commonly in the diabetic, when the upper femoral artery or common iliacs are occluded, or after a sudden severe arterial occlusion.

Paresthesias and Anesthesia

These are common and are probably due to ischemic neuritis. A complete stocking type of anesthesia of the toes or the foot or the entire leg develops after extensive acute arterial occlusion. It is a grave prognostic sign that indicates that gangrene will develop.

Cold Sensitivity

The patient complains of excessive coldness, even with slightly lowered environmental temperature.

The findings are the following:

Impaired Arterial Pulsations

These are determined by palpation. The dorsalis pedis is normally absent in 8% of patients and of itself is not necessarily significant. Regardless of the degree of atherosclerosis, reduction or absence of arterial pulsations is necessary to the diagnosis of arterial occlusion.

Color Changes

The toes may be red, bluish, or pale. Following recent acute occlusion, the foot may be extremely pale. Changes in color denote severe degrees of arterial occlusion.

Postural Color Changes

Abnormal pallor on elevation and delay of return of color followed by rubor on dependency, associated with delay in venous filling, are pathognomonic of occlusive arterial disease.

Temperture Changes

Lowered skin temperature, especially if a difference between the two feet is noted, is significant.

Trophic Changes, Ulceration, Gangrene, and Infection

The toes are scarred and shrunken. Ulceration and gangrene are often the result of avoidable trauma. When spontaneous, ulceration and gangrene usually develop in the terminal portions of the toes about the nails but may extend to involve the entire toe, occasionally the foot, and rarely the leg. Extensive gangrene denotes an acute or extensive occlusion without sufficient collaterals.

Ordinarily, ulceration and gangrene are of the dry type without systemic reaction. In diabetics, however, the lesions are often moist and infected, with rapid spread through the lymphatics and septicemia.

Minor infected lesions, such as paronychias, occur frequently. They may heal, or they may develop into gangrenous or ulcerative lesions, particularly if subjected to surgical interference.

Atrophy of Muscles, Skin, and other Soft Tissues
Osteoporosis
Edema of the Foot and the Leg

LABORATORY FINDINGS

Roentgenographic Findings. Calcification of the arteries is visualized, one being the diffuse regularly distributed type of Mönckeberg's calcification (in the medial coat). The second type is the localized patchy dense deposits of calcium usually located at the base of large atheromas. It more often is found in the midportion of the femoral artery, a common site for initial arterial occlusion.

Diabetes Mellitus Studies. Diabetes studies include urinalysis, fasting blood sugar, and the glucose tolerance test.

It is important to note certain characteristics of occlusive disease in the diabetic as compared with the nondiabetic:

1. The incidence of occlusive disease is similar in the femoropopliteal area.
2. The incidence of involvement of the three main vessels below the knee is significantly higher in the diabetic.
3. The incidence in the aorto-iliac region is lower in the diabetic.[15] This is revealed by noting an abnormal pressure gradient, by function studies, from below the knee to the ankle.

The diabetic has essentially reduced or absent vasomotor tone of the lower extremity. A significant number of patients fail to respond to sympathetic block.

Determination of Plasma Lipoids. When differentiation from TAO in the middle-aged patient is difficult, elevated values for plasma lipoids favor a diagnosis of ASO.

Skin Temperature. Elevation of skin temperature in response to sympathetic block indicates the benefit to be derived from a sympathectomy.

Noninvasive Functional Studies. The Doppler ultrasonic velocity detector is most commonly used to measure the pressure gradients and to localize the sites of occlusion. It is particularly valuable for detecting blood flow when pulses are not palpable.

Arteriography. Injection of a contrast medium provides the roentgenographic outline and localizes the point of occlusion but is advisable only in patients who are candidates for vascular reconstruction. It may also be useful in determining the appropriate level of amputation.

DIAGNOSIS

The features of occlusive arterial disease are absent pulsations, postural color changes, intermittent claudication, and, in the advanced stages, rest pain, ulceration, or gangrene. The patient often is over 50 years of age, and both sexes are affected. Calcification of large arteries is often visible in roentgenograms, and the plasma lipoids may be elevated. Diabetes mellitus is strong evidence in favor of ASO.

PROGNOSIS

In this progressive, degenerative vascular disease, the outlook for survival of the extremity is not good. However, if arterial occlusions are not too extensive or too frequent, it is possible for adequate collateral circulation to develop and compenste for loss of the main artery. If a large occlusion develops suddenly and involves a large main vessel such as the superficial femoral, the collaterals are inadequate and gangrene is inevitable.

Once gangrene develops, the chances for saving the extremity are poor, especially when diabetes is associated. The life expectancy is shortened, many die of coronary occlusion. The mortality rate following amputation varies from 4% to 20%; the rate is lowered by higher levels of amputation. These figures have been improved recently by improved surgical techniques, and the rate of success of below-knee amputations has increased.

Modern methods of early diagnosis of progressive occlusive vascular disease and improved techniques of vascular reconstruction have greatly improved the outlook. By vascular flow studies it is possible to determine whether a critical localized area of involvement is amenable to bypass or endarterectomy. When functional studies reveal extensive involvement by multiple levels of occlusion, occlusion of all three vessels below the knee and of the plantar and digital arteries, resulting in absent digital pulses, collateral circulation is insufficient, and the prognosis is ominous. It is thus possible to categorize cases into those deserving of vascular reconstruction and those requiring primary amputation.

CHRONIC AORTO-ILIAC OCCLUSION

Pain about the lower back, buttocks, thighs, and hips can arise as a result of ischemia due to occlusive arterial disease of the terminal portion of the abdominal aorta and the common iliac arteries. Chronic aorto-iliac occlusion (Leriche's syndrome) is becoming an increasingly recognized condition, mainly affecting middle-aged men in whom slowly progressive occlusion is produced by an increasing thromboatheromatous mass. The atheromatous changes at first are most pronounced about the terminal aorta and common iliacs, whereas the large vessels within the lower extremities remain relatively unaffected until a late date. Consequently, overt typical symptoms and findings of ASO may not be manifest until years later. The importance of this syndrome to the orthopaedic surgeon lies in the necessity of considering it in the differential diagnosis of pain referable to the lower back, hips, and thighs.[26]

PATHOLOGY

Early atheromatous plaques and intimal sclerosis form in the arterial wall and are followed by an organizing thrombus. The mass of organizing thrombus and atheroma is intimately connected to the arterial wall and gradually encroaches on the lumen; on operative exposure the thromboatheromatous mass partially or completely fills the lumen and is difficult to dissect free. In most instances, the changes develop initially in one of the common iliac arteries and spread proximally to the terminal aorta and the opposite common iliac. Less often it forms initially within the terminal portion of the abdominal aorta and spreads to both iliacs. Rarely, the occlusive process remains confined to one artery. In any event, despite the intensity of the process about the aorto-iliac segment, the distal arterial bed beyond the common iliacs or common femoral arteries remains relatively unaffected or minimally involved. Within the terminal aorta, the occluding thromboatheromatous mass increases in size and may extend proximally to the level of origin of the renal arteries.

Development of the occlusion is gradual, usually taking place over a period of 5 to 10 years; therefore, the collaterals that form may be sufficient to maintain nutrition of the lower extremities. The circuitous route takes place through the lumbar arteries and by way of the cruciate anastomosis about the hip to the femoral artery.

Associated with the progressive occlusive arterial disease, an intense periaortic inflammatory reaction produces extensive fibrous adhesions that make surgical dissection difficult.

CLINICAL PICTURE

Men are predisposed in a ratio of 9:1, most commonly during the fifth decade, although cases are recognized at any time from the third to the eighth decade. In the early case, pain develops insidiously, is often described as a sensation of extreme fatigue, appears after exercise and subsides after a few minutes of rest, reappearing as exercise is resumed, and is situated about the lower back, the buttocks, the hips, and the thighs.[18,26] Likened to ischemic pain in the calf, the amount of exercise necessary to produce the feeling of intense fatigue or low back pain is identical in each instance but is modified by condition. For example, if symptoms are produced by walking three blocks at a slow pace, increasing the pace or walking up a hill will lessen the distance at which the symptom will appear. The site of the symptom varies in different subjects. It may be limited to the lower back when the terminal aorta is the site of obstruction. Discomfort in the buttock generally signifies occlusion of the common iliac artery. Both lower extremities exhibit an unusual degree of pallor, which becomes pronounced in the horizontal or elevated position. Both femoral pulses are absent. The lower extremities appear atrophied. The most significant physical signs are systolic murmurs over the lower part of the abdomen and inguinal regions.

In late advanced cases, when the occlusive disease has extended to involve the common femoral, pain becomes typically ischemic in character, trophic changes develop, intermittent claudication of the calves is usual, limb pallor is replaced by cyanosis or dependent rubor, and rest pain is added. Sometimes, ischemic neuritis of the sciatic nerve is superimposed.

Leriche described five specific manifestations in the early stages of the disease: (1) sexual impotence (inability to maintain a penile erection), (2) extreme fatigability of the legs on walking, (3) gradual atrophy of both lower extremities, (4) absence of trophic disturbances, and (5) pallor of the legs.[22–24] He also noted absence of femoral and pedal pulses. In the terminal stages, cyanosis develops and is followed by ischemic changes and gangrene of the toes associated with severe rest pain. The diagnosis is established by aortography (Fig. 20-14).

In addition to aortography to define the site and extent of the disease both proximally and distally, Doppler readings at the upper thigh compare the systolic pressure at this site with the brachial systolic pressure, or the absence of sounds of blood flow over the common femoral artery signifies a complete occlusion.

TREATMENT

Chronic aorto-iliac occlusion is not a surgical emergency. Blockage takes place so slowly that an adequate collateral circulation can develop, obviating the need for vascular reconstruction. This is in direct contrast to an acute arterial occlusion caused by an embolus or an acute thrombosis.

In the early stages of the disease, conservative treatment will often suffice to control symptoms while gaining time for the formation of collaterals. Smoking is forbidden. The patient is advised to walk slowly and stop at

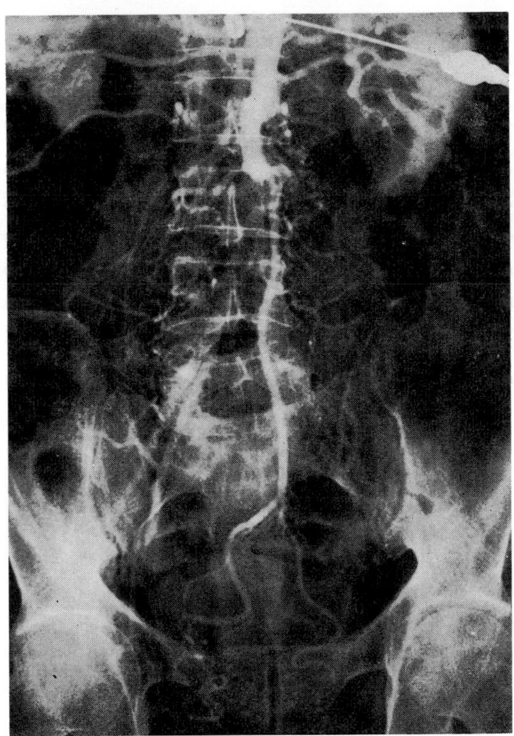

FIG. 20-14. Chronic aorto-iliac occlusion. The aortogram shows a complete occlusion of the abdominal aorta at the level of the inferior mesenteric artery. This patient had low-back claudication as well as claudication located in both buttocks. Note the profuse collateral circulation. (DeWolfe VG et al: Intermittent claudication of the hip and the syndrome of chronic aorto-iliac thrombosis. Circulation 9:1, 1954)

the first sign of distress. The head of the bed is elevated a few inches. Reflex heat is applied to the abdomen for 20 minutes twice a day. Caudal blocks using a diluted local anesthetic every 3 or 4 days are helpful.

Sympathetic blocks may alleviate symptoms temporarily and should define the result to be expected of sympathectomy. However, sympathectomy of itself is of little benefit and at the most may increase tolerance to exercise.

When symptoms persist despite conservative treatment, extension of the thombosis to the femoral arteries progressing to gangrene becomes a definite threat, and surgical intervention is indicated. Procedures to restore adequate blood flow should be undertaken while the peripheral large arteries are relatively uninvolved.

Restoration of blood flow can be achieved by excision of the aorto-iliac segment and replacement with a Dacron bifurcation graft, which has supplanted homograft replacement; thromboendarterectomy and repair with a patch graft; and a bypass graft (Fig. 20-15).[19,21,25] Whenever possible, the bypass Dacron graft is preferred.[17]

In some patients in whom the thrombotic occlusive process affects the entire abdominal aorta up to the origin of the renal arteries, it is necessary to first perform a thromboendarterectomy of this portion of the terminal aorta before the proximal end of the graft is attached. The distal ends of the bifurcation graft are then attached to the external iliac or common femoral arteries, depending on the extent of the occlusive disease.

When the process is extremely well localized to the abdominal aorta, endarterectomy with patch-graft angioplasty is performed.[16] When the aorto-iliac area is extensively diseased and associated with an intense periaortic fibrosis or aneurysmal dilatation, the aorto-

FIG. 20-15. Aorto-iliac occlusion, operative treatment. (*Left*) Diagrammatic sketch shows the type of atheromatous occlusion of the abdominal aorta with patent distal arteries below the level of the external iliac arteries. The impaired blood flow produces not only intermittent claudication of the legs and impotence in the male but also low back pain and hip pain. (*Right*) The surgical procedure consists in insertion of a Dacron bypass graft from the abdominal aorta to both external iliac arteries.

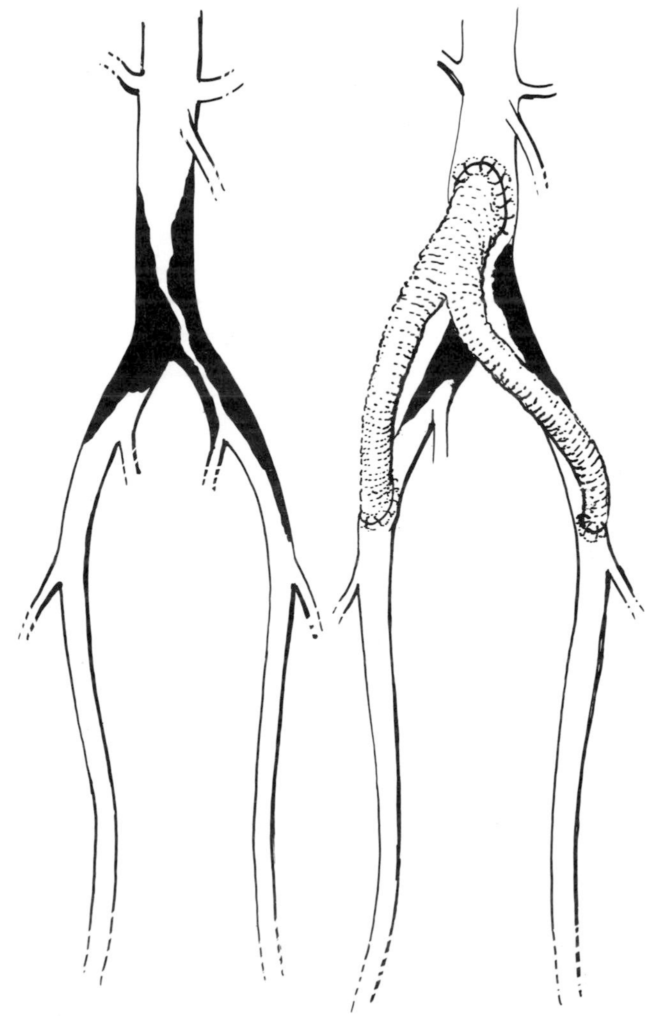

iliac segment should be removed and replaced by a bifurcation Dacron graft.[20]

As pointed out by Leriche, despite the slow course, procrastination in the face of the progressive disease will ultimately lead to extensive, often bilateral, gangrene, which is severely painful, requiring a double midthigh amputation in rather poor tissue and eventuating fatally.

THROMBOANGIITIS OBLITERANS

Thromboangiitis obliterans (Buerger's disease) is a disease of unknown origin, occurring predominantly in young and middle-aged men, often heavy smokers.[27,29] It is characterized pathologically by recurring episodes of inflammation and thrombosis in medium-sized arteries, principally in the lower extremities but also in the distal portions of the upper extremities in which ASO is never seen. Clinically, there are symptoms and findings of sudden or chronically progressive arterial occlusion. The condition frequently comes to the attention of the orthopaedic surgeon attempting to define the cause of pain in the lower extremities and in the hand. Recognition at an early stage is important in halting progression and its serious complications.

ETIOLOGY

Although the exciting cause is unknown, the predisposing factors are the following:

Age. Mainly in young or middle-aged adults between 25 and 45 years of age

Sex. Males almost exclusively. Experimental work has shown that estrogenic hormone prevents ergotamine-induced gangrene in rats.[28]

Type. Persons of Semitic extraction predisposed

Tobacco. Majority heavy smokers. The disease progresses if smoking is continued; if smoking is discontinued, new vascular lesions are diminished in frequency. Nicotine causes vasoconstriction and occlusion.[30]

Weather. Condition is worse in winter months when cold increases vasoconstriction

Blood Changes. An increased tendency to coagulation in many patients

Infection. Various investigators have recovered organisms which, when injected into experimental animals, occasionally produce intimal proliferation and thrombosis. Removal of foci of infection often reduces the pain of intermittent claudication.

PATHOLOGY

Medium-sized or small arteries, especially of the lower extremities, are involved. The large arteries are affected late and only in the severely progressive case. Less often the small and medium-sized veins are affected. The lesions are segmental and are sharply demarcated from intervening normal vessel. At the site of pathology, artery, vein, and nerve are often intimately bound together by fibrous tissue. Microscopically, an inflammatory panarteritis or panphlebitis with thrombosis is seen. The adventitia displays aggregations of lymphocytes about the vasa vasorum, an occasional giant cell, and fibrous hyperplasia. The muscle layer is atrophic. The intima is thickened by endothelial proliferation. The lumen is filled with a thrombus, which varies from a fresh clot to one that is completely organized. Openings in the occluding mass reflect an attempt at recanalization. Extensive collaterals develop about the lesion.

This lesion is distinguished from periarteritis nodosa by the greater extent of the lesion, the absence of necrosis in the media, the absence of aneurysms, and the invariable presence of an occluding mass.

In Buerger's disease, in contrast to ASO, involvement is more distal and extensive in vessels below the knee, thus explaining the frequency of foot claudication. Hand and upper extremity involvement is common, whereas in ASO this is rare.

CLINICAL PICTURE

Symptoms and findings involve the distal portions of the extremities, most often the lower leg and foot.

Symptoms

Symptoms include pain, a sensation of coldness, and abnormal sensitivity to cold temperatures.

Pain. Various types of pain are experienced, as follows:

Intermittent claudication is the most common and often the earliest complaint. It is produced by exercise, relieved by rest, and accentuated by cold and always occurs distal to the point of occlusion, typically in the arch of the foot and occasionally in the calf.

Rest pain consists of a severe gnawing ache in the toes, usually appearing after an acute occlusion and remaining severe for days or weeks. It is worse at night, aggravated by elevation, and reduced by dependency (the reverse may occur). It is caused by ischemia of tissues, including the sensory nerve terminals. Because it is often a prelude to ulceration or gangrene, frequently it is termed pretrophic pain.

Pain of ulceration or gangrene often becomes intense and persistent.

Thrombophlebitic pain is usually mild and aggravated by use of the limb or pressure on the vein. It disappears with subsidence of the inflammation.

Coldness, Sensitivity to Cold. The toes and the foot are subjectively cold and numb. These symptoms are accentuated by slightly cold temperatures, which at the same time cause blanching and cyanosis.

Findings

Objective findings pertain to identifiable arterial occlusion and the effects of circulatory insufficiency.

Impaired Arterial Pulsation. The dorsalis pedis and the posterior tibial pulsations are reduced or absent in a majority of patients. One must remember that the dorsalis pedis is normally absent in 8% of people, and its absence alone does not necessarily imply occlusive disease.

Absence of popliteal and femoral pulsations is less frequent. Radial or ulnar pulsations are absent in 40% of patients.

Occlusion can occur distal to the ankle or the wrist beyond the point of palpable pulsations. This can be determined as follows: Inquiring, for example, into the patency of the ulnar artery, the radial artery is lightly compressed. The patient clenches the fist, squeezing out the blood, then opens the fist. Normal color should return immediately. In ulnar occlusion, the pallor persists. The radial, the dorsalis pedis, and the posterior tibial arteries can be tested similarly.

Presently it is more convenient to determine arterial flow by using the ultrasonic velocity detector or the mercury strain gauge. Doppler readings at the lower thigh and at the ankle may show a marked drop in systolic pressure between these two points, indicating extensive occlusive disease of the three main vessels. A mercury strain gauge plethysmograph applied to any digit may measure blood flow distal to the ankle or wrist.

Color Changes. With elevation, the part is abnormally blanched. With dependency, after a delay of 5 to 30 seconds, color returns, and an abnormal rubor appears (R-P sign). The postural color changes are typically asymmetrical.

Temperature Changes. Asymmetrical coldness is palpable. The temperature may vary from toe to toe.

Ulceration and Gangrene. This may develop spontaneously or may follow mechanical, chemical, or thermal trauma. A small ulceration commonly appears about the nail margins. Gangrene is commonly dry and involves one digit, less often the foot. Cellulitis and spreading infection are uncommon.

Edema. This may be caused by thrombophlebitis and ischemic necrosis of small digital vessels.

Trophic Changes. Nails are thick and deformed, and digits are shrunken. Thin atrophic skin is more common in ASO. Bony structures are osteoporotic.

Superficial Thrombophlebitis. This is nodular and migratory. It occurs in 40% of patients and lasts from 1 to 3 weeks. Thrombophlebitis when seen in association with occlusive arterial disease definitely identifies the latter as TAO.

SPECIAL TESTS

Arteriography. Anteriography is indicated when a major vessel occlusion is suspected along with the smaller vessel involvement. Location of correctible points of obstruction is essential, because correction of these occlusions may increase perfusion of the diseased smaller vessels and thus relieve peripheral signs and symptoms.

Noninvasive Tests of Arterial Flow. Doppler ultrasonic readings at various levels, particularly in the lower extremity, will show that the most extensive occlusive involvement is distal to the knee. Distal to the ankle, mercury strain gauge plethysmography demonstrates the degree of digital blood flow. In TAO, this is characteristically asymmetrical and patchy. Measurement of digital blood flow and its response to temporary compression of arterial flow at the ankle (normal = vasodilatation) indicates the degree of arteriolar spasm that contributes to the ischemia. This also indicates the improvement to be expected from sympathectomy.

Sympathetic Block. This is an effective method for producing vasodilatation in the extremity. An abnormal degree of arteriolar spasm exists early in the course of the disease. A rise in temperature of the part to 86° F indicates a good response and very little organic obstruction. Lesser degrees of response relate to the severity of occlusion.

Oscillometry. This can be used to estimate arterial pulsation but has largely been replaced by Doppler readings.

Claudication Time. This also determines the effect of treatment. The standard treadmill test can be compared from time to time. The rate of walking, the grade of uphill walking, and the time of appearance of claudication are noted.

COURSE

Episodes of new occlusions, alternating with periods of remissions, take place. Between attacks, collaterals develop. There is a tendency toward improvement, and, in most cases, the disease ultimately becomes inactive. Even after gangrene develops, return to normal activity is possible. The course varies from mild and nonprogressive to severe and slowly progressive.

DIAGNOSIS

Early diagnosis may prevent gangrene. Significant signs include intermittent claudication, particularly in the foot; superficial, migratory, nodular thrombophlebitis; abnormally cold extremities with asymmetrical color changes; occurrence in a man who is usually a heavy smoker; and evidence of occlusion.

PROGNOSIS

The outlook is good. Probability of loss of limb is indefinite but is favorably influenced by discontinuance of smoking.

TREATMENT OF CHRONIC OCCLUSIVE ARTERIAL DISEASE

RECOMMENDED MEASURES

The aim of treatment is to prevent progression while collaterals develop. Recommended measures are as follows:

1. Bed rest reduces oxygen need and permits healing of ischemic neuritis, ulcers, and gangrene.
2. A warm environment encourages vasodilatation.
3. Smoking is forbidden.
4. Protection against injury includes avoidance of constricting clothing, tight shoes.
5. Extremes of temperature are avoided.
6. Exercise within limits, especially in buoyant water or in a whirlpool, encourages blood flow and reduces thrombotic episodes. Exercise reduces blood cholesterol and encourages the formation of collaterals.
7. Vasodilator drugs include alcoholic drinks and papaverine. The various preganglionic sympatholytic drugs, such as tetraethylammonium chloride, in effective doses may cause dangerous hypotensive levels.

   Other currently used drugs include *Isoxuprine* (Vasodilan), given orally, 10 mg to 20 mg three or four times a day, and tolazoline hydrochloride (Priscoline), 25 mg four times a day. This has an adrenergic blocking action as well as acting directly on the vessel. Other than causing increased gastric secretion, it is well tolerated. Nicotinyl alcohol (Roniacol), 50 mg to 100 mg three times a day acts directly on the vessel. It is also available in a prolonged-release form.

   In chronic occlusive arterial disease, the improvement effected by these drugs is unpredictable, but an occasional favorable response warrants a trial.
8. Reflex heat by placing the hands in hot water or on an electric pad on the abdomen effects vasodilatation in the lower extremities.
9. Postural exercises have a remedial effect. The extremity is elevated until pallor appears; it is kept horizontal for about 30 seconds and is held dependent until rubor appears. The exercise is repeated a number of times at each of several sessions per day.
10. Constant elevation must be avoided since it may cause dangerous ischemia.
11. Sander's oscillating bed gives postural exercise without effort by the patient.
12. Sympathetic blocking with a local anesthetic in oil or in solution by continuous drip through a polyethylene tube relieves vasospasm and ischemic pain and may prevent gangrene. Permanent blocking can be secured by injecting 6% phenol.
13. Sympathectomy is recommended in most cases. It permanently abolishes vasoconstriction and sweating and may delay or prevent the development of gangrene. It does not prevent the development of new occlusive lesions. Before sympathectomy can be considered, vasodilatation by sympathetic block or the reactive hyperemia test using the mercury strain gauge plethysmograph must be clearly demonstrable.
14. Anticoagulant treatment is begun with heparin and dicumarol at the same time; heparin is discontinued when the prothrombin time is sufficiently elevated. These measures are used only during an acute episode, because reflex arterial spasm distal to the point of occlusion is a favorable site for thrombosis.
15. Local treatment of ulcers, gangrene, and infections is at a minimum. The intact skin in the neighborhood of the lesion is extremely vulnerable. Warm boric soaks will encourage drainage, and local antibiotic ointments or powders, such as tetracycline or neosporin, may be used.
16. Removal of foci of infection has a favorable effect in reducing arterial spasms.
17. Intermittent claudication should be treated surgically. Weakening of the muscle affected by the pain reduces its oxygen demand and lessens ischemic pain. An internal popliteal neurectomy divides the branches of supply to the calf muscles. An external popliteal neurectomy paralyzes the foot dorsiflexors, which the patient accepts in preference to the pain.

    Subcutaneous tenotomy of the Achilles tendon is probably best. It weakens rather than paralyzes and effectively relieves pain in many instances. One must be reasonably certain that the inadequately nourished foot will tolerate surgery.[32]
18. Inevitable loss of a portion of a limb, when ischemia is irremediable, should be recognized and dealt with

at the earliest opportunity. By conserving as much of the limb as possible, a more functional stump can be obtained.

A gangrenous toe must be allowed to separate spontaneously. Separation may take a long time, but conservatism is safer. After a surgical attempt to remove a toe, the wound may not heal, and gangrene may extend. Amputation through the foot rarely heals.

One should seize the earliest moment to perform an amputation distal to the knee, because this provides the maximal rehabilitation potential.

The site of election is 6 inches below the knee, where modern surgical techniques have increased the chances for success. A failed femoropopliteal reconstructive procedure or bypass may reduce the rate of success of below-knee amputations, so that the risks of vascular surgery versus immediate amputation must always be carefully considered. The selection of the appropriate level for amputation can be determined preoperatively by measurement of segmental pressure gradients. A systolic pressure of 80 mm Hg at the thigh is compatible with a successful below-knee amputation. The final determination of the appropriate level is made at the time of surgery by noting the amount of bleeding and the appearance of the tissues. (See Chapter 33.)

19. Miscellaneous procedures are described, although their benefits are questionable:
    a. *Intermittent venous compression.* Theoretically, this causes venous congestion which, when released, produces reactive vasodilatation encouraging arterial and capillary flow. The mechanical compression can seriously traumatize already damaged vessels.
    b. *Intermittent suction and pressure* (passive vascular exercise—pavex). The limb is encased in a boot that by alternate suction and compression supposedly opens blood channels and encourages blood flow. It may produce dilatation of blood vessels and capillary atony and is definitely contraindicated in thrombophlebitis and ulcerative lesions.
    c. *Tissue extracts.* Occasionally, claudication seems to be abolished by pancreatic extract: 5 ml of deproteinated pancreatic tissue extract is given intramuscularly daily for about 2 weeks, then twice weekly for 4 weeks, and finally once weekly for 4 weeks.
    d. *Vitamin E* in high dosage (1600 mg daily) supposedly improves the nutritional appearance of the feet.
    e. *Intravenous hypertonic sodium chloride solution.* A low incidence of amputations with this treatment has been reported: 300 ml of a 3% to 5% solution is given three times weekly for 6 months, then twice a week for 6 months, and finally once weekly for 6 months.[37] Decreased blood viscosity and increased blood volume is the explanation of its effect. A disadvantage is thrombosis at the site of injection.

DIRECT SURGICAL ATTACK ON VESSELS

It is possible to remove an obstructing lesion or detour the flow of blood around the point of occlusion (Fig. 20-16).[36] This is especially true in cases of ASO in which arterial occlusion most frequently takes place in the superficial femoral and popliteal arteries, whereas the distal smaller vessels are relatively uninvolved. The most desirable situation is a relatively recent occlusion in a young person with a minimum of arterial disease. Another desirable set of circumstances is that in which the occlusion is limited to one segment, preferably between the upper and lower thigh, and develops slowly so that adequate collaterals can form and the main vessels distal to the knee are relatively uninvolved. Aortography and arteriography localize the obstruction and outline the internal vascular anatomy. The degree of blood flow is measured at multiple levels to ensure adequate runoff and distal vascularity. A sympathectomy may often be used in conjunction with direct vascular procedures to increase peripheral outflow.

Replacement Grafts. The reversed saphenous vein is used. Synthetic prostheses and bovine heterografts may be used as substitutes for bypassing the occluded arterial segment. The necessary prerequisites for this operation follow:

1. Arteriographic evidence of block
2. Distal vessels adequately patent to permit outflow after grafting
3. Removal of thrombus or intimal plaque insufficient for providing an adequate channel
4. Inadequate collateral circulation
5. Probability of gangrene without this procedure
6. Patient an adequate medical risk for the procedure

Procedures. The segment is bridged without destroying the collaterals. Therefore, the blocked arterial segment must not be removed. The saphenous vein is removed and reversed in direction (because of the valves), and its ends are anastomosed to the side of the artery. If the vein is not adequate, a bovine heterograft or synthetic prosthesis of suitable size and length is chosen.

The artery is opened and the ends of the vein are anastomosed to the proximal and distal arteriotomy with 4-0 or 5-0 synthetic suture. Silk must not be used because of the high incidence of suture fatigue and false aneurysm resulting from suture breakdown. Intravenous heparinization or local heparinization is essential during arterial surgery.[34–36]

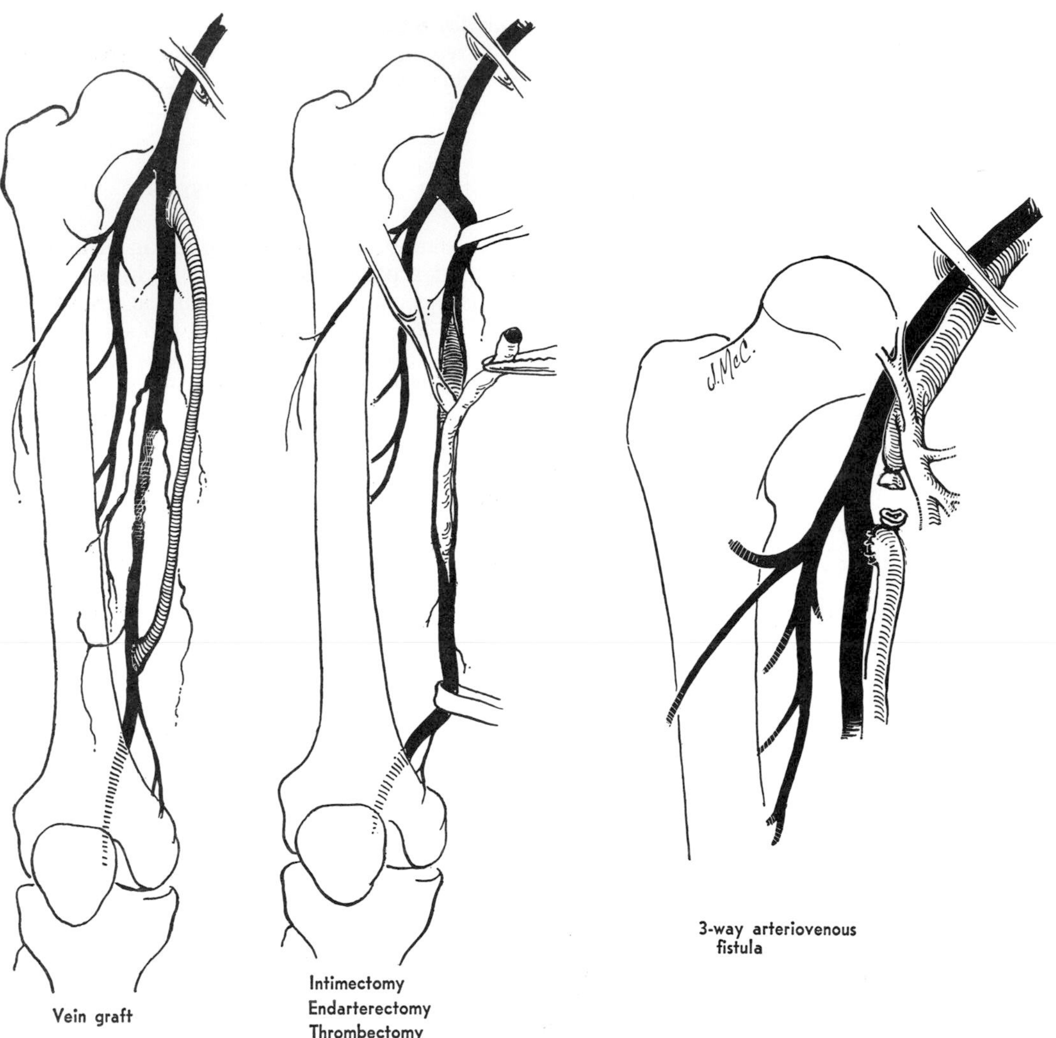

FIG. 20-16. Surgical procedures for overcoming occlusion of a large artery in an extremity. Such surgery is especially reserved for a recent occlusion in a vessel affected by arteriosclerosis obliterans, the distal small vessels being relatively unaffected. (Redrawn from Pratt GI: Cardiovascular Surgery. Philadelphia, Lea & Febiger, 1954).

Intimectomy, Thrombectomy, Endarterectomy. Intimectomy, thrombectomy, and endarterectomy have recently been more successful, perhaps because of anticoagulants.[31,33] Heparinization, either intravenously or locally, is essential. This type of surgery has a limited field of usefulness. Requisites for surgery are as follows:

1. Traumatic thrombosis of the normal limb
2. An acute area of thrombosis, especially with undermining of an atheromatous plaque
3. Failure of conservative treatment
4. Signs of progressive inadequacy of circulation in the extremity and previous loss of the opposite extremity
5. TAO in the young person with failure of conservative treatment. (This indication may be questioned because Buerger's disease involves the larger arteries late after the smaller arteries distally are already extensively involved.)
6. Arteriogram or aortogram showing a localized obstruction of short length.

Contraindications are a spreading infection, extensive involvement, or multiple areas widely separated from each other.

The obstructive site is localized by aortography or arteriography. Anesthesia, either spinal or general, is chosen on the basis of the patients's medical status. The artery is incised over the obstruction. A point of cleavage is found between the inner hard sclerotic cuff containing calcium deposits and the media. The internal substance appears like a sequestrum. The external coat is sutured with fine arterial synthetic suture, and clotting is prevented by using anticoagulants. A patch of vein or synthetic material may be interposed to prevent narrowing of the operative site. The inner lining soon endothelializes. Surgical sympathectomy may or may not be done simultaneously.

When clinically one can determine that an acute occlusion has occurred, the block is localized by aortography. The thrombus, if movable like an embolus, is removed. If the thrombus is fixed and attempted removal might invite further clots, thromboendarterectomy is advised.

Creation of Arteriovenous Fistula. An arteriovenous shunt encourages the development of tremendous collateral circulation in an effort to get blood to the periphery. A three-way lateral fistula can be created by anastomosing the superficial femoral artery to the distal component of its accompanying vein. Theoretically, and in experimental animals, such a fistula has an adverse effect on the heart and kidneys. Therefore, it should be reserved for those patients in whom gangrene is imminent and no one point of occlusion can be localized. Approximately 12% to 20% of cases can be salvaged by this therapy.[38] If this is successful, the fistula should be closed later.

Intra-arterial Dilatation by the Dotter Technique. The Dotter technique may be used in poor-risk patients when the risk of surgery exceeds the chance for success and when amputation is inevitable without attempt at arterial reconstruction.

ANGIOSPASTIC CONDITIONS

Spasm of an artery or a segment of an artery is a feature of many diseases and syndromes. Active arterial contraction occurs in response to a tactile, thermal, emotional, or chemical stimulus. Two theories explain the mechanism of spasm:

Neurogenic Theory
The stimulus acts centrally to effect a nerve impulse that excites spasm peripherally.

Chemical Theory
As a result of the stimulus, adrenaline, sympathin, or some unknown substance called spastin is liberated into the bloodstream and acts directly on the arterial muscle.

Arterial spasm may be part of a condition without an organic basis (*e.g.*, Raynaud's disease) or may complicate occlusive arterial disease (atherosclerosis, TAO, arterial embolism). Regardless of the initiating cause, unrelieved spasm can develop into a permanent organic occlusion. When arterial spasm is linked with a definite etiologic factor, sometimes it is called secondary Raynaud's phenomenon to distinguish it from the primary or functional type of Raynaud's disease.

RAYNAUD'S DISEASE

Raynaud's disease is characterized by recurrent attacks of spasm of peripheral arteries, especially the arterioles, without organic basis, predominantly and symmetrically affecting the upper extremities of women. Color changes accompany each attack, and eventually, after months or years, trophic skin changes appear.[49]

ETIOLOGY

The actual cause is unknown. Women between the ages of 18 and 35 are predisposed in a ratio of 5:1, and a nervous temperament is characteristic. Stimuli that most frequently excite spasm are cold and emotional stress. An endocrine relationship is suggested by the frequent association with menstrual dysfunction and relief with restoration of normal menses.

PATHOLOGY

The early pathology is unknown. In advanced stages, intimal thickening and thrombotic occlusion in digital arteries cause small regions of ulceration and necrosis at the fingertips.[52]

PHYSIOLOGY

Spasm of the arterioles prevents blood from entering the capillaries, observed clinically as pallor. Eventually, the capillaries and the venules become widely dilated, and reflux of blood may occur from the venules to the capillaries where the stagnant blood appears as cyanosis. Either the vasomotor system is at fault, as evidenced by relief with sympathetic ganglionectomy, or an abnormal sensitivity to direct stimuli exists in the digital arteries.[39,44]

CLINICAL PICTURE

On exposure to the stimulus the fingers become blanched and waxy, especially at their tips, accompanied by a sensation of numbness (the dead finger phenomenon). After a variable period, the spasm relaxes, cyanosis may appear, and the fingers develop a rubor, a bright red hue associated with an intense paresthesia of tingling, "pins and needles," or even pain. The frequency of attacks varies from many times a day to very infrequently. At first the color changes affect only the fingertips. Later, the changes extend more proximally to involve the hands.

If the attacks continue over a number of months, trophic changes develop. The skin becomes thin, smooth and glistening, and easily traumatized. The subcutaneous tissue atrophies and hardens, so the finger tapers toward the tip. Extremely painful ulcers and small areas of necrosis may develop over the fingertips. The lesions are often symmetrical. Between attacks the hands have a cyanotic hue. Sclerodermatous skin changes may permanently restrict use of the fingers.

DIAGNOSIS

The main clinical features include predominance in the female, a young age, bilateral and symmetrical involvement of the upper extremities, and response to exciting stimuli, especially cold. The diagnosis is confirmed by exposing the part to cold and noting the color changes.

A sympathetic block should relieve spasm. Blood flow studies and arteriogram may help to rule out occlusive arterial disease. Postural color changes and absent arterial pulsations are indicative of organic disease being primary and Raynaud's phenomenon being secondary. The cervicobrachial area is examined especially for compression at the thoracic outlet.

TREATMENT

Prophylaxis is mainly the avoidance of the exciting stimulus. General-acting vasodilating drugs, such as the nitrites, alcohol, and papaverine, are occasionally helpful in aborting an attack. Local vasodilatation is effected by "Mecholyl" given by iontophoresis. Usually, simple warming of the hands and the body is effective in terminating the attack. In mild cases associated with menopausal symptoms or aggravated during the menstrual period, relief of symptoms may follow administration of estrogens. Smoking is prohibited. Repeated sympathetic blocks are of temporary value in an acute phase and will indicate the effect of a sympathectomy. Surgical treatment is indicated only in those cases with progression of symptoms and threatened trophic changes. Surgical resection of the second and third thoracic ganglia, their rami, and accompanying intercostal nerves is advised.

When Raynaud's syndrome complicates an organic arterial disease, the factor of spasm may adversely affect the outcome. Even in the absence of clinically demonstrable spasm, sympathectomy will effect capillary dilatation and should be done wherever possible.

Gangrene generally never affects more than the tip of the finger. Rarely is amputation indicated, and then only a portion of the finger is removed.

RAYNAUD'S PHENOMENON

Raynaud's phenomenon is the symptom complex (female, provoked by cold and emotion, affecting fingers, acute episodes of blanching, cyanosis, rubor, painful paresthesias) for which an etiologic factor can be identified. True Raynaud's disease, on the other hand, is idiopathic but should never be classified as such unless no cause can be found after several years have elapsed. Following are the most common causes:

Post-traumatic

Occupational

In pneumatic hammer disease, repetitive trauma is produced by the percussion of pneumatic tools. The attack is not initiated by the percussion but sensitizes the digital vessels, so that Raynaud's phenomenon occurs on exposure to cold. The course is benign and trophic changes are rare.

In occupational occlusive arterial disease, repeated trauma with tools requiring a squeezing action can produce arterial occlusion and Raynaud's phenomenon in the hands and fingers.[40] Symptoms uniformly affect the dominant hand, and painful ulcers and scarring of the fingertips develop in many. The affected fingers and hand show occlusive arterial disease without involvement elsewhere.

In occupational acro-osteolysis, Raynaud's phenomenon occurs in workmen exposed to certain chemicals such as vinyl chloride. Radiologic evidence of resorption of the distal phalanges is characteristic (see Acro-osteolysis).[54]

Postsurgical

Raynaud's phenomenon forms part of the post-traumatic neurovascular syndrome. The vasomotor changes are persistent. Severe causalgiclike pain, edema, tenderness, hyperesthesia, or osteoporosis is present.

Thoracic Outlet Syndrome

This is caused by compression of subclavian vessels and the brachial plexus: cervical rib and scalenus anticus, hyperabduction syndrome, costoclavicular syndrome (narrowing of the costoclavicular interval by downward and backward rotation of the arm), bony abnormalities (clavicle, first rib).

In the thoracic outlet syndrome, Raynaud's phenomenon tends to be more persistent. Permanent cyanosis, coldness, or pallor indicates arterial occlusion. Diminished pulse volume is demonstrated by Doppler studies, and gangrene of one or more fingers may follow. When this condition is suspected, angiography is indicated.

Diseases of the Nervous System

Such diseases may be of either the central nervous system (tumor, disk) the peripheral nerves (carpal tunnel syndrome, causalgic state due to irritation of peripheral nerve).

Occulsive Arterial Disease

This is seen in TAO and should be suspected when Raynaud's phenomenon occurs in a male. Angiography is diagnostic.

Intoxication with Heavy Metals and Ergot

Excessive use of ergotamine tartrate for migraine headache may cause prolonged arterial spasm.

Miscellaneous

Raynaud's phenomenon may occur in association with various diseases. It is commonly seen in collagen diseases, particularly scleroderma, and may precede the sclerodermatous changes by several months.[1]

TRAUMATIC ARTERIAL SPASM

An artery is capable of active sustained contraction in response to trauma acting on, or in the vicinity of, the vessel. The trauma is either a single, severe blow, acutely affecting a single large artery, or a frequently repeated series of minor traumas, chronically affecting many of the minute vessels. The degree of arterial constriction is greater than that produced by sympathetic stimulation alone. Therefore, the mechanisms by which traumatic arterial spasm is brought about are direct trauma to the adventitia and reflex sympathetic stimulation.

The degree of arterial spasm may be greater in situations in which there are prolonged indirect traumas rather than a single direct trauma to a single artery.

Chronic

Frequently repeated minor blows occur in certain occupations such as those requiring the use of a pneumatic tool.[41,42] The traumas are inflicted mainly in the hands, where, owing to constriction of the arterioles, Raynaud's phenomenon appears. Attacks of pallor followed by cyanosis, numbness, paresthesias, pain, and perspiration usually are confined to one hand and are precipitated by cold, emotional stress, and, occasionally, the use of the tool. Attacks are pronounced in the morning or late in the day. When Raynaud's syndrome appears in a man, a source of trauma should be sought.

Treatment. The treatment includes changing the occupation, securing vasodilatation by warmth and alcohol, and removing vasoconstricting influences, namely, tobacco, cold, and excitement. The outlook for improvement is excellent once the cause is eliminated.

Acute

The most common cause of acute traumatic arterial spasm (arterial segmental spasm, arterial stupor) is a fracture occurring at certain situations where the artery is bound closely to the bone. An example is at the elbow where the artery may be angulated over and compressed against the upper fragment of a supracondylar fracture of the humerus. On exposure, the artery and frequently its accompanying vein are found to be contracted down to a matchstick size. Spasm of a large artery is associated with widespread spasm of the collaterals distal to the point of trauma. No pulsation is palpable, and the distal end of the limb is pale or cyanotic, cold, anesthetic, and painful. After arterial spasm has persisted for some time, muscular weakness and paralysis develop distally.

Acute arterial spasm (and collateral spasm) is rarely sufficient to cause gangrene. However, persisting relative ischemia thus produced causes parenchymatous necrosis and scar tissue replacement of muscles, particularly those in the forearm.

Treatment. The relief of spasm of a large artery constitutes a surgical emergency. In certain situations, one recognizes the possibility of an embolus or a thrombus occluding the vessel. Although differentiation between these conditions is impossible, it is unnecessary because treatment is almost identical. Obstruction of the main vessel in itself may be harmless, provided that the collaterals are opened.

Delay for a few hours is permissible to observe the effects of nonsurgical measures, reduction of the fracture, lessening the angle of the adjacent joint (especially important at the elbow), sympathetic block, and vasodilators (alcohol, papaverine intravenously). Anticoagulants are started immediately inasmuch as thrombosis often follows spasm.

Failure to restore circulation within a few hours is sufficient indication for exploration. Overlying fasciae are resected, the fracture is reduced under direct vision, and the vessels are freed. A warm solution of normal saline containing a local anesthetic is poured into the wound to bathe the vessels. If vasodilatation cannot be secured in this manner, it is advisable to resect the affected segments of both vessels. Ordinarily, this removes the reflex constriction of the collaterals. Nevertheless, a sympathectomy must follow this procedure.

When resection of an arterial segment would threaten viability of the part (as in organic occlusive disease), alternatives are resection with end-to-end anastomosis, resection and artery or vein graft, or bridging with a graft without resection. (See Acute Arterial Injuries.)

SUDECK'S ATROPHY

In 1900 Sudeck first described an acute atrophy of bone (reflex sympathetic dystrophy, post-traumatic painful osteoporosis) with characteristic spotty decalcification, developing after trauma, and associated with pain, edema, tenderness, cyanosis, coldness, sweating, and stiffness of the part.[53] He attempted to define a specific disease entity. However, these changes are a result of vasospasm of terminal portions of the arterioles, which develops in response to various stimuli and is found in a variety of conditions, usually traumatic in origin. Therefore, Sudeck's type of spotty osteoporosis is one manifestation of a physiological response of the sympathetics to an irritative focus.

PHYSIOLOGICAL-PATHOLOGIC MECHANISM

The irritative stimulus, often traumatic in origin (*e.g.*, fracture, incomplete nerve injury), reflexly provokes continuous vasospasm of the terminal arterial channels. Larger vessels remain unaffected; therefore, oscillometric readings remain unchanged. Because vasospasm and its resultant changes usually develop around and distal to the site of injury, irritation of sympathetic fibers in the peripheral nerves and the perivascular coats seems highly probable. Capillaries and venules become distended with sluggishly flowing blood, lacking the propulsive pressure transmitted from the arterioles. This explains cyanosis and coldness of the part. Slowly moving blood develops a low *p*H, which promotes dissolution of mineral salts of bone. The spotty arrangement of decalcification may be explained by a similar distribution of capillary beds within the bone. Arteriolar spasm effects a relative ischemia of all tissues. As a consequence, increased permeability of capillaries and venules permits diffusion of plasma and its fibrin content into the tissue spaces, manifest clinically as edema. Fibrin deposits are followed by fibrous tissue replacement. Finally, as vascular channels are reopened, bone minerals are redeposited. Fibrosis throughout the soft tissues retards vascularization so that color and temperature are slowly restored. In addition, mobility of joints is restricted and never fully recovered. Hyperhidrosis is a result of overstimulation of the sympathetics. All the described changes may be appropriately termed a reflex sympathetic dystrophy.

CLINICAL PICTURE

Trauma varying from a trivial to a severe injury precedes the appearance of symptoms. The injury often occurs about a joint, especially the wrist and the ankle. The following changes develop in the hand or the foot: swelling; edema; tenderness; cold, moist, slightly cyanotic glossy skin; and limitation of motion of the digits. Pain on movement of the part encourages immobilization and further restiction of motion. When pain becomes intense, persistent, often burning in nature, and aggravated by certain stimuli (heat, emotion, touching the part), this symptom becomes the eminent part of the syndrome, which is then designated causalgia. Symptoms and findings in the average case last a period varying from weeks to months and then gradually subside, leaving a hand or a foot that is stiff, cold, or slightly cyanotic. In the hand, fibrotic contracture of the metacarpophalangeal joints in the extended position constitutes a severe disability.

ROENTGENOGRAPHIC FINDINGS

Spotty decalcification develops throughout bones distal to the site of injury. For example, in a fracture of the lower third of the tibia, osteoporosis develops in the distal fragment and all the bones of the foot. A diffuse deossification of disuse may be superadded (Fig. 20-17).

TREATMENT

During the actively vasospastic phase, blood flow is encouraged by elevation and active exercise of the extremity. In the hand, attention is directed to preserving the full range of motion in the metacarpophalangeal and the interphalangeal joints. When pain is severe and persistent and marked swelling threatens function, sympathectomy will effect rapid recovery. This surgical procedure must be performed early, before fibrotic contractures have supervened. Persistent stiffening of the metacarpophalangeal joints in extension will require multiple capsulotomies.

The pain of causalgia is due frequently to a partial nerve injury. Relief may require not only sympathectomy but also resection and repair of the traumatized nerve. (See below.)

CAUSALGIA

Causalgia is a condition characterized by post-traumatic pain that is persistent, diffuse, and burning, occurring in paroxysms and provoked by various stimuli. Its relief by interruption of sympathetic impulses classifies it as a

FIG. 20-17. Reflex sympathetic dystrophy. The spotty osteoporosis distal to the fracture site is typical.

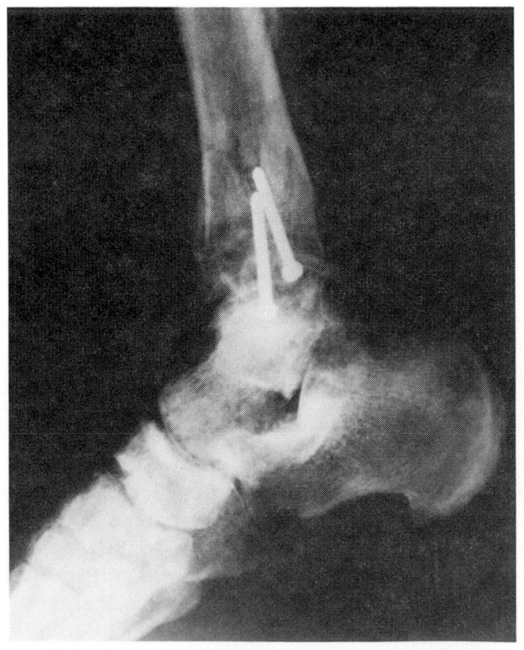

sympathetic dystrophy, and as such it is related to other conditions of sympathetic origin (*e.g.*, Sudeck's atrophy, trophic edema, and reflex arterial spasm).[44–48,51]

ETIOLOGY AND PATHOLOGIC PHYSIOLOGY

The cause is usually trauma, which is often trivial in nature. In severe injuries the pathologic feature is a partial lesion of a peripheral nerve, most commonly of the median or the sciatic nerve or the brachial plexus. When paralysis is complete and associated with causalgia, one finds at surgery a neuroma with the nerve in continuity; electric stimulation of this nerve fails to evoke a motor response.[51] Never do division and separation of nerve ends occurs.

Sympathetic dysfunction is evidenced by vasodilatation and vasoconstriction. Various theories have been advanced to explain the mechanism. A plausible theory states that efferent sympathetic impulses are shunted into sensory fibers of a mixed nerve. This explains the fact that anesthetic blocking of posterior root inflow will abolish causalgia without affecting sympathetic outflow. The spread of pain probably takes place in the internuncial pool.

CLINICAL PICTURE

The onset of pain varies from immediately after injury to several weeks later. The injury is often trivial in nature, such as a sprain, although any type of trauma is causative. The more severe injuries most frequently are those that cause a partial lesion to a peripheral nerve. The pain is constant, intense, and burning; rarely, it is knifelike, crushing, or paresthetic. It is distributed diffusely over the distal portion of a limb not related to a nerve distribution, frequently over the palm of the hand and the plantar aspect of the foot. Various stimuli that intensify the pain include touching or tapping the part, noises, dependent position, and emotional disturbance. Usually the discomfort is worsened by dryness and heat and eased by moisture and coolness; not uncommonly the opposite effect is obtained. The skin over the affected area is exquisitely hyperalgesic. Within the first few weeks the appearance of the part is normal, but eventually manifestations of autonomic disturbance appear. The skin becomes reddened, blotchy, dry, edematous, and warm, a picture of vasodilatation. The skin temperature is elevated. Later, sometimes without the antecedent vasodilatation, the skin becomes cold, pale, cyanotic, perspiring, thin, and glossy and nails are brittle and ridged. Blood flow studies are usually equal to those in the uninvolved extremity. This is surprising when vasodilatation and elevated skin termperature are present. This suggests that interruption of sensory nerves can cause only surface vasodilatation and not constriction or dilatation of the large vessels.

DIAGNOSTIC SYMPATHETIC BLOCK

Interruption of sympathetic impulses by infiltration of local anesthetic about the sympathetic chain will reduce or completely eliminate the pain. For the upper extremity, the needle is inserted between the first and second ribs. For the lower extremity, the anesthetic is injected adjacent to the first and second lumbar vertebrae. Failure to obtain relief may be due to improper technique, and the procedure should be repeated.

COURSE

With passage of time, the pain may spread upward or to the opposite limb. The patient becomes emotionally unstable and hyperirritable and, if the pain persists, may even develop suicidal tendencies. It is said that if the pain is allowed to spread centrally, it may become permanently implanted in the central nervous system and be completely unresponsive to treatment.

TREATMENT

Very rarely does the condition subside spontaneously. When it does so, the diagnosis is in doubt.

Conservative

Conservative treatment often includes warm applications, which often help the vasoconstrictor type, or cool wet applications, which may relieve discomfort of the vasodilated type. Rest and elevation reduce the hyperemia and the edema. Preganglionic blocking agents are effective occasionally.

Tetraethylammonium chloride (Etamon Chloride) is given intramuscularly every 6 hours in a dose not exceeding 20 mg/kg of body weight; the block should not be continued for more than 36 hours. Contraindications are severe hypertension, impaired renal function, a high diastolic pressure, and a recent coronary occlusion.

Tolazoline hydrochloride (Priscoline) is given orally in a dosage up to 50 mg six times daily. Because it also has a local effect in causing vasodilatation, it may accentuate symptoms in the vasodilated type of causalgia.

Nylidrin hydrochloride (Arlidin). This agent has a minimum of side-effects. Its dose is 6 mg three times a day.

Procaine injections of the sympathetic trunk are effective in many cases. It is done daily, and the relief obtained varies from an hour to permanent cure even on one injection. For the upper extremity, 0.5% procaine with Adrenalin is injected into the paravertebral space between the first and second dorsal vertebrae. An effective block is indicated by Horner's syndrome, cessation of sweating, and vasodilatation. For the lower extremity, the injection is made between each pair of vertebrae.

Surgical

Surgical treatment consists of sympathectomy. When done at an early age, the results are almost invariably good: The pain is greatly reduced or entirely eliminated. Before surgery, it is necessary to perform a procaine block to note the effect of interrupting sympathetic impulses. Delay in performing surgery is unwise, since permanent trophic changes and deformity may develop.

Upper extremity causalgia is treated by sectioning the thoracic trunk below the third ganglion and removing the gray and the white rami to the second and the third ganglia.

Lower extremity causalgia requires removal of several upper lumbar ganglia, from the first to the fourth. Results are better when the first lumbar ganglion is included.

When a partial nerve lesion can be identified, neurolysis, resection of the neuroma, and neurorrhaphy are necessary, in addition to sympathectomy, to eliminate residual partial pains and paresthesia. These procedures in themselves are of no value in eliminating the severe causalgic pain. Very late cases of causalgia rarely require cordotomy or lobotomy, but the results leave much to be desired.

FROSTBITE

Frostbite is defined as ischemic destruction of superficial soft tissues as a result of exposure to cold. Vasoconstriction plays a prominent part initially, but arteriole thrombosis and increased capillary permeability cause later damage.

ETIOLOGY

Cold produces vasoconstriction locally and reflexly. The resultant ischemia, if severe and prolonged, leads to thrombosis of the arterioles with gangrene. Death of tissue is also caused by direct freezing to a solid state of cellular fluids. Although the true freezing point of the skin is between −2°C (28.4°F) and 0°C (32°F), the skin has the ability, because of the phenomenon of supercooling, to go below its freezing point without solidifying. Therefore, freezing of the skin does not occur until −10°C (14°F) or lower. The application of oils to the skin increases the capacity for supercooling.

Factors contributing to freezing so that pathologic changes develop at a higher temperature are moisture, wind, inactivity (immobility encourages venous stasis), occlusive arterial disease, tobacco excess, and anoxemia (high altitude flying, anemia).

PATHOLOGY

On exposure to cold, vasoconstriction takes place, principally in the arterioles, and may persist for a day or more. In mild frostbite a low-grade inflammatory reaction takes place in the vessels and the surrounding tissues. On prolonged exposure to cold and persistent vasoconstriction, inflammation develops in the intima of small arteries and arterioles. The endothelium of capillaries is damaged, permitting abnormal permeability. In the process of thawing, on exposure to higher temperatures, a reactive hyperemia occurs. Thrombi form in the terminal arterioles, and blood and plasma extravasate through the damaged capillary walls, causing edema and blood-filled blisters. The fluid accumulation is rather superficial, splitting the epidermis and the dermis. Superficial necrosis develops because the increased oxygen requirements by the normal tissue are not fulfilled by the inadequate blood supply.

The basic pathogenetic factors, therefore, include the following:

1. *Vasospasm*, during exposure to cold
2. *Capillary stasis*
3. *Increased capillary permeability* with loss of intravascular fluid, resulting in
4. *Sludging and aggregation of red blood cells.* The thrombi seen within the early hours after warming consist of agglutinated clumps of red cells but no fibrin. These intravascular occlusions may regress.

CLINICAL PICTURE

Frostbite can be classified according to the severity of tissue changes.

Mild Form (First-Degree). With vasoconstriction, a dull pallor develops in the skin, accompanied by numbness and a prickling sensation. On warming the part, mild erythema or normal color returns without damage to the tissues. The affected area may remain unusually hypersensitive to subsequent exposure for a considerable time.

Moderate Form (Second-Degree). Exposure to cold of a more extreme degree or for a longer period causes actual solidifying by freezing of the part, which appears white, rigid, and insensitive. On thawing, a severe reactive hyperemia develops, starting in the vicinity of, and gradually spreading over, the ischemic, pale skin. The entire involved part is red, tender, and edematous, and blisters soon appear. Burning pain and paresthesias are often intense. Superficial sloughs of skin occur, and the part recovers.

Severe Gangrenous Form (Third-Degree). The appearance is that of the second-degree type, but it progresses to gangrene, usually of the superficial tissues. Gangrene is more likely to develop when exposure to severe cold is prolonged, trauma is inflicted (*e.g.*, an enforced march), or the part is kept immobile. Thrombosis develops, and, on warming of the part, gangrene appears.

TREATMENT

Prophylactically, the main factors to be emphasized are that clothing is loose, light, warm, and windproof; that feet are cleaned and cared for daily and kept dry and oiled; and that moderate activity is desirable but prolonged marches in cold weather should be avoided.

Active treatment aims at relief of ischemia as a vascular emergency. Mild frostbite requires only warming by any means at hand. Avoiding trauma (*e.g.*, vigorous rubbing of the affected part) and maintaining asepsis are mandatory to prevent more severe involvement.

Severe degrees of frostbite require gentle, atraumatic, and aseptic handling and administration of antibiotics and anticoagulants to combat thrombosis.[43] Compressing clothing is removed, and the involved region is exposed and protected. Smoking is forbidden. Intravenous administration of low-molecular-weight dextran will disaggregate the red corpuscles, decrease blood viscosity, and increase blood flow through the peripheral small blood vessels, thereby increasing tissue survival.

A controversy exists as to the benefits of maintaining a warm environment to warm the part rapidly or a cold environment with slowly rising temperature to warm the part gradually.

Slow-Warming Method. The slow-warming method is based on the fact that the venous and the lymphatic vessels suffer the greatest damage and are incapable of draining the blood brought in by the newly opened arteries. Blebs, edema, ecchymosis, and gangrene are evidence of excessive fluid supply. If the arteries are only partially dilated by maintaining the part in a cool tent (55°F–60°F), drainage of blood from the area is adequate. Ice bags, which cool the tent, are gradually decreased over a period of several weeks. The patient is generally more comfortable in cool surroundings, and the amputation rate by this method is extremely low.

Rapid-Warming Method. Theoretically, warming a part to the point where its increased metabolic demands cannot be satisfied by inadequate oxygen supply results in death of tissue. This explains why, on exposure to cold, gangrene is more likely under anoxemic conditions. However, experimental work on animals has demonstrated that rapid warming of the part, but not heating, resulted in no more tissue loss than slow warming.[50] The procedure merely requires immersing in mildly warm water.

After the first week, the degree of tissue destruction will become apparent. The black, dry, gangrenous tissue becomes sharply delimited and should be allowed to separate and slough spontaneously. A "hands-off" surgical policy is best. The gangrene is superficial, involving mainly the skin and the superficial tissues, and, when shed, leaves a bed of healthy granulations that can be covered with skin grafts. Surgical trauma imposed prematurely will only intensify the extent of destruction. While awaiting spontaneous separation, use of sterile dressings, antibiotics, and anticoagulants is continued. Accumulation of infective material will usually drain in a warm saline soak.

Sympatholytic drugs and surgical sympathectomy may be beneficial in patients with antecedent organic arterial occlusive disease.

TRENCH FOOT AND IMMERSION FOOT

Trench foot and immersion foot are the military and naval counterparts of frostbite. The vascular changes, because of moisture, take place at temperatures above those required to cause freezing or frostbite. Moisture acts to carry away the heat more rapidly from the affected part. Edema is more pronounced than in frostbite because of prolonged dependency. Under conditions of starvation and hypoproteinemia, edema is greater in degree. Edema implies deposition of fibrin throughout the soft tissues, leading eventually to fibrosis and stiffness of the part. In addition to moisture, immobility such as occurs in trench warfare encourages pathologic responses to less than freezing temperatures.

PATHOLOGY

Damage to capillary and venous channels (which may be ischemic in origin as a result of prolonged arteriolar spasm) results in pathologic permeability of the vessel walls. Red blood cell diapedesis and plasma diffusion into the surrounding tissues occur. Thrombosis develops, particularly in venous channels, the clot appearing to be a concentration of red corpuscles rather than actual coagulation with fibrin. Multiple areas of ischemic necrosis develop throughout the soft tissues and are replaced by scarring, particularly in muscle and nerve structures and vessel walls. When necrosis is extensive, it is usually confined to the skin and the superficial tissues.

CLINICAL PICTURE

Several stages may be identified, including the following:

Stage of Vasospasm. The first symptoms are numbness, coldness, and a sensation of "feet made of wood." Pain is usually minimal during the anesthetic period. Both feet are pale or cyanotic, often mottled and cold. After the boots are removed, swelling occurs, and intense pain and paresthesia develop.

Stage of Hyperemia. As the extremities are exposed to warmth, the feet become red and hot, edema increases, and blebs containing a hemorrhagic fluid appear. An intense burning pain is often associated. Occasionally, a shooting, stabbing pain characteristic of ischemic neuritis is experienced. This stage lasts about 2 weeks and may heal completely. Frequently, such feet remain somewhat cyanotic and cold and are hypersensitive to ordinary cold weather, the Raynaud's phenomenon being manifest. On the other hand, this stage may progress further to that of frank gangrene.

Stage of Gangrene. This varies from small blisters and ulcers to gangrene. Although the skin alone appears necrotic, diffuse ischemic degenerative changes followed by fibrous replacement are taking place throughout the deeper tissues. Muscles become fibrotic, and contractures of the joints of the foot develop. The gangrene is usually superficial and separates as healthy granulations form beneath the crust. The final result is an atrophic, contracted foot that appears dusky, cold, and hyperhidrotic as manifestations of sympathetic overactivity in response to cool temperatures.

TREATMENT

Prevention demands avoiding exposure for prolonged periods to cold and wet, engaging in activity, and changing shoes and socks frequently.

General treatment includes administration of antibiotics, prohibition of smoking, and administration of anticoagulants.

Local treatment aims at reestablishing vasomotor tone and keeping the tissues at a low metabolic level in the hyperemic stage. The legs must be elevated at intervals to reduce edema, which may interfere with circulation directly or at a later time by resulting scarring. Probably it is best to keep the feet cooled by a blowing fan or refrigeration with ice bags until vasodilatation can be overcome. Sympathectomy is not indicated at this stage, because the capillaries and the venules are incapable of handling an increased inflow of blood.

Surgical restraint is adhered to strictly during the process of separation of the superficial gangrenous crust. Later, the granulating surface may be covered with skin grafts.

The sequelae, namely, such symptoms as paresthesias, anesthesias, cold sensitivities, a feeling of the foot being cold, and hyperhidrosis, are symptoms of sympathetic overstimulation. The circulation may be improved by, for example, a warm climate, avoidance of smoking, and sympatholytic drugs, but surgical sympathectomy is best.

When frostbite, trench foot, or immersion foot develops at temperatures far above those at which changes might be expected to occur, arterial occlusive disease should be suspected. Gangrene is generally more likely and extensive and often requires amputation.

PERNIO

Pernio (chilblain, dermatitis hemialis) is a vasospastic disease affecting the smaller vessels of the skin and resulting in necrosis and ulceration.[45] Although the chief manifestations affecting the skin of the leg, and less commonly the dorsum of the foot and the hand, cause the case to come under the care of the dermatologist, eventually the cause is traced to exposure to cold and wet. Sympathectomy results in a complete cure.

CLINICAL PICTURE

Acute

Acute pernio (chilblains) is often seen in children or women without adequate protection for their feet and legs and who are exposed to cold wet weather. When the legs are affected, the shins are usually involved. The lesions of acute pernio are characterized by dermatitis with edema and a violaceous hue. The associated intense itching and burning is aggravated on exposure to warmth and these symptoms are usually present in unaffected regions. The acute manifestations generally last a few days, then gradually clear up in a week to 10 days, leaving a brownish pigmentation. The lesions are almost invariably bilateral and symmetric.

Chronic

On repeated exposure to cold, recurring crops of cutaneous lesions appear, but they disappear in the warmer months. Red, elevated, painful, small lesions appear on the lower portions of both legs anteriorly and posteriorly, accompanied by an itching and burning sensation. On the surface of the erythematous lesions, blisters form and break down, leaving hemorrhagic ulcers, each with a violaceous base. Pain subsides with appearance of ulceration. The ulcerative lesions heal in 3 to 5 weeks, leaving permanent scarring and pigmentation. No clinical evidence of arterial occlusive disease can be found, but biopsy of the lesions will reveal angiitis with low-grade inflammation in the subcutaneous tissue. Absence of tubercles rules out Koch's infection.

TREATMENT

Acute and chronic pernio may be prevented by a continual warm environment. An acute lesion requires protection from trauma and infection because the local area is ischemic. Adequate clothing covering the legs may reduce the possibility of recurrence.

Chronic pernio is often typified by progressively increasing susceptibility to cold. Eventually, the lesions, which at first develop only during the cooler months, may appear after several years during cooler days of summer months. Treatment is directed toward increasing peripheral arterial circulation. Administration of sympatholytic drugs orally or acetyl-β-methylcholine chloride (mecholyl chloride) by iontophoresis may be tried. A surgical sympathectomy will heal the lesions promptly and prevent further recurrences.

CONDITIONS CHARACTERIZED BY VASODILATATION

The following described conditions, erythromelalgia and acrocyanosis, display capillary vasodilatation as part of the pathologic physiology. However, this does not imply that dilatation of the minute vessels is the cause of symptoms. In erythromelalgia, the reddening and the warmth indicate that the arterial blood supply is normal and, although the capillaries are distended, the rate of blood flow is adequate. Therefore, sympathectomy is of no value. In acrocyanosis, coldness and cyanosis indicate sluggish blood flow. Arteriolar spasm satisfactorily explains this condition as evidenced by diminution of cyanosis during sleep and after sympathectomy.

These diseases, although not common, must be differentiated from the more common vascular diseases. Erythromelalgia must be distinguished from the painful dependent rubor of occlusive arterial disease and from the burning distress of peripheral neuritis. Acrocyanosis must be differentiated from Raynaud's disease and from pulmonary and cardiac causes of cyanosis.

ERYTHROMELALGIA

Erythromelalgia (erythermalgia) is a condition characterized clinically by paroxysms of reddening and warming of the skin in an area of an extremity associated with burning distress. Attacks are invariably provoked by heating the extremity.

Two types may be recognized, primary and secondary. The primary type is idiopathic; there is no evidence of vascular or nervous disease. Usually, both lower extremities are involved.

The secondary type is usually part of hypertension or polycythemia vera; it also occurs in gout, organic nervous disease, and heavy metal poisoning. As a rule, only one extremity is involved.

PATHOLOGIC PHYSIOLOGY

Vasodilatation is the cause of warming of the skin. The skin must be warmed above a certain minimum, the "critical point," usually between 32°C and 36°C (85° to 96°F), to induce a burning distress. Symptoms may be provoked more easily by increasing the hydrostatic pressure, such as by compressing the veins proximally or by lowering the extremity. Conversely, elevating the extremity or applying direct pressure over the painful area will lessen the distress. Incomprehensible is the difficulty of producing pain by immersing the extremity in warm water.

CLINICAL PICTURE

Adults are affected most commonly. The hands or the feet are involved and often only a small portion of the foot. The patient may state that painful burning arises while walking or at night when the foot is placed beneath the covers. An attack lasts from minutes to hours. Symptoms are more intense in the warm summer months. Relief is obtained by exposure to cold.

Examination during the paroxysm reveals the painful part to be reddened or cyanotic and warm. Some swelling may be noted. Trophic changes are absent except in the secondary type. Because of its frequent association with polycythemia vera, an enlarged spleen should be sought. The peripheral pulses are intact. Veins are distended owing to the greatly increased blood flow through the extremity. Increasing the venous dilatation by obstructing venous outflow with a lightly applied tourniquet intensifies the pain. Elevating the extremity or applying cold or direct pressure over the painful part relieves the pain.

LABORATORY FINDINGS

During the attack a sample of venous blood removed from a vein proximal to the reddened area will reveal an increased oxygen saturation. The blood count is checked for polycythemia vera.

DIFFERENTIAL DIAGNOSIS

Similar symptoms are associated with arteriosclerosis and peripheral neuritis. However, the skin is not warm, and symptoms are not induced by exposure to heat.

TREATMENT

No specific treatment is available at present. Ordinary acetylsalicylic acid often gives relief for several days. Marked relief may be obtained from epinephrine. Prophylactically, warm environments must be avoided, and light clothing should be worn. During an attack, the extremity is elevated and surrounded by cold packs. Surgically, one may try peripheral nerve section. It may be possible to desensitize the extremity gradually to warmth. The part is exposed to controlled heat, which at first is well below the critical point. Each day the temperature is raised 1° until the critical point is greatly exceeded.

ACROCYANOSIS

Acrocyanosis is a condition characterized by painless, persistent cyanosis and swelling of the hands and the feet. It occurs most commonly in females. The cause is unknown. The most plausible theory is that of arteriolar spasm causing anoxemic dilatation of the capillaries and the venules. The fact that during sleep the hands of the acrocyanotic patient become warm and red suggests a hyper-reactive sympathetic nervous system.

CLINICAL PICTURE

The patient is often female. The coldness and the bluish discoloration of the hands and to a lesser degree of the feet have been present for many years. The discoloration is more marked during the winter when the affected parts may be swollen, painful, and tender. During the summer the color is less cyanotic. No episodes of blanching occur, and trophic changes, ulceration, and gangrene are absent, thereby distinguishing this condition from Raynaud's disease and occlusive arterial disease.

TREATMENT

No treatment is necessary for this relatively asymptomatic condition. In severe cases sympathectomy is indicated.

ACUTE ARTERIAL INJURIES

A laceration of a major artery may occur during surgery and from other trauma.[55] When the involved vessel is an end-artery (*e.g.*, the popliteal), ligation will be followed by gangrene. Interruption of any large artery at least will cause ischemic changes in soft tissues, such as the development of Volkmann's contracture. The fate of the extremity depends on collateral circulation, the site of ligation, and the possibility of reconstruction. Ligation should be done only if adequate collateral circulation can be preserved. If the point of ligation is proximal to the collaterals, such as the superficial femoral, or popliteal artery, a prosthetic or venous substitute must be used to bridge the defect produced by the trauma. If this is not technically feasible, a bypass procedure may be used as an alternative. Ligation alone should never be considered as definitive, because loss of perfusion may result in distal thrombosis and precludes secondary reconstructive procedures.

If an artery is ligated at some distance distal to the main collateral branch, a blind arterial pouch remains into which the arterial blood is directed and its pressure is needlessly dissipated. As a result, arterial pressure within the collateral is insufficient. Ligation should be done immediately distal to the collateral branch so that the incidence of ischemic changes or gangrene is lessened.[56]

When a major normal artery is damaged, its collaterals undergo spasm. This physiological spasm may be nature's method of reducing hemorrhage.

ETIOLOGY

Consideration is given to wounds, fractures, and crushing injuries.

TYPES

Complete Division. Exsanguinating hemorrhage is not always a sequela, because the vessel ends retract, the artery undergoes spasm, and thrombosis seals the lumen.

Partial Division. Hemorrhage is severe, and secondary hemorrhage is likely, because the arterial ends cannot retract. A large blood clot may accumulate over the opening, forming a pulsating hematoma. The arterial pressure develops a cavitation within the hematoma, while the outer wall of the mass becomes organized, resulting in a false aneurysm.

Simultaneous partial division of the accompanying vein allows arterial blood to track from artery to vein. A definite connecting channel forms, and an arteriovenous fistula results.

Contusion. Spasm not only of the damaged vessel but also of the collaterals frequently follows injury. This type of spasm is intense and only partially relieved by sympathetic block. Thrombosis is not necessarily a sequela, because this requires damage to the intima, plus slowed blood flow.

Compression. A bone fragment is the usual cause of compression. The main danger is thrombosis. Vascular compression occurs, especially at the elbow or knee, where the vessels are held fixed close to the bone.

CLINICAL PICTURE

Hemorrhage may or may not be evident. The distinguishing features follow:

1. Extreme pallor due to spasm of the artery and its collaterals
2. Loss of pulsations
3. Glovelike anesthesia and paresis or paralysis due to ischemia of nerves and muscles
4. Severe pain

5. Bruit. A bruit, on auscultation, indicates false aneurysm; a continuous to-and-fro bruit indicates an arteriovenous aneurysm. The distinction between the two is important. In the false aneurysm, arterial pressure is high and the mass tends to expand; also, it compresses adjacent structures. Rarely, it may rupture. On the other hand, the intrasaccular pressure in an arteriovenous aneurysm is low. The lesion stimulates the development of collaterals; therefore, operation may be advantageously postponed.

   The Doppler test will ascertain the patency of distal vessels even while pulses are impalpable.

TREATMENT

In most cases diagnosis and treatment are urgent. Delay may result in thrombosis, occlusion of collaterals, and irreversible nerve and muscle changes.

Immediate treatment aims at arresting the hemorrhage and restoring blood volume, hemoglobin, and protein.

To arrest the hemorrhage, direct pressure is applied to the bleeding point with gauze, forceps, and hemostatic material (Gelfoam, fibrin foam, Oxycel). A tourniquet should be avoided, if possible, because it cuts off the collaterals.

Early operative treatment aims at restoring blood flow through the original channel. It includes the following:

1. Débridement
2. Arterial clamps placed proximally and distally. Proximal ligation is avoided because it needlessly sacrifices the collaterals.
3. Damaged portion of vessel excised
4. Anticoagulants. The vessel is irrigated with a solution containing 10 mg heparin per 100 ml saline. Intravenous heparinization should be used if no threat to hemorrhage exists elsewhere.
5. Defect closed with everting mattress suture (Fig. 20-18)
6. Vein graft replaced if destruction extensive. A bovine heterograft or a synthetic graft may be used if a vein is unavailable.

General treatment of an ischemic extremity aims at maximal arterial inflow and minimal metabolic demand. It includes the following:

1. Limb kept horizontal or dependent, never elevated
2. Cool environment desirable. (Avoid refrigeration unless amputation is inevitable.)
3. Sympathetic block or sympathectomy
4. Vasodilating agents (*e.g.*, whiskey, papaverine)
5. Fasciotomy to prevent ischemic necrosis of muscles. (This procedure is indicated only for the compartment syndrome when relative ischemia is temporary.)

ARTERIAL ANEURYSM

An arterial aneurysm is an abnormal outpouching from an artery, causing a pulsating tumor. This dilatation may

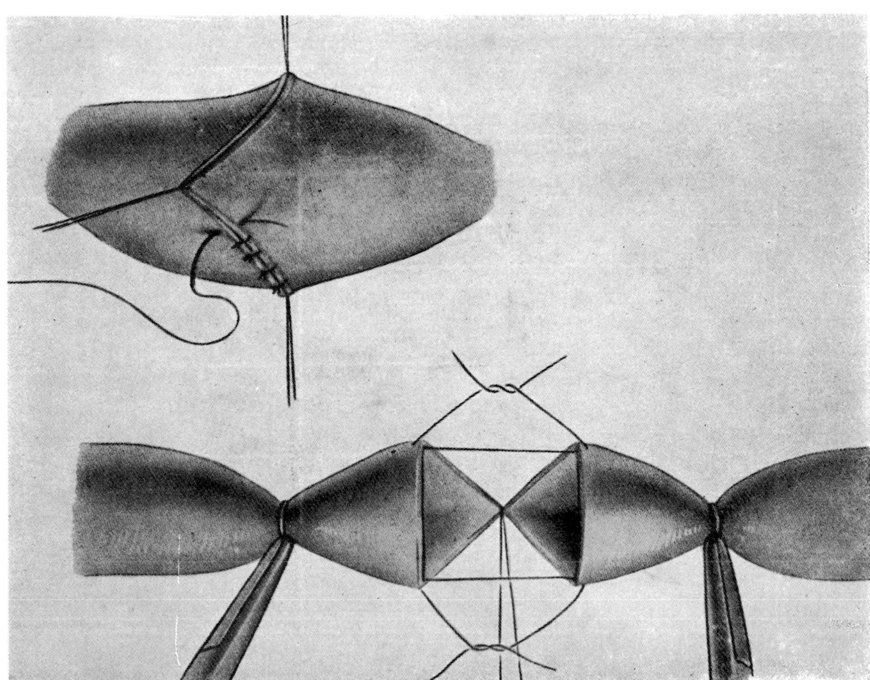

FIG. 20-18. Triangularization technique. Three sutures are inserted at equidistant points. Tension on these sutures makes suturing technically simple. Simple ligation techniques illustrated. (Bowers WF: Surgery of Trauma. Philadelphia, JB Lippincott, 1953)

occur as a gradual enlargement over an extensive area (the fusiform type of aneurysm), or it may be localized to a small segment as an abrupt enlargement (the saccular type of aneurysm). If the wall of the sac is made up of vessel structure itself, it is designated a true aneurysm. If the vessel wall is destroyed and the wall of the sac is composed of a blood clot, fibrous tissue, or surrounding structures, it is termed a false aneurysm (Fig. 20-19).

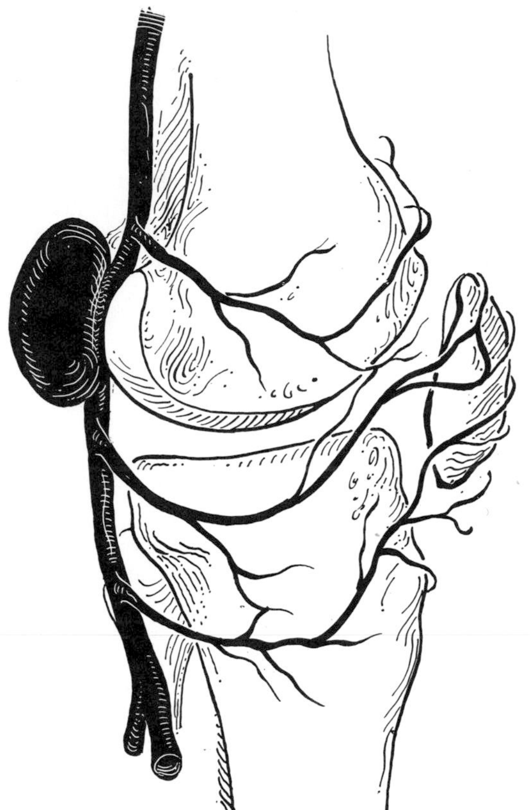

FIG. 20-19. Popliteal aneurysm.

ETIOLOGY

Aneurysms are congenital or acquired.

Congenital Arterial Aneurysm. This is rare. It is a result of an underdeveloped or absent muscle layer, the tunica media. It is found most frequently intracranially at the base of the brain where rupture causes fatal hemorrhage.

Acquired Arterial Aneurysm. This results from trauma or disease weakening the arterial wall. In the presence of a diseased vessel, trauma often precipitates the formation of an aneurysm.

Traumatic Aneurysm. Laceration of the vessel is caused from without by a penetrating wound or from within by a fracture. Only a portion of the circumference of the vessel is involved. When the laceration penetrates only the outer layers, arterial pressure dilates the inner layer. When the laceration extends through all the coats but the artery is held in continuity by part of the wall, there develops a large hematoma that temporarily obstructs the arterial flow. The pulsations of arterial pressure are transmitted by the hematoma and penetrate and enlarge the interior of the soft clot until the blood flows into the distal arterial component. Eventually, the distended clot becomes endothelialized on its inner surface, and the wall is reinforced by fibrous tissue and surrounding structures. The cavity becomes part of the peripheral artery circulation. Laminations of blood clot, as they deposit on the wall, become organized and thicken the wall to a leatherlike consistency.

Disease Causing Aneurysms. The majority of aneurysms (80%) are the result of arterial disease. (Under conditions of war, however, trauma is the main cause.)

Arteriosclerosis is the disease most commonly causing aneurysms. A calcium deposit is the usual site of rupture. Slight trauma to a sclerotic vessel is often the precipitating cause. The most common sites of saccular arteriosclerotic aneurysms are the popliteal arteries and the abdominal aorta; less commonly, the femoral artery just beyond the groin is affected.

The usual site of an arteriosclerotic aneurysm is an artery not surrounded by skeletal muscles and subject to frequent bending. They usually develop after the age of 60, and men are favored in the ratio of 10:1. Complete rupture is rare, especially in the extremities. Complete thrombosis often occurs in popliteal aneurysms.

Infections. The arterial wall may be weakened by an infection involving the vasa vasorum, particularly at sites subject to stress and strain, such as the knee. The infection arises from adjacent structures (*e.g.*, actinomycosis or mycotic aneurysm) or, more commonly, from an infective embolus (*e.g.*, subacute bacterial endocarditis). The aneurysm favors an artery unprotected by surrounding muscle and subjected to frequent bending.

Partial arterial occlusion. Poststenotic dilatation occurs typically in the subclavian artery beyond a point of compression. (See Chapter 22.)

Syphilis. Syphilitic aneurysm results as a late manifestation of untreated syphilis. It occurs predominantly in the aorta and rarely in the extremities. Present-day antibiotic therapy is making the conditon extinct.

Arteritis. Multiple areas of inflammation and necrosis cause countless numbers of small sacculations that are often identified as nodes in periarteritis nodosa.

Less common causes include burns, roentgen rays, radium, radioactive isotopes, invasion by malignancy, diabetes, lead poisoning, gout, tuberculosis, and surgical removal of overlying tissue.

PATHOLOGY

Two types of aneurysm can be identified: traumatic and nontraumatic.

Traumatic Type. If the wall is partially lacerated, the thin residual wall balloons out and is supported by the surrounding tissue. More often the entire thickness of the wall is divided, and a large hematoma forms within which arterial pressure creates a progressively increasing cavity or sac. Surrounding structures and reactive fibrosis reinforce and fix the walls from without. Laminations of clot are deposited repeatedly on the walls from within and become organized. The thick, leatherlike, endothelium-lined sac may be fusiform or saccular. A true aneurysm microscopically will show the remains of its own thinned-out layers with reactive fibrosis about it. A false aneurysm shows multiple laminations which vary from recent blood clot superficially to older deep layers of fibrous tissue. Aneurysmal pulsations will erode adjacent bone.

Nontraumatic Type. Ballooning takes place progressively thinning the wall until rupture occurs, and the surrounding tissues become the sac walls. Laminations of clot organize and thicken the walls. The wall tends to calcify, especially in arteriosclerotic aneurysms.

Pressure Effects. The accompanying vein may become occluded and thrombosed. Nerves are destroyed. Bone is eroded. Adhesions interfere with adjacent muscle movement.

Effects on Circulation. Blood supply distal to this area is diminished. The effect is accentuated by a reflex spasm of collateral vessels or an embolus thrown off from the aneurysmal clot.

PATHOGENESIS

The factors necessary for the production of an aneurysm are a weakened blood vessel wall (especially the muscular coat) and increased intraluminal pressure. A vessel wall that has been weakened by antecedent injury or disease may nøt develop an aneurysm until trauma, even of a trivial type, further weakens the wall, or when a rise in blood pressure overcomes resistance of the wall. Thus, an emotional upset or a lifting strain by increasing intra-arterial tension may cause an aneurysm to appear suddenly.

Constriction of an artery often causes an aneurysm to develop just beyond the point of narrowing. An example is compression of the subclavian artery by a cervical rib. Theories of pathogenesis include interruption of sympathetic constrictor impulses to the local segment and abnormal blood currents just beyond the stenosed channel.[57]

CLINICAL PICTURE

Symptoms will vary with the vessel involved. Collateral circulation in the upper extremity is excellent, and symptoms of peripheral ischemia are negligible. On the other hand, in the lower extremity claudication is evidencce of lesser collaterals.

Tumor Mass. This may be soft and cystic or somewhat indurated. If not obscured by a contained blood clot or by surrounding tissues, it may exhibit expansible pulsations synchronous with systole.

Pain. This occurs locally owing to pressure on adjacent structures or distally because of nerve compression (neuritic pain) and ischemic claudication.

Pressure Signs. In addition to pain, nerve compression results in paresis or paralysis; venous compression causes dependent edema.

Signs of Circulatory Insufficiency. The pulse volume is diminished or absent, Doppler readings and blood pressure are reduced, and skin temperature is lowered, as compared with the opposite extremity.

Congestion and Edema of the Parts Beyond. The veins are engorged with blood, which flows sluggishly because the arterial pressure is insufficient to move the blood along.

Bruit. A characteristic sound perceived early on auscultation is due to whirling of blood within the sac. As clotting and fibrosis reduce the size of the cavity, the bruit may disappear. In arterial aneurysms, the bruit is synchronous with systole, in contradistinction to arteriovenous aneurysms, in which there is a to-and-fro murmur.

Trophic Changes. These occur distal to the aneurysm.

Arteriogram. This reveals the size and the position of the aneurysm and the extent of collateral circulation. A normal arteriogram does not definitely exclude the possibility of an aneurysm, because the dye column may appear normal in a large aneurysm that has clotted except for the lumen.

PROGNOSIS

Aneurysms in the extremities, in contrast to those elsewhere, have an excellent outlook, because sufficient time has elapsed to develop a collateral circulation and the pathology is readily accessible to surgical therapy.

TREATMENT

Small aneurysms occasionally are obliterated spontaneously by filling with blood clot followed by fibrous organization. Otherwise, the following surgical measurements are indicated:

1. *Excision of aneurysm with end-to-end anastomosis* is the procedure of choice when continuity of circulation is vital and it is possible to appose vessel ends by stretching, rerouting, or flexion of adjacent joints. It is especially indicated in young people whose vessels are not diseased but whose collateral circulation is inadequate.
2. *Excision of aneurysm with repair of the artery* is applicable especially to traumatic aneurysms. The artery is compressed proximally and distally. The aneurysm is opened widely, and clots are removed. Often the arterial opening is found to be small. The defect is sutured with fine arterial silk, reinforced with a layer of the sac, and the remainder of the sac is excised.
3. *Excision with an autologous venous or bovine heterograft or synthetic substitute* bridges a large gap. The saphenous vein is readily available and thickens like the host artery. However, the vein selected should be comparable in size with the artery. The vein should be so placed that its distal end joins the proximal end of the artery and vice versa because of the valvular system in the veins.

   If the saphenous vein is unavailable, substitution for the aneurysmal area can be accomplished in a similar manner by using a bovine heterograft or a synthetic prosthesis to bridge the resulting defect.
4. *Perianeurysmal irritation.* In certain locations, because of its size or risk to life or limb by resection, the aneurysms can instead be wrapped in a coating of Dacron tailored to conform to its size and shape. This will produce scarring and prevent rupture but will not reduce the incidence of thrombosis or embolism and should therefore be reserved for the most complicated situations.[58]

Preoperative Management. Arteriographic and blood flow studies should clearly outline the adequacy of the distal arterial circulation preoperatively, and this should establish whether resection and substitute procedures are indicated. Sympathectomy may be considered.

Aneurysms of the Extremities. These aneurysms are the interest of the vascular surgeon, but the orthopaedic surgeon must be constantly alerted of their presence in any differential diagnosis. An attempt must be made to reestablish continuity of the artery by end-to-end anastomosis, removal of the sac with repair of the opening, a graft of autologous vein, or bovine heterograft or synthetic prosthetic replacement.

Complications of aneurysm surgery include hemorrhage, arterial or pulmonary embolism, and infection. Later, deficient blood supply is evidenced chiefly by claudication on exercise. The patient must be taught to live within the limits of his circulation until adequate collaterals develop.

ARTERIOVENOUS FISTULA

An arteriovenous fistula is an abnormal communication between an artery and a vein proximal to the capillary bed. It is congenital or acquired. The acquired type is caused almost invariably by penetrating wounds, is usually single, and occurs anywhere in the extremities. The congenital type consists of a tremendous number of communicating channels and is most common about the forearm and the hand. The following discussion is limited to the acquired type of fistula. Congenital arteriovenous fistula is covered in Chapter 25 (The Hand).[59]

PATHOLOGY

The fistulous channel is either short or long and narrow or broad and distended so as to constitute an aneurysmal sac. Locally, the vein is distended and hypertrophied and, if the fistula is small, gradually assumes the appearance of an artery. If the caliber of the fistula is large, the vein becomes greatly distended and simulates a false aneurysmal sac. The artery proximal to the fistula becomes dilated and the walls thinned. Distal to the site of communication, the artery is narrowed. The artery and the vein may enter the fistula or sac separately or through a common opening.

CLINICAL PICTURE

The typical characteristics are as follows:

1. *Profuse but controlled hemorrhage.* This appears early after an injury.
2. *Thrill and bruit.* These are continuous throughout the cardiac cycle and develop within a few hours or days. (The murmur of an aneurysm is a soft systolic "whish," whereas that of an arteriovenous fistula is a noisy "machinery" to-and-fro bruit.)
3. *Venous insufficiency.* Consequent varices, edema, stasis pigmentation, ulceration, and chronic indurative cellulitis are complications that involve the extreme distal parts of the extremity in contrast with the chronic venous insufficiency of thrombophlebitis or primary varicose veins, which causes stasis ulceration at or above the malleoli of the ankle.

4. *Gangrene.* Gangrene of digits or distal parts of the extremity is due to ischemia.
5. *Increased limb length.* This occurs if the fistula is acquired before the epiphyseal lines close.
6. *Increased skin temperature.* This occurs about and just distal to the fistula.
7. *Cardiac enlargement.* This is due to increased pressure of return blood flow. It occurs only in large-caliber communicating channels and may result in congestive heart failure.
8. *Increased oxygenation of venous blood.* A blood sample taken from a vein proximal to the fistula is bright red and arterial as compared with a sample from the opposite extremity. Actual measurement of oxygen content reveals the increase.
9. *Branham's sign.* A sharp decrease in pulse rate occurs when the fistula is closed by digital pressure. The systolic and the diastolic pressures increase at the same time.

ARTERIOGRAPHY

Injection of a contrast medium into the artery proximal to the anastomosis, and while the blood flow in the artery is stopped by a tourniquet, reveals the artery to be enlarged and tortuous proximal to the fistula. Distally, the artery is narrowed or not visualized. Locally, at the anastomotic site the vein displays a rounded saccular bulge, and the veins distally are well seen and enlarged, tortuous, and multiple.

DOPPLER STUDIES

When the fistula is large and the blood flow is easily short-circuited, Doppler readings will show a marked pressure gradient drop immediately beyond the level of the arteriovenous communication. When measured at the distal portion of the extremity, palpable pulsations may be diminished or absent and pressure readings are quite low.

TREATMENT

The surgical indications include chronic venous insufficiency, cardiac enlargement, and prevention of growth increase. A period of at least 6 months' waiting is allowed for establishment of collateral circulation. Before repair, the adequacy of collateral circulation should be tested.

Moszkowicz Test. The extremity is elevated, and a tight bandage is applied for 5 minutes, after which the extremity is placed in a horizontal position and the bandage is removed quickly. When circulation is adequate, a hyperemic blush occurs promptly. When arterial insufficiency exists, the blush is absent or slight and progresses slowly toward the periphery.

If collateral circulation is found to be inadequate, a further waiting period will eventually prove to be profitable. Occasionally, it may be necessary to relieve vascular spasm by sympathectomy after prelimnary testing by procaine block.

Technique

The inflatable tourniquet is placed and held in readiness. It is advantageous to have continuous blood flow, which permits localization of the abnormal communication by detecting the bruit. The artery is dilated proximally; the vein is dilated both proximally and distally. Then the lowest point at which Branham's bradycardia phenomenon can be elicited is determined. The fistulous area is usually engulfed by scar tissue resulting from the original injury.

The ideal procedure is to dissect out the site of the fistula connection and repair the artery and vein directly. This may be possible in the simplest of cases. In more complicated cases, scar tissue will prevent adequate dissection of the fistula site, and it is advisable to ligate the artery proximal and distal to the fistula and reestablish arterial continuity with a reverse saphenous vein graft or a bovine or synthetic substitute.

GLOMUS TUMOR

Throughout the body, lying in the stratum reticulare between the skin and the subcutaneous layer, are innumerable specialized direct connections between terminal arteries and veins. Each arteriovenous anastomosis or shunt, the glomus or neuromyoarterial glomus, is under the direct control of the sympathetic nervous system and serves the functions of local and general regulation of heat and the regulation of blood pressure. The structure of the normal glomus was first described by Sucquet and Hoyer.[60] The glomus is an arteriovenous anastomosis with thick tortuous walls. Its canal is lined with several rows of cuboid endothelial cells beneath which the elastic layer is absent. A thick muscular coat of smooth muscle surrounds the endothelium. Within and around the muscle cells are large epithelioid cells with clear or vacuolar cytoplasm and vesicular nuclei. They constitute the typical glomus cells, whose origin is unknown. Closely associated with the glomus cells is an abundance of nonmyelinated nerve fibers, which are demonstrable by special stains. The tortuous anastomotic channel is designated the Sucquet-Hoyer canal (Fig. 20-20*C* and *D*).

PATHOLOGY

The glomus tumor is probably a hypertrophy of the normal glomus. Grossly, the tumor is encapsulated, a few millimeters in diameter, and deep red or purple; and on cutting, it exudes blood, following which it assumes a gray color (Fig. 20-20*B*). Microscopically, an overgrowth of the cellular constituents, particularly the epithelioid cells, is noted.

CLINICAL PICTURE

Trauma often precedes the tumor. Although glomus tumors may appear anywhere in the body, they are most frequent on the hands and the feet, particularly beneath the fingernails. The glomus tumor typically appears as a small, painful, purplish nodule in the skin or under the nail. A severe neuralgic type of pain may be present for some time before the bluish spot just a few millimeters in diameter appears. The spot or nodule is excruciatingly tender and when pressed on may become blanched. The lesion can be localized accurately by careful testing with the point of a pin. The normal or surrounding skin is not excessively sensitive, but as soon as the glomus tumor is touched excruciating pain is provoked. The application of cold to the lesion will produce a paroxysm. Occasionally associated with the severe pain are vasomotor changes that may involve the extremity or the entire half of the body. The lesion may occur at any age.

ROENTGENOGRAPHIC FINDINGS

Because the tumor is pulsatile, when it is situated in a finger it may cause a smooth saucer-shaped erosion of the adjacent phalanx (Fig. 20-20*A*).

TREATMENT

Complete excision will effect a cure. To ensure complete removal, the phalanx should be curetted thoroughly. When using a local anesthetic, infiltration must avoid the vicinity of the tumor where swelling incident to the injection would blanch the tumor and make its identification difficult.

PERIARTERITIS NODOSA

Periarteritis nodosa (polyarteritis) is a progressive, usually fatal disease of protean manifestations secondary to widespread focal involvement of the walls of medium- and small-sized arteries. Fibrinoid degeneration in the walls of blood vessels is characteristic and classifies this as a collagen disease. It can involve any region of the

FIG. 20-20. Glomus tumor. (*A*) Roentgenogram demonstrating severe erosion of the distal phalanx. (*B*) Operative appearance at typical site. (*C*) Photomicrograph of encapsulated tumor (×90). (*D*) Higher magnification of microscopic section (×430). Note the vessel and glomus cells. The blood vessel is lined with endothelial cells, and the surrounding epithelioid cells have large, oval, darkly stained nuclei. The cytoplasm is faintly stained. (Posch JL: Tumors of the hand. J Bone Joint Surg 38A:527, 1956) (*Figure continues on facing page.*)

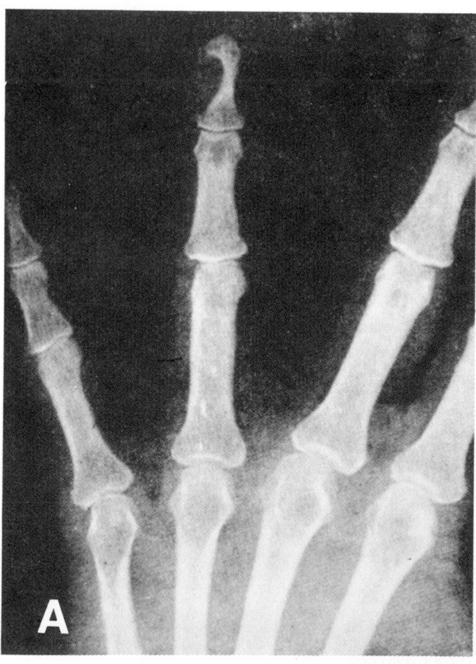

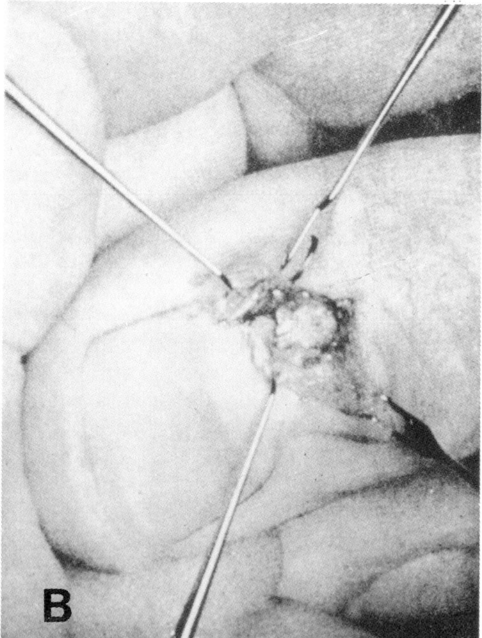

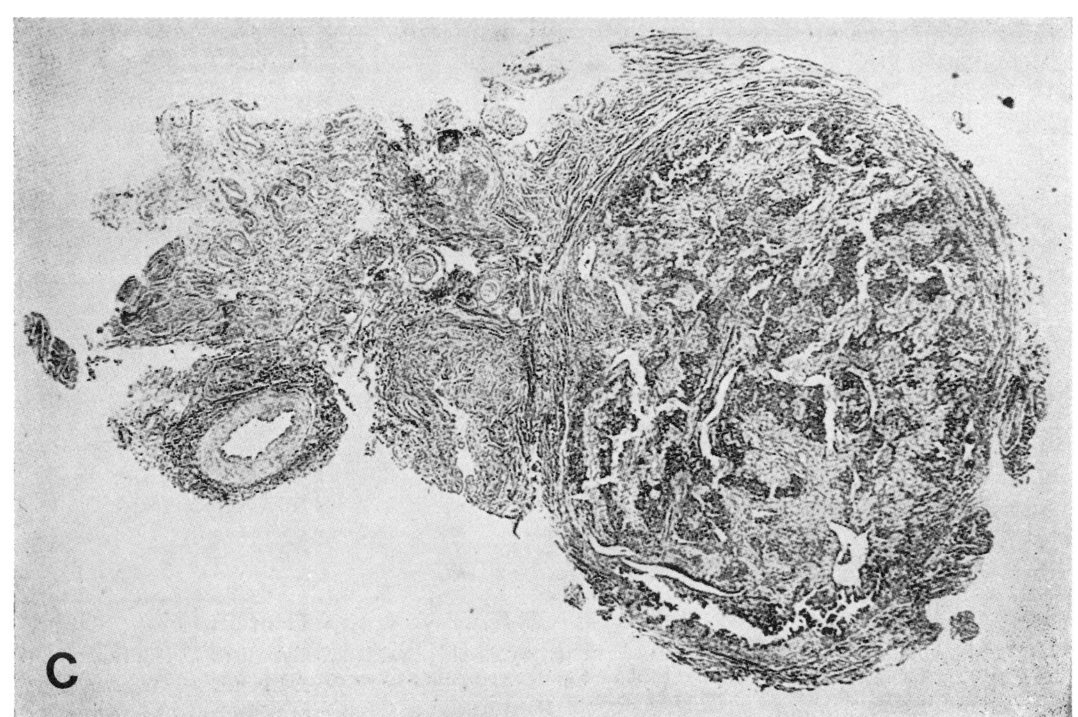
C

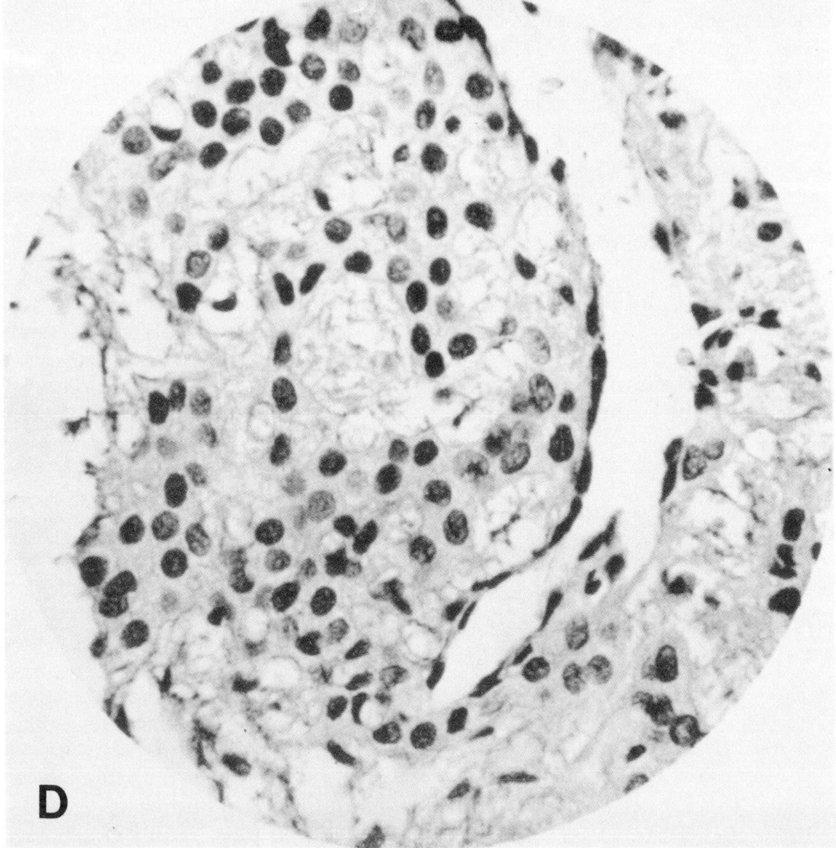
D

body. Its importance to the orthopaedic surgeon lies in differentiating it from conditions, which it may imitate, in and about the musculoskeletal system. For example, periarteritis in the neck may suggest lesions of the cervical spine; involvement of a plantar digital artery in the foot may be confused with Morton's toe. Eventually, multifocal involvement may clarify the diagnosis, but a correct antemortem interpretation is unusual.

ETIOLOGY

The cause is unknown. The affliction favors males in the ratio of 2:1. No age-group is spared, but people in the third and fourth decades are predisposed.

EXPERIMENTAL WORK

Polyarteritis can develop in patients during a serum sickness type of anaphylactic reaction.[62] It can be produced experimentally by subjecting animals to serum sickness.[63] The frequency of the condition has increased coincident with the advent and the widespread use of sulfa drugs. Many sensitizing drugs used to reproduce the disease, associated allergic conditions, and eosinophilia in many patients suggest but do not prove an allergic origin. It is now considered an autoimmune disorder, one of the entities included under collagen diseases (see text).

PATHOLOGY

The basic lesion is a necrotizing, inflammatory, obliterative process involving the small arteries, the arterioles, and, occasionally, the veins.[61] The following stages delineate the process (Fig. 20-21):

1. *Edema, eosinophilic fibrinoid necrosis* of the inner media and collagenous tissue in the subendothelial and adventitial areas of the arterial wall. Necrosis of the media leads to aneurysmal dilatation.
2. *Mononuclear cellular infiltration* of the adventitia and media occurring coincident with fibrinoid necrosis. In early stages, eosinophils appear in large numbers.
3. *Endothelial destruction leading to thrombosis and infarction,* especially seen in kidneys, intestines, liver, spleen, and myocardium. The thrombus becomes organized and eventually recanalized.
4. *Healing stage* of fibroblastic repair of damaged periarterial tissues.

FIG. 20-21. Periarteritis nodosa. Typical appearance of lesion in biopsied muscle specimen.

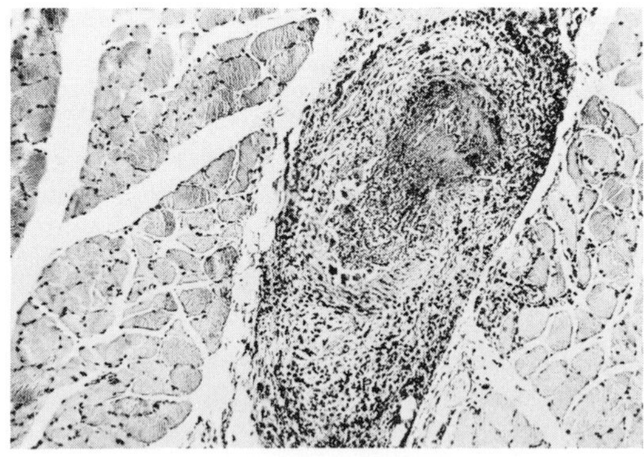

Grossly, minute and microscopic nodules along the course of the vessel consist of periarterial inflammation and fibrosis or aneurysm formation. Widespread involvement of organs and tissues is usual.

CLINICAL PICTURE

Symptoms include those of a systemic inflammation plus those specific for the affected regions. The main features are fever, weakness, and prostration; leukocytosis with a shift to the left, often an eosinophilia; albuminuria and microscopic hematuria; abdominal pain; signs and symptoms of polyneuritis; and hypertension.

The onset is insidious, with vague symptoms of fever and malaise. At first fever may persist without other symptoms. Later, symptoms appear in various, widely spread, unrelated areas.

Renal involvement consists in albuminuria, microscopic hematuria, and cylindruria. Glomerulonephritis, when present, causes generalized edema. Renal insufficiency leads to progressive intractable hypertension.

Myocardial involvement, by fibrinoid degeneration of myocardial collagen, causes abnormalities of cardiac function. Pericarditis and coronary symptoms may occur.

Pulmonary involvement causes diffuse pulmonary infiltrations. Intractable asthma may dominate the picture.

Gastrointestinal symptoms include persistent abdominal pain, anorexia, and vomiting. Hemorrhagic lesions of stomach, bowel, pancreas, liver, and spleen produce symptoms referable to these organs.

Polyneuritis symptoms are conspicuous in many cases and include hyperesthesias, numbness, and muscle weakness.

Central nervous system symptoms include convulsions, meningitis, and paralysis, as a result of ischemic foci.

Cutaneous manifestations are extremely variable. Occasionally, hemorrhagic lesions may ulcerate.

Muscle and joint pains are characteristic. Although nodules are not palpable, multiple tender spots are identified. Discomfort is persistent and accentuated by active and passive motion. Extensive involvement with multiple foci of ischemic necrosis may materially weaken the muscle.

Cutaneous nerve pain in any specified area is often severe, lancinating, and obstinate. It is due to an arteritic process in nutrient vessels of the nerve.

LABORATORY FINDINGS

Leukocytosis is moderate, and the sedimentation rate is elevated. Eosinophilia, when present, may be quite high. Antinuclear antibodies in the serum are found in most cases.

DIAGNOSIS

The disease is suspected in a prolonged systemic illness in which several unrelated organs are involved. Biopsy of muscle tissue at a tender site may reveal the characteristic vascular lesion and a sharply circumscribed area of swollen, hyalinized, disintegrating muscle fibers. When a well-localized point of tenderness can be identified beneath the skin proximal to a persistently painful part, one should not hesitate to explore, resect, and examine microscopically the cutaneous nerve.

PROGNOSIS AND TREATMENT

Until recently the prognosis was grave; most patients die of renal or cardiac insufficiency or intercurrent infection. A sensitizing antigen should be sought and eliminated. Cortisone and ACTH dramatically suppress and prevent the development of further clinical manifestations. However, if treatment has been started after irreversible damage has occurred in vital organs, the outlook continues to be serious. Some cases become permanently arrested spontaneously and undergo complete healing.

THERAPEUTIC SYMPATHETIC PARALYSIS

ANATOMICAL FACTS

The sympathetic portion of the autonomic nervous system consists of two chains of ganglia, each of which lies on the anterolateral aspect of the spine. Each chain is composed of 24 ganglia, 3 cervical (superior, middle, inferior), 12 thoracic, 4 lumbar, and the rest sacral. The white rami communicantes, which contain the efferent fibers from the cord, and the gray rami communicantes, which contain the afferent fibers to the cord, connect the spinal nerve root with its corresponding ganglion in the chain. The cervical ganglia are exceptions. They have no connection with the cervical nerves and instead reach the spinal cord through the upper thoracic nerves, by way of the thoracic ganglia. The upper three thoracic ganglia are therefore the sympathetic supply stations for the upper extremity. Occasionally, the inferior cervical ganglion is fused with the first thoracic forming the stellate ganglion. In the thoracic area, the thoracic chain lies in relation to the heads of the ribs. In the lumbar area, the chain lies between the medial border of the psoas muscle and the spine. On the right side it is overlapped medially by the vena cava. Also on the right side, the lower lumbar veins pass anterior to the lower segment of the trunk. Elsewhere they pass behind the trunk. The first lumbar ganglion lies at the margin of the diaphragmatic crura. The fourth lumbar ganglion lies just above the sacral promontory.

INDICATIONS

The orthopaedic surgeon is concerned mainly with interrupting sympathetic function to the extremities. The sympathetic fibers pass distally through the extremities through the peripheral nerves, supplying vasomotor, sudomotor, and pilomotor impulses and returning visceral painful impulses to the spinal cord. Therefore, the main uses for sympathetic interruption are reduction of sweating, effecting vasodilatation, and relieving sympathetic pain. The following conditions are benefited:

Vasospastic Conditions

Raynaud's disease, Raynaud's phenomenon as a result of such causes as the use of high-frequency vibrating tools, acrocyanosis, frostbite, trench foot or immersion foot, causalgia, livedo reticularis, segmental arterial spasm, postparalytic cold extremities, and thrombophlebitis

Arterial Obstructive Conditions

Chronic obliterative arterial disease (ASO, TAO, periarteritis nodosa), acute arterial obstruction (embolism, thrombosis, injury, surgical division). The aim is to improve the collateral circulation.

Sympathetic Pain

Ischemic pain, causalgic burning pain, and minor causalgic states, as in thrombophlebitis and arthritis, are alleviated.

TEST OF EFFECTIVENESS OF SYMPATHETIC INTERRUPTION

The degree of vasodilatation to be obtained can be evaluated by anesthetic injection of the peripheral nerve, spinal anesthesia, or general anesthesia, but it is best to determine this by anesthetization of the sympathetic trunk, which also relieves pain of sympathetic origin. Vasodilatation can be measured by comparing the rise of digital skin temperature with that in the opposite limb. In obliterative arterial disease, lack of significant alteration is not unusual; however, improvement of symptoms by sympathetic interruption is often obtained. The cessation of sweating and increase in cutaneous electric resistance in a part is proof that the sympathetic trunk has been anesthetized. These tests are useful when no vasodilatation is demonstrable. Autonomic blocking agents, such as tetraethylammonium chloride, are of no value because they effect a varying degree of vasodilation and in effective doses often cause a fall in blood pressure.

TECHNIQUE OF SYMPATHETIC BLOCKS

Injection of a local anesthetic along the side of the spinal column blocks the nerve roots at their point of emergence from their foramina and the sympathetic chain (Figs. 20-22 through 20-25). This is known as a paravertebral block. By blocking one nerve and its corresponding sympathetic ganglion, one visceral and somatic segment of the body is anesthetized (segmental block). The technique of paravertebral block is such that it is almost impossible to block the nerve root without similarly affecting its rami to the sympathetic trunk. On the other hand, the sympathetic ganglion may be blocked without affecting the nerve root. The following description pertains to thoracic and lumbar paravertebral blocks, the technique being varied as indicated to obtain sympathetic blocks. For the upper extremity, the lowest cervical and the upper three thoracic ganglia are infiltrated. All four lumbar ganglia must be blocked to deprive the lower extremity of sympathetic innervation.[66]

Landmarks. In the thoracic spine, the emerging nerve lies at the level of the tip of the spinous process of the vertebra directly above it. For example, the foramen of the first thoracic nerve will be found directly opposite the tip of the spinous process of the seventh cervical vertebra.

In the lumbar spine, the foramen is directly opposite the center of its corresponding spinous process.

The foramen in the thoracic spine lies about 1¼ inches deep to the posterior surface of the transverse process. In other words, when the needle point contacts the posterior surface of the transverse process and then is directed deeply below the inferior margin of the trans-

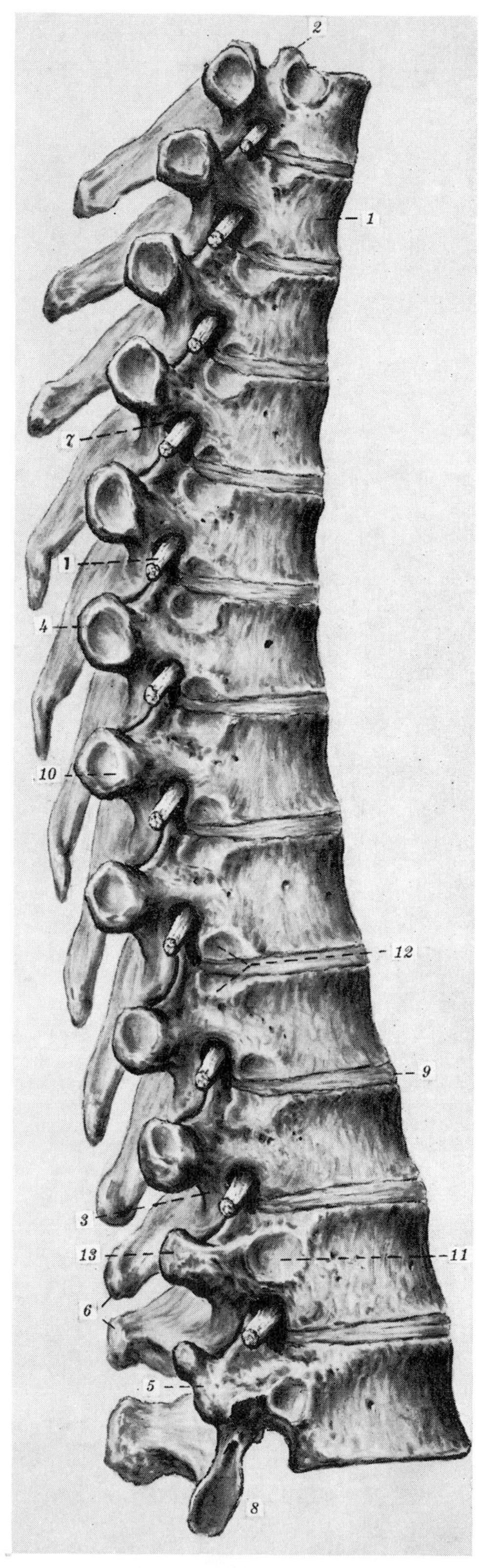

FIG. 20-22. Thoracic vertebrae as seen from the right side.
Nerve: (*1*) spinal nerve emerging from the intervertebral foramen
Tissues: (*1*) body, (*2*) superior articular surface, (*3*) lamina, (*4*) transverse process, (*5*) mamillary process, (*6*) spinous process, (*7*) intervertebral foramen, (*8*) inferior articular surface, (*9*) intervertebral cartilage, (*10*) facet on transverse process for articular part of tubercle of rib, (*11*) facet for head of rib, (*12*) demifacet for articular head of rib, (*13*) no facet on transverse process. (Southworth JL, Hingson RA, Pitkin WM (eds): Pitkin's Conduction Anesthesia. Philadelphia, JB Lippincott, 1946)

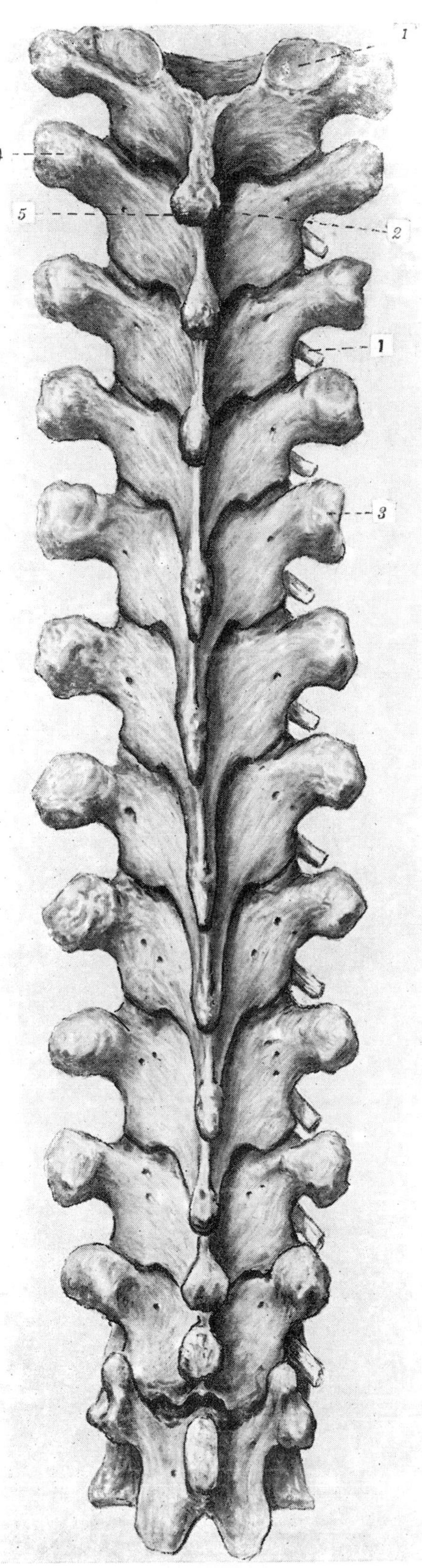

FIG. 20-23. Posterior view of the thoracic vertebrae; spinal nerves emerge from the foramina on the right side.
Nerve: (*1*) spinal
Tissues: (*1*) superior articular surface, (*2*) lamina, (*3, 4*) transverse processes, (*5*) spinous process. (Southworth JL, Hingson RA, Pitkin WM (eds): Pitkin's Conduction Anesthesia. Philadelphia, JB Lippincott, 1946)

FIG. 20-24. Lumbar vertebrae as seen from the right side.
Nerve: (*1*) first lumbar nerve emerging from the intervertebral foramen
Tissues: (*1*) body, (*2*) superior articular surface, (*3*) lamina; (*4*) transverse process, (*5*) mamillary process, (*6*) spinous process, (*7*) intervertebral foramen, (*8*) inferior articular surface, (*9*) intervertebral cartilage. (Southworth JL, Hingson RA, Pitkin WM (eds): Pitkin's Conduction Anesthesia. Philadelphia, JB Lippincott, 1946)

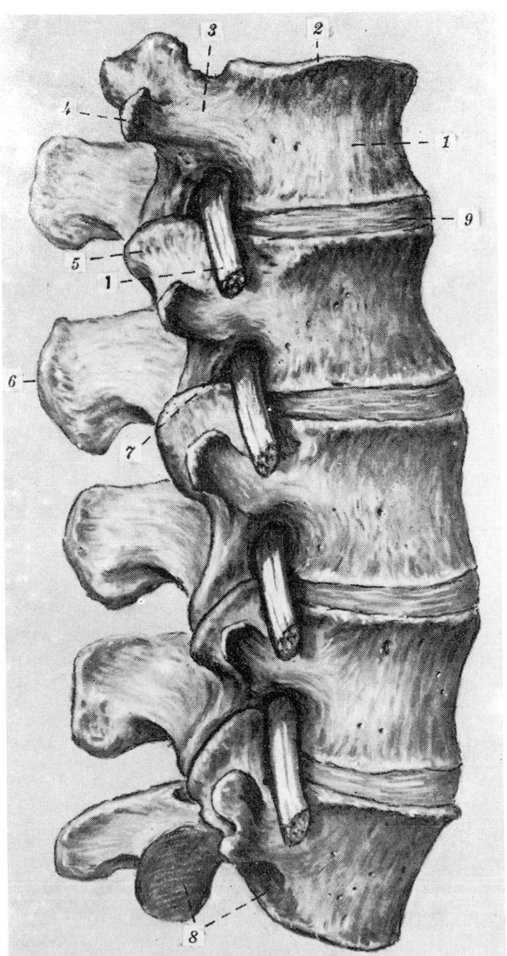

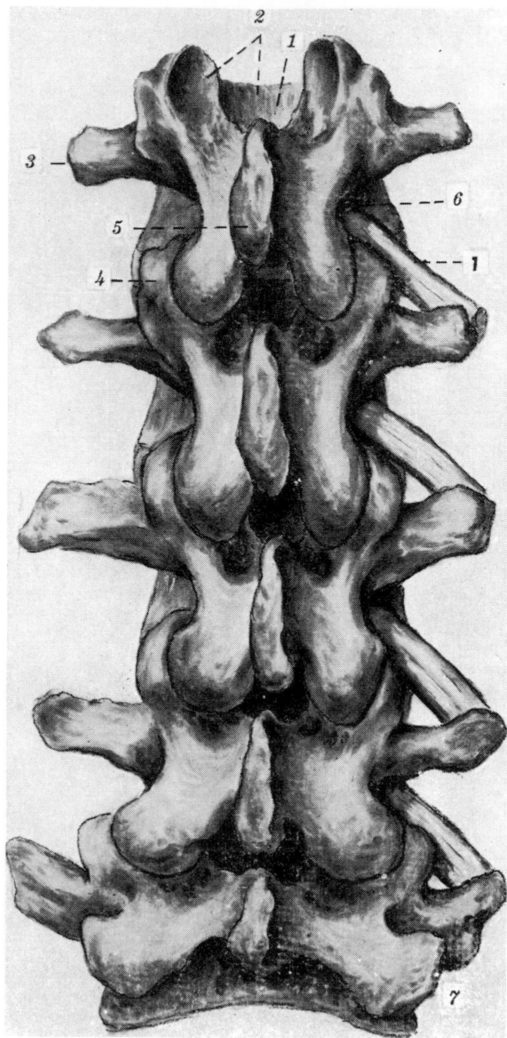

FIG. 20-25 Lumbar vertebrae, posterior view. Note that in blocking near the midline (1½ inches) as described in the text the needle glides off the inferior border of the transverse process to touch the posterior surface of the body of the vertebra at or near the intervertebral foramen. (see Figure 20-27).

Nerve: (*1*) first lumbar nerve emerging from the intervertebral foramen

Tissues: (*1*) body, (*2*) superior articular surface, (*3*) transverse process, (*4*) mamillary process, (*5*) spinous process, (*6*) intervertebral foramen, (*7*) inferior articular surface. (Southworth JL, Hingson RA, Pitkin WM (eds): Pitkin's Conduction Anesthesia. Philadelphia, JB Lippincott, 1946)

verse process, it is inserted to a depth of 1¼ inches before it contacts the nerve, the foramen, or the posterolateral aspect of the body of the vertebra. In the lumbar spine, the distance from the transverse process to the foramen is about one fourth of an inch less.

In the upper thorax, the ganglia lie beneath the necks of the ribs and near the thoracic roots, along the sides of the vertebral bodies. In the lumbar area, the ganglia lie a little deeper along the lateral surfaces of the vertebral bodies. The right sympathetic chain is covered anteriorly by the vena cava, and to the left lies the aorta.

Needle Insertion. The patient is placed in the lateral recumbent position with knees flexed on the abdomen and head bent forward, with the chin on the chest to make the spinous processes more prominent posteriorly. A wheal is made 1½ inches lateral to the selected spinous process. (In the thoracic spine, the landmarks for the upper three sympathetic ganglia are the seventh cervical and first and second thoracic spinous processes; in the lumbar spine, the first to fourth spinous processes identify the correspondingly numbered lumbar ganglia.) A 3½- or 4-inch blunt-pointed needle is inserted through the wheal inward and medially until it contacts the posterior surface of the transverse process (Figs. 20-26 and 20-27). Then it is withdrawn slightly and directed downward at an angle of 15° to 20°, tilted laterally 15° to 20°, and advanced again to pass below the inferior margin of the transverse process. It is advanced farther until it contacts the posterior surface of the body of the vertebra at the outer border of the intervertebral foramen. Contact with the nerve root may evoke paresthetic sensations. This is the position for injecting the nerve root.

If the needle angulation is reduced, that is, the needle hub is moved slightly nearer to the midline, the needle may be made to advance farther along the side of the vertebral body to the sympathetic chain. If the injection of the sympathetics is proper, it will be evidenced clinically by vasodilatation, redness, warmth, and dryness of the part. When infiltration of the first thoracic ganglion spreads to involve the inferior cervical ganglion, Horner's syndrome will be produced.

Stellate Ganglion Block. Occasionally, it is desirable to block the inferior cervical ganglion. This ganglion, when combined with the first thoracic ganglion, is known as the stellate ganglion. The inferior cervical ganglion lies immediately in front of the transverse process of the seventh cervical vertebra and in front of the first rib and just behind the vertebral artery. It may be approached in the same manner as described for paravertebral block of the first thoracic nerve and first thoracic ganglion. Occasionally, it may be easier, particularly in the obese patient, to approach it from the side (Figs. 20-28 and 20-29).

Technique. A point is selected on the lateral aspect of the neck even with the transverse process of the sixth cervical vertebra, if it is palpable, or a fingerbreadth above the seventh cervical spinous process. Anterior to the trapezius the needle is inserted and directed downward and medially at an angle of about 90° with the midline to touch the transverse process of the seventh cervical vertebra. Then the needle is withdrawn slightly and advanced more anteriorly until it contacts the body of the vertebra, where the injection is made. Proper response is indicated by Horner's syndrome and vasodilatation and dryness of the upper extremity.

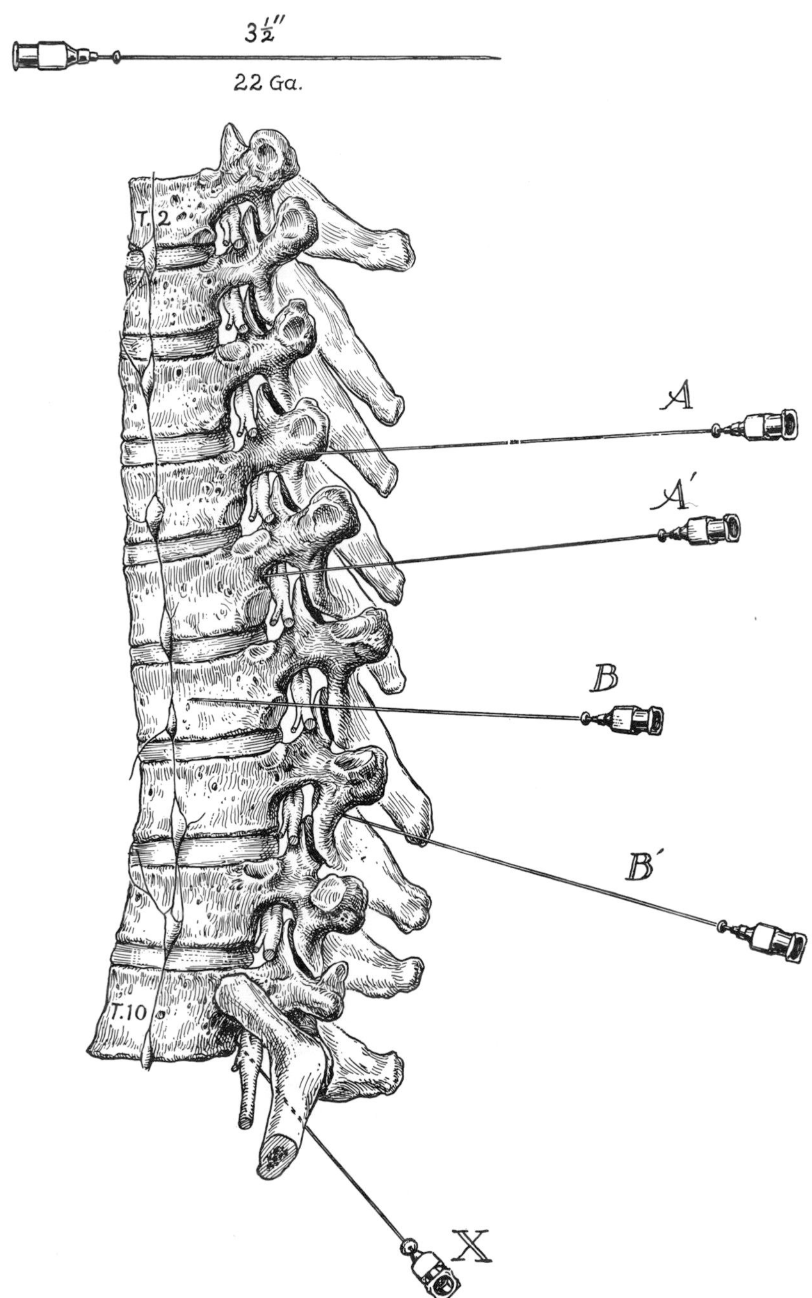

FIG. 20-26. Techniques of paravertebral block. (For explanation see text.) (Southworth JL, Hingson RA, Pitkin WM (eds): Pitkin's Conduction Anesthesia. Philadelphia, JB Lippincott, 1946)

The dangers of this method include puncture of the vertebral or subclavian artery, the pleura, or even the dura.

TECHNIQUE OF SYMPATHECTOMY

Sympathetic Denervation of the Upper Extremity. Removal of, or decentralization of, the upper dorsal ganglia below the level of the first will effect sympathetic paralysis of the upper extremity and half of the head without production of Horner's syndrome (Figs. 20-30 and 20-31). The operation not only aims at preganglionic denervation of the sympathetics but also at measures that avoid postoperative regeneration, namely, removal of the second and third spinal ganglia and a segment of two intercostal nerves, intradural section of the roots, and a silk cylinder to enclose the remaining cut chain ends.[65]

Endotracheal anesthesia is used. The patient lies in

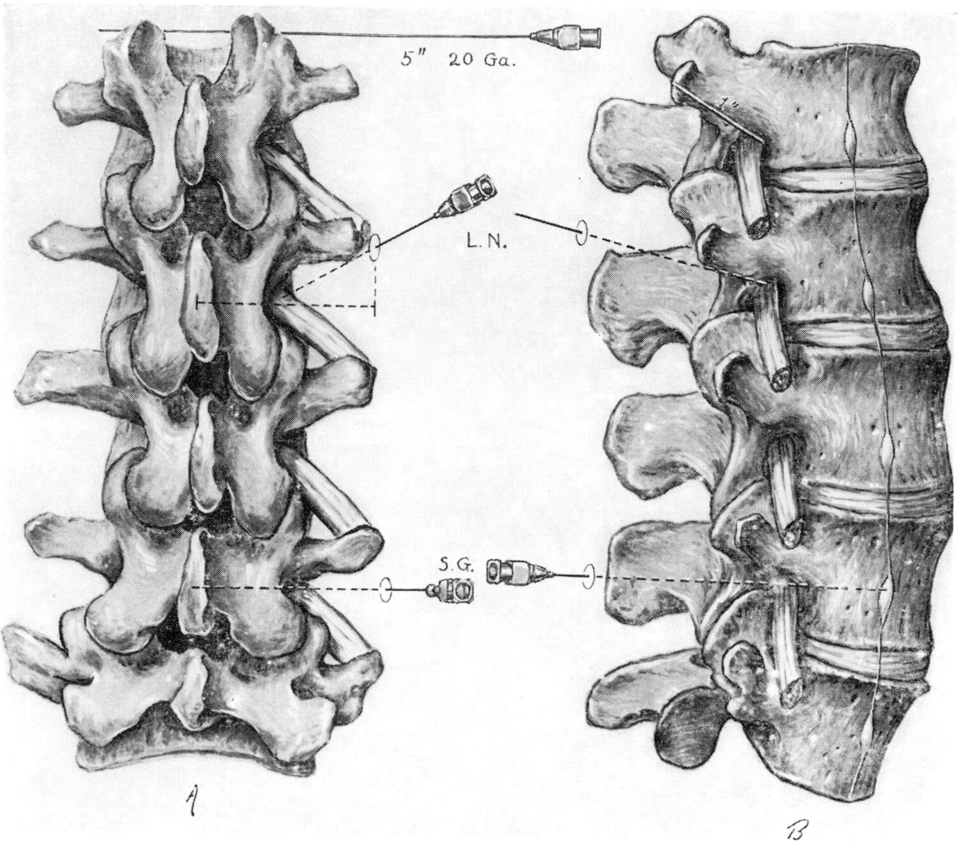

FIG. 20-27. Technique of paravertebral block in the lumbar region. (*A*) Upper needle shows the correct approach, the needle having glided off the transverse process to the intervertebral foramen (upper needle in *B*), where 5 ml of solution will block the somatic nerve and its connections in the upper lumbar region. To block the sympathetic ganglion alone, the needle approach may be made from a site a little more lateral and without downward angulation to bypass the transverse process until the point comes to rest on the anterolateral aspect of the body of the vertebra. (Southworth JL, Hingson RA, Pitkin WM (eds): Pitkin's Conduction Anesthesia. Philadelphia, JB Lippincott, 1946)

the prone position with arms alongside the body. A pillow is placed beneath the sternum so that the scapulae fall away from the midline. An incision is made from the interval between the first and second thoracic spinous processes to the spine of the scapula. The trapezius and the underlying rhomboid muscles are split. This exposes the lowermost fibers of the serratus posterior superior, at the lower margin of which attaches the lumbodorsal fascia. The fascia is incised obliquely, and the serratus is retracted superiorly. Next the lateral portion of the deep muscles is elevated from the third transverse process and retracted mesially. It is important to identify accurately the third rib by passing the finger cephalad between the rhomboids and the serratus, locating the uppermost rib and counting downward. The subclavian artery is always palpable above the first rib. The third rib is exposed subperiosteally, and the transverse process is freed of muscular attachments. An inner segment of rib is removed with the transverse process. The underlying endothoracic fascia must be removed carefully, starting the dissection medially near the vertebral body where the pleura is less intimately associated with the rib than more laterally. By blunt finger dissection, the pleura is pushed away before the rib is excised. Should the pleura be torn, the lung is kept inflated by positive pressure. At the end of the operation the lungs are kept properly inflated as the wound is closed, and no effort is made to close the perforation.

After the rib and the transverse process are removed, the third intercostal nerve is seen lying on the endothoracic fascia just above the upper margin of the fourth rib. It is picked up, separated from underlying tissues and intercostal vessels, clamped and divided laterally, and traced centrally to the spinal ganglion. The outermost rami communicantes are divided. Next, the posterior branch of the spinal ganglion is isolated and divided,

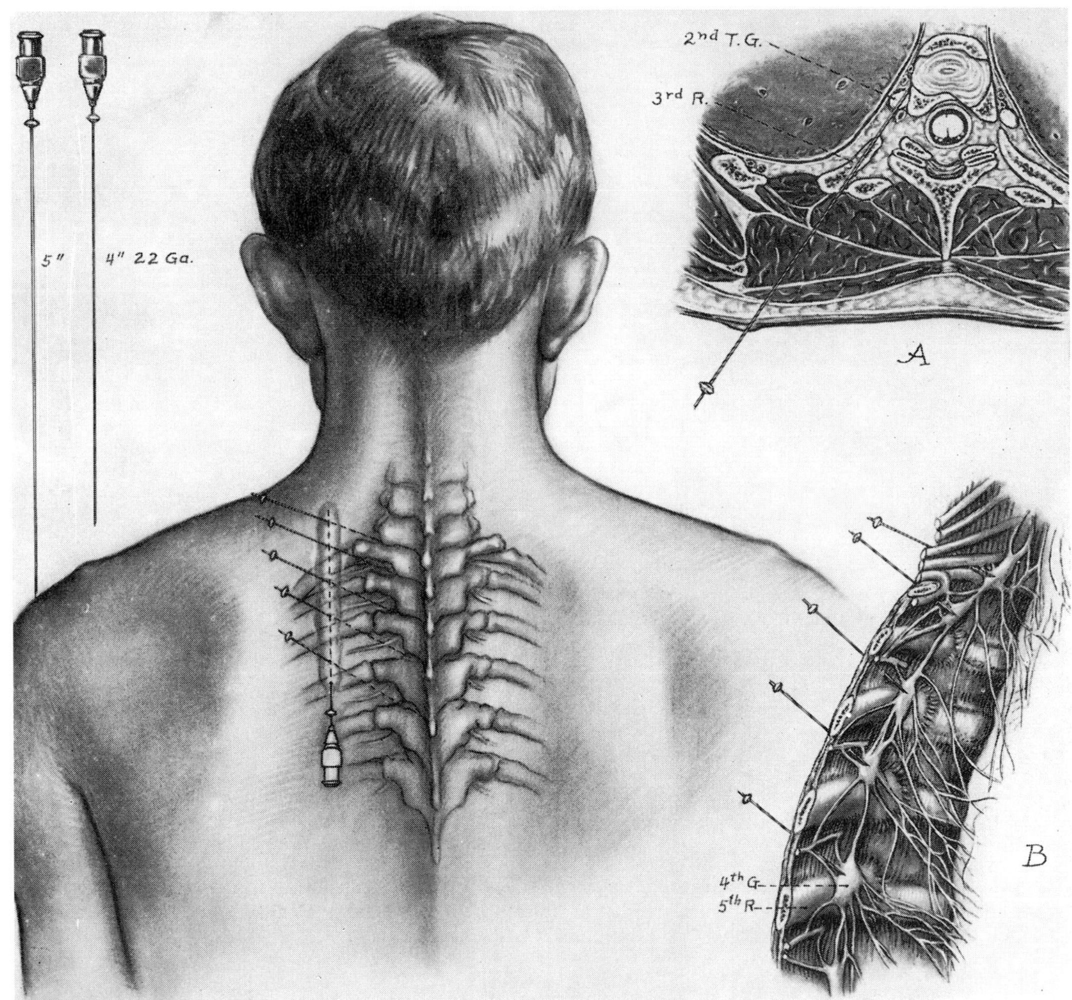

FIG. 20-28. Thoracic sympathetic ganglion block. (Southworth JL, Hingson RA, Pitkin WM (eds): Pitkin's Conduction Anesthesia. Philadelphia, JB Lippincott, 1946)

thereby freeing the ganglion and its roots. The ganglion can be easily delivered thereby so as to expose the remaining rami communicantes and the dorsal and anterior roots. The remaining rami and the dorsal root are severed. Only the anterior root remains connected with the ganglion. By pulling gently on the nerve, the glistening intradural portion of the root is pulled outside the dura. This is divided. Spinal fluid leakage is controlled with a fibrin foam packing.

The second intercostal nerve lies beneath the lower border of the second rib. This is freed from its vessels and traced centrally, and the rami communicantes, the dorsal branch, and the roots are divided . Then the pleura is separated farther from the vertebral bodies until the sympathetic chain is isolated, freed, and divided between the third and fourth ganglia. The distal end of the proximal portion of the chain is ligated. A silk cylinder is passed over it and ligated gently at its upper end and about the chain above the second ganglion. This ligature must be loose, to avoid traumatizing the chain, but tight enough to permit its slipping downward. The distal end of the cylinder is ligated firmly about the end of the freed chain, which is then sutured into the adjoining muscles. The wound is closed in layers.

Sympathetic Denervation of the Lower Extremity. Spinal anesthesia provides good muscular relaxation. Curare is administered just before the incision. When sympathectomy is unilateral, the patient is placed on his back, and the side to be operated on is elevated. The lower extremity is placed with the hip flexed to relax the iliopsoas. For bilateral sympathectomy, the patient lies flat on his back with both hips flexed, the table being tilted first to one side and then to the other.

A 10-cm incision extends obliquely from the back at the tip of the twelfth rib downward and forward to a

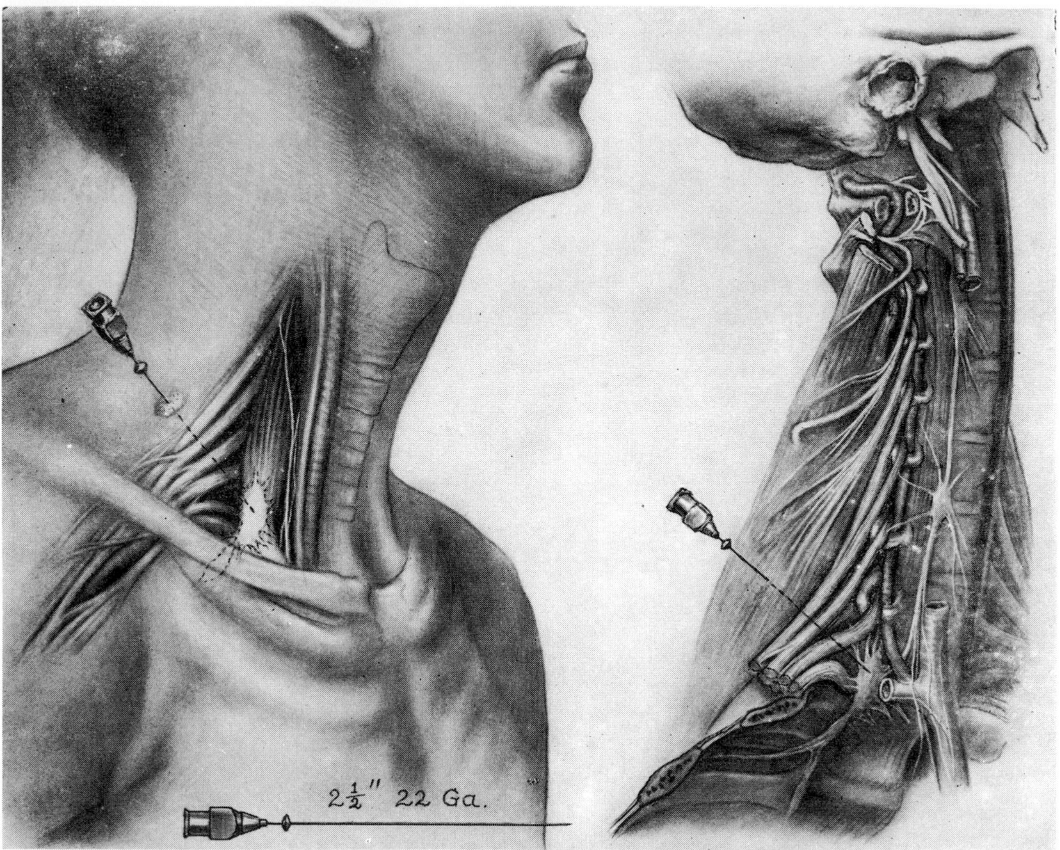

FIG. 20-29. Lateral approach to the stellate ganglion, indicating the similarity of this technique to that of brachial plexus block by the lateral route. (Southworth JL, Hingson RA, Pitkin WM (ed): Pitkin's Conduction Anesthesia. Philadelphia, JB Lippincott, 1946)

point just below and lateral to the umbilicus, following the direction of fibers of the external oblique (Fig. 20-32). The external oblique is split from the mesial to the outer margin of the wound. The internal oblique is exposed at the upper end at its point of fusion with the rectus sheath. It is split from this point downward and posteriorly and bluntly freed from the transversus beneath it. The latter is split and spread far laterally where there is less intimate contact with the peritoneum and less likelihood of tearing the latter. The opening laterally is enlarged by introducing and separating the two index fingers, at the same time displacing the peritoneum anteriorly and medially away from the flank and the retroperitoneal tissues. No retractors are used. The dissection must stay close to the peritoneum; otherwise, one may strip off with it a thick layer of retroperitoneal fat and may inadvertently begin dissecting posterior to, rather than anterior to, the iliopsoas muscle. The fingers readily pass over the iliopsoas muscle to the vertebral bodies. Almost invariably at this point one can identify by palpation the sympathetic chain, which is felt as a fixed cord of variable size running along the anterolateral aspect of the vertebral bodies.

A broad Dever retractor is introduced in the mesial portion of the wound. The areolar tissue passing from the vena cava or the aorta to the vertebral bodies is incised and lifted away from the vertebral bodies. The retractor is reinserted, and its point is held firmly against the vertebral body, thus displacing the vena cava and the aorta mesially and exposing the sympathetic chain. The genitofemoral nerve is seen lying posteriorly on the iliopsoas muscle. The ureter is visualized as adherent to and elevated with the peritoneum. It contracts when pinched. The lower pole of the kidney is seen and felt in the upper and the outer portion of the wound. The chain is picked up with a long smooth forceps between two ganglia, and a loop of silk is passed beneath it for traction. Elevation of the chain exposes the rami communicantes, which are divided. Before this is done, the position of the lumbar veins is ascertained. Except for one small vein that crosses the right chain at the level of the fourth lumbar ganglion, the veins usually, but not always, pass posteriorly. Anterior lying veins must be ligated and divided.

The aortic chain of lymph nodes or fascial bands from the iliopsoas to the vertebral bodies can be mistaken for

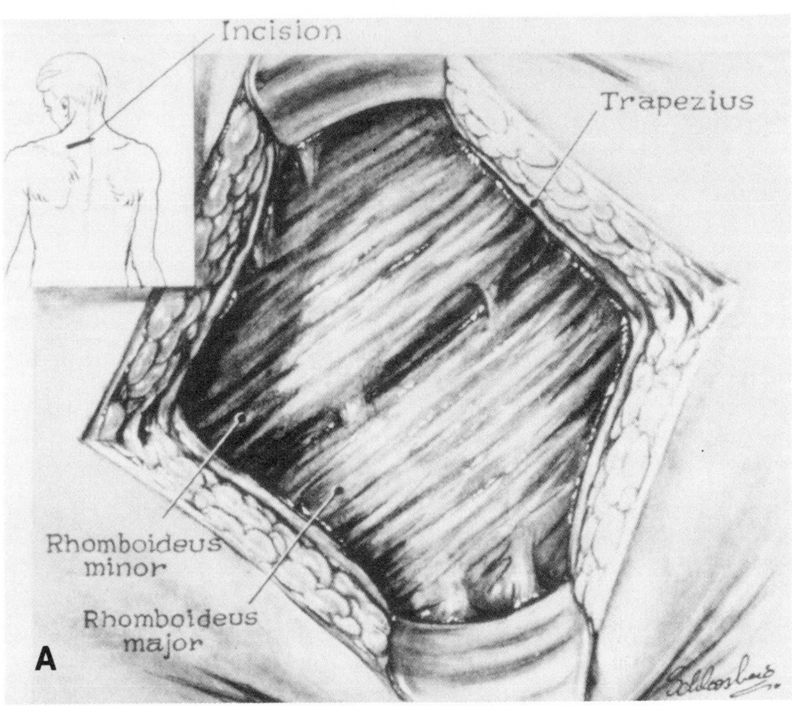

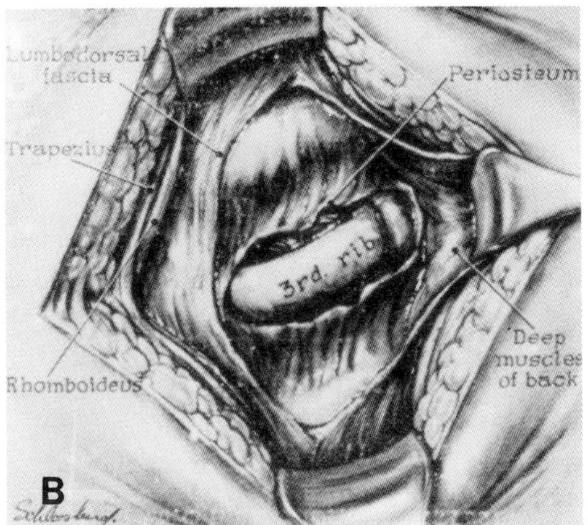

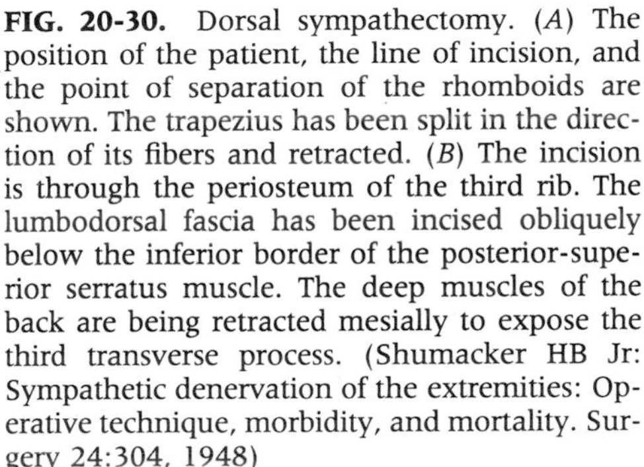

FIG. 20-30. Dorsal sympathectomy. (*A*) The position of the patient, the line of incision, and the point of separation of the rhomboids are shown. The trapezius has been split in the direction of its fibers and retracted. (*B*) The incision is through the periosteum of the third rib. The lumbodorsal fascia has been incised obliquely below the inferior border of the posterior-superior serratus muscle. The deep muscles of the back are being retracted mesially to expose the third transverse process. (Shumacker HB Jr: Sympathetic denervation of the extremities: Operative technique, morbidity, and mortality. Surgery 24:304, 1948)

the sympathetic chain. The chain and the ganglia vary greatly in size but can be identified with certainty by the tell-tale rami communicantes, the position of the fourth lumbar ganglion just above the promontory, and the position at the first ganglion at the lowermost margin of the diaphragmatic crura at its attachment to the vertebral bodies. The third and second ganglia vary in size, shape, and position and sometimes are fused. The chain is exposed more readily on the left side. On the right side, the vena cava overlies the chain.

The first to fourth ganglia are removed for sympathetic denervation of the lower extremity. In men, the first ganglia are not routinely removed bilaterally unless the patient has first given permission, because of interference with ejaculation. The cut ends of the chain may be left undisturbed.[64]

CHEMICAL DESTRUCTION OF SYMPATHETIC GANGLIA

When surgical sympathectomy is refused or is contraindicated for some reason, such as poor general condition, one may resort to chemical destruction of the ganglia. A 6% to 10% aqueous solution of phenol is used, since it has a selective action on the sympathetic ganglia, causing complete destruction without affecting the spinal nerves. The procedure is generally limited to the lumbar area.

Procedure. The second lumbar vertebral body is selected as the site of injection. First, a paravertebral injection of a local anesthetic, as described above, is carried out to confirm accurate placement of the needle. This is followed by injection of 10 ml to 15 ml of the aqueous phenol

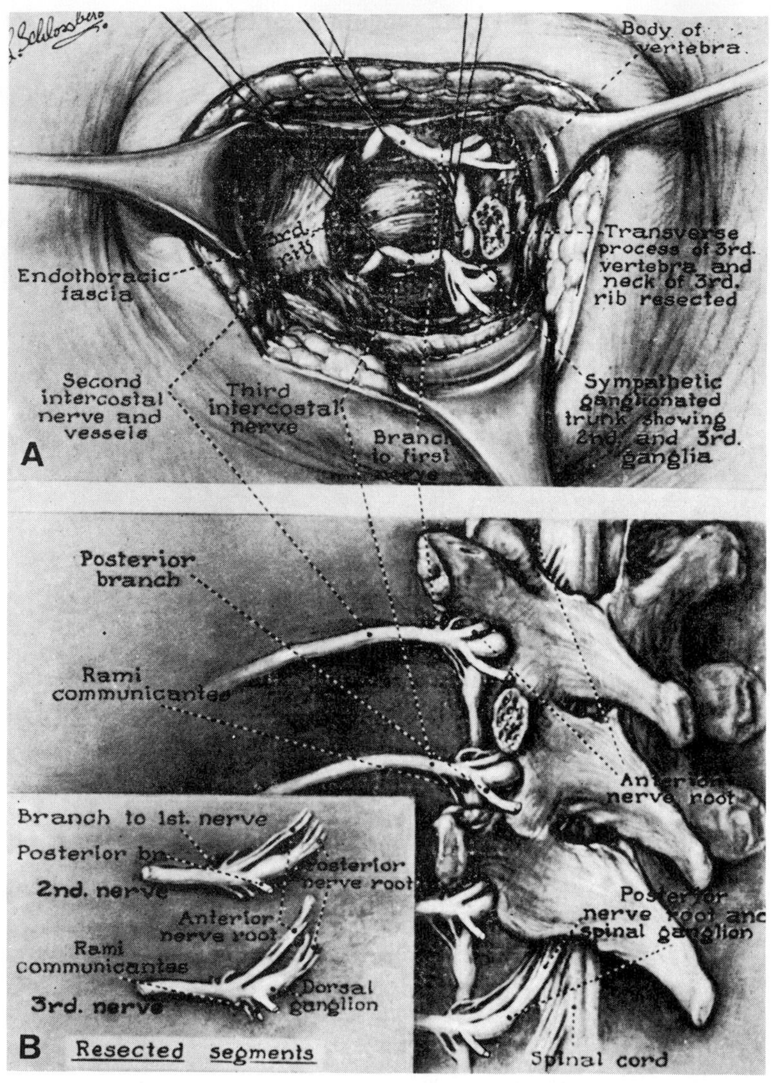

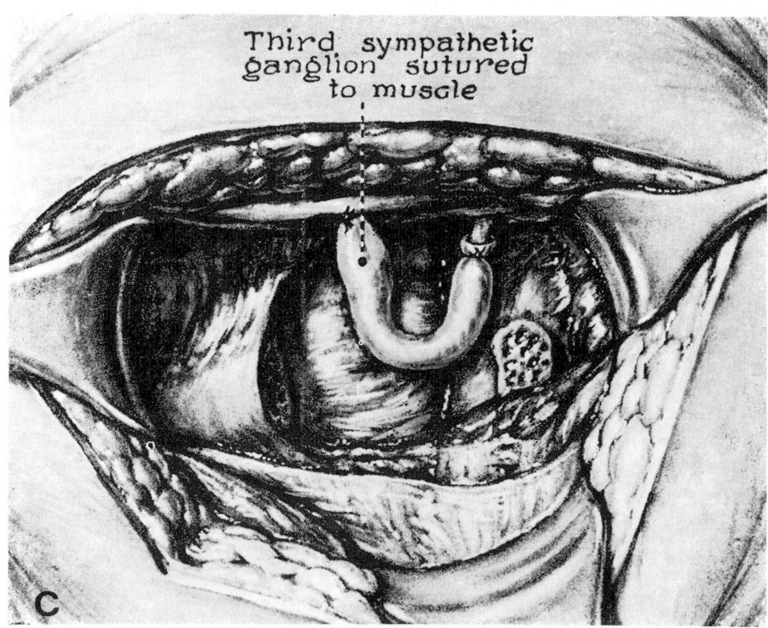

FIG. 20-31. Dorsal sympathectomy. (*A* and *B*) The third rib and the transverse process have been resected. The intercostal nerves, the dorsal ganglia, and the sympathetic chain are exposed. Attention is called to the posterior branches, which fix the dorsal ganglia centrally. (*C*) The decentralized chain is covered with a silk cylinder and sutured to the muscle. (Shumacker HB, Jr: Sympathetic denervation of the extremities: Operative technique, morbidity, and mortality. Surgery 24:304, 1948)

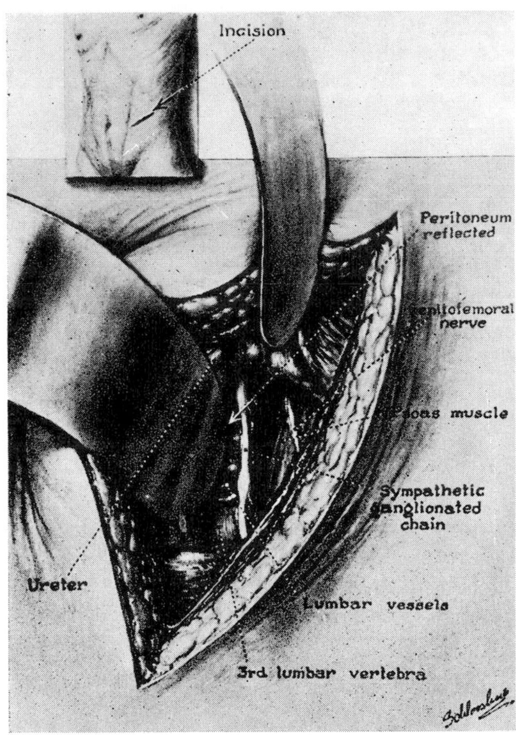

FIG. 20-32. Lumbar sympathectomy. Anterior muscle-splitting extraperitoneal incision. The retroperitoneal tissues are retracted medially and superiorly to afford exposure as high as the first lumbar ganglion. (Shumaker HB Jr: Sympathetic denervation of the extremities: Operative technique, morbidity, and mortality. Surgery 24:304, 1948)

solution. The phenol should be thoroughly dissolved by warming the solution before injection. Finally, the foot of the bed is elevated to encourage the solution to seep upward so as to reach the first lumbar and the lowermost dorsal ganglia. The patient remains horizontal in the lateral position for 20 minutes to keep the pool of phenol in contact with the lumbar ganglia.

Alcohol should never be injected about a peripheral nerve, because it damages the nerve and produces severe intractable neuralgia and paralysis.

ANTICOAGULANT THERAPY

Anticoagulant drugs are used to delay the coagulation of blood so as to prevent intravascular clotting and, once arterial or venous thromboses have developed, to retard their propagation and promote their recanalization. The impetus for anticoagulant therapy originated from the discovery of two phosphatides, cuorin and heparphosphatide, by McLean in 1916, which retarded clotting.[71] Subsequently, the properties of these drugs were further elucidated, and it was found that, in addition to increasing the clotting time, they acted to recanalize already existing thromboses, lessen platelet adhesiveness, and reduce clumping.[72,73] Two types of anticoagulants are now used: the injectable, rapid-acting ones, of which heparin is mainly used, and the oral, slower-acting ones, of which coumarin and warfarin sodium are the prime examples.

In orthopaedic surgery, the main fields of usefulness of anticoagulant therapy are prophylactically, to prevent intravascular clotting, particularly in situations with a known propensity for developing thromboses (hip and thigh operations, previous thrombophlebitis, occlusive arterial disease) for active treatment of deep venous thrombosis, to prevent thromboembolism, and for an acute arterial occlusion, until reestablishment of peripheral blood flow. Since the administration of anticoagulants is not without considerable risk, each case must be individually assessed before prophylactic anticoagulant therapy can be considered.

HEPARIN

Heparin inactivates thromboplastin so that thrombin is unavailable for combining with fibrinogen to form fibrin.[68] It acts rapidly and is administered either intravenously or subcutaneously, and its effectiveness is brief. Heparin sodium solutions are labeled in terms of United States Pharmacopeia (U.S.P.) units rather than milligrams, 1 mg being the equivalent of 100 U.S.P. units. Oral anticoagulants are started simultaneously and, when the prothrombin time has increased to the desired level, heparin is discontinued.

The indications for heparin therapy are pulmonary embolism, sudden arterial occlusion, acute venous thrombosis, cerebral arterial insufficiency (of certain types), and during and following operations on blood vessels; prophylactically, it can be administered in small doses when the potential for venous thrombosis is high (*e.g.*, total hip replacement procedures).

The common methods of administration follow:

Continuous Intravenous Infusion

Normal saline containing 1000 U.S.P. units in each 100 ml of diluent flows at 25 drops per minute. The effect on the coagulation time is variable and must be frequently monitored, and the objective is to increase the coagulation time to two to three times the normal. When intravenous administration is stopped, the anticoagulant effect disappears within 2 to 3 hours.

Intermittent Intravenous Injection

Immediately after a diagnosis of thrombosis or embolism, an intravenous injection of 5,000 to 15,000 U.S.P. units is given through the rubber cap of an indwelling intravenous catheter (Minicath—PRN, Deseret) and thereafter at 4-hour intervals. On the second day, heparin is given three times a day, and if anticoagulant therapy must be continued more than a few days, coumarin therapy is started early and continued until the desired prothrombin deficiency is reached, and heparin is then discontinued.[67]

Subcutaneous Injection

This is effective for long-term therapy but requires periodic monitoring. The heparin is contained in a gelatin-dextrose menstruum (Depo-Heparin), thereby prolonging its absorption and effect over 12 to 24 hours. The dose is 20,000 U.S.P. units every 12 hours. Because this manner of administration produces highly variable effects on coagulation, and because of pain at the injection site, subcutaneous injection is rarely used. The preferable method of administering heparin is through a heparin-lock needle by which repeated doses can be given without the need for repeatedly puncturing the vein; 5,000 to 7,500 U.S.P. units given quickly usually prolongs the prothrombin time from the normal of about 19 to 30 seconds.

Because of the frequency of allergic reactions to heparin (erythema, hives, fever, skin eruption, bronchospasm, shock), a preliminary test dose of 1000 U.S.P. units should be given subcutaneously. Osteoporosis develops in patients on long-term heparin therapy and predisposes them to compression fractures of the spine.[69]

During heparinization, hemorrhage or other complications can be controlled by protamine sulfate. Intravenous administration of 50 mg neutralizes the effect of 5000 U.S.P. units (50 mg). Protamine sulfate should be administered slowly, and no more than 50 mg should be given over any 10 minute interval.

DICUMAROL

Dicumarol is but one of the class of coumarin drugs whose active substance, dicoumarin, is obtained from sweet clover. Coumarin reduces factor VII (stable factor), factor IX (PTC), factor X (Stuart-Prower factor), and factor II (prothrombin), in that order. Its main action is to increase the prothrombin time. It is mainly used for long-term anticoagulant therapy of chronic occlusive arterial disease, repeated pulmonary and systemic emboli, recurrent thrombophlebitis, and cerebral arterial insufficiency. In orthopaedic surgery, it is often used prophylactically to prevent deep venous thrombosis and pulmonary embolic phenomena.

When an immediate anticoagulant effect is desired, heparin is given simultaneously with dicumarol. When the prothrombin time is elevated to 1½ to 2½ times the normal, heparinization is discontinued and only dicumarol is continued. The latter may be given over any period of time provided that regular prothrombin time determinations are made. A desirable prothrombin time is about 27 seconds, which is equivalent to a prothrombin level of 30%. A rise of prothrombin time over 35 seconds demands temporary stoppage of the drug. A suggested dosage of dicumarol is 300 mg the first day, 200 mg the second day, and 100 mg/day thereafter. People vary in their response, and the correct dosage is that which will keep the prothrombin time at the required level.

Vitamin K is the antidote for coumarin drugs. In the event of hemorrhage, 60 mg of synthetic vitamin K (menadione bisulfite) is given intravenously. Whole fresh blood should be given.

Other drugs may potentiate (antibiotics, acetylsalicylic acid, quinidine) or antagonize (barbiturates, meprobamate) the coumarin effect.[70]

Warfarin sodium is a coumarin drug that is also effective when administered intravenously or intramuscularly; it is used when gastrointestinal conditions will not permit oral therapy. The standard dose is 1 mg warfarin sodium per kilogram of body weight. Little or no response occurs for 12 hours, and it therefore cannot be substituted for heparin. Its maximal response is noted at 48 hours; it subsides, after a single dose, in 3 to 8 days. In poorly nourished, debilitated patients, its effect may be profound, producing an excessive hypoproteinemia. Its dosage should therefore be lowered.

COMBINED TREATMENT

When a quick and sustained anticoagulant effect is desired, 5000 to 7500 U.S.P. units (50 mg–75 mg) heparin is injected intravenously and at the same time an initial dose of coumarin is administered orally. Injections of heparin are continued every 4 hours, and prothrombin time determinations are made every 24 hours. A maintenance dose of coumarin is given orally on the second day provided that prothrombin deficiency is not excessive. When prothrombin times are sufficiently prolonged, heparin administration is stopped. Usually this is possible within 24 to 48 hours. Dicumarol is given in a single oral dose each day: 300 mg is given the first day, and subsequent doses are given in steady decrements while the prothrombin time is greater than normal (*e.g.*, 200 mg the second, 100 mg the third day, and so forth). The dosage is then regulated to maintain the desired level of anticoagulation.

CONTRAINDICATIONS

Contraindications to anticoagulant therapy are the following:

1. *Vitamin C and K deficiency and hepatic disease* (anticoagulants unnecessary)
2. *Renal insufficiency*—retention enhances the effect by an abnormal accumulation.
3. *Blood dyscrasias* which impair the clotting mechanism.

4. *Recent brain and spinal cord operations*—hemorrhage is disastrous.
5. *Ulcerative lesions or open wounds* in which a tendency to bleeding exists. However, in surgical repair of arterial wounds heparin is indispensable and may be continued for about 3 days or until the danger of clotting at the suture site has passed.

DIFFERENTIAL DIAGNOSIS OF ARTERIAL OBSTRUCTION IN AN EXTREMITY

OCCLUSIVE ARTERIAL DISEASES

Arteriosclerosis Obliterans. The onset usually occurs after 40 years of age. Men are affected more commonly but not exclusively. The upper extremities are rarely involved (40% in TAO); thrombophlebitis is never associated. The arteries are calcified, and hypertension and diabetes are often associated. In younger patients the plasma lipoids are frequently elevated.

Simple Arterial Thrombosis. Simple thrombosis is rare. It is often a complication of severe infectious disease, blood dyscrasia, congestive heart failure, or trauma. The first manifestation is often an acute, extensive arterial occlusion with a large area of gangrene.

Arterial Embolism. Embolism is a complication of bacterial endocarditis, atrial fibrillation, or myocardial infarction with a mural thrombosis. It is characterized by sudden arterial occlusion.

Compression at the Cervicobrachial Junction. Cervicobrachial compression involves one or both hands. The pulse is reduced or obliterated by various movements of the arms or the head. Peripheral nerve involvement is frequent, and a cervical rib is often present.

OTHER VASCULAR CONDITIONS

Raynaud's Disease. Raynaud's disease is rare in men. The upper extremities are involved more often. Color changes are bilateral and symmetrical. Pulsations are present, and mass gangrene of digits does not occur.

Acroscleroderma (Acrosclerosis). Acroscleroderma may produce gangrene and, rarely, occlusion of large arteries. The upper extremities are involved more extensively than the lower. It is bilateral and symmetrical. Sclerodactylia is present. (No such skin changes appear in Buerger's disease or ASO.)

Livedo Reticularis. Arterial occlusion and gangrene rarely occur. The skin is extensively involved, with a livid, reticulated mottling.

Erythromelalgia. The affected parts of the extremity are very warm during painful episodes. Pulsations are normal.

Pernio. The affected part is hot and swollen. Pulsations are normal. The condition develops after exposure to cold. The ulceration is small in extent and situated on the legs rather than the toes and the feet.

Ergotism. A rare type of arterial occlusion, ergotism is associated with a history of medication or food containing ergot. The lesions are symmetrical, and often the eyes are involved.

Acute Thrombophlebitis of Large Veins. The extremity is swollen, the veins are distended, the pulsations may be absent temporarily but soon return, and there are tenderness, redness, and pain along the course of a thickened cordlike vein. If pulsations are persistently absent, TAO is invariably an associated disease.

Venous Insufficiency. Venous insufficiency is due to varicose veins or thrombophlebitis. A congestive pain develops while standing, more so than when walking (in contrast with arterial occlusive disease, which is worse when walking) and is relieved by recumbency. Arterial pulsations are normal.

REFERENCES

Diagnosis of Vascular Disease of the Extremities

1. Allen EV, Barker NW, Hines EA Jr: Peripheral Vascular Diseases, 3rd ed. Philadelphia, WB Saunders, 1962
2. Pratt GH: Test for incompetent communicating branches in the surgical treatment of varicose veins. JAMA 117:100, 1941

Special Tests of Peripheral Circulation

3. Kincaid OW, et al: Angiography. In Juergens JL, Spittell JA Jr, Fairbairn JF II (eds): Allen–Barker–Hines Peripheral Vascular Diseases. Philadelphia, WB Saunders, 1980
4. Lang EK: A survey of the complications of percutaneous retrograde arteriography: Seldinger technique. Radiology 81:257, 1963
5. Seldinger SI: Catheter placement of needle on percutaneous arteriography: A new technique. Acta Radiol 39:368, 1953
6. Welch EE, Faxon HH, McGahey CE: The application of phlebography to the therapy of thrombosis and embolism. Surgery 12:163, 1942

Vascular Function Studies

7. Carter SA: Indirect systolic pressures and pulse waves in arterial occlusive disease of the lower extremities. Circulation 37:624, 1968
8. Carter SA: Response of ankle pressure to leg exercise in mild or questionable arterial disease. N Engl J Med 287:578, 1972

9. Strandness DE Jr, Bell JW: Peripheral vascular disease: Diagnosis and objective evaluation using a mercury strain gauge. Ann Surg (Suppl) 161(4):3, 1965
10. Strandness DE Jr, et al: Ultrasonic flow detection. Am J Surg 113:311, 1967
11. Strandness DE, Radke HM, Bell JW: Use of a new simplified plethysmograph in the clinical evaluation of patients with arteriosclerosis obliterans. Surg Gynecol Obstet 112:751, 1961
12. Strandness DE Jr, McCutcheon EP, Rushmer RF: Application of transcutaneous Doppler flowmeter in evaluation of occlusive arterial disease. Surg Gynecol Obstet 122:1039, 1966
13. Yao ST: Haemodynamic studies in peripheral arterial disease. Br J Surg 57:761, 1970
14. Yao ST, Bergan JJ: Application of ultrasound to arterial and venous diagnosis. Surg Clin North Am 54:23, 1974

Arteriosclerosis Obliterans

15. Strandness DE Jr, et al: A combined clinical and pathologic study of diabetic and non-diabetic peripheral arterial disease. Diabetes 13:366, 1964

Chronic Aorto-Iliac Occlusion

16. DeBakey ME, et al: Patch graft angioplasty in vascular surgery. J Cardiovasc Surg 3:106, 1962
17. DeBakey ME, et al: Late results of vascular surgery in the treatment of arteriosclerosis. J Cardiovasc Surg 5:473, 1964
18. DeWolfe VG, et al: Intermittent claudication of the hip and the syndrome of chronic aorto-iliac thrombosis. Circulation 9:1, 1954
19. dos Santos JC: Sur la désobstruction des thromboses artérielles anciennes. Mem Acad Chir 73:409, 1947
20. Garrett HE, et al: Surgical considerations in the treatment of aorto-iliac occlusive disease. Surg Clin North Am 46:949, 1966
21. Kunlin J: Le traitement de l'ischémie artéritique par la greffe veineuse longue. Rev Chir 70:206, 1951
22. Leriche R: Des oblitérations artérielles hautes (oblitération de la terminaison de l'aorte) comme causes des insuffisances circulatoires des membres inférieurs. Bull Mem Soc Chir (Paris) 49:1404, 1923
23. Leriche R: De la résection du carrefour aortico-iliaque avec double sympathectomie lombaire pour thrombose artéritique de l'aorte; le syndrome de l'oblitération termino-aortique par artérite. Presse Med 48:601, 1940
24. Leriche R, Morel A: The syndrome of thrombotic obliteration of the aortic bifurcation. Ann Surg 127:193, 1948
25. Oudet J: La greff vasculaire dans les thromboses du carrefour aortique. Presse Med 59:234, 1951
26. Phalen GS: Backache caused by vascular disease. Clin Orthop 5:149, 1955

Thromboangiitis Obliterans

27. Buerger L: The Circulatory Disturbances of the Extremities. Philadelphia, WB Saunders, 1924
28. McGrath EJC: Experimental peripheral gangrene; effect of estrogenic substance and its relation to thrombo-angiitis obliterans. Arch Intern Med 55:942, 1935
29. von Winiwarter F: Ueber eine eigenthumliche form von endarteritis und endophlebitis mit gangrene des fusses. Arch Chir 23:202, 1879
30. Winrath LA, Herzstein J: Relation of tobacco smoking to arteriosclerosis obliterans in diabetes mellitus. JAMA 131:205, 1940

Treatment of Chronic Occlusive Arterial Disease

31. Bazy L, et al: L'endarterectomie pour arterite obliterente des membres inferieurs. J Int Chir 9:45, 1949
32. Boyd AM, et al: Intermittent claudication. J Bone Joint Surg 31B:325, 1949
33. dos Santos JC: Note sur la désobstruction de anciennes thromboses artérielles. Presse Med 39:544, 1949
34. Kunlin J, et al: Le traitment de l' ischémie artéritique par le greffe veineuse longue. Rev Chir (Paris) 70:206, juillet–aôut 1951
35. Leriche R, Kunlin J: Possibilité de greffe veineuse de grande dimensions (15 á 47 cm) dans les thromboses artérielles etendues. Compt Rend Acad Sci 227:939, 1948
36. Pratt GH: Cardiovascular Surgery. Philadelphia, Lea & Febiger, 1954
37. Silbert S: Thromboangiitis obliterans: Results of treatment with repeated injections of hypertonic sodium chloride. JAMA 94:1730, 1930
38. Winfield JM, Ruggiero WF: Evaluation of arteriovenous shunt and the treatment of its ischemic extremity due to arteriosclerosis. Meeting of New York Surgical Society, February 1951

Angiospastic Conditions

39. Adson AW, Brown GE: The treatment of Raynaud's disease by resection of the upper thoracic and lumbar sympathetic ganglia and trunks. Surg Gynecol Obstet 48:577, 1929
40. Barker NW, Hines EA: Arterial occlusion in the hands and fingers associated with repeated occupational trauma. Proc Staff Meet Mayo Clin 19:345, 1944
41. Drenckhahn CH: Vasospastic diseases of the hands of miners due to vibration. Ill Med J 70:354, 1936
42. Hardgrove MAF, Barker NW: Pneumatic hammer disease. Proc Staff Meet Mayo Clin 8:345, 1933
43. Lange K, Boyd LF: The functional pathology of experimental frost-bite and the prevention of subsequent gangrene. Surg Gynecol Obstet 80:346, 1945
44. Lewis T: Vascular Disorders of the Limbs, p 111. New York, Macmillan, 1936
45. McGovern T, Wright IS: Pernio: A vascular disease. Am Heart J 22:583, 1941
46. Mayfield FH: Causalgia. Am J Surg 74:522, 1947
47. Miller DS, deTakats G: Posttraumatic dystrophy of the extremities. Surg Gynecol Obstet 75:558, 1942
48. Mitchell SW, Moorehouse GR, Keen WW: Gunshot and Other Injuries of Nerves. Philadelphia, JB Lippincott, 1864
49. Raynaud AGM: De L'asphyxie Locale et de la Gangrene Symetrique des Extremities, p 177. Paris, Rignoux, 1862
50. Shumacker HB, Kunkler AW: Studies in experimental frostbite. IX. Rapid thawing and prolonged cooling in the treatment of frostbite resulting from exposure to low ambient temperature. Surg Gynecol Obstet 94:475, 1952
51. Shumacker HB, Spiegel IJ, Upjohn RH: Causalgia. Surg Gynecol Obstet 86:76, 452, 1943
52. Spurling RG, Jelsma F, Roger JB: Observations in Raynaud's disease with histopathologic studies. Surg Gynecol Obstet 54:584, 1932
53. Sudeck P: Über die akute (reflectorische) Knochinatrophie Nach Entzündungen und Verletzungen An den Extremitäten

und ihre klinischen Erscheinungen. Fortschr Geb Röntgenstr 5:277, 1901–1902
54. Wilson RH, et al: Occupation acro-osteolysis. JAMA 201:577, 1967

Acute Arterial Injuries

55. Freeman ND: Acute arterial injuries. JAMA 139:1125, 1949
56. Holman E: Further observations on surgery of the large arteries. Surg Gynecol Obstet 78:275, 1944

Arterial Aneurysm

57. Holman E: On circumscribed dilatation of artery distal to partially occluding band: Poststenotic dilatation. Surgery 36:3, 1954
58. Pratt GH: Surgical treatment of aneurysm. Am Heart J 38:43, 1949

Arteriovenous Fistula

59. Fairbairn JF II, Bernatz PE: Arteriovenous fistulas. In JL Juerqens, Spittell JA Jr, Fairbairn JF II (eds): Allen–Barker–Hines Peripheral Vascular Diseases, 5th ed, p 441. Philadelphia, WB Saunders, 1980

Glomus Tumor

60. Popoff NW: The digital vascular system; with reference to the state of glomus. Arch Pathol 18:295, 1934

Periarteritis Nodosa

61. Arkin A: A clinical and pathological study of periarteritis nodosa. Am J Pathol 6:401, 1930
62. Rich AR: Role of hypersensitivity in periarteritis nodosa. Bull Johns Hopkins Hosp 71:123, 1942
63. Rich AR, Gregory JE: Experimental demonstration that periarteritis nodosa is a manifestation of hypersensitivity. Bull Johns Hopkins Hosp 72:65, 1943

Therapeutic Sympathetic Paralysis

64. Shumacker HB Jr: Sympathetic denervation of the extremities; operative technique, morbidity, and mortality. Surgery 24:304, 1948
65. Smithwick RH: Modified dorsal sympathectomy for vascular spasm (Raynaud's disease) of the upper extremity. Ann Surg 104:339, 1936
66. Southworth JL, Hingson RA, Pitkin WM (eds): Pitkin's Conduction Anesthesia, 2nd ed. Philadelphia, JB Lippincott, 1946

Anticoagulant Therapy

67. Bauer G: 9 years experience with heparin in acute venous thrombosis. Angiology 1:161, 1950
68. Fairbairn JF II, Juergens JL, Spittell JA Jr: Allen–Barker–Hines Peripheral Vascular Diseases, 5th ed. Philadelphia, WB Saunders, 1980
69. Griffith, GC: Heparin osteoporosis. JAMA 193:91, 1965
70. Kazmier FJ, Spittell JA Jr: Coumarin drug interaction. Mayo Clin Proc 45:249, 1970
71. McLean J: Thromboplastic action of cephalin. Am J Physiol 41:250, 1916
72. Murphy EA, Mustard JF: Dicumarol therapy: Some effects of platelets and their relationship to clotting tests. Circ Res 8:1187, 1960
73. Wright HP, Kubik MM: Recanalization of thrombosed arteries under anticoagulant therapy. Br Med J 1:1021, 1953

Index

INDEX

Numbers followed by an *f* indicate a figure; *t* following a page number indicates tabular material; pages in **boldface type** indicate color plates.

ISBN 0-397-50604-X